Obstetric Anesthesia

Second Edition

Obstetric Anesthesia

Second Edition

Edited by

Mark C. Norris, M.D.
Department of Anesthesiology
Washington University
St. Louis, Missouri

LIPPINCOTT WILLIAMS & WILKINS
A **Wolters Kluwer** Company
Philadelphia • Baltimore • New York • London
Buenos Aires • Hong Kong • Sydney • Tokyo

Acquisitions Editor: R. Craig Percy
Developmental Editor: Ellen DiFrancesco
Manufacturing Manager: Kevin Watt
Production Manager: Robert Pancotti
Production Editors: Jonathan Geffner and Thomas Boyce
Cover Designer: Cambria Kahoud
Indexer: Deana Reese Fowler
Compositor: Lippincott Williams & Wilkins Desktop Division
Printer: Courier–Kendallville

Printed in the United States of America

9 8 7 6 5 4 3 2 1

Library of Congress Cataloging-in-Publication Data

Obstetric anesthesia / edited by Mark C. Norris — 2nd ed.
p. cm.
Includes bibliographical references and index.
ISBN 0-7817-1017-0
1. Anesthesia in obstetrics. 2. Pregnant women—Surgery. 3. Pregnancy—Complications.
4. Labor (Obstetrics)—Complications.
I. Norris, Mark C.
[DNLM: 1. Anesthesia, Obstetrical. 2. Pregnancy Complications—surgery. 3. Surgical Procedures, Operative—in pregnancy. WO 450014232 1998]
RG732.0263 1998
617.9'682—dc21
DNLM/DLC 98-27543
for Library of Congress CIP

To my children: Julia, Benjamin, and Daniel.

No father could be more proud.

Contents

Contributing Authors

George Allen III, M.D. *Instructor, Department of Anesthesiology, University of Tennessee, Memphis, 800 Madison Avenue, Memphis, Tennessee 30103*

Audrey S. Alleyne, M.D. *Staff Anesthesiologist, Department of Anesthesiology, Emory University School of Medicine, Thomas K. Glenn Memorial Building, 69 Butler Street, SE, Atlanta, Georgia 30303*

Valerie A. Arkoosh, M.D. *Associate Professor, Department of Anesthesiology, Allegheny University Hospital for Women, 4150 City Line Avenue, Philadelphia, Pennsylvania 19131*

James A. Bartelsmeyer, M.D. *Assistant Professor, Department of Obstetrics and Gynecology, Washington University School of Medicine, 3015 North Ballas Road, Ground Floor, St. Louis, Missouri 63131*

Richard B. Becker, M.D. *Assistant Professor, Department of Anesthesiology and Critical Care Medicine, George Washington University Medical Center, Suite 2500, 901 23rd Street, NW, Washington, DC 20037*

Yaakov Beilin, M.D. *Assistant Professor, Departments of Anesthesiology and Obstetrics, Gynecology and Reproductive Sciences, Associate Director, Obstetric Anesthesiology, Mount Sinai Medical Center, 1 Gustave Levy Place, New York, New York 10029-6574*

Howard H. Bernstein, M.D. *Clinical Assistant Professor, Departments of Anesthesiology and Obstetrics, Gynecology and Reproductive Sciences, Director, Obstetric Anesthesiology, Mount Sinai School of Medicine, 1 Gustave Levy Place, New York, New York 10029-6574*

David J. Birnbach, M.D. *Director of Obstetric Anesthesiology, St. Luke's–Roosevelt Hospital Center, 1000 Tenth Avenue, New York, New York 10019*

Walter U. Brown, M.D. *Associate Clinical Professor, Department of Anesthesiology, Vanderbilt University, Middle Tennessee Anesthesiology Associates, Baptist Hospital, Nashville, Tennessee 37236*

Sherrie Buchmeier, R.D.M.S., R.T., L.P.N. *Ultrasound Technician, Department of Obstetrics and Gynecology, Washington University School of Medicine, St. Louis, Missouri 63130*

Linda Chan, M.D. *Associate Professor, Division of Maternal-Fetal Medicine, Department of Obstetrics and Gynecology, Temple University School of Medicine, 3401 North Broad Street, 7-OPB, Philadelphia, Pennsylvania 19140*

Steven L. Clark, M.D. *Department of Obstetrics and Gynecology, University of Utah, 50 North Medical Drive, Salt Lake City, Utah 84132*

John G. D'Alessio, M.D. *Assistant Clinical Professor, Department of Anesthesiology, University of Tennessee, Memphis, 800 Madison Avenue, Memphis, Tennessee 30103*

M. Joanne Douglas, M.D. *Head of Department of Anesthesia, British Columbia Women's Hospital, 4500 Oak Street, Vancouver V6H 3N1, Canada*

John W. Downing, M.B. *Professor, Department of Anesthesiology and Obstetrics and Gynecology, Vanderbilt University School of Medicine, Nashville, Tennessee 37232-2125*

Robert L. Eberle, M.D. *Assistant Professor, Departments of Anesthesiology and Obstetrics and Gynecology, A-131, Albany Medical Center, 47 New Scotland Avenue, Albany, New York 12208-3412*

Fazeela Ferouz, M.D. *Assistant Professor, Department of Anesthesiology, St. Luke's–Roosevelt Hospital Center, 1000 Tenth Avenue, New York, New York 10019*

Steven T. Fogel, M.D. *Assistant Professor, Department of Anesthesiology, Washington University School of Medicine, 660 South Euclid Avenue, St. Louis, Missouri 63110*

Robert R. Gaiser, M.D. *Assistant Professor, Department of Anesthesia and Pharmacology, Hospital of the University of Pennsylvania, 3400 Spruce Street, 1110 Penn Tower, Philadelphia, Pennsylvania 19104*

Raphael Y. Gershon, M.D. *Assistant Professor, Department of Anesthesiology, Emory University School of Medicine, Thomas K. Glenn Memorial Building, 69 Butler Street, SE, Atlanta, Georgia 30303*

Beth Glosten, M.D. *Associate Professor, Department of Anesthesiology, University of Washington Medical Center, Seattle, Washington 98195*

Evan Goodman, M.D. *Department of Anesthesia, Case Western Reserve University/University Hospitals of Cleveland, 11100 Euclid Avenue, Cleveland, Ohio 44106-5007*

Holly C. Gunn, M.D. *Acting Assistant Professor, Department of Anesthesiology, University of Washington Medical Center, Seattle, Washington 98195*

Joy Hawkins, M.D. *Associate Professor, Department of Anesthesiology, University of Colorado School of Medicine, 4200 East 9th Avenue, B-113, Denver, Colorado 80262*

Norman L. Herman, M.D., Ph.D. *Assistant Professor, Department of Anesthesiology, New York Presbyterian Hospital–Cornell Medical Center, 525 East 68th Street, New York, New York 10021*

Quinn Hogan, M.D. *Associate Professor, Department of Anesthesiology, Medical College of Wisconsin, Milwaukee, Wisconsin 53226*

William L. Holcomb Jr., M.D. *Assistant Professor, Department of Obstetrics and Gynecology, Washington University School of Medicine, St. Louis, Missouri 63110*

H. Jane Huffnagle, D.O. *Assistant Professor, Department of Anesthesiology, Thomas Jefferson University Hospital, 111 South 11th Street, Philadelphia, Pennsylvania 19107*

Suzanne Lynne Huffnagle, D.O. *Assistant Professor, Department of Anesthesiology, Jefferson Medical College, Thomas Jefferson University, 11th and Walnut Streets, Philadelphia, Pennsylvania 19107*

BettyLou Koffel, M.D. *7276 Southwest Beaverton: Hillsdale Highway, Suite 361, Portland, Oregon 97225*

Jacob C. Langer, M.D. *Associate Professor, Department of Surgery, Division of Pediatric Surgery, Washington University School of Medicine, 660 South Euclid Avenue, St. Louis, Missouri 63110*

Gabriela Rocha Lauretti, M.D., M.Sc., Ph.D. *Assistant Professor of Anesthesiology, Department of Surgery, Orthopedics, and Traumatology, Faculty of Medicine of Ribeirão Preto, University of São Paulo, Rua Mantiqueira, 460, Ribeirão Preto, São Paulo 14048-900, Brazil*

Kathleen A. Leavitt, M.D. *Assistant Professor, Codirector of Obstetric Anesthesia, George Washington University Hospital, 901 23rd Street, NW, Washington, DC 20037*

Sung-Hee Rhim Lee, M.D. *Fellow, Department of Anesthesiology, Thomas Jefferson University Hospital, 834 Chestnut Street, #1508, Philadelphia, Pennsylvania 19107*

Barbara L. Leighton, M.D. *Associate Professor, Department of Anesthesiology, Allegheny University of the Health Sciences, City Avenue Hospital, 4150 City Line Avenue, Philadelphia, Pennsylvania 19131*

Carol Ann Lennon, M.D. *Fellow, Department of Maternal-Fetal Medicine, Washington University, 1 Barnes Hospital Plaza, St. Louis, Missouri 63110*

Ji-Bin Liu, M.D. *Research Assistant Professor, Department of Radiology, Thomas Jefferson University Hospital, 132 South 10th Street, Philadelphia, Pennsylvania 19107*

Andrew M. Malinow, M.D. *Associate Professor, Department of Anesthesiology, University of Maryland, 22 South Greene Street, Baltimore, Maryland 21201*

Beth H. Minzter *Assistant Professor, Department of Anesthesiology and Obstetrics, Division of Ob/Gyn Anesthesia and IPC, 1313 21st Avenue South, 504 Oxford House, Nashville, Tennessee 37232-4125*

Holly A. Muir, M.D. *Assistant Professor, Department of Anesthesiology, Division of Women's Anesthesia, Duke University Medical Center, Durham, North Carolina 27701*

L Michael Newman, M.D., Ph.D. *World Wide Medical Director, Anesthesia & Surgical Systems, Becton Dickinson and Company, 1 Becton Drive, MC211, Bldg. II, Franklin Lakes, New Jersey 07417*

Mark C. Norris, M.D. *Professor of Anesthesiology and Obstetrics and Gynecology, Department of Anesthesiology, Washington University School of Medicine, 660 South Euclid Avenue, St. Louis, Missouri 63110-1083*

C. E. P. Orlikowsky, M.D. *Professor of Anesthesiology, University of Natal, P.O. Box 17039, Congella 4013, Durban, South Africa*

Craig M. Palmer, M.D. *Associate Professor, Department of Anesthesiology, University of Arizona Health Sciences Center, 1501 North Campbell, Tucson, Arizona 85724*

Jaya Ramanathan, M.D. *Professor, Department of Anesthesiology, Obstetrics, and Gynecology, University of Tennessee, Memphis, 800 Madison Avenue, Memphis, Tennessee 30103*

Ramiah Ramasubramanian, M.D. *Assistant Professor, Department of Anesthesiology, Vanderbilt University School of Medicine, Nashville, Tennessee 37232-2125*

Edward T. Riley, M.D. *Assistant Professor, Department of Anesthesia, Stanford University School of Medicine, 300 Pasteur Drive, Stanford, California 94305-5640*

David Anthony Rocke, F.C.A.(SA.), *Professor, Department of Anaesthetics, University of Natal, Private Bag 7, Congella 4013, Durban, South Africa*

C. C. Rout, M.D. *Lecturer, Department of Anesthesiology, University of Natal, P.O. Box 17039, Congella 4013, Durban, South Africa*

Divina Juson Santos, M.D. *Director of Obstetrical Anesthesia, Department of Anesthesiology, Columbia Hospital for Women, 2425 L Street, NW, Washington, DC 20037*

Jaye M. Shyken, M.D. *Assistant Professor, Department of Obstetrics and Gynecology, Washington University School of Medicine, 4911 Barnes Hospital Plaza, St. Louis, Missouri 63110*

Baha M. Sibai, M.D. *Professor, Department of Obstetrics and Gynecology, University of Tennessee, Memphis, 800 Madison Avenue, Memphis, Tennessee 30103*

Christopher M. Viscomi, M.D. *Assistant Professor, Department of Anesthesiology, University of Utah, 50 North Medical Drive, Salt Lake City, Utah 84132*

Richard N. Wissler, M.D., Ph.D. *Assistant Professor, Departments of Anesthesiology and Obstetrics and Gynecology, University of Rochester Medical Center, 601 Elmwood Avenue, Rochester, New York 14642*

Mark I. Zakowski, M.D. *Director of Obstetric Anesthesia, Department of Anesthesiology, Cedars–Sinai Medical Center, 8700 Beverly Boulevard, #8211, Los Angeles, California 90048*

Barbara Zucker-Pinchoff, M.D. *370 Central Park West, Apartment 501, New York, New York 10025-6521*

Preface

This book is organized the way an anesthesiologist approaches a patient: preoperative evaluation, intraoperative management, and postoperative care.

The aim of the chapters in the first section of the book is to provide background information about both normal and high-risk pregnancies. In addition to chapters discussing the physiologic changes that accompany normal gestation, there are chapters that examine how the woman with significant coexisting disease adapts to pregnancy and parturition. In these chapters, the authors provide the information needed to evaluate and prepare a woman for obstetric anesthesia. Other chapters in this section focus on the fetus. Here the reader will learn about routine fetal evaluation and surveillance, as well as the in utero diagnosis and management of fetal anomalies and complications.

The next section covers intraoperative management of the parturient throughout gestation and into the postpartum period. Although several of these chapters cover problems discussed in the first section of the book, the focus now shifts to anesthetic planning and management. Then follow two chapters covering postoperative analgesia and complications that arise after an anesthetic has been completed. In the final chapters, two important topics are discussed. Chapter 40 examines issues surrounding the provision of optimal obstetric anesthetic care in both community and university settings. Pertinent legal and ethical issues that the obstetric anesthesiologist may confront are discussed in the last chapter.

I hope that this book will be useful to both the anesthesiology resident in training and the practitioner who frequently or occasionally cares for parturients. For the trainee, I hope that this text fulfills several needs. First, it should explain how to prepare and anesthetize the healthy and complicated gravida. More importantly, however, it should explain why a given course of action is appropriate. For the practitioner, I hope that this book will serve as a review of obstetric anesthesia and a reference when she or he is faced with an unusual or difficult patient.

I thank all of the contributors to this book. I value each of their efforts. Without them, this book would never have happened. In addition, I extend my deepest thanks to Ruthann Griffin for her tireless help and support.

Mark C. Norris, M.D.
St. Louis, Missouri

Obstetric Anesthesia

Second Edition

PART I

Preoperative Assessment

Obstetric Anesthesia, second edition,
edited by Mark C. Norris.
Lippincott Williams & Wilkins, Philadelphia © 1999.

CHAPTER 1

Physiologic Adaptation to Pregnancy

The Healthy Parturient

BettyLou Koffel

The pregnant woman experiences physiologic changes in every organ system. Her body begins its transformation in the early weeks after conception and continues changing into the postpartum period. Understanding the progressive nature of this metamorphosis helps the obstetric anesthesiologist approach with confidence not only the peripartum gravida but also the pregnant surgical patient. This chapter will review pregnancy-related physiologic changes and consider their hormonal, metabolic, or mechanical basis and their anesthetic implications.

CARDIOVASCULAR SYSTEM

Physical Examination

Heart sounds not routinely heard in healthy young women appear during gestation (Fig. 1). Even S_1 and S_2 change. Pregnancy amplifies the first heart sound as early as 12 weeks estimated gestational age (EGA). Nearly all parturients have exaggerated splitting of the first heart sound. Respiratory variation of the second heart sound decreases. By 20 weeks' gestation, auscultation often (84%) reveals a third heart sound. The volume of S_3 peaks by 30 weeks. Ninety-six percent of pregnant women have a systolic murmur, most frequently of the ejection type. A diastolic flow murmur may be heard in 18% of patients (1,2). The onset of these murmurs correlates most closely with rises in blood volume, not cardiac output (1). Despite having normal electrocardiograms and systolic function, 9% of parturients will have a detectable pericardial effusion (by echocardiography) in the third trimester (3). The changes in heart sounds usually resolve within 4 weeks after delivery. A third heart sound, if present, usually disappears within 8 days of delivery (1,2). Although an audible S_3, a diastolic murmur, or a pericardial effusion should not be overlooked during pregnancy, they may be normal and not signify cardiac pathology.

Hemodynamic Measurements

The cardiovascular system changes significantly within the first 8 weeks of gestation. Heart rate increases and mean arterial pressure (MAP) decreases (4). Heart rate may rise as soon as 4 weeks after conception (5).

Longitudinal studies that evaluate the same women before and after they conceive provide particularly valuable information about the physiologic changes of pregnancy (Table 1). (Many studies use postpartum measurement as a basis of comparison when evaluating the hemodynamic changes of pregnancy. Weight and activity changes influence control data obtained after delivery. The preconception state provides a more accurate comparison for the early weeks of gestation.)

Clapp et al. (4) examined gravidae before conception and early in pregnancy. They found significant changes in heart rate (+17.5%) and MAP (−11%) by 7 weeks EGA. The heart rate and MAP did not change further through the end of the first trimester (4). Interestingly, pregnancies destined to fail did not exhibit these alterations at 8 weeks EGA (4).

Early elevations in stroke volume (6,7) and cardiac output (7,8) (20% to 40%) also have been noted. Walters et al. (6) studied women at monthly intervals beginning in the first trimester and found greater increases in stroke volume than in heart rate. Capeless and Clapp (7)

B. Koffel: Northwest Permanente, P.C., Portland, Oregon 97225.

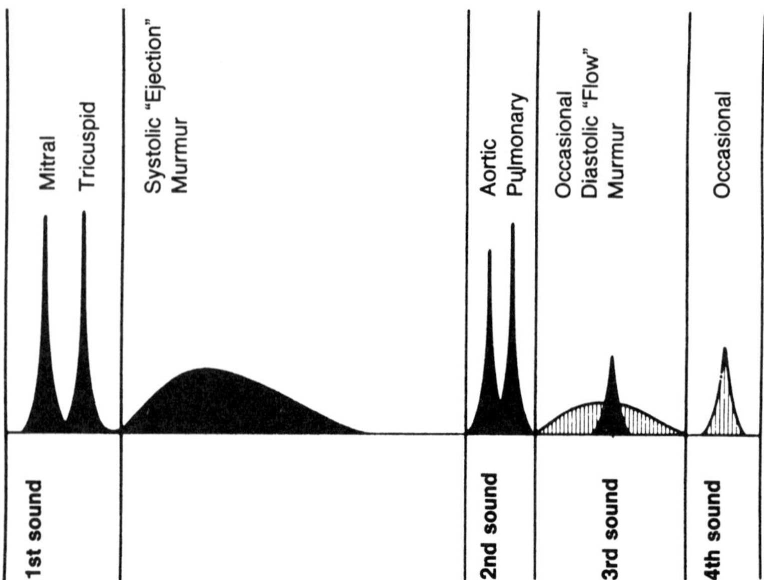

FIG. 1. Auscultatory findings of the heart during pregnancy. (From ref. 310, with permission.)

confirmed the greater stroke volume using M-mode echocardiography.

Cardiac Output

Cardiac output progressively increases throughout pregnancy (6,9,10). Most reports show cardiac output peaking between 24 and 32 weeks EGA (6,11,12). However, early investigators often failed to consider the effects of maternal position on cardiac output. In the supine position, the enlarging uterus compresses the aorta and inferior vena cava (IVC). Decreased venous return then limits cardiac output. When measured in the supine position, cardiac output peaks in the late second trimester and then falls to nonpregnant levels by term. Today, investigators and clinicians routinely attempt to limit aortocaval compression. Even so, cardiac output may peak before term. Recent measurements using pulsed and continuous-wave Doppler demonstrate further increases in cardiac output throughout the third trimester (13).

TABLE 1. *Maternal hemodynamic changes with pregnancy*

Variable	Percent change compared to nonpregnant value
Cardiac output	↑ 14%–50%
Heart rate	↑ 17%–26%
Stroke volume	No change–↑ 32%
Mean arterial pressure	No change–↓ 11%
Systemic vascular resistance	↓ 21%
Central venous pressure	No change
Pulmonary artery occlusion pressure	No change
Pulmonary vascular resistance	↓ 34%
Colliod oncotic pressure	↓ 14%

Table excludes values obtained in the supine position.
Data from refs. 6, 8, 10, 12, 15, 24, 31.

Left ventricular function (as measured by shortening characteristics) remains unchanged at term in spite of left ventricular enlargement (14). Contractility decreases in the postpartum period, suggesting augmentation at term (15). Left ventricular mass increases due to increased wall thickness (13). Echocardiography reveals increased (16) or decreased (17) myocardial contractility independent of the loading conditions of the left ventricle. Additional studies may resolve this conflict.

Measurement Techniques

Pulsed-Doppler (18) or suprasternal window continuous-wave ultrasound measurements (19) correlate reasonably well with thermodilution cardiac output. However, during periods of hemorrhage this consistency disappears (20), making noninvasive measurements difficult during parturition.

Accurate Doppler ultrasound cardiac output estimates require a constant aortic cross-sectional area. Variations in aortic area modify the estimated velocity of flow. Elevations in cardiac output detected by Doppler ultrasound could, then, be artifacts of an increasing aortic area. But, to mimic the changes in cardiac output reported during pregnancy, aortic cross-sectional area would have to expand by 30% to 45% (10). Various studies do not agree about pregnancy-related changes in aortic compliance and cross-sectional area (13,14).

During the late third trimester, thoracic electrical bioimpedence correlates well with standard oxygen extraction (Fick) measurements of cardiac index *only* in the left and right lateral positions. Poor correlation exists in all other positions (21); thus, thoracic electrical bioimpedence measurements must be interpreted with caution. Reports of these measurements with unspecified maternal position cannot be accurately interpreted.

Pressures

Maternal systemic blood pressure reaches a nadir at 16 to 20 weeks' gestation and then increases toward term (22,23). Diastolic pressure rises less than systolic pressure (23). Central venous pressure (24) and pulmonary artery occlusion pressure (24,25) remain stable throughout pregnancy. Colloid oncotic pressure decreases 14% (24). Lower colloid oncotic pressure may predispose the gravida to pulmonary edema in the face of elevated pulmonary artery occlusion pressure.

Etiology

In pregnancy, the heart must supply both the mother and fetus. Augmented cardiac output improves peripheral and uteroplacental oxygen delivery. During most of pregnancy, however, oxygen delivery exceeds fetal metabolic needs. During the first trimester, cardiac output increases 30% to 40%, whereas oxygen consumption grows only 10% (8,26). The smaller a–v O_2 difference of early pregnancy also shows that oxygen delivery exceeds oxygen consumption (9,27). Thus, the metabolic needs of the pregnancy do not provide an adequate explanation for these cardiovascular changes.

In early pregnancy, systemic vascular resistance decreases before stroke volume and cardiac output increase. This finding suggests that the fall in peripheral vascular resistance triggers the plasma volume increase, which then increases cardiac output. The decreased resistance persists throughout pregnancy (28). Perhaps the hormonal changes of early pregnancy are the true triggers. Estrogen production rises rapidly after conception. Experimentally, estrogens modulate the cardiovascular system. In sheep, infusing conjugated estrogens for 4 hours elevates cardiac output (+32%) and heart rate (+50%), and lowers MAP (−10%) and systemic vascular resistance (−19%). Thus, even a brief exposure to estrogenic hormones can significantly modify the cardiovascular system and mimic term pregnancy (29). In addition, estrogen enhances myocardial contractility (30,31). Other hormones also may play a role. Digitalis-like factor (DLIF) concentration increases during pregnancy. Interestingly, DLIF activity increases even more, suggesting that receptor function also changes (32). Relaxin, known to rise early in pregnancy, increases heart rate, left ventricular systolic pressure, and contractility in rats (33).

Effects of Positioning

In 1953, Howard (34) described a tachycardiac and hypotensive supine multigravida at term who complained of abdominal pain. The patient underwent emergency laparotomy and delivery for suspected ruptured uterus. A normal uterus and intrauterine pregnancy were found. Interestingly, a few days later, Howard observed another patient with the same syndrome of "postural shock." His investigation in dogs revealed that hypotension developed after IVC occlusion only during pregnancy. Howard believed that caval occlusion deprived the pregnant dog of a greater proportion of her total blood volume compared to the nonpregnant dog. During the third trimester, the supine, lithotomy (8,35,36), and even the right lateral (36) positions reduce maternal cardiac output, stroke volume, and systolic and diastolic blood pressure (8,35,36). Peripheral vascular resistance increases significantly in these positions (Figs. 2 and 3) (31).

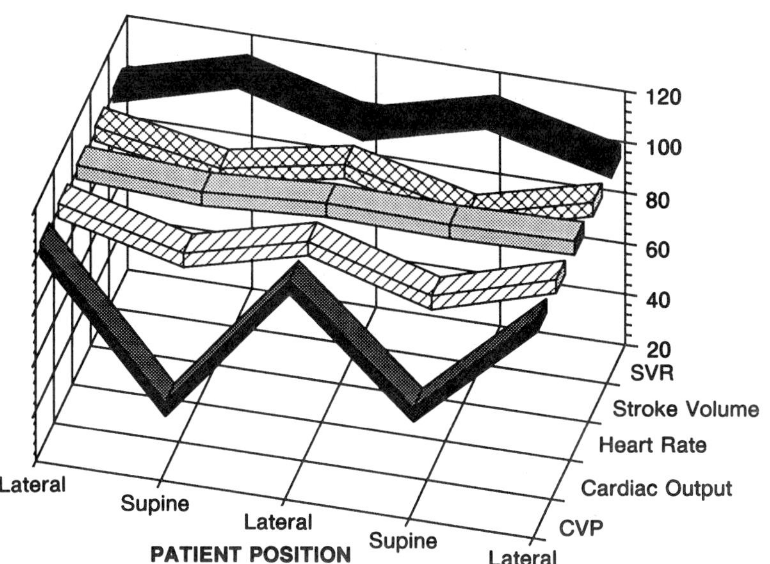

FIG. 2. Changes in central venous pressure, cardiac output, heart rate, stroke volume, and systemic vascular resistance with successive position changes. (Data from ref. 37.)

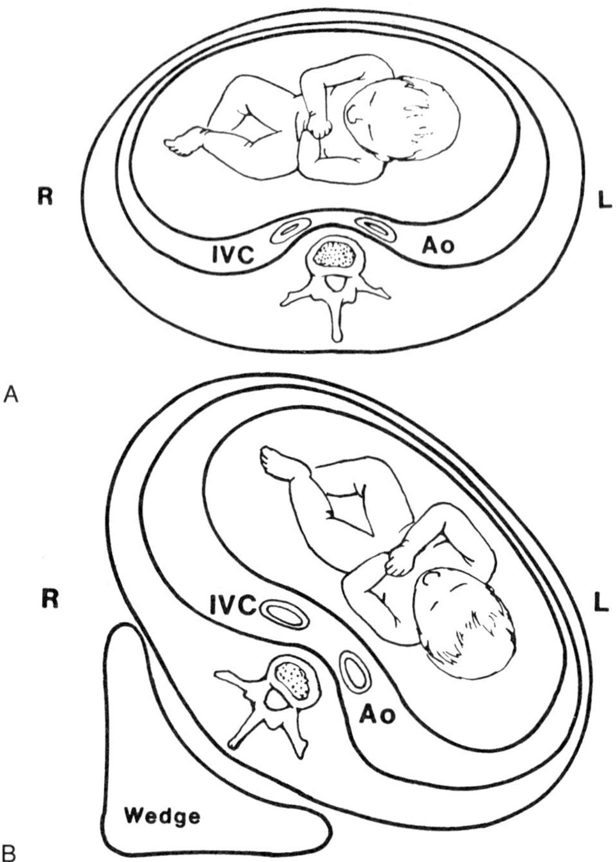

FIG. 3. A: Inferior vena cava *(IVC)* and aorta *(Ao)* compressed by the enlarged uterus when the gravida lies supine. (From ref. 311, with permission.) **B:** Lack of *IVC* and *Ao* compression with a wedge under the gravida's hip. (From ref. 311, with permission.)

Incompletely answered questions still exist regarding this phenomenon now called the supine hypotensive syndrome or aortocaval compression:

- Why do some patients exhibit the syndrome more often or more severely than others?
- What are the effects of labor on the syndrome?
- How can one prevent its occurrence?

Incidence and Etiology

Right atrial pressure declines in the supine position, limiting stroke volume and subsequently cardiac output (Fig. 2). Hypotension follows unless compensatory tachycardia or peripheral vasoconstriction ensue. An increment in systemic vascular resistance offsets the decrement in cardiac output, and most patients maintain systolic blood pressure. In some patients, however, bradycardia or a decrease in systemic vascular resistance leads to significant hypotension (37). Fifteen to twenty percent of third trimester patients exhibit hypotension or tachycardia when lying supine (37,38).

Interestingly, not all investigators have reported this syndrome (10,39). For example, McLennan and co-workers (10) evaluated gravidae at 36 and 40 weeks' gestation. In this study, position did not affect minute distance (a linear correlate of cardiac output) in any of 45 patients. These results show the inherent ability of many, but not all, parturients to compensate for aortocaval compression. Regional or general anesthesia compromise the gravida's ability to compensate for a fall in venous return. Labor, uteroplacental insufficiency, and fetal size also may affect the incidence and severity of supine hypotension.

Both occlusion of the IVC and compression of the aorta play a role in the development of the aortocaval compression syndrome. At term, the gravid uterus obstructs the IVC when the parturient lies supine. The uterus commonly completely obstructs the IVC at its bifurcation. Blood returns to the heart through the azygous and vertebral veins. After delivery, angiography demonstrates a normal IVC. The previously large azygous and vertebral veins contain only minimal dye (40). Nuclear magnetic resonance imaging documents the dilated epidural veins (41).

Supine hypotension can occur without IVC obstruction (34). In addition, IVC obstruction does not invariably lower blood pressure and cardiac output. In gravid ewes, when heart rate rose after IVC obstruction, MAP remained stable. In contrast, when the ewe became bradycardic, MAP declined (42). In chronically instrumented gravid ewes, cardiac output fell 37% and systemic blood pressure decreased 24% with suprarenal occlusion of the IVC. Infrarenal occlusion diminished cardiac output only (34). In humans, immediately after abdominal delivery, occlusion of the IVC lowered right atrial pressure but did not alter heart rate, blood pressure, or pulse pressure (37). Thus, although IVC occlusion decreases right atrial pressure, hypotension does not always follow.

Even in absence of hypotension, IVC compression may have adverse effects. Obstruction of the IVC decreases uterine artery perfusion pressure and uterine artery blood flow by raising venous pressure (43). IVC obstruction also may elevate uterine vascular resistance (44). In gravid ewes, occlusion of the uterine veins without occlusion of the IVC did not alter stroke volume or cardiac output; maternal arterial pressure actually rose (42). Thus, it is unlikely that the effects of IVC obstruction are the result of decreased uterine venous blood flow.

Simultaneous or isolated compression of the aorta also may play a role in the supine hypotensive syndrome. Femoral artery hypotension occurs earlier and more often than brachial artery hypotension (45). Usually femoral artery systolic pressure decreases more than diastolic pressure (46). Angiograms show the uterus displacing the subrenal aorta laterally, cranially and dorsally (47,48).

Other work, however, suggests that aortic compression does not play a role in the genesis of supine hypotension.

Kinsella et al. (49) measured plethysmographic leg blood flow, continuous-wave Doppler ultrasound arterial flow, leg mean arterial blood pressure, and heart rate in 20 gravidae. Heart rate increased in each position compared to the left lateral. Leg blood flow was less in the supine position, left pelvic tilt, and right pelvic tilt compared to full left lateral position. However, position did not change leg MAP or arterial flow (49). Acute aortic compression as an etiology of decreased leg blood flow is unlikely in the presence of normal leg MAP. IVC compression explains the diminished leg blood flow and tachycardia.

Labor and Aortocaval Compression

Uterine contractions may be necessary to elicit the signs of aortic compression. In 70 angiograms, Bieniarz et al. (47) showed that the relaxed uterus produced less aortic compression than the contracted uterus. During a contraction, this compression, mostly limited to L_4–L_5, can completely occlude the aorta (47). Contractions seen during a nonstress test eliminated both foot pulse and oximeter tracings in 2 of 42 parturients (38). In actively laboring women, dorsalis pedis artery ultrasound flow velocities decreased by 80% in both the supine and the lateral position during contractions (50). Painful uterine contractions may cause aortic compression through vasoconstriction by endogenous catecholamines. In 14 of 16 patients with continuous lumbar epidural analgesia, dorsalis pedis artery flow velocity remained high during contractions (50). Although these observations strongly suggest that uterine contractions worsen aortic compression, others have reported an ameliorating effect of contractions (34).

Labor also may alter IVC obstruction. In the supine position, uterine contractions augment cardiac output (25%) and stroke volume (33%) while lowering heart rate (15%). In contrast, in the lateral position, these values change very little with each contraction. These findings suggest that, in the supine position, uterine contractions relieve IVC occlusion (51).

Perhaps IVC occlusion does not occur during contractions because the uterus is more easily supported by the vertebral column in the contracted state. In effect, the contraction lifts the body of the uterus off the inferior cava. Yet the firmly contracted uterus more readily obstructs aortic flow than the relaxed uterus does.

Prevention

Although nearly all obstetric anesthesiologists routinely advocate left uterine displacement (Fig. 3), the standard pelvic tilt position does not consistently relieve IVC compression (39,52). Even the lateral position does not totally relieve compression of the IVC, at least as demonstrated by venogram (40). The lateral position does completely prevent aortic compression as measured by angiography (48). On magnetic resonance imaging, the lateral position relieves IVC compression and the associated engorgement of the epidural venous plexus (41).

We can conclude that the supine position may harm some gravidae; perhaps up to 20% will experience hypotension or decreased uterine blood flow. IVC compression impairs venous return and consequently cardiac output. These changes ultimately decrease uterine blood flow and fetal oxygen delivery. Uterine contractions may alleviate IVC compression, but exacerbate aortic compression. A 10 degree lateral tilt will eliminate aortocaval compression in most gravidae. Some will be asymptomatic only when completely on their side. Depending in part on the position of the fetal body within the uterus, a given gravida may respond better in the left or right lateral position.

Anesthetic Implications

Normal cardiac output and uterine artery perfusion depend on adequate venous return. Regional anesthesia causes peripheral vasodilation and venous pooling secondary to the loss of sympathetic tone. Vasodilation increases the likelihood of supine hypotension. Acute intravenous hydration before induction may increase blood volume and help maintain maternal cardiac output.

Aortocaval compression may complicate maternal and fetal resuscitation. Partial IVC occlusion makes resuscitation of dogs given 20 mg/kg of intravenous bupivacaine more difficult and prolonged (53). Adequate maternal resuscitation may require delivery to completely eliminate the deleterious effects of aortocaval compression (54).

Receptors and Reflexes

Pregnancy blunts vasoconstriction and vasodilation in response to α- and β-adrenergic stimulation (55,56). Whether this effect is due to changes in α- and β-adrenergic receptor number and function is not clear. Concurrent study of both receptor systems in 21 women at 10, 20, 30, and 37 weeks of pregnancy and 3 to 4 months postpartum did not reveal statistically significant changes (57). However, pregnancy attenuates catecholamine secretion in response to physiologic stress (58).

Nitric oxide release in subcutaneous blood vessels remains normal during pregnancy (59). Concentration of nitrite (a metabolite of nitric oxide) in maternal blood markedly decreases at delivery, suggesting that nitric oxide has some role in the decreased vascular resistance of pregnancy (60).

Pregnancy blunts parasympathetic responsiveness, particularly during the second trimester (61,62). Pregnancy markedly inhibits the chronotropic response to isoproterenol (63). The degree of this effect greatly exceeds that expected due to the increased plasma volume. The chron-

TABLE 2. *Maternal hemodynamic changes with labor*

	Cardiac output	Stroke volume	Heart rate
Early first stage			
Basal[a]	No change	No change	No change
Contraction[c]	↓ 15%–↑ 15%	No change–↓ 8%	No change–↑ 10%
Late first stage			
Rest[b]	No change–↑ 14%	No change–↑ 12%	No change–↑ 13%
Contraction[c]	↑ 20%	↑ 6%	↑ 13%
Second stage			
Without expulsive efforts[a]	No change	↓ 13%	↑ 27%
With expulsive efforts[a]	↓ 23%	↓ 49%	↑ 48%

[a]Compared to resting values before labor; [b]compared to basal labor values; [c]compared to between contraction values in the same stage of labor.
Data from refs. 51, 71–74.

otropic response to 15 μg of intravenous epinephrine also decreases at term (64). A pregnancy-related inhibitory circulating factor may cause this effect. Cultured rat myocardial cells (a model of β-adrenergic receptors) do not exhibit an isoproterenol-induced chronotropic effect when exposed to sera from term gravidae (65).

The altered response to sympathetic stimulation has two significant anesthetic implications. Decreased responsiveness to α- and β-adrenergic agonists limits the precision of a chronotropic intravenous test dose. And, β-Adrenergic agents are preferable for the treatment of maternal hypotension because α-adrenergic agents constrict the uterine arteries and impair uteroplacental blood flow.

Uterine Artery

Uterine artery blood flow increases from 3.5% of cardiac output in early pregnancy to 12% at term. Uterine artery blood flow rises from 50 mL/min at 10 weeks' gestation to 200 mL/min at 28 weeks and 500 mL/min at term (26). The resistance of the uterine artery to blood flow steadily declines during pregnancy (66,67). Both direct arteriovenous anastomoses in the uterus and uterine artery vasodilation secondary to estrogens and angiotensin II account for this fall. The uterine artery dilates normally in response to sodium nitroprusside and hydralazine (68) and constricts normally with norepinephrine (69).

Effects of Labor

Labor further modifies the cardiovascular system (Table 2). Each contraction squeezes about 300 mL of blood from the uterus into the central circulation (70). Uterine contractions also relieve IVC compression. Cardiac output (22%) and stroke volume (27%) rise during contractions in the first stage of labor. Maternal systolic and diastolic blood pressure increase 10 to 20 mm Hg during a contraction (51). Cardiac output reaches an apex 18 seconds before the uterus attains maximum amniotic fluid pressure (70). Both autotransfused blood and augmented venous return with each uterine contraction may explain these changes.

Both the process of labor and individual contractions affect cardiac output. Caudal analgesia prevents the progressive rise in cardiac output during labor but not the increases that coincide with each contraction (71). Robson and colleagues (72) measured stroke volume throughout labor using noninvasive techniques. All women labored in the left semilateral position with meperidine and nitrous oxide analgesia. Basal cardiac output increased 13% by 8-cm cervical dilation. Stroke volume, not heart rate, produced most of this change. Uterine contractions increased cardiac output in all patients throughout labor. The increment in cardiac output was greater at 8-cm and 4- to 7-cm cervical dilation than at 3 cm (Fig. 4). Beyond 4-cm dilation, the change in cardiac output with each contraction depended on significant increases in both heart rate and stroke volume (Figs. 5 and 6). Earlier, stroke volume changes predominated (72).

Maruta (73) confirmed increased cardiac output during contractions but found more significant increases in heart rate. In addition, expulsive efforts in the second stage of labor impaired cardiac output and stroke volume due to hypovolemia from a decrease in venous return.

We can conclude that labor increases cardiac output with changes in both heart rate and stroke volume. Adequate analgesia may limit, but not prevent, these changes. Gravidae with limited cardiac reserve frequently benefit from early labor analgesia and limited expulsive efforts.

Effects of Delivery

Cardiac output, stroke volume, and heart rate all increase immediately after delivery (Tables 3 and 4) (73,74). By 24 hours, MAP and stroke volume decline to their prelabor values (72). Cardiac output rapidly increases due to a central shift of blood from the now empty uterus and a marked decrease in IVC compression. Reports that compared hemodynamics after delivery to predelivery values measured in the supine position found greater changes in cardiac output, heart rate, and stroke volume (+80%, +50%, and +80%, respectively) (71,75). The absolute value of postpartum cardiac output is the same regardless of maternal position before delivery (71–76). Cardiac output returns to prelabor values within the first hour (76).

During abdominal delivery, cardiac output, stroke volume, and heart rate change less than with vaginal delivery (Table 3). The greater blood loss that occurs with cesarean section explains these differences (73,76). The type of anesthesia does not influence the cardiac changes associated with cesarean delivery (Table 4) (76).

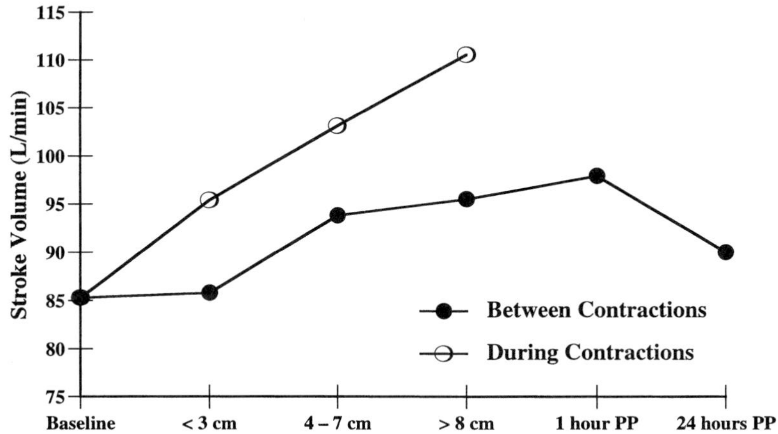

FIG. 4. Cardiac output during labor. (Data from ref. 72.)

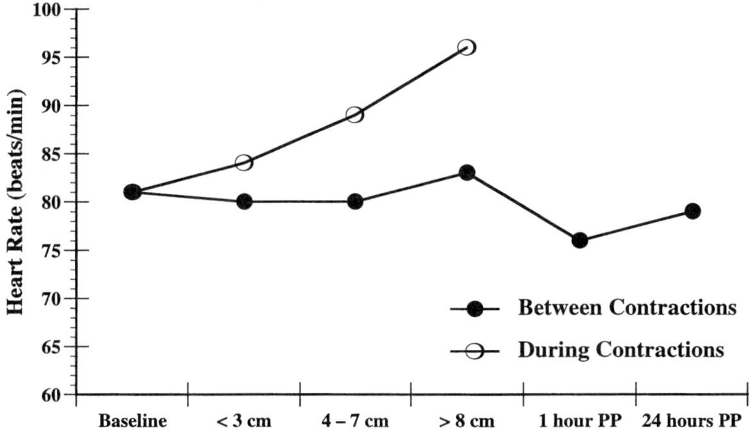

FIG. 5. Stroke volume during labor. (Data from ref. 72.)

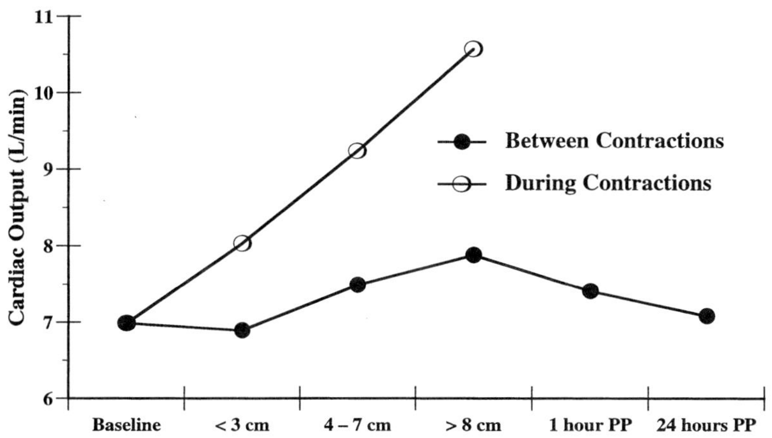

FIG. 6. Heart rate during labor. (Data from ref. 72.)

TABLE 3. *Maternal hemodynamic changes at delivery compared to late in pregnancy*

	Cardiac output	Stroke volume	Heart rate
Vaginal delivery			
Immediate	↑ 23%–25%	↑12%	↑ 12%–18%
1 h	No change	No change	No change
24 h	No change	No change	No change
Cesarean delivery			
Immediate	↑ 9%–15%	No change	↑ 12%–16%
15–30 min	↑ 17%–37%		
1 hr	No change		
24 h	No change		

No change means values reported do not differ significantly from resting values obtained late in pregnancy. Table does not include any parturients studied in the supine position.
Data from refs. 72, 73, 76.

Although postpartum hemodynamics return to term values within an hour, these are *not* nonpregnant values. Cardiac output remains increased for the first 24 hours postpartum and then progressively falls by the tenth postnatal day (25% decrease from term) (77). By 2 weeks after delivery, heart rate (20%), stroke volume (18%), cardiac output (28%), and contractility all decrease (15). Clark et al. (24) measured pulmonary artery pressures and cardiac output at term and again 11 to 13 weeks postpartum (in only the left lateral position). Cardiac output was 43% greater at term, heart rate 17% higher, systemic vascular resistance 21% lower, and pulmonary vascular resistance 34% lower (24). Maternal systolic and diastolic pressure may decrease for the first 2 days postpartum (77). They significantly increase by the fourth to sixth day postpartum (77,78). Central venous pressures rise in the first 24 hours postpartum if oxytocic drugs are given (79). If excessive blood loss (>500 mL) occurs, heart rate increases and stroke volume falls for 48 hours (77). Again, the type of anesthesia does not alter the effects of delivery on maternal hemodynamics (Table 4) (76,80).

In summary, the immediate postpartum period brings the greatest cardiac output of pregnancy. Although well tolerated by most gravidae, this stress may necessitate close surveillance in women with preeclampsia or heart disease.

Plasma Volume

Plasma volume increases during the first 24 weeks of gestation (81). Although some increment in plasma volume takes place by the end of the first trimester, most of this change occurs during the second trimester (82,83). The third trimester brings only a slight further rise (82,83). By 24 weeks, the plasma volume is 1,500 mL or 50% larger than before conception (81,84,85). Plasma volume, when expressed in milliliters per kilogram, plateaus between 24 and 40 weeks' gestation at 70 mL/kg (Fig. 7, Table 5) (81).

The expanded plasma volume enhances circulation to the uterus, meets excretory needs of the kidneys, and helps to radiate body heat produced by the elevated metabolic rate (84). The increased volume also serves to protect the fetus from the impaired venous return and decreased cardiac output of aortocaval compression. In addition, it provides a safeguard against blood loss at delivery.

The rise of plasma volume with pregnancy has several possible etiologies. The fall in systemic vascular resistance and blood pressure produce a reflex rise in blood volume (86). Estrogens also stimulate the renin-angiotensin system resulting in sodium and water retention (86,87). The influence of estrogens (whose precursors are formed in the fetal adrenal glands) has prompted Longo to say that the fetus through regulation of the hormonal milieu and in concert with the placenta, controls the maternal hematologic and cardiovascular adaptations to pregnancy (86).

TABLE 4. *Maternal hemodynamic changes with elective cesarean delivery*

Time after delivery	Cardiac output	Stroke volume	Heart rate
Epidural anesthesia			
15 min	↑ 37%	↑ 27%	No change
30 min	↑ 26%	No change	No change
60 min	No change	No change	No change
24 h	No change	No change	No change
General anesthesia			
15 min	↑ 28%	↑ 17%	↑ 11%
30 min	↑ 17%	↑ 14%	No change
60 min	No change	No change	No change
24 h	No change	No change	No change

No change means values obtained did not differ from baseline values obtained before induction of anesthesia.
Data from ref. 76.

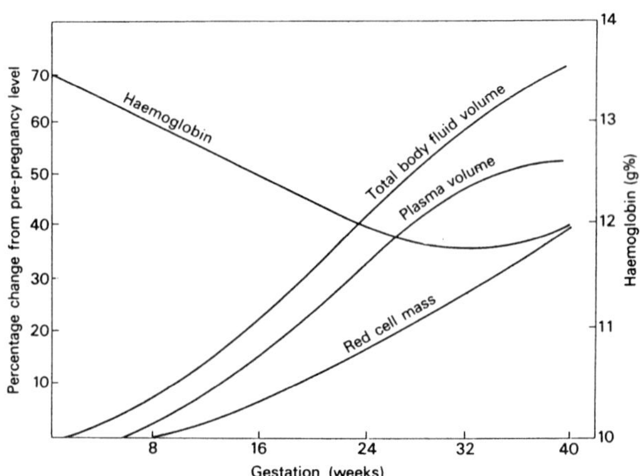

FIG. 7. Progressive changes in hemoglobin, total body fluid, plasma volume, and red cell mass throughout pregnancy. (From ref. 312, with permission.)

TABLE 5. *Plasma and red cell volume changes with pregnancy*

	Change at term
Plasma volume	↑ 25%–80%
Red cell volume	↑ 20%

Data from refs. 81–84.

Red Cells

During pregnancy, red cell mass increases by 18% (83). Red cell mass and plasma volume exhibit no fixed relation to each other (84). Red blood cell volume rises more slowly and to a lesser extent than plasma volume. This discrepancy causes the well-known decrease in hematocrit with pregnancy (81,83,84,88). A normal or elevated hematocrit during pregnancy may signify intravascular volume depletion. However, when measured on a milliliter per kilogram basis, mean red cell volume remains constant at 27 mL/kg. Plasma volume changes from 50 to 70 mL/kg (81).

Erythropoietin, synthesized by the kidneys, stimulates red cell production (89). Urinary excretion of erythropoietin peaks between 20 and 28 weeks' gestation. Human placental lactogen augments the action of erythropoietin (89). Chorionic somatotropin, prolactin, and progesterone also stimulate erythropoiesis (86).

White Cells

White blood cell counts also increase during pregnancy (88,90). Neutrophils make up most this elevation. Monocytes may contribute, but lymphocytes, eosinophils, and basophils generally decline (90).

Delivery

A gravida normally loses about 500 mL of blood at vaginal delivery and close to 1,000 mL at abdominal delivery (91). In response to the hemorrhage of delivery, blood volume rapidly decreases to normal and hematocrit changes very little (83). This response to hemorrhage in the parturient differs from that of the nonpregnant patient in whom blood volume increases and hematocrit decreases (91). Although total red blood cell volume falls rapidly (91), red cell volume per kilogram of body weight remains stable (81). Plasma volume declines over 3 to 5 days and reaches preconception levels by 8 weeks postpartum (81).

Blood loss at delivery rarely necessitates transfusion due to the rapid decrement in plasma volume that helps maintain a normal hematocrit. Postpartum, a drop in hematocrit suggests continuing blood loss.

RESPIRATORY SYSTEM

Physical Examination

The increased volume of the intraabdominal contents at term elevates the gravida's diaphragm and widens the transverse diameter of her chest 2 cm (Fig. 8). Gestation does not impair diaphragmatic motion. Roentgenograms reveal increased lung markings and a widened subcostal angle (92). Hyperemia of the nasal turbinates and facial edema commonly complicate the airway (93,94). A parturient may have severe laryngeal edema without stridor (95).

Lung Volumes

Elevation of the diaphragm and changes in the chest diameter may alter dynamic lung volumes and gas flow in the airways, but, like the cardiovascular system, hormonal and metabolic factors also play a major role. The progression of respiratory changes throughout gestation is not well understood. In one study, lung volumes did not change between the first and the third trimester (96). These results reflect the early onset of the respiratory changes of pregnancy.

Tidal volume increases, beginning in the first trimester, to 28% above nonpregnant values at term (97). Functional residual capacity (FRC) is progressively compressed throughout gestation (97–100). Residual volume and expiratory reserve volume (ERV) also fall (100–102). Total lung capacity and vital capacity change little with pregnancy (92,100). Inspiratory capacity rises 10% at term, whereas expiratory capacity decreases 20% (Fig. 9, Table 6) (100).

Airway closure occurs during normal tidal breathing if closing volume exceeds ERV. This event adversely affects gas exchange. One study reported a rise in closing volume with pregnancy (103), whereas another found no

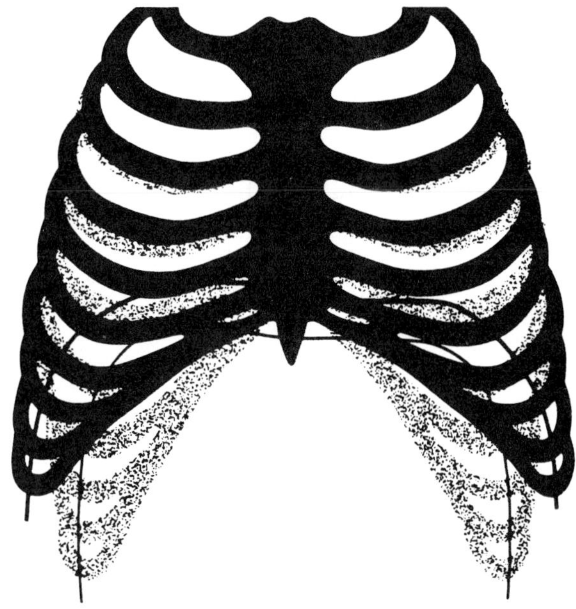

FIG. 8. The normal rib cage (*stippled,* nonpregnant) showing raised diaphragm, increased diameter, and subcostal angle as seen with pregnancy *(black).* (From ref. 310, with permission.)

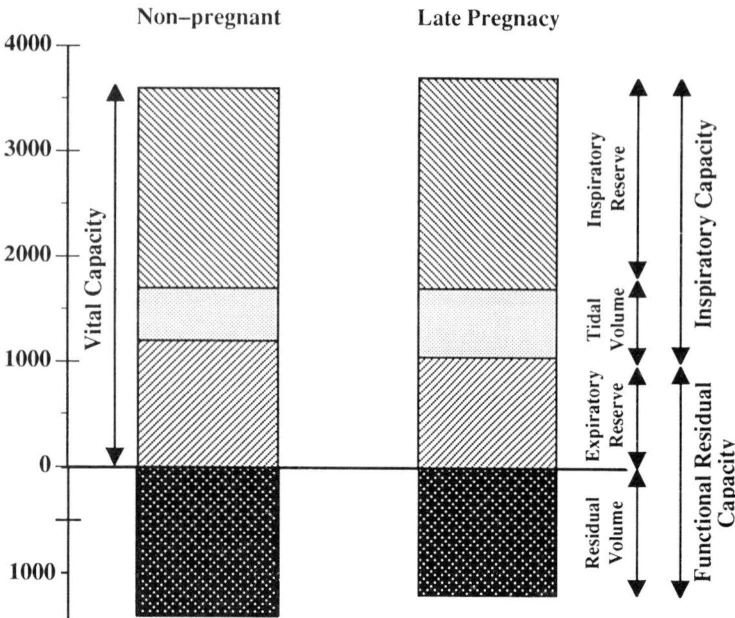

FIG. 9. Lung volumes and capacities as altered by pregnancy. (Redrawn from ref. 310.)

change (99). Closing volume at term measures 8% of vital capacity, significantly higher than the 4.8% found 4 to 5 days postpartum (103). Other investigators report closing volume to comprise 10% to 11% of vital capacity when measured both in the third trimester and 2 days postpartum (99). Perhaps the comparison to measurements made later in the postpartum period better reflect the nonpregnant (baseline) state.

The relationship between FRC and closing volume may explain the mild supine hypoxemia often seen in term parturients (103). Airway closure can adversely affect gas exchange. Late in gestation, airway closure occurs above or closer to FRC than it does in the nonpregnant state (104,105). This change may reflect not so much an alteration in closing volume as the smaller FRC (104). In most patients, position does not alter closing volume, but FRC falls further in the supine position. Hypoxemia often follows. Indeed, episodes of nocturnal hypoxemia (SpO_2 <95) occur more often during pregnancy. Even the mean SpO_2 decreases compared with nonpregnant values (95.2% vs 98.5%). In one study, airway obstruction or apnea did not occur (106).

Pregnancy does not change anatomic dead space but decreases physiologic dead space (V_D/V_T). Therefore, pregnancy must considerably reduce alveolar dead space (107). Wide variations in normal values of V_D/V_T make interpretation of this data difficult (108). A smaller alveolar dead space improves the efficiency of ventilation and lowers the gradient between alveolar and end-tidal CO_2. Intrapulmonary shunt increases from 2% to 5% in nonpregnant subjects to 13% to 15% in term gravidae. This increased shunt may explain some of the dyspnea reported on exertion during pregnancy, as patients with shunt fractions of 5% to 15% often exhibit shortness of breath with exertion (109).

TABLE 6. *Changes in lung volumes and capacities during pregnancy*

	Change at term
Tidal volume (TV)	↑ 19–28%
Expiratory reserve volume (ERV)	↓ 17%
Residual volume (RV)	No change–↓ 22%
Functional residual capacity (FRC)	↓ 12%–25%
Vital capacity (VC)	No change–↑ 6%
Inspiratory capacity (IC)	↑ 10%–19%
Expiratory capacity (EC)	↓ 20%
Total lung capacity (TLC)	No change–↓ 5%

Data from refs. 92, 97–103, 107, 111, 115.

Flow

FEV_1 does not change (100–103,110,111). Pregnancy also does not alter flow measured at various lung volumes (flow–volume loops) (99). Lung compliance also remains unaffected by gestation. Total pulmonary resistance (made up of airways resistance and tissue resistance) falls significantly. Decreased airway resistance predominates. Specific airway conductance rises during pregnancy, suggesting increased cross-sectional area of the airway (Table 7). (98).

TABLE 7. *Ventilation parameters at term*

	Change at term
Respiratory rate (RR)	↑ 8.5%
Minute ventilation (MV)	↑ 19%–50%
Forced expiratory volume (FEV_1)	No change

Data from refs. 97, 99, 100, 113, 115.

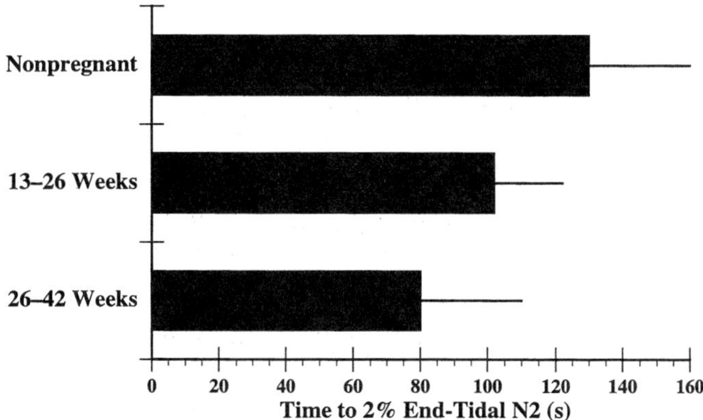

FIG. 10. Time to 2% end-tidal nitrogen concentration in three groups of women. Pregnancy progressively shortens the time needed to attain adequate preoxygenation. (Data from ref. 119.)

Normally, bronchial muscle constricts in response to hypocapnia. Therefore, a bronchodilating mechanism must exist during pregnancy to explain bronchodilation in the face of hyperventilation (112). Progesterone increases β-adrenergic activity (112) and smooth muscle relaxation occurs (102). For a given alveolar pressure, there is a significantly higher flow of air during pregnancy due to smooth muscle relaxation (102).

Minute Ventilation

Minute ventilation rises 19% to 50% by term (97,100, 113). The increment in alveolar ventilation begins very soon after conception (97,98,110,114). Respiratory rate increases 9% and tidal volume 28% (Tables 6 and 7) (100,115). Together they elevate minute ventilation to above the level required by changes in oxygen consumption and carbon dioxide production (114). Exercise further increases minute ventilation (111,114,116) and oxygen consumption (113). With greater work, however, a decrease in pulmonary reserve becomes apparent (117).

The alveolar hyperventilation of pregnancy reflects hypersensitivity of the respiratory centers. Progesterone acts as a respiratory stimulant without changing the basal metabolic rate (110). Carbon dioxide sensitivity curves shift to the left during pregnancy (100). A parturient can hold her breath only until she attains a p_aCO_2 of 39.2 versus 48.2 mm Hg in nonpregnant subjects (118). Progesterone administration to males and postmenopausal women duplicates these changes (118). Sensitivity to CO_2 does not differ between the first and third trimester but falls dramatically after delivery (96).

Nitrogen washout times also reflect alveolar hyperventilation. The time needed to reach an end-tidal nitrogen of 2% when breathing 100% oxygen falls from 130 seconds before conception to 108 seconds at 13 to 26 weeks EGA to only 80 seconds at 26 to 42 weeks (Fig. 10) (119). Clinically, rapid nitrogen washout allows adequate maternal denitrogenation with four vital capacity breaths of 100% oxygen (120). Four vital capacity breaths and 3 minutes of breathing 100% oxygen yield similar p_aO_2 values (121).

Oxygen Consumption

At term, the parturient consumes 20% to 30% more oxygen than at 12 to 14 weeks postpartum (113). Most of this oxygen goes to supply the fetus. Demands by the placenta, uterus, and breasts account for most of the remainder of the augmented oxygen need (Fig. 11) (122).

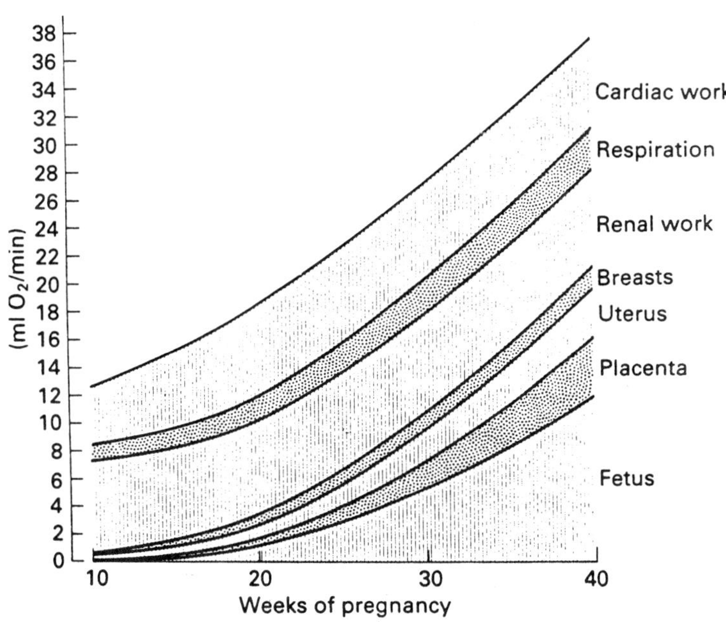

FIG. 11. Partition of the increased oxygen consumption of pregnancy. (From ref. 310, with permission.)

Pulmonary Gas Exchange

Diffusion capacity does not change (123) or increases early in gestation (105). Later decreases return the diffusion capacity at term to nonpregnant values (105). The alveolar–arterial gradient (p_AO_2–p_aO_2) does not differ between the first trimester and term (96). The p_AO_2–p_aO_2 gradient increases in the supine position compared to the sitting position (20.0 vs 14.3 mm Hg, respectively) (103). This effect most likely represents the relationship between a diminished FRC and a slightly elevated closing volume. At term, under general anesthesia for abdominal delivery, mean p_AO_2–p_aO_2 gradient is 138 mm Hg at an inspired oxygen concentration of 67.5% (108).

The hyperventilation of pregnancy lowers end-tidal CO_2 (113). Gestation also affects the arterial to end-tidal CO_2 difference. In anesthetized, nonpregnant women, arterial CO_2 (p_aCO_2) is 3.5 to 5.3 mm Hg higher than the end-tidal CO_2. After conception, this gradient narrows. Even early in gestation, p_aCO_2 is only 0.5 mm Hg higher than end-tidal CO_2 (124). By the end of the first trimester the end-tidal CO_2 approximates p_aCO_2 (124). At term, under general anesthesia, the gradient can reverse and 50% of parturients have a higher end-tidal CO_2 than arterial CO_2. The capnogram shows a steep phase III slope (Fig. 12) (101,125,126). This trend reverses with delivery and mean p_aCO_2 rises from 0.03 to 0.78 mm Hg above end-tidal CO_2 by 25 minutes postpartum (125). Still, up to 31% of postpartum patients have higher end-tidal than arterial CO_2 (126). During general anesthesia for postpartum tubal ligation, the mean p_aCO_2 gradient remains low at 0.6 mm Hg. Regression analysis suggests the relationship between arterial and end-tidal CO_2 returns to normal by 8 days after delivery (126).

Greater minute ventilation, cardiac output, and blood volume as well as the fall in alveolar dead space contribute to the smaller arterial to end-tidal CO_2 difference in pregnancy. End-tidal CO_2 values can accurately predict the degree of maternal hyperventilation and prevent uterine vasoconstriction-induced hypocarbia.

Maternal–Fetal Gas Exchange

The placenta consumes oxygen and produces carbon dioxide. Placental metabolism contributes to a considerable maternal–fetal carbon dioxide gradient. Fetal pCO_2, but not pO_2, correlates with maternal p_aCO_2. Fetal pCO_2 averages 11.3 mm Hg higher than maternal p_aCO_2 (127). The carbon dioxide gradient does not correlate with maternal p_aO_2. Maternal–fetal oxygen gradient varies with maternal p_aO_2. Umbilical vein pO_2 rises moderately in response to maternal hyperoxia (127,128). Fetal oxygen uptake and uterine blood flow do not relate to maternal p_aO_2 (128). These relationships allow administration of high oxygen concentrations to the mother without exposing the fetus to the hazards of hyperoxia.

The oxygen hemoglobin dissociation curves of normal gravidae overlap the normal range (129,130), but most lie to the right of their position if not pregnant (129). p_{50} increases significantly during gestation, allowing more oxygen delivery at the tissue level (131,132). The nonpregnant female and first, second, and third trimester values of p_{50} reflect the right-shifted oxygen hemoglobin dissociation curve (26.7, 27.8, 28.8, and 30.4, respectively) (133). The elevated p_{50} aids oxygen delivery to the uteroplacental unit.

The respiratory alkalosis of pregnancy pushes the oxygen hemoglobin dissociation curve to the left, serving as an

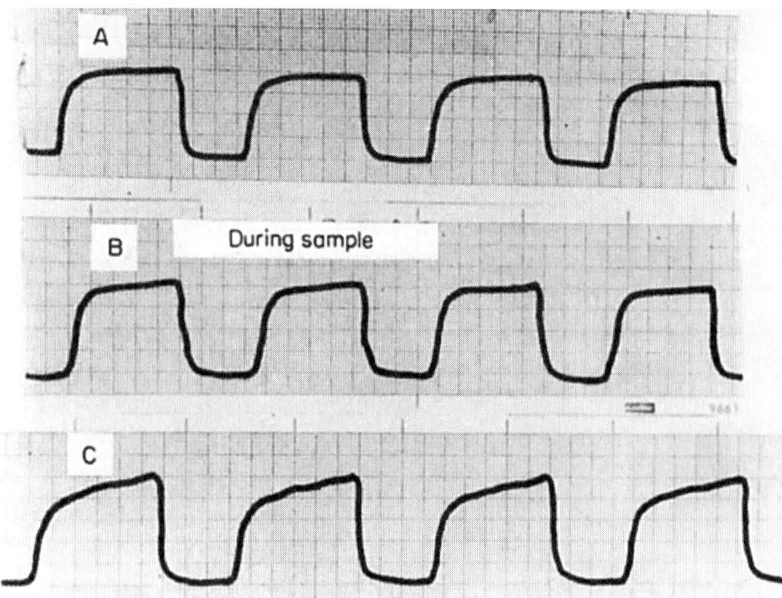

FIG. 12. Capnograms during general anesthesia in a nonpregnant female *(A)* and gravidae *(B and C)*. Capnogram *C* demonstrates a steep phase III slope, resulting in a negative arterial to end-tidal difference. (From ref. 126, with permission.)

impetus to increased 2,3-diphosphoglycerate (DPG) production. Maternal 2,3-DPG levels rise by 30% above nonpregnant values (134,135). However, some investigators report no change in 2,3-DPG (131,136). The higher concentration of 2,3-DPG pushes the dissociation curve back to the right. Intracellular acidosis, even in the face of extracellular alkalosis favors oxygen delivery to the fetus (137).

In sum, with pregnancy, the oxyhemoglobin dissociation curve moves slightly to the right but remains within the range of normal. This shift increases p_{50} and allows more oxygen delivery at the tissue level. This adaptation augments oxygen delivery to the uteroplacental unit. High-risk pregnancy also may alter these values. Preeclampsia shifts the oxygen hemoglobin dissociation curve to the left with a p_{50} of 25.1 (136).

Blood Gas Analysis

The hyperventilation of pregnancy decreases the p_aCO_2 to 26 to 32 mm Hg (96,114,138–141). The supine position does not change p_aCO_2 (103). With pregnancy, p_aO_2 rises slightly to 92 to 106 mm Hg (mean O_2 saturation 97.2%) (96,103,105,138–140). The supine position impairs oxygen exchange and average p_aO_2 falls from 101.2 to 94.6 mm Hg (103). Capillary pO_2 also is higher (13 mm Hg) in the sitting versus the supine position (141). This mild supine hypoxemia may relate to the increased volume of abdominal contents and elevated closing volume (103). Aortocaval compression also could contribute by hindering venous return and widening the arteriovenous oxygen difference.

The metabolic compensation to this respiratory alkalosis induces a fall in plasma bicarbonate concentration to 16 to 21 mEq/L, maintaining a near normal or slightly elevated pH (7.405 to 7.42) (96,105,114,138–141,143, 144). This adjustment begins early in pregnancy (110, 114). Persistently low intracellular pH values provide a continual stimulus to hyperventilation (137).

Etiology

When significant respiratory changes arise, they usually begin early in gestation, before the uterus becomes an abdominal organ (100). This trend suggests that hormonal or metabolic events instead of mechanical developments induce the transformation. Oxygen consumption escalates more gradually than cardiac output (26). Unlike cardiac output, which probably rises in response to hormonal stimuli, oxygen consumption seems to increase in concert with the metabolic needs of the mother and her fetus.

Acid–base changes begin immediately after conception. They resemble acclimatization to high altitude (110). A hormonal basis seems likely (105,145). Both progesterone and estrogens may be involved. The production of various prostaglandins, cyclic guanine monophosphate, and cyclic adenosine phosphate increases during pregnancy. These compounds may ultimately prove to be important mediators of some of the respiratory changes of pregnancy (105).

Progesterone augments the respiratory response to hypercarbia. Progesterone may modify the permeability of chemoreceptor cells or directly stimulate the central respiratory or hypothalamic neurons in contact with the blood (146). When given to male volunteers, progesterone increases tidal volume, respiratory rate, and minute ventilation with a resultant rise in pH and fall in p_aCO_2 and bicarbonate (118).

Effects of Labor

Forced vital capacity, FEV_1, and maximum voluntary ventilation do not change in labor (147). Pain induces maternal hyperventilation. Uterine contractions increase oxygen consumption (63%) and minute ventilation (74%) during the first stage of labor (148). Gravidae hyperventilate during early labor out of proportion to the increased metabolic demand (149). Adequate analgesia eliminates these changes. Contractions do not significantly modify respiratory measurements in women receiving lumbar epidural analgesia (148,149). Therefore, epidural block effectively decreases the work of breathing during labor. Even during expulsive efforts of the second stage, analgesia minimizes oxygen consumption and minute ventilation (148).

Hypoxemia also may arise during labor. Oxygen saturation fell below 90% in 49% of laboring women. Systemic narcotics and inhalation analgesia increased the frequency of low oxygen saturations (150).

In the first stage of labor, women hyperventilate during painful contractions and p_aCO_2 falls 6 to 7 mm Hg. This effect persists throughout parturition. In the second stage of labor, mean p_aCO_2 is 22.3 mm Hg between contractions and declines to 16.2 mm Hg during contractions. The pH and p_aO_2 increase during the second stage (151). Maternal hyperventilation can modify fetal acid–base status. The most alkalotic mothers (p_aCO_2 <17 mm Hg) deliver acidotic infants (152). Uterine blood flow decreases if p_aCO_2 reaches a critical level (152).

Effects of Delivery

Alveolar hyperventilation and sensitivity of respiratory centers to carbon dioxide suddenly decrease after delivery (96). Carbon dioxide production and oxygen consumption approach normal 1 to 2 weeks postpartum (115). Minute ventilation and oxygen uptake remain elevated for up to 2 weeks (97,114,115). Vital capacity, total lung capacity, and maximum breathing capacity fall markedly in the early postpartum period (92,97). Tidal volume begins to decline within 5 days (100,115). FRC and residual volume return to normal within 48 hours (100).

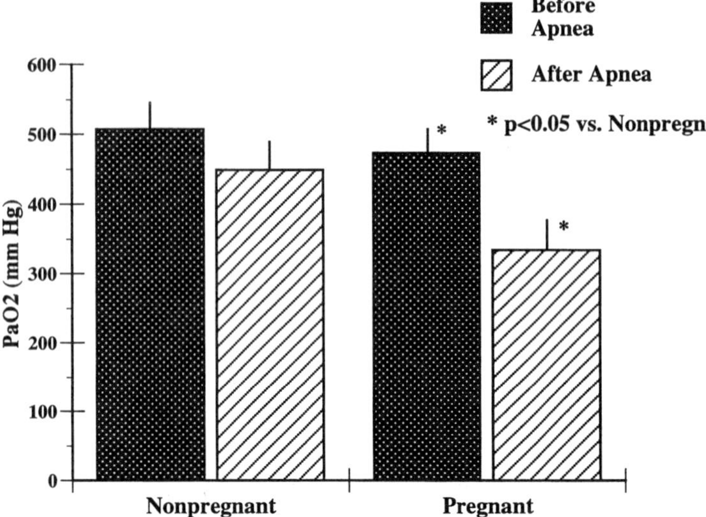

FIG. 13. Fall in p_aO_2 after 60 seconds of apnea in 12 pregnant and 8 nonpregnant women. All patients were intubated and ventilated with 97.5% O_2. The endotracheal tube was then disconnected from the anesthetic machine and exposed to room air. (Data from ref. 153.)

Anesthetic Implications

The smaller FRC and increased oxygen consumption limit the gravida's oxygen reserve. With maternal apnea, p_aO_2 falls rapidly (Fig. 13) (153). Critical hypoxemia can occur with alarming speed during induction of general anesthesia. Rapid intubation or oxygenation (by mask with cricoid pressure) by experienced personnel prevent disaster. Short-handled laryngoscopes and a range of endotracheal tube sizes may facilitate tracheal intubation.

Mechanical hyperventilation to a p_aCO_2 of 22 mm Hg in anesthetized gravid ewes lowers fetal carotid artery pO_2 by 8 mm Hg. Prolonged maternal hyperventilation may produce fetal asphyxia with severe hypoxia and metabolic acidosis (154). Maintaining maternal arterial and end-tidal CO_2 near 30 mm Hg will avoid the deleterious effects of mechanical hyperventilation on fetal oxygenation. Mechanical hyperventilation also can worsen fetal acid–base status by limiting maternal cardiac output and, therefore, placental blood flow (155). Although maternal hypercapnia may increase oxygen supply to the fetus above normal, it is not clinically indicated (154).

Due to the differences between fetal and maternal hemoglobin, raising maternal F_IO_2 from 50% to 100% elevates maternal p_aO_2 but does not change fetal pO_2 (127). High inspired concentrations of oxygen can safely maximize maternal oxygenation without compromising the fetus.

The sitting position minimizes the negative effects of pregnancy on the respiratory system. Gravidae with significant respiratory disease can best be evaluated and cared for when upright.

RENAL SYSTEM

Physical Changes

The gravid uterus and progesterone cause ureteral dilatation during pregnancy (156–161) not accompanied by an elevation in intrarenal resistivity index (162). The widening occurs above the pelvic brim (163). Ureteral dilatation manifests early in pregnancy and may persist up to 12 weeks postpartum, making a solely mechanical explanation unlikely (157,160–162). Postpartum intravenous pyleograms reveal a mean kidney length 1.5 cm greater than that measured in nonpregnant women (156).

Glomerular Filtration

Glomerular filtration increases 50% during pregnancy (156,160,161,164–167), lowering blood urea nitrogen (BUN) and creatinine to 6 to 8 mg/100 mL and 0.4 to 0.6 mg/100 mL, respectively (Fig. 14, Table 8) (160,161). Effective renal plasma flow (ERPF) significantly increases during the first two trimesters (164,166,168). The third trimester brings a fall in ERPF (as measured by para-aminohippurate [PAH] clearance) but not in glomerular filtration rate (GFR) (167,169). Also in the third trimester, creatinine production must increase. Serum creatinine concentration rises but clearance does not change (167).

Serial measurements of creatinine clearance reveal the early and progressive nature of the changes in GFR (170).

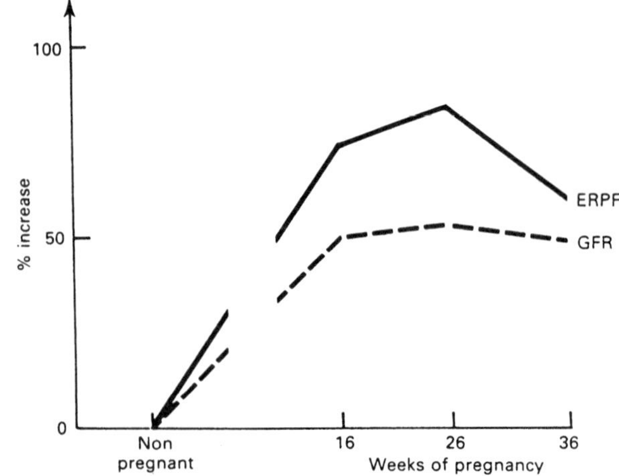

FIG. 14. Relative changes in effective renal plasma flow *(ERPF)* and glomerular filtration rate *(GFR)* during pregnancy. (From ref. 310, with permission.)

TABLE 8. *Renal changes during pregnancy*

	Change at term
Glomerular filtration rate (GFR)	↑ 50%
Effective renal plasma flow (ERPF)	↑ 25%–90%
Blood urea nitrogen (BUN)	↓ 40%
Serum creatinine	↓ 40%

Data from refs. 166, 168.

Creatinine clearance approximates GFR (171) and increases 25% by the fourth week of gestation (170). By the ninth week, clearance rises 45% (170). Despite these increases, the kidney retains the capacity to vasodilate and increase GFR in response to an acute protein load. This effect suggests that GFR can increase by more than one mechanism (172,173).

Elevated blood volume contributes to this augmented glomerular filtration (165). However, the rise in plasma volume fails to explain the early changes in renal function (170). A hormonal mechanism seems likely, as changes in creatinine clearance also occur during the normal menstrual cycle. In addition, women destined to have spontaneous abortions do not show sustained changes in creatinine clearance (170).

Harder to explain is the third trimester decrease in ERPF. Maternal position strongly influences renal blood flow (26). Similar measurements of ERPF in the left lateral (169,174) or sitting (167,174) position make aortocaval compression an unlikely but still possible explanation. Prolonged measurement of ERPF in one position yields declining values (174). Plasma volume changes provide another possible explanation. But, plasma volume continues to increase, albeit only minimally, in the third trimester (82,83).

Tubular Function

Although pregnancy does not alter the tubular handling of some substances (175), the ability to reabsorb glucose universally declines (166,176,177). In women who develop minor degrees of glycosuria, tubular function returns to normal after delivery. Parturients who exhibit more glycosuria have postpartum evidence of tubular damage (177). The mechanism of glucosuria is unclear. The presence of persistent tubular damage suggests involvement of more than just a larger filtered glucose load presented to the tubules by volume expansion and elevated GFR. Glycosuria normally resolves within 1 week of delivery, faster than carbohydrate metabolism normalizes, suggesting an alteration of tubular function (177).

To increase plasma volume, total body sodium also must rise. The body retains 500 to 850 mEq of sodium during pregnancy (161). Increased renin and aldosterone contribute to sodium retention (160). The uteroplacental unit contributes to elevated prorenin production (160,178). Aldosterone secretion compensates for natriuretic effects of pregnancy (179). Both the increased GFR and progesterone's competitive inhibition of aldosterone's action at distal tubular sites promote sodium loss (179–182). Pregnant women retain 300 mEq of potassium (183). Progesterone inhibits potassium excretion by antagonizing aldosterone (179,183). Plasma potassium concentration decreases 10% (168).

Bicarbonate reclamation remains normal during pregnancy in spite of lowered serum bicarbonate values. The gravida retains the normal renal acidifying mechanisms (184).

Plasma osmolality decreases an average of 8 to 10 mOsm/kg by the tenth week of gestation (185). The osmotic threshold for thirst declines, as does the threshold for arginine vasopressin (AVP) secretion. The parturient drinks more to maintain the lower osmolality (185). Endorphins may alter AVP secretion (185). Relaxin lowers osmolality in the pregnant rat. However, a study comparing human pregnancy conceived via ovum donation (with undetectable relaxin throughout pregnancy), in vitro fertilization and embryo transfer (elevated relaxin), or natural conception (normal relaxin) found no correlation between relaxin and plasma osmolality (186).

Renin activity remains elevated for 2 to 7 days after delivery. Umbilical venous blood contains high concentrations of prorenin (178). Thus, the placenta may be the source of extra renin during gestation. However, the lack of change in renin activity with delivery casts doubt on this explanation (187). At term, the gravida's position uniformly affects renin activity (163) so interpretation of renin data requires care.

Implications

Pregnancy modifies the interpretation of diagnostic studies that detect dilated ureters or increased kidney size. Ureteral dilatation contributes to frequent urinary tract infection. The risk of preterm labor increases with infection. A gravida with significant renal disease may maintain a somewhat normal BUN and creatinine. Slight elevation of these values suggests a need for diagnostic evaluation. Glycosuria may be normal during pregnancy. Pregnancy modifies renal handling of drugs and may have significant effects on pharmacokinetics.

GASTROINTESTINAL SYSTEM

Progesterone, as a smooth muscle relaxant, decreases gastric motility during pregnancy. Progesterone-treated male rats have impaired esophageal, antral, and colonic contractile activity (188). Progesterone and estradiol treatment inhibit the gastrointestinal contractile response elicited by acetylcholine and gastrin (189).

Esophagus

At 16 weeks EGA, pregnancy does not lower basal lower esophageal sphincter (LES) tone when measured by a three-lumen tube (190). However, the response to agents that normally increase LES tone is attenuated (190). LES becomes progressively weaker during pregnancy (191). LES pressure reaches its nadir at 36 weeks (192). Intragastric pressure rises during gestation, whereas lower intraesophageal pressure falls (193,194). Thus, pregnancy narrows the pressure difference between the stomach and esophagus from 7 mm Hg in nonpregnant women to 3.4 mm Hg (194). In addition, peristaltic speed and amplitude decline in the gravida. Elevated abdominal pressure and changes in the position of the stomach contribute to a higher incidence of hiatal hernia in parturients (194). Heartburn and associated esophagitis become quite common (up to 70% of gravidas) (195). Esophagitis correlates with the lowest gradients across the LES (193) and pyloric sphincter relaxation (196).

Stomach

Gastric Emptying

A variety of methods reveal conflicting results regarding gastric emptying. The first evaluations with barium meals (197) and induced vomiting (198) showed no delay in gastric emptying during labor without sedation. In contrast, a double-sampling technique revealed a longer total mean emptying time in term pregnant women than in nonpregnant subjects. However, the gastric volume present 30 minutes after a meal was not significantly different between the two groups (199). As measured by this technique, labor (without analgesics or sedatives) further slows emptying of the final 100 to 200 mL of test solution. During labor, gastric volume at 30 minutes is greater than in nonpregnant women (199).

Paracetamol (acetominophen) absorption also measures gastric emptying. Paracetamol is absorbed only in the small bowel. Thus, the blood concentration of paracetamol correlates with gastric emptying (200). Some have documented the earliest delay in gastric emptying at 12 to 14 weeks (201), but others demonstrate delay as early as 8 to 12 weeks (202). Studies during the third trimester and in the first 24 to 48 hours postpartum do not demonstrate delayed gastric emptying (203). The use of systemic opioids significantly slows paracetamol absorption in laboring patients (204). Interestingly, although metoclopramide does not accelerate gastric emptying in nonpregnant patients given systemic narcotics (204,205), it does during pregnancy (206). Ranitidine appears to decrease gastric volume, whether or not opioids have been given (207). These studies have generated much debate without complete resolution (208–210).

Technologic advances have provided another technique to evaluate gastric emptying. Noninvasive gastric impedance can measure gastric emptying in both pregnant and nonpregnant volunteers. Pregnancy alone, even in the third trimester, does not slow gastric emptying. Postpartum patients who had received opiate analgesia had significantly prolonged 70%, 50%, and 30% emptying times (211). However, O'Sullivan and colleagues (211) caution that the impedance technique does not always permit measurement of the final 20% to 30% of gastric fluid. That volume approximates the final 100 to 200 mL portion of the 750-mL test volume used in the double-sampling technique. Therefore, even this most recent report does not really disprove the possibility of rapid initial emptying followed by delayed complete emptying with pregnancy. Opiates significantly prolong both emptying phases in pregnant patients (205,212).

Motilin stimulates gastrointestinal smooth muscle contraction. Pregnancy markedly decreases both fasting and glucose-induced motilin secretion. Motilin may partially mediate the smooth muscle relaxation attributed to progesterone (213).

Gastric Secretions

The hormone gastrin partially controls gastric acid secretion. Gastrin also tends to promote elevated tone of the LES and inhibit the pyloric sphincter (214). Early pregnancy does not modify serum gastrin concentration. The fetus, the placenta, or both produce gastrin. So, gastrin production rises progressively throughout the second and third trimesters, as well as during labor. The volume of acid secreted by the stomach, pancreas, and small intestine increases (214). Pregnancy does not modify basal or pentagastrin-stimulated acid secretion (192).

Postpartum

Administration of systemic opioids during the puerperium also delays gastric emptying after delivery (211). Both paracetamol absorption (209) and the double-sampling technique (199) show normal emptying times by 4 to 5 days postpartum. However, these data should not suggest an absent risk of gastric acid aspiration. Postpartum studies of volume and pH suggest that 33% to 73% of patients undergoing postpartum tubal sterilization still meet at-risk criteria for aspiration pneumonitis (215,216). (For a more detailed discussion of regurgitation and aspiration risk after delivery, see Chapter 37.)

Gallbladder

Progesterone inhibits cholecystokinin release from the intestinal mucosa (217). In addition, the contractile response to cholecystokinin diminishes during pregnancy (218). The gallbladder incompletely empties, particularly in the second and third trimesters (217,219,220). These factors may contribute to the pathogenesis of cholesterol gallstones during pregnancy (220).

Liver

Certain signs of pregnancy mimic liver disease. Spider angiomata and palmar erythema proliferate due to increased estrogens (221). Eighty percent of normal parturients have prolonged retention of bromsulphalein (222). The concentration of plasma proteins, particularly albumin, falls 20% to 30% and remains low for 6 to 7 weeks postpartum (221,223). Still, the total amount of some proteins increases during pregnancy (221,224).

Smooth endoplasmic reticulum proliferates, indicating a rise in hepatic microsomal activity (225). Steroid hormones function as competitive inhibitors of enzymes involved in oxidative reactions but do not impair conjugation (223). Certain liver enzymes show higher activities, particularly after the fifth month of gestation (226). These include glucose-6-phosphate dehydrogenase and aminolevalinic acid synthetase (223). Placental production raises the serum concentration of alkaline phosphatase by 200% to 400% (221). Transferase (AST and ALT), lactic dehydrogenase, and gammaglutamyl transpeptidase (GGT) activity may rise (226). Production of GGT also increases (227). Liver ribonucleic acid content markedly increases (223).

Implications

Increased gastric volume (due to delayed emptying and a larger volume of secretions), decreased LES tone, and elevated intragastric pressure require careful attention to acid aspiration prophylaxis. Avoidance of general anesthesia limits the population at risk for aspiration. Early institution of adequate regional anesthesia can help meet this goal. When general anesthesia is required, nonparticulate antacids, H_2-receptor antagonists, metoclopramide, and rapid sequence induction with cricoid pressure may help to limit the risk of pulmonary damage.

Pregnancy complicates the diagnosis of hepatic disease by imitating certain signs. Although mild to moderate elevation of liver enzymes may be normal in pregnancy, they should not be overlooked. Protein drug binding may increase or decrease, depending on the specific drugs involved.

COAGULATION

Pregnancy activates the clotting system. All factors except XI and XIII increase during gestation (228). The most significant elevations occur with factors VII, VIII, X, and fibrinogen (221,223,229–232). Mean platelet volume rises, although platelet count either remains unchanged or falls (88,230,233–237). Platelet intracellular free calcium increases in the third trimester, mirroring increased activity (238). Pregnancy lowers plasma fibrinolytic activity (229), although plasminogen concentration increases as early as 4 months' gestation (228,232).

A compensated, accelerated state of fibrinolysis may occur during late pregnancy (232,239). Such activity at the placental–uterine interface seems possible (228,232). There, localized fibrin formation from platelet activation and coagulation occur. Active fibrinolysis follows. Measuring indices of fibrinolysis in the peripheral blood may not detect uterine fibrinolysis.

Delivery accelerates platelet activation, coagulation, and fibrinolytic activity (Fig. 15) (240–242). Twenty-one

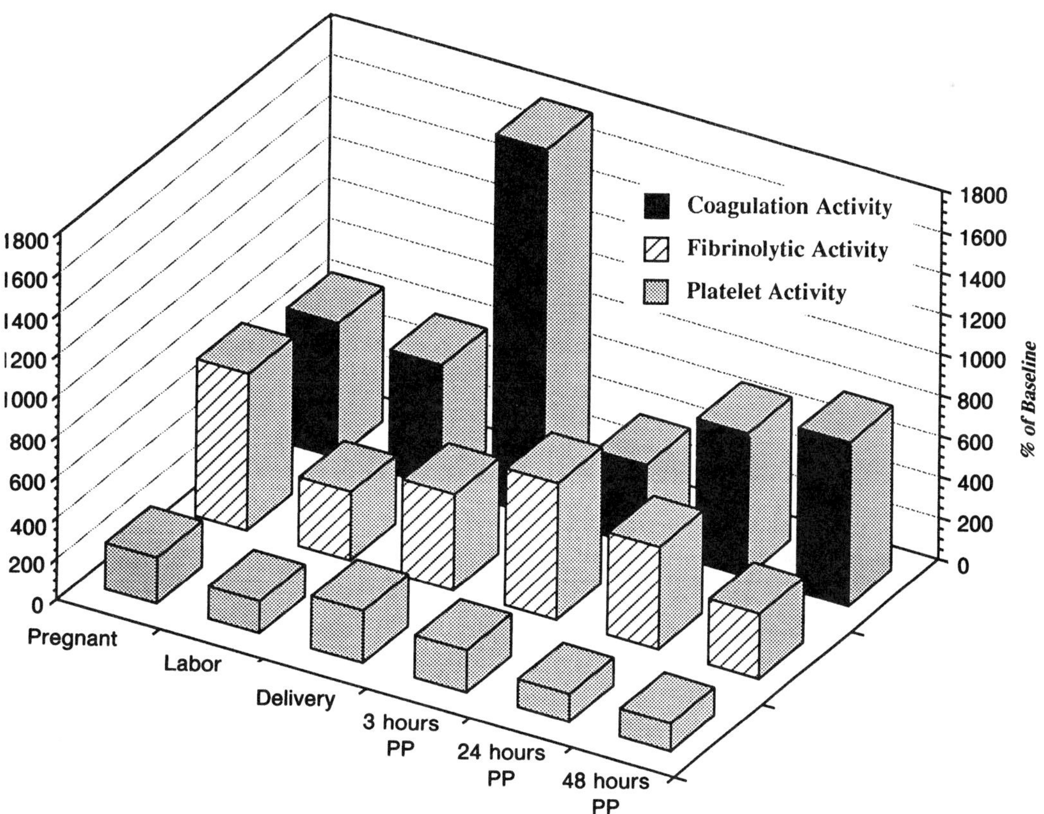

FIG. 15. Relative changes in coagulation, platelet, and fibrinolytic activity during the puerperium. (Data from refs. 232 and 242.)

percent of patients exhibit significant increases in fibrin degradation products during labor, with 32% showing the same immediately postpartum. Fibrin degradation remains elevated in only 10% of women 24 to 72 hours after delivery (243). Platelet count also returns to normal 24 to 72 hours postpartum (234). Fibrinolytic activity rapidly declines (229,234,242,244). Placental separation activates the clotting mechanism (242,245). Factor VIII activity transiently increases in uterine vein blood after delivery, shortening measured coagulation times (242, 245).

The coagulation system seems to prepare for the blood loss of delivery by increasing factors throughout pregnancy. At the same time, this hypercoagulable state complicates pregnancy and postpartum with thromboembolic events. Regional anesthetic techniques that allow early ambulation (and thus limit venous stasis) may minimize maternal morbidity and mortality.

ENDOCRINE

Glucose/Insulin

Pregnancy lowers fasting glucose concentration (246,247). Insulin secretion rises throughout gestation (247–251). At the same time, the tissue sensitivity to insulin diminishes (249–253). Insulin degradation does not vary (254). Pregnancy-specific hormonal factors cause insulin resistance (250,251,255). Human placental lactogen (HPL) has antiinsulin activity (246,253,255–257). Insulin secretion precipitously declines after delivery, suggesting that the placenta holds the stimulus for insulin release (248). Speroff et al. (253) describe HPL as a "major force in the diabetogenic effects of pregnancy." Progesterone alone does not cause the changes in glucose and insulin metabolism. In males, progesterone administration elevates fasting plasma insulin but does not lower fasting glucose as pregnancy does (246). Decreased buffering capacity predisposes the gravida to ketoacidosis.

Thyroid

Total serum thyroxine concentrations rise during gestation (258). Thyroid-binding globulin concentration peaks in the third trimester (223). The percentage of free thyroxine in the serum falls (258). Progesterone administration replicates this situation (258). Early in pregnancy, serum chorionic gonadotropin, with its intrinsic thyroid-stimulating activity, activates the thyroid gland (258–260). Human chorionic gonadotropin concentration peaks between 9 and 18 weeks of gestation. Human chorionic gonadotropin suppresses thyroid-stimulating hormone production (261,262). The thyroid gland grows larger (263). Pituitary sensitivity to thyroid-stimulating hormone remains constant (263). In spite of elevated total serum thyroxine and triiodothyronine measurements, most parturients remain euthyroid. Increased thyroid size may hinder rapid sequence induction.

Progesterone

Progesterone garners much interest as an explanation for various physiologic adaptations to pregnancy. Plasma progesterone concentration progressively rises throughout pregnancy (264,265) and abruptly declines after delivery of the placenta (264,266). This time course alone makes progesterone a likely mediator in many physiologic alterations seen in pregnancy.

Prostaglandins

Peripheral concentrations of prostaglandins also increase during pregnancy. Prostaglandin A compounds multiply most dramatically. Early in gestation, prostaglandin A–like material rises by 300%. Typical effects of prostaglandin A compounds include decreased systemic vascular resistance and increased cardiac output. Both changes occur early in pregnancy and correlate with the elevation in prostaglandin A activity (267).

Prostaglandin E does not significantly increase until the third trimester (267). A possible explanation is production in the peripheral arterial/venous system stimulated by angiotensin II. Prostaglandin E–induced vasodilation prevents angiotensin II from causing a hypertensive state (267). Prostacyclin production also may mediate vasodilatation (265).

MUSCULOSKELETAL

The corpus luteum initially secretes relaxin. During the first trimester, relaxin concentration rises dramatically. Then, the amount of relaxin declines to a stable level throughout the third trimester (268). Relaxin softens the cervix, inhibits uterine contractions, and relaxes the pubic symphysis (253). Peripheral joints become lax during the last trimester of pregnancy (269). Ligamentous laxity may contribute to the high incidence of lower back pain with pregnancy (270) and vulnerability to injury during the mechanical stress of labor (271).

CENTRAL NERVOUS SYSTEM

The placenta produces endorphins and enkephalins that may function to provide a naturally occurring analgesia during pregnancy (253,272). Pregnant animals are more tolerant to aversive stimuli (273–275). The antinociceptive threshold abruptly rises 1 to 2 days before parturition (273). Intrathecal or systemic opioid antagonists reverse this pregnancy-mediated analgesia (273–275). Systemic β-endorphin secretion increases during labor and correlates with patient perceived pain intensity (276); however, β endorphin is a large molecule that does not cross the blood–brain barrier. If this compound is important in mediating the changes in pain sensitivity in pregnancy or labor, its cerebrospinal fluid (CSF) concentrations also should rise. They do not (277).

CSF 5-HIAA, a major metabolite of serotonin, increases with gestational age (278). Plasma and CSF concentrations of progesterone significantly rise with pregnancy (279). An earlier report suggested an effective blood–brain barrier for progesterone (280). CSF progesterone concentration falls rapidly in the postpartum period (279).

Pregnant women require less spinal or epidural local anesthetic per spinal segment blocked than nonpregnant controls (281,282). This change arises early in gestation and persists into the postpartum period (282). Although higher dermatomal levels develop as soon as 5 minutes after injection, pregnancy prolongs the time to complete epidural spread (281). Pregnancy also increases the interpatient variation in the spread of caudal anesthesia (283). Both mechanical and biochemical factors may have a role in producing this change (281). Investigation of mechanical factors reveals conflicting data. Abdominal compression, which mimics the effects of the gravid uterus, increases IVC pressure to 25 cm H_2O. Intrathecal tetracaine 4 mg spreads further in women wearing an abdominal binder (284). This dose of drug spreads further still in parturients. In addition, the gravid uterus elevates epidural but not CSF pressure (285,286). These data suggest that mechanical factors may explain some, but not all, of the altered sensitivity to local anesthetics seen in pregnancy. α_1-Acid glycoprotein (AAG) CSF concentrations decrease during pregnancy. However, the decrease in AAG concentration is not likely to increase free bupivacaine concentrations in a clinically relevant manner (287). Another minor factor (at least for dextrose-free local anesthetic solutions) is the lower density of CSF during pregnancy (288).

Increased sensitivity to local anesthetics likely plays the largest role. Peripheral nerves also are more vulnerable to local anesthetics during pregnancy (289). Pregnancy hastens the onset of 50% block with bupivacaine 0.35 mmol/L in A, B, and C vagal fibers (290). This change relates to more than just altered diffusion of local anesthetic. The dose–response curve to conduction blockade in isolated A and C nerve fibers from pregnant animals also shifts to the left (291). As with many other physiologic changes, progesterone's influence predominates. Prolonged (4 days), but not acute, exposure to progesterone makes nerve fibers more susceptible to local anesthetics (292,293).

Pregnancy in ewes, and exogenous progesterone in rabbits, decreases the minimum alveolar concentration (MAC) for halothane and isoflurane (294,295). Pregnancy does not alter MAC in rats and mice (296). Gin and Chan (297) have conducted a series of studies examining the effects of pregnancy on MAC in humans. Isoflurane MAC (using transcutaneous tetanic electrical stimulus) is 0.775% at 8 to 12 weeks' gestation versus 1.075% in non-

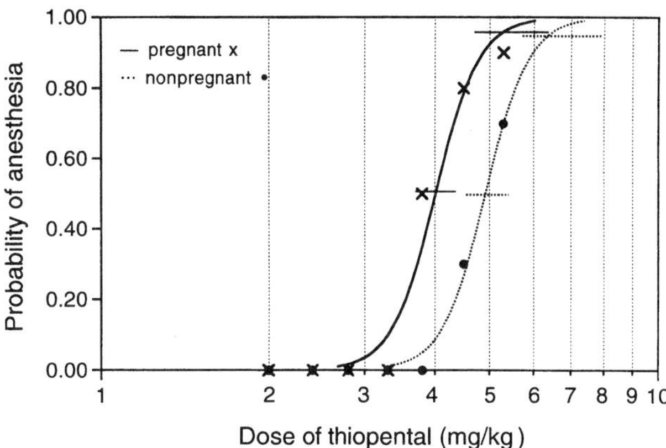

FIG. 16. Calculated dose–response curves (log dose scale) for anesthesia in pregnant and nonpregnant women. The 95% confidence intervals also are displayed. Raw data: x, pregnant; •, nonpregnant. (From ref. 300, with permission.)

pregnant women (297). Isoflurane MAC remains decreased 24 to 36 hours after delivery, but equals nonpregnant values when measured more than 72 hours after delivery (298). Pregnancy also decreases halothane and enflurane MAC by 27% and 30%, respectively (299).

By 7 to 13 weeks' gestation, parturients are more sensitive to thiopental. Gin et al. (300) gave a single dose of thiopental (2.0 to 5.3 mg/kg) to pregnant and nonpregnant women. Two minutes later, patients were asked to open their eyes to test for hypnosis. Unresponsive women were then given a transcutaneous tetanic electrical stimulus to test for anesthesia. The dose for thiopental for hypnosis and anesthesia was 17% to 18% lower in pregnant compared to nonpregnant women (Fig. 16) (300).

Increased sensitivity to local and general anesthetics requires dosage adjustments for the gravida. Careful assessment of the patient's response allows one to minimize drug exposure and obtain the desired effects without excessive maternal or fetal side effects.

PHARMACOKINETICS

Pregnancy alters drug binding and drug elimination. Albumin concentration falls, and hepatic microsomal activity rises. The larger plasma volume increases renal blood flow and augments glomerular filtration. Pharmacokinetic parameters do not show any consistent trend with pregnancy. The rate of elimination of various drugs can either rise or fall (301). Gestation prolongs the elimination of bupivacaine, diazepam, thiopental, and theophylline (225,301). The volume of distribution of thiopental and theophylline enlarges (225,301). The unbound fraction of diazepam, phenytoin, phenobarbital, and lidocaine increases with pregnancy (302).

Plasma pseudocholinesterase activity rapidly declines 24% during pregnancy and up to 60% after delivery (303–308). Structural abnormality of pseudocholinesterase has not been found (305). The augmented plasma volume inflates the volume of distribution of succinylcholine and counterbalances the fall in pseudocholinesterase activity. Postpartum, when plasma volume decreases before pseudocholineterase activity recovers, succinylcholine paralysis persists about 3 minutes longer than in nonpregnant patients (309).

CONCLUSION

Adaptations to pregnancy affect every organ system, usually within several weeks of conception. These adaptations should be viewed as continually evolving from the first weeks after conception. Change continues during and after parturition.

The cardiovascular system must adapt to the increasing demands of the growing uterus and fetus. Increases in plasma volume and cardiac output alter the hemodynamic responses to anesthetic interventions. Beginning in the second trimester, aortocaval compression can hinder uterine blood flow and maternal cardiac output. The larger plasma volume allows the parturient to tolerate greater blood loss than her nonpregnant counterpart.

The changes in the respiratory system that accompany gestation significantly narrow the parturient's margin of safety during general anesthesia. A smaller FRC and a higher oxygen consumption render her more susceptible to hypoxemia during periods of apnea. Mechanical hyperventilation can lower uterine blood flow and incite fetal acidosis.

Gastric emptying slows while acid secretion increases. In combination with a higher intraabdominal pressure, these changes place the parturient at greater risk of regurgitation and aspiration should her airway reflexes become impaired.

Pregnancy-induced alterations in the central nervous system increase the parturient's sensitivity to all anesthetics. Understanding the extent and progressive nature of the body's response to pregnancy helps the anesthesiologist approach any gravida with confidence.

REFERENCES

1. Cutforth R, MacDonald CB. Heart sounds and murmurs in pregnancy. *Am Heart J* 1966;71:741.
2. De Swiet M. The cardiovascular system. In: Hytten F, Chamberlain G, eds. *Clinical physiology in obstetrics,* 2nd ed. Oxford: Blackwell Science, 1991:3.
3. Enein M, Zina AAA, Kassem M, El-Tabbakh G. Echocardiography of the pericardium in pregnancy. *Obstet Gynecol* 1987;69:851.
4. Clapp JF III, Seaward BL, Sleamaker RH, Hiser J. Maternal physiologic adaptations to early human pregnancy. *Am J Obstet Gynecol* 1988;159:1456.
5. Clapp JF III. Maternal heart rate in pregnancy. *Am J Obstet Gynecol* 1985;152:659.
6. Walters WA, MacGregor WG, Hills M. Cardiac output at rest during pregnancy and the puerperium. *Clin Sci* 1966;30:1.
7. Capeless EL, Clapp JE. Cardiovascular changes in early phase of pregnancy. *Am J Obstet Gynecol* 1989;161:1449.
8. Lees MM, Taylor SH, Scott DB, Kerr MG. A study of cardiac output at rest throughout pregnancy. *J Obstet Gynaecol Br Commonw* 1967; 74:319.
9. Bader RA, Bader ME, Rose DJ, Braunwald E. Hemodynamics at rest and during exercise in normal pregnancy as studied by cardiac catheterization. *J Clin Invest* 1955;34:1524.
10. McLennan FM, Haites NE, Rawles JM. Stroke and minute distance in pregnancy: a longitudinal study using Doppler ultrasound. *Br J Obstet Gynaecol* 1987;94:499.
11. Ueland K, Novy MJ, Metcalfe J. Cardiorespiratory responses to pregnancy and exercise in normal women and patients with heart disease. *Am J Obstet Gynecol* 1973;115:4.
12. Ueland K, Novy MJ, Peterson EN, Metcalfe J. Maternal cardiovascular dynamics: IV. The influence of gestational age on the maternal cardiovascular response to posture and exercise. *Am J Obstet Gynecol* 1969;104:856.
13. Mabie WC, DiSessa TG, Crocker LG, Sibai BM, Arheart KL. A longitudinal study of cardiac output in normal human pregnancy. *Am J Obstet Gynecol* 1994;170:849.
14. Katz R, Karliner JS, Resnik R. Effects of a natural volume overload state (pregnancy) on left ventricular performance in normal human subjects. *Circulation* 1978;58:434.
15. Robson SC, Hunter S, Moore M, Dunlop W. Haemodynamic changes during the puerperium: a Doppler and M-mode echocardiographic study. *Br J Obstet Gynaecol* 1987;94:1028.
16. Gilson GJ, Samaan S, Crawford MH, Qualls CR, Curet LB. Changes in hemodynamics, ventricular remodeling, and ventricular contractility during normal pregnancy: a longitudinal study. *Obstet Gynecol* 1997;89:957.
17. Mone SM, Sanders SP, Colan SD. Control mechanisms for physiological hypertrophy of pregnancy. *Circulation* 1996;94:667.
18. Lee W, Rokey R, Cotton DB. Noninvasive maternal stoke volume and cardiac output determinations by pulsed Doppler echocardiography. *Am J Obstet Gynecol* 1988;158:505.
19. Easterling TR, Carlson KL, Schmucker BC, Brateng DA, Benedetti TJ. Measurement of cardiac output in pregnancy by Doppler technique. *Am J Perinatol* 1990;7:220.
20. Kamal GD, Symreng T, Starr J. Inconsistent esophageal Doppler cardiac output during acute blood loss. *Anesthesiology* 1990;72:95.
21. Clark SL, Southwick J, Pivarnik JM, Cotton DB, Hankins GDV, Phelan JP. A comparison of cardiac index in normal term pregnancy using thoracic electrical bio-impedance and oxygen extraction (Fick) techniques. *Obstet Gynecol* 1994;83:669.
22. Ihrman K. A clinical and physiological study of pregnancy in a material from Northern Sweden: VI. The arterial blood pressures at rest and in orthostatic test during and after pregnancy. *Acta Soc Med Upsaliensis* 1960;65:315.
23. MacGillivray I, Rose GA, Rowe B. Blood pressure survey in pregnancy. *Clin Sci* 1969;37:395.
24. Clark SL, Cotton DB, Lee W, et al. Central hemodynamic assessment of normal term pregnancy. *Am J Obstet Gynecol* 1989;161:1439.
25. Mashini IS, Albazzaz SJ, Fadel HE, et al. Serial noninvasive evaluation of cardiovascular hemodynamics during pregnancy. *Am J Obstet Gynecol* 1987;156:1208.
26. Ueland K, Metcalfe J. Circulatory changes in pregnancy. *Clin Obstet Gynecol* 1975;18:41.
27. Guzman CA, Caplan R. Cardiorespiratory response to exercise during pregnancy. *Am J Obstet Gynecol* 1970;108:600.
28. Duvekot JJ, Cheriex EC, Pieters FAA, Menheere PPCA, Peeters LLH. Early pregnancy changes in hemodynamics and volume homeostasis are consecutive adjustments triggered by a primary fall in systemic vascular tone. *Am J Obstet Gynecol* 1993;169:1382.
29. Ueland K, Parer JT. Effects of estrogens on the cardiovascular system of the ewe. *Am J Obstet Gynecol* 1966;96:400.
30. King TM, Whitehorn WV, Reeves B, Kubota R. Effects of estrogen on composition and function of cardiac muscle. *Am J Physiol* 1959;196: 1282.
31. Rubler S, Damani PM, Pinto ER. Cardiac size and performance during pregnancy estimated with echocardiography. *Am J Cardiol* 1977;40:534.
32. Gilson GJ, Graves SW, Qualls CR, Curet LB. Digoxin-like immunoreactive substance and sodium-potassium-adenosine triphosphatase inhibition in normal pregnancy: a longitudinal study. *Obstet Gynecol* 1997;89:743.
33. Coulson CC, Thorp JM Jr, Mayer DC, Cefalo RC. Central hemody-

namic effects of recombinant human relaxin in the isolated, perfused rat heart model. *Obstet Gynecol* 1996;87:610.
34. Howard BK, Goodson JH, Mengert W. Supine hypotensive syndrome in late pregnancy. *Obstet Gynecol* 1953;1:371.
35. Vorys N, Ullery JC. The cardiac output changes in various positions in pregnancy. *Am J Obstet Gynecol* 1961;82:1312.
36. Milsom I, Forssman L. Factors influencing aortocaval compression in late pregnancy. *Am J Obstet Gynecol* 1984;148:764.
37. Lees MM, Scott DB, Kerr MG, Taylor SH. The circulatory effects of recumbent postural change in late pregnancy. *Clin Sci* 1967;32:453.
38. Calvin S, Jones OW III, Knieriem K, Weinstein L. Oxygen saturation in the supine hypotensive syndrome. *Obstet Gynecol* 1988;71:872.
39. Ellington C, Katz VL, Watson WJ, Spielman FJ. The effect of lateral tilt on maternal and fetal hemodynamic variables. *Obstet Gynecol* 1991;77:201.
40. Kerr MG, Scott DB, Samuel E. Studies of the inferior vena cava in late pregnancy. *Br Med J* 1964;1:532.
41. Hirabayashi Y, Shimizu R, Fukuda H, Saitoh K, Igarashi T. Effects of the pregnant uterus on the extradural venous plexus in the supine and lateral positions, as determined by magnetic resonance imaging. *Br J Anaesth* 1997;78:317.
42. Wood CE, Keil LC, Rudolph AM. Hormonal and hemodynamic responses to vena caval obstruction in fetal sheep. *Am J Physiol* 1982; 243:E278.
43. Lotgering FH, Wallenburg HCS. Hemodynamic effects of caval and uterine venous occlusion in pregnant sheep. *Am J Obstet Gynecol* 1986;155:1164.
44. Pirhonen JP, Erkkola RU. Uterine and umbilical flow velocity waveforms in the supine hypotensive syndrome. *Obstet Gynecol* 1990;76: 176.
45. Marx GF, Husain FJ, Shiau HF. Brachial and femoral blood pressures during the prenatal period. *Am J Obstet Gynecol* 1980;136:11.
46. Bieniarz J, Maqueda E, Caldeyro-Barcia R. Compression of aorta by the uterus in late human pregnancy: I. Variations between femoral and bracheal artery pressure with changes from hypertension to hypotension. *Am J Obstet Gynecol* 1966;95:795.
47. Bieniarz J, Crottogini JJ, Curuchet E, et al. Aortocaval compression by the uterus in late human pregnancy: II. An arteriographic study. *Am J Obstet Gynecol* 1968;100:203.
48. Ohlson L. Effects of the pregnant uterus on the abdominal aorta and its branches. *Acta Radiol Diagn* 1978;19:369.
49. Kinsella SM, Spencer JAD, Whitwam JG. Use of digital arterial pressure to detect aortic compression during labour. *Lancet* 1989;23:714.
50. Janbu T. Blood velocities in the dorsal pedis and radial arteries during labour. *Br J Obstet Gynaecol* 1989;96:70.
51. Ueland K, Hansen JM. Maternal cardiovascular dynamics. II. Posture and uterine contractions. *Am Obstet Gynecol* 1969;103:1.
52. Kinsella SM, Lee A, Spencer JAD. Maternal and fetal effects of the supine and pelvic tilt positions in late pregnancy. *Eur J Obstet Gynecol Reprod Biol* 1990;36:11.
53. Kasten GW, Martin ST. Resuscitation from bupivacaine-induced cardiovascular toxicity during partial inferior vena cava occlusion. *Anesth Analg* 1986;65:341.
54. DePace NL, Betesh JS, Kotler MN. 'Postmortem' cesarean section with recovery of both mother and offspring. *JAMA* 1982;248:971.
55. Nisell H, Hjemdahl P, Linde B. Cardiovascular responses to circulating catecholamines in normal pregnancy and in pregnancy-induced hypertension. *Clin Physiol* 1985;5:479.
56. Hardebo JE, Edvinsson L. Reduced sensitivity to alpha- and beta-adrenergic receptor agonists of intra- and extracranial vessels during pregnancy. Relevance to migraine. *Acta Neurol Scand* 1977;64:204.
57. Pantuck CB, Smiley RM. Longitudinal study of beta- and alpha-adrenergic receptor properties during human pregnancy. *Am J Obstet Gynecol* 1997;177:234.
58. Barron WM, Mujais SK, Zinaman M, Bravo EL, Lindheimer MD. Plasma catecholamine responses to physiologic stimuli in normal human pregnancy. *Am J Obstet Gynecol* 1986;154:80.
59. McCarthy AL, Taylor PT, Graves J, Raju SK, Poston L. Endothelium-dependent relaxation of human resistance arteries in pregnancy. *Am J Obstet Gynecol* 1994;171:1309.
60. Okutomi T, Nomoto K, Nakamura K, Goto F. Nitric oxide metabolite in pregnant women before and after delivery. *Acta Obstet Gynecol Scand* 1997;76:222.
61. Elkholm EMK, Piha SJ, Antila KJ, Erhhola RU. Cardiovascular autonomic reflexes in mid-pregnancy. *Br J Obstet Gynaecol* 1993;100: 177.
62. Ekholm EMK, Piha SJ, Erkkola RU, Antila KJ. Autonomic cardiovascular reflexes in pregnancy. *Clin Auton Res* 1994;4:161.
63. DeSimone CA, Leighton BL, Norris MC, Chayen B, Menduke H. The chronotropic effect of isoproterenol is reduced in term pregnant women. *Anesthesiology* 1988;69:626.
64. Leighton BL, Norris MC, Sosis M, Epstein R, Chayen B, Larijani GE. Limitations of epinephrine as a marker of intravascular injection in laboring women. *Anesthesiology* 1987;66:688.
65. Carli A, Auclair MC, Bleichner G, Weber S, Monsallier JF, Lechat P. Inhibitory action of human serum on the isoprenaline-induced chronotropic effect in cultured rat heart cells. Influence of sex and pregnancy. *Biomedicine* 1977;27:166.
66. Dilts PV Jr, Brinkman CR III, Kirschbaum TH, Assali NS. Uterine and systemic hemodynamic interrelationships and their response to hypoxia. *Am J Obstet Gynecol* 1969;103:138.
67. Thaler I, Manor D, Itskovitz J, et al. Changes in uterine blood flow during human pregnancy. *Am J Obstet Gynecol* 1990;162:121.
68. Nelson SH, Suresh MS. Comparison of nitroprusside and hydralazine in isolated uterine arteries from pregnant and nonpregnant patients. *Anesthesiology* 1988;68:541.
69. Suresh MA, Nelson SH, Nelson TE, Steinsland OS. Pregnancy: increased effect of verapamil in human uterine arteries. *Eur J Pharmacol* 1985;112:387.
70. Hendricks CH. The hemodynamics of a uterine contraction. *Am J Obstet Gynecol* 1958;76:969.
71. Ueland K, Hansen JM. Maternal cardiovascular dynamics. III. Labor and delivery under local and caudal analgesia. *Am J Obstet Gynecol* 1969;103:8.
72. Robson SC, Dunlop W, Boys RJ, Hunter S. Cardiac output during labour. *Br Med J* 1987;295:1169.
73. Maruta S. The observation of the maternal hemodynamics during labor and cesarean section. *Acta Obstet Gynaecol JPN* 1982;6:776.
74. Hendricks CH, Quilligan EJ. Cardiac output during labor. *Am J Obstet Gynecol* 1956;71:953.
75. Hansen JM, Ueland K. The influence of caudal analgesia on cardiovascular dynamics during normal labor and delivery. *Acta Anaesthesiol Scand Scand* 1966;23[Suppl]:449.
76. James CF, Banner T, Caton D. Cardiac output in women undergoing cesarean section with epidural or general anesthesia. *Am J Obstet Gynecol* 1989;160:1178.
77. Robson SC, Boys RJ, Hunter S, Dunlop W. Maternal hemodynamics after normal delivery and delivery complicated by postpartum hemorrhage. *Obstet Gynecol* 1989;74:234.
78. Walters BNJ, Thompson ME, Lee A, DeSweit M. Blood pressure in the puerperium. *Clin Sci* 1986;71:589.
79. Brown E, Sampson JJ, Wheeler EO, Gundelfinger BF, Giansiracusa JE. Physiologic changes in the circulation during and after obstetric labor. *Am Heart J* 1947;34:311.
80. Newman B. Cardiac output changes during caesarean section. *Anaesthesia* 1982;37:270.
81. Lund CJ, Donovan JC. Blood volume during pregnancy. *Am J Obstet Gynecol* 1967;98:393.
82. Hytten FE, Paintin DB. Increase in plasma volume during normal pregnancy. *J Obstet Gynaecol Br Commonw* 1963;70:402.
83. Pritchard JA. Changes in the blood volume during pregnancy and delivery. *Anesthesiology* 1965;26:393.
84. Pirani BBK, Campbell DM. Plasma volume in normal first pregnancy. *J Obstet Gynaecol Br Commonw* 1973;80:884.
85. Hytten F. Blood volume changes in normal pregnancy. *Clin Haematol* 1985;14:601.
86. Longo LD. Maternal blood volume and cardiac output during pregnancy: a hypothesis of endocrinologic control. *Am J Physiol* 1983;14:R720.
87. Walters WAW, Lim YL. Cardiovascular dynamics in women receiving oral contraceptive therapy. *Lancet* 1969;2:879.
88. Sill PR, Lind T, Walker W. Platelet values during normal pregnancy. *Br J Obstet Gynaecol* 1985;92:480.
89. Jepson JH. Endocrine control of maternal and fetal erythropoiesis. *Can Med Assoc J* 1968;98:844.
90. Pitkin RM, Witte DL. Platelet and leukocyte counts in pregnancy. *JAMA* 1979;242:2696.
91. Pritchard JA, Baldwin RM, Dickey JC, Wiggins KM. Blood volume

changes in pregnancy and the puerperium. II. Red blood cell loss and changes in apparent blood volume during and following vaginal delivery, cesarean section, and cesarean section plus total hysterectomy. *Am J Obstet Gynecol* 1962;84:1271.
92. Thomson KJ, Cohen ME. Studies on the circulation in pregnancy. II. Vital capacity observation in normal pregnant women. *Surg Gynecol Obstet* 1938;66:591.
93. Fabricant ND. Sexual functions and the nose. *Am J Med Sci* 1960;239: 498.
94. Wong RC, Ellis CN. Physiologic skin changes in pregnancy. *Sem Dermatol* 1989;8:7.
95. Brock-Utne JG, Downing JW, Seedat F. Laryngeal oedema associated with pre-eclamptic toxaemia. *Anaesthesia* 1977;32:556.
96. Liberatore SM, Pistelli R, Potalano F, Moneta E, Incalzi RA, Ciappi G. Respiratory function during pregnancy. *Respiration* 1984;46:145.
97. Cugell DW, Frank NR, Gaensler EA, Badger TL. Pulmonary function in pregnancy. I. Serial observations in normal women. *Am Rev Tuberc* 1953;57:568.
98. Gee JBL, Packer BS, Millen JE, Robin ED. Pulmonary mechanics during pregnancy. *J Clin Invest* 1967;46:6.
99. Baldwin GR, Moorthi DS, Whelton JA, MacDonnell KF. New lung functions and pregnancy. *Am J Obstet Gynecol* 1977;127:255.
100. Alaily AB, Carrol KB. Pulmonary ventilation in pregnancy. *Br J Obstet Gynaecol* 1978;85:518.
101. Eng M, Butler J, Bonica JJ. Respiratory function in pregnant obese women. *Am J Obstet Gynecol* 1975;123:241.
102. Rubin A, Russo N, Goucher D. The effect of pregnancy upon pulmonary function in normal women. *Am J Obstet Gynecol* 1956;72:963.
103. Awe RJ, Nicotra B, Newsom TD, Viles R. Arterial oxygenation and alveolar-arterial gradients in term pregnancy. *Obstet Gynecol* 1979; 53:182.
104. Bevan DR, Holdcroft A, Loh L, MacGregor WG, O'Sullivan JC, Sykes MK. Closing volume and pregnancy. *Br Med J* 1974;1:13.
105. Weinberger SE, Weiss ST, Cohen WR, Weiss JW, Johnson TS. Pregnancy and the lung. *Am Rev Respir Dis* 1980;121:559.
106. Bourne TJ, Ogilvy AJ, Vickers R, Williamson K. Nocturnal hypoxaemia in late pregnancy. *Br J Anaesth* 1995;75:678.
107. Shankar KB, Moseley H, Vemula V, Kumar Y. Physiological dead space during general anaesthesia for caesarean section. *Can J Anaesth* 1987;34:373.
108. Lyons G, Tunstall ME. Maternal blood-gas tensions (p_AO_2-p_aO_2), physiological shunt and VD/VT during general anaesthesia for caesarean section. *Br J Anaesth* 1979;51:1059.
109. Hankins GDV, Harvey CJ, Clark SL, Uckan EM, Van Hook JW. The effects of maternal position and cardiac output on intrapulmonary shunt in normal third-trimester pregnancy. *Obstet Gynecol* 1996;88: 327.
110. Prowse CM, Gaensler EA. Respiratory and acid-base changes during pregnancy. *Anesthesiology* 1965;26:381.
111. Knuttgen HG, Emerson K Jr. Physiological response to pregnancy at rest and during exercise. *J Appl Physiol* 1974;36:549.
112. Milne JA, Mills RJ, Howie AD, Pack AI. Large airways function during normal pregnancy. *Br J Obstet Gynaecol* 1977;84:448.
113. Pernoll ML, Metcalfe J, Kovach PA, Wachtel R, Dunham MJ. Ventilation during rest and exercise in pregnancy and postpartum. *Respir Physiol* 1975;25:295.
114. MacRae DJ, Palavradji D. Maternal acid-base changes in pregnancy. *J Obstet Gynaecol Br Commonw* 1967;74:11.
115. Plass ED, Oberst FW. Respiration and pulmonary ventilation in normal nonpregnant, pregnant and puerperal women. *Am J Obstet Gynecol* 1938;35:441.
116. Pernoll ML, Metcalfe J, Schlenker TL, Welch E, Matsumoto JA. Oxygen consumption at rest and during exercise in pregnancy. *Respir Physiol* 1975;25:285.
117. Artal R, Wiswell, Romem Y, Dorey F. Pulmonary responses to exercise in pregnancy. *Am J Obstet Gynecol* 1986;154:378.
118. Lyons HA, Antonio R. The sensitivity of the respiratory center in pregnancy and after the administration of progesterone. *Trans Assoc Am Physicians* 1959;72:173.
119. Byrne F, Oduro-Dominah A, Kipling R. The effect of pregnancy on pulmonary nitrogen washout: a study of pre-oxygenation. *Anaesthesia* 1987;42:148.
120. Norris MC, Kirkland MR, Torjman MC, Goldberg ME. Denitrogenation in pregnancy. *Can J Anaesth* 1989;5:523.
121. Norris MC, Dewan DM. Preoxygenation for cesarean section: a comparison of two techniques. *Anesthesiology* 1985;62:827.
122. De Swiet M. The respiratory system. In: Hytten F, Chamberlain G, eds. *Clinical physiology in obstetrics,* 2nd ed. Oxford: Blackwell Science, 1991:83.
123. Gazioglu K, Kaltreider NI, Rosen M, Yu PN. Pulmonary function during pregnancy in normal women and in patients with cardiopulmonary disease. *Thorax* 1970;25:445.
124. Shankar KB, Moseley H, Ramasamy M. Arterial to end-tidal carbon dioxide tension difference during anaestheia in early pregnancy. *Can J Anaesth* 1989;36:124.
125. Shankar KB, Moseley H, Kumar Y, Vemula V. Arterial to end tidal carbon dioxide tension difference during Caesarean section anaesthesia. *Anaesthesia* 1986;41:698.
126. Shankar KB, Moseley H, Kumar Y, Vemula V, Krishnan A. Arterial to end-tidal carbon dioxide tension difference during anaesthesia for tubal ligation. *Anaesthesia* 1987;42:482.
127. Baraka A. Correlation between maternal and foetal pO_2 and pCO_2 during caesarean section. *Br J Anaesth* 1970;42:434.
128. Behrman RE, Peterson EN, De Lannoy CW. The supply of O_2 to the primate fetus with two different O_2 tensions and anesthetics. *Respir Physiol* 1969;6:271.
129. Darling RC, Smith CA, Asmussen E, Cohen FM. Some properties of human fetal and maternal blood. *J Clin Invest* 1941;20:739.
130. Prystowsky H, Hellegers A, Bruns P. Fetal blood studies. XIV. A comparative study of the oxygen dissociation curve of nonpregnant, pregnant and fetal human blood. *Am J Obstet Gynecol* 1989;78:489.
131. Bauer C, Ludwig M, Ludwig L, Bartels H. Factors governing the oxygen affinity of human adult and foetal blood. *Respir Physiol* 1969;7: 271.
132. Kambam JR, Handte RE, Brown WU, Smith BE. Effect of normal and preeclamptic pregnancies on the oxyhemoglobin dissociation curve. *Anesthesiology* 1986;65:426.
133. Leibson RG, Likhnitzky II. Oxygen transport of the foetal and maternal blood during pregnancy. *J Physiol* 1936;87:97.
134. McCullogh JC, Kelly AM. Investigation of pregnancy-related changes in red cell 2,3-diphosphoglycerate. *Clin Chim Acta* 1979;98:235.
135. Hess W. Pregnancy and oxygen dissociation. *Anesthesiology* 1987;66: 854.
136. Kambam JR. In *reply. Anesthesiology* 1988;69:801.
137. Bardicef O, Bardicef M, Sorokin Y, Cotton DB, Resnick LM. Physiologic intracellular acidosis in pregnancy. *Am J Obstet Gynecol* 1995; 173:879.
138. Blechner JN, Cotter JR, Stenger VG, Hinkley CM, Prystowsky H. Oxygen, carbon dioxide, and hydrogen ion concentrations in arterial blood during pregnancy. *Am J Obstet Gynecol* 1968;100:1.
139. Anderson GJ, James GB, Mathers NP, Smith EL, Walker J. The maternal oxygen tension and acid-base status during pregnancy. *J Obstet Gynaecol Br Commonw* 1969;76:16.
140. Lucius H, Gahlenbeck H, Kleine HO, Fabel H, Bartels H. Respiratory functions, buffer system, and electrolyte concentrations of blood during human pregnancy. *Respir Physiol* 1970;9:311.
141. Oberst FW, Plass ED. The acid-base balance in the plasma and blood cells of normal nonpregnant, pregnant and puerperal women. *J Lab Clin Med* 1940;26:513.
142. Ang CK, Tan TH, Walters WAW, Wood C. Postural influence on maternal capillary oxygen and carbon dioxide tension. *Br Med J* 1969;4:201.
143. Oard HC, Peters JP. The concentration of acid and base in the serum in normal pregnancy. *J Biol Chem* 1929;81:9.
144. Prystowsky H, Hellegers AE, Bruns PD. A comparative study of the alkali reserve of normal and pregnant women. *Am J Obstet Gynecol* 1961;82:1295.
145. Tyler JM. The effect of progesterone on the respiration of patients with emphysema and hypercapnia. *J Clin Invest* 1960;39:34.
146. Novy MJ, Edwards MJ. Respiratory problems in pregnancy. *Am J Obstet Gynecol* 1967;99:1024.
147. Ramanathan J, Sibai BM, Duggirala V, Maduska AL. Pulmonary function in preeclamptic women receiving $MgSO_4$. *J Reprod Med* 1988; 33:432.
148. Hagerdal M, Morgan CW, Sumner AE, Gutsche BB. Minute ventilation and oxygen consumption during labor with epidural analgesia. *Anesthesiology* 1983;59:425.
149. Fisher A, Prys-Roberts C. Maternal pulmonary gas exchange. A study

during normal labour and extradural blockade. *Anaesthesia* 1968; 23:350.
150. Reed PN, Colquhoun AD, Hanning CD. Maternal oygenation during normal labour. *Br J Anaesth* 1989;62:316.
151. Andersen GJ, Walker J. The effect of labour on the maternal blood-gas and acidbase status. *J Obstet Gynaecol Br Commonw* 1970;77:289.
152. Moya F, Morishima HO, Shnider SM, James LS. Influence of maternal hyperventilation on the newborn infant. *Am J Obstet Gynecol* 1965;91:76.
153. Archer GW Jr, Marx GF. Arterial oxygen tension during apnoea in parturient women. *Br J Anaesth* 1974;46:358.
154. Motoyama EK, Rivard G, Acheson F, Cook CD. Adverse effect of maternal hyperventilation on the foetus. *Lancet* 1966;1:286.
155. Morishima HO, Moya F, Bossers AC, Daniel SS. Adverse effects of maternal hypocapnea on the newborn guinea pig. *Am J Obstet Gynecol* 1964;88:524.
156. Bailey RR, Rolleston GL. Kidney length and ureteric dilatation in the puerperium. *J Obstet Gynecol Br Commonw* 1971;78:55
157. Dure-Smith P. Ureters in pregnancy. *N Engl J Med* 1971;284:395.
158. Rubi RA, Sala NL, Althabe O. Ureteral function in pregnant women. IV. Ureteral peristalsis during normal pregnancy, in patients with empty and physiologically refilled bladder. *J Reprod Med* 1972;8:29.
159. Katz AI, Lindheimer MD. Renal handling of acute sodium loads in pregnancy. *Am J Physiol* 1973;25:696.
160. Berman LB. The pregnant kidney. *JAMA* 1974;230:111.
161. Lindheimer MD, Katz AI. Pregnancy and the kidney. *J Reprod Med* 1973;11:14.
162. Hertzberg BS, Carroll BA, Bowie JD, et al. Doppler US assessment of maternal kidneys: analysis of intrarenal resistivity indexes in normal pregnancy and physiologic pelvicaliectasis. *Radiology* 1993;186:689.
163. Weinberger MH, Petersen LP, Herr MJ, Wade MB. The effect of supine and lateral recumbency on plasma renin activity during pregnancy. *J Clin Endocrinol Metab* 1973;36:991.
164. Rudolph JH, Wax SH. The ^{131}I renogram in pregnancy. II. Normal pregnancy. *Obstet Gynecol* 1967;3:386.
165. Shirley RL. The kidney in pregnancy. *N Engl J Med* 1970;284:107.
166. Davison JM, Dunlop W. Renal hemodynamics and tubular function in normal human pregnancy. *Kidney Int* 1980;18:152.
167. Dunlop W. Serial changes in renal haemodynamics during normal human pregnancy. *Br J Obstet Gynaecol* 1981;88:1.
168. Brown MA, Sinosich MJ, Saunders DM, Gallery EDM. Potassium regulation and progesterone-aldosterone interrelationships in human pregnancy: a prospective study. *Am J Obstet Gynecol* 1986;155:349.
169. Ezimokhai M, Davison JM, Philips PR, Dunlop W. Non-postural serial changes in renal function during the third trimester of normal human pregnancy. *Br J Obstet Gynaecol* 1981;88:465.
170. Davison JM, Noble MCB. Serial changes in 24 hour creatinine clearance during normal menstrual cycles and the first trimester of pregnancy. *Br J Obstet Gynaecol* 1981;88:10.
171. Berliner RW, Grebisch G, eds. Body fluids and the excretion of urine. In: Brobeck JR, ed. *Best and Taylor's physiological basis of medical practice,* 10th ed. Baltimore: Williams & Wilkins, 1979:53.
172. Gaboury CL, Woods LL. Renal reserve in pregnancy. *Sem Nephrol* 1995;15:449.
173. Sturgiss SN, Wilkinson R, Davison JM. Renal reserve during human pregnancy. *Am J Physiol* 1996;271:F16.
174. Dunlop W. Investigations into the influence of posture on renal plasma flow and glomerular filtration rate during late pregnancy. *Br J Obstet Gynaecol* 1976;83:17.
175. Kelly AM, McNay MB, McEwan HP. Renal tubular function in normal pregnancy. *Br J Obstet Gynaecol* 1978;85:190.
176. Davison JM, Lovedale C. The excretion of glucose during normal pregnancy and after delivery. *J Obstet Gynaecol Br Commonw* 1974; 81:30.
177. Davison JM, Hytten FE. The effect of pregnancy on the renal handling of glucose. *Br J Obstet Gynaecol* 1975;82:374.
178. Brar HS, Do YS, Tam HB, et al. Uteroplacental unit as a source of elevated circulating prorenin levels in normal pregnancy. *Am J Obstet Gynecol* 1986;155:1223.
179. Ehrlich EN, Lindheimer MD. Effect of administered mineralocorticoids or ACTH in pregnant women. *J Clin Invest* 1972;51:130.
180. Landau RL, Bergenstal DM, Lugibihl K, Kascht ME. The metabolic effects of progesterone in man. *J Clin Endocrinol Metab* 1955;15: 1194.
181. Landau RL, Lugibihl K. Inhibition of the sodium-retaining influence of aldosterone by progesterone. *J Clin Endocrinol Metab* 1958;18: 1237.
182. Landau RL, Lugibihl K. The catabolic and natriuretic effects of progesterone in man. *Recent Prog Hormone* 1961;17:249.
183. Lindheimer MD, Richardson DA, Ehrlich EN, Katz AI. Potassium homeostasis in pregnancy. *J Reprod Med* 1987;32:517.
184. Lim VS, Katz AI, Lindheimer MD. Acid-base regulation in pregnancy. *Am J Physiol* 1976;231:1764.
185. Davison JM, Valotton MB, Lindheimer MD. Plasma osmolality and urinary concentration and dilution during and after pregnancy: evidence that lateral recumbency inhibits maximal urinary concentrating ability. *Br J Obstet Gynaecol* 1981;88:472.
186. Johnson MR, Brooks AA, Steer PJ. The role of relaxin in the pregnancy associated reduction in plasma osmolality. *Human Reprod* 1996;11:1105.
187. Geelhoed GW, Vander AJ. Plasma renin activities during pregnancy and parturition. *J Clin Endocrinol* 1968;28:412.
188. Bruce LA, Behsudi FM. Progesterone effects on three regional gastrointestinal tissues. *Life Sci* 1979;25:729.
189. Fisher RS, Roberts GS, Grabowski CJ, Cohen S. Inhibition of lower esophageal spinchter circular muscle by female sex hormones. *Am J Physiol* 1978;23:E243.
190. Fisher RS, Roberts GS, Grabowski CJ, Cohen S. Altered lower esophageal sphincter function during early pregnancy. *Gastroenterology* 1978;74:1233.
191. Nagler R, Spiro HM. Heartburn in late pregnancy. Manometric studies of esophageal motor function. *J Clin Invest* 1961;40:954.
192. Van Thiel DH, Gavaler JS, Joshi SN, Sara RK, Stremple J. Heartburn of pregnancy. *Gastroenterology* 1977;72:666.
193. Lind JF, Smith AM, McIver DK, Coopland AT, Crispin JS. Heartburn in pregnancy: a manometric study. *Can Med Assoc J* 1968;98:571.
194. Ulmsten U, Sundstrom G. Esophageal manometry in pregnant and nonpregnant women. *Am J Obstet Gynecol* 1978;132:260.
195. Hart DM. Heartburn in pregnancy. *J Int Med Res* 1978;6:1.
196. Atlay RD, Gillison EW, Horton AL. A fresh look at pregnancy heartburn. *J Obstet Gynaecol Br Commonw* 1973;80:63.
197. LaSalvia LA, Steffen EA. Delayed gastric emptying time in labor. *Am J Obstet Gynecol* 1950;59:1075.
198. Crawford JS. Some aspects of obstetric anaesthesia. *Br J Anaesth* 1956;28:201.
199. Davison JS, Davison MC, Hay DM. Gastric emptying time in late pregnancy and labour. *J Obstet Gynaecol Br Commonw* 1970;77:37.
200. Nimmo WS. The measurement of gastric emptying during labour. *J Int Med Res* 1978;6:52.
201. Simpson KH, Stakes AF, Miller M. Pregnancy delays paracetamol absorption and gastric emptying in patients undergoing surgery. *Br J Anaesth* 1988;60:24.
202. Levy DM, Williams DA, Magides AD, Reilly CS. Gastric emptying is delayed at 8–12 weeks gestation. *Br J Anaesth* 1994;73:237.
203. Whitehead EM, Smith M, O'Sullivan G. An evaluation of gastric emptying times in pregnancy and the puerperium. *Soc Obstet Anesth Perinatol Proc* 1990;22:F1.
204. Nimmo WS, Wilson J, Prescott LF. Narcotic analgesics and delayed gastric emptying during labour. *Lancet* 1975;1:890.
205. Wilson J. Gastric emptying in labour: some recent findings and their clinical significance. *J Int Med Res* 1978;6:54.
206. Howard FA, Sharp DS. Effect of metoclopramide on gastric emptying during labour. *Br Med J* 1973;1:446.
207. Colman RD, Frank M, Loughnan BA, Cohen DG, Cattermole R. Use of I.M. ranitidine for the prophylaxis of aspiration pneumonitis in obstetrics. *Br J Anaesth* 1988;61:720.
208. Dundee JW, Gamble JAS. Narcotic analgesics and delayed gastric emptying during labour. *Lancet* 1975;1:1032.
209. Davison JS. Gastric emptying in labour. *Lancet* 1975;2:227.
210. Davison JS. Gastric emptying in labour. *Lancet* 1975;2:930.
211. O'Sullivan GM, Sutton AJ, Thompson SA, Carrie LE, Bullingham RE. Noninvasive measurement of gastric emptying in obstetric patients. *Anesth Analg* 1987;66:505.
212. Holdsworth JD. Relationship between stomach contents and analgesia in labour. *Br J Anaesth* 1978;50:1145.
213. Christofides ND, Ghatel MA, Bloom SR, Borberg C, Gillmer MDG. Decreased plasma motilin concentrations in pregnancy. *Br Med J* 1982;285:1453.

214. Attia RR, Ebeid AM, Fischer JE, Goudsouzian NG. Maternal fetal and placental gastrin concentrations. *Anaesthesia* 1982;37:18.
215. Blouw R, Scatliff J, Craig DB, et al. Gastric volume and pH in postpartum patients. *Anesthesiology* 1976;45:456.
216. James CF, Gibbs CP, Banner T. Postpartum perioperative risk of aspiration pneumonia. *Anesthesiology* 1984;61:756.
217. Braverman DZ, Johnson ML, Kern F Jr. Effects of pregnancy and contraceptive steroids on gallbladder function. *N Engl J Med* 1980;302: 362.
218. Ryan JP. Effect of pregnancy on gallbladder contractility in the guinea pig. *Gastroenterology* 1984;87:674.
219. Kern F Jr, Everson GT, DeMark B, et al. Biliary lipids, bile acids, and gallbladder function in the human female. *J Clin Invest* 1981;68:1229.
220. Everson GT, McKinley C, Lawson M, Johnson M, Kern F Jr. Gallbladder function in the human female: effect of the ovulatory cycle, pregnancy, and contraceptive steriods. *Gastroenterology* 1982;82:711.
221. Cruikshank DP, Hays PM. Maternal physiology in pregnancy. In: Gabbe SG, Niebyl JR, Simpson JL, eds. *Obstetrics, normal and problem pregnancies.* New York: Churchill Livingstone, 1986:137.
222. Smith B, Moya F, Shnider S. The effects of anesthesia on liver function during labor. *Anesth Analg* 1962;41:24.
223. Song CS, Kappas A. The influence of estrogens, progestins, and pregnancy on the liver. *Vitam Horm* 1968;26:147.
224. Flynn RJ, Moore J, Dwyer R, Duly E, Dundee JW. Changes in alpha 1 acid glycoprotein during labor. *Anesth Analg* 1988;67:S61.
225. Corke BC. Drugs and obstetric anesthesia. In: Wood M, Wood AJJ, eds. *Drugs and anesthesia pharmacology: pharmalcology for the anesthetist.* Baltimore: Williams & Wilkins, 1990:347.
226. Cerutti R, Ferrari S, Grella P, Castelli, GP, Rizzotti P. Behavior of serum enzymes in pregnancy. *Clin Exp Obstet Gynecol* 1976;3:22.
227. Walker FB IV, Hoblit DL, Cunningham FG, Combes B. Gamma glutamyl transpeptidase in normal pregnancy. *Obstet Gynecol* 1974;43: 745.
228. Laros RK Jr, Alger LS. Thromboembolism and pregnancy. *Clin Obstet Gynecol* 1979;22:872.
229. Letsky E. The haematological system. In: Hytten F, Chamberlain G, eds. *Clinical physiology in obstetrics,* 2nd ed. Oxford: Blackwell Science, 1991:39.
230. Bonnar J, McNicol GP, Douglas AS. Fibrinolytic enzyme system and pregnancy. *Br Med J* 1969;3:387.
231. Hellgren M, Blomback M. Studies on blood coagulation and fibrinolysis in pregnancy, during delivery and in the puerperium. 1. Normal condition. *Gynecol Obstet Invest* 1981;12:141.
232. Gerbasi FR, Bottoms S, Farag A, Mammen E. Increased intravascular coagulation associated with pregnancy. *Obstet Gynecol* 1990;75:385.
233. Nilsson IM, Kullander S. Coagulation and fibrinolytic studies during pregnancy. *Acta Obstet Gynecol Scand* 1967;46:273.
234. Shaper AG, Path MC, Kear J, Macintosh DM, Kyobe J, Njama D. The platelet count, platelet adhesiveness and aggregation and the mechanism of fibrinolytic inhibition in pregnancy and the puerperium. *J Obstet Gynaecol Br Commonw* 1968;75:433.
235. Sejeny SA, Eastham RD, Baker SR. Platelet counts during normal pregnancy. *J Clin Pathol* 1975;28:812.
236. Wallenburg HCS, Van Kessel PH. Platelet lifespan in normal pregnancy as determined by a nonradioisotopic technique. *Br J Obstet Gynaecol* 1978;85:33.
237. Pekonen F, Rasi V, Ammala M, Viinikka L, Ylikorkala O. Platelet function and coagulation in normal and preeclamptic pregnancy. *Thromb Res* 1986;43:553
238. Kilby MD, Pipkin FB, Symonds M. Changes in platelet intracellular free calcium in normal pregnancy. *Br J Obstet Gynaecol* 1993;100: 375.
239. Woodfield DG, Cole SK, Allan AGE, Cash JD. Serum fibrin degradation products throughout normal pregnancy. *Br Med J* 1968;4:665.
240. Bonnar J, Davidson JF, Pidgeon CF, McNicols GP, Douglas AS. Fibrin degradation products in normal and abnormal pregnancy and parturition. *Br Med J* 1969;3:137.
241. Bonnar J, McNicol GP, Douglas AS. Coagulation and fibrinolytic mechanisms during and after normal childbirth. *Br Med J* 1970;2:200.
242. Gerbasi FR, Bottoms S, Farag A, Mammen EF. Changes in hemostasis activity during delivery and the immediate postpartum period. *Am J Obstet Gynecol* 1990;162:1158.
243. Stiehm ER, Kennan AL, Schelble DT. Split products of fibrin in maternal serum in the perinatal period. *Am J Obstet Gynecol* 1970; 108:941.
244. Ygge J. Changes in blood coagulation and fibrinolysis during the puerperium. *Am J Obstet Gynecol* 1969;104:2.
245. Bonnar J, Prentice CRM, McNicol GP, Douglas AS. Haemostatic mechanism in the uterine circulation during placental separation. *Br Med J* 1970;2:564.
246. Kalkhoff RK, Jacobson M, Lemper D. Progesterone, pregnancy and the augmented plasma insulin response. *J Clin Endocrinol* 1970;31: 24.
247. Buch I, Hornnes PJ, Kuhl C. Glucose tolerance in early pregnancy. *Acta Endocrinol* 1986;112:263.
248. Spellacy WN, Carlson KL, Birk SA. The fetus and the placenta as a source of insulin during pregnancy. *Obstet Gynecol* 1967;29:74.
249. Burt RL, Davidson IWF. Insulin half-life and utilization in normal pregnancy. *Obstet Gynecol* 1974;43:161.
250. Kuhl C. Glucose metabolism during and after pregnancy in normal and gestational diabetic women. *Acta Endocrinol* 1975;79:709.
251. Nordlander E, Hanson U, Persson B, Stangenberg M. Pancreatic B-cell function during normal pregnancy. *Diabetes Res* 1987;6:133.
252. Fisher PM, Sutherland HW, Bewsher PD. The insulin response to glucose infusion in normal human pregnancy. *Diabetologia* 1980;19:15.
253. Speroff L, Glass RH, Kase NG. *Clinical gynecologic endocrinology and infertility.* Baltimore: Williams & Williams, 1989:317.
254. Lind T, Bell S, Gilmore E, Huisjes HJ, Schally AV. Insulin disappearance rate in pregnant and in non-pregnant women given GHRIH. *Eur J Clin Invest* 1977;7:47.
255. Samaan N, Yen SCC, Gonzalez D, Pearson OH. Metabolic effects of placental lactogen (HPL) in man. *J Clin Endocrinol* 1968;28:485.
256. Beck P, Daughaday WH. Human placental lactogen: studies of its acute metabolic effects and disposition in normal man. *J Clin Invest* 1967;46:103.
257. Kalkhoff RK, Richardson BL, Beck P. Relative effects of pregnancy, human placental lactogen and prednisolone on carbohydrate tolerance in normal and subclinical diabetic subjects. *Diabetes* 1969;18:153.
258. Malkasian GD, Mayberry WE. Serum total and free thyroxine and thyrotropin in normal and pregnant women, neonates, and women receiving progestogens. *Am J Obstet Gynecol* 1971;108:1234.
259. Harada A, Hershman JM, Reed AW, et al. Comparison of thyroid stimulators and thyroid hormone concentrations in the sera of pregnant women. *J Clin Endocrinol Metab* 1979;48:793.
260. Kimura M, Amino N, Tamaki H, et al. Physiologic thyroid activation in normal early pregnancy is induced by circulating hCG. *Obstet Gynecol* 1990;75:775.
261. Glinoer D, De Nayer P, Robyn C, Lejeune B, Kinthaert J, Meuris S. Serum levels of intact human chorionic gonadotropin (HCG) and its free alpha and beta subunits, in relation to maternal thyroid stimulation during pregnancy. *J Endocrinol Invest* 1993;16:881.
262. Kol S, Karnieli E, Kraiem Z, Itskovitz-Eldor J, Lightman A, Ish-Shalom S. Thyroid function in early normal pregnancy: transient suppression of thyroid-stimulating hormone and stimulation of triiodothyronine. *Gynecol Obstet Invest* 1996;42:227.
263. Kannan V, Sinha MK, Devi PK, Rastogi GK. Plasma thyrotropin and its response to thyrotropin releasing hormone in normal pregnancy. *Obstet Gynecol* 1973;42:547.
264. Yannone ME, McCurdy JR, Goldfien A. Plasma progesterone levels in normal pregnancy, labor, and the puerperium. II. Clinical data. *Am J Obstet Gynecol* 1968;101:1058.
265. Greig M, Coyle MG, Cooper W. Plasma progesterone in mother and foetus in the second half of human pregnancy. *J Obstet Gynaecol* 1962;69:772.
266. Deshpande GN, Turner AK. Plasma progesterone and pregnanediol in human pregnancy, during labour and post-partum. *J Obstet Gynaecol Br Emp* 1960;67:954.
267. Whalen JB, Clancey CJ, Farley DB, Van Orden DE. Plasma prostaglandins in pregnancy. *Obstet Gynecol* 1978;51:52.
268. Quagliarello J, Szlachter N, Steinetz BG, Goldsmith LT, Weiss G. Serial relaxin concentrations in human pregnancy. *Am J Obstet Gynecol* 1979;135:43.
269. Calguneri M, Bird HA, Wright V. Changes in joint laxity occurring during pregnancy. *Ann Rheum Dis* 1982;41:126.
270. Berg G, Hammar M, Moller-Nielsen J, Linden U, Thorblad J. Low back pain during pregnancy. *Obstet Gynecol* 1988;71:71.

271. O'Connell JEA. Lumbar disc protrusions in pregnancy. *J Neurol Neursurg Psychiatry* 1960;23:138.
272. Akil H, Watson SJ, Barchas JD, Li CH. β-endorphin immunoreactivity in rat and human blood: radioimmunoassay, comparative levels and physiological alterations. *Life Sci* 1979;24:1659.
273. Gintzler AR. Endorphin-mediated increases in pain threshold during pregnancy. *Science* 1980;210:193.
274. Sander HW, Gintzler AR. Spinal cord mediation of the opioid analgesia of pregnancy. *Brain Res* 1987;408:389.
275. Sander HW, Portoghese PS, Gintzler AR. Spinal κ-opiate receptor involvement in the analgesia of pregnancy: effects of intrathecal norbinaltorphimine, a κ-selective antagonist. *Brain Res* 1988;474:343.
276. Bacigalupo G, Riese S, Rosendahl H, Saling E. Quantitative relationships between pain intensities during labor and beta-endorphin and cortisol concentrations in plasma. Decline of the hormone concentrations in the early postpartum period. *J Perinat Med* 1990;18:289.
277. Steinbrook RA, Carr DB, Datta S, Naulty JS, Lee C, Fisher J. Dissociation of plasma and cerebrospinal fluid beta-endorphin-like immunoactivity levels during pregnancy and parturition. *Anesth Analg* 1982;61:893.
278. Spielman FJ, Mueller RA, Corke BC. Cerebrospinal fluid concentration of 5-hydroxyindoleactic acid in pregnancy. *Anesthesiology* 1985;62:193.
279. Datta S, Hurley RJ, Naulty JS, et al. Plasma and cerebrospinal fluid progesterone concentrations in pregnant and nonpregnant women. *Anesth Analg* 1986;65:950.
280. Lurie AO, Weiss JB. Progesterone in cerebrospinal fluid during human pregnancy. *Nature* 1967;215:1178.
281. Fagraeus L, Urban BJ, Bromage PR. Spread of epidural analgesia in early pregnancy. *Anesthesiology* 1983;58:184.
282. Abouleish EL. Postpartum tubal ligation requires more bupivacaine for spinal anesthesia than does cesarean section. *Anesth Analg* 1986;65:897.
283. Crawford OB, Chester RV. Caudal anesthesia in obstetrics: a combined procainepontocaine single injection technic. *Anesthesiology* 1949;10:473.
284. Barclay DL, Renegar OJ, Nelson EW Jr. The influence of inferior vena cava compression on the level of spinal anesthesia. *Am J Obstet Gynecol* 1968;101:792.
285. Marx GF, Zemaitis MT, Orkin LR. Cerebrospinal fluid pressure during labor and obstetrical anesthesia. *Anesthesiology* 1961;22:348.
286. Galbert MW, Marx GF. Extradural pressures in the paturient patient. *Anesthesiology* 1974;40:499.
287. Sonnenschein C, Bonsing E, Jorgensen J, Hemmingsen L. Alpha$_1$-acid glycoprotein and albumin in the spinal fluid of pregnant women. *Int J Obstet Anesth* 1996;5:165.
288. Richardson MG, Wissler RN. Density of lumbar cerebrospinal fluid in pregnant and nonpregnant humans. *Anesthesiology* 1996;85:326.
289. Butterworth JF IV, Walker FO, Lysak SZ. Pregnancy increases median nerve susceptibility to lidocaine. *Anesthesiology* 1990;72:962.
290. Datta S, Lambert DH, Gregus J, Gissen AJ, Covino BG. Differential sensitivities of mammalian nerve fibers during pregnancy. *Anesth Analg* 1983;62:1070.
291. Flanagan HL, Datta S, Lambert DH, Gissen AJ, Covino BG. Effect of pregnancy on bupivacaine-induced conduction blockade in the isolated rabbit vagus nerve. *Anesth Analg* 1987;66:123.
292. Bader AM, Datta S, Moller RA, Covino BG. Acute progesterone treatment has no effect on bupivacaine-induced conduction blockade in the isolated rabbit vagus nerve. *Anesth Analg* 1990;71:545.
293. Flanagan HL, Datta S, Moller RA, Covino BG. Effect of exogenously administered progesterone on susceptibility of rabbit vagus nerves to bupivacaine. *Anesthesiology* 1988;69:A676.
294. Palahniuk RJ, Shnider SM, Eger EI II. Pregnancy decreases the requirement for inhaled anesthetic agents. *Anesthesiology* 1974;41:82.
295. Datta S, Migliozi RP, Flanagan HL, Krieger NR. Chronically administered progesterone decreases halothane requirements in rabbits. *Anesth Analg* 1989;68:46.
296. Mazze RI, Rice SA, Baden JM. Halothane, isoflurane, and enflurane MAC in pregnant and nonpregnant female and male mice and rats. *Anesthesiology* 1985;62:339.
297. Gin T, Chan MTV. Decreased minimum alveolar concentration of isoflurane in pregnant humans. *Anesthesiology* 1994;81:829.
298. Chan MTV, Gin T. Postpartum changes in the minimum alveolar concentration of isoflurane. *Anesthesiology* 1995;82:1360.
299. Chan MTV, Mainland P, Gin T. Minimum alveolar concentration of halothane and enflurane are decreased in early pregnancy. *Anesthesiology* 1996;85:782.
300. Gin T, Mainland P, Chan MTV, Short TG. Decreased thiopental requirements in early pregnancy. *Anesthesiology* 1997;86:73.
301. Cummings AJ. A survey of pharmacokinetic data from pregnant women. *Clin Pharmacokinet* 1983;8:344.
302. Perucca E, Crema A. Plasma protein binding of drugs in pregnancy. *Clin Pharmacokinet* 1982;7:336.
303. Blitt CD, Petty WC, Alberternst EE, Wright BJ. Correlation of plasma cholinesterase activity and duration of action of succinylcholine during pregnancy. *Anesth Analg* 1977;56:78.
304. Shnider SM. Serum cholinesterase activity during pregnancy, labor and puerperium. *Anesthesiology* 1965;36:335.
305. Hazel B, Monier D. Human serum cholinesterase: variations during pregnancy and post-partum. *Can Anaesth Soc J* 1971;18:272.
306. Whittaker M. Plasma cholinesterase variants and the anaesthetist. *Anaesthesia* 1980;35:174.
307. Evans RT, Wroe JM. Plasma cholinesterase changes during pregnancy. *Anaesthesia* 1980;35:651.
308. Whittaker M, Crawford JS, Lewis M. Some observations of levels of plasma cholinesterase activity within an obstetric population. *Anaesthesia* 1988;43:42.
309. Leighton BL, Cheek TG, Gross JB, et al. Succinycholine pharmacodynamics in peripartum patients. *Anesthesiology* 1986;64:202.
310. Hytten F, Chamberlain G, eds. *Clinical physiology in obstetrics,* 2nd ed. London: Blackwell Science, 1991.
311. Stoelting RK, Miller RD, eds. *Basics of anesthesia.* New York: Churchill Livingstone, 1989, p370.
312. Crawford JS. *Principles and practice of obstetric anesthesia,* 5th ed. Oxford: Blackwell Science, 1984.

Obstetric Anesthesia, second edition,
edited by Mark C. Norris.
Lippincott Williams & Wilkins, Philadelphia © 1999.

CHAPTER 2

Preoperative Evaluation of the Parturient with Coexisting Disease

Part I: Diseases of the Cardiac, Renal, and Hematologic Systems

Raphael Y. Gershon and Audrey S. Alleyne

Major changes in physiology accompany pregnancy. The healthy parturient adapts well to these changes; yet the additional stress of coexisting disease may contribute to significant maternal and fetal morbidity and mortality. To evaluate and treat these challenging patients, anesthesiologists must understand the normal, pregnancy-related alterations in physiology and the pathophysiologic changes related to the coexisting disease process. Ultimately, preoperative evaluation of pregnant patients with coexisting disease requires answers to these questions:

- How does the disease affect the pregnancy?
- How does the pregnancy affect the disease?

Only then can a safe anesthetic be planned and administered. The next several chapters of this book discuss the preoperative evaluation of parturients with a variety of medical and obstetric problems. They focus on the pathophysiology of the disease process and the management of these high-risk parturients before and during parturition. The goal of these chapters is to provide the information needed for the initial evaluation of these women. With this background, the obstetric anesthesiologist can then formulate an appropriate anesthetic plan. Later chapters in this book will discuss specific anesthetic options and how to modify them for women with significant disease.

Disorders considered in this chapter involve the cardiac and renal systems. We also will discuss problems related to hematology and coagulation.

R. Y. Gershon and A. S. Alleyne: Department of Anesthesiology, Emory University School of Medicine, Atlanta, Georgia 30303.

CARDIAC DISEASE

Diagnostic technology, medical and surgical management, and pharmacologic therapies of cardiac disease have advanced significantly over the past decades. With improved techniques, many women with cardiac abnormalities not only survive to child-bearing age but successfully complete pregnancy. Although there are certain recognized risks (Table 1), the majority of women with mild disease or with well-repaired cardiac defects tolerate pregnancy without increased morbidity and mortality (1,2).

Heart disease complicates 0.5% to 4% of pregnancies worldwide (3,4). Recently, the incidence of rheumatic heart disease has declined, but increasing numbers of parturients present with congenital heart disease due to improved surgical corrective techniques (5). Despite improved prognosis, normal hemodynamic changes associated with pregnancy may greatly increase the risk of morbidity and mortality in the parturient with cardiac

TABLE 1. *Recognized risks for parturients with heart disease and their fetuses*

An inability of the mother to meet the physiologic demands of pregnancy
An inadequate supply of well-oxygenated maternal blood for fetal nourishment
A worsening of maternal disease
Hereditary transmission to offspring from mothers with congenital heart disease
Additional complications such as infection, hemorrhage, or thromboembolism

disease. The maternal mortality associated with pregnancy approaches 50% in women with pulmonary hypertension, complicated coarctation of the aorta, and Marfan's syndrome with aortic involvement. However, uncomplicated atrial septal defect, ventricular septal defect, patent ductus arteriosus, corrected tetralogy of Fallot, porcine valve replacement, and mitral valve stenosis [New York Heart Association (NYHA) class I or II] correlate with a maternal mortality less than 1% (6).

Normal Physiologic Changes of Pregnancy

The normal changes in the cardiovascular system during pregnancy (see Chapter 1) can simulate organic heart disease (7). To review briefly, a 35% increase in blood volume and a 45% increase in plasma volume generates the "physiologic anemia of pregnancy." A 30% rise in stroke volume plus a 15% increase in heart rate augments cardiac output by 40% (8). The great veins of the pelvis and lower extremities hold a large portion of this expanded blood volume. Aortocaval compression by the enlarging uterus can significantly impair venous return by the mid-second trimester. Total peripheral resistance decreases by 15%. Diastolic blood pressure declines by 10 to 20 mm Hg. Systolic blood pressure may decrease by up to 15 mm Hg, and mean arterial blood pressure drops by 15 mm Hg. Cardiac output progressively rises until it peaks at 28 to 32 weeks' gestation and again in the third stage of labor with placental expulsion, uterine contraction, and autotransfusion. Because of the acute changes in blood volume, the reduction in aortocaval compression, and the loss of progesterone and other hormones with fetal and placental expulsion, cardiac output remains elevated for several hours after delivery.

As a result of these normal changes, the parturient often complains of fatigability, dyspnea, orthopnea, chest discomfort, or palpitations (Table 2). An increase in total body sodium and water combined with compression of the inferior vena cava by the gravid uterus may result in edema. However, paroxysmal nocturnal dyspnea, syncope with exertion, activity-related chest pain, and anasarca warrant investigation (Table 3) (9).

A nonpathologic diastolic murmur is heard in up to 10% of parturients. Higher blood flow across the atrioventricular valves during gestation probably causes this murmur. Bruits also may be normal variants if they originate from the internal mammary artery (the "mammary soufflé"). Venous hums from increased flow and the internal mammary bruit both have diastolic components. One may mistake them for a diastolic murmur signifying cardiac pathology (10).

Cardiac Disease and Pregnancy

Successful management of parturients with moderate to severe cardiac disease requires close cooperation between obstetrician, anesthesiologist, cardiologist, perinatologist, and nursing staff. Timely evaluation and frequent monitoring throughout pregnancy are needed to follow the mother's ability to adapt to the progressively increasing cardiac stresses of gestation. The personnel involved should meet early to define the severity of the disease, discuss options, and formulate plans to cope with a variety of clinical contingencies.

TABLE 2. *Normal physical findings in pregnancy*

Signs
Peripheral edema (up to 80% of parturients)
Distended neck veins (not throughout cardiac cycle)
Laterally displaced point of maximum impulse
Symptoms
Dyspnea
Reduced exercise tolerance
Auscultation
Increased splitting of the first and second heart sounds
A third (S_3) heart sound (up to 75% of parturients)
Systolic ejection murmur (left sternal border, grades I and II)
Continuous venous murmur
Neck bruits (originating from the internal mammary artery)
Electrocardiogram
Left-axis deviation
Nonspecific ST- and T-wave changes
Chest Radiograph
Straightening of the left heart border
Heart position more horizontal
Increased vascular markings (from elevation of diaphragm)

Classification

A valuable way to assess severity of underlying heart disease is the NYHA classification of functional impairment (Table 4). Approximately 5% to 10% of pregnant cardiac patients fall into NYHA class III or IV. These women have a 75% to 90% risk of maternal mortality. Patients with cardiac disease who are in NYHA class I and II have less than a 1% mortality rate with pregnancy. In the absence of pulmonary hypertension, complicated congenital heart disease and Marfan's syndrome with aortic involvement, patients who are in class III and IV have a 5% to 15% mortality and a 20% to 30% risk of fetal loss (11,12).

TABLE 3. *Signs and symptoms of maternal heart disease*

Signs	Symptoms
Cyanosis	Severe dyspnea
Clubbing	Paroxysmal nocturnal dyspnea
Persistent neck vein distention	Hemoptysis
Systolic murmur >grade II/VI	Syncope with exertion
Diastolic murmur	Stress-related chest pain
Cardiomegaly	
Arrhythmia	
Loud P_2	

TABLE 4. *New York Heart Association functional classification*

Class I	Asymptomatic
Class II	Slight limitation of physical activities; comfortable at rest
Class III	Marked limitation with less than ordinary activity causing fatigue, palpitation, dyspnea, or angina; remains comfortable at rest
Class IV	Symptomatic at rest

Diagnosis and Management During Pregnancy

Sole reliance on subjective signs and symptoms may lead to erroneous diagnosis of cardiac disease in the parturient (13). Serial measurement of a host of noninvasive, objective parameters can provide information about the maternal ability to cope with impending parturition. Intermittent measurements of peripheral oxygen saturation with a pulse oximeter may provide an early indication of cardiac failure. Vital capacity measurement may detect increases in blood volume that produce pulmonary vascular engorgement. Electrocardiograms (ECGs) and Holter monitors can detect ischemia, arrhythmias, conduction defects, and axis deviations.

Chest films, repeated as necessary, can diagnose or confirm progressive congestive heart failure, cardiomegaly, and pleural or pericardial effusions. A chest radiograph exposes the mother to a maximum of 80 mrad of radiation, with approximately 50 mrad to the chest and 5 mrad to the gonads (14). A dose of 0.5 rad is the recommended maximal radiation exposure to the pregnant woman (15), although some authors have suggested that even 10-rad exposure is safe (16,17). A detailed analysis of prenatal radiation exposure and subsequent malformations or cancer suggests that fetal risk is very low. Fewer than 1 case of malformation or cancer is expected per 1,000 patients irradiated by 1 rad in utero during the first 4 months of pregnancy (18). So, no measurable risk is associated with a chest radiograph during pregnancy.

Radionuclide techniques expose the mother to 500 to 800 mrad (19), and cardiac catheterization exposes the patient to as much as 28,000 mrad of radiation. Flow-directed right heart and pulmonary artery catheterization without fluoroscopy can assess valvular function and chamber pressures. Two-dimensional contrast echocardiography can evaluate valve and ventricular function. Both alternatives help limit maternal and fetal exposure to radiation.

Echocardiography (two-dimensional and M-mode) generates high-frequency sound waves and records signals reflected from the blood–tissue interfaces. Assessment of cardiac chamber motion, myocardial contractility, and ejection fraction aid in patient evaluation. Doppler echocardiography detects the change in sound-wave frequency reflected from moving targets such as red blood cells. This technique can provide information about abnormal blood flow, transvalvular pressure gradients, valve area, and cardiac output.

Management at Term

Good communication between the obstetric anesthesiologist and the obstetrician facilitates the care of these high-risk parturients. Invasive monitoring, antibiotic regiments, anticoagulation, termination of pregnancy, the route of delivery, anesthetic management, maternal–fetal priorities, and the effects of various cardiac and uterine therapeutic modalities should all be discussed before parturition.

Monitoring

Clark et al. (20) used thermodilution to assess cardiac output in ten primiparous volunteers. The women were studied at 36 to 38 weeks of gestation and again between 11 and 13 weeks postpartum. By late in the third trimester, parturients had significantly lower systemic vascular resistance, peripheral vascular resistance, and colloid osmotic pressure. Both cardiac output and heart rate were elevated. Left ventricular stroke work index remained unchanged. These investigators concluded that the third trimester of normal pregnancy is not associated with hyperdynamic left ventricular function. Lee and co-workers (21) prospectively compared pulsed-Doppler and thermodilution-derived estimates of left ventricular stroke volume and cardiac output in 16 gravidae. These women had undergone right heart catheterization for several reasons (severe preeclampsia, eclampsia, hemorrhagic shock, and renal failure). The authors found a good correlation between cardiac output measurements made by pulsed-Doppler and thermodilution (Fig. 1) (21). A critical literature review (22) revealed that although cardiac output during the third trimester was widely divergent, the accuracy of Doppler echocardiography and thoracic electrical bioimpedance cardiography are similar to that of invasive techniques. These results should minimize the need for invasive modalities to measure maternal cardiac function.

There are few strict rules about when to insert a pulmonary artery (PA) catheter in the obstetric patient. The PA catheter may be contraindicated in some patients with Eisenmenger's syndrome, because in these patients, the risks (arrhythmias, passing a catheter through an atrial or septal defect in the cardiac circulation, trauma, infection and embolism) far outweigh the benefits (23–28). Some suggest that aortic stenosis in the absence of other lesions may very well be managed without PA catheter because volume status can be easily assessed with a central venous pressure catheter (5). Cardiac arrhythmias are poorly tolerated by these patients, and some choose to avoid PA catheter insertion. Others find PA catheters

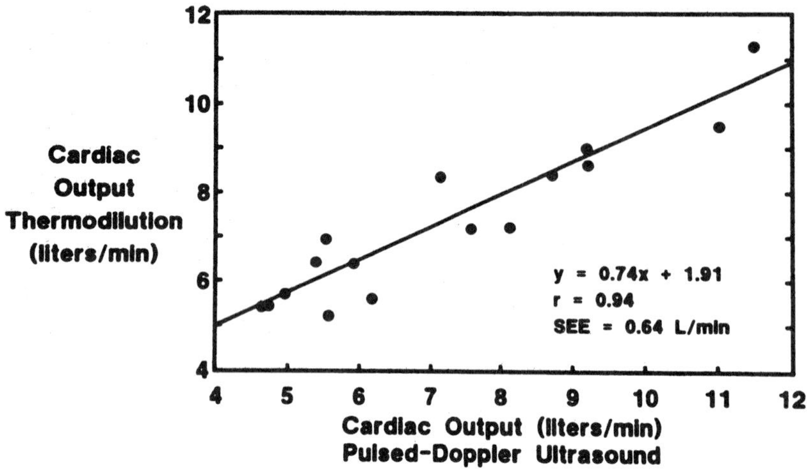

FIG. 1. Correlation between pulsed-Doppler and thermodilution cardiac output in parturients. *r*, slope correlation between the techniques; *SEE*, standard error; *x*, cardiac output, Doppler technique; *y*, cardiac output, thermodilution technique. (From ref. 21, with permission.)

extremely helpful in managing labor-related hemodynamic alterations in these patients. In general, PA catheterization is reserved for pregnant women with NYHA class III and IV cardiac disease (29). In addition, patients with severe preeclampsia/eclampsia with end-organ disease, septic shock, hypovolemic shock, or thyroid storm may benefit from a PA catheter (Table 5).

Endocarditis Prophylaxis

The genitourinary tract is second only to the oral cavity as a portal of entry for organisms that cause endocarditis. Yet, according to the recent American Heart Association guidelines (30), endocarditis prophylaxis is optional for high-risk patients undergoing vaginal delivery or vaginal hysterectomy. High-risk patients include those with prosthetic valves, previous history of bacterial endocarditis, complex cyanotic congenital heart lesions (tetralogy of Fallot), and surgically constructed shunts. Furthermore,

TABLE 5. *Clinical indications for insertion of pulmonary artery catheters during pregnancy*

Recent myocardial infarction or significant coronary artery disease
Severe left ventricular dysfunction (left ventricular ejection fraction <0.4, left ventricular end-diastolic pressure >18 torr, cardiac index <2, wall-motion abnormalities on echocardiogram)
Severe preeclampsia/eclampsia with oliguria or pulmonary edema
Class II or III rheumatic or congenital cardiac disease with severe preeclampsia in labor
Class III or IV rheumatic or congenital cardiac disease in labor
Septic shock
Adult respiratory distress syndrome
Amniotic fluid embolism
Hypovolemic shock unresponsive to fluid replacement
Thyroid storm

prophylaxis is not recommended for cesarean delivery. In the absence of localized infection, prophylaxis also is not recommended for urethral catheterization, uterine dilatation and curettage, therapeutic abortion, sterilization procedures, and insertion or removal of intrauterine devices. If the clinician decides to give endocarditis prophylaxis, the recommended regiment for these high-risk adults is ampicillin 2 g intramuscularly (IM) or intravenously (IV) plus gentamicin 1.5 mg/kg IM or IV (not to exceed 120 mg) 30 minutes before start of the procedure followed by a dose of ampicillin 1 g IM/IV or amoxicillin 1 g orally 6 hours after the procedure. For high-risk patients allergic to ampicillin or amoxicillin, vancomycin 1 g IV over 1 to 2 hours plus gentamicin 1.5 mg/kg IV or IM is recommended 30 minutes before the start of the procedure.

Anticoagulants

All patients with mechanical valve prostheses must receive anticoagulants. Those with cardiac valve disease, chronic atrial fibrillation, and a history of systemic emboli also should take these drugs. Warfarin (Coumadin) crosses the placenta and increases the danger of abnormal fetal development and congenital malformations, as well as abortion, stillbirth, and hemorrhage (31–33). It has been suggested by several retrospective European studies that these complications are due to high-dose warfarin and that in low doses (5 mg or less daily) there is minimal risk (33–35). In the United States, heparin is the preferred anticoagulant used during gestation because it does not cross the placenta. Heparin carries the risk of maternal thrombocytopenia, thromboembolism (36,37), osteoporosis (38,39), and rare hypersensitivity reactions. There also is a risk of retroplacental hemorrhage and abruptio-placentae, which can result in prematurity, stillbirth, and spontaneous abortion. Several studies have shown that heparin therapy is safe for the fetus (40,41). Low-molecular-weight heparins have been shown to cause less platelet aggregation (42), do not cross the placenta (43–45), and have a reduced association with osteoporosis (46,47); however, their safety in pregnancy has not been clearly elucidated.

Some physicians begin heparin therapy after conception and through the first trimester (to avoid embryopathy) and resume warfarin therapy in mid-pregnancy (32). Others believe that fetal bleeding may occur at all stages of development and avoid warfarin throughout the pregnancy (48). At term, discontinue heparin therapy 24 hours before elective induction of labor or cesarean section to avoid increased hemorrhage to the parturient and neonate during delivery (33). Should spontaneous labor occur in a heparinized parturient, carefully monitor the activated thromboplastin time. If it is prolonged near delivery, consider protamine sulfate (32).

Chronic Medications

Pregnant cardiac patients may arrive for delivery taking a host of medications. Digoxin appears safe during pregnancy, with therapeutic serum concentrations having no apparent toxic effects on the fetus (49). Lidocaine appears safe in the therapeutic range (50); however, apnea, hypotonia, dilated pupils, seizures, and fetal bradycardia can occur with higher serum concentrations. Quinidine and procainamide may induce premature labor. In addition, chronic use of procainamide may result in a lupus-like syndrome due to the development of maternal antinuclear antibodies. Diuretics may reduce uteroplacental blood flow and yield fetal electrolyte imbalance, neonatal jaundice, thrombocytopenia, liver damage, and fetal death.

The β-adrenergic blocking drugs—propranolol, labetalol, and esmolol, cross the placenta. These drugs, particularly esmolol (51–53), may cause fetal bradycardia, neonatal hypoglycemia, and intrauterine growth retardation (IUGR) (54,55). Nonselective β-adrenergic receptor antagonists may increase uterine tone by blocking the inhibitory effect of epinephrine on myometrium; thus, some clinicians prefer the use of selective β_1-adrenergic receptor blocking agents such as metoprolol and atenolol (55). Although these drugs do not present the same risks as their nonselective counterparts, they are still associated with growth restriction and low birth weight when used early in pregnancy (56).

Short-term use of calcium channel blockers has not been associated with demonstrable adverse effects in the fetus or newborn infant. These drugs, however, can exert a tocolytic effect (57,58). In combination with magnesium sulfate, calcium channel blockers, particularly nifedipine, have been associated with hypotension and pronounced muscle weakness (59).

Amiodarone has been associated with preterm delivery, IUGR, and neonatal hypothyroidism (60,61). Angiotensin-converting enzyme (ACE) inhibitors, such as captopril and enalapril, have been used during pregnancy. Use of ACE inhibitors during the second or third trimester has been associated with fetopathy. ACE inhibitor fetopathy is characterized by renal tubular dysplasia, hypocalvaria, IUGR, and patent ductus arteriosus (62). These drugs also increase the risk of preterm labor, oligohydramnios, and neonatal renal failure (62–64).

Specific Lesions

The parturient tolerates valvular regurgitation better than valvular stenosis. In fact, multivalvular regurgitation is not uncommon in normal pregnancy (65). Serial clinical examinations and pulsed-continuous Doppler echocardiography throughout pregnancy reveal that, as the parturient approaches term, multivalvular regurgitation is common and occasionally persists into the early postpartum period. These changes were mainly right-sided (tricuspid, 94.4%; pulmonary, 94.4%; mitral, 27.8%; aortic, 0%). Furthermore, chamber enlargement and valve annular dilation also were common findings. Remember these results when interpreting Doppler echocardiographic data and clinically evaluating the parturient with heart disease.

Mitral Stenosis

The most common acquired valvular disease presenting in pregnancy is mitral valve stenosis of rheumatic origin. The obstructing lesion usually develops 10 to 20 years after the initial infection. These women may not tolerate the normal cardiovascular changes of pregnancy. Previously asymptomatic patients, unaware that they have heart disease, may experience sudden life-threatening pulmonary edema during pregnancy (66). Symptoms occur in as many as 25% of gravidae with mitral stenosis (Table 6).

TABLE 6. *Mitral valve disease: severe mitral stenosis*

Symptoms
- Shortness of breath, dyspnea on exertion, orthopnea
- Recurrent bronchitis
- Hemoptysis
- Systemic embolism
- Acute pulmonary edema may occur with the onset of atrial fibrillation or acute pulmonary infection

Physical Findings
- First heart sound and mitral opening snap are loud with pliable valve, faint with calcific valve
- Diastolic murmur: low-frequency apical murmur is longer with more severe stenosis; may be very faint in the elderly
- ECG: left atrial enlargement or atrial fibrillation; right-axis deviation; rarely, right ventricular hypertrophy
- Chest radiograph: increased cardiac size, especially left atrium, calcification in mitral valve, pulmonary congestion
- Echocardiogram: left atrial dilation, decreased left ventricular performance, characteristic valve changes, whether pliable or rigid

Hemodynamic Findings
- Diastolic gradient between the pulmonary wedge pressure and left ventricular diastolic pressure

After ref. 269, with permission.

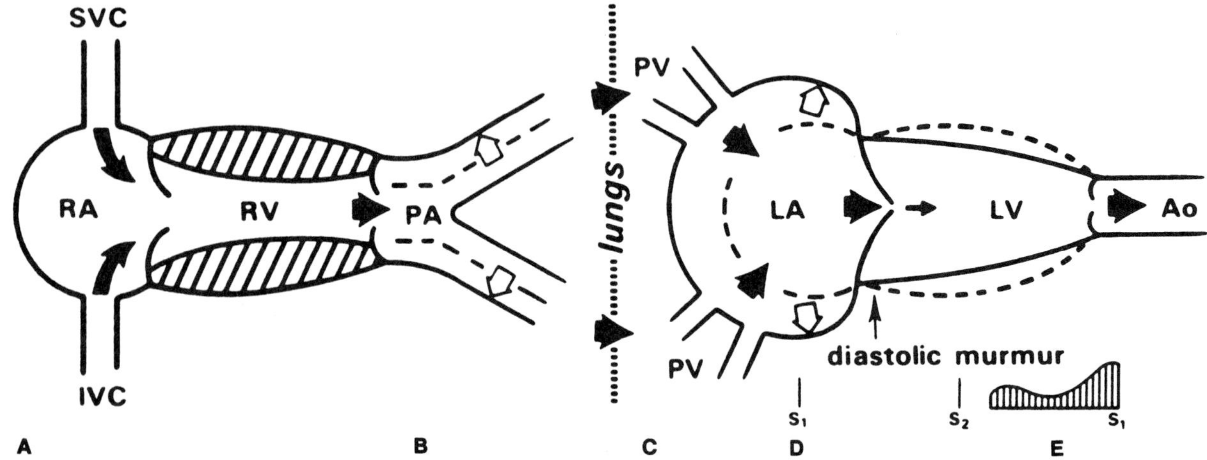

FIG. 2. Pathophysiology of mitral stenosis. **A:** Increased right atrial *(RA)* pressures reflect right-sided failure. **B:** Degree of elevation in pulmonary artery *(PA)* pressure reflects the severity of increase in pulmonary venous *(PV)* pressure. **C:** Increased PV pressure. **D:** Enlarged left atrium *(LA)*, increased left atrial pressure; diastolic gradient between LA and left ventricle *(LV)* reflects severity of stenosis. **E:** Low cardiac output with severe stenosis. *Ao,* aorta; *IVC,* inferior vena cava; *SVC,* superior vena cava. (From ref. 269, with permission.)

In progressive mitral stenosis, left ventricular volume decreases, whereas the left atrium, pulmonic system, and right heart face an increase in both pressure and volume (Fig. 2). Normal adult mitral valve area varies from 4 to 6 cm^2. Stenotic lesions are graded as follows:

- Mild: 1.5 to 2.5 cm^2
- Moderate: 1.0 to 1.5 cm^2
- Severe: less than 1 cm^2

Distal to the valve, the left ventricle is small to normal in size. Left ventricular end-diastolic pressure is in the normal range. However, approximately one third of patients with mitral valve disease have a depressed ejection fraction from either a chronic decrease in left ventricular volume or residual scarring from rheumatic myocarditis (67). A dilated left atrium may predispose to left lower lobe pulmonary infections. Severe left atrial dilation can cause left recurrent laryngeal nerve paralysis and dysphagia.

On auscultation, classic findings include an accentuated first heart sound, an "opening snap," an early diastolic sound heard best over the lower left sternal border, and a low-pitched apical diastolic "rumble" (Fig. 3) (9). Evidence of mitral regurgitation, as well as involvement of other valves, is not uncommon. The ECG and chest radiograph will detect signs of advanced disease, such as atrial fibrillation or right ventricular hypertrophy. Tachycardia, atrial fibrillation, or junctional rhythm may decrease stroke volume.

The Gorlin equation (Eq. 1) aids in the understanding of valvular disease hemodynamics. If valve area remains constant, the pressure gradient (Eq. 2) across the valve will increase by the square of any rise in flow rate (cardiac output). Left atrial pressure rises in relation to orifice size, atrial size, heart rate, cardiac compliance, and output.

The Gorlin equation:

$$\text{Valve area} = \frac{\text{Flow}}{\text{K} \times \text{pressure gradient}} \qquad [1]$$

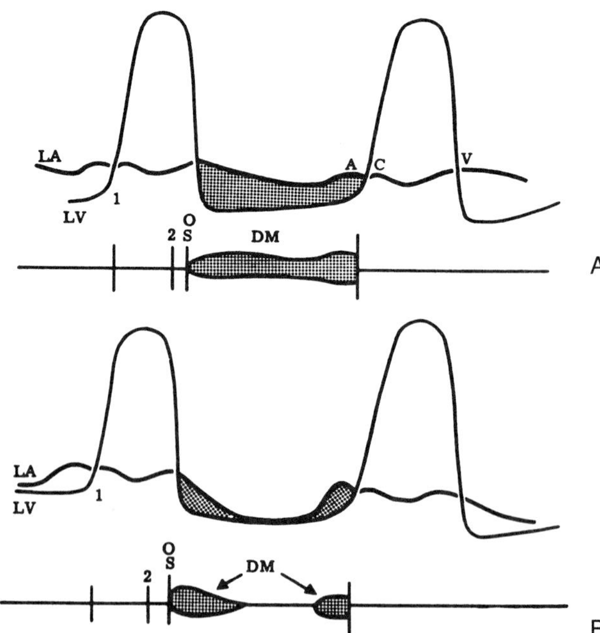

FIG. 3. Schematic representation of the duration of the diastolic murmur *(DM)* of mitral stenosis and its relationship to intracardiac pressures. The DM persists as long as there is a significant diastolic pressure gradient across the mitral valve and is, therefore, longer in more severe grades of stenosis. *A, C,* and *V* are central venous pulsation waves; *OS* is an opening snap. **A:** Severe stenosis. **B:** Mild stenosis. *LA,* left atrium; *LV,* left ventricle. (From ref. 270, with permission.)

TABLE 7. *Etiology of mitral valve insufficiency*

Rheumatic fever
Mitral valve prolapse
Chordae tendineae dysfunction and/or rupture
Cardiac trauma
Endocarditis
Papillary muscle dysfunction and/or rupture
Cardiac trauma
Endocarditis
Spatial disorientation
Cardiomyopathy with left ventricular enlargement
Idiopathic hypertrophic subaortic stenosis

Pressure gradient, mitral valvular disease:

$$\text{Pressure gradient} = \text{Left atrial pressure} - \text{Left ventricular end-diastolic pressure}$$

$$\text{Pressure gradient} = \frac{\text{Cardiac output}^2}{\text{Diastolic filling time}} \quad [2]$$

Cardiac decompensation is most likely to occur at 28 to 32 weeks' gestation, during the onset of labor, or early postpartum. These are times of maximal increase in heart rate, systemic blood volume, cardiac output, and pulmonary blood volume. With a valvular pressure gradient greater than 25 mm Hg, acute cardiac decompensation may arise, accompanied by atrial fibrillation, paroxysmal tachycardia, pulmonary vascular congestion, and infarction (68). In late-stage mitral stenosis, elevated pulmonary pressures produce persistent pulmonary hypertension and irreversible pulmonary arterial hyperplasia. Right heart failure, peripheral edema, hepatomegaly, ascites, and distended neck veins may occur. Ventilation–perfusion mismatching, which worsens in the Trendelenburg position, is not uncommon.

Mitral Insufficiency

Mitral insufficiency is often due to rheumatic fever and is usually associated with mitral stenosis (69). However, there are other causes of regurgitant flow (Table 7).

Mitral insufficiency generally is better tolerated than mitral stenosis during pregnancy. Failure of valve closure permits left ventricular blood to flow into the left atrium during ventricular systole. Regurgitant flow depends on the ventriculoatrial pressure gradient, regurgitant orifice size, and heart rate. Heart rate affects both time for ventricular filling and duration of ventricular ejection. Regurgitant blood raises left atrial pressure and may produce pulmonary vascular congestion and pulmonary edema.

The increased left ventricular diastolic volume is generally tolerated. As ventricular compliance increases, a larger left ventricular end-diastolic volume does not raise left ventricular end-diastolic pressure and oxygen consumption is not initially prohibitive. When the regurgitant fraction is greater than 60% of left ventricular volume, congestive heart failure develops. Left ventricular failure with reduced left ventricular output may cause pulmonary hypertension and ultimately right ventricular failure (Table 8).

When insufficiency of the mitral valve is combined with stenosis, both pressure and volume work increase. Symptoms are generally more severe and occur earlier than in pure insufficiency. Fatigue is the most typical early symptom. On physical examination, an apical holosystolic murmur radiating to the left axilla is common (Fig. 4). The ECG may show evidence of left atrial enlargement or fibrillation, and left ventricular hypertrophy. With significant insufficiency, chest radiograph may show cardiomegaly and pulmonary vascular congestion.

The mild tachycardia of pregnancy may benefit the gravida with mitral regurgitation, as the area of the regurgitant orifice may decrease in the faster heart. Mitral valve prolapse with regurgitation is the exception to this principle. Prolapse of redundant mitral leaflets worsens with a smaller ventricular valve orifice as caused by tachycardia. The lower systemic vascular resistance of the gravida allows her to improve forward flow. Conversely, any increase in systemic vascular resistance may cause worsening regurgitation.

TABLE 8. *Mitral valve insufficiency*

	Chronic	Acute
Symptoms	Long-standing exertional dyspnea	Acute pulmonary edema, cardiogenic shock with papillary muscle rupture
Rhythm	Usually atrial fibrillation	Usually sinus rhythm
First heart sound	Faint	Faint
Third heart sound (S_3)	May be audible	May be audible
S_4 gallop	No	Very common
Heart size	Large	Normal or slightly enlarged
Left atrial size	Markedly increased	Slightly increased
Left ventricular hypertrophy on ECG	Common	Uncommon
Echocardiogram	Chamber size, valve characteristics depend on etiology	Chamber size, typical changes of flail valve leaflet
Left atrial pressure	Not considerably increased	Very prominent V wave may approach aortic diastolic pressure

After ref. 269, with permission.

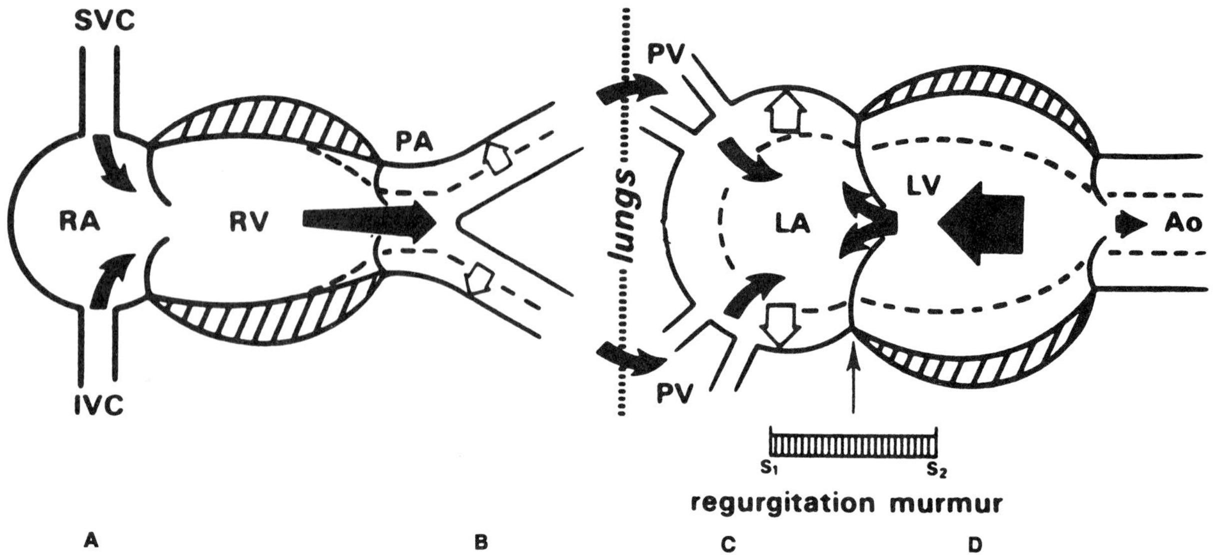

FIG. 4. Pathophysiology of mitral insufficiency. **A:** Changes in the right atrium *(RA)* and right ventricle *(RV)* depend on the degree of pulmonary hypertension. **B:** Increased pulmonary artery *(PA)* pressure reflects the increased pulmonary venous *(PV)* pressure. **C:** Dilation and increased pressure in the left atrium *(LA)* reflect severity of the disease. Dilation is more pronounced in chronic insufficiency. Increased pressure is more pronounced in acute incompetence. **D:** Degree of left ventricular *(LV)* dilation usually reflects the severity of the disease. *Ao*, aorta; *IVC*, inferior vena cava; *SVC*, superior vena cava. (From ref. 269, with permission.)

Mitral Valve Prolapse

Mitral valve prolapse affects 5% to 10% of young adults and is encountered mainly in women of child-bearing age (70). A mid- to late systolic click followed by a systolic murmur, heard best at the lower left sternal border or cardiac apex, is typical. The ECG and chest radiograph are generally nonspecific. Echocardiography reveals pathologic protrusion of the mitral leaflet into the left atrium during systole (71). Symptoms range from atypical chest pain, dyspnea, fatigue, dizziness, palpitations, and anxiety, to syncope and sudden death. Structural abnormalities in primary mitral valve prolapse consist of elongated chordae tendineae with large redundant mitral leaflets. Histologically, the familial form of mitral valve prolapse shows myxomatous degenerative changes.

The valve in primary mitral valve prolapse is functionally too large for the ventricle. This mismatch causes the redundant leaflets to prolapse into the left atrium as ventricular volume decreases in mid- and late systole. Severity of prolapse depends on ventricular volume. Increased myocardial contractility, decreased preload, tachycardia, straining, and excessive airway pressure decrease ventricular volume and worsen symptoms.

Pregnancy may change the physical signs of mitral valve prolapse, either enhancing or diminishing them, depending on changes in vascular resistance and blood volume (72–74). One large series evaluated 3,582 parturients. Forty-three patients had documented mitral valve prolapse (1.2%). All 43 had pregnancies complicated by cardiac compromise but with good fetal outcome. Neither spontaneous abortion nor premature delivery seemed higher in the women with mitral valve prolapse (75).

Aortic Stenosis

The basic pathophysiology of aortic stenosis is the development of obstruction to left ventricular outflow. Normal aortic valve area is approximately 2.5 to 3.5 cm^2. In advanced stages of aortic stenosis, when the valve area is less than 0.75 cm^2, stroke volume is decreased and fixed (Fig. 5). Concentric left ventricular hypertrophy and elevated left ventricular chamber pressure reduce subendocardial blood flow. Ischemia and ventricular failure follow. The increased oxygen required by the noncompliant, hypertrophied left ventricle doing pressure work, combined with reduced coronary artery blood flow caused by a decreased cardiac output, worsen the ischemia. Although pregnancy outcome is generally satisfactory in patients with congenital aortic stenosis (76), maternal mortality in patients with severe aortic stenosis can be high due to the dependency of cardiac output on adequate circulatory blood volume. A sudden maternal blood volume loss, such as may occur at delivery, can have catastrophic consequences. Thus, valvular surgery has been advised during pregnancy when the aortic valve gradient is 70 mm Hg or greater (77).

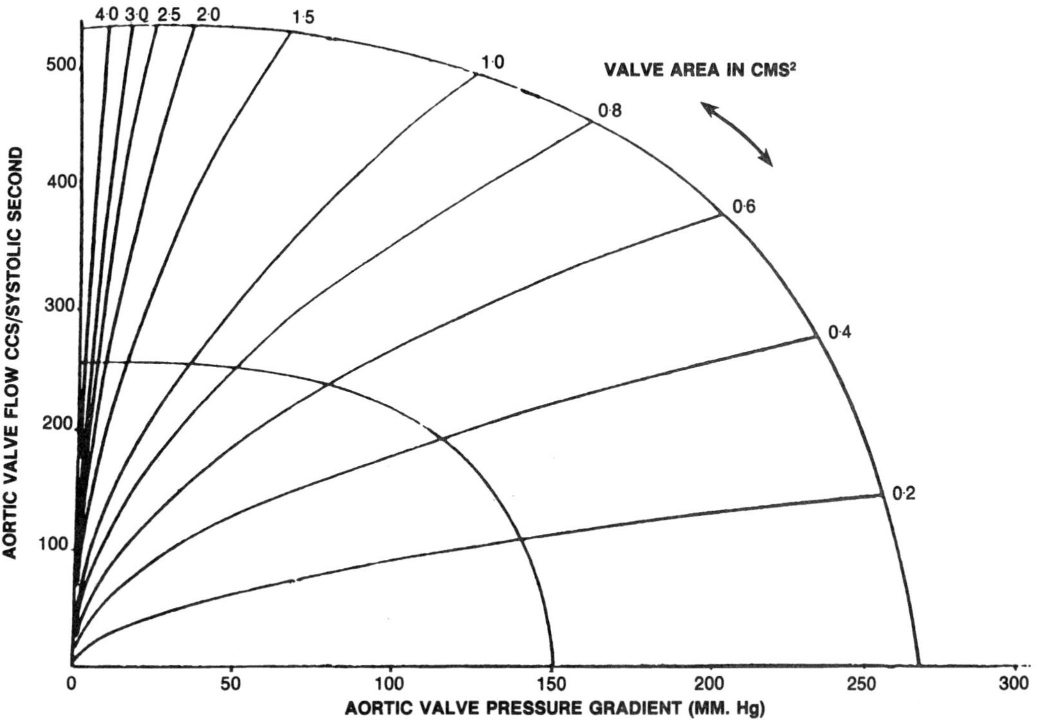

FIG. 5. Interrelation of aortic valve pressure gradient, aortic valve flow, and aortic valve area. This diagram shows the theoretic pressure and flow curves for different aortic valve cross-sectional areas (in square centimeters). (From ref. 271, with permission.)

Patients with aortic stenosis increasingly rely on atrial contraction to maintain cardiac output. Normally, atrial contraction augments stroke volume by 20%. In women with aortic stenosis, atrial contraction may contribute as much as 40% of stroke volume (78). Therefore, a loss of atrial function, whether through atrial fibrillation or junctional rhythms, may be lethal.

The classic physical finding of aortic stenosis is a harsh systolic ejection murmur, heard at the base of the heart, that radiates to the carotid arteries (Fig. 6). Other

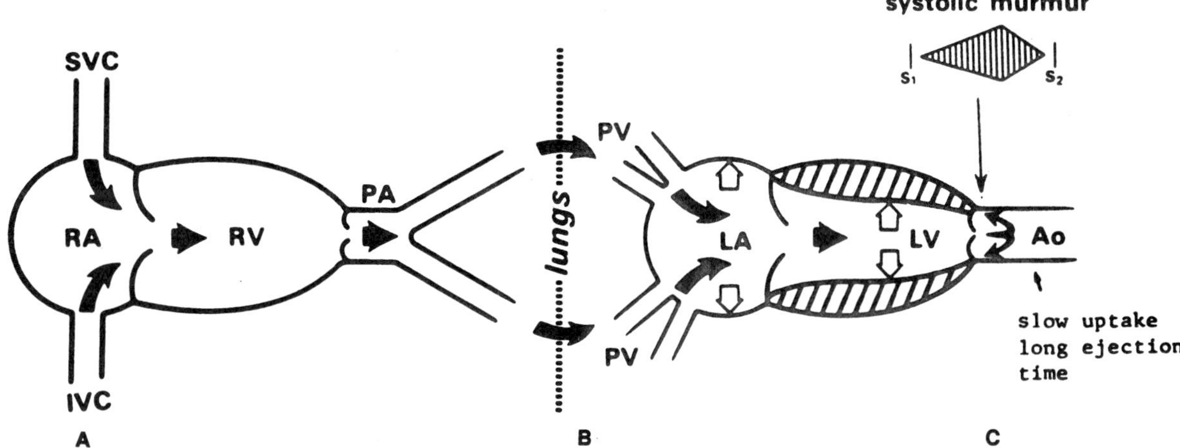

FIG. 6. Pathophysiology of aortic stenosis. **A:** The degree of right atrial *(RA)* and right ventricular *(RV)* pressure increase reflects the increase in left atrial *(LA)* pressure. **B:** Degree of increase in pulmonary venous *(PV)* pressure reflects the degree of left ventricular *(LV)* failure or decreased LV compliance. **C:** Systolic pressure increases. Degree of increase reflects the severity of aortic stenosis. A systolic gradient greater than 50 mm Hg indicates severe stenosis. Diastolic pressure decreases. *Ao*, aorta; *IVC*, inferior vena cava; *PA*, pulmonary artery; *SVC*, superior vena cava. (From ref. 269, with permission.)

TABLE 9. *Severe aortic stenosis*

Symptoms	Angina; syncope; paroxysmal nocturnal dyspnea; congestive heart failure (rare)
Physical findings	Slow carotid upstroke; left ventricular enlargement, if marked, signifies poor left ventricular performance; faint or absent aortic closure sound in calcific aortic stenosis; long ejection murmur that peaks in mid-systole heard maximally over the second space to the right of the sternum
Chest radiograph	Left ventricular enlargement; pulmonary congestion possible; aortic valve calcification
Electrocardiogram	Left ventricular hypertrophy and "strain"
Echocardiogram	Thickened valve with limited mobility; increased left-ventricular wall thickness and decreased left ventricular performance
Cardiac catheterization	Large systolic gradient across aortic valve (>50 mm Hg)

After ref. 269, with permission.

findings may include a slowly rising and prolonged arterial pulse, a fourth heart sound, or a paradoxically split second heart sound. History may reveal syncope, angina, or dyspnea on exertion (Table 9).

The increased oxygen requirements of pregnancy and labor make the myocardium of these women vulnerable to ischemic injury. The increased plasma volume of pregnancy may further elevate pressure in the noncompliant left ventricle, increasing myocardial oxygen demand and encouraging pulmonary transudation of fluid. If hemodynamically severe aortic stenosis is diagnosed before pregnancy, surgical correction in advance is advisable. Parturients with aortic stenosis have reported mortality rates as high as 17% (79). Diminished stroke volume and cardiac output may place uteroplacental blood flow at jeopardy, with possible IUGR and congenital anomalies. A fetal mortality rate of 32% has been reported in women with uncorrected aortic stenosis (80). Correction of a maternal outflow obstruction before conception reduces the fetal mortality rate to about 12% (80).

Aortic Insufficiency

Although more common than stenosis, aortic insufficiency remains unusual in pregnant women. Regurgitation often develops as the result of rheumatic disease, but also is found as a congenital abnormality or in relationship with either rheumatoid arthritis or systemic lupus erythematous. Marfan syndrome causes aortic root dilatation and subsequent regurgitation. Preconception dilation of the ascending aorta is an important predictor of aortic dissection (55). This risk increases steadily when the aortic diameter is 4.0 cm or greater (81). These high-risk parturients should have monthly transthoracic echocardiographic assessment (82). In patients with progressive aortic dilatation, some suggest surgical correction during gestation when or before the aortic root reaches 5.5 cm (55), whereas others advise an elective cesarean delivery (82). Acute regurgitation also may follow trauma and dissection.

With chronic insufficiency, symptoms follow a latent period of approximately 20 years. Fatigue and dyspnea may be worse at rest than during exercise. Pulse pressure may be increased with a rapid upstroke and rapid decline. The bisferious pulse, a double impulse during systole, may be seen. A high-pitched blowing diastolic decrescendo murmur along the sternal border is heard best with the patient sitting upright during end-expiration. The ECG, chest radiograph, and echocardiogram may help make the diagnosis (Table 10).

TABLE 10. *Aortic insufficiency*

Severe	
Symptoms	Left ventricular failure; uncommonly angina or syncope
Physical findings	Wide pulse pressure; aortic diastolic pressure <40 mm Hg; enlarged left ventricle; typical auscultatory findings
Chest radiograph	Left ventricular enlargement; pulmonary congestion possible
Electrocardiogram	Left ventricular hypertrophy with T-wave inversion in severe cases
Echocardiogram	Shows left ventricular dimensions, wall thickness, and performance
Acute	
Symptoms	Recent history of pulmonary edema, features of low cardiac output
Physical findings	Frequently not prominent; aortic diastolic pressure is not considerably reduced, and the pulse pressure is not distinctly wide; left ventricular enlargement may not be impressive; aortic diastolic murmur may be short and faint; loud S_3 common
Chest radiograph	Pulmonary edema with only slightly enlarged heart
Electrocardiogram	May be normal
Echocardiogram	May provide important clues to the diagnosis; diastolic mitral valve closure; high-frequency diastolic vibrations of the mitral leaflet and hyperkinetic left ventricle

After ref. 269, with permission.

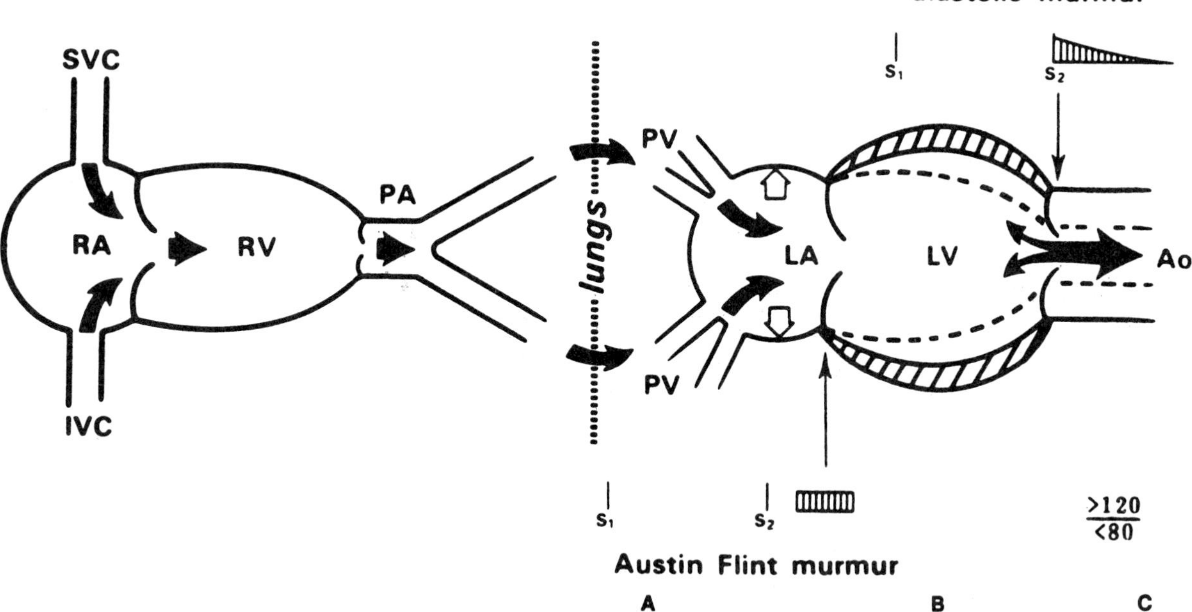

FIG. 7. Pathophysiology of aortic insufficiency. **A:** Pulmonary venous *(PV)* pressure increases only with left ventricular *(LV)* failure. **B:** Dilated left ventricle. Diastolic pressure increases with LV dysfunction or acute aortic incompetence. **C:** Wide pulse pressure reflects the severity of aortic valve incompetence. Diastolic pressure less than 40 mm Hg usually means severe insufficiency. *Ao*, aorta; *IVC*, inferior vena cava; *LA*, left atrium; *PA*, pulmonary artery; *RA*, right atrium; *RV*, right ventricle; *SVC*, superior vena cava. (From ref. 269, with permission.)

An incompetent aortic valve allows regurgitation of blood into the left ventricle, causing ventricular strain, dilatation, and ultimately, an abatement in contractile force and cardiac output (Fig. 7). The regurgitant blood adds to normal ventricular filling. The left ventricle sees a chronically elevated volume. A larger chamber size and eccentric wall thickening follow. As with all left-sided valvular lesions, in the most advanced state, pulmonary hypertension and right ventricular failure arise.

The changes wrought by aortic insufficiency are usually well tolerated in pregnancy. The parturient's increased plasma volume may help maintain cardiac output. A decreased maternal systemic vascular resistance and a faster pulse encourage forward flow. Bradycardia incites ventricular distention, increased left atrial pressure, and pulmonary congestion (82).

Idiopathic Hypertrophic Subaortic Stenosis

Idiopathic hypertrophic subaortic stenosis (IHSS) is an uncommon autosomal dominant inherited disorder that causes disproportionate hypertrophy of the intraventricular septum. The abnormally large septum bulges into the left ventricular chamber and obstructs the ventricular outflow tract in mid- to late systole. Tachycardia, increased myocardial contractility, or hypovolemia increases the degree of outflow obstruction. A systolic ejection murmur is heard at the base of the heart. The murmur increases with maneuvers that lower left ventricular volume. The ECG may show left ventricular hypertrophy with large septal Q waves. The echocardiogram shows thickening of the ventricular septum and abnormal anterior movement of the mitral valve during systole. Symptoms include dyspnea, chest pain, and palpitations. Stress, exercise, excitement, or anxiety, all conditions that increase catecholamine secretions, worsen symptoms of IHSS. There is a 1% to 3% chance of sudden death per year.

Although a worsening of symptoms of IHSS has been reported during pregnancy (Table 11), the elevated plasma volume and autotransfusion of blood from the contracting

TABLE 11. *Pregnancy and idiopathic hypertrophic subaortic stenosis: symptom exacerbation*

Increase in contractility
Hypovolemia
Tachycardia
Decreased left ventricular end-diastolic volume
Decreased left atrial pressure
Increased left ventricular ejection velocity
Vasodilator agents
Decreased peripheral vascular resistance of pregnancy
Inferior vena caval obstruction
Increased catecholamine production with labor
Acute blood loss at delivery
Digitalis, ketamine, epinephrine, ephedrine, calcium chloride

uterus at placental delivery tend to maintain maternal blood pressure. Despite potential fetal hazards of IUGR and newborn bradycardia, β blockade usually is continued throughout gestation (83,84).

Congenital Heart Disease

Congenital heart disease occurs in approximately 1% of live births in the United States (85). Women with congenital heart lesions are reaching child-bearing age in increasing numbers. Many have partially or fully corrected lesions. Even after years of apparently good health, functional deterioration may occur during pregnancy, especially in those with a history of cyanotic heart defects or other lesions that lead to pulmonary hypertension (86). Corrected maternal congenital heart lesions that result in a residual hypoxemia have been associated with a high rate of spontaneous abortion, poor fetal growth, and premature delivery (87,88). Corrective maternal cardiac surgery is most often done before conception to optimize the condition of both mother and fetus. The obstetric anesthesiologist needs to know both the medical and surgical history of the mother. Procure any other data to aid in understanding the pathophysiology of a parturient's particular lesion. These data may include ECG, chest radiograph, echocardiogram, or cardiac catheterization.

Left-to-right Shunts

Atrial Septal Defect

Atrial septal defects include ostium primum, ostium secundum, and sinus venosus. The majority are discovered and repaired in childhood. The long-term prognosis after repair is good. Ostium secundum, a defect located in the area of the foramen ovale and adjacent tissue, occurs more often in women. Supraventricular arrhythmias are common, especially if repair occurred after the onset of atrial fibrillation or flutter (88). A persistently split second heart sound associated with a systolic ejection murmur is best heard at the base of the heart (Fig. 8). The ECG shows right-axis deviation, and chest radiograph may show prominent pulmonary vasculature. Increases in systemic vascular resistance and decreases in pulmonary vascular resistance allow worsening of the left-to-right shunt and hinder in cardiac output. A higher pulmonary vascular resistance may promote acute right-to-left shunting. In the absence of large left-to-right shunting or secondary pulmonary hypertension, parturients with atrial septal defects tolerate pregnancy well (80).

Ventricular Septal Defect

More common than atrial septal defects, ventricular septal defects occur as either membranous or muscular. They appear during embryogenesis and are of different sizes and have multiple locations. Most close spontaneously in childhood. Remaining lesions are generally surgically corrected before conception. Surgical repair can damage the bundle of His, which lies at the posterior margin of the ventricular septum, producing arrhythmias (88). On physical examination, a loud holosystolic murmur is heard best along the left sternal border (Fig. 9). In the absence of symptomatic pulmonary congestion, a parturient with a ventricular septal defect may complain of fatigue and malaise but will usually tolerate pregnancy well. The predominant risk is endocarditis. Whittemore et al. (80) reviewed 98 pregnancies in 50 women with ven-

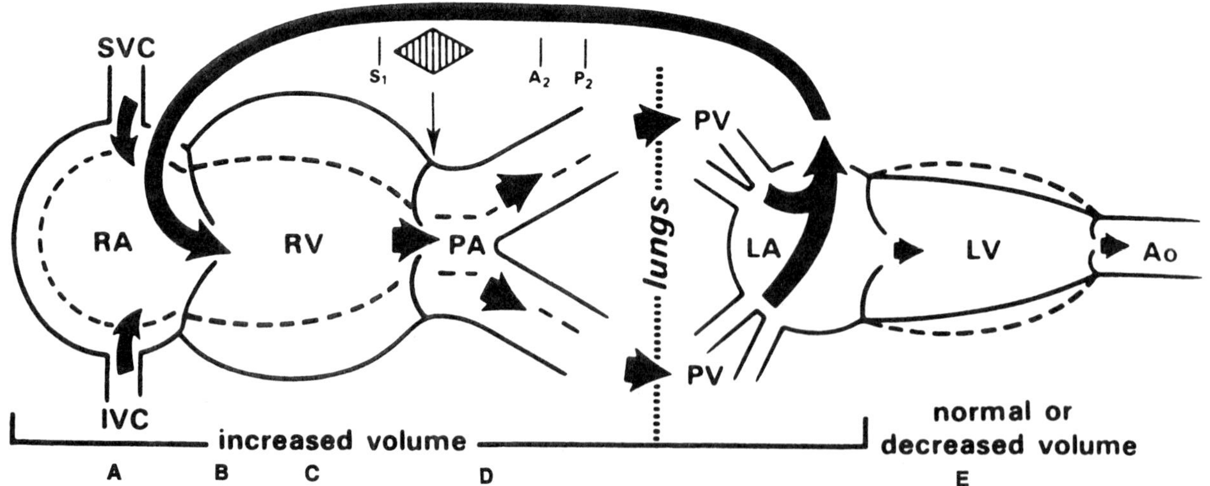

FIG. 8. Hemodynamic characteristics of atrial septal defect and anomalous pulmonary venous drainage (pretricuspid shunt). **A:** Pressures in the left atrium *(LA)* and right atrium *(RA)* are equal. **B:** There is increased diastolic flow through the tricuspid valve, often producing a diastolic tricuspid flow murmur. **C:** The right ventricle *(RV)* is considerably dilated. **D:** Pulmonary flow is increased, producing a short ejection systolic murmur and a wide split second sound. Pulmonary vasculature is exaggerated. *Solid arrow* indicates flow. **E:** The left ventricle *(LV)* and aorta *(Ao)* are small. *IVC*, inferior vena cava; *PA*, pulmonary artery; *PV*, pulmonary vein; *SVC*, superior vena cava. (From ref. 269, with permission.)

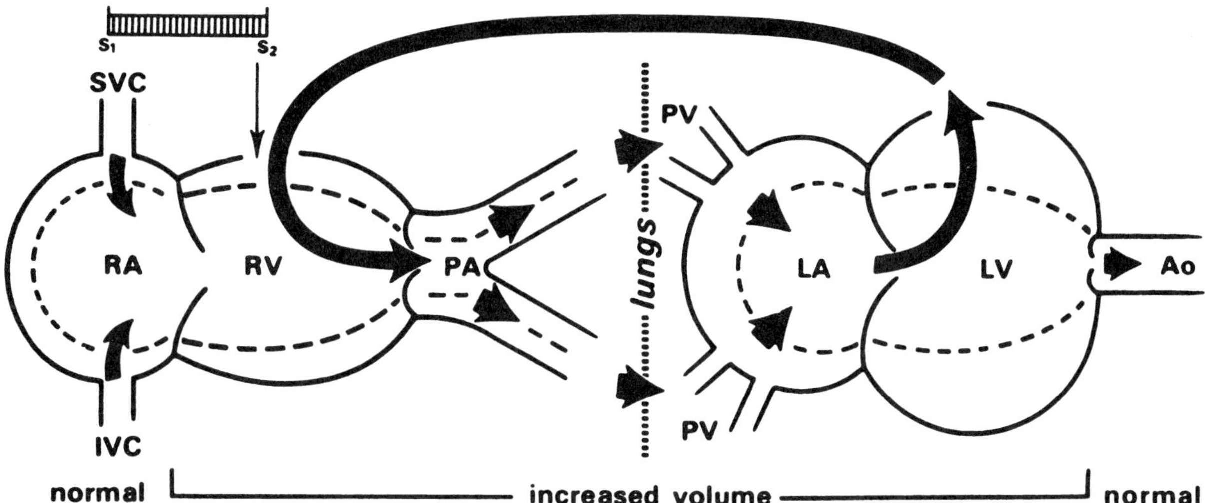

FIG. 9. Hemodynamic characteristics of ventricular septal defect. Flow increases to the right ventricle *(RV)*, pulmonary artery *(PA)*, left atrium *(LA)*, and left ventricle *(LV)*. With very large defects, the pressure in the two ventricles becomes equal, but in most cases, the pressure in the LV exceeds that in the RV. The shunt causes a holosystolic murmur, best heard over the third and fourth costal interspaces to the left of the sternum. Also, a mitral diastolic flow murmur may be audible. *Ao*, aorta; *IVC*, inferior vena cava; *PV*, pulmonary vein; *RA*, right atrium; *SVC*, superior vena cava. (From ref. 269, with permission.)

tricular septal defects. Complications included congestive heart failure, arrhythmias, and hypertension. There were 78 live births, 15 spontaneous abortions or stillbirths, and 6 interrupted pregnancies.

The parturient with an uncorrected ventricular septal defect does not tolerate large increases of systemic vascular resistance well. The subsequent increase in left-to-right shunting of blood will cause pulmonary hypertension and an increase in right ventricular work. An acute decrease in systemic vascular resistance also causes problems. With pulmonary hypertension, lower systemic vascular resistance may allow right-to-left shunting, which causes both maternal and fetal hypoxemia. It is unclear whether the fall in both systemic and pulmonary vascular resistance and rise in cardiac output and blood volume during normal pregnancy worsen atrial and ventricular septal defect symptoms.

Hypoxia and hypercarbia increase pulmonary vascular resistance. Whether the typical p_aO_2 of 105 mm Hg and p_aCO_2 of 33 mm Hg relieve pulmonary and right ventricular strain also is unclear.

Right-to-left Shunts

Tetralogy of Fallot

Tetralogy of Fallot is the most common cause of right-to-left shunt. Tetralogy of Fallot is anatomically characterized by the following:

- A ventricular septal defect,
- An aorta that overrides the pulmonary outflow tract,
- Infundibular pulmonary artery stenosis with obstruction to outflow from the right ventricle, and
- Right ventricular hypertrophy.

Seventy percent of patients have a bicuspid aortic valve, and the distal pulmonary artery may be hypoplastic or absent (Fig. 10).

The predominant anatomic anomaly that determines the physiologic state is the degree of right ventricular and pul-

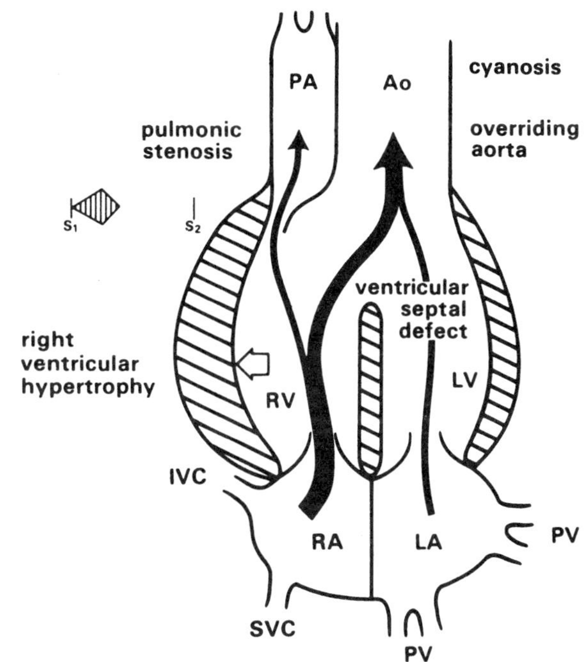

FIG. 10. Hemodynamic characteristics of tetralogy of Fallot. Note that the four defects in this disease result from abnormal development of the pulmonary infundibulum. Right ventricular *(RV)* hypertrophy is due to the fact that pressures are equal in both ventricles. *Ao*, aorta; *IVC*, inferior vena cava; *LA*, left atrium; *LV*, left ventricle; *PA*, pulmonary artery; *PV*, pulmonary vein; *RA*, right atrium; *RV*, right ventricle; *SVC*, superior vena cava. (From ref. 269, with permission.)

monary artery hypertrophy. Right-to-left shunting occurs after pulmonary vascular resistance exceeds systemic vascular resistance. Blood following the path of least resistance is shunted through an atrial or septal defect before oxygenation in the lung. Cyanosis due to arterial hypoxemia is apparent by 6 months of age. Hypercyanotic attacks, or "tet spells," are classically treated with β-adrenergic blockade to decrease spasm of the pathologic infundibular cardiac muscle. Recurrence of attacks is an indication for surgical correction. Survival to child-bearing age requires corrective surgery that usually includes closure of the ventricular septal defect and resection of the infundibular stenosis, or pulmonary valvulotomy.

In uncorrected tetralogy of Fallot, the most common auscultatory finding is an ejection murmur heard over the left sternal border resulting from blood flow across the infundibular pulmonary stenosis. One may appreciate a right ventricular heave. Chest radiograph shows a diminished pulmonary vasculature. The ECG shows right-axis deviation and right ventricular hypertrophy. Arterial blood gas determination usually reveals a normal pH and p_aCO_2. In contrast, regardless of inspired oxygen tension, these women have a markedly reduced p_aO_2. A hematocrit greater than 60% combined with an arterial oxygen saturation less than 80%, syncopal episodes, and right ventricular hypertension are all poor prognostic indicators (89). The echocardiogram reveals an aorta overriding the ventricular septum.

The risk of fetal morbidity and mortality increases with the severity of maternal cyanosis approaching a perinatal mortality rate of 20% or more (90). Spontaneous abortions, prematurity, and IUGR are common. Congenital heart defects approach 15% to 20% in the offspring of mothers with tetralogy of Fallot. Palliation or surgical correction improves outcome for both mother and fetus (91). In a series of 309 women who had surgical correction of tetralogy of Fallot, 40 pregnancies in 18 women resulted in 30 live-born children. Of the ten abortions, five were "therapeutic" (92).

There often is a dynamic element to the right ventricular outflow obstruction. The muscular infundibular area dilates or constricts, depending on the inotropic state of the myocardium and the volume of the central circulation. A drop in peripheral vascular resistance, as occurs throughout pregnancy and after acute blood loss at delivery, will increase outflow obstruction and increase right-to-left intracardiac shunt. Similarly, compression of the vena cava decreases venous return and right heart volume, which also may increase outflow obstruction and worsen the right-to-left intracardiac shunt. On the other hand, autotransfusion associated with each uterine contraction during labor and after delivery will improve venous blood return and may diminish the magnitude of this shunt postpartum.

Eisenmenger's Syndrome

The development of a pulmonary vascular resistance that exceeds systemic vascular resistance, reversing intracardiac shunt and producing cyanosis, is called Eisenmenger's syndrome (Fig. 11). This reversal may occur in up to 50% of untreated patients with a large ventricular septal defect and in 10% of patients with an atrial septal defect. A left-to-right intracardiac shunt initiates a progressive increase in right heart volume. As the pulmonary vascular resistance and right-sided pressures increase over time, some bidirectional or right-to-left shunting begins (93). Presence of this syndrome contraindicates surgical correction of the underlying congenital heart defect because pulmonary vascular resistance is irreversibly elevated.

The incidence of Eisenmenger's syndrome during pregnancy in the patient with a long-standing ventricular septal defect is approximately 2% to 4%. Maternal mortality may exceed 50% and fetal mortality may approach 30% (94). Prognosis is worse in the face of advanced medial and intimal pulmonary vascular thickening. Although pregnancy is generally discouraged in these women, prolonged bed rest, anticoagulation, and oxygen therapy has been shown to positively influence maternal and fetal outcomes (95).

Pregnancy aggravates Eisenmenger's syndrome. While systemic vascular resistance decreases, pulmonary vascu-

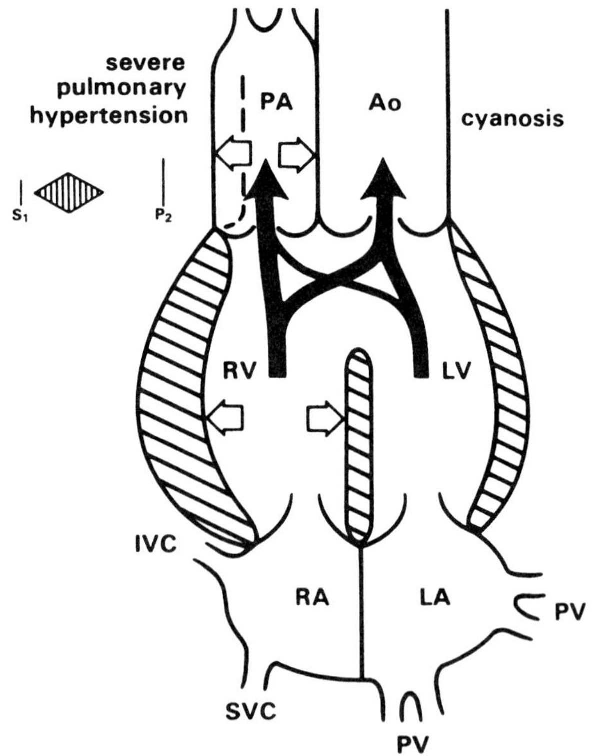

FIG. 11. Eisenmenger's syndrome. Note that Eisenmenger hemodynamics may result when severe pulmonary hypertension complicates any form of intracardiac shunt and produces shunt reversal. The defect itself does not produce a murmur. Only features of severe pulmonary hypertension and cyanosis are seen. *Ao*, aorta; *IVC*, inferior vena cava; *LV*, left ventricle; *PA*, pulmonary artery; *PV*, pulmonary vein; *RA*, right atrium; *RV*, right ventricle; *SVC*, superior vena cava. (From ref. 269, with permission.)

lar resistance remains fixed, progressively increasing the degree of right-to-left shunting, hypoxemia, and cyanosis. The physiologic changes of pregnancy, including an increased cardiac output, heart rate, blood volume, and oxygen consumption, combined with the pain and stress of labor, acute blood loss at delivery, and autotransfusion of uterine blood in the third stage of labor, put these patients at very high risk. Expulsive efforts may overload the right heart and increase the right-to-left shunt, or cause complete right heart failure.

Finger pulse oximetry may be an ideal noninvasive indicator of changes in shunt fraction and direction (96). Reversibility of the shunt may be assessed with oxygen therapy. The pulmonary vasculature may respond to oxygen or be irreversibly fixed (97). These parturients are at greatest risk late in pregnancy, when supine without uterine displacement, during labor and delivery or surgery, and in the early postpartum period. These women have little cardiac reserve. Sudden death may occur. Causes include embolism, arrhythmia, myocardial infarction, right heart overload, and sudden decreases in systemic vascular resistance. Emboli may affect the coronary or cerebral circulation.

Peripartum Cardiomyopathy

This uncommon phenomenon has a reported incidence of 1 in 1,300 to 15,000 pregnancies (98). The overall mortality rate is between 30% and 60% (99). Demakis and Rahumtoola (100) characterized peripartum cardiomyopathy as follows:

- Development of cardiac failure in the last month of pregnancy or within 5 months after delivery,
- Absence of a defined etiology for the cardiac failure, and
- Absence of demonstrable heart disease before the last month of gestation.

Outcome from peripartum cardiomyopathy relates to recovery of left ventricular function (98). Patients whose ventricular failure does not resolve within 6 months have an especially poor prognosis (101). The recurrence risk in subsequent pregnancies is at least 50%, with a 60% mortality. Heart transplantation is an option for patients with severe disease unresponsive to conventional treatment (102). There are reports of patients having undergone heart transplantation after an episode of severe peripartum cardiomyopathy who later became pregnant, delivered, and survived (103,104).

Signs and symptoms are of left ventricular failure. Early diagnosis is difficult because many women complain of fatigue, dyspnea on exertion, and edema while pregnant (see Table 2). The increased blood volume and cardiac output at term and peripartum may raise pulmonary capillary pressure and incite congestive heart failure in women with impaired ventricular function. The differential diagnosis must include amniotic fluid or pulmonary embolism, β-mimetic tocolytic therapy, or preeclampsia. Central and systemic emboli occur in up to 25% of cases (105). The final diagnosis is one of exclusion.

Echocardiography may show a dilated hypokinetic left ventricle (106). Endomyocardial biopsy reveals fibrous deposition, mural thrombi, and generalized degenerative changes. Postulated etiologies of peripartum cardiomyopathy include inadequate nutrition, viral agents, preeclampsia, immunologic disorders, advanced maternal age, multiple gestation, obesity, and breast-feeding.

In 1986, O'Connel et al. (107) reviewed 14 patients with peripartum cardiomyopathy who underwent right heart catheterization, echocardiography, radionuclide ventriculography, and right ventricular endomyocardial biopsy 1 week after onset of symptoms. They found that affected parturients are younger and have a shorter duration of symptoms than nonpregnant patients with idiopathic cardiomyopathy. Peripartum patients also have a higher incidence of myocarditis (29% vs 9%). Still, these authors concluded that patients with peripartum cardiomyopathy have no detectable pathophysiologic differences compared to those with nonpregnancy-related idiopathic cardiomyopathy and subsequent left ventricular failure (107). A more recent retrospective study of 34 patients (108) found a lower incidence of myocarditis than previously reported (8.8% compared to 9.1% of age- and sex-matched control population with idiopathic cardiomyopathy). Van Hoeven et al. (109) compared the clinicopathologic features of 13 women with peripartum cardiomyopathy to 13 women with idiopathic dilated cardiomyopathy. They concluded that the clinical course of peripartum cardiomyopathy is distinct from that of idiopathic dilated cardiomyopathy, although presenting clinical and pathologic variables may be similar.

Myocardial Infarction

The relative incidence of acute myocardial infarction during pregnancy is 1 in 10,000 (110,111). The increasing incidence of myocardial infarction in pregnancy may be related to advanced maternal age, hypertension, and smoking (112). Use of bromocriptine, collagen vascular disease, Kawasaki's disease, cocaine abuse (113,114), aortic valve disease, sickle cell chronic lung disease, hyperlipidemia, diabetes mellitus, and pheochromocytoma also have been implicated as risk factors (115). The vasospastic effect of cocaine on the coronary vasculature (116) or increased serum renin-angiotensin levels due to diminished venous return at the end of pregnancy may lead to an increased susceptibility to coronary vasospasm and subsequent ischemia. The development of thromboembolic phenomena from the hypercoagulable state of pregnancy also has been postulated as an important pathophysiologic mechanism in the genesis of acute myocardial infarction (112).

The mortality rate of acute myocardial infarction during pregnancy ranges from 21% to 50% (111,114). Poor prognostic factors are:

- Occurrence of the infarct in the third trimester,
- Age of the patient less than 35 years,
- Delivery within 2 weeks of infarct, and
- Delivery by cesarean section (111,114,117).

It is difficult to pinpoint the etiology of myocardial infarction in the parturient, but coronary artery disease is involved in the vast majority of cases. Atherosclerosis, thrombosis, aneurysm, spasm, obstruction, or dissection of the coronary vasculature may occur as well (112,114, 118,119). Cardiac risk to the patient in subsequent pregnancies is associated with residual left ventricular dysfunction, underlying coronary anatomy, and the presence of ongoing ischemia (111).

Diagnostic workup includes an extensive history. Elicit information about obesity, smoking, hyperlipidemia, hypertension, arrhythmias, angina, heart disease, obstetric history, and drug usage. On physical examination, look for carotid bruit, arrhythmia, extra heart sounds, or pulmonary congestion. Serial 12-lead ECG and cardiac isoenzymes are standard. Hematocrit, serum electrolytes, blood urea nitrogen and creatinine, coagulation profile and baseline arterial blood gas will provide relevant information. Echocardiography can evaluate left ventricular function.

The determinants of myocardial oxygen supply in pregnant woman are the same as in nonpregnant patients. Adequate coronary artery blood flow and oxygen content are required to avert myocardial injury. Mean aortic root diastolic pressure minus the left ventricular end-diastolic pressure determines coronary blood flow or perfusion pressure to the left ventricle. Many factors affect the oxygen content of blood perfusing the coronary arteries. Among them are hemoglobin, arterial oxygen saturation, pH, temperature, and 2,3-diphosphoglyceric acid (2,3-DPG). The major determinant of myocardial oxygen demand is heart rate. Other factors include preload, afterload, and contractility. The increased heart rate, stroke volume, plasma volume, metabolic rate, V/Q mismatching, and oxygen consumption of the term parturient allow her myocardium little reserve.

Primary Pulmonary Hypertension

Primary pulmonary hypertension is a very lethal, uncommon disorder that occurs most often in young women. Death often takes place within 2 years of onset of symptoms (120). Pregnancy and primary pulmonary hypertension combined produce a maternal mortality rate of 50% (121). In the later stages of the disease, a fixed, nonreactive pulmonary vasculature increases right ventricular work, leading to muscular hypertrophy. With a fixed, noncompliant right ventricle, the left heart eventually supplies an inadequate cardiac output. The end is cardiac failure. Signs and symptoms include syncope, hemoptysis, and chest pain. A right ventricular heave and a loud second heart sound are present. Peripheral cyanosis and clubbing are not uncommon.

As pregnancy progresses, plasma volume, cardiac output, and oxygen consumption rise, increasing the workload of the already strained right heart. Uterine compression of the vena cava and acute blood loss at delivery decrease venous return, left ventricular filling, and cardiac output. Despite these physiologic changes, which often result in maternal death, several cases with positive outcome have been reported (122–124). Encourage these patients to avoid pregnancy.

RENAL DISEASE

Renal Function and Pregnancy

During pregnancy, the renal calyces, pelvis, and ureters dilate as ureteral smooth muscle hypertrophies, creating a physiologic hydroureter (125,126). Dextrorotation of the gravid uterus can worsen the dilation on the right side of the urinary collecting system. The physiologic mechanism responsible for ureteral smooth muscle hypertrophy during pregnancy is unknown; however, increased circulating progesterone, gonadotropins, and prostaglandin E_1 have been suggested (125). Compression of the ureters by the iliac artery and enlarged uterine veins also play a role. These changes may allow stasis, leading to bacteriuria, and can make renal obstruction difficult to diagnose.

Glomerular filtration rate increases 30% to 50%, and renal plasma flow rises 60% to 80% above nonpregnant values (Fig. 12) (127,128). Animal studies have postulated that vasodilation of preglomerular and postglomerular resistance vessels increases renal blood flow and glomerular filtration rate (129). Progesterone-mediated changes in pressor receptors and altered responses to renin-angiotensin control also have been suggested (129,130). This reduction in vascular tone also may reset volume and osmoreceptors that help maintain volume homeostasis during pregnancy (131). Creatinine and urea nitrogen production remain unchanged, so their serum concentrations fall in comparison to prepregnancy values (132,133). Values considered normal in the nonpregnant state may suggest renal dysfunction in the parturient.

Osmoregulation is altered. There is an average 8 to 10 mOsm/kg decrease in plasma osmolality (P_{osm}) during gestation (Fig. 13) (134). This decrement in the nonparturient would produce a significant diuresis, yet the gravida appears to adjust both vasopressin secretion and thirst to maintain this lower osmolality (135,136).

Water regulation also changes over the course of pregnancy. The gravida retains approximately 2 L of intravascular water, 290 mEq of sodium, and 155 mEq of potas-

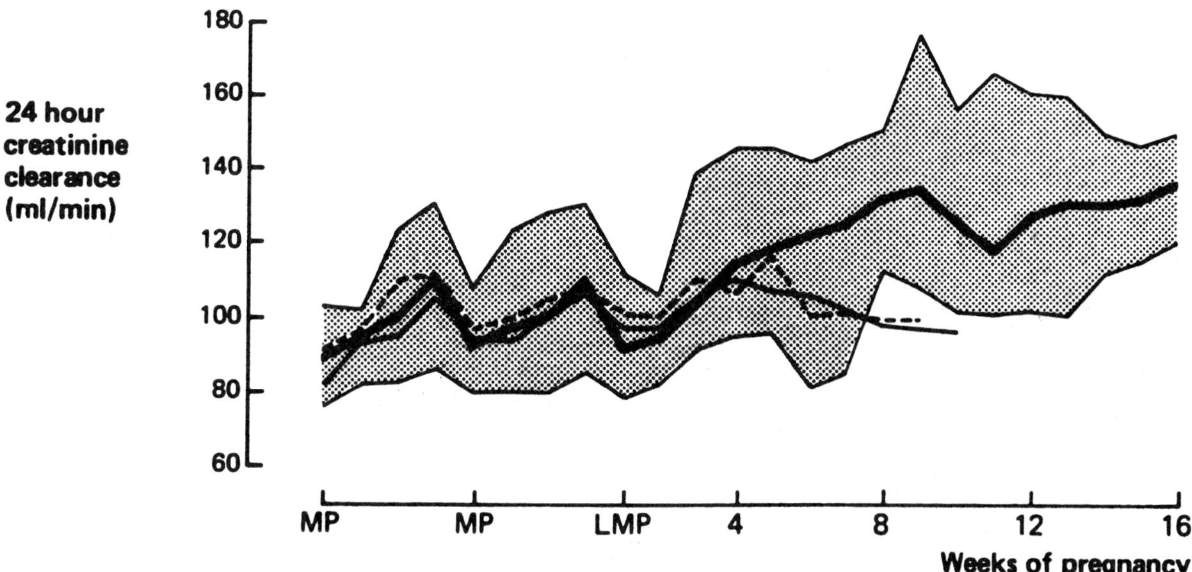

FIG. 12. Changes in 24-hour creatinine clearance measured weekly before conception and through to uncomplicated spontaneous abortion in two women (*solid* and *dashed lines*). *Thick solid line* represents the mean, and the *stippled area* represents the range for nine women with successful obstetric outcome. *LMP*, last menstrual period; *MP*, menstrual period. (From ref. 272, with permission.)

sium (137). At term, there is 1.2 L of amniotic fluid, 700 mL of water in the uterus, 300 mL in the placenta, and 400 mL in the breasts. In all, the parturient retains 7 to 8 L of total body water. Water excretion is reduced in late gestation. This effect may relate to the hemodynamic effects of maternal posture (138). The clinical usefulness of random specific gravity measurements in the supine third-trimester gravida is questionable.

Glucose

Glucosuria occurs frequently. The parturient cannot increase glucose reabsorption in parallel with the larger amount of filtered glucose. More than 30 years ago, Welsh and Sims (139) evaluated tubular maximum (T_m), a measure of renal glucose handling, in normal nonpregnant women, as compared to nonglycosuric and normoglycemic glycosuric pregnant patients. T_m was lower in the latter group than in the nonglycosuric gravidae. Therefore, urinary glucose sampling may be unreliable in evaluating pregnant diabetic patients. Also, changes in renal handling of glucose may not indicate renal pathology in the parturient.

Sodium

Sodium is the principal regulator of volume homeostasis. Its reabsorption accounts for the largest major renal adjustment in pregnancy. Total body sodium increases by 1,000 mEq, 60% of which remains maternal (Table 12) (136). Hormonal factors that increase sodium excretion generally work by competitive inhibition of aldosterone (Table 13) (137).

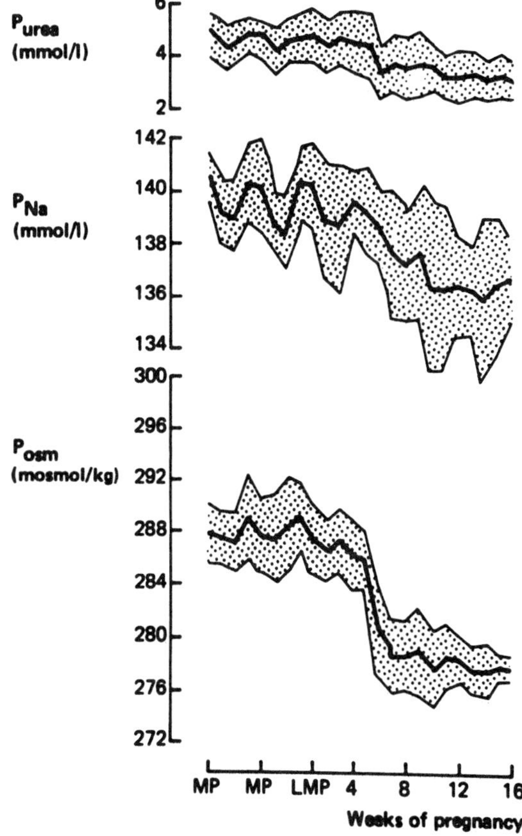

FIG. 13. Plasma osmolality (O_{osm}), sodium (P_{Na}), and urea (P_{urea}) measured weekly from before conception through the first trimester in nine women who subsequently had successful obstetric outcomes. *Solid line* is the mean, and *stippled area* is + 1 SD. *LMP*, last menstrual period; *MP*, menstrual period. (From ref. 134, with permission.)

TABLE 12. *Storage of minerals during pregnancy*

Storage Site	Sodium (mEq)	Potassium (mEq)	Calcium (g)
Fetus	290	154	28.00
Placenta	57	42	0.65
Amniotic fluid	100	3	Negligible
Uterus	80	50	0.22
Breast	35	35	0.06
Plasma	140	4	0.12
Red cells	5	8	0.25
Edema fluid	240	8	0.25
Total	947	320	29.68

After from ref. 277, with permission.

Acid–Base Balance

Plasma bicarbonate concentration decreases 4 mEq/L in response to maternal respiratory alkalosis. The average p_aCO_2 is 31 mm Hg; pH, 7.44; and serum bicarbonate, 20 mEq/L. The reduced total buffering capacity raises the risk of severe acidosis during pregnancy.

Evaluation

The initial workup for renal dysfunction includes history, physical examination, and laboratory data. A reliable diagnosis of underlying renal disease can be easily accomplished during pregnancy. Clues in the history may include hematuria, polyuria, nocturia, and enuresis. Symptoms of urinary tract infection include dysuria, urgency, and foul-smelling urine. A history of hypertension, diabetes, gout, or renal disease in both the patient and her family also is helpful. Electrolyte disturbances may present as weakness, paresthesia and areflexia, or as cardiac problems.

The first voided urine in the morning is usually concentrated and requires careful examination. Proteinuria is an important sign of renal disease because it generally indicates a derangement in glomerular permeability. With pregnancy, daily protein excretion may reach 250 mg. Proteinuria between 150 mg and 2 g daily may signal chronic interstitial nephritis or nephrosclerosis, whereas heavy proteinuria, more than 2 g daily, may occur in chronic glomerulonephritis, diabetic nephropathy, systemic lupus erythematosus, membranous glomerulonephritis, lipoid nephrosis, and focal glomerulosclerosis (140). Tubular epithelial cells are seen, particularly in tubular necrosis and nephrotoxic nephritis. The Maltese cross of epithelial cells filled with lipid is typical of the nephrotic syndrome.

TABLE 13. *Sodium excretion and reabsorption: hormonal factors in pregnancy*

Excretion	Reabsorption
Progesterone	Aldosterone
Natriuretic hormone	Deoxycorticosterone
Vasodilating prostaglandins	Angiotensin
Vasopressin	Estrogen
	Renin

When red and white blood cell casts are found in the urinalysis, there is primary renal pathology. On the other hand, microscopic hematuria may be induced by exercise, acute febrile illness, or kidney trauma. Hematuria may suggest glomerulonephritis, systemic lupus erythematosus, and periarteritis. White blood cells and casts do not necessarily indicate an infectious process but simply an inflammatory response. Sterile pyuria can accompany acute glomerulonephritis and chronic interstitial nephritis. Nonbacterial renal disease involving the interstitium may present with pyuria and white blood cell casts. Generally, a significant bacteriuria is necessary to diagnose pyelonephritis (140).

Laboratory data should include hematocrit, serum blood urea nitrogen and creatinine, electrolytes, and uric acid as well as creatinine clearance. In pregnancy, both the serum blood urea nitrogen and creatinine concentration decrease. Normal concentrations found in the parturient are suspicious. Abdominal radiographs are usually avoided, and an intravenous pyelogram is seldom needed. It is technically difficult to perform a renal biopsy in the pregnant patient, and the increase in renal blood flow presents a further risk (141).

Uremia affects multiple organ systems. The patient is immunologically compromised, and the obstetric anesthesiologist must treat her accordingly. Platelet function may be depressed; however, a recent prospective study, using viscoelastic measures of blood coagulation (thromboelastography and Sonoclot analysis), found that perioperative uremic patients were hypercoagulable (142). Autonomic neuropathies and central nervous system irritability are not uncommon (143). A uremic patient with erythropoietin deficiency anemia has less 2,3-DPG than an otherwise normal anemic patient. Compromise of fetal oxygen delivery may subsequently occur. Uremia further prolongs gastric emptying (144).

Prognosis

The most important outcome determinants in both mother and child are the presence of either preexisting chronic hypertension or onset of hypertension during pregnancy (Table 14). Outcome varies greatly according

TABLE 14. *Chronic renal disease in pregnancy: effect of level of blood pressure on pregnancy complication in 123 pregnancies in 86 women*

	Renal Deterioration	Small-for-date Babies	Preterm Delivery
Normotension	3.0%	2.3%	11.4%
Hypertension[a]	15.0%	15.6%	20.0%

[a]Blood pressure consistently 140/90 mm Hg or greater.
After ref. 278, with permission.

to the extent of the preexisting renal disease and the etiology, type, and severity of disease (Table 15) (145). Patients with glomerular disease may experience a worsening of their renal status with the increased glomerular filtration of pregnancy (146). Uncontrolled hypertension concurrent with renal insufficiency during pregnancy can cause progression to end-stage renal disease (147). The presence of hypertension before conception increases the risk of IUGR fivefold and doubles the premature delivery rate (148). Uterine artery Doppler waveforms at 19 to 24 weeks' gestation predict maternal and fetal complications in parturients with renal disease (149). Unfortunately, in one study, treatment did not alter the clinical course of women with abnormal uterine artery waveforms (147).

Hematocrit affects oxygen delivery to the fetus. The anemia of renal disease, secondary to a depression in erythropoietin production, will decrease oxygen-carrying capacity. The incidence of infants with IUGR may increase.

Women with severe renal insufficiency (serum creatinine greater than 2.5 mg/dL or creatinine clearance less than 50 mL/min) usually do not become pregnant. If they do conceive, 50% have poor fetal outcomes and will exhibit end-stage renal disease within 1 year (150). An increased rate of spontaneous abortion, hypertension, worsening renal function, and obstetric complications is associated with moderate renal insufficiency (151,152). Women with mildly depressed renal function have better fetal outcomes, and fewer advance to end-stage renal disease.

Pyelonephritis

Pyelonephritis occurs frequently during pregnancy. It has been postulated that dilatation of the collecting system as well as *Escherichia coli* virulence factor and host ligands all contribute to gestational pyelonephritis (153). If managed improperly, pyelonephritis can produce considerable morbidity in both mother and fetus. It is associated with low birth weight, increased perinatal mortality, anemia, preeclampsia, and premature rupture of membranes (154). Presentation is generally a combination of fever, chills, nausea, vomiting, costovertebral angle tenderness, and urinary symptoms. Untreated, pyelonephritis may lead to adult respiratory distress syndrome and death.

Glomerulonephritis

Gram-positive or gram-negative bacterial pathogens trigger the immune syndrome of glomerulonephritis. The condition may present as focal, diffuse, proliferative, or lupus type and may lead to the nephrotic syndrome in the presence of sufficient proteinuria. Edema and hypertension are not uncommon. Microscopic hematuria with red blood cell casts, low serum complement, and a rising antistreptolysin titer suggest the diagnosis of acute poststreptococcal glomerulonephritis. Significant proteinuria is a risk factor for impaired renal function in the postpartum period (155).

Berger's disease or IgA nephropathy also may present with hematuria but minimal proteinuria. Prognosis is generally good in these patients in the absence of hypertension. Pregnancy does not adversely influence the natural course of IgA nephropathy (156). The fetus seems protected from the maternal glomerulonephritides. Possible explanations of the phenomenon include the following:

- The antigen–antibody complexes are too large to cross the placental circulation.

TABLE 15. *Pregnancy and renal disease: functional renal status and prospects*[a]

	Severity of Renal Disease		
Prospects	Mild (%)	Moderate (%)	Severe (%)
Pregnancy complications	22	41	84
Successful obstetric outcome	95	90	47
Long-term sequelae	<5	25	53

[a]Based on literature survey of 1162 pregnancies in 804 women in reports published between 1973 and 1987. These data do not include collagen diseases.
After ref. 279, with permission.

- The fetal glomeruli do not react in the same manner to the complexes.
- The glomerular pressure (a possible factor in the development of this disease) is too low in the fetus.

Perinatal mortality may reach 18%, however (157).

Systemic Lupus Erythematosus

Systemic lupus erythematosus complicates 1 in 1,600 to 5,000 pregnancies (158). It is an autoimmune disorder in which antigen–antibody complexes form and deposit in tissues. Its etiology is unknown. In pregnancy, the most common clinical manifestations include arthralgias, fever, skin lesions, and renal disease (159). Serum complement concentration falls, antibodies against DNA arise, and the lupus anticoagulant appears. Whether pregnancy exacerbates systemic lupus erythematosus is controversial. A prospective case-controlled study found no significant increase in symptoms with pregnancy (160). On the other hand, Burkett (161) states that the disease will worsen in 50% of patients who experience exacerbations in the 6 months preceding conception. Others have reported significant morbidity and mortality for both mother and fetus with an increased risk of obstetric complications, fetal loss, prematurity, and IUGR (162,163).

The lupus anticoagulant might bind with platelet membranes, inciting aggregation and an increased incidence of thrombosis (164). This thrombosis occurs in the deep veins, peripheral arteries, retinal vessels, placenta, pulmonary vessels, and brain (165,166). The partial thromboplastin time, and rarely the prothrombin time, may be prolonged. Changes in these tests do not correlate with clinical hemorrhage. Furthermore, anticardiolipin antibodies may be detected, often with thrombocytopenia and thrombocytopathy. Antibodies can make blood crossmatching difficult. A transient or permanent deterioration in renal function may occur. Proteinuria, hypertension, and reduced creatinine clearance correlate with a poor prognosis.

Immunoglobulin-complement deposition in trophoblastic tissue may lead to fetal compromise. Congenital anomalies such as heart block and endocardial fibroelastosis are not infrequent. The risks of abortion, perinatal mortality, and premature delivery increase (167). There are reports of infants of women with systemic lupus erythematosus born with congenital anomalies even though the maternal disease appeared quiescent for years before delivery (168,169).

Diabetic Nephropathy

Glomerulosclerosis, or thickening of the glomerular basement membrane, whether localized nodular or diffuse, is the primary characteristic of diabetic nephropathy. Vascular disease of both large and small renal vessels can cause severe scarring of the renal interstitium. In the presence of proteinuria and diminished renal function, most parturients are hypertensive (140). The hypertension associated with diabetic nephropathy is probably secondary to renal vascular disease. The prognosis of patients with diabetic nephropathy relates to the degree of proteinuria. More than 3 g in a 24-hour period correlates with a rapid progression to renal insufficiency (140). Several investigators have studied the effect of pregnancy on the development or progression of diabetic nephropathy. No increased risk or acceleration of renal failure was noted in patients with mild to moderate disease (170–172). However, patients with moderate to severe disease had a greater than 40% chance of disease acceleration associated with pregnancy (133). Preeclampsia occurs more often in these women, and, when severe, perinatal mortality may approach 25% (144).

Calculi

The incidence of renal calculi does not rise during pregnancy and remains between 0.1% and 1% (173). This fact is remarkable considering the parturient's anatomy, which encourages urinary stasis. Intestinal absorption of calcium increases during pregnancy, and urinary calcium excretion usually exceeds 250 mg in a 24-hour period. Hypercalciuria accounts for more than 40% of calculi in the parturient. Urinary tract infections predispose to recurrent stone formation. Urease-containing organisms alkalinize the urine, allowing precipitation of calcium. Although incidence remains the same, dilation of the gravida renal pelvis and ureter may ease passage of any calculi.

Nephrotic Syndrome

Proteinuria, hypoalbuminemia, hyperlipidemia, and edema characterize this syndrome. Normal physiologic changes of pregnancy may be confused with an exacerbation of the underlying disease causing the nephrotic syndrome. Increases in urinary protein may simply be a consequence of the increments in renal hemodynamics, changes in the glomerular barrier, or rise in renal vein pressure. Serum albumin decreases 0.5 to 1.0 g/dL in normal gestation. Edema may follow. More cholesterol and other circulating lipids are found in both normal pregnancy and in nephrotic syndrome.

The most common cause of nephrotic syndrome in late gestation is preeclampsia. Additional etiologies include diabetic glomerulosclerosis, lupus nephritis, lipoid nephrosis, renal vein thrombosis, amyloidosis, and drug reaction. Edema results from the reduced plasma oncotic pressure. The patient may be effectively hypothyroid or immunodeficient with the total body protein loss. The parturient with nephrotic syndrome is intravascularly depleted. With uteroplacental blood flow at risk, patient positioning is crucial.

Hemodialysis

There are a few reports of conception and parturition with chronic maternal hemodialysis (174,175). These women are at greater risk of spontaneous abortion, delivery of a low-birth-weight infant, and premature labor and delivery. Risk of premature labor, vaginal bleeding, and systemic hypotension is greatest immediately at the cessation of dialysis. Ultrafiltration needs to be monitored carefully in the parturient. Dialysates containing both glucose and bicarbonate have been recommended for the gravida in renal failure. The pregnant patient may exhibit both hypoxemia and hypercarbia secondary to hypoventilation after excessive HCO_3 removal. Both intravascular volume depletion and acetate in the dialysate can cause hypotension. Bleeding may occur from heparinization. Retention of platelets on the dialysis membrane increases the risk of thrombocytopenia and bleeding. Pseudocholinesterase concentrations and platelet function may be altered (176). Premature contractions secondary to the depletion of progesterone by hemodialysis have been reported (175). In early gestation, or in the presence of IUGR or oligohydramnios, care must be taken to limit the volume of maternal fluid removed as hemodialysis results in amniotic fluid shifts (177).

Peritoneal Dialysis

The information on pregnancy in women undergoing continuous ambulatory peritoneal dialysis (CAPD) is limited. A recent survey of dialysis units caring for women aged 14 to 44 years receiving CAPD in the United States showed a conception rate of 0.2% per year (178). Pregnancy in CAPD patients is associated with hypertension, bleeding, anemia, peritonitis, and premature delivery (179). Only 40% of these pregnancies result in surviving infants (180). Interestingly, hemodialysis patients become pregnant about twice as often as CAPD women. Whether this is due to mechanical obstruction by the peritoneal dialysate interfering with ovum transport to the fallopian tube, recurrent peritonitis, or differences in hormonal milieu between the two patient subsets is unknown (178).

In 1988, Redrow et al. (181) presented the management of eight women treated with CAPD. Volume and frequency of exchanges were adjusted to achieve a total creatinine clearance of greater than 15 mL/min. Although not completely substantiated in the literature, this clinical practice has been associated with a higher likelihood of successful pregnancy (178). CAPD may offer a more constant biochemical and extracellular environment for the fetus with fewer episodes of hypotension (181).

Acute Renal Failure

Many complications may cause acute renal failure in the gravida (Table 16). Although acute renal failure in pregnancy historically accounts for 50% of cases of acute renal failure in young women (182), an epidemiologic study by Stratta et al. (183) reports a decline in the incidence and mortality of pregnancy-related acute renal failure. They attribute this decline to improved medical care and more effective preventative measures.

The most common etiology of acute renal failure is hypovolemia, renal hypoperfusion, and subsequent ischemia. With persistent hypovolemia, a reduced cortical blood flow and acute tubular necrosis may develop. Disseminated intravascular coagulation may result from amniotic fluid embolism, intrauterine fetal death, placental abruption, or major transfusion reaction and lead to acute renal failure. The increased renal vascular resistance and decreased renal blood flow in preeclampsia coincide with a fall in urinary prostaglandin E_2 and may incite acute renal failure. Renal vascular injury, especially that resulting from cortical necrosis and hemolytic uremia syndrome, has been associated with poor prognosis in the past (184). Recently, preeclampsia/eclampsia complicated by abruptio placentae has carried a worse maternal and renal prognosis (183).

Nephrotoxic renal failure may occur after the use of exogenous toxins, such as radiographic contrast media, antibiotics, and nonsteroidal antiinflammatory drugs. Nephrotoxic renal failure, which is nonischemic in origin, may cause an interstitial nephritis as well. Endogenous toxins include hemoglobin, myoglobin, uric acid, oxalic acid, and myelomatous proteins from multiple myeloma. Urinary tract obstruction secondary to the gravid uterus, polyhydramnios, nephrolithiasis, pelvic and broad ligament hematoma, or surgical damage also can cause acute renal failure.

Diagnosis must separate prerenal, intrinsic renal, or postrenal causes. History may reveal use of nephrotoxic agents. Elicitation of cardiac disease, hepatic disease, or recent muscle damage will aid in diagnosis. Physical examination should concentrate on signs and symptoms

TABLE 16. *Causes of acute renal failure in obstetrics*

Antepartum	Postpartum
Abortion	Uterine atony
Placenta previa	Retained placenta
Placenta abruption	Amniotic fluid embolism
Hyperemesis gravidarum	Uterine rupture
Pregnancy-induced hypertension	Vaginal/cervical tear
Preeclampsia	Hemolytic uremic syndrome
Chorioamnionitis	Septic abortion
Acute fatty liver	
Pyelonephritis	

TABLE 17. *Urinary findings: prerenal and intrinsic renal disease*

	Prerenal	Intrinsic Renal
Urine sediment	Not remarkable	Renal epithelial cells and casts; granular, muddy, pigmented cells
Urine osmolality (mOsm/kg)	>500	<350
Urine sodium (mEq/L)	<20	>40
Urine specific gravity	>1.020	<1.015
Urine: plasma creatinine concentration ratio	>40	<20

of dehydration and hypovolemia. Urinalysis, hematocrit, and serum blood urea nitrogen/creatinine ratio will aid in the diagnosis as well (Table 17).

The cortical necrosis that can follow acute renal failure in the gravida usually results from fibrin deposits in the renal vasculature. The outcome of acute tubular necrosis ranges from mild and short-lasting tubular damage to chronic renal failure from sclerosis of any remaining nephrons.

HEMATOLOGIC DISEASE

Anemia

Anemia is the most common hematologic complication of pregnancy. The incidence of anemia during pregnancy ranges from 20% to 80% (185). The risk is much higher than the 5% incidence in nonpregnant women of reproductive age. Data from the Center for Disease Control's Pregnancy Nutritional Surveillance System (185) suggest a prevalence of 20% to 40% in low-income women in the United States. The incidence is highest in the 15- to 19-year age group and in black women of all ages.

Anemia may present with fatigue, dyspnea, palpitations with mild physical activity, intolerance to exertion, dizziness, headache, irritability, difficulty sleeping, anorexia, and bowel irregularities (186). However, patients often are asymptomatic. The medical evaluation of anemia in the pregnant patient is as per the nongravida. Patients may show pallor or tachycardia yet, typically, physical examination does not detect anemia.

Anemia is most commonly found on routine laboratory testing. The average red blood cell size [mean corpuscular volume (MCV)] provides useful information regarding the mechanism of anemia. Macrocytosis coincides with both folate and vitamin B_{12}-deficiency anemia. Microcytosis occurs with iron deficiency, thalassemia, and lead poisoning. Hemoglobin content, red cell size distribution, reticulocyte count, and iron stores also may provide useful diagnostic information in determining the extent and source of anemia.

Physiology

Pregnancy is associated with several hematologic changes. Maternal blood volume begins to increase by the sixth to tenth week and peaks at the thirty-second week, when it exceeds the nonpregnant level by 40%. Plasma volume increases by 50% to 55% and red cell mass by 20% to 30%. Because of these changes, a physiologic anemia of pregnancy occurs (hemoglobin less than 11 g/dL in the first and third trimester, and a hemoglobin less than 10.5 g/dL during the second trimester) (187–190). Erythropoietin secretion by the kidney controls the red blood cell production. Increased red cell mass occurs primarily in the latter half of pregnancy, in contrast to the increased plasma volume early in pregnancy. Progesterone, testosterone, and thyroxine stimulate erythropoietin production. Prolactin also may have a significant role in increasing the red cell mass (188). It remains unclear the degree of maternal anemia that results in risk to the fetus or neonate. Although reports of decreased birth weight, prematurity, and perinatal death exist (191), it is difficult to control for poor nutrition and low socioeconomic status. One report suggests a progressive increase in fetal risk as hemoglobin falls below 10 g/dL (189). High-output congestive heart failure with intravascular volume overload is common in severe anemia. The gravida is therefore at an even greater risk of this complication.

Iron-deficiency Anemia

The majority of the body's iron is stored in hemoglobin. During pregnancy, the demands on iron stores are increased and iron deficiency anemia results when these stores become depleted (192). Approximately 1,000 mg of additional iron is needed during pregnancy. Most adult women maintain a 500-mg iron storage pool. Furthermore, iron is preferentially delivered to the fetus secondary to the heavy concentration of transferrin receptors on the placental trophoblastic membranes (193). Although the lack of bleeding due to amenorrhea during pregnancy saves approximately 200 mg of iron, there remains a maternal deficiency. Bleeding, multiple gestation, chronic illness, poor appetite, poor nutrition, and nausea and vomiting can cause further iron depletion. There tends to be a decrease in fetal iron when maternal iron stores are depleted (194). Maternal and fetal effects of iron-deficiency anemia, particularly when developing early in pregnancy, may include preeclampsia, low birth weight, premature labor, and stillbirth (189,191,195).

Iron-deficiency anemia may be difficult to diagnose during pregnancy. The characteristic microcytic, hypochromic red blood cell smear is a late finding (Fig. 14). The MCV typically increases during the first 2 months of gestation. Transferrin and total iron binding capacity rise during pregnancy, making the iron to transferrin ratio low, even in gravid women without iron deficiency. The most sensitive test in the parturient for iron-deficiency anemia is measurement of serum ferritin (190).

Oral iron replacement with 30 to 120 mg of elemental iron daily remains the treatment for iron-deficiency anemia. The rate of absorption varies and is reduced by 40% to 50% when iron is taken with meals. The most common untoward effect from oral iron preparations is gastrointestinal irritation. The reticulocyte count increases by the second week of treatment with iron supplementation. Iron replacement has been given parenterally; however, there are significant possible untoward reactions, such as anaphylaxis, headache, malaise, fever, arthralgias, lymphadenopathy, phlebitis, dizziness, and nausea and vomiting (192,196,197). Hallak et al. (186) studied 26 patients with severe anemia (serum hemoglobin less than 8.5 g/dL with serum iron and ferritin levels below normal) who received intravenous iron because they could not tolerate or did not respond clinically to oral preparations. There was one allergic reaction. Other mild dose-dependent side effects included flushing, headache, arthralgia, and lymphadenopathy. All patients who completed the course of therapy had significantly increased serum hemoglobin and regeneration of iron stores. They concluded that intravenous iron therapy during pregnancy may be an effective method of regenerating iron stores in severely iron-deficient patients who cannot use oral preparations.

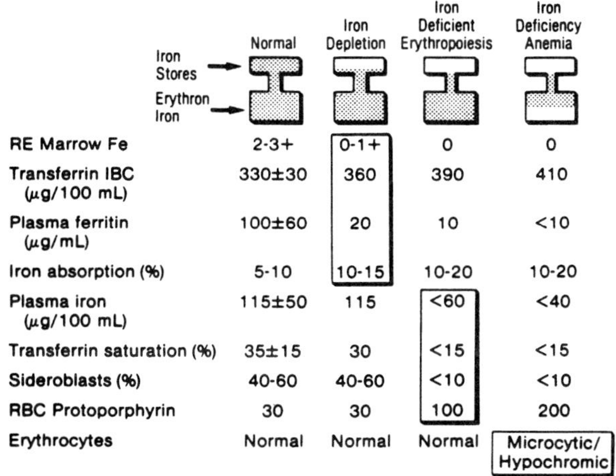

	Normal	Iron Depletion	Iron Deficient Erythropoiesis	Iron Deficiency Anemia
RE Marrow Fe	2-3+	0-1+	0	0
Transferrin IBC (μg/100 mL)	330±30	360	390	410
Plasma ferritin (μg/mL)	100±60	20	10	<10
Iron absorption (%)	5-10	10-15	10-20	10-20
Plasma iron (μg/100 mL)	115±50	115	<60	<40
Transferrin saturation (%)	35±15	30	<15	<15
Sideroblasts (%)	40-60	40-60	<10	<10
RBC Protoporphyrin	30	30	100	200
Erythrocytes	Normal	Normal	Normal	Microcytic/ Hypochromic

FIG. 14. Sequential changes in the development of iron deficiency. Indicators of iron store depletion include the visual inspection of marrow reticuloendothelial iron stores, the total iron-binding capacity, the plasma ferritin level, and the percent iron absorbed from an oral iron test dose. With the onset of iron-deficient erythropoiesis, the serum iron, percent saturation of transferrin, percent sideroblasts observed on the marrow stain, and the red cell protoporphyrin become abnormal. The anemia appears. When anemia has been present for some time, red cells become microcytic/hypochromic. (From ref. 273, with permission.)

Megaloblastic Anemia

Megaloblastic anemia is a commonly acquired nutritional anemia. Folic acid and vitamin B_{12} deficiencies are the usual causes of megaloblastic anemia. The pregnant patient is unlikely to develop a vitamin B_{12} deficiency for two reasons. Vitamin B_{12} has an integral role in all DNA replication, and a significant deficiency should result in sterility. Furthermore, normally there are large stores of vitamin B_{12}, making this an unlikely source of anemia.

Folic acid, an essential cofactor in nucleic acid synthesis, is the most likely source of megaloblastic anemia in the gravida. During pregnancy, the growing fetus induces a 50% rise in folate requirements (198). The main dietary source of folate is green leafy vegetables. Excessive cooking of vegetables decreases available folate. Some drugs, such as oral contraceptives and phenytoin, hinder the absorption of folic acid. The total body stores of this vitamin are small and short-lived. Nausea and vomiting may significantly impair its intake. Unless the diet is supplemented, pregnancy is associated with a negative folate balance, which usually arises in the third trimester. Megaloblastic changes are most common in countries or socioeconomic groups with poor nutrition.

Most patients present clinically with a significant anemia (Hb = 6 to 9 g/dL) and symptoms consistent with both a decreased intravascular volume and a diminished oxygen-carrying capacity. These may include weakness, dizziness, light-headedness, and palpitations. Common physical findings are pale skin, tachycardia, and a systolic flow murmur. Not uncommonly, patients with long-standing disease may complain of diarrhea, as well as sore tongue and mouth. Patients with vitamin B_{12} deficiency, because it is associated with demyelination of peripheral nerves, may manifest numbness and paresthesia of the extremities, ataxia, poor coordination, and eventually mental status changes, which range from minimal forgetfulness to dementia and psychosis (199).

The diagnosis of megaloblastic anemia should be considered when a low erythrocyte count and significant macrocytosis (MCV greater than 100) occur with a low reticulocyte count (199). Peripheral blood smear usually reveals anisocytosis, poikilocytosis, and macroovalocytis. Definitive diagnosis frequently requires a bone marrow aspirate, which characteristically appears cellular with a decreased myeloid to erythroid ratio (199). Other findings may include purpura, hemolytic jaundice, thrombocytopenia, and bleeding diathesis. When the diagnosis is confirmed, rapid reversal can occur with appropriate therapy (199). Pure folate deficiency results in a macrocytic anemia or may even cause pancytopenia. Iron-deficiency

TABLE 18. *Composition of hemoglobins found in normal human development and abnormal hemoglobins found in thalessemia*

Globin Chains	Hemoglobin	State
$\alpha_2\beta_2$	A	Adult
$\alpha_2\delta_2$	A_2	Adult
$\alpha_2{}^A\gamma_2$	F	Fetus
$\alpha_2{}^G\gamma_2$	F	Fetus
$\alpha_2\varepsilon_2$	Gower 2	Embryo
$\xi_2\varepsilon_2$	Gower 1	Embryo
$\xi_2\gamma_2$	Portland	Embryo
β_2	H	α thalassemia
γ_4	Bart's	α thalassemia
α_2 precipitate	—	β thalassemia

anemia frequently complicates folate deficiency, making examination of a peripheral smear difficult to interpret. Megaloblastic anemia has been linked to prematurity, low birth weights, preeclampsia, and abruptio placenta.

Thalassemias

Normal adult hemoglobin is 95% hemoglobin A and consists of two α and two β chains that form a tetramine protein. Of the six different possible globin chains in the human genome, the α and β chains are affected most in the thalassemias (Table 18). All forms of thalassemia are autosomal recessive traits (200). With suppression or absence of α- or β-chain synthesis, hemoglobin precipitation and shortened red blood cell lifespan occur. The alpha-hemoglobin monomer is encoded on four genes. The absence of all four α-globin chains is incompatible with life and results in hydrops fetalis (Fig. 15A). The gamma tetramers that form have such high oxygen affinity that release to tissues does not occur. High-output congestive heart failure and end-organ ischemia cause fetal death. In the absence of three α chains, hemoglobin H is formed (Fig. 15B). The presence of two normal α chains result in α-thalassemia minor, and these patients usually have a mild anemia. The presence of three normal α chains generally does not cause anemia at all (201). Patients with α-thalassemia trait and hemoglobin H disease have no increased incidence of fetal wastage with normal hemoglobin. However, maternal splenomegaly and bone marrow hyperplasia are not uncommon.

The β chain is encoded by only two genes. β-Thalassemia major is homozygous, whereas β-thalassemia minor is heterozygous. β-Thalassemia major is detected several months after birth as a severe anemia (Fig. 16). This condition results in infants who will require frequent transfusions. Complications of excessive iron may result in death by the second or third decade. β-Thalassemia minor produces either a mild anemia or a completely normal hemoglobin. Few women with β-thalassemia major reach reproductive age. At puberty, these women are fre-

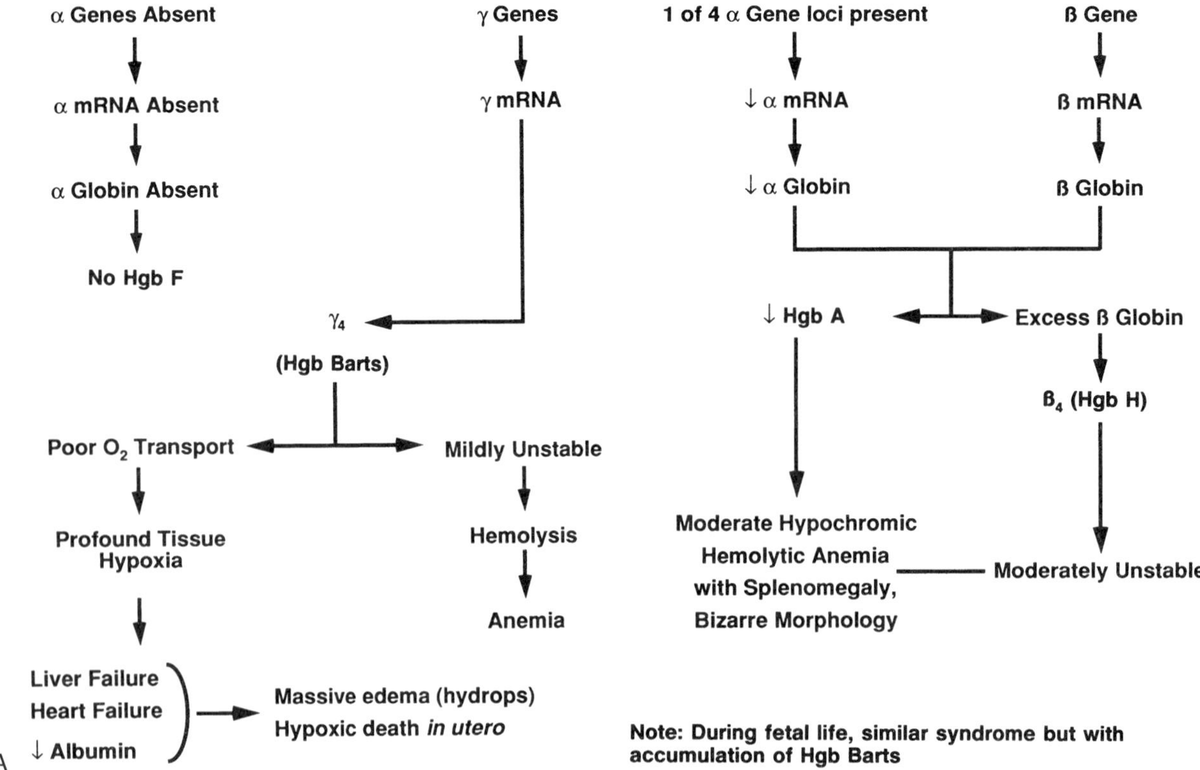

FIG. 15. The pathophysiology of hydrops fetalis with hemoglobin (Hgb) Barts **(A)** and Hgb H **(B)** disease. (From ref. 274, with permission.)

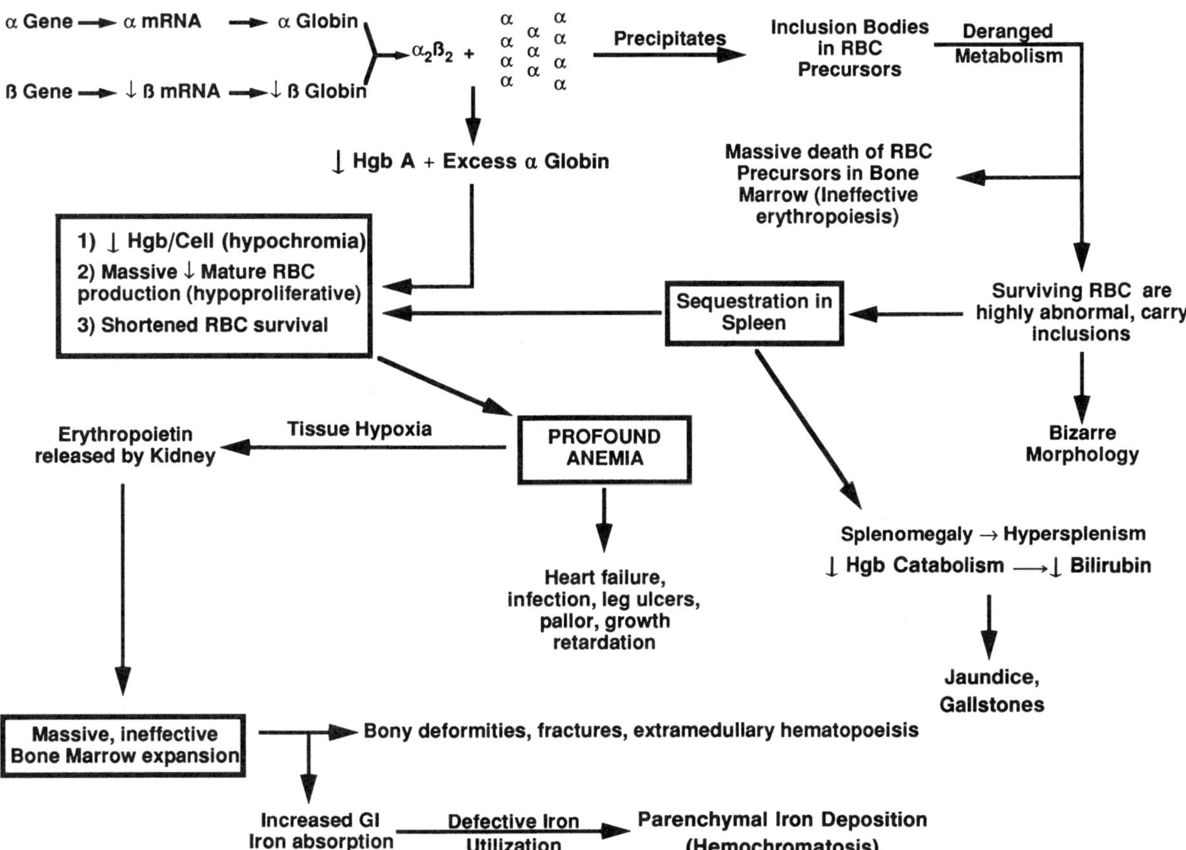

FIG. 16. Pathophysiology of severe forms of β thalassemia. The diagram outlines the pathogenesis of clinical abnormalities from the primary defect in β-globin synthesis. *GI*, gastrointestinal; *Hgb*, hemoglobin; *RBC*, red blood cells. (From ref. 274, with permission.)

quently amenorrheic due to hypogonadotrophic hypogonadism and, thus, may require ovulation induction to conceive. In an observational study of 16 women with β-thalassemia major, Jenson et al. (202) found that pregnancy, when it does occur, does not have a deleterious effect on the course of thalassemia. Even β-thalassemia major patients who are transfusion dependent have been shown to have a successful pregnancy outcome without a deleterious effect on the course of their disease (203). Anemia, hepatosplenomegaly, bone deformities, and cardiomyopathy, however, may complicate pregnancy (204). A higher rate for cesarean birth is common due to cephalopelvic disproportion from the short stature and small pelvis characteristic of many thalassemia patients (202,203).

Sickle Cell Anemia

Sickle cell anemia is the result of an error in the sixth position on the β-globin chain, with valine substituted for glutamic acid. This change produces instability of the β chain and decreased solubility of the hemoglobin molecule. When oxygen tension falls, the hemoglobin molecule will precipitate and produce the characteristic sickle-shaped red blood cells. Heterozygous sickle cell patients have 25% to 40% hemoglobin S. Patients with sickle cell trait are unlikely to have hemoglobin polymerize and precipitate unless hypoxia is severe (p_aO_2 less than 20 mm Hg). Homozygous patients may have 75% to 100% hemoglobin S. Patients with sickle cell anemia will develop sickling at a p_aO_2 of 60 mm Hg. By shifting the oxyhemoglobin dissociation curve to the right, acidosis worsens sickling. The p_{50} of the parturient is shifted to the right at term secondary to 2,3-DPG and also may potentiate maternal sickling.

The combination of hemoglobin S with other abnormal hemoglobins produces sickle cell disease. In the United States, the most frequent types are hemoglobin SS, hemoglobin SC, and hemoglobin S/β thalassemia. Pregnancy, with its increased oxygen consumption, may be associated with significant morbidity in women with abnormal hemoglobin (201). Pregnant women with sickle cell disease increase cardiac output by changing left ventricular end-diastolic volume rather than increasing heart rate or fractional shortening (205). In the face of additional physiologic stressors, these patients could be at risk for cardiovascular compromise during labor or postpartum if significant diastolic dysfunction occurs. Parturients with sickle cell trait tend to have a benign course, and the disease poses little risk to mother or fetus (206). These infants have normal intrauterine growth and birth weight (206). In contrast, a woman with homozygous sickle cell anemia (hemoglobin SS) is likely to have impaired fertility and limited survival. The mortality rate of the homozygous gravida has decreased in recent years with comprehensive and aggressive prenatal care. A recently published, large prospective multicenter study reported nonsickle-related antepartum and intrapartum complication rates comparable to those of African-American women who did not have sickle cell disease (207). Furthermore, the rate of maternal morbidity from sickle cell disease was the same during pregnancy as during the nonpregnant state. Although favorable obstetric outcomes often occur in patients with sickle cell disease, these patients are at high risk for vasoocclusive (208) and aplastic crises (Fig. 17). Thrombotic events in the placenta may lead to fetal loss and IUGR (209). The parturient with sickle cell disease has a high incidence of thrombotic events, neurological sequelae, infection, and preeclampsia, but with proper management and prompt intervention during acute episodes they tolerate pregnancy well (210).

Dysplasias

Leukemia

Leukemia, although rare, has been well described during pregnancy. Malignancy complicates an estimated 1 in 1,000 pregnancies, but the incidence of leukemia is less

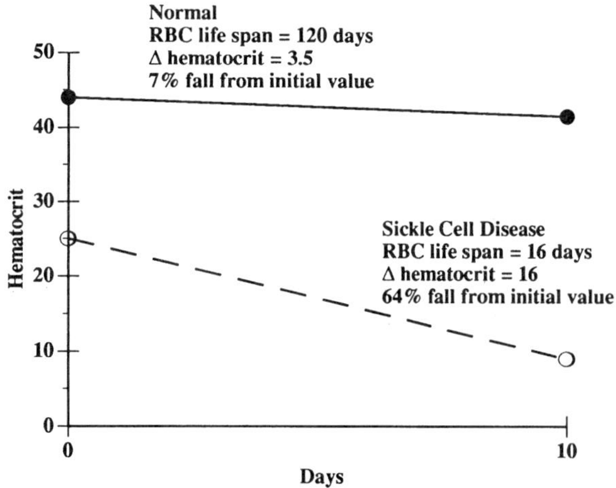

FIG. 17. Aplastic crisis. Hemolysis in patients with sickle cell anemia results in a substantial fall in hematocrit when erythroid production is suppressed. In normal individuals, the decrease in hematocrit during a similar time interval is insignificant. *RBC*, red blood cells. (From ref. 275, with permission.)

than 1 in 75,000 pregnancies (211,212). This low rate may reflect the relative infertility of women with leukemia. The diagnosis of acute leukemia during pregnancy usually requires immediate and aggressive treatment as mean survival without treatment is approximately 2 months. Many agents used to treat leukemia are relatively safe during the second and third trimesters of pregnancy; however, some antileukemic cytotoxic drugs can produce teratogenicity, IUGR, and premature birth (213). Although pregnancy tends not to alter the course of leukemia, leukemia can have a detrimental effect on pregnancy. Not infrequently, fetal death, prematurity, and teratogenesis may occur. Aggressive and appropriate management of some patients with acute leukemia (promyelocytic disease) can result in live births with complete remission of disease (214,215). Unfortunately, complications such as cardiac or pulmonary sequelae, as well as thrombocytopenia, disseminated intravascular coagulation, and opportunistic infection, often produce significant mortality (216).

Chronic myeloid leukemia tends to have a slow, indolent course, frequently allowing a delay in aggressive treatment (217). Optimal management and prognosis are unclear. Pregnancy lacks effect on the course of chronic leukemia, with more than 90% of women and 80% of fetuses surviving to delivery (212). Because of the small number of reported cases and the varied treatment options utilized, it is difficult to obtain accurate data upon which to base definitive conclusions about the effect and outcome of pregnancy.

The main defect in the leukemias is deregulation of precursor cell differentiation (212). Subsequently, one cell line proliferates in the bone marrow at the expense of other cell lines (218). Hemolysis, diminished red blood cell replacement, thrombocytopenia, and granulocytopenia cause maternal anemia, hemorrhage, and an increased susceptibility to infection. The gravida's liver, spleen, kidney, lymph node, skin, brain, and meninges may be affected.

Lymphoma

The incidence of lymphoma in pregnancy is unknown. From case reports, pregnancy does not adversely affect the course of disease (217). Prognosis of non-Hodgkin's lymphoma in pregnancy is poor due to the insidious nature of the tumor, and treatment during pregnancy has a tendency toward adverse outcomes (217).

Thrombocytopenia

Idiopathic Thrombocytopenia Purpura

Idiopathic thrombocytopenia purpura (ITP) is an autoimmune disease caused by an immunoglobulin G (IgG) antibody resulting in a low platelet count with an otherwise normal peripheral blood smear and normal complete blood count. ITP, most common in young women, is not uncommon in the parturient. The IgG antibody can cross the placenta and produce thrombocytopenia in the fetus. Placental receptors for the F_c portion of the IgG molecule allow the antibody to enter the fetal circulation. Maternal mortality may be as high as 5%, and perinatal mortality ranges from 6% to 17% (219,220). No strong correlation exists between maternal and infant platelet counts (221). Mothers with a previous splenectomy are at a reduced risk of having thrombocytopenic infants. The severity of infant thrombocytopenia may be proportional to the amount of antiplatelet antibody that is transferred across the placenta (220). A relationship between IgG antibody protein binding in the maternal serum and infant thrombocytopenia also may exist. Intracranial hemorrhage is a major risk for both mother and fetus.

Chronic ITP may present with easy bruising and petechiae, menorrhagia, or epistaxis. If the diagnosis has been made, the parturient may present to the obstetric anesthesiologist already undergoing treatment. According to the clinical guidelines proposed by the American Society of Hematology (222), pregnant women with ITP and platelet counts greater than 50×10^9/L do not routinely require treatment. Treatment is reserved for women with platelet counts less than 10×10^9/L and women with platelet counts of 10 to 30×10^9/L who are bleeding or are in the second or third trimester of pregnancy (223). Intravenous IgG is the recommended initial treatment for women with platelet counts less than 10×10^9/L in the third trimester and for those with platelet counts of 10 to 30×10^9/L who are bleeding. Glucocorticoid therapy, usually 1 to 2 mg/kg per day of oral prednisone or pulsed high-dose oral dexamethasone, also may be started (224). Because of concerns of hyperglycemia, increased blood pressure, and osteoporosis, medication is usually tapered when the platelet count begins to rise. IgG raises the patient's serum IgG concentration and impairs reticuloendothelial cell function, sparing the sensitized platelets from clearance (225). The platelet-elevating effect generally lasts less than 3 weeks, and treatment is repeated several times throughout the pregnancy.

If the parturient is resistant to steroids and intravenous IgG, splenectomy has been advocated, preferentially during the second trimester, when the risk of preterm labor is reduced and the gravid uterus does not interfere with surgical exposure. With the availability of the preceding treatment modalities, splenectomy is usually avoided in asymptomatic parturients with platelet counts greater than 10×10^9/L. Immunosuppressive therapy should be reserved for the most refractory cases, and administration should be limited to after fetal organogenesis. Platelet transfusions are only effective for several hours, and usage is reserved for severe bleeding or when surgery is planned.

To elevate both the maternal and fetal platelet counts, parturients with low platelet counts have their steroid regimens increased in the final weeks of gestation (226). Because placental enzymes inactivate most of the administered prednisone, some substitute dexamethasone or betamethasone. Treatment is not without risk. Along with possible maternal hyperglycemia, hypertension, and postpartum psychosis, fetal adrenal suppression remains a concern. Platelet transfusion may place the parturient at risk for a transfusion-related complication. Splenectomy during pregnancy has high risk of fetal loss.

Although platelet count falls in the face of autoimmune hyperdestruction, the platelets present are usually younger, larger, and superfunctional. Bleeding time in the parturient with ITP may not rise above 10 minutes until the platelet count drops below 50,000/mL^3 (227).

Gestational Thrombocytopenia

Gestational or incidental thrombocytopenia occurs in approximately 5% of parturients (228). It is often discovered incidentally during the late third trimester and is not normally associated with increased bleeding or adverse maternal or fetal outcomes (228–230). A normal pregnant platelet count may drop to as low as 80,000/mL (231). Other screening coagulation tests and bone marrow examination usually prove normal. Platelet count returns to normal in the postpartum period. No specific therapy is recommended as there is no increased risk of bleeding (228). Patients with idiopathic immune thrombocytopenia cannot be distinguished from those with gestational thrombocytopenia by the platelet antiglobulin test currently used. Glycogen-specific assays may be more useful (232).

Human Immunodeficiency Virus

Human immunodeficiency virus (HIV)-positive parturients may manifest thrombocytopenia in the early asymptomatic stage, as well as in the advanced acquired immunodeficiency syndrome (AIDS)-related complex stage. Several theories have been suggested to explain this association, including accelerated platelet destruction by autoantibodies resulting in platelet sequestration in the spleen, a production defect from bone marrow suppression, or infection of megakaryocytes (233–235). Maternal hemorrhage and fetal thrombocytopenia are potential complications that can influence obstetric outcome. As early HIV infection develops into clinical AIDS, the platelet count and function may normalize. In fact, one prospective study comparing non–HIV-infected parturients to asymptomatic HIV-infected patients, regardless of zidovudine treatment, revealed no differences in either platelet count or function (236). Zidovudine has been prescribed during pregnancy to attenuate perinatal AIDS transmission as well as to diminish the untoward effects of HIV infection on pregnancy (234). However, this drug may further compromise bone marrow function and production of platelets despite its role in decreasing platelet destruction (237).

Preeclampsia and Eclampsia

The most common cause of thrombocytopenia in pregnancy is preeclampsia (238). Approximately 15% of parturients with preeclampsia will have some form of consumptive thrombocytopenia. The incidence is even greater in the patient with eclampsia. Patients with preeclampsia who have a platelet count less than 100,000/mL also may have other abnormal coagulation tests (239,240). Platelet dysfunction may occur despite a normal platelet count (239). Platelet aggregation studies find both activated, hyperaggregable platelets and exhausted, hypoaggregable platelets in the circulation of patients with preeclampsia (241). This finding suggests that platelet aggregating factor may play a role in the mechanism of platelet dysfunction in the parturient with preeclampsia. The use of thromboelastagraphy in pregnancy is somewhat controversial, but there is some evidence that clot formation (k) time and maximum amplitude (MA) correlate strongly with platelet count and may be used to determine overall clotting ability in the presence of reduced platelet counts (242).

Drug-induced Thrombocytopenia

An extensive list of drugs can act as antigenic stimuli, resulting in an autoimmune thrombocytopenia. These purpurae are indistinguishable from those in idiopathic thrombocytopenia. Resolution occurs with cessation of the offending agent. The typical drugs include aspirin, penicillin, streptomycin, sulfa drugs, phenobarbital, heparin, and isoniazid. Aspirin irreversibly acetylates cyclooxygenase, a thromboxane precursor, and impairs platelet function. Nonsteroidal antiinflammatory agents competitively inhibit cyclooxygenase reversibly.

Heparin-induced thrombocytopenia may have both immunologic and nonimmunologic mechanisms (243). Life-threatening arterial and venous thrombosis may occur in patients taking heparin, and platelet transfusions can worsen the clinical picture. The fetus is not directly affected, as heparin does not cross the placenta. Platelet function usually recovers within 5 days after termination of heparin therapy, causing some clinicians to recommend a delay in delivery to await platelet recovery (244).

Thrombocytopenia associated with cocaine has been reported in the literature (245–247). Several mechanisms have been postulated, including α-adrenergic receptor platelet activation (248,249), bone marrow suppression, autoimmune-mediated response, hypersplenism, infection, and sepsis (250,251). However, data from retrospective and prospective studies have demonstrated that cocaine-abusing parturients are not at increased risk for thrombocytopenia (252,253). Qualitative (thromboelastography) and quantitative (platelet count) tests found no clinically significant differences in platelet count or function in this population.

Hemophilias

von Willebrand Disease

von Willebrand disease (vWD) is the most common congenital hemorrhagic disorder and results from a qualitative or quantitative defect of von Willebrand factor (vWF). vWF serves as a molecular bridge between platelets and damaged subendothelium on the vessel wall (Figure 18). In addition, it modulates circulation of factor VIII. Therefore, defects in vWF are characterized by abnormal platelet function and a decrease in factor VIII. Classic, type 1 vWD has an autosomal dominant inheritance pattern with variable penetrance resulting in manifestations ranging from patients with no evidence of disease to those with a moderate reduction in hemostatic function (254). Type 2 vWD is usually associated with a qualitative defect in vWF. The recessively inherited type

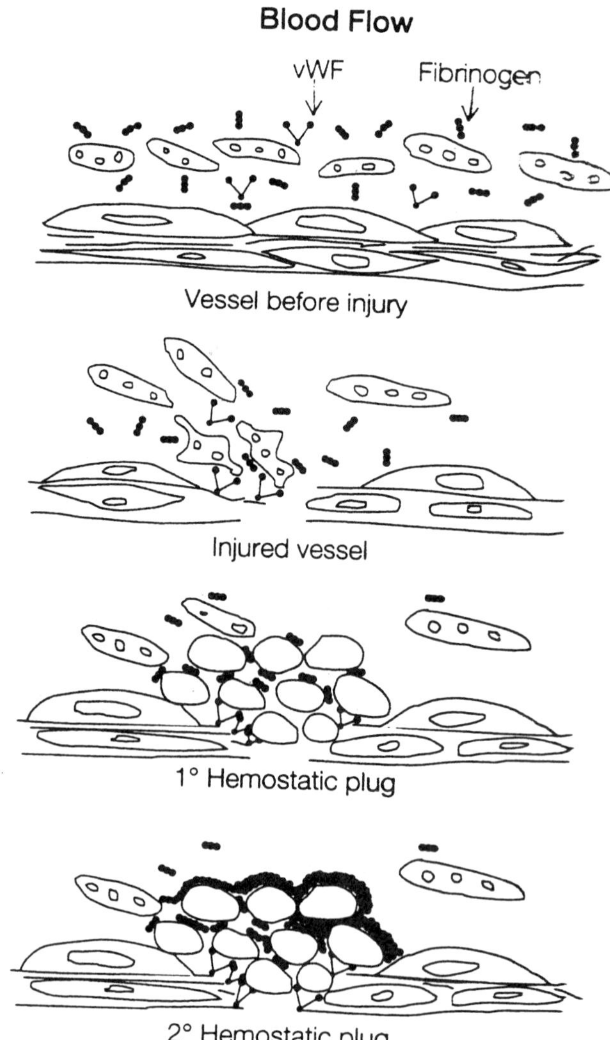

FIG. 18. Primary and secondary hemostasis in flowing blood after vessel injury. (From ref. 276, with permission.)

3 vWD is characterized by a quantitative defect in vWF and results in severely decreased levels of factor VIII.

Factor VIII is a protein complex consisting of von Willebrand factor (VIII:vWF) and factor procoagulant activity (VIII:C). Factor VIII:C measures the biologic activity of factor VIII. This factor is part of the intrinsic coagulation cascade. It is needed for the formation of a definitive hemostatic plug. Factor VIII:vWF, a large glycoprotein, allows aggregation of platelets to proceed. This is essential for the formation of a primary hemostatic plug after injury. Factor VIII:vWF also regulates the production and release of factor VIII:C. Factor VIII-related antigen (VIIIR:Ag) represents the antigenic determinants of vWF (255,256).

Although not a primary platelet disorder, because vWF is essential for platelet aggregation, the pattern of bleeding is similar to that found in patients with dysfunctional platelets (Table 19). Patients with vWD may present with menorrhagia, epistaxis, and bleeding from mucous membranes or intravenous sites. Mildly afflicted patients may have no symptoms. The diagnosis is often made following excessive surgical bleeding after dental extractions or minor surgery. Patients have an abnormal partial thromboplastin time because of the decreased coagulant activity of factor VIII, and a prolonged bleeding time secondary to the decrease in factor VIII:vWF. Giving plasma with factor VIII:vWF corrects the platelet aggregation defect.

In normal pregnancy, factor VIII:C and factor VIIIR:Ag increase 200% and 375%, respectively (257). Parturients with vWD also show an increased in factor concentration, but, by term, they have only half the normal amounts when pregnant. Bleeding may range from moderate to severe, depending on the degree of factor deficiency. With mild forms of the disease, bleeding time ranges from 12 to 24 minutes. Women with severe vWD may have bleeding times longer than 30 minutes. The increase in factor concentrations with gestation may improve the bleeding time in these women (258,259). There is no increase in maternal mortality or fetal loss. These women are at high risk for postpartum hemorrhage as factor VIII:C and factor VI''R:Ag concentrations fall precipitously (within a few hours) to nonpregnant levels. Bleeding problems tend to recur about 1 week postpartum, or at the time of abortion (260).

Hemophilia

Hemophilia A is a sex-linked recessive disorder characterized by a lack of procoagulant activity of factor VIII. Female carriers have a genetic defect on one X chromosome and a second normal gene. As a result, clotting factor level is approximately 50% of normal. In general, patients with factor VIII levels of at least 25% of normal clot without difficulty. Patients with hemophilia A become symptomatic when factor VIII activity falls below 5%. Patients with less than 1% factor VIII activity have severe disease. They bleed frequently without evidence of trauma. Those with activity greater than 5% have mild disease. They bleed infrequently, most often after trauma. Hemophiliac bleeding may occur up to days after injury, involve any organ, and, left untreated, may continue for days or weeks. Compartment syndromes, pseudophlebitis, or ischemic damage to compressed nerves may follow. Most often, these patients bleed into soft tissues, muscles, and weight-bearing joints.

Phenotypic hemophilia in women is extremely rare and acquired hemophilia is an unusual cause of postpartum hemorrhage (261). Pregnancy increases the concentration of factor VIII:C. Carrier gravidae may reach normal levels by term (262). With the rapid fall of factor VIII activity postpartum, abnormal bleeding following delivery may resume. Hemophiliacs may develop femoral neu-

TABLE 19. *Composition of hemophilia A and classic von Willebrand disease*

	Hemophilia A	von Willebrand
Deficiency	VIII:C, VIII:AHF	VIII:vWF, VIII:R
Inheritance	Recessive, X-linked	Dominant, autosomal
Clinical bleeding	Hemarthosis, muscle, soft tissue, viscera	Gums, gastrointestinal tract, mucous membranes
Bleeding disorder	Moderate to severe (60% severe)	Mild to moderate
Laboratory tests		
Bleeding time	N	A
Clot retraction	N	N
Glass bead retraction	N	A
Platelet count	N	N
Ristocetin aggregation	N	A
Prothrombin times	N	N
Partial thromboplastin time	A	A
Factor VIII	A	A
VWF:Ag	N	A

A, abnormal; N, normal.

ropathy due to pressure from an unsuspected retroperitoneal hematoma. The parturient with symptomatic disease requires a careful preanesthetic neurologic assessment. Affected male fetuses are at risk for scalp and intracranial hemorrhage during labor and delivery from the use of invasive monitoring techniques, prolonged labor, and instrumental deliveries (263).

Autologous Blood Donation

In recent years, concerns about the risk of blood transfusion have led to a significantly increased use of autologous blood donation in the nonobstetric population. In the obstetric population, premature delivery and preexisting anemia may limit autologous blood donation (264). The relative anemia of pregnancy may result in a hemoglobin below the minimal concentration for nonobstetric autologous donation guidelines (12.5 g/dL) (265). For patients undergoing elective cesarean sections, the donation procedure has been well tolerated with infrequent donor reactions (266). A hemoglobin of 11 g/dL is a predonation level for inclusion in autologous donation (265,267,268). With a predonation level higher than 11 g/dL, there have been no adverse effects reported to either mother or fetus.

REFERENCES

1. Perloff JK. Congenital heart disease and pregnancy. In: Gleicher N, ed. *Principles of medical therapy in pregnancy.* New York: Plenum Publishing, 1985:665.
2. Whittemore R. Congenital heart disease: its impact on pregnancy. *Hosp Pract* 1983;18:65.
3. McFaul PB, Dornan JC, Lamki H, Boyle D. Pregnancy complicated by maternal heart disease: a review of 519 women. *Br J Obstet Gynaecol* 1988;95:861.
4. Sullivan JM, Ramanathan KB. Management of medical problems in pregnancy: severe cardiac disease. *N Engl J Med* 1985;313:304.
5. Johnson MD, Saltzman DH. Cardiac disease. In: Datta S, ed. *Anesthetic and obstetric management of high-risk pregnancy.* St. Louis: Mosby-Year Book, 1996:200.
6. Clark SL, Phelan JP, Cotton DB, eds. *Critical care obstetrics.* Oradell, NJ: Medical Economics Books, 1987:93.
7. Nolan TE, Hankins GD. Myocardial infarction in pregnancy. *Clin Obstet Gynecol* 1989;32:68.
8. Cheek TG, Gutsche BB. Maternal physiologic alterations during pregnancy. In: Shinder SM, Levinson G, eds. *Anesthesia for obstetrics*, 3rd ed. Baltimore: Williams & Wilkins, 1993:7.
9. McAnulty JH, Metcalfe J, Cleland K. Cardiovascular disease. In: Burrow GN, Ferris TF, eds. *Medical complications during pregnancy.* Philadelphia: WB Saunders, 1988:185.
10. Cutforth R, MacDonald C: Heart sounds and murmurs in pregnancy. *Am Heart J* 1966;71:741.
11. Hess DB, Hess WL. Cardiovascular disease and pregnancy. *Obstet Gynecol Clin North Am* 1992;19:679.
12. *American College of Obstetrics and Gynecology Technical Bulletin Number 168-June 1992. Cardiac disease in pregnancy. Int J Gynaecol Obstet* 1993;41(3):298–306.
13. Rahimtoola SH. The need for cardiac catheterization and angiography in valvular heart disease is not disproven. *Ann Intern Med* 1982; 97:433.
14. Swartz HM, Reichling BA. Hazards of radiation exposure for pregnant women. *JAMA* 1978;239:1907.
15. Presbitero P, Prever SB, Brusca A. Interventional cardiology in pregnancy. *Eur Heart J* 1996;17:182.
16. Gray JE. The radiation hazard. Let's put it in perspective. *Mayo Clin Proc* 1979;54:809.
17. Deluca S, Castronovo F. Radiation exposure in diagnostic studies. *Am Fam Physician* 1987;36:101.
18. Mole RH. Radiation effects on prenatal development and their radiological significance. *Br J Radiol* 1979;52:89.
19. Elkayam U, Kawanishi D, Reid CL, et al. Contrast echocardiography to reduce ionizing radiation associated with cardiac catheterization during pregnancy. *Am J Cardiol* 1983;52:213.
20. Clark SL, Cotton DB, Lee W, et al. Central hemodynamic assessment of normal term pregnancy. *Am J Obstet Gynecol* 1989;161:1439.
22. Lee W, Rokey R, Cotton DB. Noninvasive maternal stroke volume and cardiac output determinations by pulsed Doppler echocardiography. *Am J Obstet Gynecol* 1988;158:505.
23. Van Oppen A, Stigter RH, Bruinse HW. Cardiac output in normal pregnancy: a critical review. *Obstet Gynecol* 1996;87:310.
24. Thornhill ML, Camann WR. Cardiovascular disease. In: Chestnut DH, ed. *Obstetric anesthesia principles and practice.* St. Louis: Mosby-Year Book, 1994:746.
25. Pollack KL, Chestnut DH, Wenstrom KD. Anesthetic management of a parturient with Eisenmenger's syndrome. *Anesth Analg* 1990;70:212.
26. Devitt JH, Noble WH, Byrick RJ. A Swan-Ganz catheter related complication in a patient with Eisenmenger's syndrome. *Anesthesiology* 1982;57:335.
27. Robinson S. Pulmonary artery catheters in Eisenmenger's syndrome: many risks, few benefits. *Anesthesiology* 1983;58:588.
28. Schwalbe SS, Deshmukh SM, Marx GF. Use of pulmonary artery catheterization in parturients with Eisenmenger's syndrome. *Anesth Analg* 1990;71:442.

28a. Atanassoff P, Alon E, Schmid ER, Pasch TH. Epidural anesthesia for cesarean section in a patient with severe pulmonary hypertension. *Acta Anaesthesiol Scand* 1990;34:75–77.

29. Clark SL, Horenstein JM, Phelan JP. Experience with the pulmonary artery catheter in obstetrics and gynecology. *Am J Obstet Gynecol* 1985;152:374.
30. Dajani AS, Taubert KA, Wilson W, et al. Prevention of bacterial endocarditis recommendation by the American Heart Association. *JAMA* 1997;277:1794.
31. Stevenson RE, Burton M, Ferlauto GJ, Taylor HA. Hazards of oral anticoagulants during pregnancy. *JAMA* 1980;243:1549.
32. Ginsberg JS, Hirsh J. Use of antithrombotic agents during pregnancy. *Chest* 1995;108:305S.
33. Oakley CM. Clinical perspective: anticoagulation and pregnancy. *Eur Heart J* 1995;16:1317.
34. Cotrufo M, de Luca TSL, Calabro R, et al. Coumarin anticoagulation during pregnancy in patients with mechanical valve prostheses. *Eur J Cardiothorac Surg* 1991;5:300.
35. Hirsh J. Is the dose of warfarin prescribed by American physicians unnecessarily high? *Arch Intern Med* 1987;147:769.
36. Sbarouni E, Oakley CM. Outcome of pregnancy in women with valve prostheses. *Br Heart J* 1994;71:196.
37. Hirsch J. Heparin. *N Engl J Med* 1991;324:1565.
38. Ginsberg JS, Kowalchuk G, Hirsh J, et al. Heparin effect on bone density. *Thromb Haemost* 1990;64:286.
39. Dahlman T, Lindvall N, Hellgren M. Osteopenia in pregnancy during long-term heparin treatment: a radiological study post-partum. *Br J Obstet Gynaecol* 1990;97:221.
40. Barbour LA, Kick SD, Steiner JF, et al. A prospective study of heparin-induced osteoporosis using bone densitometry. *Am J Obstet Gynecol* 1994:170:862.
41. Dahlman TC. Osteoporotic fractures and the recurrence of thromboembolism during pregnancy and the puerperium in 184 women undergoing thromboprophylaxis with heparin. *Am J Obstet Gynecol* 1993;168:1265.
42. Gingsberg JS, Hirsh J, Turner DC, et al. Risks to the fetus of anticoagulant therapy during pregnancy. *Thromb Haemost* 1989;61:197.
43. Ginsberg JS, Kowalchuk G, Hirsh J, et al. Heparin therapy during pregnancy: risks to the fetus and mother. *Arch Intern Med* 1989;149: 2233.
44. Shaughnessy SG, Young E, Deschamps P, et al. The effects of low molecular-weight and standard heparin on calcium loss from fetal rat calvaria. *Blood* 1995;86:1368.
45. Forestier F, Daffos F, Capella-Pavlovsky M. Low molecular weight heparin (PK10169) does not cross the placenta during the second trimester of pregnancy: study by direct fetal blood sampling under ultrasound. *Thromb Res* 1984;34:557.

46. Forestier F, Daffos F, Rainaut M, Toulemond F. Low molecular weight heparin (CY 216) does not cross the placenta during the third trimester of pregnancy. *Thromb Haemost* 1987;57:234.
47. Omri A, Delaloye JF, Anderson H, Bachmann F. Low molecular weight heparin (NOVO ILHN-1) does not cross the placenta during the second trimester of pregnancy. *Thromb Haemost* 1989;61:55.
48. Iturbe-Alessio I, Fonseca MC, Mutchinik O, et al. Risks of anticoagulant therapy in pregnant women with artificial heart valves. *N Engl J Med* 1986;315:1390.
49. Elkayam U. Pregnancy and cardiovascular disease. In: Braunwald E, ed. *Heart disease.* Philadelphia: WB Saunders, 1992:1790.
50. Cox JL, Gardner MJ. Treatment of cardiac arrhythmias during pregnancy. *Prog Cardiovasc Dis* 1993;36:137.
51. Eisenach JC, Castro MI. Maternally administered esmolol produces fetal beta-adrenergic blockade and hypoxemia in sheep. *Anesthesiology* 1989;71:718.
52. Ducey JP, Knape KG. Maternal esmolol administration resulting in fetal distress and cesarean section in a term pregnancy. *Anesthesiology* 1992;77:829.
53. Fairley CJ, Clarke JT. Use of esmolol in a parturient with hypertrophic obstructive cardiomyopathy. *Br J Anaesth* 1995;75:801.
54. Page RL. Treatment of arrhythmias during pregnancy. *Am Heart J* 1995;130:871.
55. Elkayam U, Ostrzega E, Shotan A, Mehra A. Cardiovascular problems in pregnant women with the Marfan syndrome. *Ann Intern Med* 1995;123:117.
56. Lip GYH, Beevers M, Churchill D, et al. Effect of atenolol on birth weight. *Am J Cardiol* 1997;79:1436.
57. Rotmensch HH, Elkayam U, Frishman W. Antiarrhythmic drug therapy during pregnancy. *Ann Intern Med* 1983;98:487.
58. Wolff F, Breuker KH, Schlensker KH, Bolte A. Prenatal diagnosis and therapy of fetal heart rate anomalies: with a contribution on the placental transfer of verapamil. *J Perinat Med* 1980;8:203.
59. Lindheimer MD. Hypertension in pregnancy. *Hypertension* 1993;22:127.
60. Laurent M, Betremieux P, Biron Y, Lellelloco A. Neonatal hypothyroidism after treatment with amiodarone during pregnancy. *Am J Cardiol* 1987;60:942.
61. Nademanee K, Piwonka RW, Singh BN, Hershman J. Amiodarone and thyroid function. *Prog Cardiovasc Dis* 1989;6:427.
62. Feldkamp M, Jones KL, Ornoy A, et al. Postmarketing surveillance for angiotensin-converting enzyme inhibitor use during the first trimester of pregnancy—United States, Canada, and Israel, 1987–1995. *MMWR* 1997;46:240.
63. Lavaratti G, Seracini D, Fiorini P, et al. Neonatal anuria by ACE inhibitors during pregnancy. *Nephron* 1997;76:235.
64. Shotan A, Widerhorn J, Hurst A, Elkayam U. Risks of angiotensin-converting enzyme inhibition during pregnancy: experimental and clinical evidence, potential mechanisms, and recommendations for use. *Am J Med* 1994;96:451.
65. Campos O, Andrade JL, Bocanegra J, et al. Physiologic multivalvular regurgitation during pregnancy: a longitudinal Doppler echocardiographic study. *Int J Cardiol* 1993;40(3):265.
66. Oakley CM. Valvular disease in pregnancy. *Curr Opin Cardiol* 1996;11:155.
67. Jackson JM. Valvular heart disease. In: Thomas SJ, ed. *Manual of cardiac anesthesia.* New York: Churchill Livingstone, 1984:220.
68. Joyce TH, Palacios Q. Cardiac disease. In: James FM III, Wheeler AS, Dewan DM, eds. *Obstetric anesthesia: the complicated patient*, 2nd ed. Philadelphia: FA Davis, 1988:163.
69. Stoelting RK, Dierfdorf SF. *Anesthesia and coexisting disease,* 3rd ed. New York: Churchill Livingstone, 1993:28.
70. Barlow JB, Popcock WA. The problem of nonejection systolic clicks and associated mitral systolic murmurs: emphasis on the billowing mitral leaftlet syndrome. *Am Heart J* 1975;90:636.
71. Degani S, Abinader EG, Scharf M. Mitral valve prolapse and pregnancy: a review. *Obstet Gynecol Surv* 1989;44:642.
72. Hass JM. The effect of pregnancy on the midsystolic click and murmurs of the prolapsing posterior leaflet of the mitral valve. *Am Heart J* 1976;92:407.
73. Cowles T, Gonik B. Mitral valve prolapse in pregnancy. *Semin Perinatol* 1990;14:34.
74. Shapiro EP, Trimble EL, Robinson JC, et al. Safety of labor and delivery in women with mitral valve prolapse. *Am J Cardiol* 1985;56:806.
75. Rayburn WF, Fontana ME. Mitral valve prolapse and pregnancy. *Am J Obstet Gynecol* 1981;141:9.
76. Lao TT, Sermer M, MaGee L, et al. Congenital aortic stenosis and pregnancy—a reappraisal. *Am J Obstet Gynecol* 1993;169:540.
77. Sullivan HJ. Valvular heart surgery during pregnancy. *Surg Clin North Am* 1995;75:59.
78. Kroetz FW, Leonard JJ, Shaver JA, et al. The effect of atrial contraction on left ventricular performance in valvular aortic stenosis. *Circulation* 1967;35:852.
79. Arias F, Pineda J. Aortic stenosis and pregnancy. *J Reprod Med* 1978;20:229.
80. Whittemore R, Hobbins JC, Engle MA. Pregnancy and its outcome in women with and without surgical treatment of congenital heart disease. *Am J Cardiol* 1982;50:641.
81. Lipscomb KJ, Smith JC, Clarke P, et al. Outcome of pregnancy in women with Marfan's syndrome. *Br J Obstet Gynaecol* 1997;104:201.
82. Thomas SJ. *Anesthetic management of the patient with valve disease and other unusual cardiac problems. ASA refresher course lectures.* Philadelphia: JB Lippincott, 1989:311.
83. Datta S, Kitzmiller JL, Ostheimer GW, Shoenbaum SC. Propranalol and parturition. *Obstet Gynecol* 1978;51:577.
84. Oakley GDG, McGarry K, Limb DG, Oakley CM. Management of pregnancy in patients with hypertrophic cardiomyopathy. *Br Med J* 1979;1:1749.
85. Hoffman JL, Christianson R. Congenital heart disease in a cohort of 19,502 births with long-term follow-up. *Am J Cardiol* 1978;42:641.
86. Jackson DM, Dildy GA, Varner MW, Clark SL. Severe pulmonary hypertension in pregnancy following successful repair of ventricular septal defect in childhood. *Obstet Gynecol* 1993;82[Suppl]:680.
87. Presbitero P, Somerville J, Stone S, et al. Pregnancy in cyanotic congenital heart disease. Outcome of mother and fetus. *Circulation* 1994;89:2673.
88. Findlow D, Doyle E. Congenital heart disease in adults. *Br J Anaesth* 1997;78:416.
89. Weiss BM, Atanassoff PG. Cyanotic congential heart disease and pregnancy: natural slection, pulmonary hypertension, and anesthesia. *J Clin Anesthesiol* 1993;5:322.
90. Gleicher N. *Principle and practice of medical therapy in pregnancy,* 2nd ed. Norwalk: Appleton & Lange, 1992:792.
91. Morris CD, Menashe VD. Recurrence of congenital heart disease in offspring of parents with surgical correction. *Clin Res* 1985;33:68A.
92. Singh H, Bolton PJ, Oakley CM. Pregnancy after surgical correction of tetralogy of Fallot. *Br Med J* 1982;285:168.
93. Alpert JS. *Physiopathology of the cardiovascular system.* Boston: Little, Brown and Company, 1984:122.
94. Gleicher R, Midwall J, Hochberger D, et al. Eisenmenger's syndrome and pregnancy. *Obstet Gynecol Surv* 1979;34:721.
95. Avila WS, Grinberg M, Snitcowsky R, et al. Maternal and fetal outcome in pregnant women with Eisenmenger's syndrome. *Eur Heart J* 1995;16:460.
96. Garber SZ, Choi HJ, Tremper KK, et al. Use of a pulse oximeter in the anesthetic management of a pregnant patient with Eisenmenger's syndrome. *Anesthesiol Rev* 1988;15:59.
97. Midwall J, Jaffin H, Herman MV, Kupersmith J. Shunt flow and pulmonary hemodynamics during labor and delivery in the Eisenmenger syndrome. *Am J Cardiol* 1978;42:299.
98. Lampert MB, Lang RM. Peripartum cardiomyopathy. *Am Heart J* 1995;130:860.
99. Homans DC. Current concepts: peripartum cardiomyopathy. *N Engl J Med* 1985;312:1432.
100. Demakis JG, Rahimtoola SH. Peripartum cardiomyopathy. *Circulation* 1971;44:964.
101. Demakis JG, Rahimtoola SH, Sutton GC, et al. Natural course of peripartum cardiomyopathy. *Circulation* 1971;44:1053.
102. Rickenbacher PR, Rizeq MN, Hunt SA, et al. Long-term outcome after heart transplantation for peripartum cardiomyopathy. *Am Heart J* 1994;127:1318.
103. Camann WR, Goldman GA, Johnson MD, et al. Cesarean delivery of a patient with a transplanted heart. *Anesthesiology* 1989;71:618.
104. Liljestrand J, Lindstrom B. Childbirth after post partum cardiac insufficiency treated with cardiac transplant. *Acta Obstet Gynecol Scand* 1993;72:406.
105. Hodgman MT, Pessin MS, Homans DC, et al: Cerebral embolism as the

initial manifestation of peripartum cardiomyopathy. *Neurology* 1982; 32:668.

106. Silverman RI, Ribner II. Peripartum cardiomyopathy. Cardiac problems in pregnancy. In: Elkayam U, Gleicher N, eds. *Diagnosis and management of maternal and fetal disease.* New York: Alan R. Liss, 1982:115.
107. O'Connell JB, Constanzo-Nordu MR, Subramamian R, et al. Peripartum cardiomyopathy: clinical, hemodynamic, histologic and prognostic characteristics. *J Am Coll Cardiol* 1986;8:52.
108. Rizeq MN, Rickenbacher PR, Fowler MB, Billingham ME. Incidence of myocarditis in peripartum cardiomyopathy. *Am J Cardiol* 1994;74:474.
109. Van Hoeven KH, Kitsis RN, Katz SD, Factor SM. Peripartum versus idiopathic dilated cardiomyopathy in young women—a comparison of clinical, pathologic and prognostic features. *Int J Cardiol* 1993;40:57.
110. Hankins GD, Wendell GD Jr., Leveno KJ, Stoneham J. Myocardial infarction during pregnancy: a review. *Obstet Gynecol* 1985;65:139.
111. Webber MD, Halligan RE, Schumacher JA. Acute infarction, intracoronary thrombolysis, and primary PTCA in pregnancy. *Cathet Cardiovasc Diagn* 1997;42:38.
112. Badui E, Enciso R. Acute myocardial infarction during pregnancy and puerperium. *Angiology* 1996;47:739.
113. Howard RE, Hueter DC, Davis GJ. Acute myocardial infarction following cocaine abuse in a young woman with normal coronary arteries. *JAMA* 1985;254:95.
114. Mehta PM, Grainger TA, Lust RM, et al. Effect of cocaine on left ventricular function. *Circulation* 1995;91:3002.
115. Roth A, Elkayam U. Acute myocardial infarction associated with pregnancy. *Ann Intern Med* 1996;125:751.
116. Pasternack PF, Colvin SB, Bauman FG. Cocaine-induced angina pectoris and acute myocardial infarction in patients younger than 40 years. *Am J Cardiol* 1985;55:847.
117. Trouton TG, Sidhu H, Adgey AJ. Myocardial infarction in pregnancy. *Int J Cardiol* 1988;18:35.
118. Laughlin MP, From RP, Choi W. Recent myocardial infarction in a parturient. *Anesthesiol Rev* 1986;8:43.
119. Roberts SL, Chestnut DH. Anesthesia for the obstetric patient with cardiac disease. *Clin Obstet Gynecol* 1987;30:601.
120. Weir EK. Diagnosis and management of primary pulmonary hypertension. In: Weir EK, Reeves JT, eds. *Pulmonary hypertension.* Mount Kisco, NY: Futura Publishing, 1984:115.
121. Slomka F, Salmeron S, Zetlaoui P, et al. Primary pulmonary hypertension and pregnancy: anesthetic management for delivery. *Anesthesiology* 1988;69:959.
122. Rich S, Kaufman L, Levy P. The effects of high doses of calcium-channel blockers on survival in primary pulmonary hypertension. *N Engl J Med* 1992;327:76.
123. Nootens M, Rich S. Successful management of labor and delivery in primary pulmonary hypertension. *Am J Cardiol* 1993;71:1124.
124. Kiss H, Egarter C, Asseryanis E, et al. Primary pulmonary hypertension in pregnancy: a case report. *Am J Obstet Gynecol* 1995;172;1052.
125. Freidman AJ. The urinary tract in pregnancy. *Am Urol-Gynecol Soc Rep* 1987;7:1.
126. Beydoun SN. Morphologic changes in the renal tract in pregnancy. *Clin Obstet Gynecol* 1985;28(2):249.
127. Davison JM. Overview: kidney function in pregnant women. *Am J Kidney Dis* 1987;9:248.
128. Davison JM, Dunlop W. Renal hemodynamics and tubular function in normal human pregnancy. *Kidney Int* 1980;18:152.
129. Conrad KP. Possible mechanisms for changes in renal hemodynamics during pregnancy: studies from animal models. *Am J Kidney Dis* 1987;9:253.
130. Gant HF, Whalley PJ, Everet RB, et al. Control of vascular reactivity in pregnancy. *Am J Kidney Dis* 1987;9:303.
131. Duvekot JJ, Peeters LL. Renal hemodynamics and volume homeostasis in pregnancy. *Obstet Gynecol Surv* 1994;49:830.
132. Marchant DJ. Alterations in anatomy and function of the urinary tract during pregnancy. *Clin Obstet Gynecol* 1978;21:855.
133. Purdy LP, Hantsch CE, Molitch ME, et al. Effect of pregnancy on renal function in patients with moderate-to-severe diabetic renal insufficiency. *Diabetes Care* 1996;19:1067.
134. Davison JM, Vallotton MB, Lindheimer MD. Plasma osmolality and urinary concentration and dilution during and after pregnancy. *Br J Obstet Gynaecol* 1981;88:472.
135. Davison JM, Gilmore EA, Durr J, et al. Altered osmotic thresholds for vasopressin secretion and thirst in human pregnancy. *Am J Physiol* 1984;246:F105.
136. Lindheimer MD, Barron WM, Durr J, Davidson JM. Water homeostasis and vasopressin release during rodent and human gestation. *Am J Kidney Dis* 1987;9:270.
137. Gallery ED, Brown MA. Control of sodium excretion in human pregnancy. *Am J Kidney Dis* 1987;9:290.
138. Weinberger MH, Kramer NJ, Petersen P, et al. Sequential changes in renin-angiotensin-aldosterone systems in normal and abnormal pregnancies. In: Lindheimer MD, Katz AI, Zuspan FP, eds. *Hypertension in pregnancy.* New York: John Wiley and Sons, 1976:264.
139. Welsh GW, Sims EAH. The mechanisms of renal glucosuria in pregnancy. *Diabetes* 1960;9:363.
140. Ferris TF. Renal disease. In: Burrow GN, Ferris TF, eds. *Medical complications during pregnancy,* 3rd ed. Philadelphia: WB Saunders, 1988:277.
141. Packham D, Fairley KF. Renal biopsy: indications and complications in pregnancy. *Br J Obstet Gynaecol* 1987;94:935.
142. Pivalizza EG, Abramson DC, Harvey A. Perioperative hypercoagulability in uremic patients: a viscoelastic study. *J Clin Anesth* 1997;9:442.
143. Reese GN, Appel SH. Neurological complications of renal failure. *Semin Nephrol* 1981;1:137.
144. Zelnick EB, Goyal RK. Gastrointestinal manifestations of renal failure. *Semin Nephrol* 1981;1:124.
145. Lindheimer MD, Katz AI. Gestation in women with kidney disease: prognosis and management. *Baillieres Clin Obstet Gynaecol* 1987:1: 921.
146. Katz AI, Lindheimer MD. Does pregnancy aggravate primary glomerular disease? *Am J Kidney Dis* 1985;6:261.
147. Jungers P, Forget D, Henry-Amar M, et al. Chronic renal disease and pregnancy. *Adv Nephrol from Necker Hosp* 1986;15:103.
148. Davison JM, Katz AI, Lindheimer MD. Kidney disease and pregnancy: obstetrics outcome and long-term renal prognosis. *Clin Perinatol* 1985;12:497.
149. Ferrier C, North RA, Becker G, et al. Uterine artery waveform as a predictor of pregnancy outcome in women with underlying renal disease. *Clin Nephrol* 1994;42:362.
150. Katz AI, Lindheimer MD. Effects of pregnancy upon the natural course of kidney disease. *Semin Nephrol* 1984;4:252.
151. Holley JL, Bernardini J, Quadri KHM, Greenberg A, Laifer SA. Pregnancy outcomes in a prospective matched control study of pregnancy and renal disease. *Clin Nephrol* 1996;45(2):77.
152. Jones DC, Hayslett JP. Outcome of pregnancy in women with moderate or severe renal insufficiency. *N Engl J Med* 1996;335:226.
153. Nowicki B, Martens M, Hart A, Nowicki S. Gestational age-dependent distribution of Escherichia coli fimbriae in pregnant patients with pyelonephritis. *Ann N Y Acad Sci* 1994;730:290.
154. Klein EA. Urologic problems of pregnancy. *Obstet Gynecol Surv* 1984;39:605.
155. Hemmelder MH, de Zeeuw, Fidler V, de Jong PE. Proteinuria: a risk factor for pregnancy-related renal function decline in primary glomerular disease. *Am J Kidney Dis* 1995;26:187.
156. Abe S. The influence of pregnancy on the long-term renal prognosis of IgA nephropathy. *Clin Nephrol* 1994;41:61.
157. Gabert HA, Miller JM Jr. Renal disease in pregnancy. *Obstet Gynecol Surv* 1985;40:449.
158. Estes D, Larson DC. Systemic lupus erythematous and pregnancy. *Clin Obstet Gynecol* 1965;8:307.
159. Syrop CH, Varner MW. Systemic lupus erythematosus. *Clin Obstet Gynecol* 1983;26:547.
160. Lockshin MD, Reinitz E, Druzin ML, et al. Lupus pregnancy case control prospective study demonstrating absence of lupus exacerbation during or after pregnancy. *Am J Med* 1984:77:893.
161. Burkett G. Lupus nephropathy and pregnancy. *Clin Obstet Gynecol* 1985;28:310.
162. Huong D, Wechsler B, Piette JC, Bletry O, Godeau P. Pregnancy and its outcome in systemic lupus erythematosus. *Q J Med* 1994;87:721.
163. Julkunen H, Kaaja R, Palosuo T, Gronhagen-Riska C, Teramo K. Pregnancy in lupus nephropathy. *Acta Obstet Gynecol Scand* 1993;72:258.
164. Malinow AM, Rickford WJ, Moriski BL, et al. Lupus anticoagulant: implications for obstetric anaesthetists. *Anaesthesia* 1987;42:1291.
165. Jungers P, Dougados M, Pelissier C, et al. Lupus nephropathy and pregnancy: report of 104 cases in 36 patients. *Arch Int Med* 1982;142:771.

166. Lubbe WF, Liggins GC. Lupus anticoagulant and pregnancy. *Am J Obstet Gynecol* 1985;153:322.
167. Gimovsky ML, Montoro M, Paul RH. Pregnancy outcome in women with systemic lupus erythematosus. *Obstet Gynecol* 1984;63:686.
168. McCune AB, Weston WL, Lee LA. Maternal and fetal outcome in neonatal lupus erythematosus. *Ann Intern Med* 1987;106:518.
169. Anonymous. Neonatal lupus syndrome [Editorial]. *Lancet* 1987; ii:489.
170. Miodovnik M, Rosenn BM, Khoury JC, et al. Does pregnancy increase the risk for development and progression of diabetic nephropathy. *Am J Obstet Gynecol* 1996;174:1180.
171. Kaaja R, Sjoberg L, Hellsted T, et al. Long-term effects of pregnancy on diabetic complications. *Diabet Med* 1996;13:165.
172. Mackie ADR, Doddridge MC, Gamsu HR, et al. Outcome of pregnancy in patients with insulin-dependent diabetes mellitus and nephropathy with moderate renal impairment. *Diabet Med* 1996;13:90.
173. Horowitz E, Schmidt JD. Renal calculi: pregnancy. *Clin Obstet Gynecol* 1985;2:324.
174. Cameron JS, Hicks J. Pregnancy in patients with pre-existing glomerular disease. *Contrib Nephrol* 1984;37:149.
175. Johnson TR, Jr., Lorenz RP, Menon KMJ. Successful outcome of a pregnancy requiring dialysis: effects on serum progesterone and estrogens. *J Reprod Med* 1979;22:217.
176. Weir PH, Chung FF. Anesthesia for patients with chronic renal disease. *Can Anaesth Soc J* 1984;31:468.
177. Brost BC, Newman RB, Fries M, Calhoun BC. The effects of hemodialysis on total intrauterine volume. *Ultrasound Obstet Gynecol* 1996;8:34.
178. Okundaye I, Hou S. Management of pregnancy in women undergoing continuous ambulatory peritoneal dialysis. *Adv Perit Dial* 1996;12: 151.
179. Hou S. Pregnancy and birth control in CAPD patients. *Adv Perit Dial* 1993;9:173.
180. Hou S. Pregnancy in women treated with peritoneal dialysis: viewpoint 1996. *Perit Dial Int* 1996;16:442.
181. Redrow M, Cherem L, Elliott J, et al. Dialysis in the management of pregnant patients with renal insufficiency. *Medicine* 1988;67:199.
182. Knuppel RA, Montenegro R, O'Brien WF. Acute renal failure in pregnancy. *Clin Obstet Gynecol* 1985;28:288.
183. Stratta P, Besso L, Canavese C, et al. Is pregnancy-related acute renal failure a disappearing clinical entity. *Ren Fail* 1996;18(4):575.
184. Alexopoulos E, Tambakoudis P, Bili H, et al. Acute renal failure in pregnancy. *Ren Fail* 1993;15:609.
185. Centers for Disease Control. Anemia during pregnancy in low income women—United States 1987. *MMWR* 1990;39:73.
186. Hallak M, Sharon A, Diukman R, et al. Supplementing iron intravenously in pregnancy. *J Reprod Med* 1997;42:99.
187. Goodlin RC. Maternal hematocrit and premature labor. *Am J Obstet Gynecol* 1989;161:1750.
188. Longo LD. Maternal blood volume and cardiac output during pregnancy: a hypothesis of endocrinologic control. *Am J Physiol* 1983;83: R720.
189. Garn SM, Ridella SA, Petzold AS, Falkner F. Maternal hematologic levels and pregnancy outcomes. *Semin Perinatol* 1981;5:155.
190. Romslo I, Haram K, Sagen N, Augensen K. Iron requirement in normal pregnancy as assessed by serum ferritin, serum transferrin, saturation and erythrocyte protoporphyin determinations. *Br J Obstet Gynaceol* 1983;90:101.
191. Murphy JF, Newcomber RG, O'Riordan J, et al. Relation of haemoglobin levels in the first and second trimester to outcome of pregnancy. *Lancet* 1986;I:992.
192. Schwartz WJ, Thurnau GR. Iron deficiency anemia in pregnancy. *Clin Obstet Gynecol* 1995;38:443.
193. Okuyama T, Tawada F, Furuya H, Villee CA. The role of transferrin and ferritin in the fetal-maternal placental unit. *Am J Obstet Gynecol* 1985;152:344.
194. Milman N, Agger AO, Nielson OJ. Iron status markers and serum erythropoietin in 120 mothers and newborn infants: effect of iron supplementation in normal pregnancy. *Acta Obstet Gynecol Scand* 1994; 73:200.
195. Scholl TO, Hediger ML. Anemia and iron deficiency anemia: compilation of data on pregnancy outcome. *Am J Clin Nutr* 1994;59:492S.
196. Hamstra RD, Block MH, Schocket AL. Intravenous iron dextran in clinical medicine. *JAMA* 1980;243:1726.
197. Kumpf VJ. Parenteral iron supplementation. *Nutr Clin Prac* 1996;11: 139.
198. Taylor DJ. Prophylaxis and treatment of anaemia during pregnancy. *Clin Obstet Gynaecol* 1981;8:297.
199. Campbell BA. Megaloblastic anemia in pregnancy. *Clin Obstet Gynecol* 1995;38:455.
200. Kilpatrick SJ, Laros RK. Thalassemia in pregnancy. *Clin Obstet Gynecol* 1995;38:485.
201. American College of Obstetricians and Gynecologists Technical Bulletin Number 200—February 1996. Hemoglobinopathies in pregnancy. *Int J Gynecol Obstet* 1996;53:184.
202. Jenson CE, Tuck SM, Wonke B. Fertility in β thalassaemia major: a report of 16 pregnancies, preconceptual evaluation and a review of the literature. *Br J Obstet Gynaecol* 1995;102:625.
203. Kumar RM, Rizk DEE, Khuranna A. β-Thalassemia major and successful pregnancy. *J Reprod Med* 1997;42:294.
204. Alger LS, Golbus MS, Laros RK. Thalassemia and pregnancy: results of an antenatal screening program. *Am J Obstet Gynecol* 1979;134: 662.
205. Veille JC, Hanson R. Left ventricular systolic and diastolic function in pregnant patients with sickle cell disease. *Am J Obstet Gynecol* 1994; 170:107.
206. Baill IC, Witter FR. Sickle cell trait and its association with birth weight and urinary tract infection in pregnancy. *Int J Fed Obstet Gynecol* 1990;33:19.
207. Smith JA, Espeland M, Bellevue R, et al. Pregnancy in sickle cell disease: experience of the cooperative study of sickle cell disease. *Obstet Gynecol* 1996;87:199.
208. Howard RJ. Management of sickling conditions in pregnancy. *Br J Hosp Med* 1996;56:7.
209. Danzer BI, Birnbach DJ, Thys DM. Anesthesia for the parturient with sickle cell disease. *J Clin Anesth* 1996;8:598.
210. Koshy M. Sickle cell disease and pregnancy. *Blood Rev* 1995;9:157.
211. McLain C. Leukemia in pregnancy. *Clin Obstet Gynecol* 1974;17:185.
212. Siddiqui T, Elfenbein GJ, Noyes WD, et al. Myelodysplastic syndromes presenting in pregnancy. *Cancer* 1990;66:377.
213. Reynoso EE, Huerta F. Acute leukemia and pregnancy—fatal fetal outcome after exposure to idarubicin during the second trimester. *Acta Oncol* 1994;33:709.
214. Harrison P, Chipping P, Fothergill GA. Successful use of all-trans retinoic acid in acute promyelocytic leukemia presenting during the second trimester of pregnancy. *Br J Haematol* 1994;86:681.
215. Stenloft J, Lanng Nielsen J, Hvidman LE. All-trans retinoic acid in acute promyelocytic leukemia in late pregnancy. *Leukemia* 1994;8:1585.
216. Hoffman MA, Wiernik PH, Kleiner GJ. Acute promyelocytic leukemia and pregnancy. *Cancer* 1995;76:2237.
217. Antonelli NM, Dotters DJ, Katz VL, Kuller JA. Cancer in pregnancy: a review of the literature. Part II. *Obstet Gynecol Surv* 1996; 51:135.
218. Aitchison RG, Marsh JCW, Hows JM, et al. Pregnancy-associated aplastic anemia: a report of 5 cases and review of current management. *Br J Haematol* 1989;73:541.
219. Flessa HC. Hemorrhagic disorders and pregnancy. *Clin Obstet Gynecol* 1974;17:236.
220. Kelton JG. Management of the pregnant patient with idiopathic thrombocytopenia purpura. *Ann Intern Med* 1983;99:796.
221. Iyori H, Fujisawa K, Akatsuka J. Thrombocytopenia in neonates born to women with autoimmune thrombocytopenic purpura. *Ped Hematol Oncol* 1997;14:367.
222. George JN, Woolf SH, Raskof GE, et al. Idiopathic thrombocytopenic purpura: a practice guideline developed by explicit methods for the American Society of Hematology. *Blood* 1996;88:3.
223. The American Society of Hematology ITP Practice Guideline Panel. Diagnosis and treatment of idiopathic thrombocytopenic purpura: recommendations of the American Society of Hematology. *Ann Intern Med* 1997;126:319.
224. Byrne JD, Incerpi MH, Goodwin TM. Idiopathic thrombocytopenic purpura in pregnancy treated with pulsed high-dose oral dexamethasone. *Am J Obstet Gynecol* 1997;177:468.
225. Lavery JP, Koontz WL, Liu YK, Howell R. Immunologic thrombocytopenia in pregnancy: use of antenatal immunoglobulin therapy. Case report and review. *Obstet Gynecol* 1985;66:415.
226. Hedge UM. Immune thrombocytopenia in pregnancy and the newborn. *Br J Obstet Gynaecol* 1985;92:657.

227. Thompson AR, Harker LA. *Manual of hemostasis and thrombosis,* 3rd ed. Philadelphia: FA Davis, 1983.
228. Burrows RF, Kelton JG. Fetal thrombocytopenia and its relation to maternal thrombocytopenia. *N Engl J Med* 1993;329:1463.
229. Matthews JH, Benjamin S, Gill DS, Smith NA. Pregnancy associated thrombocytopenia: definition, incidence and natural history. *Acta Haematol* 1990;84:24.
230. Anteby E, Shaley O. Clinical relevance of gestational thrombocytopenia of <100000/microliters. *Am J Hematol* 1994;47:118.
231. Bell WR, Kickler TS. Thrombocytopenia in pregnancy. *Rheum Dis Clin North Am* 1997;23:183.
232. Lescale KB, Eddleman KA, Cines DB, et al. Antiplatelet antibody testing in thrombocytopenic pregnant women. *Am J Obstet Gynecol* 1996;174:1014.
233. Bierling P, Bettaieb A, Oksenhendler E. Human immunodeficiency virus-related immune thrombocytopenia. *Semin Thromb Hemost* 1995;21:68.
234. Mandelbrot L, Schlienger I, Bongain A, et al. Thrombocytopenia in pregnant women infected with human immunodeficiency virus: maternal and neonatal outcome. *Am J Obstet Gynecol* 1994;171:252.
235. Ballem PJ, Belzberg A, Devine DV, et al. Kinetic studies of the mechanism of thrombocytopenia in patients with human immunodeficiency virus infection. *N Engl J Med* 1992;327:1779.
236. Gershon RY, Dolak J, Board E, et al. Platelets and the HIV-infected parturient (abstract). *Anesth Analg* 1998;86[Suppl]:S368.
237. Najean Y, Rain JD. The mechanism of thrombocytopenia in patients with HIV infection. *J Lab Clin Med* 1994;123:415.
238. Kelton JG, Hunter DJ, Neame PB. A platelet function defect in preeclampsia. *Obstet Gynecol* 1985;65:107.
239. Ramanathan J, Sibai BM, Vu T, Chauhan D. Correlation between bleeding times and platelet counts in women with preeclampsia undergoing cesarean section. *Anesthesiology* 1989;71:188.
240. Leduc L, Wheeler JM, Kirshon B, Mitchell P, Cotton DB. Coagulation profile in severe preeclampsia. *Obstet Gynecol* 1992;79:14.
241. Ahlawat S, Pati HP, Bhatla N, et al. Plasma platelet aggregating factor and platelet aggregation studies in pre-eclampsia. *Acta Obstet Gynecol Scand* 1996;75:428.
242. Orlikowski CEP, Rocke DA, Murray WB, et al. Thrombelastography changes in pre-eclampsia and eclampsia. *Br J Anaesth* 1996;77:157.
243. Aster RH, George JN. Thrombocytopenia due to enhanced platelet destruction by immunologic mechanisms. In: Williams WJ, Beutler E, Ersley AJ, Lichtman MA, eds. *Haematology.* New York: McGraw-Hill, 1991:1370.
244. Biswas A, Arulkumaran, Ratnam SS. Disorders of platelets in pregnancy. *Obstet Gynecol Surv* 1994;49:585.
245. Kain ZN, Mayes LC, Pakes J, et al. Thrombocytopenia in pregnant women who use cocaine. *Am J Obstet Gynecol* 1995;173:885.
246. Birnbach DJ, Stein DJ, Fogelberg R, et al. Thrombocytopenia in the cocaine abusing parturient. *Anesthesiology* 1994;81[Suppl]:1181.
247. Kain ZN, Mayes L, Pakes J, Schottenfield R. Thrombocytopenia in cocaine abusing parturients: a case control study. *Anesthesiology* 1994;81[Suppl]:1182.
248. Abramowicz JS, Sherer DM, Woods JR. Acute transient thrombocytopenia associated with cocaine abuse in pregnancy. *Obstet Gynecol* 1991;78:499.
249. Burday MJ, Martin ES. Cocaine induced thrombocytopenia. *Am J Med* 1991;91:656.
250. Leissinger CA. Severe thrombocytopenia associated with cocaine abuse. *Ann Intern Med* 1990;112:708.
251. Orser B. Thrombocytopenia and cocaine abuse. *Anesthesiology* 1991;74:195.
252. Gershon RY, Fisher AJ, Graves WL. The cocaine-abusing parturient is not at an increased risk for thrombocytopenia. *Anesth Analg* 1996; 82:865.
253. Gershon RY, Dolak J, Stack K, et al. The cocaine-abusing parturient is not at an increased risk for thrombocytopathy. *Anesthesiology* 1997; 87:A875.
254. Ewenstein BM. The pathophysiology of bleeding disorders presenting as abnormal uterine bleeding. *Am J Obstet Gynecol* 1996;175:770.
255. Writer WDR. Hematologic disease. In: James FM III, Wheeler AS, Dewan DM, eds. *Obstetric anesthesia: the complicated patient*, 2nd ed. Philadelphia: FA Davis, 1988:267.
256. Ellison N. Hemostasis and hemotherapy. In: Barash PG, Cullen BF, Stoelting RK, eds. *Clinical anesthesia.* Philadelphia: JB Lippincott Co., 1989:707.
257. Hanna W, McCarroll D, McDonald T, et al. Variant von Willebrand's disease and pregnancy. *Blood* 1981;58:873.
258. Lipton RA, Ayromlooi J, Coller BS. Severe von Willebrand's disease during labor and delivery. *JAMA* 1982;248:1355.
259. Nishino M, Nishino S, Sugimoto M, et al. Changes in factor VIII binding capacity of von Willebrand factor and factor VIII coagulant activity in two patients with type 2N von Willebrand disease after hemostatic treatment and during pregnancy. *Int J Hematol* 1996;64:127.
260. Ito M, Yoshimura K, Toyoda N, Wada H. Pregnancy and delivery in patients with von Willebrand's disease. *J Obstet Gynaecol Res* 1997; 23:37.
261. Kadir RA, Koh MB, Lee CA, Pasi KJ. Acquired haemophilia, an unusual cause of severe postpartum haemorrhage. *Br J Obstet Gynaecol* 1997;104:854.
262. Caldwell DC. Williamson RA, Goldsmith JG. Hereditary coagulopathies in pregnancy. *Clin Obstet Gynecol* 1985;28:53.
263. Kadir RA, Economides DL, Braithwaite J, et al. The obstetric experience of carriers of haemophilia. *Br J Obstet Gynaecol* 1997;104:803.
264. Dinsmoor MJ, Hogg BB. Autologous blood donation with placenta previa: it is feasible? *Am J Perinatol* 1995;12:382.
265. Kruskall MS, Leonard S, Klapholz H. Autologous blood donation during pregnancy: analysis of safety and blood use. *Obstet Gynecol* 1987; 70:938.
266. O'Dwyer G, Mylotte M, Sweeney M, Egan EL. Experience of autologous blood transfusion in an obstetrics and gynaecology department. *Br J Obstet Gynaecol* 1993;100:571.
267. McVay PA, Hoag RW, Hoag MS, Toy PT. Safety and use of autologous blood donation during the third trimester of pregnancy. *Am J Obstet Gynecol* 1989;160:1479.
268. Druzin ML, Wolf CF, Edersheim TG, et al. Donation of blood by the pregnant patient for autologous transfusion. *Am J Obstet Gynecol* 1988;159:1023.
269. Basta LL. *Cardiovascular disease.* New York: Medical Examination Publishing Co., 1983.
270. Tavel ME. *Clinical phonocardiography and external pulse recording,* 4th ed. Chicago: Year-Book Medical Publishers, 1985:169.
271. Grossman W. *Cardiac catheterization and angiography,* 2nd ed. Philadelphia: Lea & Febiger, 1980:124.
272. Davison JM, Noble MCB. Serial changes in 24-hour creatinine clearance during normal menstrual cycles and the first trimester of pregnancy. *Br J Obstet Gynaecol* 1981;88:10.
273. Hillman RS, Finch CA. *Red cell manual,* 5th ed. Philadelphia: FA Davis, 1985:60.
274. Schwartz E, Benz EJ. The thalassemia syndromes. In: Hoffman R, Benz E, eds. *Hematology: basic principles and practice*. London: Churchill Livingstone, 1991.
275. Lubin B, Vichinsky F. Sickle cell disease. In: Hoffman R, Benz E, eds. *Hematology: basic principles and practice*. London: Churchill Livingstone, 1991:4591.
276. Hawiger J. Formation and regulation of platelet and fibrin hemostatic plug. *Hum Pathol* 1987;18:111.
277. Hytten FE, Leitch I. *The physiology of pregnancy,* 2nd ed. Oxford: Blackwell Science, 1971.
278. Svrian M. Glomerular disease and pregnancy: a study of 123 pregnancies in patients with primary and secondary disease. *Nephron* 1984;36:101.
279. Lindheimer MD, Katz AI. The kidney and hypertension in pregnancy. In: Brenner BM, Rector FL, eds. *The kidney,* 4th ed. Philadelphia: WB Saunders, 1991:1551.

Obstetric Anesthesia, second edition,
edited by Mark C. Norris.
Lippincott Williams & Wilkins, Philadelphia © 1999.

CHAPTER 3

Preoperative Evaluation of the Parturient with Coexisting Disease

Part II: Pulmonary and Neuromuscular Disease, Acquired Immunodeficiency Syndrome, and Substance Abuse

Richard B. Becker

This chapter explores the preanesthetic evaluation of parturients who have common respiratory or neurological diseases. We also examine, from a preanesthetic point of view, the more specific topic of substance abuse among pregnant women and the increasingly prevalent human immunodeficiency virus (HIV)-positive parturient with acquired immunodeficiency syndrome (AIDS).

RESPIRATORY DISEASE

Changes in Respiratory Physiology in Pregnancy

Figure 1 reviews the major respiratory changes in pregnancy (1–3).

Asthma

Asthma, which complicates approximately 1% of pregnancies, is the most common pulmonary disease in women of child-bearing age (4). In asthmatic patients, the tracheobronchial tree is more sensitive to a variety of stimuli. In response to provocation, bronchospasm and the major symptoms of asthma (dyspnea, wheezing, and cough) occur. Asthmatic symptoms vary from mild and almost undetectable to the severe and unremitting syndrome of status asthmaticus. The primary physiologic manifestation of this hyperresponsiveness is intermittent small airway obstruction. Hypersecretion of mucus, mucosal edema, and smooth muscle hyper contractility also contribute to the obstructive physiology of this disease. Airway obstruction from smooth muscle contraction is most marked on expiration, creating air trapping and hyperinflation.

Pathophysiology

Classically, asthma has two forms: intrinsic and extrinsic. Table 1 compares intrinsic and extrinsic asthma. Extrinsic asthma tends to be a seasonal allergic response to inhaled irritants. These patients usually have a lifelong history of allergies and have elevated blood and sputum eosinophils and increased serum immunoglobulin E (IgE) concentrations (5). In contrast, patients with the intrinsic form are often older and may not have a seasonal allergic predisposition. These patients typically have normal serum IgE and eosinophils but may have increased sputum eosinophils. Because of the nonspecific nature of intrinsic asthma, it is usually more difficult to treat (6). The distinction between the two forms may not be clear, and an individual may have elements of each. Common factors that can precipitate bronchospasm include:

- IgE-mediated hypersensitivity to inhaled irritants,
- Acute inflammatory disease,
- Cold,
- Exercise,
- Aspirin,

R. B. Becker: Department of Anesthesia, George Washington Hospital, Washington, DC 20037.

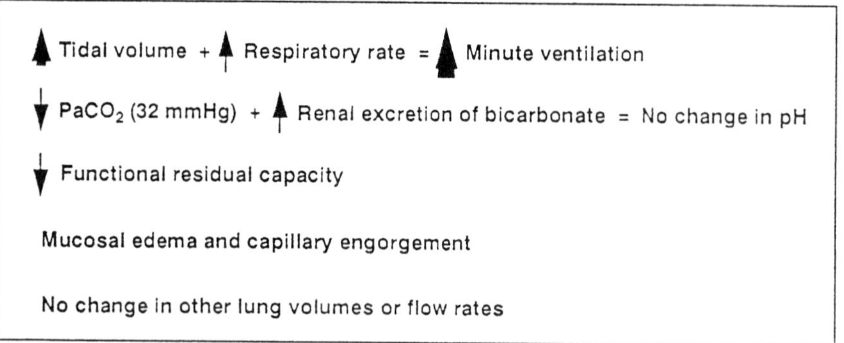

FIG. 1. Review of the major respiratory changes in pregnancy.

- Non–immune-mediated (direct) bronchoconstriction to inhaled substances (e.g., animal dander, dust, and smoke),
- Emotional stress, and
- Mechanical stimulation (e.g., intubation of the trachea).

Several theories attempt to explain the pathophysiology of asthma. One hypothesis claims that asthma represents an imbalance between the sympathetic and parasympathetic nervous systems. Vagal tone and α-adrenergic action predominate over β-adrenergic action (7). Another theory suggests that asthma patients produce autoantibodies to β-adrenergic receptors (8). A final idea proposes that various stimuli produce inflammatory pulmonary changes in susceptible individuals (9). Little definitive evidence supports most of these theories (10). However, in inflammatory-mediated asthma, evidence suggests that the process proceeds in the following manner. Upon reexposure of an individual to a particular allergen, an antigen–antibody complex forms and binds to specific mast cell receptors. This binding induces mast cell degranulation with release of vasoactive and cell-mediator biochemicals, including histamine, leukotrienes, prostaglandins, platelet-activating factor, and cell chemotactic factors. These mediators produce vascular and airway changes, causing the symptoms seen during an asthma attack. They also attract increased numbers of inflammatory cells (macrophages and esosinophils) that cause further capillary endothelial and airway epithelial cell damage. This damage increases vascular permeability and incites airway hyperreactivity, resulting in further airway compromise from mucosal edema and bronchoconstriction (10,11).

The mediators also may directly affect the autonomic control of airway tone (10). Stimulation of parasympathetic airway fibers increases intracellular cyclic guanosine monophosphate (cGMP). This increase promotes bronchial smooth muscle contraction (bronchoconstriction) and airflow obstruction.

Clinical evidence of obstruction includes wheezing, hyperinflated lung volumes, and decreased forced expiratory volume. The ultimate effects of obstruction are ventilation-perfusion abnormalities with resultant hypoxemia and hypercarbia. Bronchoconstriction reverses when sympathetic stimulation of β_2 receptors increases intracellular cyclic adenosine monophosphate (cAMP). By interfering with bronchial smooth muscle actinomyosin activity, cAMP produces muscle relaxation and bronchodilation (12). Figure 2 summarizes the pathophysiology of asthma.

TABLE 1. *Comparison of intrinsic and extrinsic asthma*

Intrinsic	Extrinsic
Seasonal allergies	Lifelong allergies
Normal serum IgE and eosinophils	Increased blood and sputum eosinophils
Increased sputum eosinophils	Increased serum IgE concentration

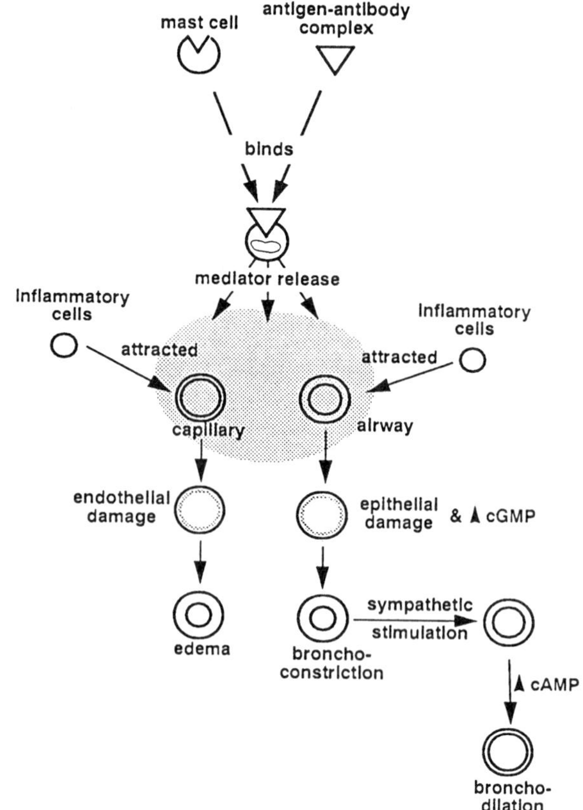

FIG. 2. The asthma process.

Interaction with Pregnancy

Effect of Pregnancy on Asthma

Few studies show a consistent effect of pregnancy on preexisting asthma. A review of 1,054 pregnancies found that half of the parturients reported no change in the severity of asthma symptoms, 29% improved, and 21% got worse (13). Recently, a small study found a strong overall decline in airway responsiveness in pregnancy. This improvement is greatest in those with the most hyperresponsive airways (14). Asthma-related changes during gestation are difficult to study. It is hard to distinguish between the changes induced by the disease and those normally caused by pregnancy. Two things seem clear:

- Patients with severe asthma before pregnancy will have the most severe exacerbations during pregnancy, and
- The course of asthma in previous pregnancies is the best predictor of the course in future pregnancies (15,16).

The most common causes for exacerbation are respiratory tract infection (59%) and noncompliance with therapeutic regimens (27%) (17).

Specific pregnancy-related changes may worsen the course of asthma. Production of prostaglandin $F_{2\alpha}$ (a known bronchoconstrictor) increases (18). Changes in cell-mediated immunity may increase the parturient's susceptibility to infection (19).

Plasma concentrations of cortisol and progesterone (which induces smooth muscle relaxation) rise during gestation and may improve asthma. Progesterone was formerly believed to be a major factor in the improvement of asthma during pregnancy. However, there is no statistically significant relationship between serum progesterone concentration and airway response. Therefore, if progesterone does improve asthma, it does not work alone (20).

Effect of Asthma on Pregnancy

Asthma may complicate pregnancy in several ways (Table 2) (21). One large study reported increases in hemorrhage, hyperemesis, and toxemia. This and other studies found an association between asthma and neonatal deaths, preterm deliveries, and low-birth-weight infants (22,23). During an acute asthma attack, maternal hypoxemia and respiratory alkalosis may severely compromise the fetus. Maternal–fetal oxygen exchange depends on, among other things, maternal arterial oxygen tension and the oxygen affinity of maternal blood.

Maternal hypoxemia lessens the maternal–fetal oxygen diffusion gradient, hindering oxygen delivery to the fetus. Maternal alkalosis causes leftward shift of the oxyhemoglobin dissociation curve, resulting in a greater affinity of maternal hemoglobin for oxygen and less exchange to the fetus. The fetus inhabits a relatively hypoxemic environment with an umbilical venous oxygen partial pressure of approximately 33 mm Hg (24). Fetal hemoglobin has a greater affinity for oxygen than maternal hemoglobin and can release oxygen more efficiently to the tissues at low partial pressures. As a consequence, the fetus rapidly develops hypoxemia and risks vital organ damage when its oxygen supply is compromised. A well-documented study of patients with severe asthma attempted to determine perinatal effects of uncontrolled asthma. It showed that status asthmaticus during pregnancy may be deleterious to both the mother and the fetus, and management of asthma to prevent episodes of status asthmaticus may result in a favorable outcome (25).

TABLE 2. *Asthma complications of pregnancy*

Hemorrhage	Neonatal deaths
Hyperemesis	Preterm deliveries
Toxemia	Low-birth-weight infants

Pharmacotherapy

Management goals in treating asthma include:

- Identification and removal of precipitating factors,
- Proper rest, nutrition, and hydration,
- Aggressive antibiotic treatment of infection, and
- Pharmacotherapy where indicated.

Strongly consider the risk–benefit ratios of therapeutic interventions. Avoid drugs that are teratogenic or otherwise harmful to the fetus. Pharmacotherapy for pregnant asthmatics differs very little from that used in the nonpregnant patient. The available evidence suggest that commonly employed drugs are safe for use in the pregnant patient. The benefits of avoiding uncontrolled asthma outweigh the risks of drug-induced fetal malformation. But, as it is impossible to eliminate all possibility of fetal hazard, avoid drug use in the first trimester if maternal condition allows.

Bronchodilator Agents

β Agonists. β-adrenergic stimulation relaxes bronchial smooth muscle by increasing intracellular concentrations of cAMP (Fig. 3). β-agonist bronchodilators are safe for use throughout pregnancy, and no reports link their use with congenital defects (26). However, use of β agonists may interfere with normal labor due to uterine relaxation and may contribute to postpartum uterine atony and hemorrhage. Choose drugs and routes of administration to maximize β_2 effects (bronchial dilation) and minimize β_1 effects (tachycardia). Terbutaline, metaproterenol, salmeterol, and albuterol are the most β_2-selective agents. Aerosol administration speeds onset, reduces the side effects from systemic absorption, and enhances β_2 specificity.

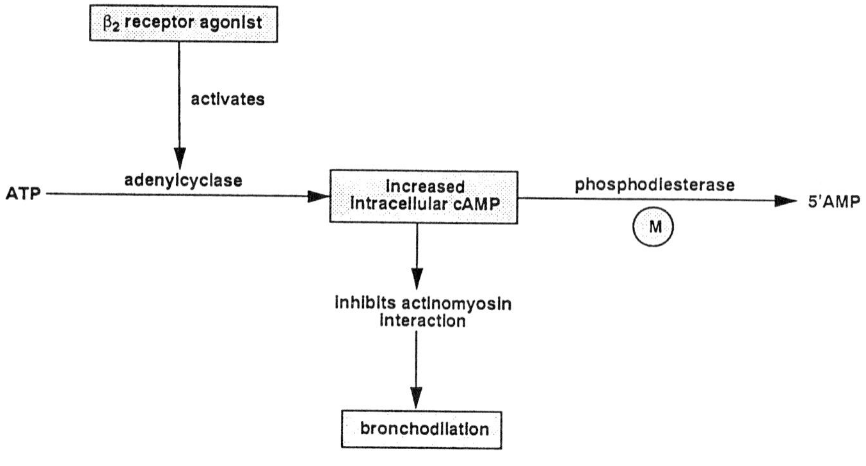

FIG. 3. Mechanisms of action of β-adrenergic bronchodilators.

Epinephrine has α-adrenergic (possible uteroplacental vasconstriction) effects along with nonspecific β-adrenergic activity. Some authors advocate its use during gestation to control acute asthma (27). Others argue against it because of possible fetal distress. In cases of life-threatening asthma refractory to other therapies, use epinephrine without hesitation because of the high risk of maternal and fetal complications resulting from respiratory failure.

Parasympatholytics. The anticholinergic agent ipratropium bromide relaxes bronchial smooth muscles by competitive inhibition of vagus-mediated bronchoconstriction. Aerosol administration minimizes systemic anticholinergic effects (e.g., tachycardia, dry mouth). Because use of this agent in pregnancy has not been well studied, avoid it unless other drugs have failed.

Methylxanthines. Theophylline and its water-soluble salt aminophylline are methylxanthines. The exact mechanism of action of these agents is unknown. The most common theory is that they inhibit phosphodiesterase, the enzyme responsible for the breakdown of cAMP. This action increases intracellular cAMP (Fig. 3). Other theories suggest that the methylxanthines modulate the interaction of actinomyosin and calcium, antagonize prostaglandins, or inhibit adenosine (28–30). Inhibition of adenosine releases endogenous catecholamines, augmenting the bronchodilatory effects of cAMP. Adenosine antagonism also attenuates the release of mast cell mediators (29).

Methylxanthines have a long record of safe use in pregnancy and have traditionally been used as adjuvants to β-agonist therapy. However, recent evidence suggests that aminophylline does not add significant improvement to the standard β-agonist–steroid therapy in adult asthma exacerbations (31).

The most common dosing regimen advises an intravenous bolus of aminophylline (85% theophylline by weight) of 5 mg/kg, followed by a maintenance dose of 0.5 to 1.0 mg/kg/hour to achieve a therapeutic plasma concentration between 10 and 20 μg/mL. Monitor theophylline concentration closely in the last half of pregnancy. Some studies have found significantly reduced theophylline clearance during the third trimester. Some patients develop signs of toxicity with their usual doses (32). The most likely mechanisms of this effect include reduced hepatic metabolism and increased theophylline absorption from the gastrointestinal tract (33). These findings contradict previous suggestions that higher theophylline doses may be needed to compensate for an increased volume of distribution in pregnancy (34).

Antiinflammatory Agents

Steroids. Glucocorticoids have potent antiinflammatory effects that are beneficial in treating asthma (35). Steroids function by altering protein production, inhibiting mediator release, and suppressing inflammatory mediator action. During an acute asthma exacerbation, steroids increase the synthesis of proteins that inhibit the production of prostaglandins and platelet-activating factor. They also increase the synthesis of new β_2 receptors (36). Steroids regulate protein synthesis through gene induction. Glucocorticoids bind to and activate cell receptors. The activated receptor complex binds to the nucleus and then to gene regulators. The regulator then activates or inhibits gene transcription and ultimately increases or decreases protein production by that gene (Fig. 4). (37).

Steroids also suppress the symptoms of asthma by mediating other processes (Table 3). They increase the responsiveness of β receptors to catecholamines, potentiate β-agonist bronchodilation, and reverse β-receptor fatigue from prolonged stimulation (31). In addition, steroids reduce airway edema by inhibiting the release of chemical mediators and suppressing their adverse effect on microvascular permeability (38). Finally, steroids inhibit the for-

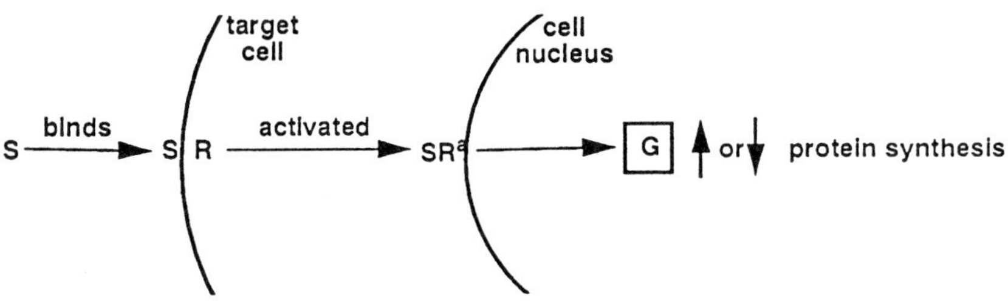

FIG. 4. Steroid regulation of protein synthesis.

mation of inflammatory cell chemotactic mediators and inactivate inflammatory cells already involved in the asthma process (39).

Steroid use in pregnancy is not greatly different from its use in treating nonpregnant asthmatics. Although high-dose systemic steroids may be lifesaving in treating acute asthma, some therapeutic actions have a lengthy onset. Use alternative therapies to medicate the attack until steroid onset. Steroid use in the chronic asthmatic is less well defined. Dunlap and Bailey (40) give the following recommendations:

- For chronic maintenance, use the lowest effective dose.
- Aerosol administration may help eliminate or reduce systemic steroid use. It also localizes the action of steroids and reduces systemic side effects, thereby minimizing the risk of adrenal suppression. If patients have used high-dose systemic steroids for 1 month or longer, adrenal suppression is possible. Taper doses when discontinuing the drug.
- During periods of increased physiologic stress, these patients may require steroid supplementation.

Cromolyn Sodium. Cromolyn sodium is an aerosol agent that prevents degranulation of mast cells by membrane stabilization. It is reasonably safe in pregnancy, but only as a prophylactic agent. Do not use it to treat acute bronchospasm because it cannot counter effects of previously released substances.

Evaluation

History is the most valuable tool in evaluating a stable asthmatic (Table 4). In an acute crisis, however, management of hypoxia and respiratory compromise take precedence over gathering history (41). In addition, asking the patient how she rates her current ability to breathe provides a rough idea of the degree of bronchospasm.

Note the patient's general appearance. Marked tachypnea, cyanosis, and fatigue signal impending respiratory failure. Wheezing is evidence of diffuse bronchoconstriction and is a sign of air exchange; lack of wheezing is more serious and demotes inability to ventilate. Increasing use of accessory muscles and nostril flaring point to worsening distress. Note the patient's ability to converse. Someone who can speak in sentences is less ill than someone working so hard to breathe that she cannot speak at all. Additionally, note heart rate. Tachycardia is a compensatory response to stress and hypoxia; bradycardia may precede hypoxic cardiac arrest. Also, a decrease in heart rate of 15 beats/min or greater with inspiration (pulsus paradoxus) is a nonspecific indication of a severe attack. An elevated temperature may signal acute infection.

Other data can be helpful in evaluating an acute asthma attack. Obtain serum electrolytes and a complete blood count. Gram stain any sputum. Take a chest radiograph with abdominal shielding to protect the fetus. Evaluate the radiograph for any acute underlying infectious

TABLE 3. *Steroid action*

Alter protein production
New β_2 receptors
Inhibit synthesis of prostaglandins and platelet-activating factor
Suppress biochemical mediator release
Augment function of β_2 receptors
Reverse β_2-receptor fatigue
Inhibit inflammatory cell function

TABLE 4. *Pertinent history in parturients with acute exacerbation of asthma*

Previous attacks
Number
Severity
Duration
Previous emergency room visits
Number
Most recent
Previous need for intubation and mechanical ventilation
Course of asthma in previous pregnancies
Current therapy
Medications
Compliance
Known precipitating factors
Environmental exposures
Recent or current upper respiratory infection
Coexisting pulmonary or cardiac problems

TABLE 5. *Treatment of acute asthma*

Unstable asthma	Stable asthma
Correct hypoxemia and acidosis	Obtain history
Support ventilation, if necessary	Remove precipitating factors
Give supplemental oxygen	Hydrate
Give bronchodilators and steroids	Obtain clinical studies (labs, arterial blood gas, chest radiograph, spirometry, sputum stain)
Treat underlying cause	Initiate pharmacotherapy
Proceed to **stable asthma** treatment when stable	Bronchodilators
	Steroids
	Consider aminophylline
	Antibiotics for infection
	Repeat clinical studies to assess efficacy of therapy

process, hyperinflation, pneumothorax, or pneumomediastinum. An arterial blood gas can be critical in evaluating severity. Remember that blood gas values normally change in pregnancy. The blood gas will uniformly show hypoxemia; therefore, this parameter is not as useful as a pH and p_aCO_2. If the patient has alkalosis and lower-than-normal pregnancy p_aCO_2 (32 mm Hg), the attack is mild, If the observed pH and p_aCO_2 are normal for pregnancy, the attack is more severe. Acidosis and hypercapnia (pH = 7.35, p_aCO_2 = 35 to 38 mm Hg) signal impending respiratory failure, especially combined with a p_aO_2 less than 60 mm Hg (42).

Spirometry also can provide useful information. A single set of values for forced expiratory volume in 1 second (FEV_1) and peak expiratory flow may not be significant because nomograms are not available for parturients. However, a series of measurements taken before and at intervals after treatment can determine the efficacy of therapy (41). For a summary of the treatment of acute asthma, refer to Table 5.

Differential Diagnosis

The initial reaction to acute respiratory distress may be to assume that its etiology is asthma. However, the following causes of respiratory distress should be eliminated:

- Acute upper airway obstruction,
- Pulmonary embolism,
- Anaphylaxis,
- Congestive heart failure,
- Acute infection,
- Chronic obstructive pulmonary disease, and
- Aspiration pneumonitis.

Cystic Fibrosis

Cystic fibrosis (CF) is a multisystem, autosomal recessive disorder that occurs in approximately 1 in 1,000 births. It is the most common lethal genetic disorder in whites. The disease is one of chronic exocrine gland dysfunction, but the underlying defect is unknown. CF shows itself through the dysfunction of several systems. These patients produce thick, tenacious mucus. They suffer pancreatic insufficiency with accompanying protein and fat malabsorption. Hepatobiliary disease with chronic cholestasis, fibrosis, and cirrhosis occurs. Last, abnormally high sweat duct excretion of sodium chloride is seen. The abnormal electrolyte content of sweat confirms the diagnosis in patients exhibiting symptoms of the disease. Patients typically are diagnosed early in childhood, but milder forms of the disease may not be recognized until much later.

The average survival of patients with CF is 20 to 30 years, with death usually from respiratory failure. Patients have persistent bronchial infections, usually with *Pseudomonas aeruginosa.* Chronic infection generates airway fibrosis and, later, parenchymal fibrosis, ventilation-perfusion mismatching, and hypoxemia.

Improved survival of CF patients has allowed women to reach child-bearing age (Fig. 5) (43). The maternal outcome of pregnancy correlates with maternal condition before conception. Pregnant women with mild disease usually do well, whereas those with moderate or severe disease may deteriorate (44). Pregnancy itself does not seem to influence the course of the disease. Patient dete-

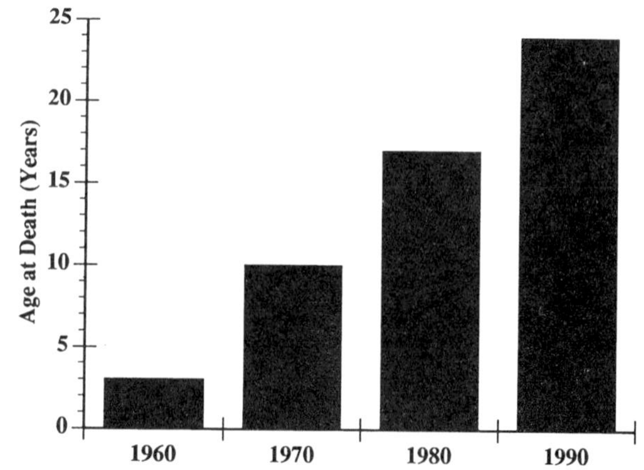

FIG. 5. Increasing survival of patients with cystic fibrosis.

rioration in pregnancy stems from natural progression of the disease (45). Maternal condition during gestation predicts perinatal outcome. Chronically, hypoxemic and malnourished mothers have increased perinatal morbidity and mortality, whereas well-managed mothers with mild disease have improved outcomes (42).

Treatment of CF aims at the reparatory system. Advances in this area are responsible for the increased survival of patients. Aggressive antibiotic therapy for infection along with avid pharmacologic and physiotherapeutic measures to facilitate removal of secretions are the mainstays of management. Additionally, pancreatic enzyme replacement will decrease gastrointestinal malabsorption, and vitamin K supplementations can correct bleeding problems that arise from poor hepatic function or malabsorption of fat-soluble vitamins.

The preanesthetic evaluation of the pregnant patient with CF focuses on the degree of respiratory compromise. Ensure that the patient is in the best possible pulmonary condition. Hydrate the patient well to help her clear secretions. If there is any suspicion of a pulmonary infection, obtain a sputum gram stain and initiate appropriate antibiotic therapy. Laboratory evaluation can detect electrolyte imbalance, acute infection, or coagulation defect. Arterial blood gas tensions or pulse oximetry will detect hypoxemia. Changes with time may help in assessing the degree of respiratory deterioration.

Cigarette Smoking

Smoking during pregnancy has many adverse maternal and fetal consequences. For the mother, smoking increases airway irritability and mucus production, and impairs respiratory tract mucociliary function. The inhalation of carbon monoxide from smoke produces carboxyhemoglobin, shifting both maternal and fetal oxyhemoglobin dissociation curves leftward. This shift limits oxygen exchange between the mother and fetus and between the fetus and its vital organs. In addition, smoking is the leading risk factor for the development of pulmonary malignancies and chronic obstructive pulmonary disease (COPD).

Increased expiratory airway resistance with air trapping complicates both forms of COPD—emphysema and chronic bronchitis. Patients with emphysema have airflow obstruction because of loss of airway elasticity. Patients with chronic bronchitis have airflow obstruction because inflammation, edema, and excessive mucus secretion shrink airway diameter. These pathologic changes then produce ventilation and perfusion abnormalities that, in turn, cause hypoxemia and carbon dioxide retention. Dyspnea in patients with COPD reflects the increased work of breathing required to compensate for these changes.

Because older women, who may have longer smoking histories, are having babies, anesthesiologists are likely to encounter COPD in the pregnant population. Superimposing the normal respiratory changes of pregnancy upon the changes induced by COPD could produce so great an increase in the work of breathing that decompensation occurs. Fortunately, however, patients with COPD usually tolerate pregnancy (46). Monitor such women closely. It may be difficult to distinguish between the pregnancy-related dyspnea and that caused by worsening pulmonary function.

Smoking can complicate pregnancy in several ways (Table 6). Smokers have a higher incidence of ectopic pregnancy (47) and placental complications, including abruption, previa, and premature calcification (45,48). Fetal hazards include growth retardation, which is directly proportional to the number of cigarettes smoked (49), prematurity, and spontaneous abortion (50). The fetal effects relate chiefly to chronic fetal hypoxemia (secondary to increased fetal carboxyhemoglobin) and uteroplacental hypoperfusion (from nicotine-induced vasospasm). Studies have not consistently demonstrated a teratogenic effect of smoking (49).

Treatment of pregnant smokers attempts to optimize pulmonary function. Cessation of smoking is paramount. In as little as 48 hours, the oxyhemoglobin dissociation curve resumes its normal configuration, increasing oxygen availability. In 2 to 3 months after stopping smoking, sputum production decreases and ciliary function improves. Acute respiratory infections occur frequently in patients with chronic bronchitis. Control such infection with antibiotics. Treat any bronchospastic component of airway disease with bronchodilators.

The preanesthetic evaluation of the pregnant smoker should determine the presence and severity of pulmonary

TABLE 6. *Consequences of smoking during pregnancy*

Maternal	Fetal
Increased airway irritability	Decreased oxygen exchange from mother
Increased mucous production	Growth retardation
Decreased mucociliary function	Prematurity
Increased dyspnea	Spontaneous abortion
Increased risk of cancer and COPD	Uteroplacental hypoperfusion
Left shift of oxyhemoglobin dissociation curve	
Increased risk of ectopic pregnancy	
Increased placental abnormalities	

disease. A history of decreased exercise tolerance and increased cough, sputum production, and dyspnea requires further evaluation. In patients with COPD, pulmonary function testing shows a decrease in FEV_1 (and a consequent decrease in FEV_1:forced vital capacity) plus an increase in total lung capacity. The results of such testing predict the patient's ability to cough and clear her airway. Laboratory evidence may be helpful. An elevated leukocyte count may indicate reparatory infection, and an arterial blood gas analysis will show hypoxemia or hypercarbia.

Sarcoidosis

Sarcoidosis is a generalized granulomatous disease with a pulmonary predilection. Resulting fibrosis and a restrictive pattern of pulmonary disease can lead to hypoxemia, pulmonary hypertension, and cor pulmonale. Steroids are often useful in the treatment of severe disease. Because of increased maternal serum cortisol concentration, pregnant patients generally tolerate existing sarcoidosis well. Monitor oxygenation closely to prevent maternal and fetal hypoxemia. A small percentage of these patients have laryngeal involvement, so anticipate airway interference.

Pulmonary Infection

Pulmonary infections occur as commonly in pregnant women as in the general population. Like the general population, pregnant women tolerate these illnesses well unless immunocompromised or otherwise afflicted with chronic disease. Treatment in these special cases must be aggressive. Prophylaxis with immunizations or pharmacologic agents may be beneficial. The etiology of acute, community-acquired respiratory infection is most often viral (influenza). Such infections are rarely from varicella. Bacterial infections are uncommon unless the patient is debilitated. Isolate the infecting organism from blood or sputum, and tailor antibiotic therapy accordingly. Fungal pulmonary infections are rare in healthy patients. With the rising number of immunocompromised patients with AIDS, the incidence of fungal infections will likely increase.

NERVOUS SYSTEM DISEASE

Neurological disease does not occur frequently in women of child-bearing age. Consequently, clinicians may be unfamiliar with the combined problems of pregnancy and neurological disorders. Pregnant women are susceptible to the same neurological illnesses as nonpregnant women. Because improved diagnosis and therapy allow women with neurological disease to survive to reproductive age, and because older women are becoming pregnant, anesthesiologists will encounter more pregnant patients with neurological disease and must prepare to care for them.

The gross neurological examination of the healthy gravida is not greatly altered from that of the nonpregnant patient. Motor function, sensation, and reflexes are the same. Edema or a changed center of gravity from pregnancy may alter gait. Cranial nerves are grossly intact, although normal pregnancy-induced hypertrophy of the pituitary gland occasionally alters visual-field examination.

Seizure Disorders

Seizure disorders complicate approximately 0.5% of pregnancies and are the most common neurological disorder encountered in parturients (48). Seizures are not themselves a disease but are the expression of an underlying neurological problem. Epilepsy is the ongoing tendency to have seizures. When excessive numbers of neurons discharge in a synchronous fashion, seizures result. This hyperexcitability can be focal or general, or may begin in a localized fashion and spread to become generalized. The cerebral cortex, thalamus, and brainstem can be involved. The most common etiology is idiopathic, but intracranial lesions, head trauma, metabolic derangement, hypoxia, cerebral inflammatory disease, and drug toxicity can cause seizures. In pregnancy, eclampsia also may account for seizures.

Traditional categories of seizure disorders are:

- Tonic-clonic (grand mal) seizures involve generalized motor activity with loss of consciousness.
- Simple partial and complex partial seizures involve brief alterations in consciousness, behavior, and motor or sensory function.
- Absence seizures (petit mal) involve brief alterations in awareness with little or no change in motor function.

Epilepsy appears to increase the risk of maternal and fetal complications, particularly congenital malformations, prematurity, low birth weight, preeclampsia, stillbirth, hemorrhage, and obstetric intervention (49,50). Most, but not all, studies support the theory that epilepsy predisposes women to purely obstetric complications (51,52). Therefore, treat epileptic gravidae as a high-risk group. Indisputably, hypoxia and acidosis incurred during a prolonged seizure or status epilepticus can precipitate fetal distress and, if uncorrected, lead to maternal and fetal demise.

Pregnancy has a variable effect on seizure frequency. In a review of 27 studies published between 1885 and 1980, Schmidt (53) found that of 2,165 women, 24% experienced an increased frequency of seizures, 22% had fewer seizures, and in 53% the frequency of seizures did not change. Patients with secondary generalized and complex partial seizures are more likely to experience increased seizure frequency during gestation than are those with primary generalized epilepsy (54). Seizure control before pregnancy seems to be the best predictor of control during pregnancy. Although the most common reason for an increase in seizure frequency during pregnancy is poor compliance with anticonvulsant therapy, pregnancy-induced changes in drug metabolism may account for some seizures (55).

Treatment

Anticonvulsants appear to act by reducing the spread of activity from hyperexcitable neurons to normal neurons. They may be used singly or in combination. The simpler the regimen, the better the compliance and the less likely are side effects and adverse drug interactions. Because all anticonvulsants commonly used in pregnancy have been variably charged with being teratogens, it is vitally important to weigh the risks and benefits of pharmacologic therapy. The American Academy of Pediatrics Select Committee on Anticonvulsants in Pregnancy has made the recommendations shown in Table 7 (56).

Phenytoin (Dilantin) is the most commonly administered antiepileptic drug. It is effective for most types of seizures except absence seizures. Its site of action is the motor cortex, where it may promote sodium efflux from neurons, thus stabilizing the membrane hyperexcitability threshold. Clearance is via the liver. Maternal side effects include gastrointestinal distress, skin rash, pancytopenia, megaloblastic anemia, systemic lupus erythematous, gingival hyperplasia, and peripheral polyneuropathy. Toxic manifestations include ataxia, nystagmus, and dysarthria progressing to reparatory and circulatory depression.

Phenytoin has been implicated as a causative factor in the increased incidence of congenital malformations in the offspring of epileptic women. In women taking anticonvulsants, however, it is difficult to determine the teratogenic role of the drug because of the difficulties in collecting human data. In addition, genetic factors in epileptic women may contribute more strongly to birth defects than any drug. Fetal malformations associated with phenytoin include craniofacial and limb malformations and fetal hydantoin syndrome. This syndrome is characterized by growth retardation, mental deficiency, and dysmorphic facial and limb features. Phenytoin also may cause deficiencies in folic acid and vitamin K-dependent clotting factors. Women should receive folic acid and vitamin K supplements during pregnancy to prevent megaloblastic anemia and hemorrhage.

TABLE 7. *Recommendations for use of anticonvulsants in pregnancy*

1. Before conception, withdraw anticonvulsant medication from women who have been seizure-free for many years.
2. A woman taking anticonvulsants should be told that if she becomes pregnant, she will have approximately a 90% chance of having a normal baby. However, the risk of having a baby with mental retardation or congenital malformations is two to three times greater than average.
3. There is no reason to switch a woman from well-known anticonvulsants, such as phenytoin or phenobarbital, to less well-known drugs.
4. Do not discontinue medication in women whose seizures are controlled by that medication because seizures may be deleterious to them and their fetuses.

After ref. 56, with permission.

Phenobarbital is a barbiturate with indications for use similar to phenytoin. Its major side effects are sedation, skin rash, and megaloblastic anemia. Toxic manifestations include nystagmus and ataxia. Phenobarbital is a potent inducer of hepatic microsomal enzymes and can enhance metabolism of other substances. Excretion is by the kidneys. In the past, because of lower suspected teratogenicity, many pregnant patients switched from phenytoin to phenobarbital. However, phenobarbital use now correlates with a syndrome similar to fetal hydantoin syndrome. Also, like phenytoin, phenobarbital may cause folate deficiency and coagulopathy. Unlike phenytoin, phenobarbital may cause neonatal depression and neonatal drub withdrawal. Primidone (Mysoline) is partly metabolized to phenobarbital. Its uses, side effects, and cautions are similar to those for phenobarbital.

Some physicians believe that carbamazepine (Tegretol) is the safest and least teratogenic of the anticonvulsants and are using it more frequently as a primary agent in treating tonic-clonic and partial seizures (57). Because much less is known about carbamazepine in pregnancy, use caution when considering prescribing it for a well-controlled pregnant epileptic who has been receiving phenytoin or phenobarbital. Side effects include dizziness, drowsiness, skin rash, and bone marrow depression with aplastic anemia and congestive heart failure. Neuromuscular symptoms are prominent at toxic drug concentrations. Elimination is mainly by the renal route.

Ethosuximide, clonazepam, trimethadione, and valproic acid are used to treat petit mal seizures. The little data that exist for ethosuximide and clonazepam show few fetal effects and suggest that their use in pregnancy is relatively safe. Trimethadione is the most potent known teratogen among the anticonvulsants, and its use is contraindicated in women of reproductive age. Also avoid valproic acid in pregnancy. It is associated with craniofacial, limb, and heart malfunctions. Women using it also show a 1% incidence of neural tube defects (58).

Anticonvulsant Pharmacokinetics in Pregnancy

Pregnancy induces several maternal pharmacokinetic changes that may significantly alter serum concentrations of anticonvulsants (Fig. 6). In plasma, total protein and albumin content falls, whereas free fatty acids rise. Fewer proteins mean less drug–protein binding, whereas rising free fatty acids displace drugs from proteins. This combi-

↑ **Unbound drug fraction**

↓ **Bowel absorption**

↑ **Volume of distribution**

\+ ↑ **Hepatic metabolism and clearance**

↑ **Dose requirement**

FIG. 6. Anticonvulsant pharmacokinetic changes in pregnancy.

nation allows a higher concentration of pharmacologically active free drug. Because protein binding is highly variable among individuals, the amount of free drug increase is unpredictable.

Despite the greater unbound fraction of drug, other pharmacologic changes combine to reduce the serum concentration of anticonvulsant drugs. Bowel absorption of phenytoin falls, probably as a result of decreased gastrointestinal motility and a change in gastric pH (59). This impaired uptake may hold for other anticonvulsants as well. An increase in total body water, accumulation of fat mass, and the addition of fetal, placental, and uterine tissues produce a larger volume of distribution. This increased volume dilutes the drugs in the serum. Elevated estrogen and progesterone increase hepatic metabolism of anticonvulsants drugs, speeding their clearance from the body and lowering serum concentration. In addition, the drugs themselves may induce liver enzymes to speed metabolism. These changes generally require increases in drug doses.

Monitor pregnant women taking anticonvulsants closely to ensure therapeutic drug concentrations. Estimate drug amounts from either plasma or saliva. Saliva drug concentration correlates well with plasma concentration of pharmacologically active drug. Measuring saliva concentrations is a simpler, less invasive, less expensive alternative to measuring plasma concentrations (54). After delivery, because maternal physiology rapidly reverts to its prepregnancy state, decrease anticonvulsant doses to avoid toxicity.

Status Epilepticus and Pregnancy

Status epilepticus is the repetitive occurrence of grand mal seizures during which the patient does not regain consciousness. It is a medical emergency. Without treatment, hypoxia, acidosis, and death ensue. The prognosis depends on the promptness of therapy and the etiology of the seizure. Abruptly halting anticonvulsant medication is the most common reason for seizures. Treatment involves maintaining a patent airway and administering intravenous anticonvulsants. Because of the fatal nature of this condition if left untreated, do not consider the teratogenicity of agents employed in arresting it. Initial therapy involves the administration of diazepam followed by loading and maintenance with phenytoin or phenobarbital. Ultimately, if these agents fail, induction of general anesthesia with an potent inhalation agent and the use of neuromuscular blocking agent may be needed.

The anesthetic preoperative evaluation of the stable pregnant epileptic involves early recognition. To avoid the surprise, confusion, and misdiagnosis arising from unexpected convulsions, identify epileptic patients immediately on arrival. Determine:

- Seizure type,
- Frequency of seizures during this and previous pregnancies,
- Anticonvulsant regimen, and
- Compliance.

Measure serum or saliva concentrations of drugs and adjust to therapeutic ranges, if necessary. Finally, do a brief baseline neurological examination to help assess subsequent changes.

Myasthenia Gravis

Myasthenia gravis (MG) is a chronic autoimmune neuromuscular disorder caused by a loss of functional acetylcholine receptors at the postsynaptic membrane of the neuromuscular junction. About 85% of patients have autoantibodies against acetylcholine receptors (60). In the remaining patients, autoantibodies binding to non-acetylcholine receptor neuromuscular junction determinants induce the receptor loss (61). MG usually manifests in the third decade. Its incidence is approximately 1 in 15,000 to 20,000 adults. MG affects women twice as often as men. Characteristically, the disease produces exacerbations and remissions of muscle weakness and fatigue, especially of oculomotor, facial, laryngeal, and reparatory muscles. MG may be associated with cardiomegaly or other diseases of immune origin, such as thyroid disease, lupus, or rheumatoid arthritis. Emotional or physiologic stress, infection, electrolyte imbalance, aminoglycoside antibiotics, magnesium sulfate, and neuromuscular blocking agents can precipitate or aggravate muscle weakness.

Interaction with Pregnancy

Pregnancy affects the disease process in unpredictable ways. In approximately equal numbers of patients, the disease stays the same, gets worse, or gets better during pregnancy. The course of MG in previous pregnancies does not predict the course in subsequent pregnancies. Respiratory difficulty and inadequate expulsive efforts from muscle fatigue during the second stage are the only effects on labor and delivery. Stress or infection during labor may precipitate a myasthenic crisis with severe weakness with respiratory insufficiency. Cholinergic crisis also presents with severe weakness; however, these women have evidence of muscarinic receptor stimulation with nausea, vomiting, lacrimation, and diarrhea. Because of transplacental transfer of antibodies, the newborn may show signs of neonatal MG. The symptoms may not appear for days, and although some infants require treatment, the condition usually is transient.

Treatment

The goal of treating MG is to increase the function of the acetylcholine receptors either by increasing the amount of endogenous acetylcholine or by decreasing the amount or function of acetylcholine receptor autoantibodies. There are four current approaches to therapy:

- Administration of anticholinesterase drugs,
- Immunosuppression,
- Plasmapheresis, and
- Surgical thymectomy.

The most common pharmacologic treatment is with anticholinesterase drugs such as edrophonium, neostigmine, and pyridostigmine. These drugs are quaternary ammonium structures that produce a reversible inhibition of acetylcholinesterase. By converting acetylcholine to acetic acid and choline, acetylcholinesterase terminates the action of acetylcholine. Acetylcholinesterase is found anywhere in the body there is acetylcholine. Inhibition of acetylcholinesterase increases the amount of acetylcholine available for neurotransmission and thereby augments the ability of skeletal muscle to respond to repetitive stimuli. Elevated acetylcholine levels in the vicinity of the uterus from anticholinesterase therapy theoretically increase uterine tone. In practice, however, this has not proved to be a great danger.

Edrophonium forms an electrostatic attachment to acetylcholinesterase, preventing the proper alignment of acetylcholine. Because the electrostatically bound complex is weak, acetylcholine can easily compete for binding sites, and the therapeutic effect of edrophonium is short-lived. The main use of edrophonium is in diagnosing MG and assessing the adequacy of anticholinesterase therapy. Give intravenous edrophonium in small (1 mg) doses every minute or two until weakness improves. In new-onset MG, this test is diagnostic. In treated patients, improvement shows that current therapy is inadequate. In contrast, administering edrophonium to patients with weakness from cholinergic crisis (anticholinesterase overdose) will not improve symptoms.

The other commonly used anticholinesterase agents are neostigmine and pyridostigmine. These produce reversible carbamyl-ester complexes with acetylcholinesterase. Both competitively inhibit the enzyme interaction with acetylcholine and act longer than edrophonium. The longer duration is likely due to true chemical bonding instead of relatively weak electrostatic bonding.

The pharmacologic effect of anticholinesterase agents is present at both muscarinic and nicotinic receptors. Nicotinic receptors are responsible for effects at the neuromuscular junction, whereas muscarinic receptors effect such responses as bradycardia, salivation, and emesis. If necessary, control muscarinic side effects with anticholinergic agents. When using anticholinesterase agents, consider that they impair the function of plasma cholinesterase, possibly prolonging the action of succinlycholine and ester local anesthetics.

Continue anticholinesterase therapy throughout labor and delivery. Because gastric absorption of drugs during labor may be erratic, administer these agents by intravenous or intramuscular routes. In addition, to prevent further muscle weakness, judiciously avoid agents with muscle-relaxing properties such as neuromuscular blockers, magnesium sulfate, and certain antibiotics (e.g., gentamicin and erythromycin).

When anticholinesterase drugs are inadequate, immunosuppression may prove beneficial. The common immunosuppressants (prednisone, azathioprine, and cyclophosphamide) prevent the production of, or reduce the circulating concentration of, acetylcholine receptor antibodies. No controlled data prove the efficacy of these agents in pregnancy. Because they are potentially teratogenic (especially azathioprine and cyclophosphamide), avoid their use during gestation.

Plasmapheresis is an uncommon therapy for MG that is aimed at reducing the circulating autoantibodies. Consider its use when conventional therapeutic measures have failed. Plasmapheresis may benefit the acetylcholine receptor antibody-negative subset of MG patients by removing an unspecified pathogenic substance (62).

Surgical thymectomy for the treatment of MG aims to remove the source of antibody production. Patients receiving this alternative treatment have favorable remission rates. It is not clear which patients benefit most from thymectomy. One review found that patients with moderate or advanced disease benefit more than do those with mild symptoms (27% improvement with mild disease vs 86% with moderate to advanced disease) (62). Another review found that the presence of acetylcholine receptor antibodies and thymic hyperplasia were the best indicators of a favorable response to thymectomy (63). Table 8 provides a quick reference for MG.

Preoperative Evaluation

The anesthetic preoperative evaluation of patients with MG involves assessing the degree of neuromuscular weakness. Look closely for evidence of respiratory compromise. The evaluation also should catalogue the current drug regimen and previous therapies and their efficacies.

TABLE 8. *Summary of myesthenia gravis in pregnancy*

Autoimmune	85% acetylcholine receptor 15% nonacetylcholine-receptor autoantibodies
Onset	Third decade
Epidemiology	Women two times the frequency of men
Characteristics	Exacerbations and remissions of muscle fatigue
Associated diseases	Cardiomegaly Other autoimmune diseases
Precipitators	Stress Infection Electrolyte imbalance Neuromuscular blocking agents
Interaction with pregnancy	Unpredictable Early second-stage fatigue
Interaction with neonate	Transient MG syndrome
Diagnosis	Administer edrophonium until weakness improves
Treatment	Anticholinesterase Thymectomy Plasmapheresis
Cholinergic crisis	
Symptoms	Weakness Diarrhea Excessive salivation
Treatment	Anticholinergics (atropine)

Determine the ability of the patient to maintain a patent airway (e.g., can she cough and clear secretions?). Ask about coexisting major diseases. If a patient who is treated with an anticholinesterase agent exhibits weakness, a trial of edrophonium may help determine the adequacy of her current regimen. Conversely, consider anticholinergic crisis if edrophonium fails to alleviate symptoms. Finally, a brief baseline neurologic examination may prove helpful in determining subsequent changes.

Multiple Sclerosis

Multiple sclerosis (MS) is a chronic, acquired disorder of the central nervous system (CNS) characterized by multiple, random areas of axonal demyelination (plaques) in the brain and spinal cord. MS occurs most frequently during the peak reproductive years (20 to 40 years). It affects women twice as often as men. Multiple sclerosis has a striking geographic distribution, with higher prevalence in temperate zones than in tropical or subtropical zones. MS is most likely to affect affluent urban dwellers. First-degree relatives of those affected have a 12- to 15-fold increase in incidence, pointing to a genetic predisposition. Sixty percent of patients with MS have a common histocompatibility antigen (HLA-DW2) compared to only 18% of controls.

Although some patients suffer a chronic progressive course, most individuals with MS experience periods of exacerbation and remission throughout their disease. These episodes occur at unpredictable intervals over many years. Eventually, residual symptoms persist and the patient experiences disability. Typical symptoms include visual disturbances, spastic weakness, fatigue, bowel and bladder dysfunction, sexual dysfunction, gait disturbance, and incoordination. Less common symptoms include alterations in cognitive function and affective disorders. The symptomatology is a manifestation of the area of demyelination. For example, if demyelination occurs in the motor pathways, spastic weakness can result, whereas demyelination of frontal and periventricular areas correlates with psychological disturbances (64). Mastrostefano et al. (65) report a case of partial seizures, headache, hemianopsia, apraxia, and aphasia in a woman with a focal parietal lobe mass ultimately diagnosed as MS. This presentation with intracranial symptoms and mass is rare.

Researchers have proposed several theories regarding the pathogenesis of MS. The most common theory suggests an infectious etiology. Although the identity of the agent is unknown, a virus seems the most likely culprit. Some viruses do cause human and animal demyelinating diseases. Presumably, the virus initiates an altered immune response in genetically susceptible individuals and autoimmune destruction of myelin follows. The viruses most often implicated are the measles virus and canine distemper virus.

The infectious theory seems strongest and best studied. Investigators have found a temporally related higher incidence of MS in previously low-prevalence areas upon mass entry of people from high-prevalence areas, such as in time of war (66). Also, increased blood and cerebrospinal fluid (CSF) titers of measles antibodies have been found in patients with MS when compared to controls; however, because antibody concentrations are low, the data are difficult to interpret. Furthermore, in two high-prevalence areas, there is no such measles antibody association.

Several factors relate MS and canine distemper virus. Canine distemper encephalitis, like MS, is a demyelinating disease (67). Dogs with canine distemper encephalitis, as do patients with MS, have increased CSF γ-globulin levels (68). However, whereas dogs are common almost everywhere, MS is not, and even though vaccinations have caused a decline in canine distemper encephalitis, the incidence of MS has remained unchanged.

Other theories are more controversial and less well studied. A high-fat diet may be a risk factor for the development of MS (69). The pathogenetic mechanism may relate in some way to the predominantly lipid composition of the myelin sheath. Geographic areas such as Norway and Switzerland and affluent urban areas with diets especially high in animal fat have higher rates of MS. In areas where dietary fats have become scarce, such as war-occupied countries, MS rates decline. People who migrate from areas of low-fat diets to ones of high-fat diets have higher rates of disease. However, certain populations with a low incidence of MS and high-fat diets contradict this theory.

Some researchers feel that trauma, especially of the head or spinal column, also may relate to the development of MS (70). Trauma alters the blood–brain barrier and may lead to plaque formation in vulnerable individuals. Other researchers find no evidence that trauma is a causative factor in MS.

Industrial workers exposed to zinc have an elevated incidence of MS (71). This correlation suggests that exposure to heavy metals or other toxins may be a risk factor. One proposed mechanism is that a zinc imbalance caused an immunoregulatory defect. If this were the case, these same workers also should exhibit greater numbers of other immunologically related diseases, but they do not.

Finally, Elias (72) hypothesizes that environmental exposure to an unknown agent in genetically predisposed individuals damages oligodendrocyte precursor cells. This damage prevents production of sufficient numbers of oligodendrocytes to maintain myelin.

Diagnosis

After excluding other neurological diseases, diagnose MS with clinical findings and supporting laboratory data. In addition to neurological symptoms, the patient may have evidence of demyelination with slowed nerve conduction on evoked potential testing. Computed tomography (CT) may reveal plaques that are areas of demyelination. The majority of patients will have elevated CSF immunoglobulin G (IgG) with mononuclear pleocytosis. This finding is not specific, however, and may occur with inflammatory or connective tissue diseases of the brain. Finally, elevated CSF myelin basic protein concentrations signify myelin destruction.

Treatment

There is no known cure for MS. Treatment is supportive and aims to decrease the number and duration of exacerbations, decrease disability, and limit the progression of chronic disease. Because MS may involve immunologically mediated destruction of myelin, medical management of acute exacerbations centers around immunosuppressive therapy. The most commonly used agents are adrenocorticotropic hormone (ACTH) and corticosteroids. Adrenocorticotropic hormone stimulates the adrenal cortex to secrete cortisol, corticosteroid, and aldosterone. Adrenocorticotropic hormone decreases the duration of acute exacerbations but seems to have no long-term benefit (73). Corticosteroids produce similar results more rapidly than ACTH. Both drugs decrease synthesis of CSF IgG (74). Adverse consequences of chronic steroid administration or adrenal stimulation include fluid and electrolyte disturbances, catabolism, hypertension, susceptibility to infection, poor wound healing, diabetes, peptic ulcer disease, hemorrhage, and secondary adrenocortical unresponsiveness.

Treatment of chronic progressive MS is controversial. Possible therapies include azathioprine, cyclophosphamide, plasmapheresis, intrathecal interferon-β, total lymphoid irradiation, cyclosporin A, and monoclonal antibodies.

Interaction with Pregnancy

Women with MS are justly concerned about the consequences of MS for themselves and their babies. MS does not seem to adversely affect the course of pregnancy (75) or the outcome of the fetus. There are no specific reports of MS-induced complications or malformations. MS-related symptoms such as fatigue, weakness, and incoordination may influence pregnancy. These women may tire more readily during labor and have weaker, less effective expulsive efforts. The choice of drugs used to treat MS also may affect pregnancy. Corticosteroids are safe for treating MS in pregnancy. Chronic steroid administration, on the other hand, may cause adverse effects such as hypertension, fluid and electrolyte imbalance, catabolism and muscle wasting, anemia from gastrointestinal bleeding, poor wound healing, and susceptibility to infection. ACTH use in pregnancy has not undergone controlled testing and is embryocidal (76). As with all drugs in pregnancy, use ACTH only if the potential benefits outweigh the risks. Do not use azathioprine, cyclophosphamide, and the agents under investigation because of the known or potential risk of teratogenesis. Khatri et al. report the successful use of plasmapheresis in a parturient with severely progressive MS (77). They preferred plasmapheresis because of the potential teratogenicity of immunosuppressive therapy. The mother experienced rapid reversal of her neurological decline and delivered a healthy term infant.

Unlike MG, there is no neonatal MS syndrome. Infants born to women with MS, as do other first-degree relatives, have an increased incidence of MS. This implies that even though the disease is not hereditary, there may be a genetic susceptibility.

Women with MS do not frequently suffer neurological deterioration during pregnancy. The normal, pregnancy-related hormonal changes, such as elevated plasma cortisol, may explain this phenomenon. The rate of exacerbation during the first postpartum months, however, is up to ten times the relapse rate during pregnancy. Many women deteriorate in the first 3 months after delivery (74). This relapse rate may be related to the withdrawal of pregnancy-related hormones. The number of pregnancies, exacerbation of MS in relation to pregnancy, and temporal relationship of the onset of MS to pregnancy do not influence long-term disability. Epidural or spinal anesthesia during parturition may correlate the exacerbation of MS. No study has fully elucidated the role of regional anesthesia in relapse, but a review of medical records supports this suggestion (78). Table 9 provides a quick reference for MS.

Preoperative Evaluation

The preanesthetic evaluation of patients with MS is similar to that for women with MG. Assess the degree of neuromuscular weakness and respiratory compromise. Obtain a history of concurrent major illness and current drug therapy. In those patients treated with chronic steroids, blood chemistries may be abnormal. Perform a neurological examination to aid in assessing any later exacerbation.

Neurofibromatosis

Neurofibromatosis is a chronically progressive, autosomal dominant disorder of the supportive tissues of the nervous system. It occurs in approximately 1 in 3,000 births and has diverse clinical expression. Classically, patients have diagnostic cutaneous pigmentary changes (e.g., cafe-au-lait spots or axillary freckling). Neurofibromas are tumors that arise from the Schwann cell sheaths and fibroblasts of peripheral, cranial, or autonomic nerves. The tumors can be small and discrete, or extensive masses. They usually involve the skin but also can occur in deeper nerves, blood vessels, and organs. Although usually a benign, cosmetic concern, they can cause major neurological or obstructive symptoms or undergo sacromatous degeneration. Airway compromise can occur with neurofibromas of the oropharynx, larynx, or mediastinum. Neurofibromas are often very vascular and can cause severe hemorrhage. Some patients have intracranial or spinal cord tumors and may develop intracranial hypertension, neurological compromise, or seizures. Cranial nerve involvement may lead to altered gag or swallowing reflexes. Disorders of bone growth are common. Cervical spine involvement is a major concern during positioning for laryngoscopy or surgery. Lumbar or thoracic spine involvement may make regional anesthesia impossible. Other organ involvement and associated diseases can include pulmonary parenchymal fibrosis leading to pulmonary hypertension, pheochromocytoma, hyperthyroidism, Wilm's tumor, neuroblastoma, and congenital heart lesions, especially pulmonary stenosis.

Treatment

Treatment of neurofibromatosis involves symptomatic drug therapy (e.g., anticonvulsants for seizures) and surgical removal of selected lesions. Reserve surgery for those tumors that are particularly disfiguring or associated with obstructive symptoms or neurologic compromise. Correction or amelioration of associated symptoms such as orthopedic deformity, endocrine dysfunction, or cancer also may require surgery.

Interaction with Pregnancy

During pregnancy, neurofibromas often enlarge, creating the potential for hemorrhage, increased obstruction, and neurological compromise. Laryngeal or pharyngeal tumors may obstruct the airway. Intracranial or spinal tumors may enlarge and create a mass effect or obstruct the flow of CSF. Pelvic neurofibromas may preclude vaginal delivery or create pressure symptoms. Pregnant women with neurofibromatosis also can be hypertensive, probably due to renal artery stenosis from vascular changes associated with the disease (79). Finally, patients may exhibit an altered response to muscle relaxants, with prolonged paralysis after nondepolarizing neuromuscular blocking agents. The response to succinylcholine may be either exaggerated or diminished. Generalized neurofibromatosis may induce motor end-plate denervation. However, little evidence supports this hypothesis (80,81).

TABLE 9. *Summary of multiple sclerosis and pregnancy*

Pathology	Central nervous system demyelination Genetic predisposition (HLA-DW$_2$)
Onset	20–40 yr Women affected two times more than men
Geographic distribution	Temperate zones
Pathogenic theories	Infectious agent (measles, canine distemper virus) High-fat diet Trauma Heavy metal exposure Oligodendrocyte precursor damage
Interaction with pregnancy	Nonspecific, related to MS symptoms Higher risk of relapse postpartum
Interaction with neonate	No immediate interaction
Diagnosis	Evoked potentials: slow nerve conduction Computed tomography evidence of plaques Increased CSF IgG Increased CSF myelin basic protein

Because neurofibromatosis is an autosomal dominant disorder, infants born to affected mothers have a 50% chance of developing the disease. Many of the signs and symptoms of this progressive disorder are absent at birth. Axillary freckling or the presence of five or more cafe-au-lait spots larger than 0.5 cm in diameter are diagnostic.

Preoperative Evaluation

The preanesthetic evaluation of a parturient with neurofibromatosis must include a careful search for problematic manifestations of the disease. A history of strictly cutaneous disease is not alarming, whereas a history of voice changes, symptoms of increased intracranial pressure, or neurologic changes should cause concern. A history of significant cardiopulmonary disease, endocrine dysfunction, and orthopedic malformation is important. Assess the airway carefully for possible obstruction and cervical spine involvement. Finally, as with all patients with neurological disease, perform a baseline examination.

Paraplegia and Quadriplegia

Improved treatment of spinal cord injury victims has allowed more women with these injuries to survive and bear children. Trauma, infection, tumors, and vascular lesions are the most common causes of spinal cord injury or transection. Paraplegia is paralysis of the lower extremities and quadriplegia involves all four extremities. The initial phase of an acute spinal cord transection is known as spinal shock. Characteristics of this period include flaccid paralysis and loss of sensation, temperature regulation, and spinal reflexes below the level of the lesion. Characteristically, patients experience hypotension, bradycardia, cardiac dysrhythmias (especially premature ventricular contractions), and electrocardiographic changes consistent with ischemia (82). Women are amenorrheic for 2 to 3 months following injury.

A lesion between C_2 and C_4, causing diaphragmatic denervation, may require immediate and permanent ventilatory support. With lower lesions and intact diaphragmatic innervation, the patient can probably generate adequate tidal volumes but may not be able to cough and clear her airway. The mechanism behind this impairment is probably twofold. The first reason may be that paralysis of the abdominal musculature does not allow the patient to generate the force required to cough. The second possibility is that abdominal muscle paralysis allows the intraabdominal contents to shift and displace the diaphragm. The result is altered lung volumes, particularly a decreased functional residual capacity and decreased expiratory reserve volume—the volume used to generated a cough. Another possible result of altered lung volumes is ventilation-perfusion mismatching, resulting in hypoxemia. Because of these respiratory changes, pulmonary aspiration and pneumonia are common.

Following the initial phase of injury, patients enter the chronic stage. During this stage, spinal cord reflexes generally return and the patient experiences muscle spasm and sympathetic nervous system hyperactivity. Other findings associated with chronic spinal cord injury include chronic pulmonary and urinary tract infections, anemia, thermoregulatory dysfunction, and cardiovascular instability.

Respiratory changes during the chronic stage of spinal cord injury are not greatly different from those in the acute phase. Patients with cervical transections and diaphragmatic paralysis will continue to require ventilatory support. Paralysis that spares the diaphragm, but affects the accessory respiratory muscles, may decease ventilatory reserve and lead to alveolar hypoventilation. Impairment of the ability to cough and clear the airway along with atelectasis from hypoventilation makes these patients prone to chronic pulmonary infection.

Renal failure resulting from chronic urinary tract infection or renal calculi is a major cause of morbidity and mortality in patients with spinal cord injuries. Spinal cord transection often disrupts the motor innervation of the bladder and ureters, causing urinary stasis, chronic bladder infection, and pyelonephritis. Also, chronic instrumentation for bladder elimination increases the risk of infection. Good perineal hygiene, routine bladder emptying, and chronic suppression therapy can lessen the risk of infection.

Spinal cord injury patients often have anemia. Some of the most commonly proposed causes for this anemia are iron deficiency and renal failure from chronic infection, obstruction, or renal calculi. This anemia also may be an anemia of chronic disease from chronic infection, skin ulcer, or renal failure.

Sympathetic nervous system hyperactivity can produce cardiovascular instability following the return of spinal cord reflexes after spinal shock. This syndrome, known as autonomic hyperreflexia (83), results from the dissociation of sympathetic spinal reflexes (below the level of the transection) from controlling mechanisms in the CNS. Visceral or cutaneous stimulation, most commonly by distention of a hollow viscus such as the bowel, bladder, or uterus, initiates the reflex. In neurologically intact individuals, visceral stimulation sends afferent signs that enter the spinal cord and elicit a sympathetic nervous system response. Descending impulses from the CNS normally regulate this response; however, spinal cord injury disrupts the transmission of this information, resulting in sympathetic hyperactivity. The level of the spinal cord lesion determines the incidence of autonomic hyperreflexia. Nearly all patients (85%) with transections above T_6 will experience the syndrome, whereas it is unlikely to occur in those with lesions below T_{10}. The most common manifestations are severe paroxysmal hypertension, tachycardia, bradycardia, headache, facial flushing, diaphoresis, piloerection, pupillary dilation, and nasal congestion.

Hyperreflexia requires immediate attention because severely elevated blood pressure can incite seizures and unconsciousness as well as retinal, cerebral, and subarachnoid hemorrhages (84). The treatment of autonomic hyperreflexia involves rapid measures to control the blood pressure. Removal of the initiating stimulus is important (e.g., emptying a full bladder). Initiate pharmacologic therapy with peripheral vasodilators such as ganglionic blocking drugs, α-adrenergic agonists, direct vasodilators, or general or regional anaesthesia. Because of the disruption of regulatory pathways, centrally acting agents are ineffective. Table 10 summarizes the consequences of spinal cord injury.

Spinal cord injury has several obstetric consequences. Women who suffer spinal cord injuries during pregnancy have a greater risk of stillbirth (85). The level of injury will determine the patient's response to labor pain. Women with lesions below T_{11} to L_1 will feel labor pain. Those with lesions from T_{10} to T_5 to T_6 will not have pain but can palpate contractions. Those with lesions above T_5 to T_6 are at high risk for autonomic hyperreflexia. Because women in these last two groups may find labor painless, premature, unsupervised delivery may occur. Labor also tends to progress rapidly (86). Additional problems related to pregnancy include possible respiratory embarrassment from the distended uterus, profound anemia, and urinary obstruction with increased incidence of distention, infection, and autonomic hyperreflexia.

The preanesthetic evaluation of pregnant patients with spinal cord injuries focuses on the respiratory status. The level of the lesion will provide a clue to the likelihood of the need for ventilatory support. Other important points include assessing the patient's ability to clear her airway and considering the degree of respiratory compromise due to the gravid uterus. In any event, be prepared to lend ventilatory assistance. Knowing the level of transection will also alert the anesthesiologist to the possibility of autonomic hyperreflexia. Laboratory data can help detect severe anemia or pulmonary or urinary tract infection.

Central Nervous System Neoplasms

CNS neoplasms are uncommon in women of reproductive age. Roelvink et al. (87) reviewed 223 cases of primary brain and spinal cord tumors that became symptomatic during or immediately after pregnancy. The incidence of brain tumors during pregnancy may be less than the that in nonpregnant women of the same age. This lowered risk may represent an artifact. Women with subclinical cancer may have more unnoticed, spontaneous early pregnancy losses (88). Although CNS neoplasms are not more common in pregnancy, pregnancy can precipitate or aggravate the symptoms of these lesions. The mechanism is unclear, but it is probably related to tumor enlargement due to water retention or increased vascularity (89). Tumors may be either metastatic or primary. Metastatic tumors of particular importance to women in this age group are those from breast and lung cancer and from choriocarcinoma. Except for metastatic choriocarcinoma, there is no difference in the distribution of brain tumors whose symptoms first occur in pregnant women and in nonpregnant women in the same age group. Previous authors have suggested that meningiomas are particularly predisposed to manifest symptoms during pregnancy (61,88, 90); however, other evidence does not support this theory (87).

Of spinal cord tumors, spinal hemangiomas seem to occur more frequently in the pregnant population. Certain tumors seem to manifest symptoms at different times during gestation. For example, spinal hemangiomas generally present in the third trimester, gliomas in the first trimester, and meningiomas progressively throughout pregnancy. Progesterone seems to positively correlate with tumor symptoms, but the mechanism of this effect is unknown (86).

The diagnosis of CNS tumors in pregnant patients does not differ from their diagnosis in nonpregnant patients. Signs and symptoms suggestive of a CNS space-occupy-

TABLE 10. *Consequences of spinal cord injury*

Acute	Chronic
Neural	Neural
Flaccid paralysis	Muscle spasm
Loss of sensation, temperature regulation, and spinal reflexes	Altered thermoregulation
Cardiovascular	Return of spinal reflexes
Hypotension	Cardiovascular
Bradycardia	Autonomic hyperreflexia with lesions above T_6
Dysrhythmia	Respiratory
ECG changes	C_2–C_4 lesions require ventilatory support
Respiratory	Lower lesions alter lung volumes and may impair the ability to protect the airway
C_2–C_4 lesions require ventilatory support	Renal
Lower lesions alter lung volumes and may impair the ability to protect the airway	Failure from infection or calculi
Other	Other
Amenorrhea for 3 months	Anemia

ing lesion form the basis for diagnosis. Use CT and magnetic resonance imaging without hesitation.

Tumor-related symptoms may be difficult to distinguish from some pregnancy-related complaints. Typical symptoms of CNS tumors include nausea and vomiting, headache, visual changes, altered mental status, and convulsions. Other findings may include sensory or motor deficits. These symptoms can arise because of the anatomic location of the tumor, because they obstruct the flow of CSF, or because they produce an intracranial mass effect with resultant intracranial hypertension.

Pregnancy should not alter or delay treatment of these tumors. Radiation treatment and chemotherapy (except for possible teratogens and surgery) should be used as indicated. If the mother's neurological examination is stable and she shows no evidence of increased intracranial pressure, delay treatment until after delivery. A deteriorating status due to severe, uncontrolled intracranial hypertension requires immediate therapy, with pregnancy termination and surgery as necessary. Some measures that may be needed include:

- Intubation and hyperventilation,
- Corticosteroids to reduce cerebral edema,
- Drainage of CSF via ventricular shunting or ventriculostomy, and
- Administration of barbiturates.

If possible, avoid hyperosmotic drugs such as mannitol, which may shift water from the fetus to the mother.

The preanesthetic evaluation of the parturient with known or suspected CNS lesions should focus on determining the patient's level of consciousness and assessing her ability to maintain and protect her airway. Also look for intracranial hypertension and initiate therapy as appropriate. To immediately appreciate changes in neurological status, frequent examinations are essential.

Cerebrovascular Disease

Cerebrovascular disorders are uncommon in women of reproductive age. But, when they do occur during pregnancy, they are a leading cause of maternal mortality (91). Because these disorders are unusual in this age group, it is easy to attribute their symptoms to more common diseases such as eclampsia or seizure disorders. As a consequence, crucial delays in therapy may result. The cerebrovascular diseases most commonly seen in pregnancy include intracerebral hemorrhage and subarachnoid hemorrhage.

The etiologies of intracerebral hemorrhage include hypertension, eclampsia, and metastatic choriocarcinoma. Unless associated with a complication of gestation, pregnancy does not alter the incidence of intracerebral hemorrhage. Hemorrhage is rare except when due to eclampsia or preeclampsia. The presumed causes of bleeding in these instances are hypertension and vascular changes associated with preeclampsia. A review of 533 deaths due to eclampsia and preeclampsia found that cerebral dysfunction caused 180. Almost half of these had gross evidence of intracerebral hemorrhage (92). Symptoms include headache, convulsions, mental status changes, and focal neurological findings.

Subarachnoid hemorrhage complicates fewer than 1 in 10,000 pregnancies (93). The etiologies include cerebral aneurysm, arteriovenous malformation, metastatic choriocarcinoma, eclampsia, and disseminated intravascular coagulation. Aneurysm and arteriovenous malformation are the first and second most common causes, respectively.

Gravidas with aneurysms tend to be older (30 to 35 years) than those with arteriovenous malformations (20 to 25 years). Aneurysms have a progressively increasing risk of rupture during the pregnancy, with the highest risk between 30 and 40 weeks' gestation. They rarely rupture during labor. In contrast, arteriovenous malformations may rupture at any time during pregnancy or labor or after delivery. Ruptured aneurysms are generally more fatal than ruptured arteriovenous malformations (94,95).

Symptoms of subarachnoid hemorrhage include severe headaches, nausea, vomiting, altered mental status, nuchal rigidity, and focal neurological deficit. Distinguishing a ruptured aneurysm from a ruptured arteriovenous malformation by neurological examination is difficult and may require specific testing, such as CT and cerebral angiography. The preanesthetic evaluation of the pregnant patient with cerebrovascular disorders is similar to that for a patient with CNS neoplasms.

HUMAN IMMUNODEFICIENCY VIRUS INFECTION

Epidemiology

Acquired immunodeficiency syndrome (AIDS) is a currently incurable disease complex that results from infection with the human immunodeficiency virus (HIV). By the end of 1993, more than 300,000 cases of AIDS in the United States were reported to the Centers for Disease Control, and at least 1 million individuals in the United States were thought to be infected with HIV. Approximately 6,530 HIV-infected women gave birth in the United States in 1993, and, based on a 25% vertical transmission rate, an estimated 1,630 of their infants were infected with HIV (96). This rising incidence shows no signs of slowing. In the United States, in areas with high prevalence, male-to-female HIV-seropositive ratios approach 1:1 (97). Eighty percent of reported cases of AIDS in adult women occurs among those of reproductive age (98). A majority of these cases, 53% in one study, occur in intravenous drug abusers, with another 27% resulting from heterosexual transmission (99). Several studies of HIV seroprevalence in pregnant women reveal as many as 8 to 20 per 1,000 (99,100). Many studies confirm the efficacy of routine HIV screening in areas of higher prevalence. For example, one study of 1,264 women from a multiethnic population in an inner London health district, 39% reported risk factors personally or by a partner (100). Most of these risk factors were not disclosed earlier in the routine history taking. Although several prospective studies of HIV-infected pregnant women are under way, the interaction of pregnancy and HIV remains unclear. Based upon future projections of rising incidence of AIDS in women, the number of AIDS-related complications and deaths during pregnancy, now relatively low, will rise and become a significant problem.

Pathophysiology

AIDS results from immunosuppression by HIV-1, a large family of retroviruses that use host reverse transcriptase to produce, ultimately, core viral ribonucleic acid (RNA). The virus replicates by binding to a receptor labeled CD4 on the cell membranes of T-cell lymphocytes, monocytes, macrophages, a small number of B-cell lymphocytes, glial cells, gut chromaffin cells, lymph nodes, skin, and rectal mucosal cells (101). Once inside the cell, the viral RNA is converted to DNA, which either integrates into the deoxyribonucleic acid (DNA) of the host cell (proviral DNA) or remains unintegrated. The proviral DNA may lie dormant indefinitely, but the cell is permanently infected and will reduplicate the viral DNA with each cell division. Cell-free virus is found in various body fluids—synovial, cerebrospinal, pleural, peritoneal. The primary mode of transmission is via cells containing virus. After infection with HIV, many of the CD4 lymphocytes die or become dysfunctional, probably accounting for the decrease in the absolute CD4 lymphocyte population associated with HIV disease. The mechanism of death for these cells infected with HIV is unknown, but the destruction of the helper T_4 cell ultimately leads to significant defects in cell-mediated immunity.

Infection with HIV is detected either by culture or serology. Culturing the virus yields unreliable results (102,103). Serologic tests for HIV antibodies prove reproducible, sensitive, and specific (Table 11) (104). The enzyme-linked immunosorbent assay (ELISA) and rapid latex agglutination tests are sensitive, but nonspecific. Western blot immunophoresis and cytoplasmic membrane immunofluorescence tests are very specific but more often require repeating (105). Recently, rapid diagnostic assays have been developed that directly detect HIV antigens instead of HIV antibody. Although availability of these assays is not yet widespread, it is hoped that they will prove to be a quick and reliable means to screen individuals at risk for HIV infection and help to identify those infected with HIV who have undetectable antibody levels.

Identification of the pregnant woman with HIV infection requires a high degree of clinical suspicion. Look for risk factors. Beware of the variable spectrum of disease.

TABLE 11. *Sensitivity and specificity of HIV screening tests*

	Sensitivity	Specificity
ELISA	99.3%–100%	98.1%–99.5%
Western blot	97.1%–100%	97.8%–100%

A history of intravenous drug abuse, a sexual partner who is either HIV-positive or an intravenous drug user, or blood transfusion since 1978 should heighten clinical suspicion of HIV seropositivity. Prevalence of this disease in women, as for men, is highest in lower socioeconomic groups. Whereas 63% of infected males are white, 51% of HIV positive-women are black, 28% white, and 20% Hispanic (106).

Initially, AIDS was recognized only in its end stages, when multiple opportunistic infections and unusual cancers occurred. Now, the disease is understood as a progression that depends on a multitude of factors, including extent of initial exposure. Based on the correlation between quantity of virus in the blood and severity of illness, Redfield et al. (107) proposed a six-stage classification. Stage 0 represents the initial exposure. Stage 6 is overt AIDS. This system also follows the T_4 lymphocyte count. Fewer than 400 cells/mL coincides with AIDS-related symptomatology (108). The progression of HIV-associated illness varies among individuals. The patient's own immune response to the virus may slow viral replication. Ultimately, however, the virus multiplies to a degree sufficient to overpower the host immune system. Then T_4 count becomes extremely low, and the patient develops frequent infections by opportunistic bacteria, fungi, viruses, and progression of various cancers. An in-depth discussion of AIDS and various organ systems is beyond the scope of this text, but AIDS-associated cardiomyopathy, nephropathy, and dementia may complicate the course of this disease.

Although HIV infection remains incurable, new drug therapies can slow the progression of AIDS and reduce the total viral load in HIV-infected patients. Azidothymidine (AZT), now called zidovudine (ZDV), is a thymidine analog that blocks the replication of HIV by inhibiting reverse transcriptase activity and was the first agent shown to improve the clinical and laboratory status of patients infected with HIV. An important characteristic of ZDV is its ability to penetrate the blood–brain barrier; concentrations in the CNS are approximately 30% to 50% of serum concentrations. Currently, the Food and Drug Administration recommends beginning ZDV, 200 mg by mouth three times a day, in any HIV-infected person with a CD4 count less than 500. ZDV may become less effective with long-term use.

Didanosine (ddI) is another nucleoside analog that interferes with reverse transcriptase. Patients treated with ddI have a significant delay in progression to AIDS compared with those who had received prior ZDV therapy.

Zalcitabine (ddC) is another reverse transcriptase inhibitor that is approved for use in combination with ZDV in patients with CD4 counts less than 300 and evidence of clinical progression on ZDV alone. Combination therapy with ZDV and ddI or ddC is under intense study (109) and may make an attractive approach to combating AIDS and HIV infection. Multiple other antiviral agents that act at different sites in the lifecycle of HIV also are being evaluated (110).

Interaction with Pregnancy

There is no evidence that HIV infection or AIDS affects fertility. Although one of the primary goals in counseling this patient population is prevention of pregnancy, there is no irrefutable evidence that abortion, although frequently recommended, will alter the course of disease.

Cell-mediated immunity is depressed during pregnancy, especially in the second and third trimesters (111, 112). Some evidence suggests that pregnancy accelerates the course of disease in HIV-infected women. Two studies found that 45% to 75% of asymptomatic HIV-infected parturients developed symptoms of AIDS within 28 to 60 months of delivery (113,114). However, these studies enrolled only a small number of patients and lacked controls. Other data suggest that pregnancy does not accelerate the occurrence of AIDS among HIV-positive women. Similarly, pregnancy may increase the death rate in women with AIDS. Koonin et al. (105) examined mean survival from diagnosis of AIDS to death in New York City. They compared a population of pregnant women who were intravenous drug abusers and died of *Pneumocystis carinii* pneumonia to nonpregnant but otherwise identical controls. The parturients had a much shorter survival (59 vs 187 days). Factors such as delayed diagnosis and access to health care may account for some of this difference. Other studies find no significant difference in survival among pregnant HIV-positive intravenous drug abusers versus their nonpregnant controls (115,116). These data warrant further investigation to reach a definite conclusion on the true impact of pregnancy on the course of HIV infection.

Confusion also exists about the effect of HIV infection on pregnancy. Despite a much higher incidence of complications, including premature rupture of membranes, low birth weight, and preterm birth, patient populations with risk factors such as low socioeconomic status, drug abuse, poor nutritional status, and poor prenatal care show little difference in maternal risk and outcome between HIV-seropositive and HIV-seronegative mothers (117). Women who abuse drugs in general have an increased risk of pregnancy complications (spontaneous abortion, preterm deliveries, and low-birth-weight infants) (118,119). Although the true effect of HIV infection on the course of pregnancy remains unclear, these patients are at high risk during pregnancy.

With the obstetric implications of HIV seropositivity and even AIDS still unclear, the issue of screening for HIV in pregnant women remains in the foreground of debate. A recent report attempted to calculate the national costs of reducing perinatal transmission of HIV through counseling and voluntary testing of pregnant women and ZDV treatment of infected women and their infants (120). Without intervention, there is an 25% vertical transmission rate. At the current prevalence of HIV-complicated pregnancies, 1,750 HIV-infected infants would be born annually with lifetime medical care costs estimated at $282 million. The cost of the intervention (counseling, testing, and ZDV treatment) was estimated to be $67.6 million, which would prevent 656 pediatric HIV infections with a medical care cost saving of $105.6 million. The net cost saving of the intervention was $38.1 million, absent the cost of human suffering.

Nevertheless, the debate over screening continues. The arguments for screening include:

- Voluntary testing may miss a large percentage of positive individuals.
- Perinatal transmission of the virus may be reduced.
- Health care workers may be better protected.

Those against screening point out (121):

- The high cost of an effective screening program,
- The high false-positive rates in low-prevalence populations, and
- The likelihood of discouraging prenatal care with mandatory HIV screening.

Instead of widespread testing, health care workers should rely on universal precautions for personal protection. Presuming that all patients are infected when handling blood or other body fluids should limit the risk of exposure and transmission of disease from patient to health care worker or vice versa. Testing for HIV should be limited to those patients at high risk for the disease.

Perinatal transmission of HIV is a worsening problem. In most of these cases, infants will acquire the infection through vertical transmission from their mothers. Knowing that a pregnant woman is HIV-seropositive does not necessarily indicate that her fetus is or will be infected. Testing for HIV in newborns reveals only the presence or absence of maternal antibodies, establishing the presence of the virus in the mother but not the neonate. Current estimates are that 30% of HIV-positive mothers in the United States transmit HIV to their newborn infants. Transmission may occur in utero, as virus has been isolated from an infant born by cesarean section (122,123). Exposure to maternal blood and body fluids at the time of birth is another possible route of HIV transmission. For this reason, scalp electrodes and fetal blood sampling should be avoided in the HIV-positive patient. Cesarean delivery may decrease the rate of transmission by as much as 50%, although this route of delivery is by no means completely protective (124). Maternal HIV-1 RNA levels are highly predictive of the risk of perinatal transmission. Maternal antiviral therapy (ZDV) appears to decrease the risk of vertical transmission (125,126). Finally, HIV is present in breast milk, and there are several cases in which transmission is thought to have occurred during breast-feeding (127–129).

Prenatal diagnosis of fetal HIV infection is currently not possible. Fetal dysmorphism, with characteristic findings that include growth failure, microcephaly, oblique eyes, and a flattened forehead, appear to correlate in severity with age of the child at diagnosis of AIDS (130). There is a great deal of overlap with other fetal dysmorphic syndromes attributable to other viruses or maternal substance abuse.

There is no association between risk of transmission and trimester during which exposure occurred. Absence of maternal symptoms does not appear protective (131), although, following the birth of an affected child, an infected mother may give birth to an unaffected child (132,133). The efficiency of sexual transmission varies in different risk groups. Similar stratification may exist with transmission of the virus to offspring.

SUBSTANCE ABUSE

Drug use constitutes a major public health problem in the United States today. Women of child-bearing age constitute a large portion of its population. Nicotine, alcohol, marijuana, and cocaine remain the most commonly abused substances. As many as 20% of parturients in the United States smoke cigarettes (134), 12% abuse alcohol (135), and 11% to 20% report regular use of cocaine or crack (136). The proportion of birth certificates indicating use of illicit substances rose threefold between 1981 and 1987. Such evidence suggests a significant increase in maternal drug use during pregnancy (137).

Drug use in various settings reflects factors varying from availability to social acceptance (138). The maternal drug abuser stereotypically progresses from cigarettes to alcohol to marijuana and then on to cocaine and intravenous drugs (139). With the rising prevalence of substance abuse, the anesthesiologist must understand and anticipate its various effects and consequences.

The physiologic changes of pregnancy alter pharmacokinetic and pharmacodynamic behavior and then amplify cardiovascular and respiratory depressant effects of many addictive drugs (140). The placenta is similar to the liver in its ability to metabolize drugs, but environmental factors determine the quality and quantity of enzymes present. Drug abuse may decrease the number of placental neurotransmitter receptors and generate abnormal fetal and neonatal behavioral development (141). Any substance that affects the vascular tone of the placenta may alter placental blood flow and ultimately result in placental infarction and fetal compromise.

Substances ingested, inhaled, or injected by the mother may cross the placenta and directly affect the fetus by one of several mechanisms. The drug or a metabolite may have direct fetal effects. Alternately, drugs can induce hepatic enzymes and affect development via altered synthetic and degradation pathways (142). The risk of disease transmission is greatest for the fetus of a substance abuser. Maternal malnutrition, which so often accompanies substance abuse, manifests as an increased incidence of neural tube defects and a host of peripartum complications (143).

The course of gestation for substance abusers often depends on their ability and willingness to participate in counseling and detoxification programs. Up to 25% of substance abusers who seek prenatal care deny drug use. Even so, a widely focused approach seems the best way to address the multiple problems of these women. Such a program might include:

- Counseling,
- Detoxification and substitution therapy,
- Education about nutrition, drug effects, maternal care, and HIV prophylaxis,
- Screening for hepatitis, HIV, tuberculosis, and vaginal/cervical infections, and
- Evaluation of fetal growth with ultrasound, nonstress test, biophysical profile, and phosphatidyl gylcerol (144).

Ethanol

Ethanol, a CNS depressant, may induce behavioral stimulation by depressing inhibitory control mechanisms and allowing unrestrained activity of various parts of the brain. As intoxication advances, this initial excitatory phase is succeeded by a general impairment of nervous function. A condition of general anesthesia ultimately prevails. The CNS effects of alcohol are proportional to the blood alcohol concentration. They are most marked in the face of a rising alcohol concentration (145). The rate-limiting step in alcohol metabolism is the conversion of ethanol to acetaldehyde by alcohol dehydrogenase. This enzyme has variable activity. Multiple isoenzymes coded for by five genes exist (146). Variable expression of these genes occurs between races and individuals (147). Alcohol exhibits cross-tolerance with most CNS depressant drugs. Acute intoxication increases the effects of cross-tolerant drugs. Chronic ingestion of alcohol decreases other drug effects. Tolerance does not alter the lethal blood concentration of alcohol (148).

Acquired tolerance to, and physical dependence on, ethanol results from neurophysiologic changes that compensate for the depressant effect of alcohol on neuronal excitability, impulse conduction, and transmitter release. Abrupt cessation of alcohol ingestion incites hyperactivity of all senses, hyperreflexia, muscle tension and tremor, overalertness, anxiety, insomnia, and reduction of seizure threshold, once commonly known as the withdrawal syndrome (149). Symptoms range from mild to severe and can appear as early as several hours after the last drink but more typically occur after 48 hours of abstinence. Delirium tremens is a medical emergency characterized by extreme autonomic hyperactivity and global confusion. If left untreated, it has a mortality rate greater than 40%. In contrast to opiate withdrawal, which responds immediately to administration of an opiate and is rarely fatal, delirium tremens, once established, cannot be rapidly reversed with alcohol (150). Sedative therapy in withdrawal syndrome and delirium tremens involves replacement of alcohol with a cross-tolerant drug and calming the anxious, hallucinating, or delirious patient. It is unknown which sedative best achieves these goals. In the parturient suffering withdrawal symptoms, pharmacologic substitution therapy is necessary despite the risk of further fetal drug exposure. Phenobarbital and clonidine are preferred. The teratogenicity of benzodiazepines and the acidosis associated with paraldehyde have made these drugs less useful (151).

Chronic alcohol abuse affects the function of multiple organ systems. In addition to CNS symptoms, chronic myelopathy, polyneuropathy, and myopathy may be present. These problems can complicate anesthetic management of labor and delivery or cesarean section by altering recovery from muscle relaxants and regional or general anesthesia.

Acute cardiovascular effects of ethanol include myocardial depression and altered electrophysiology, leading to atrial and ventricular dysrhythmias. Chronic consumption results in cardiomyopathy and progressive myocardial dysfunction (152). The increased cardiac demand of pregnancy may result in cardiac failure in the pregnant alcohol abuser with significant myocardial disease. Anesthetics that depress cardiac function may accelerate this process.

Respiratory complications are common among chronic alcohol abusers. These range from mild ventilation-perfusion mismatch and intrapulmonary shunting to chronic infection and aspiration pneumonia. Alcohol further compounds the already higher risk of aspiration in the term parturient because it too decreases gastric motility and lowers esophageal sphincter tone.

Liver disease is common after ethanol abuse. Fatty infiltration, cirrhosis, portal hypertension, and hepatic encephalopathy can occur. In addition, hepatocellular damage can yield hypoglycemia from impaired gluconeogenesis and induced glycogenolysis. Decreased drug metabolism and protein and coagulation factor synthesis may alter the anesthetic approach to the pregnant patient with alcoholic liver disease, either at term or upon earlier presentation.

Gastritis, esophagitis, bleeding varices, and pancreatitis are gastrointestinal manifestations of alcohol abuse and contribute to an increased risk of aspiration pneumonia either before, during, or after anesthesia. The stress response is altered. Cortisol, prolactin, epinephrine, norepinephrine, renin, angiotensin, and aldosterone rise while growth hormone decreases (153). Electrolyte abnormalities such as hyponatremia, hypokalemia, and hypomagnesemia may require correction. Correct hyponatremia slowly to avoid overcorrection and central pontine myelinolysis.

Ethanol does not affect umbilical arterial tone, confirming the absence of a direct effect of alcohol on placental blood flow (154). Alcohol consumption, however, blocks the placental transport of α-aminobutyric acid, implying that ethanol inhibits placental transfer of other nutrients (155).

Alcohol works through several mechanisms to cause fetal and subsequent neonatal morbidity. Cirrhosis, cardiomyopathy, gastritis, and pancreatitis result in the mother. Alcohol increases the conversion of dihomogammalinolenic acid (DGLA) to prostaglandin E_1 (PGE_1) In addition, ethanol inhibits δ-6-desaturase, an enzyme essential for a continued supply of DGLA. As a result, these fetuses have low concentrations of PGE_1 (156). This deficiency may account for many of the changes noted with the fetal alcohol syndrome. This syndrome consists of growth deficiency, major and minor birth defects, abnormal mental and motor performance, and fetal or neonatal wastage, which are well-documented effects of alcohol abuse during pregnancy (157).

Maternal alcoholism is not the only cause of fetal and neonatal morbidity from ethanol. Paternal exposure to ethanol also breeds fetal growth retardation and decreased DNA, RNA, and leucine synthesis (158). Maternal consumption, however, relates to fetal and neonatal morbidity in a dose-dependent and temporal fashion. More than 90 g of alcohol per day produces developmental defects with first-trimester exposure. Exposure during the third trimester can cause growth retardation and a delayed rise in the lecithin/sphingomyelin ratio (159).

Barbiturates

The barbiturates have both presynaptic and postsynaptic effects on the neurotransmitter γ-amino-butyric acid (GABA) and its receptors. They reversibly depress the activity of all excitable tissues. The CNS is most sensitive. All degrees of depression of the CNS, from mild sedation to general anesthesia, are achievable with various doses of barbiturate. Mono- and polysynaptic responses are depressed by barbiturates. Only very large doses or doses of extended duration have clinically detectable direct effects on peripheral tissues. Pharmacodynamic and pharmacokinetic tolerance can occur, with the former more responsible for the decreased effect with repetitive dosing. Despite tolerance to mood-altering and other systemic effects, the lethal dose remains the same; thus, with continued use, the therapeutic index falls and the risk of lethal overdose rises.

Barbiturates exhibit cross-tolerance with ethanol. An abstinence syndrome similar to that occurring with ethanol can develop. The severity of withdrawal relates to the degree of tolerance and, therefore, the extent, duration, and continuity of abuse. Symptomatology is very similar to the alcohol abstinence syndrome, with a range of manifestations from tremors, insomnia, and irritability to seizures, delirium, and hallucinations. Convulsions are an ominous occurrence in barbiturate withdrawal. Administration of barbiturates does not acutely reverse this syndrome.

Compromise of uteroplacental blood flow may occur during maternal intoxication or withdrawal. Behavioral and morphologic features of the fetal alcohol syndrome also appear in children of barbiturate abusers, but there is no specific fetal defect attributable to barbiturates (160). The induction of fetal hepatic enzymes tends to decrease neonatal bilirubin. Newborns of barbiturate abusers or even therapeutic users (i.e., epileptics) may be dependent on barbiturates. Depending on the half-life of the barbiturate and the length of maternal use, withdrawal symptoms may arise up to 1 week after birth.

Benzodiazepenes

Benzodiazepenes also exert their CNS effects via the GABA receptor, although they are not general neuronal depressants like the barbiturates and ethanol. There are wide differences in selectivity among this group of drugs with varying clinical usefulness, but there is cross-tolerance between benzodiazepenes and ethanol or barbiturates. Similarly, withdrawal syndromes do occur and are best managed with additional benzodiazepenes, as these drugs tend to lack cardiovascular or respiratory depressant effects when administered as single agents. Although physostigmine or naloxone partially antagonize the CNS effects of benzodiazepines, flumazenil is a specific benzodiazepine antagonist (161). Several studies attest to the teratogenicity of benzodiazepines (162,163); however, more recent studies contradict these data (164). In the neonate, benzodiazepines impair thermoregulation, resulting in hypothermia.

Cocaine

Cocaine alkaloid, an ester of benzoic acid, undergoes hydrolysis to become ecgonine, which in turn is benzoylated and methylated to the base cocaine (165). The hydrochloride salt of this base is the commercial product that, when mixed with an alkali, produces cocaine freebase, or "crack." This illicit preparation is more stable on heating, vaporizes easily, and has a high bioavailability when smoked (166). The bioavailability of topical intranasal cocaine is four to six times less than an equivalent intravenous dose, with peak plasma concentration proportional to the total dose administered (167). Time to peak concentration, however, lengthens with increasing doses, as cocaine may limit its own absorption via vasoconstriction (168).

The biologic half-life of cocaine is 0.5 to 1.5 hours. Metabolism occurs via plasma and liver esterases, with liver hydrolysis producing the only active metabolite, norcocaine (169,170). Norcocaine has been detected in primate brain, where it inhibits the reuptake of norepinephrine more than cocaine (171). Plasma from homozygotes for atypical cholinesterase has impaired in vitro decay of cocaine (172). Acquired deficiencies of the enzyme (liver disease, malnutrition, plasmapheresis, anticholinesterase medications, and pregnancy) also result in impaired plasma hydrolysis.

Changes in cocaine metabolism, alternations in central or peripheral adrenergic receptor sensitivity to norepinephrine, or differences in cocaine-induced cardiac responsiveness may individually or collectively account for the heightened sensitivity to cocaine seen in the pregnant ewe (173). Liver cytochrome P_{450} concentrations fall by as much as 25%, and activity of glucuronyl transferase and monoxygenase declines in pregnant rats and rabbits in comparison with nonpregnant animals (174,175). Progesterone treatment of nonpregnant rats increases N-demethylation of aminopyrine. This compound has almost identical kinetics as N-demethylation of cocaine to norcocaine (176). Yet another recent study shows that high concentrations of progesterone in pregnant ewes can delay cocaine metabolism or increase its bioactivity. Progesterone may either increase N-demethylation to norcocaine or enhance α-adrenergic receptor sensitivity. The fetus and newborn also are prone to altered metabolism and impaired clearance of cocaine and its metabolites. In the neonate, esterase metabolites persist as long as 4 to 5 days after maternal cocaine use (177).

Cocaine's mechanism of action, although complex and not completely understood, is one of additive effects on many neurotransmitter systems, including nerve conduction, autonomic sympathetic, and CNS functions (178). Several binding sites for cocaine exist in both central and peripheral nervous systems (179). Although the response to cocaine depends on dosage, duration of exposure, mode of administration, concurrent medications, predisposition, and environmental setting, a given dose of the drug still has predictable effects (180). The acute actions are brief and intense, resembling the neuropharmacologic and cardiovascular effects of amphetamines. Tachycardia, increased myocardial contractility, vasoconstriction, bronchodilation, pupillary dilation, muscle tremors, and elevated temperature are predictable, even with low doses of intranasal or intravenous cocaine. Arousal and euphoria proceed dysphoria, anxiety, somnolence, and drug craving (181). During gestation, cocaine may stimulate cardiac output to a greater degree than in the nonpregnant state. This effect may be mediated via a pregnancy-related increase in cardiac contractility, stroke volume, or both (173). In animals, maternal and fetal mean arterial pressure increase and uterine blood flow decreases, even with so-called "recreational" doses of cocaine (182). Such changes can result in marked fetal hypoxemia, hypertension, and tachycardia secondary to reduced uterine blood flow, direct fetal effects of cocaine, and increased fetal catecholamine concentrations (183).

Anyone using cocaine as a recreational drug may present with toxic manifestations regardless of dose or length of use. This toxicity may lead to sudden death and is characterized by its unpredictability and rapidity of onset (184). Manifestations include overstimulation of respiratory, cardiovascular, and central nervous systems. Ultimately, seizures, profound depression, and cardiovascular collapse arise. Because of enhanced maternal sensitivity to the drug, one may hypothesize that the incidence of toxic effects is higher among pregnant cocaine users versus their nonpregnant counterparts, although no data confirm this theory. The syndrome of hypertension, altered mental status, and seizures may mimic preeclampsia or eclampsia, and, in this case, history of cocaine use or urine and blood drug screening may be an important determinant of ensuing therapy and management.

Cocaine alkaloid, or "crack," is a highly potent, addictive, and relatively inexpensive form of cocaine that has more adverse perinatal effects than other forms of cocaine. Epidemic rates of maternal crack use bring national estimates of fetal cocaine exposure into the range of 91,500 to 240,000 children per year (185–187). Maternal cocaine use increases the risk of a multitude of perinatal problems, such as:

- Congenital urogenital abnormalities,
- Lower mean birth weight,
- Lower mean gestational age at delivery,
- Preterm labor and delivery,
- Abruptio placentae,
- Premature rupture of membranes, and
- Overall increased neonatal morbidity and mortality.

The maternal crack user is at greater risk for these complications than noncrack maternal cocaine users (188–194).

Fetal cocaine exposure increases both the neonatal hospital costs and length of stay. Crack exposure increases these costs far beyond those incurred with other illicit drug or noncrack cocaine exposure. At a national level, these costs add to almost $500 million per year.

Opioids

The physiologic effects of narcotics in humans are well known. Except for a steeper dose–response curve, they are the same in the pregnant population. Most maternal effects of opioids occur secondary to respiratory depression. Maternal hypercarbia and hypoxemia impair uterine blood flow. During withdrawal, heightened sympathetic tone further lowers uterine blood flow. These physiologic changes result in a placental abruption rate of 25% among opioid addicts (94).

Neonatal effects of opioids vary from an increased incidence of respiratory distress syndrome (195) and meconium aspiration to overt withdrawal syndrome (95). Symptoms of withdrawal occur in up to 80% of infants (chronically) exposed to opioids. Maternal treatment, including prenatal care through methadone clinics, markedly lowers neonatal morbidity and mortality (94). However, treatment does not preclude an extremely high incidence of neonatal withdrawal syndrome among infants of methadone-dependent mothers.

For their first 2 years of life, infants exposed to opioids are 250 to 500 g lighter and have a 1-cm smaller head circumference than controls (196). After 2 years of age, there are no growth or developmental differences (197), although an elevated incidence of central motor dysfunction persists until 5 years of age (198).

REFERENCES

1. Prowse CM, Gaensler EA. Respiratory acid-base changes during pregnancy. *Anesthesiology* 1965;36:381.
2. Cugell DW, Frank NR, Gaensler EA, et al. Pulmonary function in pregnancy; 1. Serial observations in normal women. *Am Rev Tuberc Pulmon Dis* 1953;67:568.
3. DiMarco AF. Asthma in the pregnant patient: a review. *Ann Allergy* 1989;62:527.
4. Schaefer G, Silverman F. Pregnancy complicated by asthma. *Am J Obstet Gynecol* 1961;82:182.
5. American Thoracic Society. Standards for the diagnosis and care of patients with chronic pulmonary obstructive disease (COPD) and asthma. *Am Rev Respir Dis* 1987;136:25.
6. Beck B. Pharmacologic approach to obstructed airway disease. *Primary Care Clin* 1985:12:239.
7. Szentivanyl A. The beta-adrenergic theory of the atopic abnormality in bronchial asthma. *J Allergy* 1968;42:203.
8. Ventner JC, Fraser CM, Harrison, LC. Autoantibodies to B2-adrenergic receptors: A possible cause of adrenergic hyporesponsiveness in allergic rhinitis and asthma. *Science* 1980;207:1361.
9. Holgate ST. Inflammatory cells and their mediators in the pathogenesis of asthma. *Postgrad Med J* 1988;64[Suppl 4]:82.
10. Insel PA, Wasserman SI. Asthma: a disorder of adrenergic receptors. *FASEB J* 1990;4:2732.
11. George RB, Owens NW. Bronchial asthma. In: Bone RC, ed. *Disease-a-Month.* St. Louis: Mosby-Year Book, 1991:5.
12. Popa V. Beta-adrenergic drugs. *Clin Chest Med* 1986;7:313.
13. Turner ES, Greenberger PA, Patterson R. Management of the pregnant asthmatic patient. *Ann Intern Med* 1980;6:105.
14. Juniper EF, Daniel EE, Roberts RS, et al. Effect of pregnancy on airway responsiveness and asthma severity. Relationship to serum progesterone. *Am Rev Respir Dis* 1991:143[Suppl]:78.
15. Schatz M, Harden K, Forsythe A, et al. The course of asthma during pregnancy postpartum and with successive pregnancies: a prospective analysis. *J Allergy Clin Immunol* 1988;81:509.
16. Gluck, JC, Gluck PA. The effects of pregnancy on asthma: a prospective study. *Ann Allergy* 1976;37:164.
17. Apter AJ, Greenberger PA, Patterson R. Outcomes of pregnancy in adolescents with severe asthma. *Arch Intern Med* 1989;149:2571.
18. Mathe AA, Hedqvist P. Effect of prostaglandins F2a and E2 on airway conductance in healthy subjects and asthmatic patients. *Am Rev Respir Dis* 1975;111:313.
19. Jones E, Curzen P, Gaugas JM. Suppression activity of pregnancy plasma on mixed lymphocyte reaction. *J Obstet Gynecol* 1973;80:603.
20. Gee JBL, Packer BS, Millen JE, et al. Pulmonary mechanics during pregnancy. *J Clin Invest* 1967;46:945.
21. Barslu HE. Asthma and pregnancy. A challenge for everyone concerned. *Postgrad Med* 1911;89:125.

22. Bahna SL, Bjerkdal T. The course and outcome of pregnancy in women with bronchial asthma. *Acta Allergy* 1972;27:397.
23. Schatz M, Zeiger RS, Hoffman CP. Intrauterine growth is related to gestational pulmonary function in pregnant asthmatic women. *Chest* 1990;98:389.
24. Wulf KH, Kunzel W, Lehmann V. Clinical aspects of placental gas exchange. In: Lango LD, Bartels H, eds. *Respiratory gas exchange and blood flow in the placenta.* Bethesda: National Institutes of Health, Public Health Service, US Department of Health, Education, and Welfare, 1962:505.
25. Fitzsimmons R, Greenberger PA, Patterson R. Outcome of pregnancy in women requiring corticosteroids for severe asthma. *J Allergy Clin Immunol* 1986;78:349.
26. Schatz M, Zeiger RS, Harden KM, et al. The safety of inhaled β-agonist bronchodilators during pregnancy. *J Allergy Clin Immunol* 1988; 82:686.
27. Greenberger PA, Patterson R. Current concepts. Management of asthma during pregnancy. *N Engl J Med* 1985;312:897.
28. Weinberger M. Pharmacology and therapeutic use of theophylline. *J Allergy Clin Immunol* 1984;73:525.
29. Ng WH, Polosa R, Church MK. Adenosine bronchoconstriction in asthma: investigations into its possible mechanism of action. *Br J Clin Pharmacol* 1990;30[Suppl]:89s.
30. Bukowsky M, Nakatsu K, Hunt DW. Theophylline reassessed. *Ann Intern Med* 1984;101:63.
31. Self TH, Aboul-Shalla N, Burns R, et al. Inhaled albuterol and oral prednisone therapy in hospitalized adult asthmatics. Does aminophylline add any benefit? *Chest* 1990;98:1317.
32. Gardner MJ, Schatz M, Cousins L, et al. Longitudinal effects of pregnancy on the pharmacokinetics of theophylline. *Eur J Clin Pharmacol* 1987;31:289.
33. Carter BL, Discoll CE, Smith GD. Theophylline clearance during pregnancy. *Obstet Gynecol* 1986;68:555.
34. Sutton PL, Rose JQ, Goldstein S, et al. Theophylline pharmacokinetics during pregnancy and post partum. *J Allergy Clin Immunol* 1980; 65:177.
35. Kelly HW, Murphy S. Corticosteroids for acute, severe asthma. *DICP* 1991;25:72.
36. Svedmyr N. Action of corticosteroids on β-adrenergic receptors. *Am Rev Respir Dis* 1990;141[Suppl]:31.
37. Munck A, Mendel DB, Smith LI, Orti E. Glucocorticoid receptors and actions. *Am Rev Respir Dis* 1990;141[Suppl]:2.
38. Williams TJ, Yaarwood H. Effect of corticosteroids on microvascular permeability. *Am Rev Respir Dis* 1990:141[Suppl]:39.
39. Schleimer RP. Effects of glucocorticoids on inflammatory cells relevant to their therapeutic applications in asthma. *Am Rev Respir Dis* 1990;141[Suppl]:59.
40. Dunlap NE, Bailey WC. Corticosteroids in asthma. *South Med J* 1990;83:428.
41. McDonald AJ. Asthma. *Emerg Med Clin North Am* 1989;7:219.
42. Hernandez E, Angell CS, Johnson JWC. Asthma in pregnancy: current concepts. *Obstet Gynecol* 1980;55:739.
43. Britton JR. Effects of social class, sex, and region of residence on age at death from cystic fibrosis. *Br Med J* 1989;298:483.
44. Cohen LF, di Sant Agnese PA, Friedlander J. Cystic fibrosis and pregnancy: a national survey. *Lancet* 1980;2:842.
45. Pittard WB III, Sorenson RU, Schnatz PT. Pregnancy outcome in mothers with cystic fibrosis: normal neonatal immune responses. *South Med J* 1987;80:347.
46. Longo LD. Some health consequences of maternal smoking: issues without answers. *Birth Defects* 1982;18:13.
47. Handler A, Davis F, Ferre C, Yeko T. The relationship of smoking and ectopic pregnancy. *Am J Public Health* 1989;79:1239.
48. Philbert H, Dam M. The epileptic mother and her child. *Epilepsia* 1982;23:85.
49. Bjerkdal T, Bahna SL. The occurrence and outcome of pregnancy in women with epilepsy. *Acta Gynecol Scand* 1976;55:187.
50. Niswander KR, Gordon M. The Collaborative Perinatal Study of the National Institute of Neurological Disease and Stroke. Washington, DC: Department of Health, Education, and Welfare; 1972; NIH-73-379.
51. Yerby MS. Problems and management of the pregnant woman with epilepsy. *Epilepsia* 1987;28:529.
52. Hiilesmaa VK, Bardy A, Teram K. Obstetric outcome in women with epilepsy. *Am J Obstet Gynecol* 1985;152:499.
53. Schmidt D. The effect of pregnancy on the natural history of epilepsy: review of the literature. In: Janz D, Dam M, Richens A, et al., eds. *Epilepsy, pregnancy and the child.* New York: Raven Press, 1982:3.
54. Remillard G, Dansky L, Andermann E, Andermann F. Seizure frequency during pregnancy and puerperium. In: Janz D, Dam M, Richens A, et al., eds. *Epilepsy, pregnancy and the child.* New York: Raven Press, 1982:15.
55. Knott C, Williams CP, Reynolds F. Phenytoin kinetics during pregnancy and the puerperium. *Br J Obstet Gynaecol* 1986;93:1030.
56. American Academy of Pediatrics Committee on Drugs. Anticonvulsants and pregnancy. *Pediatrics* 1979;63:331.
57. Saunders M. Epilepsy in women of childbearing age. *Br Med J* 1989;299:581.
58. Fabra S. Valproic acid and birth defects. *Reprod Toxicol Newsletter* 1983;2:9.
59. Ramsay RE, Strauss RG, Wilder BJ, Wilimore LJ. Status epilepticus in pregnancy: effect of phenytoin malabsorption on seizure control. *Neurology* 1978;28:85.
60. Vincent A. Immunology of acetylcholine receptor in relation to myasthenia gravis. *Physiol Rev* 1980;60:756.
61. Mossman S, Vincent A, Newsom-Davis J. Myasthenia gravis without acetylcholine-receptor antibody: a distinct disease entity. *Lancet* 1986;1:116.
62. Hatton PD, Diehl JT, Daly BDT, et al. Transternal radical thymectomy for myasthenia gravis: a 15-year review. *Ann Thorac Surg* 1989;47: 838.
63. Mulder DG, Graves M, Herrman C. Thymetomy for myasthenia gravis: recent observations and comparisons with past experience. *Ann Thorac Surg* 1989;48:551.
64. Reischies FM, Baum K, Brau H, et al. Cerebral magnetic resonance imaging in multiple sclerosis. *Arch Neurol* 1988:263.
65. Mastrostefano R, Occhipinti E, Bigotti G, Pompili A. Multiple sclerosis plaque-stimulating cerebral tumor: case report and review of the literature. *Neurosurgery* 1987;21:244.
66. Kurtzke JF, Hyllested K. Multiple sclerosis in the Faroe islands. II. Clinical update, transmission, and the nature of MS. *Neurology* 1986; 36:307.
67. McCullough B, Krakowka S, Koestner A. Experimental canine distemper virus-induced demyelination. *Lab Invest* 1974;31:216.
68. Cutler RWP, Averill DR Jr. Cerebrospinal fluid gamma globulins in canine distemper encephalitis. *Neurology* 1969;19:1111.
69. Swank RL. Multiple sclerosis: a correlation of its incidence with dietary fat. *Am J Med Sci* 1950;220:421.
70. Poser CM. Trauma and multiple sclerosis: an hypothesis. *J Neurol* 1987;234:155.
71. Stein EC, Schiffer RFB, Hall WJ, Young N. Multiple sclerosis and the workplace: a report of an industry-based cluster. *Neurology* 1987;37: 1672.
72. Elias SB. Oligodendrocyte development and the natural history of multiple sclerosis. *Arch Neurol* 1987;44:1294.
73. Rose AS, Kuzma JW, Kurtzke JF, et al. Cooperative study in the evaluation of therapy in multiple sclerosis: ACTH vs. placebo: final report. *Neurology* 1970;20:1.
74. Tourtellotte WW, Baumhefner RW, Pohin AR, et al. Multiple sclerosis de novo CSF IgG synthesis: effect of ACTH and corticosteroids. *Neurology* 1980;30:1155.
75. Birk K, Ford C, Smeltzer S, et al. The clinical course of multiple sclerosis during pregnancy and the puerperium. *Arch Neurol* 1990;47:738.
76. *Physician's Desk Reference,* 51st ed. Montvale: Medical Economics Co., 1997:1865.
77. Khatri BO, D'Cruz O, Priesler G, et al. Plasmapheresis in a pregnant patient with multiple sclerosis. *Arch Neurol* 1990;47:11.
78. Birnbach DJ, Bader A, Ostheimer GW. Anesthesia and multiple sclerosis. *JAMA* 1988;260:2838.
79. Swapp GH, Main RA. Neurofibromatosis in pregnancy. *Br J Dermatol* 1973;80:431.
80. Magbagbeola JAO. Abnormal responses to muscle relaxants in a patient with von Recklinghausen's disease. *Br J Anaesth* 1970;42:183.
81. Baraka A. Myasthenic response to muscle relaxants in von Recklinghausen's disease. *Br J Anaesth* 1974;46:701.
82. Schonwald G, Fish KJ, Perkesh I. Cardiovascular complications during anesthesia in chronic spinal cord injured patients. *Anesthesiology* 1981;55:550.
83. Head H, Reddoch G. The autonomic bladder, excessive sweating and

some other reflex conditions in gross injury of the spinal cord. *Brain* 1917;40:188.
84. Lambert DH, Deane RS, Mazuzan JE. Anesthesia and the control of blood pressure in patients with spinal cord injury. *Anesth Analg* 1982;61:344.
85. Goller H, Paeslack V. Our experiences about pregnancy and delivery of the paraplegic woman. *Paraplegia* 1970;8:161.
86. Greenspan JS, Paul RH. Paraplegia and quadriplegia: special considerations during pregnancy and labor and delivery. *Am J Obstet Gynecol* 1986;155:738.
87. Roelvink NC, Kamphorst W, van Alphen HA, Rao BR. Pregnancy-related primary brain and spinal tumors. *Arch Neurol* 1987;44:209.
88. Choi NW. Epidemiology of primary central nervous system neoplasms: II. Case-controlled study. *Am J Epidemiol* 1970;91:467.
89. Weyand RD, MacCarty C, Wilson RB. The effect of pregnancy on intracranial meningiomas occurring about the optic chiasm. *Surg Clin North Am* 1951;31:1225.
90. Markwalder T. Estrogen and progesterone receptors in meningiomas in relation to clinical and pathologic features. *Surg Neurol* 1983; 20:42.
91. Biller J, Adams HP. Cerebrovascular disorders associated with pregnancy. *Am Fam Physician* 1986;33:125.
92. Donnelly JF, Lock FR. Causes of death in 533 fatal cases of toxemia in pregnancy. *Am J Obstet Gynecol* 1954;68:184.
93. Reece EA, Chervenak FA, Coultrip L, Hobbins JC. The perinatal management of pregnancy complicated by massive intracerebral hemorrhage. *Am J Perinatol* 1984;1:266.
94. Robinson JL, Hall CJ, Sedizmir CB. Subarachnoid hemorrhage in pregnancy. *J Neurosurg* 1972;36:27.
95. Robinson JL, Hall CJ, Sedizmir CB. Arteriovenous malformations, aneurysms and pregnancy. *J Neurosurg* 1974;41:63.
96. Dais SF, Byers RH Jr, Lindegren ML, Caldwell MB, Karon JM, Gwinn M. Prevalence and incidence of vertically acquired HIV infection in the United States. *JAMA* 1995:274:952.
97. Burke DS, Brundage JF, Herbold JR, et al. Human immunodeficiency virus infections among civilian applicants for United States military service: October, 1985–March, 1986. *N Engl J Med* 1987;317:131.
98. Koonin LM, Ellerbrock TV, Atrash HK, et al. Pregnancy-associated deaths due to AIDS in the United States. *JAMA* 1989;261:1306.
99. Centers for Disease Control. *AIDS Weekly Surveillance Report–United States.* Atlanta: Centers for Disease Control, December 26, 1988:1.
100. Hawken J, Chard T, Costeloe K, Jeffries DJ, Hudson CN. Risk factors for HIV infection overlooked in routine antenatal care. *J R Soc Med* 1995;88:634.
101. Boylston AW, Francis ND. Does it matter which cells are infected by the immunodeficiency virus type 1? *J Pathol* 1988;156:93.
102. Albert J, Gaines H, Sunnerborg A, et al. Isolation of human immunodeficiency virus from plasma during primary HIV infection. *J Med Virol* 1987;23:67.
103. Levy JA, Shimaabukuro J. Recovery of AIDS-associated retroviruses from patients with AIDS-related conditions and from clinically healthy individuals. *J Infect Dis* 1985;152:734.
104. Schwartz JS, Dans PE, Kinosian BP. Human immunodeficiency virus test evaluation, performance and use: proposals to make food tests better. *JAMA* 1988;259:2574.
105. Koonin LM, Ellerbrock TV, Atrash HK, et al. Pregnancy-associated deaths due to AIDS in the United States. *JAMA* 1989;261:1306.
106. Guinan ME, Hardy A. Epidemiology of AIDS in women in the United States. *JAMA* 1987;257:2039.
107. Redfield RR, Wright DC, Tramont EC. Special report: the Walter Reed staging classification for HTLV III/LAV infection. *N Engl J Med* 1986;314:131.
108. Redfield RR, Burke DS. HIV infection: the clinical picture. *Sci Am* 1988;259:90.
109. Meng TC, Fischl MA, Boota AM, et al. Combination therapy with zidovudine and dideoxycytidine in patients with advanced human immunodeficiency infection: a phase I/II study. *Ann Intern Med* 1992; 116:13.
110. Hirsch MD, Martin S, D'Aquila MD, et al. Therapy for human immunodeficiency virus infection. *N Engl J Med* 1993;328:1686.
111. Baines MG, Pross HF, Miller KG. Spontaneous human lymphocyte-mediated cytotoxicity against tumor target cells; IV. The suppressive effect of normal pregnancy. *Am J Obstet Gynecol* 1978;130:741.
112. Sridama V, Pacini F, Yang S, et al. Decreased levels of helper T cells: a possible cause of immunodeficiency in pregnancy. *N Engl J Med* 1982;307:352.
113. Minkoff HL, Nanda D, Menez R, et al. Follow up of mothers of children with AIDS. *Obstet Gynecol* 1987;87:288.
114. Scott GB, Fischl MA, Klimas N, et al. Mothers of infants with the acquired immunodeficiency syndrome: evidence for both symptomatic and asymptomatic carriers. *JAMA* 1985;253:363.
115. Schoenbaum EE, Selwyn PA, Feingold AR, et al. The effect of pregnancy on progression of HIV related disease. In: *Abstracts of the 3rd International Conference on AIDS.* Washington DC: US Department of Health and Human Services and the World Health Organization, 1987:27.
116. The NYC Collaborative Study Group for Vertical Transmission of HIV. Human immunodeficiency virus infection during pregnancy: a longitudinal study. In: *Abstracts of the 3rd International Conference on AIDS.* Washington, DC: US Department of Health and Human Services and the World Health Organization, 1987:73.
117. Minkoff H, Nanda D, Menez R, et al. Pregnancies resulting in infants with AIDS or AIDS-related complex. *Obstet Gynecol* 1987;69:285.
118. Fricker HS, Segal S. Narcotic addiction, pregnancy, and the newborn. *Am J Dis Child* 1978;132:360.
119. MacGregor SW, Keith LG, Chasnoff IJ, et al. Cocaine use during pregnancy: adverse perinatal outcome. *Am J Obstet Gynecol* 1987;157:686.
120. Gorsky RD, Farnham PG, Straus WL, et al. Preventing perinatal transmission of HIV—costs and effectiveness of recommended intervention. *Public Health Rep* 1996;111:335.
121. Dinsmoor MJ. HIV infection and pregnancy. *Med Clin North Am* 1989;73:701.
122. Joviasas E, Koch MA, Schafer A, et al. LAV HTLV-III in a 20 week fetus. *Lancet* 1985;2:1129.
123. Lapointe N, Michaud J, Pekovic D, et al. Transplacental transmission of HTLV-III virus. *N Engl J Med* 1985;312:1325.
124. Caesarean section and risk of vertical transmission of HIV-1 infection. The European Collaborative Study. *Lancet* 1994;343:1464.
125. Dickover RE, Garratty EM, Herman SA, et al. Identification of levels of maternal HIV-1 RNA associated with risk of perinatal transmission. Effect of maternal zidovudine treatment on viral load. *JAMA* 1996;275:599.
126. Boyer PJ, Dillon M, Navaaie M, et al. Factors predictive of maternal-fetal transmission of HIV-1. Preliminary analysis of zidovudine given during pregnancy and/or delivery. *JAMA* 1994;271:1925.
127. Hino S, Yamaguchi K, Katamine S, et al. Mother-to-child transmission of human T-cell leukemia virus type 1. *Jpn J Cancer Res* 1985; 76:474.
128. Thiry L, Sprecher-Goldberger S, Jonckheer T, et al. Isolation of AIDS virus from cell-free breast milk of three healthy virus carriers. *Lancet* 1985;2:891.
129. Ziegler JB, Johnson RO, Cooper DA, et al. Postnatal transmission of AIDS-associated retrovirus from mother to infant. *Lancet* 1985;1:896.
130. Marion RW, Wiznia M, Hutcheon RG, et al. Fetal AIDS syndrome score. *Arch Dis Child* 1987;141:429.
131. Minkoff H, Nanda D, Menez R, Fikrig S. Pregnancies resulting in infants with AIDS or AIDS-related complex: follow-up of mothers, children and subsequently born siblings. *Obstet Gynecol* 1987;69:288.
132. Menez-Bautista R, Fikrig SM, Pahwa S, et al. Monozygotic twins discordant for the acquired immunodeficiency syndrome. *Arch Dis Child* 1986;140:678.
133. Park CL, Streicher H, Rothberg R. Transmission of HIV from parents to only one dizygotic twin. *J Clin Microbiol* 1987;25:1119.
134. Williamson DF, Surdula JS, Kendrick NF, et al. Comparing the prevalence of smoking in pregnant and nonpregnant women 1985–1986. *JAMA* 1989;261:70.
135. Rubin PC, Craig GF, Gavin K, Sumner D. Prospective survey of use of therapeutic drugs, alcohol and cigarettes during pregnancy. *Br Med J Clin Res Ed* 1986;292:81.
136. McCalla S, Minkoff HL, Feldman J, et al. The biologic and social consequences of perinatal cocine use in an inner-city population: results of an anonymous cross-sectional study. *Am Obstet Gynecol* 1991;164:625.
137. Chavkin W. Drug addiction and pregnancy—policy crossroads. Public health and the law. *Am J Public Health* 1990;80:483.
138. Kulberg A. Substance abuse: clinical identification and management. *Pediatr Clin North Am* 1986;33:325.
139. Semlitz L, Gold MS. Adolescent drug abuse: diagnosis, treatment, and prevention. *Psychiatr Clin North Am* 1986;9:455.

140. Mucklow JC. The fate of drugs in pregnancy. *Clin Obstet Gynecol* 1986;13:161.
141. Perry BD, Pesavento DJ, Kussie PH, et al. Prenatal exposure to drugs of abuse in humans: effects on placental neurotransmitter receptors. *Neurobehav Toxicol Teratol* 1984;6:295.
142. Martin JC. Irreversible changes in mature and aging animals following intrauterine drug exposure. *Neurobehav Toxicol Teratol* 1986; 8:335.
143. Milunsky A, Jick H, Jick SS, et al. Multivitamin/folic acid supplementation in early pregnancy reduces the prevalence of neural tube defects. *JAMA* 1989;262:2847.
144. Zuckerman B, Frank DZ, Hingson R, et al. Effects of maternal marijuana and cocaine use on fetal growth. *N Engl J Med* 1989;320:762.
145. Maling HM. Toxicology of single doses of ethyl alcohol. In: Tremolieres J, ed. *Alcohols and derivatives, vol. 2, international encyclopedia of pharmacology and therapeutics.* Oxford: Pergamon Press, 1970:277.
146. Li TK, Boston WF. Genetic variability of enzymes of alcohol metabolism in human beings. *Ann Emerg Med* 1986;15:997.
147. Chan AW. Racial differences in alcohol sensitivity. *Alcohol* 1986;21:93.
148. Erwin VG, McClearn GE. Genetic influences on alcohol consumption and action of alcohol. *Curr Alcohol* 1981;8:405.
149. Sellers EM, Kalant H. Alcohol intoxication and withdrawal. *N Engl J Med* 1976;294:757.
150. Thompson WL. Management of alcohol withdrawal syndromes. *Arch Intern Med* 1978;138:278.
151. Thompson WL, Johnson AD, Maddrey WL. Diazepam and paraldehyde for treatment of severe delirium tremens. A controlled trial. *Arch Intern Med* 1975;82:175.
152. Segel LD, Klausner SC, Gnadt JT, Amsterdam EA. Alcohol and the heart. *Med Clin North Am* 1984;68:147.
153. Ylikahari RH, Huttenen MU, Harkonen M. Hormonal changes during alcohol intoxication and withdrawal. *Pharmacol Biochem Behav* 1980;13:131.
154. Erksine RL, Ritchie JW. The effect of maternal consumption of alcohol on human umbilical artery blood flow. *Am J Obstet Gynecol* 1986;154:318.
155. Fisher SE, Arkinson M, Van Thiel DH. Selective fetal malnutrition: the effect of nicotine, ethanol and acetaldehyde upon in vitro uptake of alpha-aminobutyric acid by human term placental villous slices. *Dev Pharmacol Ther* 1984;7:229.
156. Horrobin DF. A biochemical basis for alcoholism and alcohol-induced damage including the fetal alcohol syndrome and cirrhosis: interference with essential fatty acid and prostaglandin metabolism. *Med Hypotheses* 1980;6:929.
157. Andres RL, Jones KL. Social and illicit drug use in pregnancy. In: Creasy RK, Resnick R, eds. *Maternal-fetal medicine. Principles and practice*. 3rd Edition. Philadelphia: WB Saunders Co., 1994:184.
158. Tanaka H, Suzuki N, Arima M. Experimental studies on the influence of male alcoholism on fetal development. *Brain Dev* 1982;4:1.
159. Smith IE, Coles CD, Lancaster J, Fernhoff PM, Falek A. The effect of volume and duration of ethanol exposure on neonatal physical and behavioral development. *Neurobehav Toxicol Teratol* 1986;8:375.
160. Fishman RH, Yanai J. Long-lasting effects of early barbiturates on central nervous system and behavior. *Neurosci Biobehav Rev* 1983; 7:19.
161. Ghoneim MM, Dembo HB, Block RI. Time course of antagonism of sedative and amnesic effects of diazepam by flumazenil. *Anesthesiology* 1989;70:899.
162. Saxen I, Saxen L. Association between maternal intake of diazepam and oral clefts. *Lancet* 1975;2:498.
163. Safra MJ, Oakley GP. Association between cleft lip with or without cleft palate and prenatal exposure to diazepam. *Lancet* 1975;2:478.
164. Rice SA, Pelligrini M. Teratology of fixed agents. In: Baden JM, Brodsky JB, eds. *The pregnant surgical patient.* Mount Kisco: Futura Publishing, 1985:53.
165. Caldwell J, Sever PS. The biochemical pharmacology of abused drugs; 1. Amphetamines, cocaine, and LSD. *Clin Pharmacol Ther* 1974;116:625.
166. Grabowski J, Dworkin SI. Cocaine: an overview of current issues. *Int J Addict* 1985;20:1065.
167. VanDyke C, Barash PG, Jatlow P, Byck R. Cocaine: plasma concentrations after intranasal application in man. *Science* 1976;191:859.
168. Wilkinson P, VanDyke C, Jatlow P, Barash PG, Byck R. Intranasal and oral cocaine kinetics. *Clin Pharmacol Ther* 1980;27:386.
169. Stewart DJ, Inaba T, Lucssen M, Kalow W. Cocaine metabolism: cocaine and norcocaine hydrolysis by liver and serum esterases. *Clin Pharmacol Ther* 1979;25:464.
170. Inaba T, Stewart DJ, Kalow W. Metabolism of cocaine in man. *Clin Pharmacol Ther* 1978;23:547.
171. Hawks RL, Kopin IJ, Colburn RW, Thoa NB. Norcocaine: a pharmacologically active metabolite of cocaine found in brain. *Life Sci* 1974; 15:2189.
172. Jatlow P, Barash PG, VanDyke C, Radding J, Byck R. Cocaine and succinylcholine sensitivity: a new caution. *Anesth Analg* 1979;58:235.
173. Woods JR Jr, Plessinger MA. Pregnancy increases cardiovascular toxicity to cocaine. *Am J Obstet Gynecol* 1990;162:529.
174. Neale MG, Parke DV. Effects of pregnancy on the metabolism of drugs in the rat and rabbit. *Biochem Pharmacol* 1973;22:1451.
175. Dean ME, Stock BH. Hepatic microsomal metabolism of drugs during pregnancy in the rat. *Drug Metab Dispos* 1973;2:325.
176. Ochs H, Dusterberg B, Schulte-Hermann R. Induction of monooxygenases and growth in rat liver by progesterone. *Arch Toxicol* 1986;59:146.
177. Chasnoff IJ, Lewis DE, Griffith DR, Willey S. Cocaine and pregnancy: clinical and toxicological implications for the neonate. *Clin Chem* 1989;35:1276.
178. Fleming JA, Byck R, Barash PG. Pharmacology and therapeutic applications of cocaine. *Anesthesiology* 1990;73:518.
179. Reith MEA. Cocaine receptors on monoamine transporters and sodium channels. *NIDA Res Monogr* 1988;88:23.
180. Adams EH, Kozel NJ. Cocaine use in America: introduction and overview. *NIDA Res Monogr* 1985;61:1.
181. Ritchie JM, Greene NM. Local anesthetics. In: Gilman AG, Goodman AF, Rall W, Murad F, eds. *Goodman and Gillman's the pharmacological basis of therapeutics,* 7th ed. New York: MacMillan, 1985:321.
182. Moore TR, Sorg J, Miller L, Dey TC, Resnik R. Hemodynamic effects of intravenous cocaine on the pregnant ewe and fetus. *Am J Obstet Gynecol* 1986;155:883.
183. Woods JR, Plessinger MA, Clark KE. Effects of cocaine on uterine blood flow and fetal oxygenation. *JAMA* 1987;257:957.
184. Cregler LL, Mark H. Medical complications of cocaine abuse. *N Engl J Med* 1986;315:1495.
185. US General Accounting Office. Drug-exposed infants: a generation at risk. Washington, DC: US General Accounting Office; 1990; GAO/HRD-90-138.
186. Gomby D, Shiono PH. Estimating the number of substance-exposed infants. *Future Child* 1991;1:17.
187. Besharov DJ. The children of crack: will we protect them? *Public Welfare* 1989;Fall:6.
188. MacGregor SN, Keith LLG, Bachicha JA, Chasnoff IJ. Cocaine abuse during pregnancy: correlation between prenatal care and perinatal outcome. *Obstet Gynecol* 1989;74:882.
189. Neerhof MG, MacGregor SN, Retzky SS, Sullivan TP. Cocaine abuse during pregnancy: Peripartum prevalence and perinatal outcome. *Am J Obstet Gynecol* 1989;161;633.
190. Chavez GF, Mulinaree J, Cordero JF. Maternal cocaine use during early pregnancy as a risk factor for congenital urogenital anomalies. *JAMA* 1989;262:795.
191. Mitchell M, Sabbagha RE, Keith L, et al. Ultrasonic growth parameters in fetuses of mothers with primary addiction to cocaine. *Am J Obstet Gynecol* 1988;159:1104.
192. Fulroth R, Phillips B, Durand DJ. Perinatal outcome of infants exposed to cocaine and/or heroin in utero. *Am J Dis Child* 1989;13:905.
193. Cherukuri R, Minkoff H, Feldman J, Parkh A, Glass L. A cohort study of alkaloidal cocaine ("crack") in pregnancy. *Obstet Gynecol* 1988;72:147.
194. Acker D, Saachs BP, Tracey KJ, et al. Abruptio placentae associated with cocaine use. *Am J Obstet Gynecol* 1983;146:220.
195. Parekh A, Mukherjee TK, Jhaveri R, et al. Intrauterine exposure to narcotics and cord blood prolactin concentrations. *Obstet Gynecol* 1981;57:477.
196. Keith LG, MacGregor S, Friedell S, et al. Substance abuse in pregnant women: recent experience at the Perinatal Center for Chemical Dependence of Northwestern Memorial Hospital. *Obstet Gynecol* 1989;73:715.
197. Chasnoff IJ, Burns KA, Burns WJ, et al. Prenatal drug exposure and effects on neonatal and infant growth and development. *Neurobehav Toxicol Teratol* 1986;8:357.
198. Dobercyzk TM, Kandall SR, Rongkapan O, et al. Peripheral nerve conduction studies in passively addicted neonates. *Arch Phys Med Rehabil* 1986;67:4.

Obstetric Anesthesia, second edition,
edited by Mark C. Norris.
Lippincott Williams & Wilkins, Philadelphia © 1999.

CHAPTER 4

Pathophysiology and Obstetric Management of Preeclampsia

Jaya Ramanathan, John G. D'Alessio, and Baha M. Sibai

Hypertension complicates 7% to 10% of pregnancies and is a major cause of maternal morbidity and mortality worldwide (1). Clinically, hypertension manifests as a wide spectrum of disorders, ranging from mildly elevated blood pressure to severe disease involving all of the major organ systems. The revised Technical Bulletin from the American College of Obstetricians and Gynecologists published in 1996 defined hypertension during pregnancy as a sustained blood pressure of 140 mm Hg systolic or 90 mm Hg diastolic (2).

HYPERTENSIVE DISORDERS OF PREGNANCY

Hypertensive disorders of pregnancy can be broadly classified as chronic hypertension and pregnancy-induced hypertension (PIH) (2). PIH encompasses several clinical subsets depending on end-organ effects (2). Table 1 shows the classification of the hypertensive disorders of pregnancy. Brief descriptions of the subsets are as follows.

Preeclampsia

Preeclampsia is the development of hypertension with proteinuria after the 20th week of gestation in a previously normotensive woman. Preeclampsia can be mild or severe (Table 2).

Eclampsia

Eclampsia is the development of convulsions or coma in women with preeclampsia without other precipitating causes of seizures.

J. Ramanathan: Departments of Anesthesiology and Obstetrics and Gynecology, University of Tennessee, Memphis, Tennessee 30103.

J. G. D'Alessio: Department of Anesthesiology, University of Tennessee, Memphis, Tennessee 30103.

B. M. Sibai: Department of Obstetrics and Gynecology, University of Tennessee, Memphis, Tennessee 30103.

HELLP Syndrome

HELLP syndrome (hemolysis, elevated liver enzymes, and low platelet count) manifests clinically with severe hematologic and hepatic dysfunction in women with PIH.

Chronic Hypertension of Pregnancy

Chronic hypertension of pregnancy is an elevated blood pressure of any etiology with no proteinuria, usually occurring before the 20th week of gestation and persisting more than 6 weeks postpartum. The development of preeclampsia in pregnant women with chronic hypertension is classified as superimposed preeclampsia.

Gestational Hypertension

Gestational hypertension develops in the second half of pregnancy or in the first 24 hours postpartum without evidence of edema or proteinuria. Blood pressure returns to normal within 10 days of delivery.

Although the terminology and the definitions are well described, the accurate diagnosis of various subsets of hypertension during pregnancy is often difficult. Poor

TABLE 1. *Classification of hypertensive disorders in pregnancy*

I. Pregnancy-induced hypertension
   A. Preeclampsia
      1. Mild
      2. Severe
   B. Eclampsia
II. Chronic hypertension preceding pregnancy (any etiology)
III. Chronic hypertension with superimposed pregnancy-induced hypertension
IV. Gestational hypertension

After ref. 9.

TABLE 2. *Clinical manifestations of severe disease in patients with pregnancy-induced hypertension*

1. Systolic pressure of 160 mm Hg, or diastolic pressure 110 mm Hg on two occasions at least 6 h apart
2. Proteinuria of at least 5 g in 24-h urine collection (3+ or 4+ on semiquantitative assay)
3. Oliguria of <400 mL in 24 h
4. Cerebral or visual disturbances such as altered consciousness, headache, scotomas, or blurred vision
5. Pulmonary edema or cyanosis
6. Epigastric or right upper quadrant pain
7. Impaired liver function of unclear etiology
8. Thrombocytopenia

After ref. 115.

documentation of blood pressures and inaccurate or insufficient assessment of renal function during earlier visits can make differentiating preeclampsia from preexisting chronic hypertension and renal dysfunction an arduous task. In addition, the nonspecific signs of preeclampsia (proteinuria and generalized edema) are often present in normal pregnancy. Lastly, there are no specific clinical or biochemical markers for the positive diagnosis of preeclampsia.

INCIDENCE AND PREDISPOSING FACTORS

Although preeclampsia is primarily a disease of the young primigravida, it also occurs in women older than 40 years. The increased occurrence in older women presumably is due to the higher incidence of chronic hypertension. Preeclampsia complicates 6% to 7% of pregnancies in the United States. The incidence among young, black primigravidae in inner-city hospitals is 20%. Risk factors include:

- Preeclampsia during previous pregnancy,
- Molar pregnancy,
- Twin gestation,
- Hydrops fetalis,
- Diabetes mellitus,
- Chronic hypertension,
- Chronic renal disease, and
- Antiphospholipid syndrome.

Other characteristic hazards include African-American race, inadequate prenatal care, poor socioeconomic background, nutritional deficiencies, and a family history of PIH (2,3).

ETIOLOGY

Preeclampsia is a disease of unknown etiology. It occurs only in human pregnancy and has yet to be reproduced in animals. Of the various theories regarding the etiology of preeclampsia, the following merit brief discussions.

Abnormal Response to Placentation

In preeclampsia, the maternal vasculature does not respond appropriately to the early implantation and growth of placenta. In the early stages of normal pregnancy, endovascular trophoblasts invade the decidual segments of the spiral arteries. A second wave of trophoblast migration follows at the 16th week of gestation (4–6). The second wave of migration invades the myometrial segments of the spiral arteries (Fig. 1). In preeclampsia, vascular changes involve only the decidual segments of the spiral arteries. The musculoelastic portions of the myometrial segments of the spiral arteries remain intact. The myometrial portion of the spiral artery is small and narrow and responds readily to vasomotor stimuli with vasoconstriction. This narrowing decreases placental perfusion, produces areas of placental infarction, and predisposes to intrauterine growth retardation (4–6). This abnormal maternal response to placentation is the earliest pathognomonic feature of preeclampsia; however, such changes are impossible to detect as the placenta is inaccessible during early pregnancy.

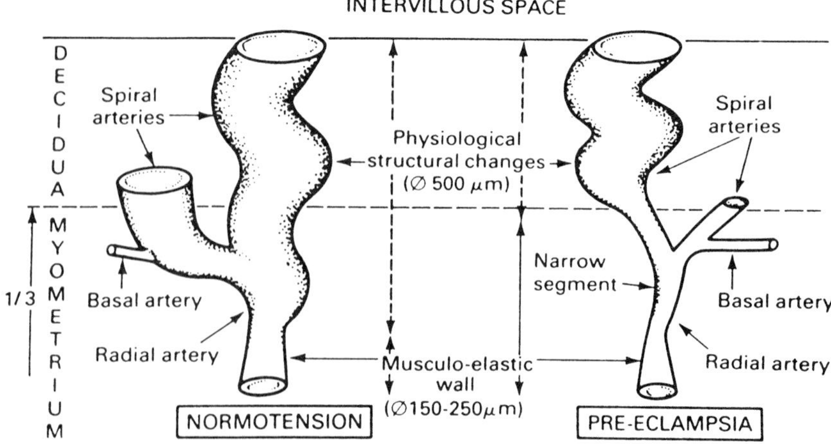

FIG. 1. Diagrammatic representation of changes in decidual vessels in normal and preeclamptic pregnancies. (From ref. 5, with permission.)

Thromboxane–Prostacyclin Imbalance

Thromboxane A_2, produced by the platelets, is a potent vasoconstrictor and induces platelet aggregation. Prostacyclin, on the other hand, is a potent vasodilator and an inhibitor of platelet aggregation. Prostacyclin is produced by the vascular endothelium and the renal cortex. Many investigators have published conflicting reports about maternal serum and urinary concentrations of these compounds in women with PIH (7–9). In general, the ratio of thromboxane A_2 to prostacyclin is consistently elevated in maternal serum, umbilical serum, amniotic fluid, and urine in women with preeclampsia compared to normotensive parturients (10–12). Therefore, it is not surprising that many authors consider the imbalance in the production of thrombaxane A_2 and prostacyclin as an important etiologic factor of PIH.

Altered Platelet Calcium Metabolism

A major determinant of vascular smooth muscle tone is the quantity of intracellular free calcium. Systemic vascular resistance is elevated in most women with preeclampsia. Increased intracellular calcium and altered calcium metabolism are frequently present in preeclampsia and other hypertensive states (13,14). Platelets and vascular smooth muscle cells have many anatomic and functional similarities. Women who subsequently develop preeclampsia have an exaggerated response of platelet intracellular calcium to arginine vasopressin (15). This dramatic platelet response occurs early in pregnancy and predicts subsequent preeclampsia (15). Others postulate that, in preeclampsia, the preexisting factors causing vascular smooth muscle constriction also may incite platelet activation (16). Preeclampsia may be a trophoblast-dependent process mediated by platelet dysfunction and may be partially prevented by antiplatelet therapy.

Renin–Angiotensin–Aldosterone System

In normal parturients, plasma concentrations of renin, angiotensin II, and aldosterone are considerably higher than in nonpregnant controls (17). In women with preeclampsia, however, the blood contains lower amounts of these compounds (18). In normal pregnancy, vascular response to pressors such as angiotensin II diminishes. In preeclampsia, despite the lower plasma concentrations, the pressor response to angiotensin II infusion increases significantly. This loss of refractoriness to angiotensin II infusions is an early finding in women with preeclampsia (19). This feature may be a marker for early diagnosis of preeclampsia. Clinical manifestations include increased vascular reactivity and increased sensitivity to pressor agents.

Sympathoadrenal Activity

The results of the many studies of adrenergic system activity, as measured by arterial and venous concentrations of epinephrine and norepinephrine, conflict. Although some investigators found higher plasma concentrations of both epinephrine and norepinephrine in PIH, others found no such differences (20–23). Due to the pregnancy-induced physiologic alterations in the metabolism and excretion of catecholamines, plasma concentrations alone may not be an accurate measure of sympathetic nervous system activity. Recent direct measurements, using microelectrodes, of postganglionic sympathetic nerve activity in skeletal muscle vasculature found that sympathetic nerve activity (expressed as bursts per minute) in women with preeclampsia was more than three times higher than in normotensive pregnant women and twice as high as in hypertensive nonpregnant women (24). This increased sympathetic nervous system activity was unrelated to maternal age, gestational age, body mass index, and heart rate. Baroreflex-mediated control of heart rate (Valsalva maneuver) and nonbaroreflex-mediated sympathoexcitatory stimulus (cold pressor test) were not significantly different between preeclamptic and normotensive women. These results suggest that, in preeclampsia, the increases in the peripheral vascular resistance and blood pressure are partly mediated by a substantial enhancement of central sympathetic vasoconstrictor activity (24).

Digoxin-like Immunoreactive Substance

Digoxin-like immunoreactive substance (DLIS) is a natriuretic and produces vasoconstriction. Several investigators have shown that the plasma concentration of DLIS rises in preeclampsia (25). Although some investigators have found a direct correlation between DLIS and diastolic pressures as well as reduced plasma volume, others report no differences in DLIS concentration between women with PIH and normotensive controls (26,27). There are many potential reasons for these conflicting results, such as the lack of proper subclassification of hypertensive disorders of pregnancy as well as inclusion of diabetic women (28). For example, nondiabetic women with preeclampsia had significantly increased serum digoxin-like immunoreactive factor (DLIF) and DLF (digitalis-like factor) compared to normotensive women. But, normotensive pregnant women with insulin-dependent diabetes mellitus also had significantly higher serum levels of DLIS and DLF than their nondiabetic counterparts. Therefore, the inclusion or exclusion of diabetic women can affect the results of such studies (28).

Atrial Natriuretic Peptides

Atrial natriuretic peptide (ANP) is a potent natriuretic, diuretic, and a vascular smooth muscle relaxant. The quantity of ANP affects plasma volume and vascular tone. The primary stimulus for ANP release is distension of atrial stretch receptors by expanded blood volume. Plasma ANP concentration increases 41% above nonpregnant values during the third trimester. An additional rise occurs the first week after delivery (29,30). ANP also increases in women with preeclampsia (31). Because the right atrial pressures are normal or reduced in preeclampsia, the increase in ANP concentration may be due to increased production or reduced clearance (32). A potent stimulus for ANP release may be the increased plasma concentration of endothelin associated with severe preeclampsia (32). The significance of elevated ANP in women with preeclampsia is unknown.

Endothelin and Nitric Oxide

Endothelin, a vasoconstrictor ten times more potent than angiotensin II, is secreted in response to endothelial injury (33). Endothelin concentrations rise in patients with acute myocardial infarction, severe hypertension, and acute and chronic renal failure (34). A significant increase in plasma endothelin occurs in women with preeclampsia and in patients with HELLP syndrome (35).

Nitric oxide (NO) also may be involved in the pathogenesis of preeclampsia. NO is synthesized in the vascular endothelium and is a potent relaxant of vascular, gastrointestinal, and bronchial smooth muscles. Studies of NO in women with PIH have yielded conflicting results (36,37). Seligman et al. (36) found that serum NO concentrations were lower in women with preeclampsia compared to normotensive pregnant women and correlated inversely with systolic and diastolic blood pressures. On the other hand, another recent study showed that the plasma NO concentrations were significantly elevated in preeclamptic women compared to normotensive controls and parturients with chronic hypertension (37). Further studies should define the role of endothelin and NO in the development of preeclampsia.

PATHOPHYSIOLOGY

Intense vasospasm is the single most important pathophysiologic change in women with PIH. This process involves all major organs, including the uterus and placenta. Generalized vasospasm in turn decreases perfusion throughout the body, causing widespread organ dysfunction.

Cardiovascular System

Blood Volume

In normal pregnancy, blood volume increases by 35%, plasma volume by 45%, and red cell volume by 20%. In contrast, in mild preeclampsia, the plasma volume is approximately 9% lower than in normotensive pregnant women (38). Plasma volume is 30% to 40% lower in women with severe preeclampsia than in normal parturients of similar gestational age (38). It is unclear if this volume contraction causes or results from generalized vasoconstriction. Preeclamptic women with fetuses that are small for gestational age also have less plasma volume expansion during pregnancy than other women (38).

Despite decreased plasma volume, extravascular and interstitial volume markedly increase in these women. Decreased plasma volume leads to hemoconcentration and increased blood viscosity. This change further reduces already compromised uteroplacental perfusion, causing areas of placental infarction. Maternal hematocrit and hemoglobin concentrations correlate directly with the frequency of placental infarction and inversely with the weight percentile of the newborn (39).

Hemodynamic Profile

Pregnancy, labor, and delivery cause major maternal cardiovascular changes (Table 3) (40). The following occur by term in normal pregnancy (Fig. 2):

- A 43% increase in cardiac output (17% increase in heart rate and 27% increase in stroke volume),
- A 21% decline in systemic vascular resistance (SVR),
- A 34% decrease in pulmonary vascular resistance (PVR),
- Pulmonary artery occlusion pressure (PAOP), central venous pressure (CVP), and mean arterial pressure (MAP) remain unchanged, and
- Left ventricular function does not change.

The hemodynamic changes that accompany severe preeclampsia are much more complex and highly variable. Several investigators have attempted to describe a characteristic hemodynamic profile in severe preeclampsia. These studies are inconsistent and sometimes conflict. The following list includes some of the confounding variables that complicate their interpretation:

- Previous administration of antihypertensive medications or fluids,

TABLE 3. *Hemodynamic findings from nonpregnant and normal-term pregnant women*

Hemodynamic variable	Nonpregnant (n=10)	Pregnant (n=10)
MAP (mm Hg)	86.4 ± 7.5	90.3 ± 5.8
Heart rate (beats/min)	71 ± 10	83 ± 10
Cardiac output (L/min)	4.3 ± 0.9	6.2 ± 1.0
SVR (dyne sec cm^{-5})	1,530 ± 520	1,210 ± 266
PCWP (mm Hg)	6.3 ± 2.1	7.5 ± 1.8
CVP (mm Hg)	3.7 ± 2.6	3.6 ± 2.5
LVSWI (g m m^2)	41 ± 8	48 ± 6
COP (mm Hg)	20.8 ± 1.0	18.0 ± 1.5

Data are expressed as mean ± SEM.

COP, colloid osmotic pressure; LVSWI, left ventricular stroke work index.

After ref. 40.

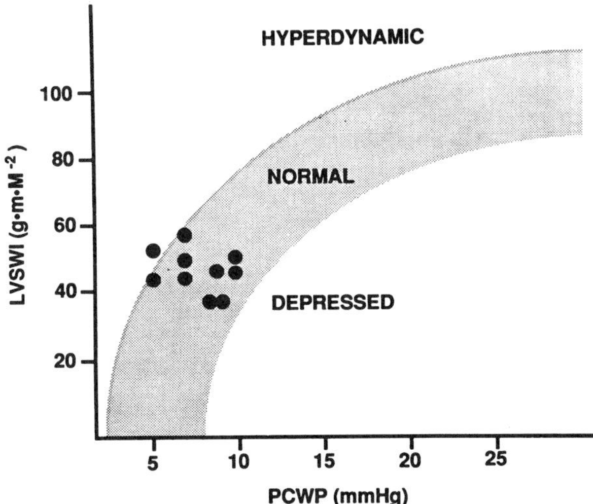

FIG. 2. Left ventricular stroke work index *(LVSWI)* versus pulmonary artery occlusion pressure *(PAOP)*. Left ventricular function is normal in healthy pregnant women. (From ref. 40, with permission.)

- Concurrent medical problems such as chronic hypertension,
- Duration and severity of preeclampsia,
- Labor,
- Mode of delivery, and
- Small number of patients studied.

Wallenburg (41) studied untreated preeclamptic women before therapeutic interventions. These patients had significantly lower cardiac output, stroke volume, and PAOP and higher SVR compared to normotensive parturients. These findings agree with the classic description of the hemodynamic profile in preeclampsia. Despite the low cardiac output, left ventricular function was hyperdynamic.

In contrast, women with severe preeclampsia who had received various forms of treatment before transfer to a major perinatal center showed a wide range of hemodynamic values. Two studies have reported hemodynamic findings from such patients (Table 4) (42,43). In general, these women have an elevated cardiac output, normal to high PAOP, and a normal to elevated SVR. Most also have hyperdynamic left ventricular function (Fig. 3). Because preeclampsia is characterized by intense vasospasm involving all the major vascular beds, one would expect a significantly elevated SVR; however, because SVR is derived by dividing MAP by cardiac output, abnormally high cardiac output can lower the calculated SVR to the normal range (43).

CVP versus PAOP

In the absence of valvular heart disease or left ventricular dysfunction, CVP correlates well with PAOP. In women with preeclampsia, however, changes in CVP often do not parallel changes in PAOP. The reasons for the disparity are unclear. Wallenburg (41) postulates that, in women with preeclampsia, a placid right atrium accommodates increased filling volume without simultaneous increases in pressure. This change would limit the sensitivity of CVP as a measure of intravascular volume. Cotton et al. (42) speculate that, in severe preeclampsia, cardiac output remains high despite the increased left ventricular afterload. This effort leads to higher left-sided intracavitary pressures compared with normal or low pressures in the right heart. Mabie et al. (43) suggest that the central redistribution of intravascular volume due to generalized vasospasm involving the capacitance vessels produces the observed changes in severe preeclampsia.

TABLE 4. *Hemodynamic variables in women with severe preeclampsia*

Hemodynamic variable	Mabie et al (43)	Cotton et al. (42)
Heart rate (beats/min)	94 ± 2	95 ± 2
MAP (mm Hg)	130 ± 2	138 ± 3
PCWP (mm Hg)	8.3 ± 0.3	10 ± 1
CVP (mm Hg)	4.8 ± 0.4	4 ± 1
Cardiac output (L/min)	8.4 ± 0.2	7.5 ± 0.2
SVR (dyne sec cm^{-5})	1,226 ± 37	1,496 ± 64
LVSWI (g m m^2)	84 ± 2	81 ± 2

Data are expressed as mean ± SEM.
LVSWI, left ventricular stroke work index.
After ref. 43.

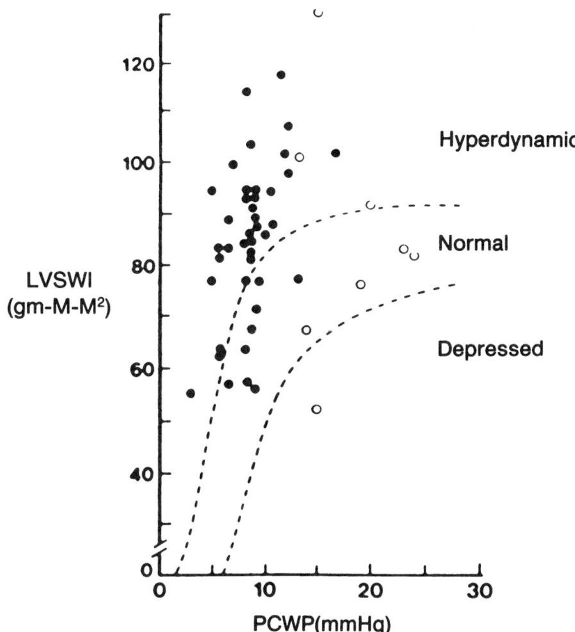

FIG. 3. Left ventricular stroke work index *(LVSWI)* versus pulmonary artery occlusion pressure *(PAOP)*. Left ventricular function is hyperdynamic in most women with severe preeclampsia. (From ref. 43, with permission.)

Pulmonary Edema

A serious complication of severe preeclampsia, pulmonary edema can be cardiogenic or noncardiogenic. Cardiogenic pulmonary edema results from left ventricular dysfunction in the face of severe increases in SVR, chronic hypertension, peripartum cardiomyopathy, and other conditions. On the other hand, increased pulmonary capillary permeability, iatrogenic fluid overload, or a reduction in plasma oncotic pressure (POP)–PAOP gradient can cause noncardiogenic pulmonary edema.

The relationship between POP and PAOP is defined by Starling's equation, as follows (44):

$$Q = k(P_c - P_i) - k(\pi_c - \pi_i)$$

where Q is fluid flux, P is hydrostatic pressure in the capillaries (P_c) and interstitial space (P_i), and π is osmotic pressure in the plasma (π_c) and interstitial space (π_i).

Clinically, PAOP reflects P_c. An oncometer will measure POP. Hydrostatic pressure in the capillaries (PAOP) facilitates outward movement of fluids from capillaries. POP ($^1{}_c$) helps retain fluid and maintain intravascular volume. Approximately 70% of POP is exerted by plasma albumin and the remaining 30% by globulins.

In nonpregnant patients, POP averages 25.4 ± 2.3 mm Hg and PAOP varies from 8 to 12 mm Hg, with a POP–PAOP gradient of about 12 mm Hg. In pregnancy, POP values range from 18 to 21 mm Hg, and PAOP averages 7.5 ± 1.8 mm Hg. The POP–PAOP gradient remains similar to nonpregnant values (44,45). In normal pregnancy, POP falls significantly after delivery, reaching its nadir 6 hours postpartum (45). This decline in POP presumably results from aggressive peripartum crystalloid therapy (45). Neither the type of anesthesia (epidural vs general) nor the mode of delivery (vaginal vs abdominal) significantly influences the reduction in POP (45,46).

Women with severe PIH have lower than normal values for POP both before and after delivery. The lower POP in preeclampsia results from either renal loss or impaired synthesis of albumin (hepatic dysfunction). After delivery, POP falls from 17.9 ± 0.3 mm Hg to 13.7 ± 0.5 mm Hg (47). Simultaneously, PAOP increases significantly owing to the mobilization of extravascular edema fluid, iatrogenic fluid overload, and diminished renal output. The lowering of POP with the simultaneous elevation of PAOP narrows the POP–PAOP gradient and may risk noncardiogenic pulmonary edema.

Recently, Mabie et al. (48) described a subset of women with pulmonary edema probably of cardiac etiology. These women were markedly obese, with chronic hypertension and superimposed preeclampsia. All had severe hypertension, elevated cardiac output, elevated PAOP, normal SVR, normal POP, and pulmonary edema. Echocardiography showed large chambers with thick walls, normal systolic function, and abnormal diastolic function. In these women, pulmonary edema resulted from intrinsic volume overload in the presence of impaired left ventricular relaxation (diastolic dysfunction). Vasodilator therapy worsened the high-output state and pulmonary edema by further increasing cardiac output without lowering MAP. All patients in this study responded well to diuretic therapy. The authors still caution that diuretic therapy should be guided by invasive monitoring to keep PAOP and cardiac output within normal limits.

Similar results were found in a recent study involving 16 preeclamptic women in hypertensive crisis (49). Hypertensive crisis is a serious complication of severe preeclampsia, often complicated by pulmonary edema. Using two-dimensional and Doppler echocardiography, Desai et al. (49) found that the majority of patients (12 of 16) with severe preeclampsia in hypertensive crisis had impaired left ventricular diastolic filling with normal systolic function. In the remaining 4 of the 16 women in hypertensive crisis, pulmonary edema was associated with impaired left ventricular systolic function.

In the 1970s, studies showed that in nonpregnant patients who developed pulmonary edema, there was a significant narrowing of POP–PAOP gradient (50,51). Others could not find any correlation between POP–PAOP gradient and x-ray evidence of pulmonary edema or intrapulmonary shunting (52,53). Although recent studies point to cardiac origin of pulmonary edema, no information exists describing the peripartum changes in POP. Further studies are needed to define the role of abnormally low POP–PAOP gradients in such situations.

Respiratory System

Upper airway edema associated with normal pregnancy worsens in preeclampsia. Occasionally the edema can be severe enough to cause total airway obstruction (54).

The maternal oxyhemoglobin dissociation curve is shifted to the left due to decreased 2,3-diphosphoglycerate concentration or increased carboxyhemoglobin concentration (55,56). Such changes, in association with the preexisting marked decrease in uteroplacental blood flow, can significantly interfere with maternal–fetal oxygen transfer.

Coagulation Abnormalities

Preeclampsia is associated with microvascular endothelial damage and enhanced clotting. Plasma concentration of fibronectin, a marker of vascular endothelial damage, increases (57). Significant reductions in antithrombin III and α_2-antiplasmin signal enhanced clotting (58). Platelet activation and platelet consumption with shortened platelet lifespan are characteristic. Increased concentration of platelet-specific proteins such as β thromboglobulin and platelet factor 4 suggest ongoing platelet aggregation and degranulation (59).

Thrombocytopenia occurs in 15% to 20% of women with preeclampsia. The incidence is as high as 50% in

TABLE 5. *Results of hemostatic assays performed on 44 nulliparous preeclamptic patients*

Test	Nonthrombocytopenic (n=22)	Thrombocytopenic (n=22)
Platelet count ($\times 10^3/\mu L$)	199.6 ± 34	79.4 ± 40.6[a]
Bleeding time (min)	7.6 ± 4.6	3.0 ± 8.3[a]
Platelet-associated IgG (fg per platelet)	3.9 ± 2.0	10.6 ± 12.2[a]
Mean platelet volume (fL)	11.5 ± 1.4	14.1 ± 6.4[a]
Prothrombin time (sec)	10.9 ± 0.6	10.5 ± 0.6
Partial thromboplastin time (sec)	30.4 ± 4.4	33.5 ± 4.3
Fibrinogen (mg/dL)	553.6 ± 199.0	452.8 ± 1.23
β-thromboglobulin (ng/mL)	5.0 ± 2.0	4.8 ± 2.9
Thromboxane B_2 (ng/mL)	1,204 ± 103.4	122.6 ± 94.3
Protamine sulfate paracoagulation assay	Negative	Negative

Data are expressed as mean ± SD.
[a]$p < 0.05$.
Reprinted from ref. 62.

those with severe disease (60). The exact mechanism of thrombocytopenia is uncertain. An earlier report suggested that thrombocytopenia occurred early in pregnancy and became evident even before the occurrence of renal dysfunction (61). To investigate the causes of thrombocytopenia in women with preeclampsia, Burrows et al. (62) did hemostatic and platelet function studies in 61 preeclamptic women and 24 healthy pregnant controls (Table 5). Half of the women with preeclampsia had thrombocytopenia and increased mean platelet (larger than normal platelets), which signified increased platelet destruction. This platelet destruction was not related to increased thrombin activity (disseminated intravascular coagulation), as prothrombin time (PT), partial thromboplastin time (PPT), and the protamine sulfate paracoagulation assay were normal. Increased platelet-associated immunoglobulin (IgG) concentrations occurred in 35% of the preeclamptic patients and correlated inversely with the severity of thrombocytopenia. The presence of platelet-associated IgG suggests autoimmune-mediated platelet destruction as the cause of thrombocytopenia in preeclampsia.

Besides affecting the number of platelets, preeclampsia also alters their function. The template bleeding time, an in vivo platelet function test, is prolonged. Synthesis of platelet thromboxane A_2, an in vitro platelet function test, also falls (62,63). Even in the presence of an adequate platelet count, women with preeclampsia may have a prolonged bleeding time (62,64).[1]

[1]The current spate of negative publicity surrounding the use of the template bleeding time is mostly limited to obstetric anesthesia lecture circuits. The principal investigator in the oft-quoted study (published in *Semin Thromb Hemost* 1990;16:1) is not even an anesthesiologist. Obstetric anesthesiologists often make the difficult day-to-day decisions regarding the use of regional anesthesia in severely preeclamptic women with compromised platelet function. They bear the consequences of these choices. Recent studies on the use of the thromboelastograph in this situation are interesting. However, the thromboelastograph does not specifically evaluate platelet function, and platelet function abnormality may be the only finding in most patients with severe preeclampsia. Until a suitable alterative laboratory test becomes available, template bleeding time is the only currently available bedside in vivo platelet function test.

Although thrombocytopenia is a common finding in women with severe preeclampsia, clinically evident disseminated intravascular coagulation (DIC) is rare. Admission platelet count is an excellent predictor of subsequent platelet counts; the lower the admission platelet count, the higher the incidence of subsequent severe thrombocytopenia (65). Signs and symptoms of DIC, such as low fibrinogen or prolonged PT and PTT, do not occur in the absence of thrombocytopenia. Serial platelet counts alone are adequate in most women with severe preeclampsia. Estimation of PT, PTT, and fibrinogen concentration should be reserved for those cases complicated by platelet count less than 100,000/μL (65).

How long does it take for the spontaneous resolution of thrombocytopenia after delivery? Ravi Chandran and others (66) studied 30 women with HELLP syndrome and found that the mean time until platelet count exceeded 100,000/μL was 67 ± 25 hours after delivery and 44 ± 17 hours from the platelet nadir. All women in this study had counts above 100,000/μL by 111 hours after delivery and by 88 hours after the platelet nadir (66).

Newer and more sensitive tests that assess the integrity of the hemostatic system and may predict subsequent development of preeclampsia have produced interesting results (67,68). Cadroy et al. (67) evaluated six markers of hemostatic system such as prothrombin fragments 1+2, thrombin–antithrombin III complexes (TAT), fibrin D-Dimers (DD), von Willebrand factor, plasminogen activator inhibitor (PAI), and platelet counts in normotensive pregnant women and those with PIH. The authors found that although all six markers increased with gestational age, TAT increased predictably in women with PIH. The authors postulate that TAT may be an useful marker for the early detection of pregnancies complicated by hypertension and preeclampsia (67).

Renal Function

In normal pregnancy, both effective renal plasma flow and glomerular filtration rate increase by 30% to 50%

(69). In contrast, both glomerular filtration rate and renal plasma flow are significantly lower in women with preeclampsia (70). In addition, intrinsic renal structural abnormalities arise. These changes include:

- Swelling of glomerular endothelial cells,
- Deposition of fibrin along the basement membrane, and
- Narrowing or complete obliteration of the capillary lumen.

Renal glomerular endotheliosis is one of the important histopathologic markers of preeclampsia (71). The extent and severity of glomerular endotheliosis correlates with protein loss (70). Significant urinary protein loss lowers POP. Diminishing the gradient between POP and capillary hydrostatic pressure leads to generalized edema. In addition, PIH impairs renal excretion of sodium, increasing total body sodium. Clearance of urea, uric acid, and creatinine decline, significantly increasing their serum concentrations.

Hepatic Function

Intense vasospasm involving the hepatic arteriolar bed can cause mid-zonal necrosis and multiple areas of hepatic infarction. Epigastric or right upper quadrant pain in women with severe preeclampsia is symptomatic of small subcapsular hepatic hemorrhages. Rarely, severe spontaneous hepatic hemorrhage and rupture with sudden cardiovascular collapse can occur (72). Hyperbilirubinemia and elevated liver enzymes, although frequently present, seldom persist after delivery. Plasma pseudocholinesterase concentrations are significantly lower compared to healthy parturients, and, therefore, the duration of succinylcholine and ester type of local anesthetics may be prolonged (73).

Central Nervous System

Neurological manifestations of preeclampsia include diffuse symptoms such as severe headache, confusion, excitability, nausea, and vomiting, as well as focal signs like blurred vision, blindness, hyperreflexia, hemiparesis, and, more importantly, seizures heralding the onset of eclampsia. Eclamptic seizures may occur at any time and can lead to severe maternal morbidity and mortality. Abnormal electroencephalographic findings are seen in 75% of eclamptic women and 50% of preeclamptic women (74). Computed tomographic (CT) and magnetic resonance imaging (MRI) studies show ischemic lesions in the parietal and occipital lobes in patients with eclampsia. Postmortem examinations of eclamptic women reveal cerebral edema and widespread hemorrhagic intracerebral lesions (75).

The etiology of eclamptic seizures is uncertain. Many authors believe that the seizures are due to widespread vasospasm of intracranial arteries resulting in focal ischemia. Others believe the syndrome may be a form of hypertensive encephalopathy (76–79). Cerebral blood flow velocity is significantly elevated in preeclamptic women compared to normotensive controls, presumably due to vasospasm of intracranial vessels (76,77). However, using a phase-contrast MRI technique, Moriss et al. (78) found no significant differences in middle and posterior cerebral artery blood flows in women with preeclampsia/eclampsia compared with controls. Despite the absence of vasospasm, T_2-weighted brain images were markedly abnormal in all women with eclampsia. Cerebral edema, due to loss of autoregulation, can occur during sudden and severe increases in MAP. Episodes of hyperperfusion, with forced overdistension of the arteries (with a preexisting damaged, leaky endothelium), may cause large areas of vasogenic edema and brain lesions in women with eclampsia (78,79). Cerebral blood flow velocities are markedly elevated in women with preeclampsia, and, interestingly, the flow velocities show significant positive correlation with systemic arterial pressures. Passive overdistension and forced vasodilation as a result of high systemic blood pressures in the presence of endothelial dysfunction and impaired autoregulation may lead to significant cerebral edema in women with severe preeclampsia and eclampsia (79).

The implications of these studies are important to anesthesiologists. Rapid sequence induction of general anesthesia and tracheal intubation can cause acute and severe elevations in maternal MAP in women with severe preeclampsia. The resultant rapid increase in the blood flow velocity or overdistension of intracerebral arteries can cause cerebral edema or hemorrhage. This risk underscores the importance of pretreatment with antihypertensive agents or β-adrenergic blocking drugs before tracheal intubation in women with severe preeclampsia.

The Uterus and Placenta

Uteroplacental blood flow is markedly decreased due to intense spasm of the uteroplacental vasculature. The uterus is hypertonic and the placenta is often small, with areas of infarction, calcification, and fibrin deposition. The incidence of placental abruption is significantly higher in women with PIH. A recent meta-analysis of the association of placental abruption with PIH showed that the risk of abruption is significantly higher in women with chronic hypertension and those with eclampsia (80).

OBSTETRIC MANAGEMENT OF PREECLAMPSIA

Mild Preeclampsia

Because of the high risk of placental abruption and eclampsia, all women with mild preeclampsia *at or near term* require immediate hospitalization for further evaluation and treatment. Because maternal or fetal condition can worsen suddenly, those with a cervix favorable for induction should be delivered without delay.

Management of mild preeclampsia detected early in pregnancy is controversial. Several prospective randomized clinical trials have examined the benefits of early and prolonged hospitalization versus ambulatory management (81,82). At the University of Tennessee, all women with mild preeclampsia enter the hospital at the time of diagnosis. Figure 4 summarizes our routine management. Any evidence of maternal or fetal deterioration results in immediate rehospitalization for further evaluation and treatment.

Severe Preeclampsia

Management of women with severe preeclampsia is more aggressive. All women with this diagnosis are admitted to the labor and delivery floor for observation regardless of gestational age. Those women with gestational age beyond 35 weeks are delivered within 24 hours of admission. Patients at 33 to 35 weeks' gestation receive steroids to accelerate fetal lung maturity and are then delivered. Women with resistant hypertension or maternal and fetal deterioration also are delivered within 24 hours regardless of gestational age and fetal lung maturity. All patients with severe preeclampsia receive 6 g of intravenous magnesium sulfate ($MgSO_4$) followed by a 2 g/hour infusion. In addition, we give hydralazine intravenously, in doses of 5 mg, to lower the diastolic pressure below 110 mm Hg. If patients presenting at less than 33 weeks' gestation respond well to therapy (as evidenced by diuresis and diastolic pressures below 110 mm Hg), we will stop $MgSO_4$ and hydralazine therapy and closely monitor both mother and fetus until the fetal lungs mature.

TREATMENT

The major goals of therapy are as follows:

- Prevention of convulsions,
- Control and stabilization of blood pressure, and
- Optimization of intravascular volume status.

Attaining these goals will contribute to safe delivery of a viable baby.

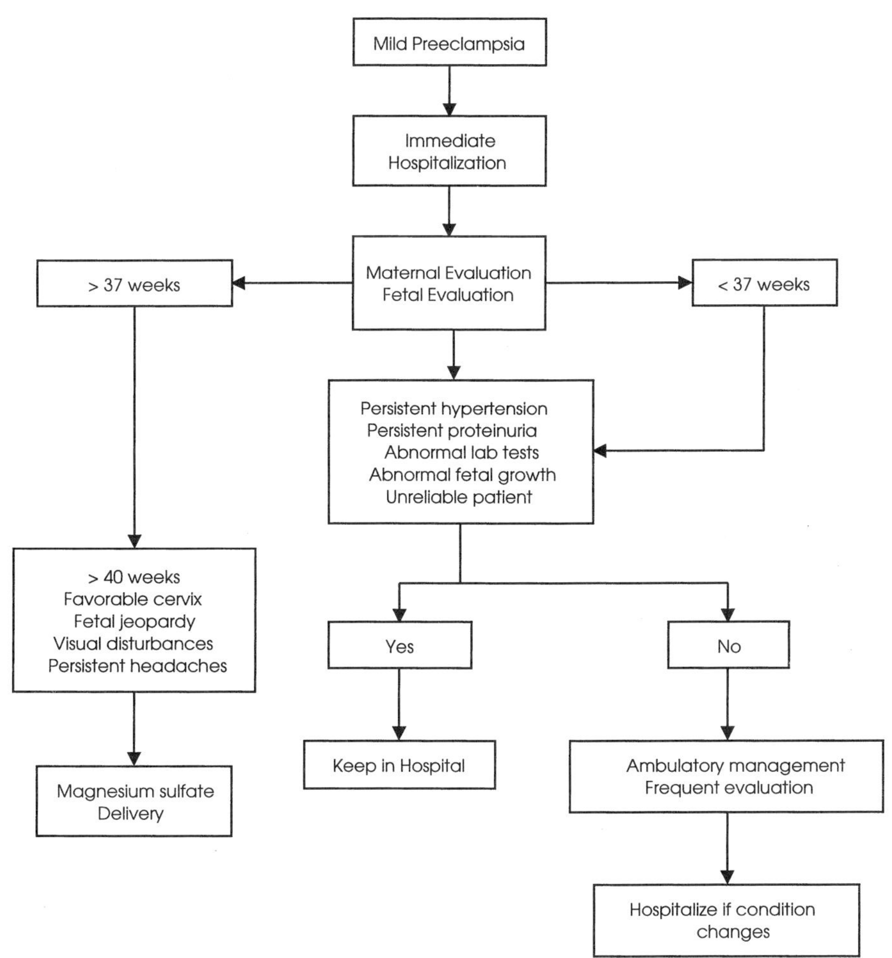

FIG. 4. Management of women with mild preeclampsia. (From ref. 3, with permission.)

Seizure Prophylaxis

Prevention of eclampsia is an important goal of the care of women with preeclampsia. In the United States, magnesium sulfate is the drug of choice for this purpose (83). Phenytoin, being the traditional anticonvulsant, is preferred by some for prophylaxis and treatment of preeclampsia (84). Others argue that appropriate treatment of maternal hypertension is sufficient to prevent eclampsia (85,86). Such controversy is expected, because the incidence of eclampsia is extremely low. Two large observational studies in the United States, involving more than 13,000 preeclamptic women receiving magnesium, showed that the incidence of eclampsia is 0.26% (83). On the other hand, in Europe, the incidence of eclampsia among 3,885 preeclamptic women not receiving any seizure prophylaxis was 0.18%, which is not significantly different than that in United States (86). Despite the controversy, in the United States, seizure prophylaxis is considered essential, and magnesium is recommended for all preeclamptic women (2).

Magnesium Sulfate

Earlier studies suggested that magnesium prevented convulsions by producing generalized depression of the central nervous system. However, animal studies have shown that magnesium ions specifically suppress experimentally induced electroencephalographic spike activity and neuronal burst response (87). Magnesium also is a cerebral vasodilator and may prevent seizures by preventing cerebral ischemia. Magnesium also impairs neuromuscular function. One of the troublesome drug interactions of magnesium is the potentiation of nondepolarizing muscle relaxants. The severity of this effect directly correlates with the serum magnesium concentration (88).

Infusion of $MgSO_4$ increases cardiac index by 12.5% and transiently lowers MAP without significantly changing other hemodynamic variables (89).

Magnesium rapidly crosses the placental barrier. With prolonged administration, fetal and maternal serum concentrations equilibrate. Neonatal hypotonia and respiratory depression may follow.

Therapeutic magnesium concentrations range from 5.0 to 7.0 mg/dL. Toxicity arises as the serum concentration approaches 9 mg/dL. Overdose, severely compromised renal function, or both can produce toxic serum concentrations of magnesium. Pulmonary function tests show transient but mild changes at serum concentrations as low as 3.0 to 4.1 mg/dL (90). In toxic doses, magnesium can cause respiratory arrest by impairing muscle strength and cardiac arrest by inducing a rapid decline in available calcium. Treatment usually involves cardiorespiratory support and administration of calcium chloride.

Magnesium sulfate is a safe and effective agent for prevention of convulsions. Still, some patients can have eclamptic seizures while receiving magnesium infusion. In such cases, give further bolus doses of intravenous magnesium or small doses of a short-acting barbiturate or midazolam. If convulsions persist, resort to tracheal intubation and artificial ventilation to prevent pulmonary aspiration of gastric contents.

Other Drugs for Prevention of Eclampsia

European obstetricians opt for conventional anticonvulsants such as diazepam, barbiturates, and chlormethiazol. Although these agents are excellent anticonvulsants, their use may produce significant maternal and neonatal sedation and respiratory depression. Administration of large doses of diazepam to the mother correlates with neonatal hypothermia, jaundice, and respiratory depression (91).

Phenytoin, a traditional anticonvulsant agent, has been used to prevent and treat convulsions in preeclampsia without adverse maternal or neonatal effects. One randomized clinical trial involving 2,137 women with mild preeclampsia compared magnesium and phenytoin for the prevention of eclampsia. Ten of the 1,089 women randomly assigned to receive phenytoin seized compared to none of the 1,049 women in the magnesium group (92). The observed superiority of magnesium may be related to other preeclampsia-specific beneficial effects, such as reversal of cerebral artery vasoconstriction, release of endothelial prostacyclin, and inhibition of platelet aggregation (92).

Treatment of Hypertension

Although $MgSO_4$ transiently lowers maternal blood pressure, other drugs are often needed to control hypertension in women with preeclampsia. Some commonly used agents are described in the following sections.

Hydralazine

Hydralazine is a commonly used antihypertensive agent in women with PIH. In pregnant ewes, hydralazine reduces maternal blood pressure and uterine vascular resistance while increasing uterine blood flow (93). Its onset is slow and unpredictable, usually peaking 20 minutes after intravenous administration. In women with preeclampsia, hydralazine significantly increases maternal heart rate and cardiac index and reduces MAP and SVR without changing PAOP (94). Hydralazine readily crosses the placental barrier. The slow onset, delayed peak effects, and compensatory tachycardia are some major disadvantages of this drug. Doppler ultrasonographic studies have shown that hydralazine does not cause any changes in the placental or maternal renal artery flow velocity waveforms, suggesting that placental and renal vascular resistance remain unaffected (95). At the University of Tennessee, we give hydralazine in bolus doses of 5 to 10 mg to lower diastolic pressure below 110 mm Hg. We adjust the dose to the maternal blood pressure response. Both maternal electrocardiogram and blood pressure are monitored continuously during administration.

Labetalol

Labetalol is a combined α- and β-adrenergic blocking agent with a β to α blockade ratio of 3:1 after oral administration and 7:1 after intravenous use. In animals, intravenous labetalol ameliorates the effects of norepinephrine on maternal MAP, uterine blood flow, and fetal pH and p_aO_2 (96). It produces less adrenergic blockade in the fetus than in the mother. In women with preeclampsia, labetalol decreases SVR without altering cardiac output. Compared with hydralazine, labetalol has a more rapid onset and provides a smoother reduction of blood pressure (97). It also crosses the placental barrier with a maternal to fetal ratio of 1:1. It does not cause any adverse neonatal effects. Infants have excellent Apgar scores and acid–base status. Hypotension and hypoglycemia do not occur (97,98). Labetalol, in doses of 1 mg/kg, safely blunts the hypertensive response to endotracheal intubation during induction of general anesthesia in women with severe preeclampsia (98). The major disadvantage of this drug is the widely varying dose requirement, which cannot be predicted by any clinical criteria.

Calcium Channel Blocking Agents

Nifedipine

Among the various types of calcium channel blocking agents, nifedipine is used most frequently for the treatment of PIH (99). Contrary to animal data, nifedipine lacks harmful maternal or fetal effects when used to treat blood pressure in parturients. Nifedipine, given orally in doses of 10 mg, lowers the blood pressure in a predictable manner. Onset is within 10 to 30 minutes and peak effect occurs in 40 to 75 minutes. The degree of blood pressure reduction is related to the pretreatment pressures; the higher the MAP, the greater the effect of the drug. Nifedipine crosses the placental barrier, but does not alter the fetal hemodynamics. Treatment of acute hypertension with immediate-release nifedipine is not recommended by the Cardiorenal Advisory Committee of the Food and Drug Administration due to the unpredictable nature of the resultant blood pressure decrease. Chronic administration of nifedipine during pregnancy is safe. Nifedipine is frequently used as a second choice for the chronic treatment of hypertension in pregnancy when other antihypertensive drugs such as methyl dopa, labetalol, and atenolol have failed. Other calcium channel blocking agents such as nicardipine are currently undergoing clinical trials.

Potent Antihypertensive Drugs

We reserve more potent antihypertensive agents such as nitroglycerin, nitroprusside, and trimethaphan for specific indications such as:

- Acute hypertensive crisis,
- Intractable hypertension unresponsive to conventional therapy, and
- Prevention of severe hypertensive response to tracheal intubation under general anesthesia.

Administration of such potent antihypertensive agents requires continuous monitoring of maternal arterial pressure (via an indwelling radial artery catheter) and maternal electrocardiogram. In addition, at our institution, we monitor the left-sided filling pressures via pulmonary artery catheters.

Sodium Nitroprusside

Sodium nitroprusside (SNP) is a potent arteriolar dilator with a rapid onset and short duration. Earlier animal studies showed that infusion of high doses of SNP caused fetal cyanide toxicity and death (100). However, other studies have shown that SNP reverses norepinephrine-induced reductions in uterine blood flow and normalizes maternal blood pressure, without any evidence of cyanide in the fetus (101). Although fetal cyanide toxicity is a cause for concern, the use of low doses of SNP for short periods is probably safe. In women with PIH complicated by pulmonary congestion and heart failure, SNP dramatically decreases in PAOP and produces significant hemodynamic improvement (102). No adverse maternal or fetal effects have been reported in humans. Significant amounts of cyanide have not been detected in either maternal or umbilical cord blood.

Nitroglycerin

Nitroglycerin (NTG) is a venodilator that reduces cardiac filling pressures by acting mainly on capacitance vessels. Like SNP, NTG reverses the uterine artery vasoconstriction, restores uterine blood flow, and counteracts maternal hypertension caused by phenylephrine (103). In women with severe preeclampsia, NTG reduces MAP, PAOP, and cardiac index. Heart rate, stroke volume, and CVP do not change. Volume expansion markedly impedes the hypotensive effects of the drug (104). NTG blunts the hypertensive response to tracheal intubation in women with severe preeclampsia undergoing cesarean delivery under general anesthesia (105). Both SNP and NTG cross the blood–brain barrier and increase cerebral blood flow and intracranial pressure (106).

Trimethaphan

Trimethaphan is an effective ganglionic blocking agent with limited placental transfer due to its high molecular weight. Still, compensatory tachycardia, tachyphylaxis, histamine release, and possible prolongation of the action of succinylcholine can complicate its use.

HELLP SYNDROME

First described by Weinstein (107) in 1982, the syndrome of hemolysis, elevated liver enzymes, and low platelet count (HELLP) is a recognized complication of severe preeclampsia. The incidence varies from 2% to 12%. HELLP syndrome can develop any time during pregnancy. Seventy percent of cases occur antepartum and 30% postpartum. The risk is highest among older (age more than 25 years), white, multiparous women with poor obstetric history (108).

Near term, diagnosis of HELLP syndrome usually is easy; however, some patients present early in pregnancy with nonspecific symptoms such as malaise, nausea and vomiting, and right upper quadrant pain. Adding to difficulty of diagnosis, hypertension and proteinuria may not be present. In fact, many women are misdiagnosed as having conditions such as viral hepatitis, gastroenteritis, peptic ulcer, cholecystitis, fatty liver of pregnancy, idiopathic thrombocytopenia, or hemolytic uremic syndrome. Controversy still surrounds the definition and obstetric management of this syndrome. At the University of Tennessee, we use the following criteria for the diagnosis of HELLP syndrome:

- Hemolysis:
  - Abnormal peripheral smear
  - Increased serum bilirubin (greater than 1.2 mg/dL)
  - Increased lactic dehydrogenase levels (greater than 600 IU/L).
- Elevated liver enzymes:
  - Serum glutamic oxalo-acetic transaminase (SGOT) greater than 70 IU/L
  - Increased lactic dehydrogenase levels (greater than 600 IU/L)
- Low platelet count: less than 100,000/mm^3.

Patients with a diagnosis of HELLP syndrome should be immediately transferred to a tertiary care center for further evaluation and treatment. Initial management resembles that for women with severe preeclampsia. First, stabilize the maternal condition, especially coagulation function. At our institution, we do not consider the presence of HELLP syndrome an indication for immediate cesarean delivery. We anticipate vaginal delivery and begin oxytocin induction of labor in all women with gestational age of 32 weeks or more. We choose cesarean section for women with gestational age less than 32 weeks and an unripe cervix. Those developing laboratory evidence of disseminated intravascular coagulation are delivered immediately, despite fetal gestational age. In these women, platelet function requires close monitoring as rapid deterioration often occurs (109). Any decrease in platelet function has significant implications for obstetric and anesthetic management.

PREVENTION OF PREECLAMPSIA

Prevention of preeclampsia is difficult, as its etiology is unknown. Earlier recommendations of dietary salt restriction and diuretics simply reduced the blood volume with little or no beneficial effect on hypertension (110). The role of low-dose aspirin therapy to reduce the incidence of preeclampsia is controversial. Two large multicenter randomized clinical trials involving thousands of nulliparous normotensive women and those at increased risk for preeclampsia failed to show any improvements in maternal and neonatal morbidity (111,112). In one of the trials, although the incidence of preeclampsia was lower in a subset of patients with systolic pressures of 120 to 130 mm Hg, the incidence of placental abruption was significantly higher in the aspirin-treated group (111). Based on the available information, the American College of Obstetricians and Gynecologists does not recommend routine use of aspirin for prevention of preeclampsia.

A recent meta-analysis of randomized controlled trials evaluating the beneficial effects of calcium supplementation reported some impressive results. The pooled analysis showed a significant reduction in systolic and diastolic pressures and in the incidence of preeclampsia. Lowered maternal and fetal major morbidity are likely, but are as yet unconfirmed (113). Unfortunately, a recent study of 4,589 healthy nulliparous women randomly assigned to receive either 2 g of elemental calcium or placebo daily throughout pregnancy arrived at different conclusions (114). Here, calcium supplementation did not significantly reduce the incidence or severity of preeclampsia or delay its onset. In addition, calcium supplementation did not prevent pregnancy-associated hypertension, preterm deliveries, and other adverse perinatal outcomes (114).

CONCLUSION

The pathophysiologic changes of preeclampsia involve every major organ system. A thorough knowledge of these complex events is essential for successful obstetric and anesthetic management of women with hypertensive disorders of pregnancy. The anesthesiologist, with knowledge and expertise in critical care and invasive monitoring, can play a vital role in the peripartum management of these severely ill parturients.

REFERENCES

1. Roberts J. Pregnancy-related hypertension. In: Creasy R, Resnik R, eds. *Maternal fetal medicine: principles and practice*. Philadelphia: WB Saunders, 1989:777.
2. American College of Obstetricians and Gynecologists. Hypertension in pregnancy. *Int J Gynecol Obstet* 1996;53:175.
3. Sibai B. Preeclampsia-eclampsia. In: Beribri R, Berek S, Creasy R, Decherney A, Ryan KJ. *Current problems in obstetrics, gynecology and fertility*. Chicago: Year Book Medical Publishers, 1990:9.
4. Brosens I, Robertson U, Dixon G. The physiologic response of the vessels of the placental bed to normal pregnancy. *J Pathol Bacteriol* 1967;93:569.
5. Brosens I. Morphological changes in the uteroplacental bed in pregnancy hypertension. *Clin Obstet Gynaecol* 1977;4:573.
6. Robertson W, Brosens I, Dixon G. Uteroplacental vascular pathology. *Eur J Obstet Gynaecol Reprod Biol* 1975;5:47.
7. Koullapis E, Nicolaides K, Collins W. Plasma prostaanoids in pregnancy-induced hypertension. *Br J Obstet Gynecol* 1982;89:617.

8. Lewis P. Does prostacyclin deficiency play a role in preeclampsia? In: Lewis P, Moncada S, O'Grady J, eds. *Prostacyclin in pregnancy.* New York: Raven Press, 1983:215.
9. Yamaguchi M, Mori N. 6-Keto prostaglandin F1a, thromboxane B2 and 13, 14-dihydro-15 keto prostaglandin F concentrations of normotensive and preeclamptic patients during pregnancy, delivery, and the postpartum period. *Am J Obstet Gynecol* 1985;151:121.
10. Walsh S. An imbalance in placental prostacyclin and thromboxane production. *Am J Obstet Gynecol* 1985;152:335.
11. Remuzzi G, Marchesi D, Zoja C. Reduced umbilical and placental vascular prostacyclin in severe preeclampsia. *Prostaglandins* 1980; 20:105.
12. Ylikorkala O, Makila U, Viinikka L. Amniotic fluid prostacyclin and thromboxane in normal, preeclamptic, and some other complicated pregnancies. *Am J Obstet Gynecol* 1981;141:487.
13. Sowers J, Zemel M, Bronsteen R. Erythrocyte cation metabolism in preeclampsia. *Am J Obstet Gynecol* 1989;161:441.
14. Sowers J, Zemel M, Standley P, Zemel P. Calcium and hypertension. *J Lab Clin Med* 1989;114:338.
15. Zemel M, Zemel P, Berry S. Altered platelet-calcium metabolism as an early predictor of increased peripheral vascular resistance and preeclampsia in urban black women. *N Engl J Med* 1990;323:434.
16. Redman C. Platelets and the beginnings of preeclampsia. *N Engl J Med* 1990;323:478.
17. Symonds E. The renin-angiotension system in pregnancy-induced hypertension. In: Sharp F, Symonds E, eds. *Hypertension in pregnancy.* Ithaca: Perinatology Press, 1987:91.
18. Broughton PF. The renin-angiotension system in normal and hypertensive pregnancies. In: Rubin P, ed. *Handbook of hypertension, vol 10, hypertension in pregnancy.* Amsterdam: Elsevier Science, 1988:118.
19. Gant N, Daley G, Chand D, Whalley P, MacDonald P. A study of angiotension II pressor response throughout primigravid pregnancy. *J Clin Invest* 1973;52:2682.
20. Oian P, Lande K, Kjeldsen S, Aakesson I, Eide I, Maltau J. Enhanced platelet release reaction related to arterial plasma adrenaline and blood pressure in preeclampsia. *Br J Obstet Gynaecol* 1986;93:548.
21. Davey D, MacNab M. Plasma adrenaline, noradrenaline and dopamine in pregnancy hypertension. *Br J Obstet Gynaecol* 1981;88:611.
22. Pedersen E, Rasmussen A, Christensen N, Johannesen P, Lauritsen J, Kristensen S. Plasma noradrenaline and adrenaline in preeclampsia, essential hypertension in pregnancy and normotensive pregnant control subjects. *Acta Endocrinol* (Copenh) 1982;99:594.
23. Nisell H, Lunell N, Hiendahl P. Catecholamines in pregnancy-induced hypertension. In: Sharp F, Symonds E, eds. *Hypertension in pregnancy.* Ithaca: Perinatology Press, 1987:187.
24. Schobel H, Fischer T, Heuszer K. Preeclampsia—a state of sympathetic overactivity. *N Engl J Med* 1996;335:1480.
25. Gudson J, Buchlew V, Henessy J. A digoxin-like immunoreactive substance in preeclampsia. *Am J Obstet Gynecol* 1984;150:83.
26. Graves S. The possible role of digitalis-like factors in pregnancy-induced hypertension. *Hypertension* 1987;10:84.
27. Gonzalez A, Phelps S, Cochran E, Sibai B. Digoxin-like immunoreactive substance in pregnancy. *Am J Obstet Gynecol* 1987;157:660.
28. Graves SW, Lincoln K, Cook SL, Seely EW. Digitalis-like factor and digoxin-like immunoreactive factor in diabetic women with preeclampsia, transient hypertension of pregnancy, and normotensive pregnancy. *Am J Hypertens* 1995;8:5.
29. Steegers E, Hein P, Tan A, Groeneveld E, Jongsma H, Benrsad T. Plasma atrial natriuretic peptide (ANP) in late pregnancy and puerperium. *Eur J Obstet Gynecol Reprod Biol* 1987;26:213.
30. Kini N, Yanaihara T, Nakayama T, Ishibashi IM, Yamaji T. Plasma levels of atrial natriuretic peptide during normal pregnancy and in pregnancy complicated by hypertension. *Am J Obstet Gynecol* 1988; 159:27.
31. Miyamoto S, Shimohwa H, Sumioki H, Touno A, Nahno H. Circadian rhythm of plasma atrial natriuretic peptide, aldosterone and blood pressure during the third trimester in normal and preeclamptic pregnancies. *Am J Obstet Gynecol* 1988;158:393.
32. Castro LC, Hobel CJ, Gornbein J. Plasma levels of atrial natriuretic peptide in normal and hypertensive pregnancies: a meta-analysis. *Am J Obstet Gynecol* 1994;171:1642.
33. Yanagisawa M, Kuvishara H, Kimura S, Tomdbobe Y, Kobayashi M, Mitsui Y. A novel potent vasoconstrictor peptide produced by vascular endothelial cells. *Nature* 1988;332:411.
34. Brenner B, Troy J, Ballermann B. Endothelium-dependent vascular responses; mediators and mechanisms. *J Clin Invest* 1973;84:1373.
35. Nova A, Sibai B, Barton J, et al. Maternal plasma endothelin is increased in preeclampsia. *Am J Obstet Gynecol* 1991;165:724.
36. Seligman S, Buyon J, Clancy M, Young B. The role of nitric oxide in the pathogenesis of preeclampsia. *Am J Obstet Gynecol* 1991;17:944.
37. Nobunaga T, Tokugawa Y, Hashimoto K, et al. Plasma nitric oxide levels in pregnant patients with preeclampsia and essential hypertension. *Gynecol Obstet Invest* 1996;41:189.
38. MacGillivary I. Preeclampsia. In: The hypertensive diseases of pregnancy. Philadelphia: WB Saunders, 1983.
39. Koller O. The clinical significance of hemodilution during pregnancy. *Obstet Gynecol Surv* 1982;37:649.
40. Clark S, Cotton D, Lee W. Central hemodynamic assessment of normal term pregnancy. *Am J Obstet Gynecol* 1989;161:1439.
41. Wallenburg H. Hemodynamics in hypertensive pregnancy. In: Rubin P, ed. *Hypertension in pregnancy.* Amsterdam: Elsevier Science, 1988:66.
42. Cotton D, Lee W, Huhta J, Dorman K. Hemodynamic profile of severe pregnancy-induced hypertension. *Am J Obstet Gynecol* 1988;158:523.
43. Mabie W, Ratts T, Sibai B. The central hemodynamics of severe preeclampsia. *Am J Obstet Gynecol* 1989;161:1443.
44. Gonik B. Intensive care monitoring of the critically ill pregnant patient. In: Creasy R, Resnik R, eds. *Maternal fetal medicine: principles and practice.* Philadelphia: WB Saunders, 1989:845.
45. Gonik B, Cotton D, Spillman T, Abouleish E, Zavisca F. Peripartum colloid osmotic pressure changes. *Am J Obstet Gynecol* 1985;151:812.
46. Cotton D, Gonik B, Spillman T, Dorman K. Intrapartum to postpartum changes in colloid osmotic pressure. *Am J Obstet Gynecol* 1984; 149:174.
47. Benedetti T, Carlson R. Studies of colloid osmotic pressure in pregnancy-induced hypertension. *Am J Obstet Gynecol* 1979;135:308.
48. Mabie W, Ratts T, Ramanathan K, Sibai B. Circulatory congestion in obese hypertensive women: A subset of pulmonary edema in pregnancy. *Obstet Gynecol* 1988;72:553.
49. Desai DK, Moodley J, Naidoo DP, Bhorat I. Cardiac abnormalities in pulmonary oedema associated with hypertensive crises in pregnancy. *Br J Obstet Gynaecol* 1996;103:523.
50. da Luz PL, Shubin H, Weil M, et al. Pulmonary edema related to changes in colloid osmotic and pulmonary artery wedge pressure in patients after acute myocardial infarction. *Circulation* 1975;51:350.
51. Stein L, Berand JJ, Morisette M, et al. Pulmonary edma during volume infusion. *Circulation* 1975;52:483.
52. Goodlin RC. Pulmonary edma in pregnant patients treated for hypertension. *Am J Obstet Gynecol* 1980;136:1087.
53. Rafferty TD, Ljunquist R, Firestone L, et al. The plasma oncotic pressure-pulmonary artery occlusion pressure gradient—a poor predictor of pulmonary edema in surgical intensive care unit patients. *Arch Surg* 1983;118:841.
54. Heller P, Scheider E, Marx G. Pharyngolaryngeal edema as a presenting symptom in preeclampsia. *Obstet Gynecol* 1983;62:523.
55. Kambam J, Handte R, Brown W. Effects of normal and preeclamptic pregnancies on oxyhemoglobin dissociation. *Anesthesiology* 1986; 65:426.
56. Kambam J, Entman S, Mouton S. Effect of preeclampsia on carboxyhemoglobin levels. *Anesthesiology* 1988;68:433.
57. Stubbs T, Lazarchick J, Horger EI. Plasma fibronectin levels in preeclampsia: A possible biochemical marker for vascular endothelial damage. *Am J Obstet Gynecol* 1984;150:885.
58. Weiner C, Brandt J. Plasma antithrombin III activity: pathophysiology and obstetric management of preeclampsia. An aid in the diagnosis of preeclampsia-eclampsia. *Am J Obstet Gynecol* 1982;142:275.
59. Socol ML, Weiner CP, Louis G, Rehnberg-Rossi EC. Platelet activation in preeclampsia. *Am J Obstet Gynecol* 1985;151:494.
60. Giles C, Inglis T. Thrombocytopenia and macrothrombocytosis in gestational hypertension. *Br J Obstet Gynaecol* 1981;88:1115.
61. Redman C, Bowman J, Berlin L. Early platelet consumption in preeclampsia. *Br Med J* 1978;1:46.
62. Burrows R, Hunter D, Andrew M, Kelton J. A prospective study investigating the mechanism of thrombocytopenia in preeclampsia. *Obstet Gynecol* 1987;70:334.
63. Kelton J, Hunter D, Neame P. A platelet function defect in preeclampsia. *Obstet Gynecol* 1985;65:107.
64. Ramanathan J, Sibai B, Vdu T, Chauhan D. Correlation between bleeding times and platelet counts in women with preeclampsia undergoing cesarean section. *Anesthesiology* 1989;71:118.
65. Leduc L, Wheeler JM, Kirshon B, Mitchell P, Cotton DB. Coagulation profile in severe preeclampsia. *Obstet Gynecol* 1992;79:14.

66. Chandran R, Serra-Serra V, Redman CW. Spontaneous resolution of pre-eclampsia-related thrombocytopenia. *Br J Obstet Gynaecol* 1992; 99:887.
67. Cadroy Y, Grandjean H, Pichon J, et al. Evaluation of six markers of haemostatic system in normal pregnancy and pregnancy complicated by hypertension or pre-eclampsia. *Br J Obstet Gynaecol* 1993;100:416.
68. Caron C, Goudemand J, Marey A, Beague D, Ducroux G, Drouvin F. Are haemostatic and fibrinolytic parameters predictors of preeclampsia in pregnancy-associated hypertension? *Thromb Haemost* 1991;66:410.
69. Lindheimer M, Katz A. The kidney in pregnancy. In: Brenner B, Rector F, eds. *The kidney.* Philadelphia: WB Saunders, 1986:1253.
70. James FI. Pregnancy-induced hypertension. In: James F, Wheeler A, Dewan D, eds. *Obstetric anesthesia: the complicated patient.* Philadelphia: FA Davis, 1988:411.
71. McCartney C. Acute hypertensive disorders of pregnancy, classified by renal histology. *Gynaecologica* 1969;167:214.
72. Dennis E, Hester L, MacFarland K. The preeclampsia-eclampsia syndrome. In: Danforth D, ed. *Obstetrics and gynecology.* New York: Harper & Row, 1982:455.
73. Kambam J, Mouton S, Entman S. Effect of preeclampsia on plasma cholinesterase activity. *Can J Anaesth* 1987;34:509.
74. Sibai B, Spinnato J, Watson D, Lewis J, Anderson G. Effect of magnesium sulfate on electroencephalographic findings in preeclampsia-eclampsia. *Obstet Gynecol* 1984;64:261.
75. Roybsurt M, Siedman DS, Serr DM, et al. Neurologic involvement in hypertensive diseases of pregnancy. *Obstet Gynecol Surg* 1991;46:656.
76. Williams K, McLean C. Peripartum changes in maternal cerebral flow velocity in normotensive and preeclamptic patients. *Obstet Gynecol* 1993;82:334.
77. Toreres P, Antolin E. Cortical blindness in preeclampsia. *Acta Obstet Gynaecol Scand* 1995;74:642.
78. Moriss CM, Twickler DM, Hatab MR, et al. Cerebral blood flow and cranial magnetic resonance imaging in eclampsia and severe preeclampsia. *Obstet Gynecol* 1997;89:551.
79. Zunker P, Ley Pozo J, Louwen F, et al. Cerebral hemodynamics in preeclampsia/eclampsia syndrome. *Ultrasound Obstet Gynecol* 1995; 6:411.
80. Ananth CV, Savitz DA, Williams MA. Placental abruption and its association with hypertension and prolonged rupture of membranes: a methodologic review and meta-analysis. *Obstet Gynecol* 1996; 88:309.
81. Gilstrap L, Cunningham G, Whalley P. Management of pregnancy induced hypertension in the nulliparous patient remote from term. *Semin Perinatol* 1978;2:73.
82. Mathews D. A randomized controlled trial of bed rest and sedation on normal activity and non-sedation in the management of hypertension in late pregnancy. *Br J Obstet Gynaecol* 1977;84:108.
83. Sibai B, Ramanathan J. The case for magnesium sulfate in preeclampsia-eclampsia. *Int J Obstet Anaesth* 1992;1:167.
84. Appleton MP, Kuehl TJ, Raebel MA, et al. Magnesium sulfate versus phenytoin for seizure prophylaxis in pregnancy-induced hypertension. *Am J Obstet Gynecol* 1991;165:907.
85. Chua S, Redman C. Are prophylactic anticonvulsants required in severe preeclampsia? *Lancet* 1991;357:250.
86. Walker J. Hypertensive drugs in pregnancy: antihypertensive therapy in pregnancy, preeclampsia-eclampsia. *Clin Perinatol* 1991;18:845.
87. Borges L, Gucer G. Effect of magnesium on epileptic foci. *Epilepsia* 1978;19:81.
88. Ramanathan J, Sibai B, Pillai R, Angel J. Neuromuscular transmission studies in preeclamptic women receiving magnesium sulfate. *Am J Obstet Gynecol* 1988;158:40.
89. Cotton D, Gonik B, Dorman K. Cardiovascular alterations in severe pregnancy-induced hypertension: acute effects of intravenous magnesium sulfate. *Am J Obstet Gynecol* 1984;148:162.
90. Ramanathan J, Sibai B, Duggviala V, Madush A. Pulmonary function in preeclamptic women receiving $MgSO_4$. *J Reprod Med* 1988;33:432.
91. McAllister C. Placental transfer and neonatal effects of diazepam when administered to women just before delivery. *Br J Anaesth* 1980; 52:423.
92. Lucas MJ, Leveno KJ, Cunningham FG. A comparison of magnesium sulfate with phenytoin for the prevention of eclampsia. *N Engl J Med* 1995;333:201.
93. Brinkman C, Assali N. Uteroplacental hemodynamic response to antihypertensive drugs in hypertensive pregnant sheep. In: Lindheimer M, Katz A, Zuspan F, eds. *Hypertension in pregnancy.* New York: John Wiley & Sons, 1976:363.
94. Cotton D, Gonik B, Dorman K. Cardiovascular alterations in severe prepregnancy-induced hypertension seen with an intravenously given hydralazine bolus. *Surg Gynecol Obstet* 1985;161:240.
95. Gudmundsson S, Gennser G, Marsal K. Effects of hydralazine on placental and renal circulation in pre-eclampsia. *Acta Obstet Gynecol Scand* 1995;74:415.
96. Eisenach J, Mandell G, Dewan D. Maternal and fetal effects of labetalol in pregnant ewes. *Anesthesiology* 1991;742:292.
97. Mabie W, Gonzalez A, Sibai B, Amon E. A comparative trial of labetalol and hydralazine in the acute management of severe hypertension complicating pregnancy. *Obstet Gynecol* 1987;70:328.
98. Ramanathan J, Sibai B, Mabie W, Chanhan D, Ruiz A. The use of labetalol for the attenuation of hypertensive response to endotracheal intubation in preeclampsia. *Am J Obstet Gynecol* 1988;159:650.
99. Levin AC, Doering PL, Hatton RC. Use of nifedipine in the hypertensive diseases of pregnancy. *Ann Pharmacother* 1994;28:1371.
100. Naulty J, Cefalo R, Lewis P. Fetal toxicity of nitroprusside in the pregnant ewe. *Am J Obstet Gynecol* 1981;139:708.
101. Ellis S, Wheeler A, James FI. Fetal and maternal effects of sodium nitroprusside used to counteract hypertension in gravid ewes. *Am J Obstet Gynecol* 1982;143:766.
102. Stempel JE, O'Grady JP, Morton MJ, Johnson KA. Use of sodium nitroprusside in complications of gestational hypertension. *Obstet Gynecol* 1982;60:533.
103. Craft JB, Co EG, Ynecura MC, et al. Nitroglycerine therapy for phenylephrine-induced hypertension in pregnant ewes. *Anesth Analg* 1980;59:494.
104. Cotton D, Longmire S, Jones M, Dorman K, Tessam J, Joyce T. Cardiovascular alterations in severe pregnancy-induced hypertension: effects of intravenous nitroglycerine coupled with blood volume expansion. *Am J Obstet Gynecol* 1986;154:1053.
105. Hood D, Dewan D, James FI, Floyd H, Bogard T. The use of nitroglycerine in preventing the hypertensive response to tracheal intubation in severe preeclampsia. *Anesthesiology* 1985;63:329.
106. Marsh ML, Aidinis SJ, Naughton KVH, et al. The technique of nitroprusside administration modifies the intracranial pressure response. *Anesthesiology* 1979;51:538.
107. Weinstein L. Syndrome of hemolysis, elevated liver enzymes and low platelet count: severe consequence of hypertension. *Am J Obstet Gynecol* 1982;142:159.
108. Sibai B, Taslimi M, El-Nazer A, Amon A, Mabie W, Ryan G. Maternal-perinatal outcome associated with the syndrome of hemolysis, elevated liver enzymes and low platelets in severe preeclampsia-eclampsia. *Am J Obstet Gynecol* 1986;155:501.
109. Ramanathan J, Khalil M, Sibai B. Anesthetic management of the syndrome of hemolysis, elevated liver enzymes and low platelet count (HELLP) in severe preeclampsia. *Reg Anaesth* 1988;13:20.
110. Sibai BM. Treatment of hypertension in pregnant women. *N Engl J Med* 1996;335:257.
111. Sibai BM, Caritis SN, Thom E, et al. Prevention of preeclampsia with low-dose aspirin in healthy, nulliparous pregnant women. The National Institute of Child Health and Human Development Network of Maternal-Fetal Medicine Units. *N Engl J Med* 1993;329:1213.
112. CLASP (Collaborative Low-dose Aspirin Study in Pregnancy) Collaborative group. A randomized trial of low-dose aspirin for the prevention and treatment of preeclampsia among 9364 pregnant women. *Lancet* 1994;343:619.
113. Bucher HC, Guyatt GH, Cook RJ, et al. Effect of calcium supplementation on pregnancy-induced hypertension and preeclampsia: a meta-analysis of randomized controlled trials. *JAMA* 1996;275:1113.
114. Levine RJ, Hauth JC, Curet LB, et al. Trail of calcium to prevent preeclampsia. *N Engl J Med* 1997;337:69.
115. American College of Obstetricians and Gynecologists. Preeclampsia. *Technical Bulletin 219.* 1996.

Obstetric Anesthesia, second edition,
edited by Mark C. Norris.
Lippincott Williams & Wilkins, Philadelphia © 1999.

CHAPTER 5

Diabetes Mellitus in Pregnancy

Pathophysiology and Obstetric Management

John G. D'Alessio, Jaya Ramanathan, and George Allen III

Diabetes mellitus is a common cause of maternal and perinatal morbidity and mortality. In the United States, this disease afflicts approximately 1.5 million women of child-bearing age. In addition, transient disturbances in glucose tolerance occur in 1% to 3% of pregnancies (1). Before the discovery of insulin, most diabetic pregnancies ended in abortion or premature labor. In those pregnancies that reached term, the incidence of maternal mortality and stillbirths reached or exceeded a staggering 50% (2,3). The availability of insulin dramatically improved both maternal and neonatal outcome. A better understanding of the pathophysiology of the disease process and advances in fetal monitoring and obstetric management also have improved the prognosis for pregnant diabetic women.

Diabetes mellitus is a chronic metabolic disorder caused by an absolute or relative lack of insulin. There are two main types of disease in pregnancy: preexisting, usually insulin dependent (IDDM), and gestational diabetes (GDM), which is carbohydrate intolerance of variable severity first recognized during pregnancy (4). Insulin deficiency causes:

- Hyperglycemia,
- Abnormal protein and lipid metabolism,
- Microangiopathy involving the retinal and renal vessels, and
- Peripheral neuropathy.

J. G. D'Alessio: Department of Anesthesiology, University of Tennessee, Memphis, Tennessee 30103.

J. Ramanathan: Departments of Anesthesiology and Obstetrics and Gynecology, University of Tennessee, Memphis, Tennessee 30103.

G. Allen III: Private practice, Glasgow, Kentucky 42141.

Severe, uncontrolled diabetes culminates in catastrophic ketoacidosis, with a perinatal mortality rate of 50% to 90% (5–7).

White's classification of diabetes mellitus in pregnancy (Table 1) is based upon the age of onset of diabetes, its duration and severity, and the occurrence of related complications (8). Table 2 shows a newer classification, revised and adopted from the National Diabetes Data Group (1). Type I diabetes accounts for approximately 10% of cases. The patients in this group are younger, usually of normal weight, dependent upon insulin, and prone to ketosis. Patients with type II diabetes are neither insulin dependent nor ketosis prone (5). They are usually obese and, although not insulin dependent, may require insulin therapy during pregnancy. Type III diabetics are gestational diabetics diagnosed by

TABLE 1. *Classification of diabetes in pregnancy*

Class	Description
A	Gestational diabetes with normal fasting plasma glucose and postprandial plasma glucose <120 mg/100 mL
B_1	Gestational diabetes with fasting hyperglycemia and/or postprandial plasma glucose >120 mg/100 mL
B_2	Overt diabetes, onset after age 20, and duration <10 yr
C	Overt diabetes, onset before age 20, or duration 10–20 yr
D	Overt diabetes, duration >20 yr, or onset before age 10; benign retinopathy
E	Calcified pelvic vessels
F	Nephropathy (proteinuria, azotemia)
R	Malignant (proliferative) retinopathy (retinitis proliferans)

TABLE 2. *Classification of glucose intolerance in pregnant women*

Nomenclature	Old names(s)	Clinical characteristics
Type I or insulin-dependent diabetes mellitus	Juvenile diabetes, juvenile-onset diabetes, ketosis prone diabetes	Ketosis-prone; insulin-deficient due to islet cell loss; often associated with specific HLA types with predisposition to viral insulitis or autoimmune (islet cell antibody phenomena); occurs at any age: common in youth; these women are usually of normal weight but may be obese
Type II or noninsulin-dependent diabetes mellitus, nonobese, obese	Adult-onset diabetes, maturity onset-diabetes, ketosis-resistant diabetes, stable diabetes	Ketosis-resistant; more frequent in adults but occurs at any age; majority are overweight; may be seen in family aggregates as an autosomal dominant genetic trait; always require insulin for hyperglycemia during pregnancy but not "insulin-dependent"; previous history of "borderline diabetes," impaired glucose tolerance, or treatment with oral hypoglycemic agents; HbA_{1c} >8% during first 20 weeks of gestation
Type III or gestational carbohydrate intolerance, nonobese, obese	Gestational diabetes	Screening tests: all pregnant women; 50 g of oral glucose given randomly (need not be fasting) at 24 and 28 weeks of gestation; a plasma glucose 1 h later >140 g/100 mL (7.8 mmol) is an indication for oral glucose tolerance test
Type IV or secondary diabetes	Conditions and syndromes associated with impaired glucose tolerance	Cystic fibrosis; endocrine disorders such as acromegaly, hyperprolactinemia, Cushing's syndrome, insulin receptor abnormalities, or aberrant forms of insulin, drugs, or chemical agents, renal dialysis, organ transplantation, certain genetic syndromes

screening tests such as the oral glucose tolerance test. Type IV, or secondary diabetes affects 5% to 10% of pregnant women with conditions such as cystic fibrosis or endocrine disorders.

EFFECTS OF DIABETES ON THE MOTHER

Major changes in glucose metabolism occur with pregnancy. Nonpregnant women, when fasted, maintain a basal plasma concentration of glucose by both the continuous release of glucose from hepatic glycogen stores and gluconeogenesis from amino acids and other glucose precursors. Insulin and glucagon control plasma glucose concentrations. In healthy, pregnant women, fasting for a duration of 12 hours (overnight) can produce a rapid fall in plasma glucose concentration to as low as 40 to 45 mg/dL (9). This rapid fall in plasma glucose reduces insulin secretion, leading in turn to ketosis (10,11). Such exaggerated response to fasting is termed accelerated starvation of pregnancy. Increases in maternal and fetal glucose utilization and in the volume of distribution for glucose apparently cause this rapid lowering of maternal plasma glucose during fasting (12). Accelerated starvation and maternal hypoglycemia increase production of ketoacids, which readily cross the placenta and accumulate in the fetus, causing acidosis.

When healthy parturients eat, their plasma glucose concentration rises (Fig. 1) (13). This exaggerated hyperglycemic response to a carbohydrate load markedly increases insulin production (13). Hypertrophy of the β cells of the islets of Langerhans yields this hyperinsulinemic response. This effect is most evident during the third trimester (14). Persistent hyperglycemia signals the development of hepatic resistance to insulin. The synergistic effects of placental hormones, human placental lactogen, estrogen, and progesterone produce the insulin resistance and decreased tissue sensitivity to insulin that are characteristic during pregnancy (15,16).

Diabetes during pregnancy exaggerates all these effects. In early pregnancy, maternal hypoglycemia frequently occurs and necessitates drastic reductions in insulin dose (17,18). During the latter half of pregnancy, however, insulin resistance develops, with a progressive increase in insulin requirements (17,18). Typical doses of insulin are 0.7 U/kg of ideal body weight in the first trimester, increasing to 0.9 U/kg by the time of delivery (19). In addition, without tight metabolic control, these women are extremely prone to ketoacidosis.

The incidence of obstetric complications such as preeclampsia, hydramnios, and preterm labor is significantly higher in pregnant women with diabetes. Other serious complications of severe diabetes mellitus during pregnancy include diabetic retinopathy, nephropathy, hypertension, and coronary insufficiency.

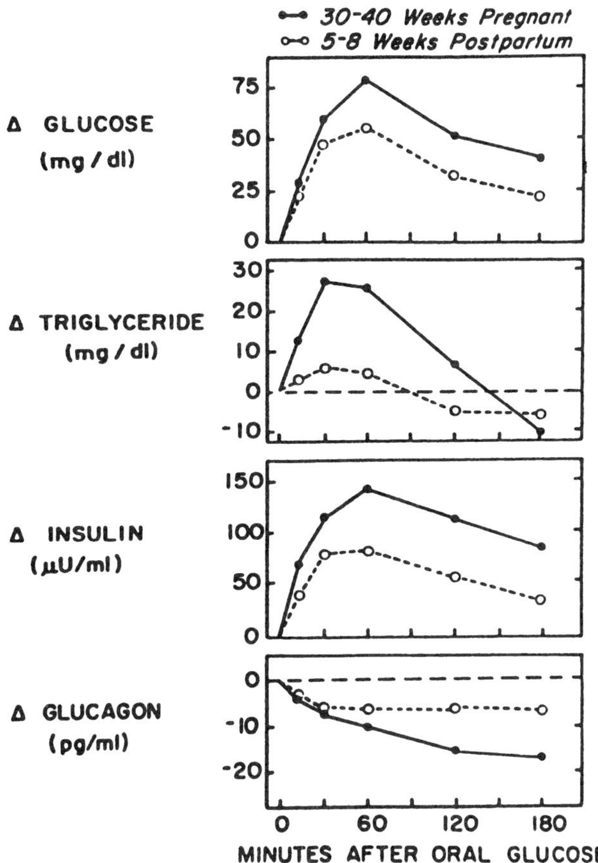

FIG. 1. Effect of pregnancy on the response of plasma glucose, triglyceride, immunoreactive insulin, and glucagon to oral glucose. Values have been expressed as changes from basal concentrations after the administration of 100 mg of oral glucose after a 14-hour overnight fast. (Reprinted from ref. 13, with permission.)

EFFECTS OF DIABETES ON THE FETUS

Congenital Anomalies

The advent of insulin therapy in pregnancy reduced perinatal mortality to less than 5% (20). Despite the general decline in perinatal morbidity and mortality, major congenital anomalies continue to occur at a rate of 6% to 12%, approximately two to four times that in the general population, and account for 40% of neonatal deaths among children of diabetic parturients (Table 3) (21). The exact mechanism of these anomalies remains a mystery. Inadequate control of diabetes during the early stages of pregnancy, particularly organogenesis, may at least partly explain the high incidence of anomalies (22,23). Strict control of diabetes and maintenance of euglycemia beginning before conception or at very early gestation can significantly lower the incidence of congenital defects (22,24). Aggressive glycemic control may reduce the incidence of such complications to nearer that of nondiabetic gravidae (25).

Macrosomia

Maternal hyperglycemia provides excessive quantities of glucose to the fetus. Glucose crosses the placenta by facilitated diffusion, a carrier-mediated and nonenergy-dependent process. Hyperglycemia in the fetus stimulates increased insulin production and fuel utilization. Insulin is a primary anabolic hormone of the fetus. Increased fat deposition, hypertrophy of visceral organs, and increased skeletal growth occur. Diabetes-induced macrosomia manifests as fetal fat deposition in the shoulders and trunk with an increased weight/length ratio, making the fetal head no longer the largest part of the delivering fetus (26). During vaginal delivery, macrosomia (fetal weight greater than 4,000 g) contributes to a high incidence of birth injuries such as shoulder dystocia, facial nerve or brachial plexus injury, and asphyxia (27). Traumatic birth also may predispose to neonatal asphyxia, subdural hematoma, clavicular fracture, and poor Apgar scores (20). Despite good metabolic control, the incidence of macrosomia may be as high as 20% to 30% (28–30).

Neonatal Hypoglycemia

In infants of healthy, nondiabetic mothers, insulin concentration falls rapidly with the separation of placenta at delivery, compensating for the sudden cessation of the fuel supply from the mother. Such rapid hormonal adaptation fails to occur in infants of diabetic women (31,32). Chronic intrauterine oversupply of glucose induces fetal pancreatic islet cell hypertrophy and hyperinsulinemia. Hyperinsulinemia persists after birth and often causes neonatal hypoglycemia, with blood sugar falling to less than 30 mg/dL. From 25% to 40% of infants of diabetic mothers will experience hypoglycemia, with macrosomic and preterm infants at the highest risk (33). Infants of diabetic mothers also secrete less glucagon and catecholamines in response to spontaneous hypoglycemia,

TABLE 3. *Congenital defects in infants of diabetic mothers*

Central nervous system
Anencephaly
Microcephaly
Neural tube defects, spina bifida
Caudal regression syndrome
Cardiac
Transposition of the great vessels
Coarctation of the aorta
Ventricular septal defect
Single or hypoplastic left ventricle
Gastrointestinal
Duodenal atresia
Anorectal atresia
Renal
Renal agenesis
Ureteral duplication
Hydronephrosis

After ref. 20.

resulting in the inability of the liver to produce glucose in response to stress (33). Therefore, it is especially important to avoid giving these women bolus infusions of dextrose-containing solutions during labor. Other neonatal metabolic derangements of both IDDM and GDM include hyperbilirubinemia, acidosis, hypocalcemia, and hypomagnesemia (20,26).

Respiratory Distress Syndrome

Respiratory distress syndrome (RDS) is a common cause of neonatal morbidity and mortality. Recent obstetric advances, including frequent evaluations of fetal lung maturity, have helped to decrease the incidence of RDS dramatically, from 30% to 3% (34). Fetal hyperinsulinemia may interfere with surfactant production and delay pulmonic maturity, leading to a five- to sixfold greater risk of RDS in the premature infant of the inadequately controlled diabetic mother (35). Frequent amniocentesis to estimate lecithin-sphingomyelin ratio (greater than 2.0) and phosphatidyl glycerol concentration (greater than 0.5%) enable the obstetrician to postpone delivery until the fetal lungs mature.

CHANGES IN UTEROPLACENTAL CIRCULATION AND FETAL OXYGENATION

Several studies have shown that diabetes significantly impairs uteroplacental perfusion (36,37). In addition, the structure of the placenta itself is modified by diabetes. The villi are enlarged, intervillous spaces are smaller, and effective uterine blood flow is reduced (36–38). The presence of increased maternal glycosylated hemoglobin (HbA_{1c}) also may compromise fetal oxygenation (39). When glucose covalently binds to the two β chains in the adult Hb (HbA), it creates HbA_{1c}, which interferes with oxygen uptake. In insulin-dependent diabetic women, HbA_{1c} interferes with hemoglobin oxygen transport and compromises fetal oxygenation (39). Serial measurements of HbA_{1c} concentration provide valuable information on the quality of maternal blood sugar control and the effectiveness of therapy.

DIABETIC KETOACIDOSIS

Diabetic ketoacidosis (DKA) remains a serious and often preventable cause of maternal and fetal morbidity and mortality. It affects up to 0.7% of pregnancies complicated by GDM and 1.7% to 9.3% of gravidas with IDDM (5).

Perinatal mortality ranges from 22% to 65% depending on the presence of coma, gestational age, serum glucose and osmolality, blood urea nitrogen, insulin requirements, and duration of the acidotic state (5–7). Fortunately, monitoring and therapy can resuscitate the fetus in utero and prevent fetal death (7,40). Maternal mortality from DKA during pregnancy can be as high as 5%, equal to mortality of ketoacidosis in the general population (7,41).

The etiology of DKA often is multifactorial (Table 4).The two largest studies examining precipitating factors identified:

- Poor patient compliance,
- Undiagnosed diabetes,
- Administration of β-mimetic agents,
- Emesis, and
- Poor physician management (7,42).

Regardless of the etiology, ketoacidosis may occur in gravid diabetics with a lesser degree of hyperglycemia (150 to 300 mg/dL) than in nongravid diabetics (7).

Symptoms of ketoacidosis include:

- Nausea and vomiting,
- Malaise,
- Altered mental status (ranging from drowsiness to lethargy and coma),
- Polydipsia,
- Polyuria, and
- Abdominal pain.

Classic signs include hyperventilation (Kussmaul respiration), a fruity or acetone breath odor, dehydration, and, occasionally, hypotension.

The diagnosis of DKA is confirmed by the following:

- Plasma glucose greater than 300 mg/dL,
- Plasma HCO_3 less than 15 mEq/L,
- pH less than 7.30, and
- Serum acetone at 1:2 dilutions.

Once the diagnosis of DKA is confirmed, prompt treatment and continuous fetal monitoring are imperative. Although serum sodium, potassium, and BUN may be low, normal, or high, virtually all patients have total body sodium and potassium deficits. During the period of active treatment, electrolytes and acid–base status should be evaluated hourly. Treatment of DKA consists of correcting volume deficit, electrolyte abnormalities, hyperglycemia, and the inciting cause of decompensation (Table 5). Fluid deficits of up to 10 L are not uncommon.

TABLE 4. *Etiologies of diabetic ketoacidosis*

	Montoro et al. (7)	Rodgers and Rodgers (42)
Patient compliance	35%	11%
New onset IDDM	30%	8%
β-mimetic use	0%	30%
Emesis/inadequate caloric intake	5%	27%
Infection	20%	5%
Poor physician management	0%	13%
Maternal drug abuse	10%	0%

After ref. 7, 42.

TABLE 5. *Treatment of diabetic ketoacidosis*

1. Monitor:	Electrolyte, blood glucose, arterial blood gases, fluid intake/out each hour. Consider intraarterial catheter for continuous measurement of blood pressure and blood sampling. Also consider central venous catheter to evaluate response to fluid therapy. Continuously monitor fetal heart rate and uterine activity.
2. Fluids:	1–2 L of isotonic saline in the first hour; 300–500 mL/h of 0.45% or 0.9% saline thereafter determined by the serum sodium via a large peripheral vein or central venous catheter.
3. Insulin:	10–20 U of regular insulin IV, then continuous infusion of 5–10 U/h until plasma glucose reaches 200 mg/dL. Then decrease to 1–2 U/h.
4. Potassium:	40 meQ KCl/L of fluid after 2–4 h of insulin therapy and establishment of urine output >0.5 mL/kg/h.
5. Sodium bicarbonate:	Administer for pH <7.1.
6. Glucose:	Begin administering IV glucose when plasma levels decline to 200–250 mg/dL.

After ref. 81.

Approximately half of the deficit should be replaced in the first 5 hours using warmed, isotonic fluids (normal saline) (43). Intravascular volume expansion improves organ and peripheral perfusion, lowers serum osmolarity, dilutes hyperglycemia, prevents metabolic acidosis, and allows peripheral uptake of exogenously administered insulin. Total body potassium deficit ranges from 3 to 10 mmol/kg and must be replaced following initiation of rehydration and concurrently with intravenous insulin. Both the increase in urine production with obligate potassium loss and the intracellular shift of potassium in the presence of glucose and insulin may lead to dramatic declines in measured potassium. Electrocardiographic monitoring is essential because the fluctuating potassium gradient can cause cardiac dysrythmias (44).

Begin insulin therapy after starting volume replacement. An intravenous bolus of 10 to 20 U of regular insulin is followed by an infusion of 5 to 10 U/hour. Aim to decrease serum glucose concentration by 30% to 40% in the first 4 hours of therapy. If there is inadequate change, rebolus the patient and double the infusion rate. When serum glucose levels reach approximately 250 mg/dL, start an intravenous dextrose infusion at 150 mg/hour and decrease the insulin infusion to 1 to 2 U/hour. Normoglycemia (80 to 120 mg/dL) is the goal of therapy. Administration of sodium bicarbonate should be reserved for patients with an arterial pH less than 7.1. Sodium bicarbonate may cause paradoxic intracerebral acidosis and hinder oxygen delivery to tissues. Limit the dosage to 100 mEq (2 amps) per liter of intravenous fluid (0.45% saline), to minimize hyperosmolarity and pain with injection. Discontinue use of sodium bicarbonate when the pH reaches 7.20 and change fluid to 0.9% saline. Any gravida in DKA during the second or third trimester should undergo continuous fetal monitoring for signs of fetal distress.

TIMING OF DELIVERY

Both maternal and fetal condition must be considered when planning delivery of the fetus of the diabetic mother (27). The parturient who has maintained normoglycemia and is carrying a healthy fetus may be allowed to progress to term and experience spontaneous labor. Fetal surveillance consists of nonstress testing, fetal biophysical profile, maternal assessment of fetal activity, and, when indicated, contraction stress testing (45). The goal of testing is to identify the fetus at risk of compromise or intrauterine death and to prevent unnecessary preterm delivery. Premature labor should be treated with bed rest, intravenous fluids, and magnesium sulfate. β-Sympathomimetic agents are contraindicated because they have direct antiinsulin effects and induce hyperglycemia and ketoacidosis (27). Likewise, corticosteroids for fetal lung maturation should be used with caution. However, their use may be justified provided glucose homeostasis is maintained (27). Fetal maturation should be confirmed before delivery if the diabetes is well controlled and the fetal parameters remain normal.

Labor is often induced at 38 to 40 weeks' gestation. Prostaglandin gel may help ripen the unfavorable cervix. If fetal surveillance, biophysical profile, or stress test suggests a compromised pregnancy, prompt delivery may be necessary even without evidence of fetal lung maturity (27). Fetal intolerance to labor or macrosomia may make successful vaginal delivery unlikely (46–48). The obese parturient with GDM is at substantially increased risk of fetal macrosomia and operative delivery (28).

Even when all factors are ideal and labor is allowed to occur, the diabetic parturient is more likely to require cesarean delivery (46,47). In patients with either IDDM and GDM, induced and spontaneous labor are equally likely to progress to operative delivery. Interestingly, GDM patients with excellent glycemic control and normosomic infants are at equal risk of cesarean section as poorly controlled parturients with macrosomic infants (29,48).

INTRAPARTUM MANAGEMENT OF THE DIABETIC PARTURIENT

Preoperative evaluation of the diabetic parturient should be directed at those organ systems most commonly affected by chronic diabetes mellitus. By knowing the classification of diabetes, it is possible to obtain a directed history quickly, if necessary, before a rapid delivery or emergency cesarean section. The presence of renal insufficiency, cardiac disease, or long-standing diabetes increases the incidence of peripartum complications. Hypertension in conjunction with diabetes mellitus significantly increases morbidity and mortality (49,50). Renal insufficiency is associated with a lower hematocrit, greater urinary protein loss, and higher serum creatinine. Cautious fluid management is necessary as the potential for renal failure is increased (51). The presence of peripheral or autonomic neuropathy must be determined and sensory or motor deficits documented.

Physical examination should include thorough evaluation of the airway for signs of stiff joint syndrome and the potential for difficult intubation (see following) (52). Look for signs of cardiac decompensation. The older parturient or one with suspected or documented cardiac disease should have a recent ECG. Baseline laboratory evaluation includes electrolytes, BUN, creatinine, and glucose.

Hypoglycemia is the most common complication in neonates of diabetic mothers. Antenatal maternal hyperglycemia also can produce neonatal acidosis (53). Maintaining maternal plasma glucose at a normal concentration (70 to 120 mg/dL) during labor significantly reduces the incidence of neonatal acidosis and hypoglycemia. Three commonly used insulin/glucose protocols can attain this goal (Table 6A–E) (19,53,54). The glucose requirement during labor is constant at 2.55 mg/kg/min, whereas insulin requirements vary (55). Frequently, insulin is not needed during the first stage of labor due to the fasting state and increased glucose utilization (19,55–57). Usual insulin requirements range from 0 to 5 U of regular insulin per hour. Glucose and insulin infusions should be maintained on separate mechanical pumps. Although preventing hyperglycemia is important, avoiding hypoglycemia with attendant ketosis also is essential, as these metabolic imbalances significantly prolong labor and induce neonatal hypoglycemia (58). During labor or cesarean delivery, all diabetic parturients should have blood sugar measured hourly.

Patients with insulin-dependent diabetes presenting for elective cesarean delivery can receive their usual insulin dosage the evening before surgery (Table 6A–E). If possible, schedule surgery in the morning. On the morning of surgery, withhold both food and the usual insulin dosage. Check a fasting plasma glucose concentration. If it is less than 120 mg/dL, use intravenous solutions without dextrose. If surgery is delayed or if plasma glucose values are greater than 120 mg/dL, give combined glucose/insulin infusions. Should plasma glucose be greater than 120 mg/dL, delivery should be delayed until the plasma glucose has remained less than 120 mg/dL for 4 hours. Management of diet-controlled, gestational diabetics is simpler. Usually, intravenous fluids without dextrose provide adequate control of maternal plasma glucose concentration while monitoring is continued, as in the IDDM parturient.

Immediately postpartum, insulin requirement drops to approximately 60% of the prepregnancy requirement

TABLE 6A. *Management of women with insulin-dependent diabetes mellitus for elective cesarean delivery or scheduled labor induction*

1. Give the usual insulin dose the evening before surgery and a small meal before midnight. In the morning, give one fourth to one half of the usual dose of the intermediate acting insulin dose. Titrate 5% glucose infusion to maintain blood glucose at 70–120 mg/dL.
2. Measure fasting glucose on the morning of surgery and obtain a finger stick glucose every 1–2 h thereafter. If fasting glucose is >120 mg/100 mL or if the surgery is delayed, start 5% glucose at 2.55 mg/kg/min and insulin at 1–5 U/h to maintain blood sugar at 70–120 mg/dL. Delay surgery until euglycemia is maintained for 4 h.
3. If fasting glucose level is <120 mg/100 mL, start intravenous fluids without dextrose. No further insulin is given.
4. Treat any blood glucose >120 mg/dL with sliding scale, intermittent, IV boluses of insulin. Dose 1–10 U of insulin for each 50 mg/dL increment >120 mg/dL.
5. Immediately postpartum, decrease insulin to 60% prepregnancy dose or one third to one half of antepartum dose. Continue frequent blood glucose monitoring.

Modified from ref. 19.

TABLE 6B. *Management of women with insulin-dependent diabetes mellitus for elective cesarean delivery or scheduled labor induction: insulin and glucose infusion*

1. Withhold all subcutaneous insulin. Measure blood sugar.
2. Begin continuous infusion insulin at 1–2 U/h and glucose at 150 mg/kg/h. Measure blood glucose each hour and modify insulin infusion.
3. Adjust insulin from 0.5–2 U/h. Treat >140 mg/dL with IV bolus insulin 2 U and increase infusion. Blood sugar <70 mg/dL, administer 2–5 g of glucose.

Modified from ref. 53.

TABLE 6C. *Management of women with insulin-dependent diabetes mellitus for elective cesarean delivery or scheduled labor induction: low-dose constant insulin infusion for the intrapartum period*

1. Finger stick blood glucose every hour.
2. Blood glucose <100 mg/dL, insulin 0 U, IV 5% dextrose lactated Ringer's solution.
3. Blood glucose 100–140 mg/dL, insulin 1 U/h, IV 5% dextrose lactated Ringer's solution.
4. Blood glucose 141–180 mg/dL, insulin 1.5 U/h, IV normal saline.
5. Blood glucose 181–220 mg/dL, insulin 2.0 U/h, IV normal saline.
6. Blood glucose >220 mg/dL, insulin 2.5 U/h, IV normal saline.

After ref. 27.

TABLE 6D. *Management of women with insulin-dependent diabetes mellitus for elective cesarean delivery or scheduled labor induction: intermittent insulin bolus*

1. No morning insulin.
2. Use nondextrose-containing fluids.
3. Measure blood sugar frequently.
4. Treat blood glucose >120 mg/dL with 1–2 U of IV insulin.

After ref. 82, with permission.

TABLE 6E. *Insulin management in labor*

1. Blood sugar <120 mg/dL: Give one third the usual daily dose of insulin subcutaneously (intermediate acting). Measure blood sugar every 1–2 h. If blood sugar increases to >120 mg/dL, begin insulin infusion of 0.5–2 U/h.
2. Blood sugar >120 mg/dL on arrival: Give one third the usual daily dose of insulin subcutaneously (intermediate acting). Measure blood sugar every 1–2 h. Begin intravenous insulin infusion immediately. Monitor as above and treat blood sugar >140 mg/dL with 1–2 U of IV insulin bolus.

After ref. 82, with permission.

(19). The dose will return to baseline in about 5 to 6 days. The purported mechanism for this response is a decrease in growth hormone secretion and a state of relative hypopituitarism (15,16,59). During this time, continue to frequently monitor blood glucose.

THE AIRWAY AND DIABETES IN PREGNANCY

The airway of the gravida with either IDDM or GDM presents several potential problems, which, if recognized, may be effectively circumvented. Insulin-dependent diabetes seen in parturients frequently begins in childhood as juvenile-onset diabetes mellitus (JODM). Associated with JODM is the syndrome of limited joint mobility (LJM) (60). First described in 1974, this syndrome consists of nonfamilial short stature; thick, tight, waxy skin; delayed sexual maturation; early microvascular complications; and limited mobility of the small joints (61). This syndrome was found in 28% of JODM patients within 5 years of diagnosis (62). Of the 28% of patients with LJM syndrome, one third will have severe manifestations including significant involvement of the cervical spine (60–62).

Impaired cervical spine movement, especially limited movement at the atlantooccipital joint, associated with diabetes, impairs the ability to intubate the trachea (63–66). There is a 26% to 41% incidence of difficult intubation in diabetic patients undergoing general anesthesia (64–66). Difficult intubation correlates with inflexibility of the joints of the hand (66). An easy bedside test for joint abnormalities is to have the patient oppose the palms of the hands and see if the proximal interphalangeal joints of the fourth and fifth fingers will touch (Fig. 2) (60,62). Patients with LJM also are likely to have microvascular, renal, and retinal changes. Therefore, parturients with Class C-R diabetes are at substantially increased risk of LJM syndrome and difficult intubation (60,62). This information, in combination with the knowledge of increased intubation difficulty in pregnancy, should prompt thorough airway evaluation, including joint mobility and cervical range of motion in all pregnant diabetics (66).

The gravida with gestational diabetes also is at risk for difficult intubation, but for different reasons. The majority of gestational diabetic women are obese (body mass index greater than 30 or greater than 150% ideal body weight) (67). Obesity is a risk factor for difficult intubation, and it increases the potential for both macrosomia and failure to delivery vaginally (68). Obesity plus pregnancy increase the likelihood of difficult intubation by tenfold. Airway complications are the leading cause of maternal morbidity and mortality associated with general anesthesia (68–70). Anticipate these difficulties. Formulate a plan for labor and delivery analgesia. Early placement of an epidural catheter

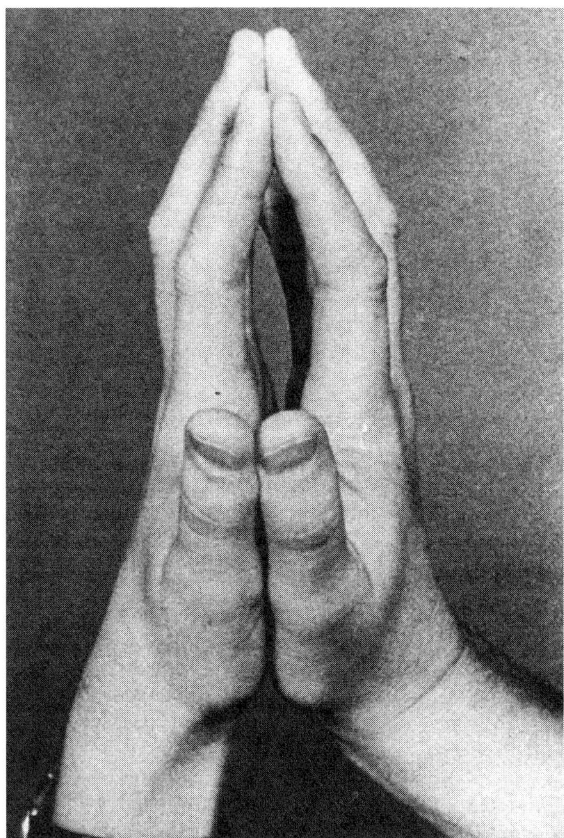

FIG. 2. Limitation of small joint mobility evidenced by inability to approximate the interphalangeal joints, "the prayer sign." Patients with this manifestation of diabetes frequently present difficulties with direct laryngoscopy and tracheal intubation. (Reprinted from ref. 62, with permission.)

and adequate analgesia may promote vaginal delivery or smooth the transition to cesarean section (68).

NEUROPATHY AND REGIONAL ANESTHESIA

Autonomic Neuropathy

Autonomic neuropathy occurs within 15 years of onset of insulin treatment in up to 30% of diabetics (71). About 23% of gravidae with IDDM have autonomic dysfunction (72). Manifestations include:

- Orthostatic hypotension or lightheadedness,
- Diarrhea or constipation,
- Bladder complaints,
- Resting tachycardia, and
- Decreased heart rate variability with deep breathing or vagal stimulation.

Interestingly, diabetic parturients experience less of an increase in resting heart rate with pregnancy than nondiabetics, and, therefore, resting tachycardia is not an appropriate marker of autonomic dysfunction in pregnancy (73). Orthostatic hypotension results from denervation of the splanchnic vasculature (74). Diabetic gastroparesis is extremely rare in pregnancy, and gastric function is not significantly different than that of the nondiabetic pregnant woman (50).

General anesthesia in the parturient with autonomic neuropathy is likely to be marked by hypotension and a significant heart rate decline during induction and less rebound following tracheal intubation than normal controls. Thirty-five percent of diabetics require vasopressor treatment (75). The fetus of the IDDM mother tolerates hypotension poorly and, therefore, any significant hemodynamic changes must be treated aggressively with fluid and vasopressors (76).

The sympathetic blockade accompanying regional anesthesia in the insulin-dependent parturient may induce a greater degree of hypotension than in the nondiabetic. Cardiac and vasoconstrictive responses to hypotension are blunted by autonomic neuropathy because the sympathetic nerves are less well supplied with norepinephrine, the primary neurotransmitter of the peripheral sympathetic nervous system (74). Therefore, changes in preload and afterload must be anticipated and treated early. Ephedrine or phenylephrine are appropriate choices as determined by the heart rate.

Peripheral Neuropathy

Distal sensory and motor lesions are the most common forms of diabetic neuropathy, which manifests as paresthesias, pain, or hypesthesia of the distal extremities. Small fiber neuropathy is less common and presents as distal burning pain or hyperalgesia. Autonomic neuropathy is more commonly associated with small fiber disease. Up to 50% of diabetics have some evidence of peripheral neuropathy (77). If regional analgesia/anesthesia is contemplated, it is essential to document the extent and type of peripheral neuropathy in advance.

Changes in nerve structure and blood supply inherent to diabetes mellitus may place the affected parturient at increased risk of all types of peripartum nerve injury. Assure careful and proper positioning during both general and regional anesthesia. The ulnar nerve, as it passes through the cubital tunnel, is most commonly affected during general anesthesia (78,79). Passage of the fetus through the pelvis, placement of forceps, and the lithotomy position may cause nerve injury during vaginal delivery. Commonly affected are the lumbosacral trunk, sacral, femoral, lateral femoral cutaneus, and lateral popliteal nerves. A regional anesthetic may be frequently, though incorrectly, implicated in postdelivery changes in neurological function (see Chapter 39) (80).

CONCLUSION

Knowledge of the pathophysiology of diabetes and its effects on mother, fetus, and neonate allows proactive, not reactive, anesthetic management. Goals of peripartum management of the diabetic patient center on maintaining euglycemia. The classification of maternal disease and preoperative evaluation will allow proper choice of fluids, glucose, and insulin. Appropriate anesthetic management can help insure maternal and neonatal well-being.

REFERENCES

1. Hollingsworth D, Moore T. Diabetes in pregnancy. In: Creasy R, Resnik R, eds. *Maternal fetal medicine: principles and practice*. Philadelphia: WB Saunders, 1989:925.
2. Craigin E, Ryder G. *Obstetrics: a practical textbook for students and practitioners*. Philadelphia: Lea & Febiger, 1916.
3. Williams J. *Obstetrics: a textbook for the use of students and practitioners*. New York: Appleton & Lange, 1925.
4. Metzger B. Summary and recommendations of the third international workshop-conference on gestational diabetes mellitus. *Diabetes* 1991; 20[Suppl 2]:197.
5. Kilvert J, Nicholson H, Wright A. Ketoacidosis in diabetic pregnancy. *Diabetic Med* 1993;10:278.
6. Kyle G. Diabetes and pregnancy. *Ann Intern Med* 1963;59[Suppl 3]:1.
7. Montoro MN, Myers VP, Mestman JH, Xu Y, Anderson BG, Golde SH. Outcome of pregnancy in diabetic ketoacidosis. *Am J Perinatol* 1993; 10:17.
8. White P. Pregnancy and diabetes. In: Marble A, White P, Bradley R, Krall L, eds. *Joslin's diabetes mellitus*. Philadelphia: Lea & Febiger, 1971:581.
9. Felig P, Lynch V. Starvation in human pregnancy: hypoglycemia, hypoinsulinemia, and hyperketonemia. *Science* 1970;170:990.
10. Kalhan S, D'Angelo L, Savin S, Adam P. Glucose production in pregnant women at term gestation. Sources of glucose for human fetus. *J Clin Invest* 1979;63:388.
11. Buchanan T, Unterman T, Metzger B. The medical management of diabetes in pregnancy. *Clin Perinatol* 1985;12:625.
12. Freinkel N. Effects of the conceptus on maternal metabolism during pregnancy. In: Leibel B, Wrenshall G, eds. *On the nature and treatment of diabetes*. Amsterdam: Excepta Medica, 1964:679.
13. Freinkel N. Of pregnancy and progeny. *Diabetes* 1980;29:1023.
14. van Assche F, Aerts L. Morphologic and ultrastructure modifications in the endocrine pancreas in pregnant rats. In: Camerini-Davalos R,

Cole H, eds. *Early diabetes in early life.* New York: Academic Press, 1975:333.
15. Coustan D, Felig P, Ferris TF. Diabetes mellitus. In: Burrow G, Ferris TF, eds. *Medical complications during pregnancy.* Philadelphia: WB Saunders, 1988:33.
16. Fisher P, Sutherland H, Bewsher P. The insulin response to glucose infusion in normal human pregnancy. *Diabetologia* 1980;19:15.
17. Landon M, Gabbe S. Diabetes and pregnancy. *Med Clin North Am* 1988;72:1493.
18. Coustan D, Berkowitz R, Hobbins J. Tight metabolic control of overt diabetes in pregnancy. *Am J Med* 1980;68:845.
19. Homko CJ, Khandelwal M. Glucose monitoring and insulin therapy during pregnancy. *Obstet Gynecol Clin North Am* 1996;23:47.
20. Tyrala EE. The infant of the diabetic mother. *Obstet Gynecol Clin North Am* 1996;23:221.
21. Reece EA, Eriksson UJ. The pathogenesis of diabetes-associated congenital malformations. *Obstet Gynecol Clin North Am* 1996;23:29.
22. Miller E, Hare J, Cloherty J. Elevated maternal hemoglobin A1c in early pregnancy and major congenital anomalies in infants of diabetic mothers. *N Engl J Med* 1988;304:1331.
23. Ylinen K, Aula P, Stenman U-H, et al. Risk of minor and major malformations in diabetes with haemoglobin A1c values in early pregnancy. *Br Med J* 1984;289:345.
24. Fuhrmann K, Reiher H, Semmler K, Glockner E. The effect of intensified conventional insulin therapy before and during pregnancy on the malformation rate in offspring of diabetic mothers. *Exp Clin Endocrinol* 1984;83:173.
25. Kitzmiller J, Gavin L, Gin G, Jovanovic-Peterson L, Main E, Zigrang W. Preconception care of diabetes. Glycemic control prevents congenital anomalies. *JAMA* 1991;265:731.
26. Ballard J, Rosen B, Khoury J. Diabetic fetal macrosomia: significance of disproportionate growth. *J Pediatr* 1993;122:115.
27. Committee on Technical Bulletins of the American College of Obstetricians and Gynecologists. ACOG technical bulletin. Diabetes and pregnancy. Number 200—December 1994. *Int J Gynaecol Obstet* 1995; 48:331.
28. Nasrat H, Fageeh W, Abalkhail B, Yamani T, Ardawi MS. Determinants of pregnancy outcome in patients with gestational diabetes. *Int J Gynaecol Obstet* 1996;53:117.
29. Naylor CD, Sermer M, Chen E, Sykora K. Cesarean delivery in relation to birth weight and gestational glucose tolerance: pathophysiology or practice style? Toronto Trihospital Gestational Diabetes Investigators. *JAMA* 1996;275:1165.
30. Coustan DR. Management of gestational diabetes mellitus: a self-fulfilling prophecy? *JAMA* 1996;275:1199.
31. Sosenko I, Kitzmiller J, Loo S, Blix P, Rubenstein A, Gabbay K. The infant of the diabetic mother: correlation of increased cord C-peptide levels with macrosomia and hypoglycemia. *N Engl J Med* 1979; 301:859.
32. Bloom S, Johnston D. Failure of glucagon release in infants of diabetic mothers. *Br Med J* 1972;4:453.
33. Kalhan S, Savin S, Adam P. Attenuated glucose production rate in the newborn infants of insulin-dependent diabetic mothers. *N Engl J Med* 1977;296:375.
34. Frantz II, Epstein M. Fetal lung development in pregnancies complicated by diabetes. In: Merkatz I, Adam P, eds. *The diabetic pregnancy: a perinatal perspective.* New York: Grune & Stratton, 1979.
35. Huffaker J. Fetal pulmonary maturation in the infant of the diabetic mother. In: Jovanovic L, Peterson C, Fuhrmann K, eds. *Diabetes and pregnancy: teratology, toxicity and treatment.* New York: Praeger, 1986:361.
36. Nylund L, Lunell N, Lewander R, Persson B, Sarby B. Uteroplacental blood flow in diabetic pregnancy: measurements with indium 113m and a computer-linked gamma camera. *Am J Obstet Gynecol* 1982;144:298.
37. Bjork O, Persson B. Placental changes in relation to the degree of metabolic control in diabetes mellitus. *Placenta* 1982;3:367.
38. Bjork O, Persson B. Villous structure in different parts of the cotyledon in placentas of insulin-dependent women. *Acta Obstet Gynecol Scand* 1984;63:37.
39. Madsen H, Ditzel J. Changes in red blood cell oxygen transport in diabetic pregnancy. *Am J Obstet Gynecol* 1982;143:421.
40. Hagay ZJ, Weissman A, Lurie S, Insler V. Reversal of fetal distress following intensive treatment of maternal diabetic ketoacidosis. *Am J Perinatol* 1994;11:430.
41. Basu A, Close C, Jenkins D, Krentz A, Nattrass M, Wright A. Persisting mortality in diabetic ketoacidosis. *Diabet Med* 1993;10:282.
42. Rodgers B, Rodgers D. Clinical variables associated with diabetic ketoacidosis during pregnancy. *J Reprod Med* 1991;36:797.
43. Siperstein M. Diabetic ketoacidosis and hyperosmolar coma. *Endocrinol Metab Clin North Am* 1992;21:415.
44. Wong K, Schafer P, Schultz J. Hypokalemia and anesthetic implications. *Anesth Analg* 1993;77:1238.
45. Landon M, Gabbe S. Fetal surveillance and timing of delivery in pregnancy complicated by diabetes mellitus. *Obstet Gynecol Clin North Am* 1996;23:109.
46. Kjos SL, Leung A, Henry OA, Victor MR, Paul RH, Medearis AL. Antepartum surveillance in diabetic pregnancies: predictors of fetal distress in labor. *Am J Obstet Gynecol* 1995;173:1532.
47. Kjos SL, Henry OA, Montoro M, Buchanan TA, Mestman JH. Insulin-requiring diabetes in pregnancy: a randomized trial of active induction of labor and expectant management. *Am J Obstet Gynecol* 1993;169:611.
48. Goldman M, Kitzmiller J, Abrams B, Cowan R, Laros R. Obstetric complications with GDM. *Diabetes* 1991;40[Suppl 2]:79.
49. Gordon MC, Landon MB, Boyle J, Stewart KS, Gabbe SG. Coronary artery disease in insulin-dependent diabetes mellitus of pregnancy (class H): a review of the literature. *Obstet Gynecol Surv* 1996;51:437.
50. Hagay Z, Weissman A. Management of diabetic pregnancy complicated by coronary artery disease and neuropathy. *Obstet Gynecol Clin North Am* 1996;23:205.
51. Landon M, Gabbe S. Diabetes mellitus and pregnancy. *Obstet Gynecol Clin North Am* 1992;19:633.
52. Hawkins J, Koonin L, Palmer S, Gibbs C. Anesthesia-related deaths during obstetric delivery in the United States, 1979–1990. *Anesthesiology* 1997;86:277.
53. Ramanathan S, Khoo P, Arismendy J. Perioperative maternal and neonatal acid-base status and glucose metabolism in patients with insulin-dependant diabetes mellitus. *Anesth Analg* 1991;73:105.
54. Jovanovic L, Peterson C. Management of the pregnant, insulin-dependant diabetic woman. *Diabetes Care* 1980;3:63.
55. Jovanovic L, Peterson C. Insulin and glucose requirements during the first stage of labor in insulin-dependent diabetic women. *Am J Med* 1983;75:607.
56. Jovanovic-Peterson L, Peterson CM. Pregnancy in the diabetic woman. Guidelines for a successful outcome. *Endocrinol Metab Clin North Am* 1992;21:433.
57. Golde S, Good-Anderson B, Montoro M, Artal R. Insulin requirements during labor: a reappraisal. *Am J Obstet Gynecol* 1982; 144:556.
58. Lean M, Pearson D, Sutherland H. Insulin management during labor and delivery in mothers with diabetes. *Diabet Med* 1990;7:162.
59. Yen S, Vela P, Tsai C. Impariment of growth hormone secretion in response to hypoglycemia during early and late pregnancy. *J Clin Endocrinol Metab* 1970;31:29.
60. Rosenbloom A. Skeletal and joint manifestations of childhood diabetes. *Pediatr Clin North Am* 1984;31:569.
61. Grgic A, Rosenbloom A, Weber F, Giordano B, Malone I, Shuster J. Joint contracture-common manifestation of childhood diabetes mellitus. *J Pediatr* 1976;88:584.
62. Kennedy L, Archer D, Campbell S, Beacom R, Carson D, Johnston P. Limited joint mobility in type I diabetes mellitus. *Postgrad Med J* 1982;58:481.
63. Salzarulo H, Taylor L. Diabetic "stiff joint syndrome" as a cause of difficult endotracheal intubation. *Anesthesiology* 1986;64:366.
64. Hogan K, Rusy D, Springman S. Difficult laryngoscopy and diabetes mellitus. *Anesth Analg* 1988;67:1162.
65. Eleborg L, Norberg A. Are diabetic patients difficult to intubate? *Acta Anaesthesiol Scand* 1988;32:508.
66. Reissell E, Orko R, Maunuksela E-L, Lindgren L. Predictability of difficult laryngoscopy in patients with long tern diabetes mellitus. *Anaesthesia* 1990;45:1024.
67. Langer O, Hod M. Management of gestational diabetes mellitus. *Obstet Gynecol Clin North Am* 1996;23:137.
68. Hood D, Dewan D. Anesthetic and obstetric outcome in morbidly obese parturients. *Anesthesiology* 1993;79:1210.
69. Rocke D, Muray W, Rout C, Gouws E. Relative risk analysis of factors associated with difficult intubation in obstetric anesthesia. *Anesthesiology* 1992;77:67.

70. Endler G, Mariona F, Sokol R, Stevenson L. Anesthesia related maternal mortality in Michigan, 1972–1984. *Am J Obstet Gynecol* 1988; 159:187.
71. Palumbo P, Elveback L, Whisnant J. Neurologic complications of diabetes mellitus: transient ischemic attack, stroke, and peripheral neuropathy. *Adv Neurol* 1978;19:593.
72. Airaksinen K, Anttila L, Linnaluoto M. Autonomic influence on pregnancy outcome in IDDM. *Diabetes Care* 1990;13:756.
73. Airaksinen K, Salmela P, Ikaheimo M. Effect of pregnancy on autonomic nervous function and heart rate in diabetic and nondiabetic women. *Diabetes Care* 1987;10:748.
74. Hilsted J, Low P. Diabetic autonomic neuropathy. In: Low P, ed. *Clinical autonomic disorders: evaluation and management*. Boston: Little, Brown and Company, 1993:423.
75. Burgos L, Ebert T, Asiddao C, et al. Increased intraoperative cardiovascular morbidity in diabetics with autonomic neuropathy. *Anesthesiology* 1989;70:591.
76. Datta S, Brown WU, Ostheimer GW, Weiss JB, Alper MH. Epidural anesthesia for cesarean section in diabetic parturients: maternal and neonatal acid-base status and bupivacaine concentration. *Anesth Analg* 1981;60:574.
77. Pirart J. Diabetes mellitus and its degenerative complications: a prospective study of 4400 patients observed between 1947 and 1973. *Diabet Med* 1977;3:245.
78. Warner M, Warner M, Martin J. Ulnar neuropathy. *Anesthesiology* 1994;81:1332.
79. Caplan R, Posner K, Cheney F. Perioperative ulnar neuropathy. *Anesthesiology* 1994;81:1321.
80. Vandam L. Complications of spinal and epidural anesthesia. In: Gravenstein N, Kirby R, eds. *Complications in anesthesiology.* Philadelphia: Lippincott-Raven Publishers, 1996:563.
81. Whiteman VE, Homko CJ, Reece EA. Management of hypoglycemia and diabetic ketoacidosis in pregnancy. *Obstet Gynecol Clin North Am* 1996;23:87.
82. Datta S. *Common problems in obstetric anesthesia,* 2nd ed. St. Louis: Mosby-Year Book, 1994:373.

Obstetric Anesthesia, second edition,
edited by Mark C. Norris.
Lippincott Williams & Wilkins, Philadelphia © 1999.

CHAPTER 6

Perinatal Physiology and Pharmacology

M. Joanne Douglas

Of necessity, there is a close relationship between a mother and her fetus. The fetus receives all its nourishment and oxygen from the mother. In addition, this intimate connection exposes the fetus to almost any substance to which the mother is exposed. Any drug given during gestation can potentially affect the fetus and the newborn.

PLACENTA

Structure

The placenta is a unique disc-shaped organ that acts as an interface between the mother and her fetus. It acts as fetal lung, gastrointestinal system, and excretory system. It permits passage of some substances while acting as a barrier to others. During gestation, the placenta grows, offering an ever larger surface area for maternal–fetal exchange. At term, the placenta weighs about 500 g.

The basic structural unit of the placenta is the chorionic villus. The villi are highly vascular projections of fetal tissue surrounded by the chorion, the outermost layer of fetal tissue. The chorion has two layers, the syncytiotrophoblast and the cytotrophoblast. The syncytiotrophoblast lies in direct contact with maternal blood within the intervillous space (Fig. 1) (1). Substances that pass from mother to fetus travel in maternal blood to the intervillous space. There, they cross the two layers of trophoblast, some fetal connective tissue, and, finally, the fetal capillary wall into the fetal blood stream (Fig. 2). No continuous direct communication exists between maternal and fetal circulations. Occasionally, however, a delicate villus may break, allowing fetal cells to enter the intervillous space and the maternal circulation (2,3). Maternal sensitization to fetal red blood cells (isoimmunization) may then occur.

M. J. Douglas: Department of Anesthesia, BC Women's Hospital, Vancouver, Canada V6H 3N1.

Uteroplacental Circulation

The blood supply to the placenta is maternal in origin. Uteroplacental blood flow near term is approximately 600 mL/min. Maternal blood spurts into the intervillous space with each heart beat. This blood is then forced upwards and laterally, bathing the chorionic villi. Continued influx of blood pushes blood already within the intervillous space toward venous openings that ultimately drain through uterine and pelvic veins (Fig. 1) (4,5).

At term, the uteroplacental circulation appears maximally vasodilated, with flow dependent mostly on maternal blood pressure (6). Changes in intrauterine pressure and the pattern of uterine contractions also can interfere with placental blood supply.

In summary, the basic site of exchange in the placenta is the intervillous space, where maternal blood contacts fetal tissue. Constant movement of blood through this space depends on the pressure of the blood entering the space. Vasoconstriction of the uterine vessels and changes in intrauterine pressure alter placental perfusion pressure (7).

Function

Synthesis and Metabolism

The placenta contains enzyme systems that synthesize hormones, including estrogen, progesterone, chorionic gonadotropin, and placental lactogen (8). The latter is abundant in the mother but not the fetus. It promotes insulin resistance in the mother by blocking the peripheral uptake and utilization of glucose. It also promotes maternal mobilization and use of free fatty acids. These actions ensure a ready supply of glucose for the fetus and placenta.

The placenta contains specialized cellular receptors and enzymes. These structures include insulin and β-adrenergic receptors as well as the enzymes adenylate cyclase, alkaline phosphatase, and pseudocholinesterase.

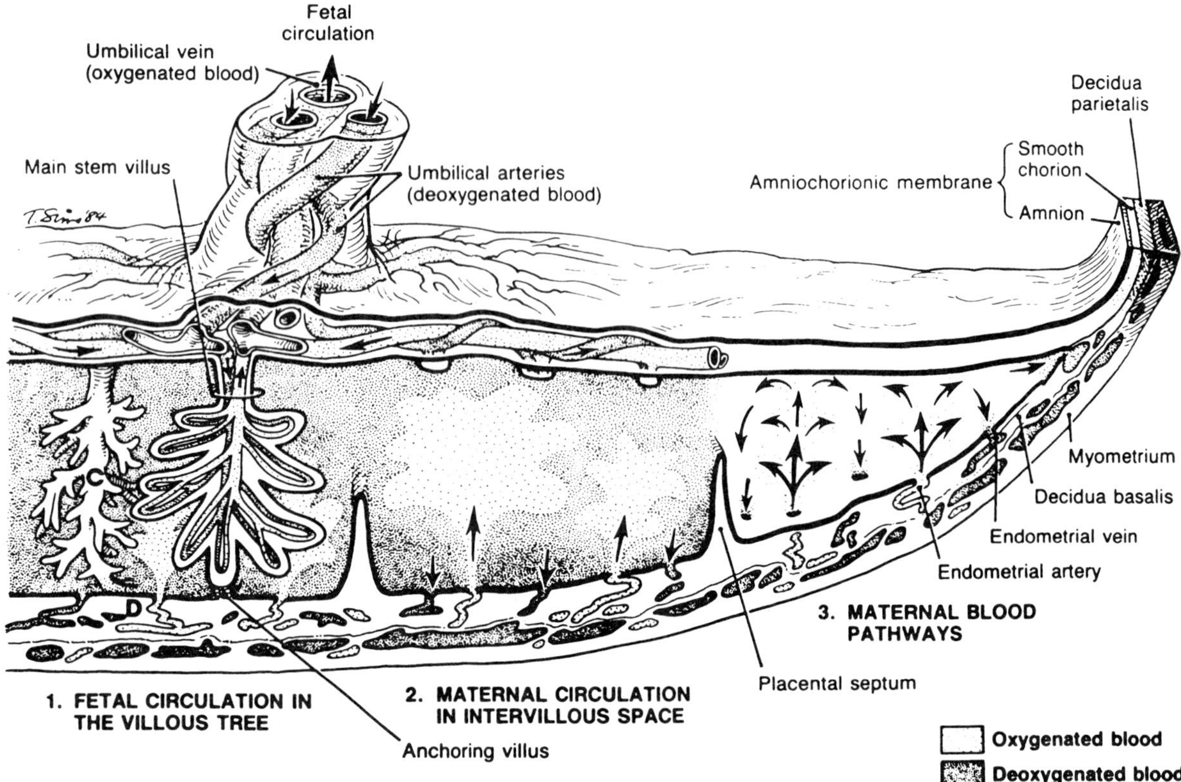

FIG. 1. Schematic drawing of a section through a full-term placenta. **1:** The relation of the villus chorion *(C)* to the decidua basalis *(D)* and the fetal placental circulation. **2:** The maternal placental circulation. Maternal blood flows into the intervillous spaces in funnel-shaped spurts, and exchanges occur with the fetal blood as the maternal blood flows around the villi. **3:** The inflowing arterial blood pushes venous blood into the endometrial veins, which are scattered over the entire surface of the decidua basalis. Note that the umbilical arteries carry deoxygenated fetal blood to the placenta and that the umbilical vein carries oxygenated blood to the fetus. Note that the cotyledons are separated from each other by placenta (decidual) septa of the materna portion of the placenta. Each cotyledon consists of two or more main stem villi and their many branches. (Reprinted from ref. 247, with permission.)

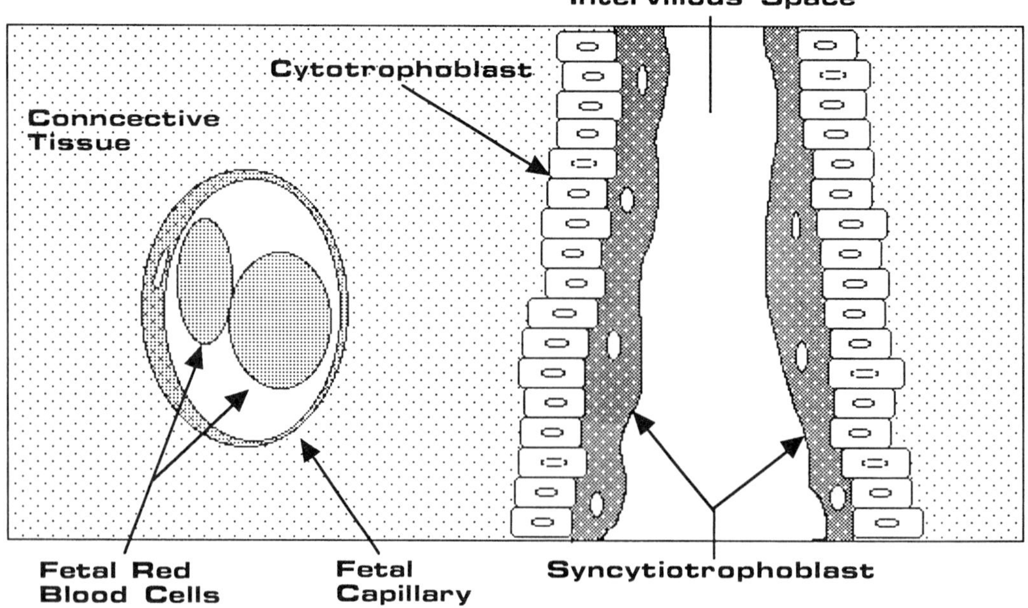

FIG. 2. Schematic representation of a fetal villous, showing the tissue layers that separate fetal and maternal blood in the human placenta. The cytotrophoblast layer is much less distinct in the third trimester than depicted here. (Drawing courtesy of M. Norris, M.D.)

Two other enzymes, catechol-O-methyl transferase and monoamine oxidase, impede the passage of catecholamines across the placenta.

The placental barrier allows the mother to accept the fetus (nonself). It also acts as a filter, permitting selective transport of maternal antibodies to the fetus. Some of these maternal antibodies help provide fetal immunity while others can cause fetal disease. In Rh isoimmunization, maternal antibodies specific for fetal red blood cells cross the placenta and produce fetal hemolytic anemia. Antibodies producing maternal autoimmune disease (e.g., thyrotoxicosis, idiopathic thrombocytopenic purpura, myasthenia gravis, and systemic lupus erythematosus) also can attack fetal tissue (9).

Placental Exchange

Functionally, the placenta is a complex organ of exchange. A variety of nutrients, waste products, and toxins continuously cross this barrier. Most substances traverse the trophoblast by simple diffusion, also known as flow-limited transfer (10). Polar (hydrophilic) substances (e.g., metabolic wastes, nutrients, and some drugs) need special help to cross the lipid membranes of the placenta. Specialized transport processes include facilitated diffusion, active transport, and pinocytosis. Unlike simple diffusion, these methods of transfer expend energy (11). Table 1 lists the modes of placental exchange and gives examples of compounds that use each approach.

Most drugs and respiratory gases cross the placenta by simple diffusion, which uses no energy. The rate at which substances pass from mother to fetus depends only on the difference in concentration of the substance in maternal and fetal blood. The Fick equation describes the factors involved in this process:

$$Q/T = k \bullet C = \left(\frac{C_m - C_f}{X}\right)$$

where Q/T represents the quantity of a substance transferred per unit time; k is the diffusion constant, which is determined by molecular weight, lipid solubility, degree of ionization, and spatial configuration; A is the area available for diffusion; C_m is the concentration in mother; C_f is the concentration in fetus; and X is the thickness of the membrane (placenta).

TABLE 1. *Mechanisms of placental exchange*

Mechanism	Example
Simple diffusion	Oxygen Carbon dioxide Sodium Chloride Fatty acids
Facilitated diffusion	Glucose Lactate
Active transport	Amino acids Calcium Phosphorus Iron Vitamins A and C
Pinocytosis	IgG

As with simple diffusion, compounds that cross the placenta through facilitated diffusion travel down a concentration gradient. Here, however, the speed of transfer is faster than predicted by the Fick equation for simple diffusion. Substances occurring in low concentration in maternal plasma that are essential to the fetus (e.g., glucose and lactate) traverse the placenta by facilitated diffusion.

Active transport involves transferring compounds against a concentration gradient. Substances actively transported include some amino acids, calcium, phosphorous, iron, and vitamins A and C.

The placenta acts as a barrier to most proteins; the most notable exception being immunoglobulin G (IgG). IgG probably crosses the placenta by pinocytosis (endocytosis), which involves specific receptors located on the trophoblast (12). Once IgG attaches to the receptor, the bound IgG is then enclosed in small vacuoles. These vacuoles then pinch off and cross to the fetal side of the trophoblast. There, they release their contents.

Respiratory Exchange

Respiratory gases pass to the fetus by simple diffusion. At the tissue level, respiratory exchange also depends upon the interaction of oxygen and carbon dioxide with hemoglobin and on the nature of blood flow in the maternal and umbilical circulations (13).

Oxygen

Multiple factors enhance fetal oxygenation. Fetal hemoglobin binds oxygen tightly, favoring oxygen uptake from maternal blood. The high concentration of fetal hemoglobin and a greater cardiac output per unit of body weight than in the adult favor efficient uptake and distribution of oxygen within the fetus. Oxygen transfer across the placenta is blood flow limited and not related to the thickness or surface area of the placenta (14). The difference between the maternal and fetal partial pressures of oxygen determines the gradient for oxygen diffusion across the placenta (15). Relative differences in the affinity of maternal and fetal hemoglobins for oxygen account for most of the difference between maternal and fetal pO_2. The oxyhemoglobin dissociation curve of fetal hemoglobin lies to the left of the dissociation curve of adult hemoglobin. As a result, fetal blood binds oxygen more tightly and has a higher oxygen content at a given pO_2 than adult blood (Fig. 3) (16).

Carbon Dioxide.

Carbon dioxide diffuses readily across the placenta. The small difference between maternal and fetal pCO_2

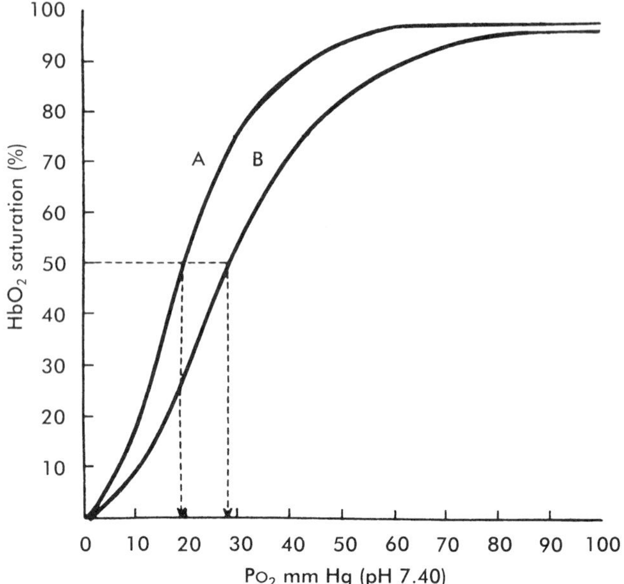

FIG. 3. Fetal *(A)* and maternal *(B)* oxyhemoglobin saturation curves. The *dashed vertical line* represents the p_{50}. (Reprinted from ref. 248, with permission.)

may result from shunting or unequal distribution of maternal and fetal blood flow within the placental vasculature. Placental metabolism also may contribute carbon dioxide. Fetal hemoglobin has a lower affinity for carbon dioxide than does maternal hemoglobin. The hyperventilation of pregnancy lowers maternal pCO_2. Both factors favor transfer of carbon dioxide from fetus to mother. In addition, both oxygen and carbon dioxide influence the binding of the other to hemoglobin. Placental transfer of one gas enhances the exchange of the other (13).

Fetal Oxygenation

The fetus obtains oxygenated blood from the mother by a unique arrangement (17). The umbilical vein carries oxygenated blood to the fetus and empties into the portal sinus. From there, most of the blood bypasses the liver by flowing through the ductus venosus to the inferior vena cava. The remainder passes through the liver by way of the portal and hepatic veins. The oxygen-rich blood in the ductus venosus enters the right atrium, and then goes through the foramen ovale into the left atrium. There it mixes with pulmonary venous blood and travels through the left ventricle and into the aorta. This arrangement ensures a well-oxygenated blood supply for the coronary and cerebral circulations. Blood returning from the head, brain, and upper body via the superior vena cava enters the right atrium. There, with blood from the inferior vena cava, it flows into the right ventricle to the pulmonary artery. Most of the blood entering the pulmonary artery skips the lungs by flowing through the ductus arteriosus directly into the descending aorta. The umbilical arteries, arising from the internal iliac arteries, carry desaturated blood out of the fetus and back to the placenta.

PHYSIOLOGIC CHANGES OF PREGNANCY THAT ALTER PHARMACOKINETICS

During pregnancy, the absorption, distribution, protein binding, and elimination of maternally administered drugs may change (18). Hyperventilation and a decreased functional residual capacity increase the maternal uptake of inhalational anesthetics during pregnancy (19). These changes, combined with an increase in cardiac output, speed anesthetic induction in the parturient. Progesterone and motilin concentrations increase during gestation. These compounds slow gastrointestinal motility, potentially altering the absorption of maternal oral medications (20,21). Opioids administered for pain relief further delay gastric emptying (22,23). Hormonal changes are thought to be responsible for the decrease in minimum alveolar concentration (MAC) seen during gestation (24) and the increased susceptibility of nerves to local anesthetics (25,26).

During pregnancy, total body water increases by up to 8 L and plasma volume increases by 50% (27). This increase in body water expands the volume of drug distribution. Serum albumin concentration falls. Free fatty acids and acidic drugs (i.e., salicylates, anticonvulsants, and benzodiazepines) compete for a reduced number of albumin binding sites. As the affected drugs are less protein bound, they may be more potent than in nonpregnant women. The serum concentration of α_1-acid glycoprotein remains stable (28). The free fraction of basic drugs, including local anesthetics and opioids that bind primarily to α_1-acid glycoprotein, does not change during gestation.

Hepatic metabolism may increase during pregnancy, as enzyme induction by progesterone speeds elimination of some drugs. Renal plasma flow and glomerular filtration rise during gestation. Clearance of drugs that are primarily renally excreted, such as pancuronium, will increase.

Transfer of Drugs

Most drugs cross the placenta by simple diffusion. The ease of passage depends on their lipid solubility. Drugs that readily cross the blood–brain barrier also freely cross the placenta (29). The concentration of drug on the maternal side of the placenta determines the degree of fetal exposure. Maternal drug delivery to the placenta depends on several of the following factors:

- Total dose and duration of administration,
- Route of administration,
- Rate of absorption,
- Uteroplacental blood flow,
- Maternal metabolism and excretion,
- Maternal protein binding, and
- Maternal pH and the pK_a of the drug.

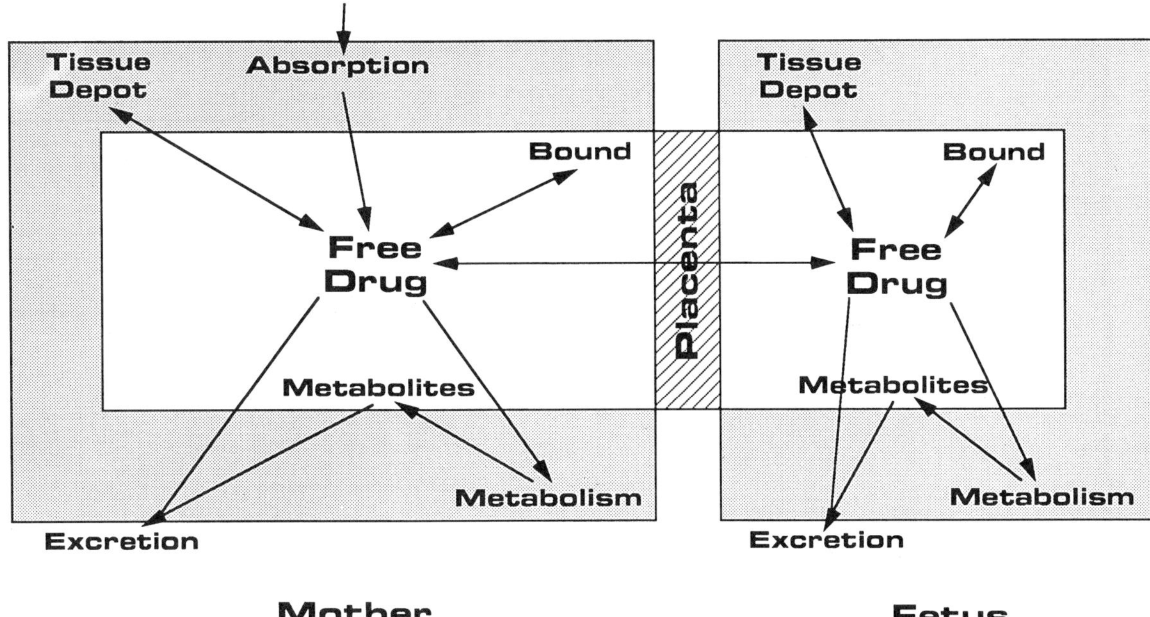

FIG. 4. Drug distribution in mother and fetus. (Drawing courtesy of M. Norris, M.D.)

Once the drug crosses the placental barrier, its concentration in fetal plasma depends on fetal protein binding, cardiac output, tissue uptake, metabolism, and excretion (Fig. 4). Knowledge of placental physiology and perfusion should enable the design of drugs specifically for use in pregnancy (30).

Measurement of Placental Drug Transfer

Much of the early work on placental drug transfer used animals (sheep and rabbits). More recently, the isolated, dual perfused, human placental lobule and placental microsome models have been used to study transfer (31).

FETAL PHYSIOLOGY AND PHARMACOKINETICS

Several aspects of the uptake, distribution, and elimination of drugs in the fetus and newborn differ from the adult. Uptake into the fetus begins as drug passes through the placenta and enters the fetal circulation by way of the umbilical vein. Once there, the extent of drug distribution depends on several factors. The drug may undergo considerable metabolism within the liver, or it may bypass the liver via the ductus venosus and directly enter the fetal arterial circulation. This "first-pass" metabolism by the fetal liver can significantly lower the amount of drug delivered to highly perfused organs such as the heart and the brain. Shunts within the fetal circulation (i.e., foramen ovale and ductus arteriosus) also alter fetal drug distribution.

The concentration of drug in fetal blood depends on the dose administered to the mother and the placental transfer rate. The rate of transfer depends primarily on differences in maternal and fetal protein binding and acid–base status (32–34). Maternal protein binding limits the amount of free (unbound) drug available for placental transport. This mechanism significantly limits fetal exposure to highly bound drugs (e.g., bupivacaine) (Fig. 5).

The pH gradient between maternal and fetal blood also can influence the extent of placental transfer of weakly acidic or basic compounds. Normally, a slight (0.1) pH gradient exists between the maternal and fetal circulations. Only un-ionized drugs cross the lipid barrier of the placenta. With acidic drugs (salicylates, anticonvulsants, barbiturates), the pH gradient limits transfer. With basic drugs (local anesthetics and opioids), the lower fetal pH favors drug transfer to the fetus (Fig. 6A). "Ion trapping" of basic drugs can occur if fetal pH falls. As un-ionized drug enters the fetal circulation, it becomes ionized, and cannot diffuse back to the maternal circulation (Fig. 6B). Both local anesthetics and opioids can become "trapped" in the fetus by this mechanism (35–43).

The fetus and newborn have a larger total body water content and a higher extracellular-to-intracellular water ratio than adults. In relation to its body weight, the fetus has a small muscle mass and a large liver and brain. In addition, the fetal brain has a low myelin content and a high cerebral blood flow (44). These factors combine to increase the potential central nervous system effects of exogenous drugs.

Drugs are eliminated from the fetus by metabolism, urinary excretion, and diffusion back to the mother. By term, most hepatic microsomal enzyme systems are present, but they are often less effective than adult enzymes (44). The

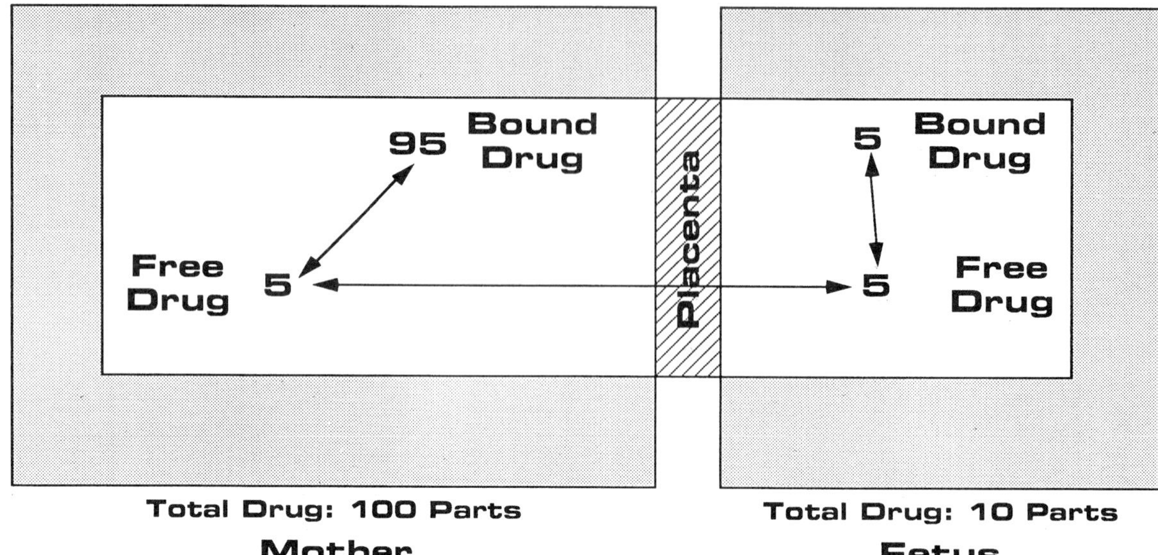

FIG. 5. Maternal protein binding can limit fetal drug exposure. In this example, maternal blood contains 100 parts of drug. In maternal blood, the drug is highly protein bound (95%) so only five parts of drug are free (unbound) and able to diffuse across the placenta. At equilibrium, the concentration of free drug is the same (5) in maternal and fetal blood. In the fetus, however, the drug is only 50% protein bound. Because of these differences in protein binding, the total amount of drug in fetal blood is only 10% of the concentration of drug in maternal blood. (Drawing courtesy of M. Norris, M.D.)

premature infant has even more limited metabolic capabilities and experiences greater drug effects than the term infant. Drug excreted in the urine in utero enters the amniotic fluid, where it may be swallowed by the fetus. Once reingested, drug may reenter the systemic circulation after being absorbed from the gastrointestinal tract.

Measuring Fetal Drug Effect

Drug Measurement

To determine the effects of a drug on the fetus or newborn, one must know the plasma concentration of drug at the time the reputed drug effect occurs. It is hard to directly measure the fetal concentration of a drug. One can sample amniotic fluid or fetal scalp blood during labor, but the information derived from such sources is limited. Before birth, maternal plasma concentration of drug provides an indirect measurement of fetal plasma concentration. Using the human placental perfusion model, researchers can examine placental drug transfer, but these studies do not reflect what happens in a dynamic system with ongoing changes in maternal and fetal distribution and elimination (31).

Testing for Intrapartum Drug Effects

Intrapartum drug effects can be evaluated indirectly by monitoring changes in fetal heart rate pattern after maternal drug exposure (45,46). Other investigators have studied the effects of anesthetic drugs and techniques on uterine, placental, and fetal blood flow (Table 2). Some of the techniques used include measuring uteroplacental blood flow with radioactive tracers (xenon^{133} or indium^{113}) (47,48) and measuring fetal umbilical and aortic blood flow velocity with Doppler ultrasonography (49,50). More recently, in utero drug concentrations have been measured by cordocentesis (51–53). This technique measures the amount of drug in the umbilical circulation at the time of funipuncture and is not linked to delivery. Unfortunately, it is unclear how umbilical blood drug concentration correlates with total fetal drug exposure. Nor does blood drug concentration predict fetal effect. Initial studies using cordocentesis suggest that animal models do not readily predict human results (52).

Postpartum (Newborn) Testing

At birth, blood from the maternal vein, umbilical vein, and umbilical artery can be analyzed for the presence of specific drugs and their metabolites. These data can provide some information about the amount of drug transferred to the fetus and its uptake by fetal tissues. The umbilical venous concentration of drug represents drug delivered to the fetus via the placenta. The ratio of umbilical venous to maternal venous drug levels (UV/MV) reflects the rate and extent of placental transfer. Umbilical arterial drug concentration is the portion of drug remaining after tissue uptake and metabolism. The ratio of drug concentration in the umbilical artery to the umbilical vein (UA/UV) shows the extent of uptake by fetal tissues

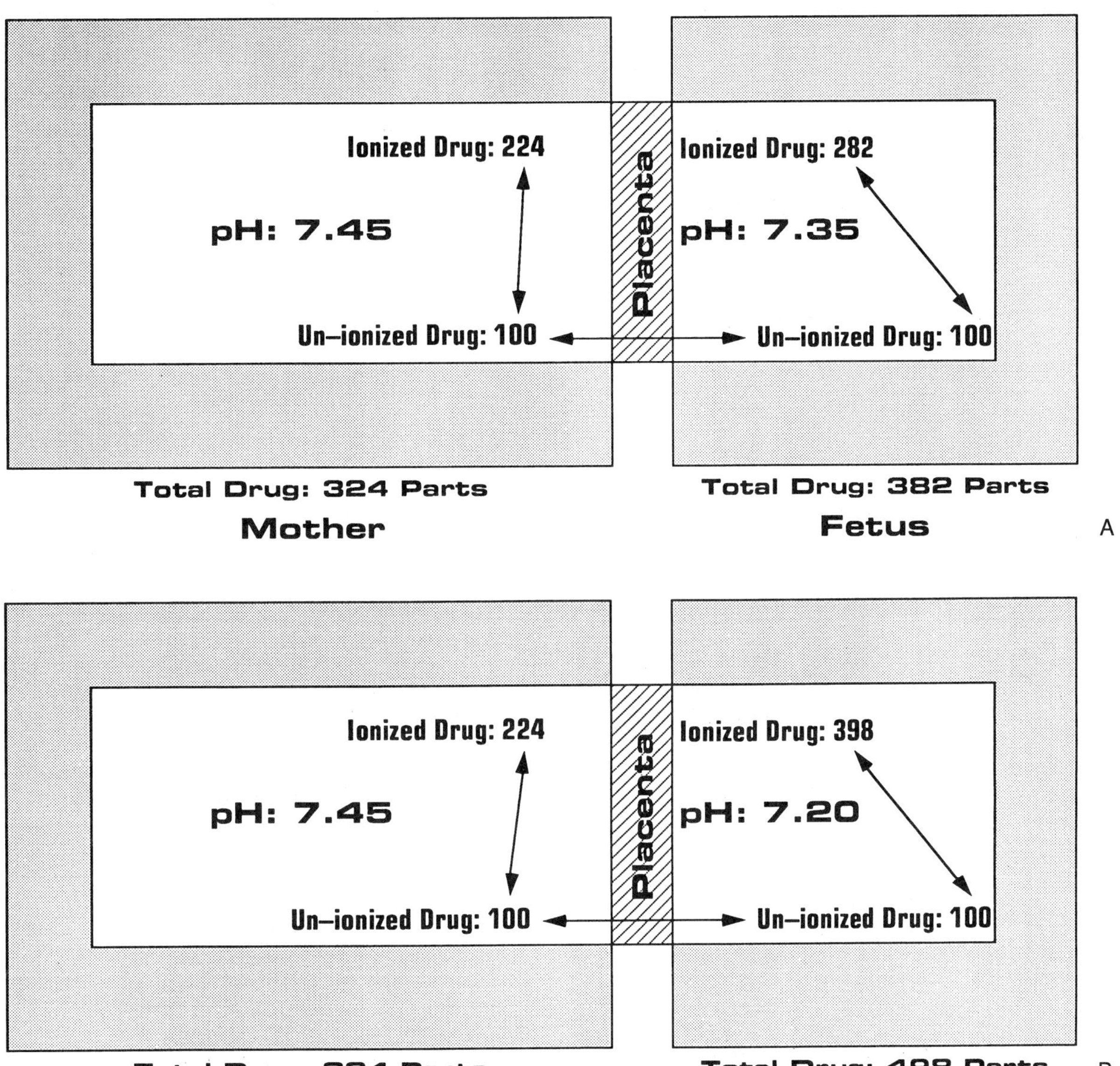

FIG. 6. The pH gradient between mother and fetus affects the placental transfer of local anesthetic drugs. In this example, lidocaine exists in equilibrium between basic (un-ionized) and cationic (ionized) forms. The relative proportion of drug in each from is determined by the drug's pK_a (7.8 for lidocaine) and the pH of the surrounding plasma ($pH = pK_a + \log base/cation$). Only un-ionized drug can cross the lipid membranes of the placenta. At equilibrium, the concentration of un-ionized drug is equal on both sides of the placenta. The lower plasma pH in the fetus causes relatively more local anesthetic to be ionized in the fetal compared to maternal blood **(A)**. In fetal acidosis, the lower fetal pH creates more ionized drug that is "trapped" on the fetal side of the placenta **(B)**. (Drawing courtesy of M. Norris, M.D.)

(Table 3). These measurements do not, however, indicate the total amount of drug present in the infant. To quantify fetal drug exposure accurately, one must repeatedly sample and analyze neonatal blood and urine.

Other methods of testing neonatal drug effects include assigning Apgar scores and measuring acid–base status. Although sometimes useful, these tests are nonspecific and their results change in response to a multitude of variables.

Several investigators have developed tests designed to look for subtle behavioral effects of drugs (Table 4). These tests examine the neonate's muscle tone and ability to do the following:

- Alter the state of arousal,
- Suppress responses to repetitive or intrusive stimuli,
- Respond appropriately to external events, and
- Initiate complex motor acts and the appropriateness of reflex motor responses (54).

The Brazelton Neonatal Behavioral Assessment Scale (BNBAS), a test favored by developmental psycholo-

TABLE 2. *Testing for fetal drug effects*

- Intrapartum
  - Maternal plasma drug concentration
  - Fetal heart rate changes
    - Variability
    - Decelerations
  - Blood flow studies
    - Uteroplacental
    - Fetal (umbilical and aortic)
- Postpartum
  - Acid–base status
  - Apgar scores
  - Drug and metabolite concentrations
    - Maternal vein
    - Umbilical vein
    - Umbilical artery
    - Neonatal (blood and urine)
  - Neonatal neurobehavioral testing

gists, looks explicitly at the mother–infant interaction (55). It requires specific training and considerable time to perform.

In 1974, Scanlon et al. (56) designed the Early Neonatal Neurobehavioral Scale (ENNS) to examine the effect of anesthetic drugs. It is done 2 to 8 hours after birth, a time that theoretically correlates with the maximum effect of prenatally administered drugs. It requires less time to perform than the BNBAS and focuses on muscle tone and the infant's response to repetitive stimuli.

Amiel-Tison et al. (57) wanted to examine muscle tone more closely. They were especially interested in differences in tone between different muscle groups (i.e., flexors and extensors of the neck). They believed that by examining these variables, they could distinguish between the effects of maternal drugs and birth trauma. The Neurologic and Adaptive Capacity Score (NACS) takes even less time to do than the ENNS and so has gained favor with many anesthesiologists.

The results of these tests pose a dilemma for the obstetric anesthesiologist: What do they mean? If specifically sought, subtle neonatal effects can be detected with most anesthetic agents and techniques. Many anesthesiologists consider these neurobehavioral changes clinically insignificant (58). However, controversy still surrounds this subject. In nonhuman primates, postnatal behavioral maturation may be altered by drug exposure at birth (59). Milestones in brain development may be delayed, but complex cognitive processes such as learning, memory, and attention are not substantially affected. Other researchers suggest that exposure to obstetric analgesia (opioids and nitrous oxide) may lead to substance abuse in the future, although socioeconomic factors and hospital of delivery are confounders that make interpretation impossible (60). The authors suggest that regional analgesia is a preferred option for labor pain (61).

TABLE 3. *Umbilical artery:umbilical vein ratios*

UA/UV Ratio	Extent of fetal uptake
1	Maternal/fetal equilibrium
<1	Continuing fetal tissue uptake
>1	Elimination of drug from fetus via diffusion into maternal blood

TABLE 4. *Neonatal neurobehavioral tests*

- Brazelton neonatal behavioral assessment scale
  - Most comprehensive
  - Forty-nine items
  - Reflects "mother–infant" interaction
  - Used mainly by developmental psychologists
  - Takes 30–45 min
  - Difficult to summarize for data analysis
- Scanlon early neonatal neurobehavioral scale
  - Designed to examine newborn changes associated with anesthesia
  - Done 2–8 h after birth
  - Fifteen observations of primary reflexes, muscle tone, and response to repeated stimuli
  - Takes <10 min
- Neurological and adaptive capacity score
  - Designed to distinguish between drug effects and birth trauma
  - Twenty criteria in five areas
    - Adaptive capacity
    - Passive tone
    - Active tone
    - Primary reflexes
    - General neurological state
  - Takes <5 min
  - Favored by anesthesiologists

Neonatal neurobehavioral testing remains an important method of determining drug effect. However, the significance of effects of medication administered during labor and delivery is unclear. Hopefully, future research will help resolve this controversy.

Specific Drugs

Induction Agents

Thiopental. Thiopental, a highly lipid-soluble drug, passes readily from mother to fetus (Table 5). Equilibrium between maternal vein and umbilical vein occurs within 3 minutes (Fig. 7) (62). Pregnancy prolongs the half-life of thiopental, probably because of an increased volume of distribution (63). In early pregnancy (7 to 13 weeks), the dose of thiopental for hypnosis is 17% less and for anesthesia is 18% less than in nonpregnant women (64). Thiopental undergoes rapid distribution in the fetus. The UA/UV ratio is 0.46 by 4 to 7 minutes after induction and 0.87 after 8 to 22 minutes (65,66). Some of the drug that crosses the placenta undergoes "first-pass" metabolism in the fetal liver. This effect decreases the amount of drug that reaches the fetal brain (67). Thiopental appears to depress the neonate only when used in large doses (8 mg/kg) (66).

TABLE 5. *Placental transfer and neonatal elimination of three intravenous induction agents*

	MV (μg/mL)	UV (μg/mL)	UV/MV	Neonatal elimination half-life
Thiopental (4 mg/kg)	4.31 (3.12–6.50)	4.65 (3.25–5.69)	0.96 (0.79–1.15)	14.7 h
Propofol (2 mg/kg)	0.87 (0.53–1.48)	0.54 (0.39–1.40)	0.65 (0.31–0.97)	
Midazolam (0.3 mg/kg)	0.34 (0.23–0.62)	0.32 (0.19–0.41)	0.66 (0.5–1.05)	6.3 h

Mean values indicated.
Range shown in parentheses.
Data from ref. 82,100.

Ketamine. Ketamine's ability to ablate awareness and provide profound analgesia has led to its use in obstetrics (68–70). In a dose of 1 mg/kg, ketamine does not commonly cause maternal dreaming (71,72). Ketamine does, however, cause maternal tachycardia and hypertension on induction. These properties make ketamine unsuitable for use in women with preeclampsia. Ketamine rapidly crosses the placenta. Umbilical cord drug concentration exceeds maternal blood ketamine concentration within 2 minutes (73,74). Ketamine induction (1 mg/kg) of general anesthesia for cesarean delivery depresses neonatal neurobehavioral (ENNS) scores (75). Epidural analgesia has less of an effect, whereas thiopental (4 mg/kg) has a greater depressant effect (74).

Propofol. Propofol is a newer intravenous induction agent. When used in a rapid-sequence induction for cesarean section, it is associated with less maternal hypertension than thiopental (76), and it attenuates the catecholamine response to laryngoscopy and tracheal intubation (77). All studies show rapid placental transfer of this drug (76,78–81). The UV/MV ratio at delivery following an induction dose of 2 mg/kg is about 0.65 (see Table 5) (82). A UA/UV ratio of 1.07 after a single maternal bolus of propofol suggests rapid fetal tissue uptake and equilibration (82). Both fetal and maternal blood concentrations fall rapidly after induction (Fig. 8) (78). When using a continuous infusion of propofol to maintain anesthesia, the UA/UV ratio is lower (0.70) than after a single bolus, suggesting continued fetal tissue uptake of drug (78). Propofol is rapidly cleared from the fetal circulation. Fetal blood concentration falls to 0.078 ng/mL by 2 hours after birth, and some propofol can be detected in breast milk (78).

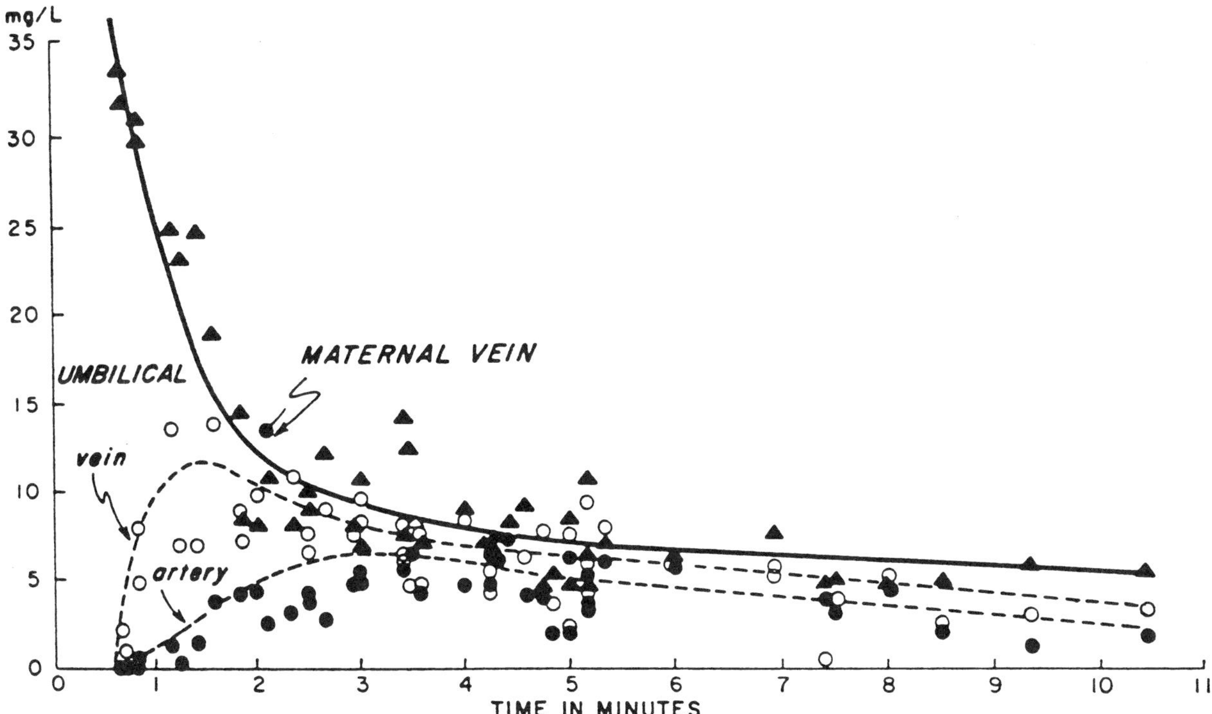

FIG. 7. Thiopental concentration in maternal vein, umbilical vein, and umbilical artery after injection of a single 4 mg/kg dose for induction of general anesthesia. Note the rapid decay of maternal venous blood concentration and the rapid transfer to the fetus. (Reprinted from ref. 66, with permission.)

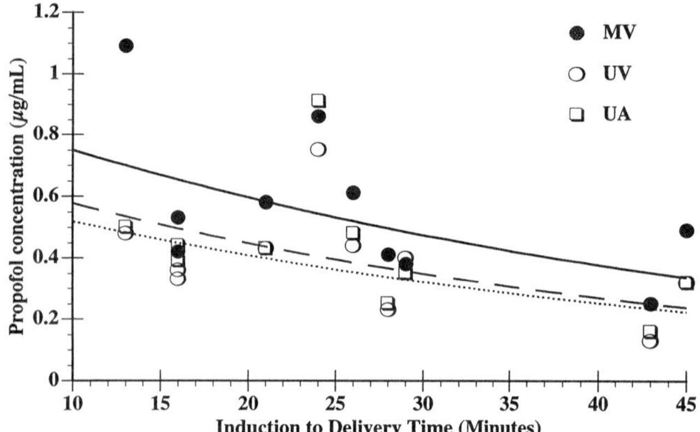

FIG. 8. Propofol concentrations at delivery versus induction to delivery interval during general anesthesia for cesarean section. Ten healthy term parturients received a single 2.5 mg/kg bolus of propofol for induction of anesthesia. The *solid regression line* describes the change in maternal venous, the *dashed line* umbilical vein, and the *dotted line* umbilical artery propofol concentrations. (Data from ref. 78.)

In the pregnant ewe, induction of anesthesia with propofol (2 mg/kg) had no adverse effects on maternal or fetal arterial pressure, heart rate, acid–base status, or uterine blood flow (79). In contrast, thiopental transiently decreases uterine blood flow. In pregnant sheep, succinylcholine, given for intubation following propofol induction, can cause transient, but severe, maternal bradycardia (79).

The neonatal effects of propofol are unclear. Dailland et al. (78) induced general anesthesia for cesarean section with 2.5 mg/kg of propofol and used either 50% nitrous oxide or a 5 mg/kg/hour propofol infusion for maintenance. Apgar scores correlated with neither the time from induction to delivery nor umbilical venous propofol concentration. Infants had good NACS scores by 2 hours with either anesthetic technique (Table 6) (78).

In contrast, Celleno and colleagues (83) compared infants whose mothers received a slightly larger induction dose of propofol (2.8 mg/kg) with two other groups. In one group, mothers who delivered abdominally received general anesthesia induced with thiopental 5 mg/kg. The third group consisted of infants born by uncomplicated and unmedicated vaginal delivery. Propofol significantly depressed both 1- and 5-minute Apgar scores (Table 7). Five infants in the propofol group were severely hypotonic at birth, and one was somnolent. The propofol infants had significantly lower ENNS scores at 1 hour but, by 4 hours, their scores were normal (83).

Gregory and colleagues (84) compared a control group (thiopental 4 mg/kg, maintenance with enflurane 1% in 50% nitrous oxide, oxygen) with two different propofol infusion groups (6 mg/kg/hour with nitrous oxide 50% in oxygen and 9 mg/kg/hour with 100% oxygen) for maintenance of anesthesia (following a propofol induction of 2 mg/kg) during cesarean section. They found that the 2-hour NACS scores were poorer in the high-dose infusion group than in the other two groups. The median NACS at 2 hours was highest in the thiopental group [32 vs 31 (low-dose propofol) vs 30 (high-dose propofol)].

Abboud and colleagues (85) compared propofol for induction (1.5 to 2.5 mg/kg) followed by a continuous infusion of propofol at a rate of 0.05 to 0.2 mg/kg/min with induction with thiopental (3 to 4 mg/kg) and maintenance with isoflurane (0.25% to 0.75%). They assessed neonatal status with Apgar scores, umbilical cord acid–base values, and NACS. The authors found no significant differences between the groups with respect to these variables. The mean induction to delivery time was equivalent between groups at 14.5 minutes for propofol and 14.9 minutes for isoflurane. Of interest, the "time to full wakefulness" in the mother tended to be shorter in the isoflurane group (6.9 vs 8.2 minutes in the propofol group) (85).

TABLE 6. *NACS scores in infants whose mothers received 2.5 mg/kg of propofol to induce and either 50% nitrous oxide or a 5 mg/kg/h propofol infusion to maintain anesthesia*[a]

Time	Induction only (n=10)	Induction and maintenance (n=11)
30 min	30% (32–36)	55% (20–37)
2 h	90% (34–38)	100% (35–39)
24 h	100% (38–40)	100% (37–40)

[a]A NACS score of > 35 was considered good (the maximum possible NACS score is 40).

Values indicated are percentages of good scores. NACS ranges are shown in parentheses.

Data from ref. 78.

TABLE 7. *Apgar scores at 1 and 5 minutes after vaginal delivery without anesthesia or cesarean section using either Thiopental (5 mg/kg) or Propofol (2.8 mg/kg)*[a]

Apgar score	Spontaneous delivery (n = 20)	Thiopental, 5 mg/kg (n = 20)	Propofol, 2.5 mg/kg (n = 20)
1 min			
6	0	0	2[b]
7	0	5	8
8	0	6	7
9	20	9	3
10	0	0	0
5 min			
6	0	0	0[b]
7	0	0	1
8	0	3	3
9	0	6	10
10	20	11	6

[a]Scores in the propofol group are significantly different from those of the spontaneous delivery group at 1 ($p < 0.002$) and 5 ($p < 0.02$) minutes.

[b]Scores in the propofol group are significantly different from those of the thiopental group at 1 and 5 minutes ($p < 0.05$).

Data from ref. 83.

Yau and colleagues (86) induced anesthesia in 20 patients with propofol 2 mg/kg, maintained anesthesia with propofol 6 mg/kg/hour, and compared these women to another 20 who received a thiopental 4 mg/kg, enflurane 1% anesthetic. Induction to delivery time for the thiopental group was 12.2 minutes versus 10.8 in the propofol group. The shortest induction to delivery times were in the propofol group (three patients less than 8 minutes) and the longest were in the thiopental group (four patients more than 14 minutes) (Fig. 9). In the propofol group, NACS decreased significantly as the time from induction to delivery time increased. These authors concluded that propofol infusion is a poor choice for maintenance of general anesthesia for cesarean section.

Other concerns about propofol include the possibility of awareness and uterine relaxation. [Propofol inhibits contractility of isolated human uterine muscle at clinically used doses (87).] On balance, there is no compelling reason to routinely use propofol as a induction agent at cesarean delivery.

Benzodiazepines. Diazepam and midazolam are the two most thoroughly studied benzodiazepines. Both drugs are used for maternal sedation and to induce general anesthesia (88,89). The pharmacokinetics of both drugs in pregnancy have been reported (90,91). Both drugs are highly protein bound but readily cross the placenta and induce neonatal effects. Oral administration produces poor sucking, whereas intravenous administration may cause hypotonia and hypothermia (92,93). In addition, their onset is too slow to be useful during a rapid sequence induction of general anesthesia.

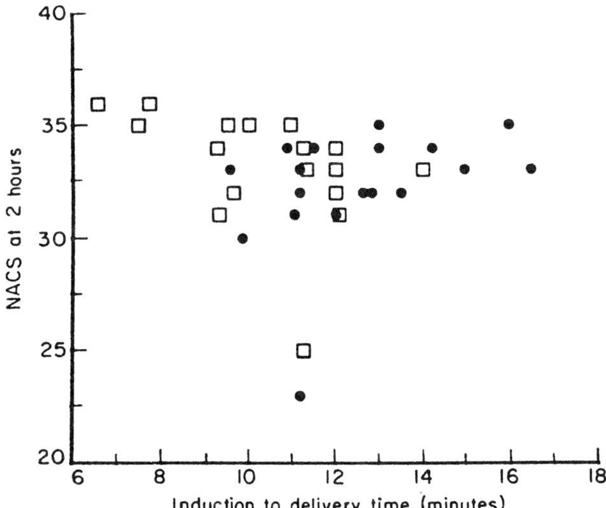

FIG. 9. Induction to delivery time vs NACS scores 2 hours after cesarean delivery with general anesthesia. Mothers received either thiopental 4 mg/kg (•) or propofol 2 mg/kg for induction plus an infusion at 6 mg/kg/hour for maintenance (□). (Reprinted from ref. 86, with permission.)

Diazepam is highly lipid soluble and has a molecular weight of 285. In labor, it can decrease beat-to-beat fetal heart rate variability (94,95). The maximum fetal blood concentration occurs 5 to 10 minutes after maternal administration. Neonatal plasma concentrations are higher than maternal concentrations at birth, possibly reflecting more rapid distribution of the drug in the mother (94).

Midazolam has a shorter half-life and produces less local tissue irritation than diazepam. It is water soluble in its injectable formulation. At physiologic pH, its structure changes and it becomes lipid soluble (96). Midazolam readily crosses the placenta (97) and, like diazepam, can cause neonatal depression. In pregnant sheep, less midazolam than diazepam crosses the placental barrier, producing lower maternal and fetal drug concentrations (98). Ravlo et al. (99) compared midazolam to thiopental for induction of general anesthesia at cesarean section. Midazolam has a slower onset than thiopental (120 vs 111 seconds). The midazolam neonates had lower ENNS scores for body temperature, general body tone, and arm recoil for the first 2 hours of life. Placental transfer was extensive with both drugs. The neonatal elimination half-life of midazolam averages 6.3 hours (Table 5) (100).

In summary, all the intravenous induction agents studied rapidly traverse the placental barrier. As yet, "no drug has been shown to offer sufficient advantages over thiopental in obstetric anaesthesia to warrant its replacement" (101).

Inhalation Agents and Muscle Relaxants

When planning a general anesthetic, the obstetric anesthesiologist hopes to choose drugs that enter the fetal circulation in the smallest possible amounts and are then rapidly eliminated (102). All the inhalational agents freely cross the placental barrier. The UV/MV ratio for nitrous oxide is 0.79 after 10 to 14 minutes. Fetal uptake also occurs rapidly, with a UA/UV ratio of 0.89 after an average of 36 minutes (103). The halogenated agents are highly lipid soluble, un-ionized, and low in molecular weight; thus, they cross the placenta rapidly. The UV/MV ratio for 0.65% halothane is 0.35; for 1% enflurane, it is 0.6 (104,105). A study by Dwyer and colleagues (106) comparing the uptake of halothane and isoflurane during cesarean section found that the uptake of isoflurane (0.44) was more rapid than halothane (0.35). The ratios of umbilical venous partial pressure to maternal arterial partial pressure for the two gases were identical (0.71). Of importance, the authors found that the partial pressure of isoflurane used was equipotent with that found to prevent recall, when combined with 40% nitrous oxide, in volunteers (106). Remember, pregnancy decreases the MAC of isoflurane. At 8 to 12 weeks' gestation, isoflurane MAC is 28% less than isoflurane MAC in nonpregnant women (107). The neonatal neurobehavioral effects of nitrous oxide, enflurane, and isoflurane are insignificant when used for cesarean section anesthesia (108–110). Studies comparing sevoflurane and desflurane to isoflurane found no significant differences among them in terms of maternal and neonatal outcome (111,112).

Muscle relaxants are highly polar compounds that do not cross the placenta easily. In monkeys, succinylcholine transfers rapidly to the fetus. However, the resulting fetal concentration is low (113). Fetal blood concentrations of nondepolarizing muscle relaxants are 5% to 20% of maternal blood concentrations (Table 8) (114–117).

Rocuronium, one of the newer nondepolarizing muscle relaxants, is an alternative to succinylcholine for rapid sequence induction and intubation in the parturient. In parturients, the effect of 0.6 mg/kg rocuronium peaks 98.1 seconds after injection, a time comparable to that in nonpregnant patients (117). Increasing the dose of thiopental from 4 to 6 mg/kg improved the intubating conditions (decreased patient movement and allowed earlier intubation) (117). The times to 50% and 100% neuromuscular block following rocuronium (0.6 mg/kg) were similar with thiopental or ketamine induction (118). However, ketamine allowed easy tracheal intubation at 50% neuromuscular block in all patients compared to only 25% with thiopental (118). In nonpregnant patients, increasing the dose of rocuronium to 0.9 mg/kg (3 × ED_{95}) made the onset equal to that of succinylcholine but increased the duration (119). Postpartum, both vecuronium (120,121) and rocuronium have a prolonged duration (122).

To date, no nondepolarizing muscle relaxant can completely match the onset and rapid recovery of succinylcholine when used for intubation in the pregnant patient.

Local Anesthetics

Local anesthetics are basic drugs that principally bind to α_1-acid glycoprotein. Placental transfer depends on:

- pK_a (pH at which 50% of a drug is ionized),
- Maternal and fetal pH, and
- Extent of protein binding.

Fetal hypoxia and acidosis accentuate the transfer of these weak bases, yielding higher fetal to maternal ratios (Fig. 6B) (36–42). Acidosis also appears to intensify the toxic effects of local anesthetics on the fetus and newborn (123). Neurobehavioral studies show varying results depending on the test used. Any effects are subtle and must be diligently sought.

Bupivacaine. Bupivacaine is more than 80% protein bound. As such, its placental transfer is limited compared with lidocaine (70% protein bound) (124). Mean UV/MV ratio for bupivacaine is approximately 0.3 (125,126). This ratio is similar whether the drug is administered in the epidural or the subarachnoid space (127). Bupivacaine's high lipid solubility encourages rapid uptake by fetal tissues. This property probably explains the increase in the elimination half-life of bupivacaine seen in pregnancy. It is metabolized to the inactive 2,6-pipecolylxylidine. Both bupivacaine and 2,6-pipecolylxylidine can be detected in the newborn urine for at least 36 hours after delivery. A study in sheep suggests that the pharmacokinetics of ropivacaine and bupivacaine are similarly altered by pregnancy (128). The authors suggest that the alterations do not confer a specific advantage of one drug over the other should intravenous injection occur.

In the 1980s, concerns were raised about the safety of bupivacaine following reports of maternal morbidity and mortality after inadvertent intravenous injection of large doses of bupivacaine for epidural anesthesia (129). Animal studies confirmed that bupivacaine had a greater toxicity than lidocaine and that its cardiac effects were of longer duration (130–134). While an early study suggested that the cardiotoxicity of bupivacaine was enhanced by pregnancy (130), a recent study by the same investigators contradicted these findings (135). Inadequate blinding in the initial study may have led the investigators to erroneous conclusions. Downing and colleagues (136) reported that peak bupivacaine maternal arterial concentrations do not approach unsafe levels when bupivacaine is injected into the epidural space for cesarean section.

Lidocaine. Lidocaine is less highly protein bound than bupivacaine, resulting in higher UV/MV ratios (0.57) in vitro (137) and after epidural administration for cesarean section (136,138). Unlike bupivacaine, the route of administration influences the UV/MV ratio of lidocaine. With local perineal infiltration, the ratio is higher (1.32) than after epidural administration (139). Recent studies have not found any adverse neonatal neurobehavioral

TABLE 8. *Placental transfer of nondepolarizing muscle relaxants*

	MV	UV	UV/MV
Atacurium (0.3 mg/kg)[a]	0.7–3.34 µg/mL	ND–0.23 µg/mL	0.05–0.2
Vecuronium (0.04 mg/kg)[b]	162.0–10.0 ng/mL	17.9–2.0 ng/mL	0.11–0.22
Pancuronium(0.04 mg/kg)[b]	115–10.5 ng/mL	21.6–4.0 ng/mL	0.19–0.03
Rocuronium (0.6 mg/kg)[b]	2,412–180 ng/mL	389.6–27.8 ng/mL	0.161

[a]Range; [b]mean ± SE.
ND, not detected.
Data from refs. 114, 115, 117.

effects of lidocaine (140–142). Placental transfer of lidocaine hydrocarbonate is similar to that of lidocaine hydrochloride (143).

2-Chloroprocaine. 2-Chloroprocaine, an ester local anesthetic, is favored by many obstetric anesthesiologists because of its rapid hydrolysis by plasma cholinesterase. Also, its metabolites, 2-chloroamino-benzoic acid and 2-diethylaminoethanol are allegedly inactive. The in vitro half-life of 2-chloroprocaine is measured in seconds. Its in vivo half-life after epidural anesthesia is measured in minutes (144). Because of this rapid clearance from maternal plasma, only small amounts cross the placenta and appear in the fetal circulation (145). In laboring parturients, 2-chloroprocaine has minimal effects on neurobehavioral scores (58). After cesarean section under epidural anesthesia, however, 2-chloroprocaine infants do less well on the BNBAS than bupivacaine infants (146). Although very little 2-chloroprocaine remains in neonatal blood after delivery, significant amounts of metabolites do. These metabolites may induce the neurobehavioral effects seen. When choosing a drug for perineal infiltration, 2-chloroprocaine is a better option than lidocaine because little, if any, pharmacologically active drug reaches the fetus (147).

Ropivacaine. Ropivacaine is an amino amide local anesthetic that is structurally related to mepivacaine and bupivacaine. In contrast to bupivacaine (a racemic mixture of R and S enantiomers), ropivacaine is being marketed as the pure S-enantiomer (148). Placental transfer of ropivacaine is similar to that of bupivacaine (149,150). In studies comparing equal concentrations of bupivacaine and ropivacaine, ropivacaine has a similar duration but it is less cardiotoxic (134,151,152). In clinical trials, it appears equipotent with bupivacaine for labor analgesia (0.25% and 0.2%) (153–157) and cesarean section (0.5%) (150,158–160). Toxicity studies in animals (134) and human volunteers (151,152) report a greater margin of safety when it is injected intravenously. After epidural injection, ropivacaine is cleared from plasma more slowly than bupivacaine (150). As a result, the free concentration of ropivacaine in maternal and umbilical cord plasma is twofold higher than that of a similar dose of bupivacaine (128,150).

The potential advantages of ropivacaine over bupivacaine include less motor block and less urinary retention. In volunteers, recovery from motor block was slower in patients receiving an epidural infusion of bupivacaine than in those receiving ropivacaine (161). Ropivacaine's sensory and motor block tended to be dose dependent (Fig. 10). Caudal spread of analgesia diminished with time in all ropivacaine groups but not with bupivacaine. This property may limit the usefulness of ropivacaine infusions in patients with a long labor.

Levobupivacaine. Levobupivacaine is the pure S-enantiomer of bupivacaine, and early studies indicate that its sensory profile is similar to that of bupivacaine (148). There are no published studies of its use in obstetrics.

Cocaine. Although not generally used as a local anesthetic during pregnancy, the widespread illicit use of this drug mandates its inclusion in this chapter. Similar to other local anesthetics, cocaine rapidly crosses the placenta (162). Its metabolites, norcocaine and cocaethyl-

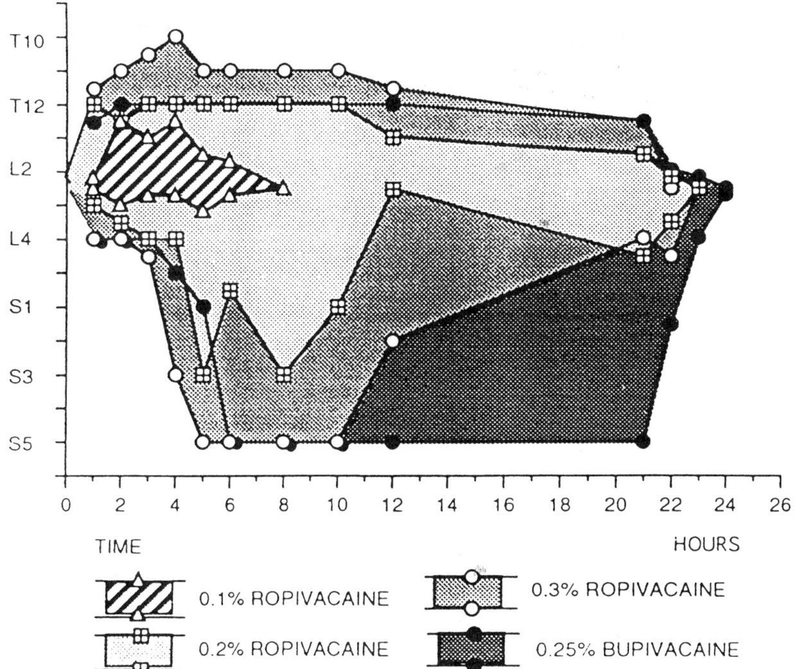

FIG. 10. Spread of sensory analgesia to pinprick with 0.1%, 0.2%, and 0.3% ropivacaine and 0.25% bupivacaine (10-mL bolus followed by 10 mL/hour infusion for 21 hours) in male volunteers. (Reprinted from ref. 161, with permission.)

ene, also are rapidly transferred (162). Using the dually perfused human term placenta model, Malek and colleagues (163) found that cocaine impairs placental permeability and could inhibit the transplacental exchange of nutrients and metabolites. Although controversial (164), this effect might explain fetal growth retardation associated with cocaine exposure.

Opioids

When given to laboring women, all opioids can cause neonatal respiratory depression. The infant is more sensitive than the adult to the central nervous system effects of opioids. Neonates have lower brain myelin content, higher cerebral blood flow, altered protein binding, and different respiratory control mechanisms than adults (44). Although these agents have long been used for labor analgesia, they are not particularly effective and cause marked maternal sedation (165).

Morphine. Many centers have abandoned morphine for labor analgesia because of concerns about neonatal depression. However, morphine is more extensively metabolized in parturients than in nonpregnant patients (166). Peak plasma concentrations occur within 15 minutes of intramuscular administration. Placental transfer is rapid. A pseudo-equilibrium occurs in 5 minutes and the fetal to maternal ratio is close to one (167). These data suggest that the duration of fetal exposure to morphine is short. Perhaps it should be reconsidered as a labor analgesic (147).

Meperidine. Until recently, meperidine was the most widely used opioid for labor analgesia. Meperidine is less likely than morphine to induce neonatal respiratory depression. Meperidine depresses the newborn's respiratory response to carbon dioxide less than morphine (168,169).

Meperidine is very lipid soluble and readily crosses to the fetus. Pregnancy does not alter the maternal pharmacokinetics of meperidine (170,171). Following intravenous injection, it appears in fetal plasma within 2 minutes. Maternal:fetal equilibrium occurs by 6 minutes (172–174). After intramuscular injection, UV/MV ratio rises as the time to delivery increases (175). After 2 to 3 hours, the concentration of meperidine is higher in fetal than in maternal blood (176–178). Larger maternal doses and repeated injections increase the fetal concentration of drug. With multiple doses, a concentration gradient persists between maternal and fetal blood, maximizing fetal exposure (179,180).

The neonate can metabolize meperidine, although not as efficiently as the adult (175). Normeperidine, the principal metabolite of meperidine, can be recovered from neonatal urine for 2 to 6 days after birth (173,178,181, 182). In animals, normeperidine depresses respiration as much as meperidine does (183).

Maternal meperidine exposure also may alter infant behavior. If given shortly before birth (1.5 to 5.3 hours), meperidine may interfere with neonatal breastfeeding (184). In one study of 34 infants whose mothers received meperidine, 15 were still not breastfeeding 2 hours after birth. In contrast, only 1 of 38 infants whose mothers received either no analgesia, epidural analgesia (medication not specified), or nitrous oxide had not breastfed within 2 hours of birth (185).

Like other opioids, meperidine decreases fetal heart rate variability during labor (45,46). Most likely, this effect is secondary to central nervous system depression and does not warrant obstetric intervention. Variability is not affected during stimulating events such as fetal movement or uterine contractions (186).

Meperidine and probably normeperidine cause changes in the neonatal electroencephalogram (187) and neurobehavior (188–190). Even low doses of meperidine (25 mg) depress BNBAS scores (191). Infants exposed to meperidine in utero had more abnormal reflexes and altered regulation of state scores. The longer the drug-to-delivery interval, the greater the impact of meperidine on neurobehavior. Naloxone reverses meperidine-induced respiratory depression (192) but only partly reverses the neurobehavioral changes (193,194). The prolonged half-life and pharmacologic actions of normeperidine in the neonate may explain the neurobehavioral changes seen after maternal meperidine administration (54).

Fentanyl. Fentanyl is more lipophilic and more protein bound (69%) than meperidine. It provides excellent labor analgesia after intravenous, epidural, or subarachnoid administration. After intravenous administration, rapid tissue uptake of fentanyl ensures a short plasma half-life. Fentanyl rapidly crosses the placenta and appears in fetal blood within 1 minute (195). When given intravenously in labor, it provokes a brief decrease in fetal heart rate variability that lasts about 30 minutes (196,197). Pain relief begins within 5 minutes and lasts less than 1 hour. In a nonrandomized, unblinded study of 50 to 600 μg intravenous fentanyl during labor, UV/MV ratios ranged from 0.05 to 0.7 (196). Umbilical venous concentrations correlated linearly with maternal fentanyl dose. Apgar scores, incidence of respiratory depression, and NACS scores did not differ compared to unmedicated control infants (196).

Two cases of patient-controlled intravenous fentanyl for labor pain in women with a platelet abnormality have been reported (198,199). The total dose of fentanyl was 400 μg over 3.5 hours of labor in one (198) and 1,025 μg over nearly 12 hours of labor in the other (199). In the latter case, free fentanyl concentrations (0.16 ng/mL) were identical in the mother and newborn at delivery (199). Neither infant had depressed respiration at birth. However, intravenous fentanyl may still produce significant neonatal respiratory depression. In an unblinded study comparing fentanyl and meperidine for labor analgesia, infants in both groups occasionally needed naloxone to treat respiratory depression (197). In a study comparing the ability of intravenous fentanyl (2.5 μg/kg) and alfentanil (10 μg/kg) to obtund the hypertensive response to intubation, 40 parturients with severe preeclampsia were randomly assigned to receive either drug during induction of general anesthesia for cesarean section (200). The induction to delivery times averaged 13.5 minutes and the uterine incision to delivery times 90 seconds. The majority of neonates in both groups had a prolonged time to sustained ventilation (Fig. 11). The authors did not report the number of infants who required naloxone therapy.

Adding fentanyl to epidural bupivacaine improves and prolongs labor analgesia (201,202). In a small study, Bader et al. (203) examined the effects of a long-term (70 minutes to 15 hours) epidural infusion of bupivacaine and fentanyl 2 μg/mL on the neonate. Apgar scores, neurobehavioral testing, and umbilical artery blood gas values were within normal limits. With time, there was no statistically significant increase in umbilical vein fentanyl concentrations. The UV/MV ratio was 0.94. Adding fentanyl to established epidural lidocaine analgesia produced similar reductions in fetal heart rate variability and fetal heart rate accelerations as epidural saline (204).

When given during epidural anesthesia for cesarean section, fentanyl improves the quality of lidocaine and bupivacaine anesthesia without producing detectable changes in neonatal neurobehavior (205–207). Giving fentanyl directly to the newborn for surgical analgesia may produce prolonged respiratory depression (208). Maternal administration of 100-μg epidural fentanyl during cesarean section produces no changes in neonatal respiratory rate, minute ventilation, or pulmonary compliance immediately after delivery. However, these authors still recommend caution when exposing premature or acidotic fetuses to fentanyl (209).

Sufentanil. Like fentanyl, sufentanil is increasingly used for spinal and epidural labor analgesia. In pregnant sheep, sufentanil 50 μg lacks effects on maternal mean arterial pressure, heart rate, and uterine blood flow; fetal mean arterial pressure and heart rate; and maternal and fetal acid–base status (210). After epidural injection of sufentanil 50 μg, maternal arterial plasma concentration peaked at 0.059 ng/mL at 25 minutes and then declined to 0.039 ng/mL by 2 hours. At no time was sufentanil detected in the fetal plasma. In contrast, with fentanyl, peak maternal concentration occurs at 60 minutes and fetal arterial concentration was 0.02 ng/mL 45 minutes after injection (196).

Others have investigated the placental transfer of sufentanil using the dual-perfused, single cotyledon placental model (43,211). Here, sufentanil crosses the placenta by passive diffusion, but the degree of transfer is affected by maternal protein binding and fetal acidosis. A clinical study by Loftus et al. (212) compared epidural bupivacaine alone or with fentanyl or sufentanil. Fentanyl and sufentanil were administered in a ratio of 5.7:1, but the MV plasma concentrations were 27:1. The UV/MV ratios were 0.37 for fentanyl and 0.81 for sufentanil. Fentanyl was found in most UA samples but sufentanil in only one sample, implying that there was less fetal exposure to sufentanil. The NACS at 24 hours were lower in the bupivacaine-fentanyl group, possibly reflecting residual fentanyl in the neonate (212).

Alfentanil. Alfentanil is a highly protein-bound (88.7%), rapidly acting opioid analgesic with a short elimination half-life. These properties suggest that it may be an ideal labor analgesic. The rapid elimination should guard against long-term effects in the neonate. Unfortunately, animal and human studies have not confirmed these advantages. The pharmacokinetics of alfentanil are similar in pregnant and nonpregnant women (213). After a 30 μg/kg dose, the UV/MV ratio of alfentanil is 0.31. Unbound alfentanil readily crosses the placenta. The fraction of unbound alfentanil is higher in the fetus than in the mother, as the fetus has a lower serum concentration of α_1-acid glycoprotein (the main site of binding of basic drugs like alfentanil) (214). In newborn monkeys, alfentanil produces longer-lasting behavioral effects than does meperidine (214). NACS testing after an epidural infusion of alfentanil for labor analgesia reveals neonatal hypotonia (215).

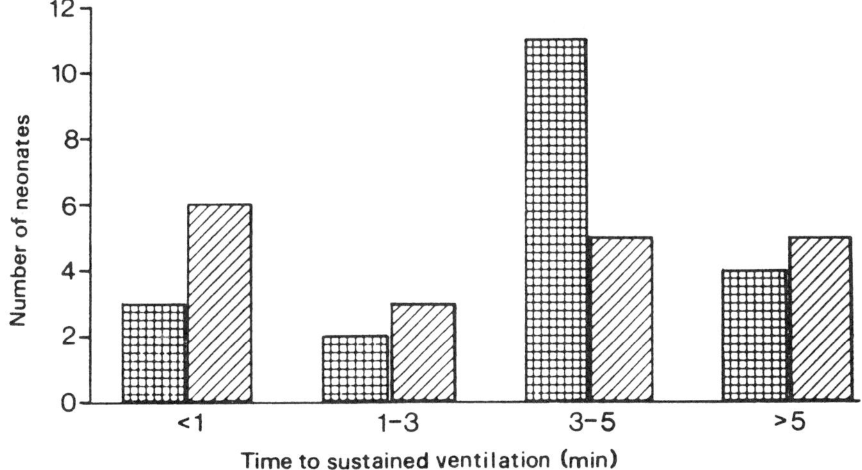

FIG. 11. Time to sustained respiration after intravenous fentanyl (2.5 μg/kg) or alfentanil (10 μg/kg) in 40 parturients with severe preeclampsia. (Reprinted from ref. 200, with permission.)

Butorphanol and Nalbuphine. Narcotic agonist–antagonist drugs often are used for maternal labor analgesia. These drugs may present less risk of respiratory depression than pure agonist agents. Both butorphanol and nalbuphine generate changes that are similar to those induced by meperidine on fetal heart rate pattern, Apgar scores, and neurobehavioral scores (216–219). On the other hand, they cause fewer maternal side effects. A recent report assessed fetal response to vibroacoustic stimulation before and after maternal labor analgesia with 5 mg of nalbuphine (220). This low dose of nalbuphine decreased the number of spontaneous reactive fetal heart rate patterns but did not alter the fetal response to vibroacoustic stimulation, suggesting no serious effect on the fetus.

Epidural butorphanol prolongs the duration of local anesthetics. However, a dose of 3 mg produces maternal sedation and a sinusoidal fetal heart rate pattern (221).

Other Drugs

Anticholinergic Agents. Atropine readily crosses the placenta and produces a fetal tachycardia (222–225). A fetal to maternal ratio of 1.0 is seen 4 hours after injection (222).

Glycopyrrolate, a quaternary ammonium compound, undergoes only limited placental transfer. In sheep, a peak UV/MV ratio of 0.13 arises 4 hours after injection (222). In humans, glycopyrrolate, unlike atropine, produces no change in fetal heart rate (226). A recent case report suggests that this failure to increase fetal heart rate could be detrimental when neostigmine (which readily crosses the placental barrier) is given with glycopyrrolate (227).

Sympathomimetic Agents. Ephedrine crosses the placenta readily, increasing fetal heart rate and beat-to-beat variability (228). Ephedrine has subtle effects on the newborn. Kangas-Saarela et al. (229) compared ephedrine and fluid for prevention of maternal hypotension during spinal anesthesia for cesarean delivery. Neonates in both treatment groups scored similarly on ENNS testing; however, spectral electroencephalogram showed significant differences within the first 2 hours of life (229).

Antihypertensive Agents. Labetalol blocks both α and β adrenoreceptors. It lowers blood pressure mostly through blockade of α adrenoreceptors in peripheral arterioles. Reflex tachycardia does not occur because of labetalol's blockade of β adrenoreceptors. Labetalol is useful in the treatment of preeclampsia and in blunting the hypertensive response to endotracheal intubation (230). Labetalol crosses the placenta with a UV/MV ratio of 0.5 (231). In mature newborns, maternal administration of labetalol produces no clinically significant sympathetic blockade (232).

Esmolol, a water-soluble β_1-adrenoreceptor antagonist, has a rapid onset and a short duration. Its distribution half-life is 2 minutes, and its elimination half-life averages 9 minutes in nonpregnant patients (233). Because of its low lipid solubility and rapid metabolism, placental passage should be minimal. A study of esmolol in pregnant ewes found that the drug rapidly crossed the placenta and quickly left both maternal and fetal circulations (234). Maternal and fetal heart rates decreased during the period of esmolol infusion. A further study by Eisenach and Castro (235) showed dose-dependent β-adrenergic blockade in both ewe and fetus (Fig. 12). With prolonged administration, esmolol decreased fetal heart rate and p_aO_2.

Case reports (236–238) underline potential problems with the use of this drug during pregnancy. In one case, esmolol was used to terminate an episode of supraventricular tachycardia, which was thought to be due to thyrotoxicosis (236). An initial bolus of 0.5 mg/kg was followed by an infusion of 50 μg/kg/min. At first, fetal heart rate was normal. Then it increased by 10 to 15 beats/min. However, fetal bradycardia necessitating cesarean section developed next. The second patient had a history of tachyarrhythmias that recurred during labor (237). Esmolol was used first to terminate the arrhythmia and then continued as a maintenance infusion (total dose: 1,060 mg). At delivery, the infant had decreased muscle tone, weak cry, and became dusky and apneic with feedings. All investigations were normal. By 60 hours of age, muscle tone, cry, and respiratory effort were normal. The authors felt that these symptoms were secondary to β blockade. In the third case (238), esmolol was used to control maternal tachycardia during a craniotomy at 29 weeks' gestation. Both maternal and fetal heart rates decreased but returned to normal once the infusion was terminated. The patient was delivered by cesarean section 12 days later due to late decelerations. The newborn made an uneventful recovery. Until further studies elucidate the safety of this agent for the fetus, I urge using it with caution.

Antiarrhythmics. The antiarrhythmic adenosine is being used increasingly to terminate narrow complex

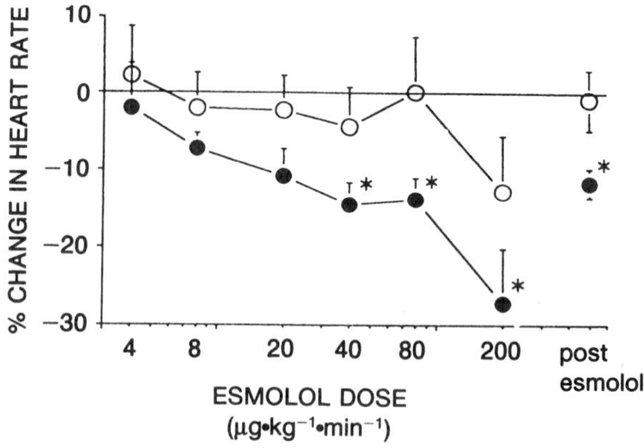

FIG. 12. Resting heart rates in ewes (○) and fetuses (•) at the end of 4, 8, 20, 40, 80, and 200 μg/kg/min maternal esmolol infusions to the ewe and at 30 minutes after stopping maternal esmolol. All values are expressed as mean (± SEM) percent change from baseline. *p <0.005 vs baseline. (Reprinted from ref. 235, with permission.)

tachycardias of supraventricular origin in nonpregnant patients. Although not extensively studied in pregnancy, there is some supportive literature. In pregnant ewes, a bolus injection of adenosine transiently produced a maternal bradycardia followed by tachycardia and decreased diastolic and mean arterial pressures (239). Adenosine altered neither maternal and fetal arterial blood gas tension nor fetal heart rate or arterial pressure. Case reports describing its use in terminating supraventricular tachycardias confirm this lack of effect on the fetal heart rate (240,241).

H_2-Receptor Agonists. The H_2-receptor antagonists, cimetidine and ranitidine, are commonly used to reduce the volume and raise the pH of maternal gastric secretions. Cimetidine has a low lipid solubility and a pK_a of 6.8 and might be expected to have limited placental transfer. However, the UV/MV ratio is 0.84 at 90 to 120 minutes after intravenous injection (242). Peak umbilical venous concentrations occur at 60 minutes. When given orally the night before cesarean section and again intramuscularly 1 to 3 hours before surgery, cimetidine has a UV/MV ratio of 0.6 (243). Evaluation of the fetus using Apgar scores and ENNS testing reveals no significant differences compared to a group that did not receive cimetidine. Rapid renal excretion plays a role in elimination from the fetus (242).

Magee and colleagues (244) prospectively examined pregnancy outcome in 178 women receiving H_2-receptor blockers during the first trimester of pregnancy matched with 178 controls. The frequency of major malformations did not increase, suggesting that H_2-receptor blockers have no major teratogenic effects.

Metoclopramide. Metoclopramide has a low molecular weight and high lipid solubility. Animal studies show rapid placental transfer (less than 1 minute after intravenous injection) (245). The mean fetal to maternal ratio is 0.6 in humans (246). Examination of the neonate using Apgar scores and NACS did not detect any observable effects.

CONCLUSION

All drugs administered to the mother cross the placenta into the fetal circulation. The extent to which passage occurs depends on the maternal:fetal concentration gradient, the lipid solubility of the drug, the amount of un-ionized drug, and the degree of protein binding. Effects on the fetus depend on the concentration of free drug present in the fetus and can only be measured indirectly. Current methods of testing the newborn (neonatal neurobehavior scores, Apgar scores, acid–base status) may not detect subtle changes. When drug effects are detected, it is difficult to assess their long-term importance.

REFERENCES

1. Morriss FH, Boyd RDH, Mahendran D. Placental transport. In: Knobil E, Neill JD, eds. *The physiology of reproduction,* vol. 2, 2nd ed. New York: Raven Press, 1994;813.
2. Beal RW. Non-rhesus (D) blood group isoimmunization in obstetrics. *Clin Obstet Gynaecol* 1979;6:493.
3. Cohen F, Zuelzer WW. The transplacental passage of maternal erythrocytes into the fetus. *Am J Obstet Gynecol* 1965;93:566.
4. Ramsey EM. Circulation in the intervillous space of the primate placenta. *Am J Obstet Gynecol* 1962;84:1649.
5. Ramsey EM. What we have learned about placental circulation. *J Reprod Med* 1985;30:312.
6. Greiss FC. A clinical concept of uterine blood flow during pregnancy. *Obstet Gynecol* 1967;30:595.
7. Borell U, Fernstrom I, Ohlson L, Wiqvist N. Influence of uterine contractions on the uteroplacental blood flow at term. *Am J Obstet Gynecol* 1965;93:44.
8. Chard T. Placental synthesis. *Clin Obstet Gynaecol* 1986;12:447.
9. Redman CWG. Immunology of the placenta. *Clin Obstet Gynaecol* 1986;13:469.
10. Faber JJ. Review of flow limited transfer in the placenta. *Int J Obstet Anesth* 1995;4:230.
11. Miller RK, Berndt WD. Mechanisms of transport across the placenta: an in vitro approach. *Life Sci* 1974;16:7.
12. Johnson PM, Brown PJ. Review article: Fcγ receptors in the human placenta. *Placenta* 1981;2:355.
13. Hill EP, Power GG, Longo LD. A mathematical model of carbon dioxide transfer in the placenta and its interaction with oxygen. *Am J Physiol* 1973;224:283.
14. Wilkening RB, Meschia G. Fetal oxygen uptake, oxygenation, and acid-base balance as a function of uterine blood flow. *Am J Physiol* 1983;244:H749.
15. Longo LD, Hill EP, Power GG. Theoretical analysis of factors affecting placenta O_2 transfer. *Am J Physiol* 1972;222:730.
16. Itskovitz J, Goetzman WS, Roman C, Rudolph AM. Effects of fetal-maternal exchange transfusion on fetal oxygenation and blood flow distribution. *Am J Physiol* 1984;247:H655.
17. Cunningham FG, MacDonald PC, Gant NF, et al. The morphological and functional development of the fetus. In: Cunningham FG, Gant NF, MacDonald PC, et al., eds. *Williams obstetrics*, 20th ed. Stamford: Appleton & Lange, 1997:151.
18. Krauer B, Krauer F. Drug kinetics in pregnancy. *Clin Pharmacokinet* 1977;2:167.
19. Cohen SE. Physiological alterations of pregnancy. *Clin Anaesthesiol* 1986;4:33.
20. Wald A, Van Thiel DH, Hoechstetter L, et al. Effect of pregnancy on gastrointestinal transit. *Dig Dis Sci* 1982;27:1015.
21. Christofides ND, Ghatei MA, Bloom SR, Borberg C, Gillmer MDG. Decreased plasma motilin concentrations in pregnancy. *Br Med J* 1982;285:1453.
22. Nimmo WS, Wilson J, Prescott LF. Narcotic analgesics and delayed gastric emptying during labour. *Lancet* 1975;1:890.
23. Whitehead EM, Smith M, Dean Y, O'Sullivan G. An evaluation of gastric emptying times in pregnancy and the puerperium. *Anaesthesia* 1993;48:53.
24. Palahniuk RJ, Shnider SM, Eger EI II. Pregnancy decreases the requirement for inhaled anesthetic agents. *Anesthesiology* 1974;41:82.
25. Datta S, Lambert DH, Gregus J, Gissen AJ, Covino BG. Differential sensitivitics of mammalian nerve fibers during pregnancy. *Anesth Analg* 1983;62:1070.
26. Butterworth JF IV, Walker FO, Lysak SZ. Pregnancy increases median nerve susceptibility to lidocaine. *Anesthesiology* 1990;72:962.
27. Hytten FE, Thomson AM, Taggart N. Total body water in normal pregnancy. *J Obstet Gynaecol Br Commonw* 1966;73:553.
28. Krauer B, Dayer P, Anner R. Changes in serum albumin and α_1 acid glycoprotein concentrations during pregnancy: an analysis of fetal-maternal pairs. *Br J Obstet Gynaecol* 1984;91:875.
29. Reynolds F, Knott C. Pharmacokinetics in pregnancy and placental drug transfer. *Oxf Rev Reprod Biol* 1989;11:389.
30. Dancis J, Liebes L. Drug delivery during pregnancy: evaluation in vitro of new drugs. *Reprod Fertil Dev* 1995;7:1485.
31. Bourget P, Roulot C, Fernandez H. Models for placental transfer studies of drugs. *Clin Pharmacokinet* 1995;28:161.
32. Kennedy RL, Bell JU, Miller RP, et al. Uptake and distribution of lidocaine in fetal lambs. *Anesthesiology* 1990;72:483.
33. Hanshaw-Thomas A, Reynolds F. Placental transfer of bupivacaine, pethidine and lignocaine in the rabbit: effect of umbilical flow rate and protein content. *Br J Obstet Gynaecol* 1985;92:706.
34. Hanshaw-Thomas A, Rogerson N, Reynolds F. Transfer of bupiva-

caine, lignocaine and pethidine across the rabbit placenta: influence of maternal protein binding and fetal flow. *Placenta* 1984;5:61.
35. Finster M, Morishima HO, Boyes RN, Covino BG. The placental transfer of lidocaine and its uptake by fetal tissues. *Anesthesiology* 1972;36:159.
36. Datta S, Brown WU, Ostheimer GW, Weiss JB, Alper MH. Epidural anesthesia for cesarean section in diabetic parturients: maternal and neonatal acid-base status and bupivacaine concentrations. *Anesth Analg* 1981;60:574.
37. Gaylard DG, Carson RJ, Reynolds F. Effect of umbilical perfusate pH and controlled maternal hypotension on placental drug transfer in the rabbit. *Anesth Analg* 1990;71:42.
38. Kennedy RL, Erenberg A, Robillard JE, Merkow A, Turner T. Effects of changes in maternal-fetal pH on the transplacental equilibrium of bupivacaine. *Anesthesiology* 1979;51:50.
39. Brown WU, Bell GC, Alper MH. Acidosis, local anesthetics and the newborn. *Obstet Gynecol* 1976;48:27.
40. Biehl D, Shnider SM, Levinson G, Callender K. Placental transfer of lidocaine: effects of fetal acidosis. *Anesthesiology* 1978;48:409.
41. Johnson RF, Herman NL, Johnson HV, Arney TL, Paschall RL, Downing JW. Effects of fetal pH on local anesthetic transfer across the human placenta. *Anesthesiology* 1996;85:608.
42. Johnson RF, Herman NL, Johnson HV, et al. Bupivacaine transfer across the human term placenta. A study using the dual perfused human placental model. *Anesthesiology* 1995;82:459.
43. Johnson RF, Herman N, Arney TL, Johnson HV, Paschall RL, Downing JW. The placental transfer of sufentanil: effects of fetal pH, protein binding, and sufentanil concentration. *Anesth Analg* 1997;84:1262.
44. Morselli PL, Franco-Morselli R, Bossi L. Clinical pharmacokinetics in newborns and infants, age-related-differences and therapeutic implications. *Clin Pharmacokinet* 1980;5:485.
45. Petrie RH, Yeh S, Murata Y, et al. The effect of drugs on fetal heart rate variability. *Am J Obstet Gynecol* 1978;130:294.
46. Petrie RH. Dose/response effects of intravenous meperidine on fetal heart rate variability. *J Matern Fetal Med* 1993;2:215.
47. Jouppila R, Jouppila P, Kuikka J, Hollmen A. Placental blood flow during Caesarean section under lumbar extradural analgesia. *Br J Anaesth* 1978;50:275.
48. Skjoldebrand A, Eklund J, Lunnell NO, Nylund L, Sarby B, Thornstrom S. The effect on uteroplacental blood flow of epidural anaesthesia containing adrenaline for caesarean section. *Acta Anaesthesiol Scand* 1990;34:85.
49. Baumann H, Alon E, Atanassoff P, Pasch T, Huch A, Huch R. Effect of epidural anesthesia for cesarean delivery on maternal femoral arterial and venous, uteroplacental, and umbilical blood flow velocities and wave-forms. *Obstet Gynecol* 1990;75:194.
50. Lindblad A, Bernow J, Vernersson E, Marsal K. Effects of extradural anaesthesia on human fetal blood flow in utero: comparison of three local anaesthetic solutions. *Br J Anaesth* 1987;59:1265.
51. Brown CEL, Christmas JT, Bawdon RE. Placental transfer of cefazolin and piperacillin in pregnancies remote from term complicated by Rh-isoimmunization. *Am J Obstet Gynecol* 1990;163:938.
52. Moise KJ Jr, Ou C-N, Kirshon B, Cano LE, Rognerud C, Carpenter RJ Jr. Placental transfer of indomethacin in the human pregnancy. *Am J Obstet Gynecol* 1990;162:549.
53. Pons JC, Taburet AM, Singlas E, Delfraissy JF, Papiernik E. Placental passage of azathiothymidine (AZT) during the second trimester of pregnancy: study by direct fetal blood sampling under ultrasound. *Eur J Obstet Gynecol Reprod Biol* 1991;40:229.
54. Kuhnert BR, Linn PL, Kuhnert PM. Obstetric medication and neonatal behavior: current controversies. *Clin Perinatol* 1985;12:423.
55. Brazelton TB. *Neonatal behavioral assessment scale,* 2nd ed. Philadelphia: JB Lippincott, 1984.
56. Scanlon JW, Brown WU, Weiss JB, Alper MH. Neurobehavioral responses of newborn infants after maternal epidural anesthesia. *Anesthesiology* 1974;40:121.
57. Amiel-Tison C, Barrier G, Shnider SM, Levinson G, Hughes SC, Stefani SJ. A new neurologic and adaptive capacity scoring system for evaluating obstetric medications in full-term newborns. *Anesthesiology* 1982;56:340.
58. Kuhnert BR, Harrison MJ, Linn PL, Kuhnert PM. Effects of maternal epidural anesthesia on neonatal behavior. *Anesth Analg* 1984;63:301.
59. Golub MS. Labor analgesia and infant brain development. *Pharmacol Biochem Behavior* 1996;55:619.
60. Jacobson B, Nyberg K, Eklund G, Bygdeman M, Rydberg U. Obstetric pain medication and eventual adult amphetamine addiction in offspring. *Acta Obstet Gynecol Scand* 1988;67:677.
61. Nyberg K, Allebek P, Eklund G, Jacobson B. Obstetric medication versus residential area as perinatal risk factors for subsequent drug addiction in offspring. *Paediatr Perinat Epidemiol* 1993;7:23.
62. McKechnie FB, Converse JG. Placental transmission of thiopental. *Am J Obstet Gynecol* 1955;70:639.
63. Morgan DJ, Blackman GL, Paull JD, Wolf LJ. Pharmacokinetics and plasma binding of thiopental. II: studies at cesarean section. *Anesthesiology* 1981;54:474.
64. Gin, T, Mainland P, Chan MTV, Short TG. Decreased thiopental requirements in early pregnancy. *Anesthesiology* 1997;86:73.
65. Schepens P, Heyndrickx A. Placental transfer of thiopental. *Eur J Toxicol* 1975;8:87.
66. Kosaka Y, Takahashi T, Mark LC. Intravenous thiobarbiturate anesthesia for cesarean section. *Anesthesiology* 1969;31:489.
67. Finster M, Morishima HO, Mark LC, Perel JM, Dayton PG, James LS. Tissue thiopental concentrations in the fetus and newborn. *Anesthesiology* 1972;36:155.
68. Schultetus RR, Hill CR, Dharamraj CM, Banner TE, Berman LS. Wakefulness during cesarean section after anesthetic induction with ketamine, thiopental, or ketamine and thiopental combined. *Anesth Analg* 1986;65:723.
69. Baraka A, Louis F, Noueihid R, Diab M, Dabbous A, Sibai A. Awareness following different techniques of general anaesthesia for caesarean section. *Br J Anaesth* 1989;62:645.
70. Baraka A, Louis F, Dalleh R. Maternal awareness and neonatal outcome after ketamine induction of anaesthesia for Caesarean section. *Can J Anaesth* 1990;37:641.
71. Meer FM, Downing JW, Coleman AG. An intravenous method of anaesthesia for caesarean section. Part II: ketamine. *Br J Anaesth* 1973;45:191.
72. Pelz B, Sinclair DM. Induction agents for caesarean section: a comparison of thiopentone and ketamine. *Anaesthesia* 1973;28:37.
73. Ellingson A, Haram K, Sagen N, Solheim E. Transplacental passage of ketamine after intravenous administration. *Acta Anaesthesiol Scand* 1977;21:41.
74. Little B, Chang T, Chucot L, et al. Study of ketamine as an obstetric anesthetic agent. *Am J Obstet Gynecol* 1972;113:247.
75. Hodgkinson R, Marx GF, Kim SS, Miclat NM. Neonatal neurobehavioral tests following vaginal delivery under ketamine, thiopental, and extradural anesthesia. *Anesth Analg* 1977;56:548.
76. Gin T, Gregory MA, Oh TE. The haemodynamic effects of propofol and thiopentone for induction of caesarean section. *Anaesth Intensive Care* 1990;18:175.
77. Gin T, O'Meara ME, Kan AF, Leung RKW, Tan P, Yau G. Plasma catecholamines and neonatal condition after induction of anaesthesia with propofol or thiopentone at caesarean section. *Br J Anaesth* 1993;70:311.
78. Dailland P, Cockshott ID, Lirzin JD, et al. Intravenous propofol during cesarean section: Placental transfer, concentrations in breastmilk, and neonatal effects: A preliminary study. *Anesthesiology* 1989;71:827.
79. Alon E, Ball RH, Gillie MH, Parer JT, Rosen MA, Shnider SM. Effects of propofol and thiopental on maternal and fetal cardiovascular and acid-base variables in the pregnant ewe. *Anesthesiology* 1993; 78:562.
80. Moore J, Bill KM, Flynn RJ, McKeating KT, Howard PJ. A comparison between propofol and thiopentone as induction agents in obstetric anaesthesia. *Anaesthesia* 1989;44:753.
81. Valtonen M, Kanto J, Rosenberg P. Comparison of propofol and thiopentone for induction of anaesthesia for elective caesarean section. *Anaesthesia* 1989;44:758.
82. Gin T, Gregory MA, Oh TE. Maternal and fetal levels of propofol at caesarean section. *Anaesth Intensive Care* 1990;18:180.
83. Celleno D, Capogna G, Tomassetti AM, Costantino P, Di Feo G, Nisini R. Neurobehavioural effects of propofol on the neonate following elective caesarean section. *Br J Anaesth* 1989;62:649.
84. Gregory MA, Gin T, Yau G, Leung RKW, Chan K, Oh TE. Propofol infusion anaesthesia for caesarean section. *Can J Anaesth* 1990; 37:514.
85. Abboud TK, Zhu J, Richardson M, Peres Da Silva E, Donovan M. Intravenous propofol vs thiamylal-isoflurane for caesarean section: comparative maternal and neonatal effects. *Acta Anaesthesiol Scand* 1995;39:205.

86. Yau G, Gin T, Ewart MC, Kotur CF, Leung RKW, Oh TE. Propofol for induction and maintenance of anaesthesia at caesarean section. *Anaesthesia* 1991;46:20.
87. Shin Y, Kim Y, Collea J. Relaxant effects of propofol on contractility in isolated human pregnancy uterine muscle. *Anesthesiology* 1997; 87:A921.
88. Haram K, Lund T, Sagen N, Boe OE. Comparison of thiopentone and diazepam as induction agents of anaesthesia for caesarean section. *Acta Anaesthesiol Scand* 1981;25:470.
89. Crawford ME, Carl P, Bach V, Ravlo O, Mikkelsen BO, Werner M. A randomized comparison between midazolam and thiopental for elective cesarean section anesthesia. I. Mothers. *Anesth Analg* 1989; 68:229.
90. Gamble JAS, Moore J, Lamki H, Howard PJ. A study of plasma diazepam levels in mother and infants. *Br J Obstet Gynaecol* 1977; 84:588.
91. Wilson CM, Dundee JW, Moore J, Howard PJ, Collier PS. A comparison of the early pharmacokinetics of midazolam in pregnant and nonpregnant women. *Anaesthesia* 1987;42:1057.
92. Cree JE, Meyer J, Hailey DM. Diazepam in labour: its metabolism and effect on the clinical condition and thermogenesis of the newborn. *Br Med J* 1973;4:251.
93. Owen JR, Irani SF, Blair AW. Effect of diazepam administered to mothers during labour on temperature regulation of neonate. *Arch Dis Child* 1972;47:107.
94. Scher J, Hailey DM, Beard RW. The effects of diazepam on the fetus. *J Obstet Gynaecol Br Commonw* 1972;79:635.
95. Yeh SY, Paul RH, Cordero L, Hon EH. A study of diazepam during labor. *Obstet Gynecol* 1974;43:363.
96. Greenblatt DJ, Arendt RM, Abernethy DR, Giles HG, Sellers EM, Shader RI. In vitro quantitation of benzodiazepine lipophilicity: relation to in vivo distribution. *Br J Anaesth* 1983;55:985.
97. Vree TB, Reekers-Ketting JJ, Fragen RJ, Arts THM. Placental transfer of midazolam and its metabolite 1-hydroxymethylmidazolam in the pregnant ewe. *Anesth Analg* 1984;63:31.
98. Conklin KA, Graham CW, Murad S, et al. Midazolam and diazepam: maternal and fetal effects in the pregnant ewe. *Obstet Gynecol* 1980; 56:471.
99. Ravlo O, Carl P, Crawford ME, Bach V, Mikkelsen BO, Nielson HK. A randomized comparison between midazolam and thiopental for elective cesarean section anesthesia. II. Neonates. *Anesth Analg* 1989;68:234.
100. Bach V, Carl P, Ravlo O, et al. A randomized comparison between midazolam and thiopental for elective cesarean section anesthesia. III: Placental transfer and elimination in neonates. *Anesth Analg* 1989; 68:238.
101. Holdcroft A, Morgan M. Intravenous induction agents for caesarean section [Editorial]. *Anaesthesia* 1989;44:719.
102. Gin T. Pharmacokinetic optimisation of general anaesthesia in pregnancy. *Clin Pharmacokinet* 1993;25:59.
103. Marx GF, Joshi CW, Orkin LR. Placental transmission of nitrous oxide. *Anesthesiology* 1970;32:429.
104. Latto IP, Waldron BA. Anaesthesia for caesarean section: analysis of blood concentrations of halothane using 0.2% or 0.65% halothane with 50% nitrous oxide in oxygen. *Br J Anaesth* 1977;49:371.
105. Coleman AJ, Downing JW. Enflurane anesthesia for cesarean section. *Anesthesiology* 1975;43:354.
106. Dwyer R, Fee JPH, Moore J. Uptake of halothane and isoflurane by mother and baby during caesarean section. *Br J Anaesth* 1995;74:379.
107. Gin T, Chan MTV. Decreased minimum alveolar concentration of isoflurane in pregnant humans. *Anesthesiology* 1994;81:829.
108. Stefani SJ, Hughes SC, Shnider SM, et al. Neonatal neurobehavioral effects of inhalation analgesia for vaginal delivery. *Anesthesiology* 1982;56:351.
109. Palahniuk RJ, Scatliff J, Biehl D, Wiebe H, Sankaran K. Maternal and neonatal effects of methoxyflurane, nitrous oxide and lumbar epidural anaesthesia for caesarean section. *Can Anaesth Soc J* 1977;24:586.
110. Warren RM, Datta S, Ostheimer GW, Naulty JS, Weiss JB, Morrison JA. Comparison of the maternal and neonatal effects of halothane, enflurane, and isoflurane for cesarean delivery. *Anesth Analg* 1983; 62:516.
111. Gambling DR, Sharma SK, White PF, Van Beveren T, Bala AS, Gouldson R. Use of sevoflurane during elective cesarean birth: a comparison with isoflurane and spinal anesthesia. *Anesth Analg* 1995;81:90.
112. Wallace DH, Armstrong A, Darras A, Gajraj N, Gambling D, White P. The effect of desflurane or low-dose enflurane on uterine tone at cesarean delivery: placental transfer and recovery. *Anesthesiology* 1993;79:A1019.
113. Drabkova J, Crul JF, Van der Kleijn E. Placental transfer of ^{14}C labeled succinylcholine in near-term macaca mulatta monkeys. *Br J Anaesth* 1973;45:1087.
114. Frank M, Flynn PJ, Hughes R. Atracurium in obstetric anaesthesia. *Br J Anaesth* 1983;55:113S.
115. Dailey PA, Fisher DM, Shnider SM, et al. Pharmacokinetics, placental transfer, and neonatal effects of vecuronium and pancuronium administered during cesarean section. *Anesthesiology* 1984;60:569.
116. Duvaldestin P, Demetriou M, Henzel D, Desmonts JM. The placental transfer of pancuronium and its pharmacokinetics during caesarean section. *Acta Anaesthesiol Scand* 1978;22:327.
117. Abouleish E, Abboud T, Lechevalier T, Zhu J, Chalian A, Alford K. Rocuronium (Org 9426) for cesarean section. *Br J Anaesth* 1994; 73:336.
118. Baraka AS, Sayyid SS, Assaf BA. Thiopental-rocuronium versus ketamine-rocuronium for rapid-sequence intubation in parturients undergoing cesarean section. *Anesth Analg* 1997;84:1104.
119. Magorian T, Flannery KB, Miller RD. Comparison of rocuronium, succinylcholine and vecuronium for rapid-sequence induction of anesthesia in adult patients. *Anesthesiology* 1993;79:913.
120. Camp C, Tessam J, Adenqala J, Joyce TH. Vecuronium and prolonged neuromuscular blockade in postpartum patients. *Anesthesiology* 1987; 67:1006.
121. Khuenl-Brady KS, Koller J, Mair P, Puhringer F, Mitterschiffthaler GI. Comparison of vecuronium- and atracurium-induced neuromuscular blockade in postpartum and nonpregnant patients. *Anesth Analg* 1991; 72:110.
122. Pühringer FK, Sparr HJ, Mitterschiffthaler G, Agoston S, Benzer A. Extended duration of action of rocuronium in postpartum patients. *Anesth Analg* 1997;84:352.
123. Morishima HO, Heyman MA, Rudolph AM, Barrett CT. Toxicity of lidocaine in the fetal and newborn lamb and its relationship to asphyxia. *Am J Obstet Gynecol* 1972;112:72.
124. Tucker GT, Boyes RN, Bridenbaugh PO, Moore DC. Binding of anilide-type local anesthetics in plasma. II. Implications in vivo, with special reference to transplacental distribution. *Anesthesiology* 1970;33:304.
125. McGuinness GA, Merkow AJ, Kennedy RL, Erenberg A. Epidural anesthesia with bupivacaine for cesarean section: neonatal blood levels and neurobehavioral responses. *Anesthesiology* 1978;49:270.
126. Scanlon JW, Ostheimer GW, Lurie AO, Brown WU, Weiss JB, Alper MH. Neurobehavioral responses and drug concentrations in newborns after maternal epidural anesthesia with bupivacaine. *Anesthesiology* 1976;45:400.
127. Kuhnert BR, Zuspan KJ, Kuhnert PM, Syracuse CD, Brown DE. Bupivacaine disposition in mother, fetus, and neonate after spinal anesthesia for cesarean section. *Anesth Analg* 1987;66:407.
128. Santos AC, Arthur GR, Lehning EJ, Finster M. Comparative pharmacokinetics of ropivacaine and bupivacaine in nonpregnant and pregnant ewes. *Anesth Analg* 1997;85:87.
129. Albright GA. Cardiac arrest following regional anesthesia with etidocaine or bupivacaine. *Anesthesiology* 1979;51:285.
130. Morishima HO, Pedersen H, Finster M, et al. Bupivacaine toxicity in pregnant and nonpregnant ewes. *Anesthesiology* 1985;63:134.
131. Kotelko DM, Shnider SM, Dailey PA, et al. Bupivacaine-induced cardiac arrhythmias in sheep. *Anesthesiology* 1984;60:10.
132. Liu P, Feldman HS, Covino BM, Giasi R, Covino BG. Acute cardiovascular toxicity of intravenous amide local anesthetics in anesthetized ventilated dogs. *Anesth Analg* 1982;61:317.
133. de Jong RH, Ronfeld RA, DeRosa RA. Cardiovascular effects of convulsant and supraconvulsant doses of amide local anesthetics. *Anesth Analg* 1982;61:3.
134. Rutten AJ, Nancarrow C, Mather LE, Ilsley AH, Runciman WB, Upton RN. Hemodynamic and central nervous system effects of intravenous bolus doses of lidocaine, bupivacaine, and ropivacaine in sheep. *Anesth Analg* 1989;69:291.
135. Santos AC, Arthur GR, Wlody D, De Armas P, Morishima HO, Finster M. Comparative systemic toxicity of ropivacaine and bupivacaine in nonpregnant and pregnant ewes. *Anesthesiology* 1995;82:734.
136. Downing JW, Johnson HV, Gonzalez HF, Arney TL, Herman NL, Johnson RF. The pharmacokinetics of epidural lidocaine and bupivacaine during cesarean section. *Anesth Analg* 1997;84:527.

137. Ala-Kokko TI, Pienimäki P, Herva R, Hollmén AI, Pelkonen O, Vähäkangas K. Transfer of lidocaine and bupivacaine across the isolated perfused human placenta. *Pharmacol Toxicol* 1995;77:142.
138. Ralston DH, Shnider SM. The fetal and neonatal effects of regional anesthesia in obstetrics. *Anesthesiology* 1978;48:34.
139. Philipson EH, Kuhnert BR, Syracuse CD. Maternal, fetal and neonatal lidocaine levels following local perineal infiltration. *Am J Obstet Gynecol* 1984;149:403.
140. Abboud TK, Kim KC, Noueihed R, et al. Epidural bupivacaine, chloroprocaine, or lidocaine for cesarean section: maternal and neonatal effects. *Anesth Analg* 1983;62:914.
141. Abboud TK, Sarkis F, Blikian A, Varakian L, Earl S, Henriksen E. Lack of adverse neonatal neuro-behavioral effects of lidocaine. *Anesth Analg* 1983;62:473.
142. Kileff ME, James FM, Dewan DM, Floyd HM. Neonatal neurobehavioral responses after epidural anesthesia for cesarean section using lidocaine and bupivacaine. *Anesth Analg* 1984;63:413.
143. Guay J, Gaudreault P, Boulanger A, Tang A, Lortie L, Dupuis C. Lidocaine hydrocarbonate and lidocaine hydrochloride for cesarean section: transplacental passage and neonatal effects. *Acta Anaesthesiol Scand* 1992;36:722.
144. Kuhnert BR, Kuhnert PM, Philipson EH, Syracuse CD, Kaine CJ, Changhyon Y. The half-life of 2-chloroprocaine. *Anesth Analg* 1986; 65:273.
145. Kuhnert BR, Kuhnert PM, Prochaska AL, Gross TL. Plasma levels of 2-chloroprocaine in obstetric patients and their neonates after epidural anesthesia. *Anesthesiology* 1980;53:21.
146. Kuhnert BR, Kennard MJ, Linn PL. Neonatal neurobehavior after epidural anesthesia for cesarean section: a comparison of bupivacaine and chloroprocaine. *Anesth Analg* 1988;67:64.
147. Philipson EH, Kuhnert BR, Syracuse CD. 2-Chloroprocaine for local perineal infiltration. *Am J Obstet Gynecol* 1987;157:1275.
148. Reynolds F. Does the left hand know what the right hand is doing? An appraisal of single enantiomer local anaesthetics. *Int J Obstet Anesth* 1997;6:257.
149. Minzter BH, Johnson RF, Arney TL, et al. A comparison of the placental transfer of ropivacaine versus bupivacaine. *Anesthesiology* 1997;87:A878.
150. Ala-Kokko TI, Alahuhta S, Jouppila P, Korpi K, Westerling P, Vähäkangas K. Feto-maternal distribution of ropivacaine and bupivacaine after epidural administration for cesarean section. *Int J Obstet Anesth* 1997;6:145.
151. Scott DB, Lee A, Fagan D, Bowler GMR, Bloomfield P, Lundh R. Acute toxicity of ropivacaine compared with that of bupivacaine. *Anesth Analg* 1989;69:563.
152. Knudsen K, Beckman Suurküla M, Blomberg S, Sjövall J, Edvardsson N. Central nervous and cardiovascular effects of i.v. infusions of ropivacaine, bupivacaine and placebo in volunteers. *Br J Anaesth* 1997; 78:507.
153. Benhamou D, Hamza J, Eledjam JJ, et al. Continuous extradural infusion of ropivacaine 2mg ml^{-1} for pain relief during labour. *Br J Anaesth* 1997;78:748.
154. Eddleston JM, Holland JJ, Griffin RP, Corbett A, Horsman EL, Reynolds F. A double-blind comparison of 0.25% ropivacaine and 0.25% bupivacaine for extradural analgesia in labour. *Br J Anaesth* 1996;76:66.
155. Stienstra R, Jonker TA, Bourdrez P, Kuijpers JC, van Kleef JW, Lundberg U. Ropivacaine 0.25% versus bupivacaine 0.25% for continuous epidural analgesia in labor: a double-blind comparison. *Anesth Analg* 1995;80:285.
156. McCrae AF, Jozwiak H, McClure JH. Comparison of ropivacaine and bupivacaine in extradural analgesia for the relief of pain in labour. *Br J Anaesth* 1995;74:261.
157. Muir HA, Writer D, Douglas J, Weeks S, Gambling D, Macarthur A. A double-blind comparison of epidural ropivacaine 0.25% and bupivacaine 0.25% for the relief of childbirth pain. *Can J Anaesth* 1997; 44:599.
158. Datta S, Camann W, Bader A, VanderBurgh L. Clinical effects and maternal and fetal plasma concentrations of epidural ropivacaine versus bupivacaine for cesarean section. *Anesthesiology* 1995;82:1346.
159. Griffin RP, Reynolds F. Extradural anaesthesia for caesarean section: a double-blind comparison of 0.5% ropivacaine with 0.5% bupivacaine. *Br J Anaesth* 1995;74:512.
160. Alahuhta S, Räsänen J, Jouppila P, et al. The effects of epidural ropivacaine and bupivacaine for cesarean section on uteroplacental and fetal circulation. *Anesthesiology* 1995;83:23.
161. Zaric D, Nydahl P-A, Philipson L, Samuelsson L, Heierson A, Axelsson K. The effect of continuous lumbar epidural infusion of ropivacaine (0.1%, 0.2%, and 0.3%) and 0.25% bupivacaine on sensory and motor block in volunteers. A double-blind study. *Reg Anesth* 1996;21:14.
162. Schenker S, Yang Y, Johnson RF, et al. The transfer of cocaine and its metabolites across the term human placenta. *Clin Pharmacol Ther* 1993;53:329.
163. Malek A, Ivy D, Blann E, Mattison DR. Impact of cocaine on human placental function using an in vitro perfusion system. *J Pharmacol Toxicol Methods* 1995;33:213.
164. Graham K, Feigenbaum A, Pastuszak, et al. Pregnancy outcome and infant development following gestational cocaine use by social cocaine users in Toronto, Canada. *Clin Invest Med* 1992;15:384.
165. Olofsson Ch, Ekblom A, Ekman-Ordberg G, Jhelm A, Irestedt L. Lack of analgesic effect of systemically administered morphine or pethidine on labour pain. *Br J Obstet Gynaecol* 1996;103:968.
166. Gerdin E, Salmonson T, Lindberg B, Rane A. Maternal kinetics of morphine during labour. *J Perinat Med* 1990;18:479.
167. Gerdin E, Rane A, Lindberg B. Transplacental transfer of morphine in man. *J Perinat Med* 1990;18:305.
168. Way WL, Costley EC, Way EL. Respiratory sensitivity of the newborn infant to meperidine and morphine. *Clin Pharmacol Ther* 1965;6:454.
169. Gerhardt R, Bancalari E, Cohen H, Macias-Loza M. Respiratory depression at birth-value of Apgar score and ventilatory measurements in its detection. *J Pediatr* 1977;90:971.
170. Kuhnert BR, Kuhnert PM, Tu AL, Lin DCK, Foltz RL. Meperidine and normeperidine levels following meperidine administration during labor. I. Mother. *Am J Obstet Gynecol* 1979;133:904.
171. Morgan D, Moore G, Thomas J, Triggs E. Disposition of meperidine in pregnancy. *Clin Pharmacol Ther* 1978;23:288.
172. Shnider SM, Way EL, Lord MJ. Rate of appearance and disappearance of meperidine in fetal blood after administration of narcotic to the mother. *Anesthesiology* 1966;27:227.
173. Crawford JS, Rudofsky S. The placental transmission of pethidine. *Br J Anaesth* 1965;37:929.
174. Szeto HH, Mann LI, Bhakthavathsalan A, Liu M, Inturrisi CE. Meperidine pharmacokinetics in the maternal-fetal unit. *J Pharmacol Exp Ther* 1978;206:448.
175. Caldwell J, Wakile LA, Notarianni LJ, et al. Maternal and neonatal disposition of pethidine in childbirth—a study using quantitative gas chromatography-mass spectrometry. *Life Sci* 1978;22:589.
176. Belfrage P, Boreus LO, Hartvig P, Irestedt L, Raabe N. Neonatal depression after obstetrical analgesia with pethidine: the role of the injection-delivery time interval and of the plasma concentrations of pethidine and norpethidine. *Acta Obstet Gynaecol Scand* 1981;60:43.
177. Shnider SM, Moya F. Effects of meperidine on the newborn infant. *Am J Obstet Gynecol* 1964;89:1009.
178. Kuhnert BR, Kuhnert PM, Tu AL, Lin DCK. Meperidine and normeperidine levels following meperidine administration during labor. II. Fetus and neonate. *Am J Obstet Gynecol* 1979;133:909.
179. Kuhnert BR, Philipson EH, Kuhnert PM, Syracuse CD. Disposition of meperidine and normeperidine following multiple doses during labor. I. Mother. *Am J Obstet Gynecol* 1985;151:406.
180. Kuhnert BR, Philipson EH, Kuhnert PM, Syracuse CD. Disposition of meperidine and normeperidine following multiple doses during labor. II. Fetus and neonate. *Am J Obstet Gynecol* 1985;151:410.
181. Hogg MIJ, Wiener PC, Rosen M, Mapleson WW. Urinary excretion and metabolism of pethidine and norpethidine in the newborn. *Br J Anaesth* 1977;49:891.
182. Cooper LV, Stephen GW, Aggett PJA. Elimination of pethidine and bupivacaine in the newborn. *Arch Dis Child* 1977;52:638.
183. Stephen GW, Cooper LV. The role of analgesics in respiratory depression: a rabbit model. *Anaesthesia* 1977;32:324.
184. Nissen E, Widström A-M, Lilja G, et al. Effects of routinely given pethidine during labour on infants' developing breastfeeding behaviour. Effects of dose-delivery time interval and various concentrations of pethidine/norpethidine in cord plasma. *Acta Paediatr* 1997;86:201.
185. Righard L, Alade MO. Effect of delivery room routines on success of first breast-feed. *Lancet* 1990;336:1105.
186. Zimmer EZ, Divon MY, Vadasz A. Influence of meperidine on fetal movements and heart rate beat-to-beat variability in the active phase of labor. *Am J Perinatol* 1988;5:197.

187. Brower KR, Crowell DH, Leung P, Cashman TM. Neonatal electroencephalographic patterns as affected by maternal drugs administered during labor and delivery. *Anesth Analg* 1978;57:303.
188. Brackbill Y, Kane J, Manniello RL, Abramson D. Obstetric meperidine usage and assessment of neonatal status. *Anesthesiology* 1974;40:116.
189. Hodgkinson R, Husain FJ. The duration of effect of maternally administered meperidine on neonatal neurobehavior. *Anesthesiology* 1982; 56:51.
190. Hodgkinson R, Bhatt M, Wang CN. Double-blind comparison of the neurobehavior of neonates following the administration of different doses of meperidine to the mother. *Can Anaesth Soc J* 1978;25:405.
191. Kuhnert BR, Linn PL, Kennard MJ, Kuhnert PM. Effects of low doses of meperidine on neonatal behavior. *Anesth Analg* 1985;64:335.
192. Gerhardt R, Bancalari E, Cohen H, Rocha LF. Use of naloxone to reverse narcotic respiratory depression in the newborn infant. *J Pediatr* 1977;90:1009.
193. Hodgkinson R, Batt M, Grewal G, Marx GF. Neonatal neurobehavior in the first 48 hours of life: effect of the administration of meperidine with and without naloxone in the mother. *Pediatrics* 1978;62:294.
194. Wiener PC, Hogg MI, Rosen M. Neonatal respiration, feeding and neurobehavioural state. *Anaesthesia* 1979;34:996.
195. Craft JB, Coaldrake LA, Bolan JC, et al. Placental passage and uterine effects of fentanyl. *Anesth Analg* 1983;62:894.
196. Rayburn W, Rathke A, Leuschen P, Chleborad J, Weidner W. Fentanyl citrate analgesia during labor. *Am J Obstet Gynecol* 1989;161:202.
197. Rayburn WF, Smith CV, Parriott JE, Woods RE. Randomized comparison of meperidine and fentanyl during labor. *Obstet Gynecol* 1989;74:604.
198. Kleiman SJ, Wiesel S, Tessier MJ. Patient-controlled analgesia (PCA) using fentanyl in a parturient with a platelet function abnormality. *Can J Anaesth* 1991;38:489.
199. Rosaeg OP, Kitts JB, Koren G, Byford LJ. Maternal and fetal effects of intravenous patient-controlled fentanyl analgesia during labour in a thrombocytopenic parturient. *Can J Anaesth* 1992;39:277.
200. Rout CC, Rocke DA. Effects of alfentanil and fentanyl on induction of anaesthesia in patients with severe pregnancy-induced hypertension. *Br J Anaesth* 1990;65:468.
201. Justins DM, Knott C, Luthman J, Reynolds F. Epidural versus intramuscular fentanyl: analgesia and pharmacokinetics in labour. *Anaesthesia* 1983;38:937.
202. Chestnut DH, Owen CL, Bates JN, Ostman LG, Choi WW, Geiger MW. Continuous infusion epidural analgesia during labor: a randomized, double-blind comparison of 0.0625% bupivacaine/0.0002% fentanyl versus 0.125% bupivacaine. *Anesthesiology* 1988;68:754.
203. Bader AM, Fragneto R, Terui K, et al. Maternal and neonatal fentanyl and bupivacaine concentrations after epidural infusion during labor. *Anesth Analg* 1995;81:829.
204. Viscomi CM, Hood DD, Melone PJ, Eisenach JC. Fetal heart rate variability after epidural fentanyl during labor. *Anesth Analg* 1990;71:679.
205. Preston PG, Rosen MA, Hughes SC, et al. Epidural anesthesia with fentanyl and lidocaine for cesarean section: maternal effects and neonatal outcome. *Anesthesiology* 1988;68:938.
206. Paech MJ, Westmore MD, Speirs HM. A double-blind comparison of epidural bupivacaine and bupivacaine-fentanyl for caesarean section. *Anaesth Intensive Care* 1990;18:22.
207. Schlesinger TS, Miletich DJ. Epidural fentanyl and lidocaine during cesarean section: maternal efficacy and neonatal safety using impedance monitoring. *Anesthesiology* 1988;69:A649(abst).
208. Koehntop DE, Rodman JH, Brundage DM, Hegland MG, Buckley JJ. Pharmacokinetics of fentanyl in neonates. *Anesth Analg* 1986;65:227.
209. Benlabed M, Dreizzen E, Ecoffey C, Escourrou P, Midgal M, Gaultier C. Neonatal pattern of breathing after cesarean section with or without epidural fentanyl. *Anesthesiology* 1990;73:1110.
210. Vertommen JD, Marcus MAE, Van Aken H. The effects of intravenous and epidural sufentanil in the chronic maternal-fetal sheep preparation. *Anesth Analg* 1995;80:71.
211. Krishna BR, Zakowski MI, Grant GJ. Sufentanil transfer in the human placenta during in vitro perfusion. *Can J Anaesth* 1997;44:996.
212. Loftus JR, Hill H, Cohen SE. Placental transfer and neonatal effects of epidural sufentanil and fentanyl administered with bupivacaine during labor. *Anesthesiology* 1995;83:300.
213. Gepts E, Heytens L, Camu F. Pharmacokinetics and placental transfer of intravenous and epidural alfentanil in parturient women. *Anesth Analg* 1986;65:1155.
214. Golub MS, Eisele JH, Donald JM. Obstetric analgesia and infant outcome in monkeys: infant development after intrapartum exposure to meperidine or alfentanil. *Am J Obstet Gynecol* 1988;159:1280.
215. Heytens L, Cammu H, Camu F. Extradural analgesia during labour using alfentanil. *Br J Anaesth* 1987;59:331.
216. Maduska AL, Hajghassemali M. A double-blind comparison of butorphanol and meperidine in labour: maternal pain relief and effect on the newborn. *Can Anaesth Soc J* 1978;25:398.
217. Hodgkinson R, Huff RW, Hayashi RH, Husain FJ. Double-blind comparison of maternal analgesia and neonatal neurobehavior following intravenous butorphanol and meperidine. *J Int Med Res* 1979;7:224.
218. Hatjis CG, Meis PJ. Sinusoidal fetal heart rate pattern associated with butorphanol administration. *Obstet Gynecol* 1986;67:377.
219. Frank M, McAteer EJ, Cattermole R, Loughnan B, Stafford LB, Hitchcock AM. Nalbuphine for obstetric analgesia. *Anaesthesia* 1987;42:697.
220. Poehlmann S, Pinette M, Stubblefield P. Effect of labor analgesia with nalbuphine hydrochloride on fetal response to vibroacoustic stimulation. *J Reprod Med* 1995;40:707.
221. Hunt CO, Naulty JS, Malinow AM, Datta S, Ostheimer GW. Epidural butorphanol-bupivacaine for analgesia during labor and delivery. *Anesth Analg* 1989;68:323.
222. Murad SHN, Conklin KA, Tabsh KMA, Brinkman CR, Erkkola R, Nuwayhid B. Atropine and glycopyrrolate: hemodynamic effects and placental transfer in the pregnant ewe. *Anesth Analg* 1981;60:710.
223. Mendez-Bauer C, Poseiro JJ, Arellano-Hernandez G, Zambrana MA, Caldeyro-Barcia R. Effects of atropine on the heart rate of the human fetus during labor. *Am J Obstet Gynecol* 1963;85:1033.
224. Kivalo I, Saarikoski S. Placental transmission of atropine at full-term pregnancy. *Br J Anaesth* 1977;49:1017.
225. Kanto J, Virtanen R, Iisalo E, Maenpaa K, Liukko P. Placental transfer and pharmacokinetics of atropine after a single maternal intravenous and intramuscular administration. *Acta Anaesthesiol Scand* 1981;25:85.
226. Abboud TK, Read J, Miller F, Chen T, Valle R, Hendriksen E. Use of glycopyrrolate in the parturient: effect on the maternal and fetal heart and uterine activity. *Obstet Gynecol* 1981;57:224.
227. Clark RB, Brown MA, Lattin DL. Neostigmine, atropine, and glycopyrrolate: does neostigmine cross the placenta? *Anesthesiology* 1996;84:450.
228. Hughes SC, Ward MG, Levinson G, et al. Placental transfer of ephedrine does not affect neonatal outcome. *Anesthesiology* 1985;63:217.
229. Kangas-Saarela T, Hollmen AI, Tolonen U, et al. Does ephedrine influence newborn neurobehavioural responses and spectral EEG when used to prevent maternal hypotension during caesarean section? *Acta Anaesthesiol Scand* 1990;34:8.
230. Ramanathan J, Sibai BM, Mabie WC, Chauhan D, Ruiz AG. The use of labetalol for attenuation of the hypertensive response to endotracheal intubation in preeclampsia. *Am J Obstet Gynecol* 1988;159:650.
231. Michael CA. Use of labetalol in the treatment of severe hypertension during pregnancy. *Br J Clin Pharmacol* 1979;8:211S.
232. MacPherson M, Broughton Pipkin F, Rutter N. The effect of maternal labetalol on the newborn infant. *Br J Obstet Gynaecol* 1986;93:539.
233. Sun CY, Yacobi A, Kartiznel R, Stampfli H, Davis CS, Lai C. Kinetics of esmolol, an ultra-short-acting β-blocker, and of its major metabolite. *Clin Pharmacol Ther* 1983;34:427.
234. Östman PL, Chestnut DH, Robillard JE, Weiner CP, Hdez MJ. Transplacental passage and hemodynamic effects of esmolol in the gravid ewe. *Anesthesiology* 1988;69:738.
235. Eisenach JC, Castro MI. Maternally administered esmolol produces fetal β-adrenergic blockade and hypoxemia in sheep. *Anesthesiology* 1989;71:718.
236. Ducey JP, Knape KG. Maternal esmolol administration resulting in fetal distress and cesarean section in a term pregnancy. *Anesthesiology* 1992;77:829.
237. Gilson GJ, Knieriem KJ, Smith JF, Izquierdo L, Chatterjee MS, Curet LB. Short-acting beta-adrenergic blockade and the fetus. A case report. *J Reprod Med* 1992;37:277.
238. Larson CP, Shuer LM, Cohen SE. Maternally administered esmolol decreases fetal as well as maternal heart rate. *J Clin Anesth* 1990;2:427.
239. Mason BA, Ogunyemi D, Punla O, Koos BJ. Maternal and fetal cardiorespiratory responses to adenosine in sheep. *Am J Obstet Gynecol* 1993;168:1558.
240. Leffler S, Johnson DR. Adenosine use in pregnancy: lack of effect on fetal heart rate. *Am J Emerg Med* 1992;10:548.

241. Mason BA, Ricci-Goodman J, Koos BJ. Adenosine in the treatment of maternal paroxysmal supraventricular tachycardia. *Obstet Gynecol* 1992;80:478.
242. Howe SP, McGowan WAW, Moore J, McCaughey W, Dundee JW. The placental transfer of cimetidine. *Anaesthesia* 1981;36:371.
243. Hodgkinson R, Glassenberg R, Joyce TH, Coombs DW, Ostheimer GW, Gibbs CP. Comparison of cimetidine (Tagamet) with antacid for safety and effectiveness in reducing gastric acidity before elective cesarean section. *Anesthesiology* 1983;59:86.
244. Magee LA, Inocencion G, Kamboj L, Rosetti F, Koren G. Safety of first trimester exposure to histamine H_2 blockers. A prospective cohort study. *Dig Dis Sci* 1996;41:1145.
245. Riggs KW, Axelson JE, Gruber NC, McErlane BA, McMorland GH, Rurak DW. Metoclopramide pharmacokinetics in pregnant and non-pregnant sheep. *J Pharmacol Sci* 1988;77:373.
246. Bylsma-Howell M, Riggs KW, McMorland GH, et al. Placental transport of metoclopramide: assessment of maternal and neonatal effects. *Can Anaesth Soc J* 1983;30:487.
247. Cunningham FG, MacDonald PC, Gant NF, et al. The placenta and fetal membranes. In: Cunningham FG, Gant NF, MacDonald PC, et al., eds. *Williams obstetrics,* 20th ed. Stamford: Appleton & Lange, 1997:116.
248. Delivoria-Papadopoulos M, DiGiacomo JE. Oxygen transport. In: Polin RA, Fox WW, eds. *Fetal and neonatal physiology, vol 1.* Philadelphia: WB Saunders, 1992:807.

Obstetric Anesthesia, second edition,
edited by Mark C. Norris.
Lippincott Williams & Wilkins, Philadelphia © 1999.

CHAPTER 7

Fetal Evaluation

Carol Ann Lennon and James A. Bartelsmeyer

The architecture of the human placenta is villous hemochorial because the maternal blood comes in direct contact with the fetal chorionic villi (1). This relation allows the placenta efficiently to exchange oxygen, carbon dioxide, nutrients, and waste products between maternal and fetal circulations. Placental transfer depends on the villous surface area, concentration gradient, placental function, and the maternal and fetal blood flow.

The maternal blood supply originates in the uterine arteries, branches into spiral arteries within the myometrium, and finally enters the intervillous space. After passing around the chorionic villi, maternal blood drains into veins within the basal plate before returning to the maternal circulation. The blood flow within the intervillous space is normally characterized by low resistance, and thus flow depends on perfusion pressure within the spiral arteries. Maternal and fetal substances are exchanged within the connective tissue of the chorionic villi. Oxygen-rich blood returns to the fetus via the umbilical vein. The rate of blood flow in the maternal and fetal circulations is important in determining the oxygen supply to the fetus. Maternal position, uterine contraction activity, anesthesia, presence of hypertension, abruptio placenta, and umbilical cord compression may alter blood flow.

Normally, the oxygen tension in fetal blood is 20 to 25 mm Hg. The fetus maintains adequate tissue oxygenation despite this low oxygen tension through several adaptations:

- High cardiac output,
- Fetal hemoglobin with a higher affinity for oxygen, and
- A higher hematocrit.

The fetus can survive temporary periods of low oxygen delivery (hypoxemia) by making a series of compensatory responses. Fetal cardiac output or umbilical blood flow to the placenta changes little, but blood flow redistributes to favor vital organs such as the brain, heart, and adrenal glands at the expense of blood flow to the intestines and kidneys (2,3). The fetus decreases its activity and thus decreases the total oxygen consumption (4). In addition, anaerobic metabolism occurs in those organs in which oxygen supply is inadequate to meet energy demands. During prolonged hypoxia with the accumulation of lactic acid, these compensatory responses are no longer maintained. There is a decrease in cardiac output, blood flow to brain and heart diminishes, and umbilical blood flow decreases. With time, there is progressive tissue damage and ultimately fetal death.

During labor, uterine contractions temporarily interrupt uterine blood flow and decrease oxygenation of fetal blood. This process is usually well tolerated. However, when it is superimposed on chronic uteroplacental insufficiency, the fetus may not compensate for the intermittent decrease in oxygenation, and hypoxemia may develop. The fetus is then more susceptible to other processes that impair oxygenation, such as maternal hypotension or cord compression.

The objective of fetal assessment, whether intrapartum or antepartum, is to identify those fetuses who are compromised or at significant risk of being compromised and to allow timely interventions. The main approach to fetal assessment has been monitoring of the fetal heart rate (FHR) by auscultation with a stethoscope or a Doppler ultrasound device or by direct fetal electrocardiogram (ECG). This chapter provides a review of not only FHR evaluation, but also other commonly used methods of fetal assessment.

Experimental models have provided insight into the regulation of the FHR (5,6). The atrial pacemaker, modulated by the autonomic nervous system, determines the baseline heart rate. Parasympathetic outflow via the vagus nerve decreases FHR, whereas sympathetic activity increases FHR and cardiac output. Baroreceptors

C. A. Lennon: Department of Obstetrics and Gynecology, Washington University in St. Louis, St. Louis, Missouri 63110.
J. A. Bartelsmeyer: Department of Obstetrics and Gynecology, Washington University in St. Louis, St. Louis, Missouri 63110.

respond to increasing blood pressure to modulate the FHR through the autonomic nervous system. Chemoreceptors respond in a similar fashion to decreasing p_aO_2 and increasing p_aCO_2. Cerebral cortical activity and hypothalamic activity affect FHR through their influence on the vasomotor center in the medulla oblongata (7).

FETAL HEART RATE EVALUATION

In the 1960s, the first electronic fetal monitors became available and were initially used solely in high-risk deliveries. By the 1970s, electronic FHR monitoring had become routine. It was hoped that such information could identify the compromised fetus and allow delivery before death or permanent damage occurred. A review by the National Institutes of Health of 11 retrospective studies suggested that monitored patients had a lower intrapartum death rate compared with those who received no fetal monitoring (8).

There have been at least seven randomized controlled studies comparing the effectiveness of auscultation or intermittent monitoring with continuous monitoring in both high- and low-risk patients. Overall, these studies showed that fetal outcome (Apgar scores, intrapartum death rates, and long-term neurological impairment) is the same with either approach (9–14). Despite these data, continuous FHR monitoring remains standard for most laboring patients in the United States. In practice, successful intermittent auscultation requires one-to-one nursing care and skilled labor attendants. These criteria may be achieved in some hospitals but are unlikely in all centers.

The choice of heart-rate monitoring method depends on the comfort level of the attendant, the degree of complicating factors in the patient, and the availability of trained staff. Intermittent auscultation of FHR is appropriate for both low- and most high-risk patients. After obtaining a 30-minute continuous recording, the FHR should be evaluated every 30 minutes during the first stage of labor and every 15 minutes during second stage, preferably before, during, and after a contraction.

The interpretation of the FHR is closely tied to the timing of the uterine contractions, and therefore uterine contraction monitoring is an integral portion of fetal assessment. Uterine contractions can be monitored externally by uterine palpation or with a tocodynamometer, or internally with an intrauterine pressure catheter. Uterine palpation allows the examiner to assess contraction onset, duration, and intensity. The uterus can be indented at the fundus if intrauterine pressure is less than 50 mm Hg. Alternatively, the external tocodynamometer allows determination of the approximate onset, duration, and offset of each contraction; however, the magnitude of the contraction cannot be assessed.

An intrauterine pressure catheter (IUPC) provides the most reliable data concerning strength of uterine contractions. The IUPC is a fluid-filled plastic catheter that is placed through the dilated cervix after amniorrhexis. Intrauterine pressure monitoring enables the obstetrician to objectively gauge the magnitude of contractions and to quantify uterine activity. An IUPC is useful during the management of labor, especially in obese patients for whom palpation may not be revealing or when a external recording of uterine contractions is poor with an FHR pattern with uniform repetitive decelerations. IUPCs also are needed for the purpose of amnioinfusion.

External or internal techniques are used to assess the FHR. Doppler ultrasound detects the changes in ventricular wall motion, blood flow in the major vessels, and movement of the cardiac valves during each cardiac cycle. The monitor calculates the FHR by measuring the interval between each fetal myocardial contraction. Alternatively, an ECG lead attached to the fetal scalp allows the cardiotachometer to calculate the FHR by measuring each successive RR interval. Both the external and internal methods allow continuous assessment of the FHR.

The purpose of describing the FHR is to recognize normal patterns as well as abnormal and ominous patterns. The end point is to recognize established fetal hypoxemia and acidosis and to allow ready treatment or delivery. Another purpose is to avoid the establishment of fetal hypoxemia and acidosis by some form of intervention, when indicated. Universal descriptive terms have been developed to facilitate communication. In general, three basic characteristics of the FHR have been described:

- Baseline rate,
- Variability, and
- Periodic changes.

Baseline

The baseline heart rate is the average rate at which the fetal heart beats most of the time. The normal baseline FHR in a term infant ranges between 110 and 160 beats/min. A new baseline rate is established when a different rate occurs for more than 10 minutes.

Fetal tachycardia is defined as a baseline FHR greater than 160 beats/min. Common associated findings with fetal tachycardia include maternal temperature elevation, maternal infection, and intra-amniotic infection. Alternative etiologies of intrapartum fetal tachycardia include fetal tachyarrhythmias, fetal hypoxemia, or maternal hyperthyroidism. Maternal medications also may cause fetal tachycardia (i.e., β-adrenergic medications such as terbutaline, or anticholinergic agents such as atropine).

Evaluation of the fetus with baseline tachycardia should include a review of maternal medications and a thorough search for evidence of intra-amniotic infection. Isolated fetal tachycardia in the presence of good short- and long-term variability and in the absence of decelerations is rarely, if ever, associated with fetal compromise. However, fetal tachycardia with other concurrent FHR abnormalities should alert the obstetrician to the possibility of fetal acidemia. Complicated tachycardia that does not respond to conservative measures may be further evaluated by fetal scalp-blood sampling.

Fetal bradycardia is defined as a baseline FHR below 110 beats/min for more than 2 minutes. The possible etiologies of acute fetal bradycardia during labor are varied. As the initial response of the fetus to hypoxemia is vagally mediated bradycardia, its etiology can include any mechanism that can acutely impair fetal oxygenation. Examples are acute prolonged umbilical cord compression, umbilical cord prolapse, abruptio placentae, acute maternal hypotension, uterine hyperstimulation, and uterine rupture. Fetal bradyarrhythmias also can be responsible for an abnormal baseline FHR. Bradycardia coexisting with an otherwise normal FHR tracing is rarely ominous. Mild bradycardia (90 to 120 beats/min) during delivery is relatively common but well tolerated. The fetus with additional abnormalities on the FHR monitor, or prolonged bradycardia, requires further evaluation and, in some situations, prompt delivery.

Fetal Heart Rate Variability

Fetal heart rate variability refers to the irregularity of the FHR baseline (Figs. 1 and 2). Two components of variability are commonly described: short-term or beat-to-beat variability and long-term variability. FHR variability results from the competing effects of the parasympathetic and sympathetic nervous systems on the heart.

Short-term or beat-to-beat variability refers to the irregular intervals between successive heartbeats. Doppler ultrasound may not always detect short-term variability accurately. The newer Doppler monitors that use autocorrelation techniques seem to provide a close approximation of short-term variability (15). A fetal ECG electrode provides the most reliable estimate of short-term variability.

Short-term variability is relatively easy to identify. If the baseline recording is jagged, the short-term variability is most likely to be adequate. The presence of FHR variability is associated with fetal normoxia and is generally indicative of a normal central nervous system (CNS), vagus nerve, and circulatory system.

Long-term variability represents the rough sine wave oscillations that commonly occur three to six times per minute. Normal long-term variability also is described as at least six beats/min variation in the baseline FHR. As gestation advances and the fetal autonomic system matures, both the long- and short-term variability increase.

The lack of variability or a smooth FHR tracing should raise concern. Multiple factors can decrease variability. The greatest cause for concern is fetal hypoxemia. Poor FHR variability with accelerations may be associated with maternal narcotic administration. However, this finding also can be associated with remote neurological injury. A fetus with a lack of variability, especially when complicated by decelerations or baseline changes, requires further evaluation.

Periodic Changes

Periodic changes are alterations of the baseline heart rate occurring in conjunction with a uterine contraction. FHR acceleration occurs when there is an increase in FHR above the baseline. With a deceleration, FHR drops below the baseline. Decelerations are generally classified as early, variable, or late depending on the shape of the deceleration and the temporal relation to uterine contractions (16).

Early Decelerations

Early decelerations begin with the onset of the contraction and are characterized by a gradual decrease in FHR, which returns slowly to baseline by the completion of the contraction. The nadir is coincident with the peak of the contraction. The deceleration is smooth, rounded, and U-shaped in configuration and mirrors the contraction shape. Early decelerations are thought to occur as result of a vagal response to head compression during labor. Early decelerations are usually benign and are associated with normal fetal pH.

Variable Decelerations

Variable decelerations of the FHR are defined as abrupt decreases from baseline of at least 15 beats/min, lasting no more than 2 minutes and with usually an abrupt return to baseline. They also are characterized by their irregular shape, reflecting rapid heart-rate fluctuation during the deceleration. They are described as severe when the nadir is 60 beats/min below the baseline and lasts more than 60 seconds. A variable deceleration lasting more than 2 minutes is called a prolonged deceleration.

Variable decelerations are the most common periodic changes (Figs. 3 and 4). These abrupt decelerations are believed to occur as result of vagal response to either umbilical cord compression or to substantial head compression during pushing. Variable decelerations do not predict fetal outcome unless accompanied by decrease in variability or baseline change. The severity of the variable decelerations can be used to gauge the potential harm to the fetus.

When repetitive severe variable decelerations are present, efforts should be undertaken to abolish them if rapid delivery is not anticipated. With persistent intermittent reduction in umbilical blood flow, the normal fetus may eventually decompensate. Amnioinfusion, the instillation of sterile crystalloid into the amniotic cavity through an intrauterine catheter, has been shown to lower the incidence of severe decelerations and may allow progression to vaginal delivery (17).

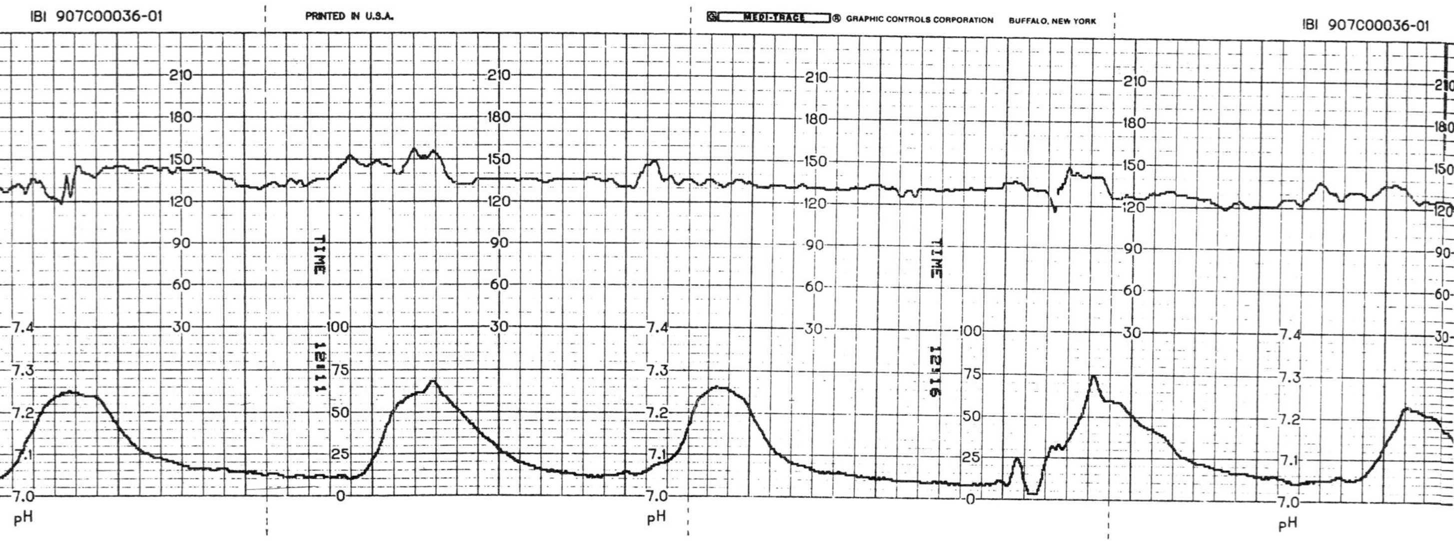

FIG. 1. This reassuring labor record demonstrates a baseline heart rate of 130 beats/min with accelerations. Contractions are occurring every 2 to 3 minutes.

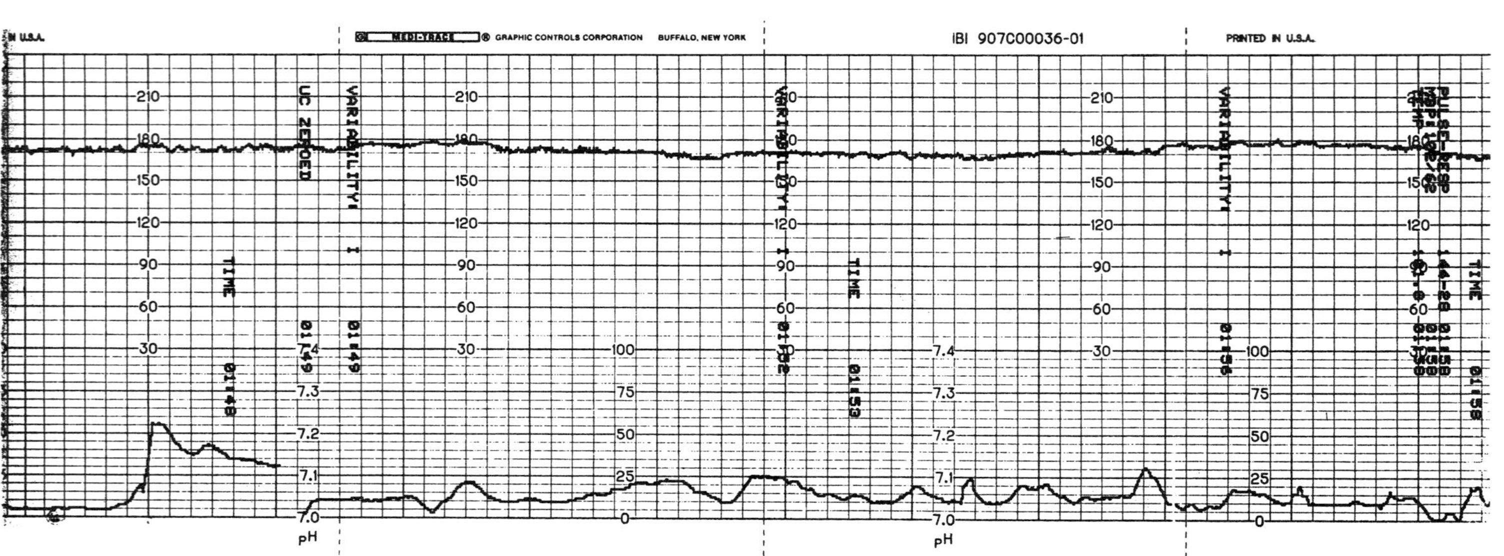

FIG. 2. This nonreassuring fetal heart record displays an elevated baseline rate (170 beats/min) and absent variability in the absence of uterine contractions.

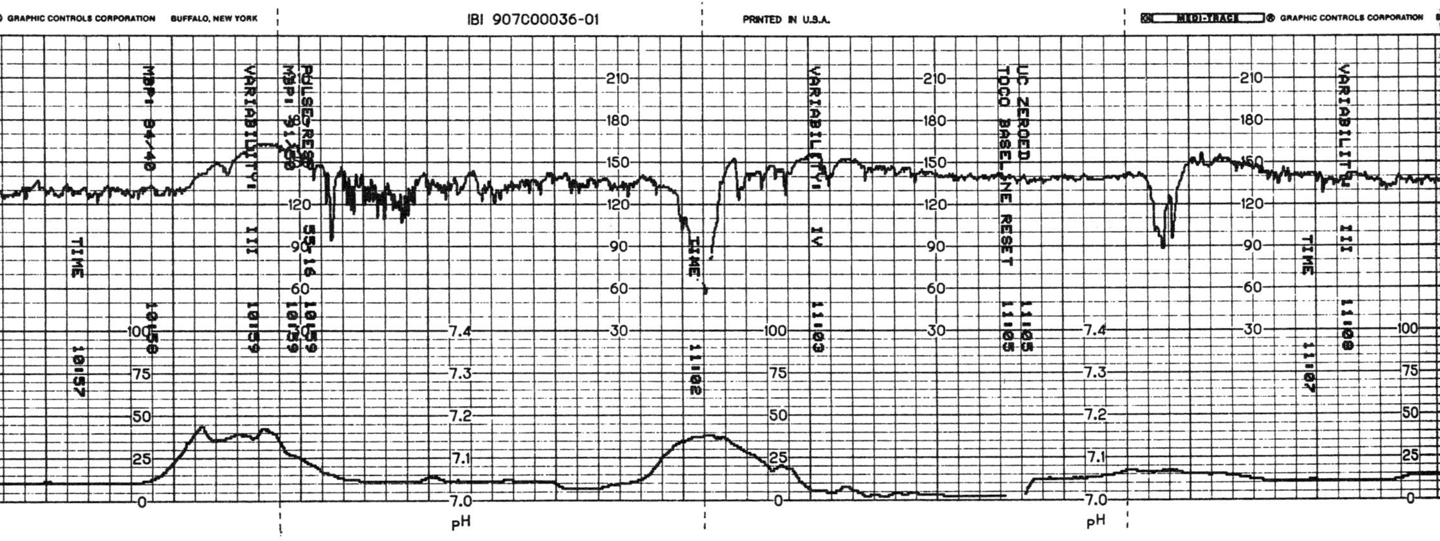

FIG. 3. This labor record demonstrates repetitive variable decelerations in conjunction with good beat-to-beat variability and accelerations.

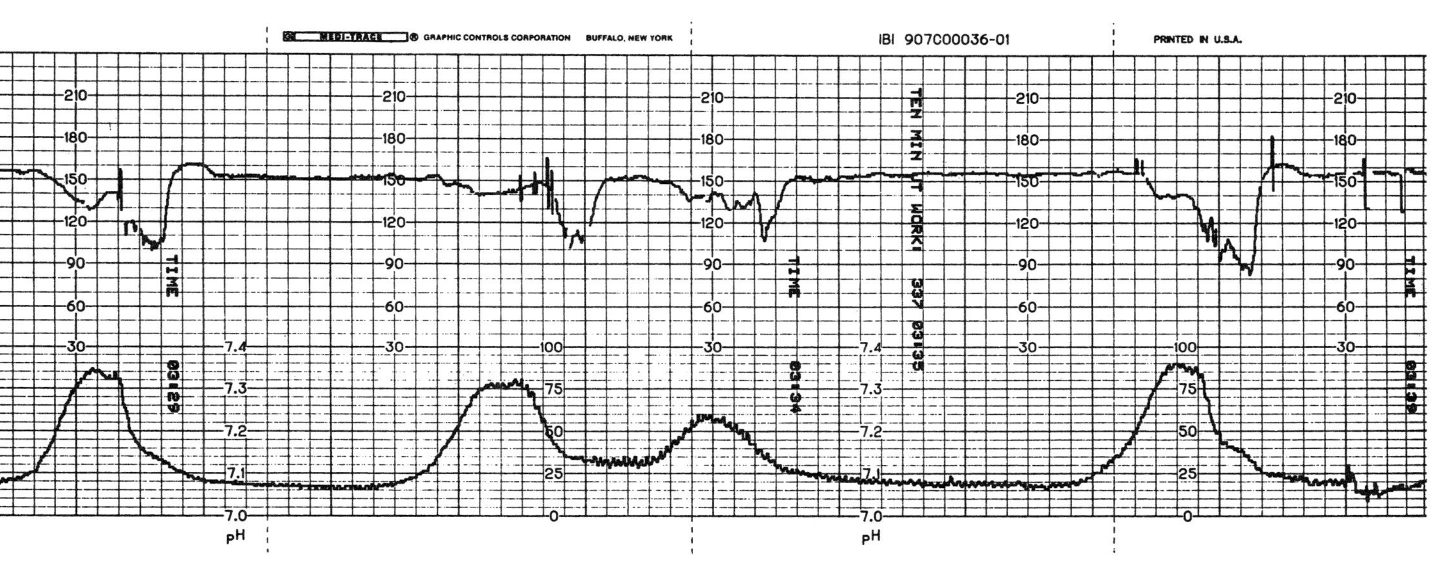

FIG. 4. This labor record demonstrates repetitive variable decelerations and absent variability. These findings should prompt assessment of fetal acid–base status or delivery.

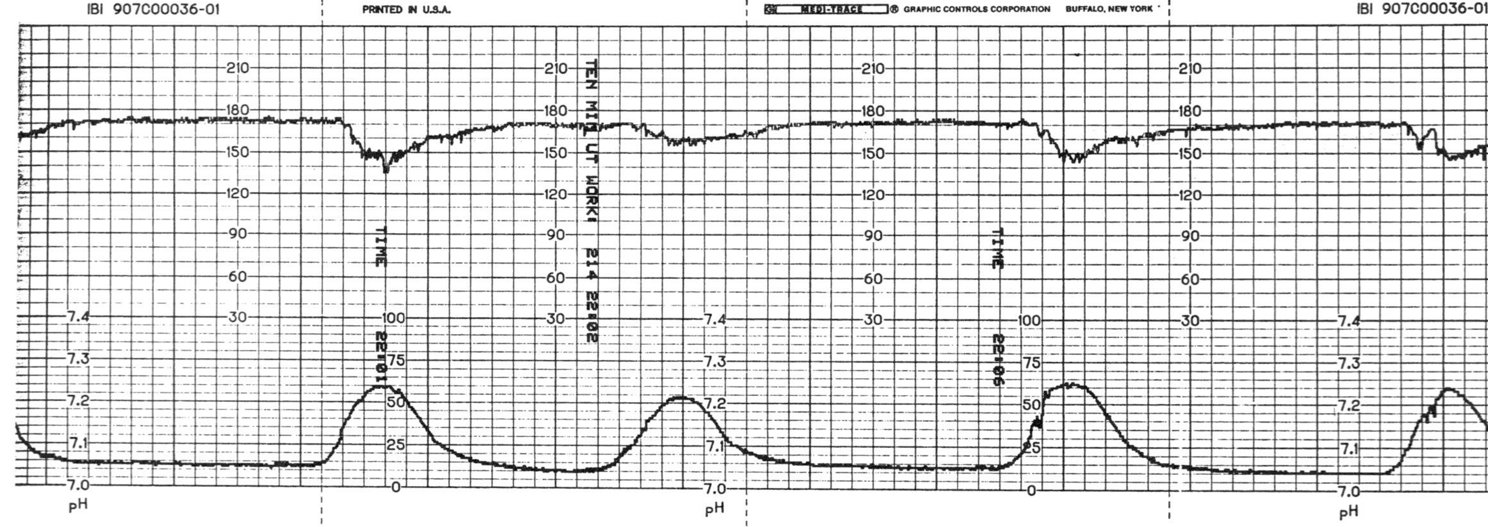

FIG. 5. This nonreassuring labor record demonstrates a fetal tachycardia (baseline of 170 beats/min) with absent variability and repetitive late decelerations. Contractions are occurring every 2 to 3 minutes. This tracing warrants prompt delivery.

Late Decelerations

Late decelerations are characterized by a smooth, gradual decrease in the FHR after the onset of the contraction, with the nadir occurring after the peak of the contraction (Fig. 5), and a smooth gradual return to baseline after the completion of the contraction. Classically, late decelerations are a sign of uteroplacental insufficiency. Late decelerations may occur as a vagal response to hypoxic stimulation of chemoreceptors or as result of direct hypoxic myocardial depression. Isolated late decelerations are not associated with poor fetal outcome but must be observed closely. Repetitive late decelerations, especially in conjunction with decreased variability or other baseline change, must be evaluated further, with consideration of delivery if they cannot be abolished.

ANTEPARTUM FETAL EVALUATION

NoninvasiveTesting

Contraction Stress Test

The contraction stress test (CST) is based on the FHR response to uterine contractions, which transiently reduce intervillous blood flow. A fetus with marginal oxygenation at rest may not tolerate uterine contractions and the subsequent decrease in oxygen availability. The transient decrease in oxygen may stimulate a vagal response. Late decelerations may occur.

The CST is performed in the semi-Fowler's position, in which external monitors may record the FHR and contractions. Contractions are elicited with oxytocin or by nipple stimulation. An adequate CST requires three uterine contractions of moderate intensity lasting approximately 40 to 60 seconds in 10 minutes. The CST is interpreted as negative if no late decelerations occur. A negative CST is associated with a good fetal outcome. A positive result occurs if late decelerations follow 50% or more of contractions, even if the contraction frequency is fewer than three in 10 minutes. A positive CST has been associated with an increased incidence of intrauterine death, late decelerations in labor, low 5-minute Apgar scores, and meconium-stained amniotic fluid. A suggestive or equivocal result occurs with intermittent late or significant variable decelerations and should be repeated in 24 hours. Up to 50% of positive CSTs are falsely positive (fetus tolerates labor well after positive test). More important, the false-negative rate, defined as stillbirths occurring within 1 week of a reassuring or negative test is 0.4/1,000 (18).

Nonstress Test

The nonstress test (NST) is based on the premise that the heart rate of a nonacidotic fetus will temporarily accelerate in response to fetal movement. The accelerations require intact neurological coupling between the fetal CNS and the fetal heart, which is dependent on normal CNS oxygenation.

The NST is usually performed in the outpatient setting with the FHR monitored by an external transducer. The most common definition of a reactive or normal NST is at least two FHR accelerations of at least 15 beats/min above the baseline and lasting 15 seconds, within a 20-minute period. A nonreactive NST is the absence of sufficient accelerations within 40 minutes. A nonreactive NST has a high false-positive rate of 75% to 85%. Common reasons for nonreactive NSTs include a quiet fetal sleep cycle, the use of CNS depressants, extreme prematurity, and the use of β-blockers. A nonreactive NST is associated with a higher perinatal mortality, and a nonreactive test should be followed up with further testing. The false-negative rate of NST is 1.4/1,000 (18).

Ultrasound

Ultrasound is a versatile tool that is frequently used to evaluate fetal health. The accepted indications for ultrasound during pregnancy are numerous:

- Gestational age assignment,
- Assessment of fetal number, lie, and presentation,
- Placental localization,
- Screening for congenital anomalies,
- Assessment of amniotic fluid volume, and
- Determination of fetal weight.

Approximately 70% to 75% of pregnant women in the United States have an ultrasound at some time during gestation (19). There are clearly many potential benefits to ultrasound. However, the ability of routine ultrasound in low-risk patients to identify fetal anomalies or other pathologic conditions and to improve perinatal outcome is controversial. Studies have not consistently shown significant improvements in perinatal outcome through the detection of life-threatening anomalies, accurate gestational age assignment, or diagnosis of other conditions. Analyses of selected at-risk groups clearly demonstrates the utility of ultrasound in many clinical situations. For instance, early detection of multiple gestations has been associated with a 50% reduction in perinatal morbidity (20).

Detection of Fetal Anomalies

A second-trimester fetal anatomic survey performed in a low-risk population will detect 17% to 74% of significant fetal anomalies (20). Ultrasounds performed later or earlier in gestation are less sensitive. The sensitivity of ultrasound to detect fetal anomalies depends on the clinical setting and the skill of the person performing the examination. The specificity of a fetal anatomic survey to detect fetal anomalies exceeds 99%. In low-risk populations, ultrasound may be helpful in ruling out anomalies, but it is not particularly reliable in detecting them.

Fetal Weight

Ultrasonic estimation of fetal weight (EFW) is frequently used to make management decisions regarding the induction of labor or route of delivery. Unfortunately, evidence does not support the notion that this management will significantly improve perinatal outcome (21). Current ultrasound weight-estimate calculations are not accurate enough to be used effectively in the detection of macrosomia by defined weight criteria. For estimating fetal weights greater than 4,500 g, the accuracy of ultrasound is less than 50%, with a tendency to overestimate the fetal weight. Even if clinicians could accurately estimate fetal weight, the frequency of persistent brachial plexus injuries associated with vaginal birth of a large-for-gestational-age nondiabetic patient is so low that induction of labor or cesarean birth can rarely be justified on the basis of fetal weight alone.

Amniotic Fluid Volume

Abnormalities of amniotic fluid volume are associated with poor pregnancy outcome. In the late second and third trimesters, amniotic fluid volume reflects fetal urine output. Placental dysfunction with hypoxemia causes a redistribution of fetal blood flow, which may decrease fetal urine function. Other pathologic conditions, such as maternal diabetes or fetal anomalies, may be associated with excessive amounts of amniotic fluid. Sonography provides a means of assessing amniotic fluid volume and indirectly evaluating the function of the uteroplacental unit and the health of the fetus.

Ultrasonographic visualization of amniotic fluid volume has been used for both subjective and semiquantitative methods of fluid estimation. The most popular method of assessing amniotic fluid volume is the amniotic fluid index (AFI). The AFI is derived by dividing the uterus into four quadrants and summing the measurements of the deepest vertical pocket in each quadrant. Normal values for each week of gestation have been published (22). Less is known about the predictive value of the AFI. Whereas normal values are reassuring and are unlikely to be associated with significant chronic problems with placental function, the ability of abnormal values to predict poor perinatal outcome has not been established.

Biophysical Profile

Ultrasound also can be used to assess fetal oxygenation and acid–base status. The presence of normal biophysical parameters (e.g., fetal movements, fetal tone) established by sonographic evaluation indicate normal neurologic function, an indirect indicator of fetal oxygenation, acid–base status, and placental function (23). Numerous biophysical parameters can be monitored by ultrasound, and at least three biophysical profiles (BPPs) have been developed (23,24). The components and scoring methods for the most commonly used BPP are shown in Table 1. With this method, a score of 8 or 10 is normal; a score of 6 is considered equivocal and generally requires repeated testing within 12 to 24 hours. A score of 4 or less is abnormal and is usually an indication for delivery. When oligohydramnios is encountered, further investigation is required.

As in all tests of fetal well-being, the BPP has a high false-positive rate. In up to 40% of instances in which test results are abnormal, fetuses tolerate labor well. The false-negative rate, defined as the incidence of a stillbirth occurring within 1 week of a reassuring or negative test, is reported as 0.6/1,000 (18).

The modified BPP has been used as a more rapid assessment of fetal health. The modified BPP includes an NST as a short-term indication of fetal acid–base status and assessment of amniotic fluid volume, generally by AFI, as an indication of long-term placental function (19,25). This easier test is apparently equivalent to the other methods of fetal assessment.

Doppler Ultrasound

Doppler ultrasound offers a noninvasive technique for evaluating fetal, fetoplacental, and uteroplacental circulations. A large body of evidence associates abnormal Doppler findings with pregnancy complications and

TABLE 1. *Five components of biophysical profile*

Test	Normal value	Scoring	
		Presence	Absence
NST	Reactive	+2	0
Fetal breathing movements	One or more episodes of rhythmic fetal breathing movements of ≥30 s[a]	+2	0
Fetal movement	Three or more discrete body or limb movements[a]	+2	0
Fetal tone	One or more episodes of extension of a fetal extremity with return to flexion[a]	+2	0
Amniotic fluid volume	One or more 2 × 2-cm pockets of amniotic fluid	+2	0

[a]Fetal breathing movements, movements, and tone are established within a 30-min period.
NST, nonstress test.
From ref. 24, with permission.

adverse perinatal outcome. The greatest value of fetal Doppler ultrasound is in conjunction with other modalities of fetal assessment.

Pulsatile movement of red blood cells within a vessel during a cardiac cycle will result in a change in the frequencies of the reflected sound waves. The change in frequency, the Doppler shift, depends on the changing velocity of blood flow during diastole and systole. Accurate measurement of velocity or volume of flow within small fetal vessels is extremely difficult. Most investigators use standard indices to compare systolic flow with diastolic flow. The most commonly reported index is the S/D ratio, which simply measures the peak systolic frequency divided by the end-diastolic frequency.

In perinatal medicine, Doppler ultrasound is most commonly used in two situations:

- To assess pregnancies with presumed uteroplacental insufficiency, such as intrauterine growth restriction (IUGR) or maternal hypertension, and
- To evaluate fetal cardiac abnormalities.

Doppler ultrasound, including color Doppler mapping, has been extremely useful in evaluation of the structural and hemodynamic characteristics of fetal cardiac abnormalities. The utility of antepartum Doppler ultrasound in the evaluation of abnormal fetoplacental circulation is less certain.

Most of the studies evaluating Doppler ultrasound as a method of detecting abnormalities of fetoplacental circulation have been observational. Only recently have well designed, prospective, randomized trials been reported (26,27). Studies of Doppler ultrasound usually assume that impaired placental blood flow, as a result of vascular constriction or destruction within the placental bed, will produce greater resistance to flow in the maternal and fetal vessels that supply the uteroplacental unit (i.e., the uterine and umbilical arteries) (28). The resultant hypoxemia will cause redistribution of fetal blood flow. Vascular beds in critical organs like the brain will dilate to allow greater flow at less resistance. Increased resistance will be seen in vessels supplying nonvital organs. Currently, umbilical artery blood-flow velocity provides the most reliable and reproducible results. Measuring umbilical artery blood-flow velocity may prove useful as a screening tool for low-risk, unselected populations and as part of the overall assessment of high-risk pregnancies.

To date, numerous reports, including observational studies, meta-analyses, and randomized controlled studies, have failed to show consistently any benefit of routine umbilical artery Doppler ultrasound velocimetry in low-risk pregnancies (29,30). Conversely, umbilical artery Doppler velocimetry is a useful adjuvant to other methods of fetal assessment in high-risk pregnancies, particularly in the presence of maternal hypertensive disorders or small-for-gestational-age fetuses. Randomized reviews and meta-analyses have revealed a statistically significant improvement in perinatal outcome, including a reduction in perinatal mortality (26,31). Absent or reversed end-diastolic umbilical artery blood flow is highly associated with adverse perinatal outcome, and when present, may be an indication for intervention or increased surveillance (32). Unfortunately, the predictive value of abnormal umbilical artery Doppler flow studies has not been established, and the exact role of Doppler ultrasound in these high-risk situations is uncertain. Doppler ultrasound has been most commonly used for antepartum fetal assessment and has not found much use as a tool to assess intrapartum fetal health.

Vibroacoustic Stimulation

A provoked FHR acceleration in response to vibroacoustic stimulation (VAS) has been used for more than 10 years as an adjunct for the assessment of fetal well-being. The majority of clinical studies have used an electronic artificial larynx applied to the maternal abdomen to deliver a short acoustic burst to the fetus. Simultaneous recording of the FHR is obtained with electronic fetal monitoring. An acceleration of the FHR after VAS indicates fetal health. The rationale for VAS is that with the appropriate stimulation, the healthy fetus, in a quiet sleep state associated with a nonreactive FHR, will change to an active state and demonstrate reassuring FHR accelerations. VAS has been found significantly to decrease the rate of false-positive NSTs and to shorten testing times (33,34). However, studies of VAS have used a variety of methods. Although most studies examining the safety of VAS have been reassuring, concern remains about short-term effects on fetal oxygenation and fetal pain perception, as well as long-term effects on hearing.

A number of studies have examined intrapartum VAS as an adjunct to continuous FHR monitoring (35,36). Reports have correlated the intrapartum FHR response after VAS to fetal scalp-blood pH, base deficit, and short-term neonatal outcome. An acceleration of the FHR after VAS is highly predictive of a normal pH from fetal scalp-blood sampling, normal Apgar scores, and normal umbilical artery acid–base values. VAS also has a reasonable ability to predict low fetal scalp-blood pH during labor. As with many methods of fetal assessment, VAS is a better predictor of fetal health than of fetal jeopardy. Although VAS has gained wide acceptance as a method of antepartum and intrapartum assessment of fetal health, the predictive nature, safety, and exact role of this test has not been fully determined.

Invasive Testing

Indirect, noninvasive methods of assessing fetal well-being are sufficient in most situations. Occasionally, the results of noninvasive testing or other risk factors necessitate that invasive tests be considered to determine fetal health. Indications for invasive testing include:

- Identification of chromosomal or Mendelian disorders,
- Direct assessment of fetal oxygenation or acid–base status,
- Identification of fetal hematologic or enzymatic abnormalities,
- Determination of fetal lung maturity, and
- Identification of intra-amniotic or fetal infections.

Chorionic Villous Sampling

Chorionic villous sampling (CVS) is a technique in which a small sample of placental tissue is obtained. Villi obtained are derived from the same embryonic origin as the fetus and reflect the genetic makeup of the fetus. CVS is generally performed between 10 and 12 weeks of gestation. Sampling can be done by either the transcervical or transabdominal route under ultrasound guidance. Chorionic villi can be analyzed to determine chromosomal, enzymatic, or DNA status of the fetus (16). CVS offers patients an earlier option for prenatal diagnosis of a genetic defect than does midtrimester amniocentesis. Chorionic villi cannot be used for prenatal diagnosis of neural tube defects, which requires analysis of amniotic fluid, or the Fragile X syndrome.

Data from large-scale collaborative studies indicate that when performed by experienced operators, transcervical or transabdominal CVS does not significantly change fetal-loss rate compared with traditional midtrimester amniocentesis (37,38). Concern has been raised about the possible association of limb-reduction defects in infants born to mothers after CVS. Numerous reports both supporting and refuting the association have been published (39,40). Further studies are needed to determine the risk of transverse digital deficiency after CVS performed at 10 to 12 weeks.

Amniocentesis

Amniocentesis is the technique of obtaining a sample of amniotic fluid by transabdominal needle insertion into the amniotic space under ultrasound guidance. Amniocentesis is primarily performed for three indications:

- Detection of genetic disorders,
- Determination of fetal lung maturity, and
- Identification of intramniotic infections.

Genetic Testing

Prenatal diagnosis of chromosomal or Mendelian disorders by amniocentesis is usually done between age 15 and 20 weeks. Fetal karyotype can be obtained from viable cells found in the amniotic fluid. As with CVS, many Mendelian disorders can be identified through amniocentesis. Amniocentesis also offers the additional ability to identify open neural tube defects by measuring amniotic fluid α-fetoprotein concentration.

Several large collaborative studies addressed the safety of amniocentesis (41,42). The loss rate after second-trimester amniocentesis, when compared with the baseline rate of fetal loss in a control population is consistently reported to be less than 1%. Smaller, more recent studies, reported even lower fetal-loss rates. Most clinicians continue to counsel patients that the risk of abortion resulting from amniocentesis is 0.5% or slightly less. Serious maternal complications or fetal injury are exceedingly rare.

Recently early amniocentesis, performed before 15 weeks' gestation, has gained popularity as an alternative to CVS and conventional second-trimester amniocentesis. Early amniocentesis appears safe and accurate for prenatal diagnosis. However, before the procedure becomes routine clinical practice, it will require appraisal by large randomized trials.

Fetal Lung Maturity

Amniocentesis remains the most accurate method of determining fetal lung maturity. The direct or indirect measurement of phospholipids in amniotic fluid is the principal means of assessing the risk of neonatal respiratory distress. The lecithin/sphingomyelin (L/S) ratio is the gold standard with which all other tests are compared. The false-negative ratio [percentage of fetuses identified as not being at risk for respiratory distress syndrome (RDS) but do develop RDS] for the L/S ratio is generally considered to be low (43). However, the test is time consuming and expensive. Several indirect measurements of amniotic fluid phospholipids have been reported in the last 10 years. Perhaps the most popular is the assessment of fetal lung maturity by measurement of the fluorescence polarization of amniotic fluid (44). The fluorescent polarization of amniotic fluid is determined by the relative binding of a fluorescent probe to either phospholipid structures or to albumin. The decrease in fluorescent polarization associated with binding to albumin can be measured and correlated with fetal lung maturity. The sensitivity, specificity, and predictive value of the test are similar to L/S ratio. The test has the advantage of requiring less sample and being quicker and less expensive than the L/S ratio.

REFERENCES

1. Ramsey EM, Martin CB Jr, Donner MW. Fetal and maternal circulation. *Am J Obstet Gynecol* 1967;98:419.
2. Itskovitz J, La Gamma EF, Rudolf AM. Effects of cord compression on fetal blood flow distribution and oxygen delivery. *Am J Physiol* 1987; 2552:H100.
3. Peeters LLH, Sheldon RE, Hones MD, et al. Blood flow to fetal organs as a function of arterial oxygen content. *Am J Obstet Gynecol* 1979; 135:637.
4. Boddy K, Dawes GS, Fisher R, Pinter S, Robinson JS. Foetal respiratory movements, electrocortical and cardiovascular responses to hypoxaemia and hypercapnia in sheep. *J Physiol (Lond)* 1974;243:599.
5. Schitterli P, Caldeyro-Barcia R. Effects of atropine and beta adrenergic drugs on the heart rate of the human fetus. In: Boreus L, ed. *Fetal pharmacology*. New York: Raven Press, 1973:259.

6. Renou P, Warnick N, Wood C. Autonomic control of fetal heart rate. *Am J Obstet Gynecol* 1969;105:949.
7. Parer JT. Physiological regulation of fetal heart rate. *J Obstet Gynecol Neonatal Nurs* 1976;5:265.
8. National Institutes of Health. *Antenatal diagnoses: report of a consensus development conference*. NIH publication 79-1973. Bethesda, MD: NIH, 1979.
9. Haverkamp AD, Orlans M, Langendoerter S, McFee J, Murphy J, Thompson HE. A controlled trial of the differential effects of intrapartum fetal monitoring. *Am J Obstet Gynecol* 1979;134:349.
10. Haverkamp AD, Thompson HE, McFee JG, Cetrulo C. The evaluation of continuous fetal heart rate monitoring in high-risk pregnancy. *Am J Obstet Gynecol* 1976;125:310.
11. Renou P, Chang A, Anderson I, Wood C. Controlled trial of fetal intensive care. *Am J Obstet Gynecol* 1976;126:470.
12. Kelso IM, Parsons RJ, Lawrence GF, Arora SS, Edmonds DK, Cooke ID. An assessment of continuous fetal heart rate monitoring in labor: a randomized trial. *Am J Obstet Gynecol* 1978;131:526.
13. Wood C, Renou P, Oats J, Farrell E, Beischer N, Anderson I. A controlled trial of fetal heart rate monitoring in a low-risk obstetric population. *Am J Obstet Gynecol* 1981;141:527.
14. MacDonald D, Grant A, Sheridan-Pereira M, Boylan P, Chalmero I. The Dublin randomized controlled trial of intrapartum fetal heart rate monitoring. *Am J Obstet Gynecol* 1985;152:524.
15. Amato J. Fetal heart rate monitoring. *Am J Obstet Gynecol* 1983; 147:967.
16. American College of Obstetricians and Gynecologists. *Antenatal diagnosis of genetic disorders.* ACOG Technical Bulletin 207. Washington DC: ACOG, July 1995.
17. Miyazaki F, Nevorez F. Saline amnioinfusion for relief of variable or prolonged decelerations. *Am J Obstet Gynecol* 1983;14:670.
18. American College of Obstetricians and Gynecologists. *Antepartum fetal surveillance.* ACOG Technical Bulletin 188. Washington DC: ACOG, January 1994.
19. American College of Obstetricians and Gynecologists. *Routine ultrasound in low-risk pregnancy.* ACOG Practice Pattern 5. Washington, DC: ACOG, 1997.
20. Ewigman BG, Crane JP, Grigoletto FD, LeFeure ML, Bain RP, McNellis D. Effect of prenatal ultrasound screening on perinatal outcome: RADIUS study group. *N Engl J Med* 1993;329:821.
21. Sandmire HF. Whither ultrasound prediction of fetal macrosomia? *Obstet Gynecol* 1993;82:860.
22. Moore TR, Cayle JE. The amniotic fluid index in normal human pregnancy. *Am J Obstet Gynecol* 1990;162:1168.
23. Vintzileos AM, Campbell WA, Ingardia CJ, Nochimson DJ. The fetal biophysical profile and its predictive value. *Obstet Gynecol* 1983;62:271.
24. Manning FA, Harman CR, Manson I, Menticoglon SM, Lange IR, Johnson JM. Fetal assessment based on fetal biophysical profile scoring. IV. An analysis of perinatal morbidity and mortality. *Am J Obstet Gynecol* 1990;162:703.
25. Clark SL, Sabey P, Jolley K. Nonstress testing with acoustic stimulation and amniotic fluid volume assessment: 5973 tests without unexpected fetal death. *Am J Obstet Gynecol* 1989;160:694.
26. Davies JA, Gallivan S, Spender JAD. Randomized controlled trial of Doppler ultrasound screening of placental perfusion during pregnancy. *Lancet* 1992;340:1299.
27. Alfireviz Z, Neilson JP. Doppler ultrasonography in high-risk pregnancies: systemic review with meta-analysis. *Am J Obstet Gynecol* 1995; 172:1379.
28. Luvrini R, Laurin J, Marsal K. Placental histology and fetal blood flow in intrauterine growth retardation. *Acta Obstet Gynecol Scan* 1994;73:529.
29. Goffinet F, Paris-Llada J, Nisand I, Breart G. Umbilical artery Doppler velocimetry in unselected and low risk pregnancies: a review of randomized controlled trials. *Br J Obstet Gynaecol* 1997;104:425.
30. Goffinet F, Paris-Llada J, Nisand I, Breart G. French Doppler study group: a randomized controlled trial of Doppler ultrasound velocimetry of umbilical artery in low risk pregnancies. *Br J Obstet Gynaecol* 1997; 104:419.
31. Pattison RC, Norman IC, Odendaal HJ. The rule of Doppler velocimetry in the management of high risk pregnancies. *Br J Obstet Gynaecol* 1994;101:114.
32. Karsdorp VH, vanVogt JM, vanGeijn HP, et al. Clinical significance of absent or reversed end diastolic velocity waveform in umbilical artery. *Lancet* 1994;344:1664.
33. Ohel G, Birkenfel A, Robinowitz R, Sadovsky E. Fetal response to vibroacoustic stimulation in periods of low heart rate reactivity and low reactivity. *Am J Obstet Gynecol* 1972;114:613.
34. Smith CV, Phelan JP, Platt LP, Brousard P, Paul RH. Fetal acoustic stimulation testing II: a randomized clinical comparison with the nonstress test. *Am J Obstet Gynecol* 1986;155:131.
35. Smith, CV, Nguyen HN, Phelan JP, Paul RH. Intrapartum assessment of fetal well-being: a comparison of fetal acoustic stimulation with acid-base determinations. *Am J Obstet Gynecol* 1986;155:726.
36. Bartelsmeyer JA, Sadovsky Y, Fleming B, Petrie RH. Utilization of fetal heart rate acceleration following vibroacoustic stimulation in labor to predict fetal acidemia and base deficit levels. *J Matern Fetal Med* 1995; 4:120.
37. Rhoads GG, Jackson JG, Schlesselman SE, et al. The safety and efficiency of chorionic villous sampling for early prenatal diagnosis of cytogenic abnormalities. *N Engl J Med* 1989;320:609.
38. Ledbetter DH, Martin AO, Verlinsky Y, et al. Cytogenic results of chorionic villous sampling: high success rate and diagnostic accuracy in the United States collaborative study. *Am J Obstet Gynecol* 1990;162:495.
39. Olney RS, Khoury MJ, Alo CT, et al. Increased risk for transverse digital deficiency after chorionic villous sampling: results of the United States multistatic case-control study, 1988-1992. *Teratology* 1995;51:20.
40. Fishman RHB. 1994 WHO on CVS safety. *Lancet* 1994;443:1420.
41. Taber A, Maldsen M, Obel E. Randomized controlled trial of genetic amniocentesis in 4606 low-risk women. *Lancet* 1986;1:1287.
42. NICHD National Registry for Amniocentesis Study Group. Midtrimester amniocentesis for prenatal diagnosis, safety and accuracy. *JAMA* 1976;236:1471.
43. Kulovich MV, Hallman MB, Gluch L. The lung profile I. Normal pregnancy. *Am J Obstet Gynecol* 1975;135:57.
44. Russel JC, Cooper CM, Ketchum CH, et al. Multicenter evaluation of TDx test for assessing fetal lung maturity. *Clin Chem* 1980;35:1005.

Obstetric Anesthesia, second edition,
edited by Mark C. Norris.
Lippincott Williams & Wilkins, Philadelphia © 1999.

CHAPTER 8

Fetal Complications

William L. Holcomb Jr., and Sherrie Buchmeier

As a rule, the fetus is the more vulnerable member of the maternal–fetal pair. When there is a threat to the pregnant woman, homeostatic mechanisms operate to preserve the life of the mother at the expense of the fetus. Situations of abnormal fetal number, growth, physiology, or structure place the fetus at particular risk. Events well tolerated by a normal singleton fetus may be devastating when there are preexisting fetal complications. The anesthesiologist, working with other members of the obstetrical team, has a unique opportunity to improve pregnancy outcome in these challenging situations. Antepartum evaluation and implications of several common fetal conditions are the focus of this chapter.

TWIN GESTATIONS

The proportion of pregnancies complicated by twin gestation has increased substantially in recent years, largely because of assisted reproductive technology (1). The magnitude of risk associated with twin gestations is unappreciated by most laypersons and many health professionals. Perinatal mortality is at least fivefold higher for a twin fetus than for a singleton (2). Fetal growth restriction, 10 times more prevalent in twins, is associated with most intrauterine deaths, whereas premature delivery, especially before 30 weeks gestation, accounts for most neonatal deaths (3). Preeclampsia and gestational diabetes also are more common during twin pregnancies and can affect fetal growth and well-being.

Risk Assessment

We can predict much of the risk in twin pregnancy when the type of placentation is known (4). The greater the extent of chorioamnionic sharing, the greater the fetal risk. Approximately 80% of twins are dizygotic, all of which are diamnionic/dichorionic. The situation is more complex for monozygotic twins. About 30% of these are dichorionic, but the remainder share a single placenta (5). As a result of placental sharing, vascular communication between the twins greatly increases the risk for both fetuses.

The clinical syndrome of twin–twin transfusion (TTTS) complicates about 20% of monochorionic twin gestations (6). It occurs when one or more placental arteriovenous anastomoses result in a net transfer of blood from one twin to the other. Interestingly, the number of vascular anastomoses with TTTS placentas is fewer than with non-TTTS monochorionic placentas, there being a paucity of artery-to-artery and vein-to-vein connections in TTTS (7). Some postulate that the bidirectional like-vessel anastomoses buffer and compensate for the unidirectional arteriovenous anastomoses, preventing TTTS (7,8). Typically, the donor twin is small for gestational age with decreased or absent amniotic fluid, whereas the recipient is normally grown, or large, with polyhydramnios. Risk of perinatal death is extremely high with TTTS. In historical series with expectant management, the perinatal survival was as low as 5% (9). The donor twin is at greater risk before delivery, but after delivery, the recipient twin is at greater jeopardy.

When the twins share a single amniotic sac, as well a single placenta, there is the additional risk of cord entanglement that may result in the death of one or both twins. About 1% of twin gestations are monoamnionic. Cord complications resulting in fetal death most often occur before 30 weeks' gestation, but, as the case Fig. 1 illustrates, they may occur at any time in gestation (10).

The most extreme degree of sharing results in conjoined twins, a usually fatal, but fortunately rare, occurrence.

W. L. Holcomb Jr.: Division of Maternal-Fetal Medicine, Department of Obstetrics and Gynecology, Washington University School of Medicine, St. Louis, Missouri 63110.
S. Buchmeier: Divisions of Genetics, Maternal-Fetal Medicine, and Ultrasound, Department of Obstetrics and Gynecology, Washington University in St. Louis, St. Louis, Missouri 63110.

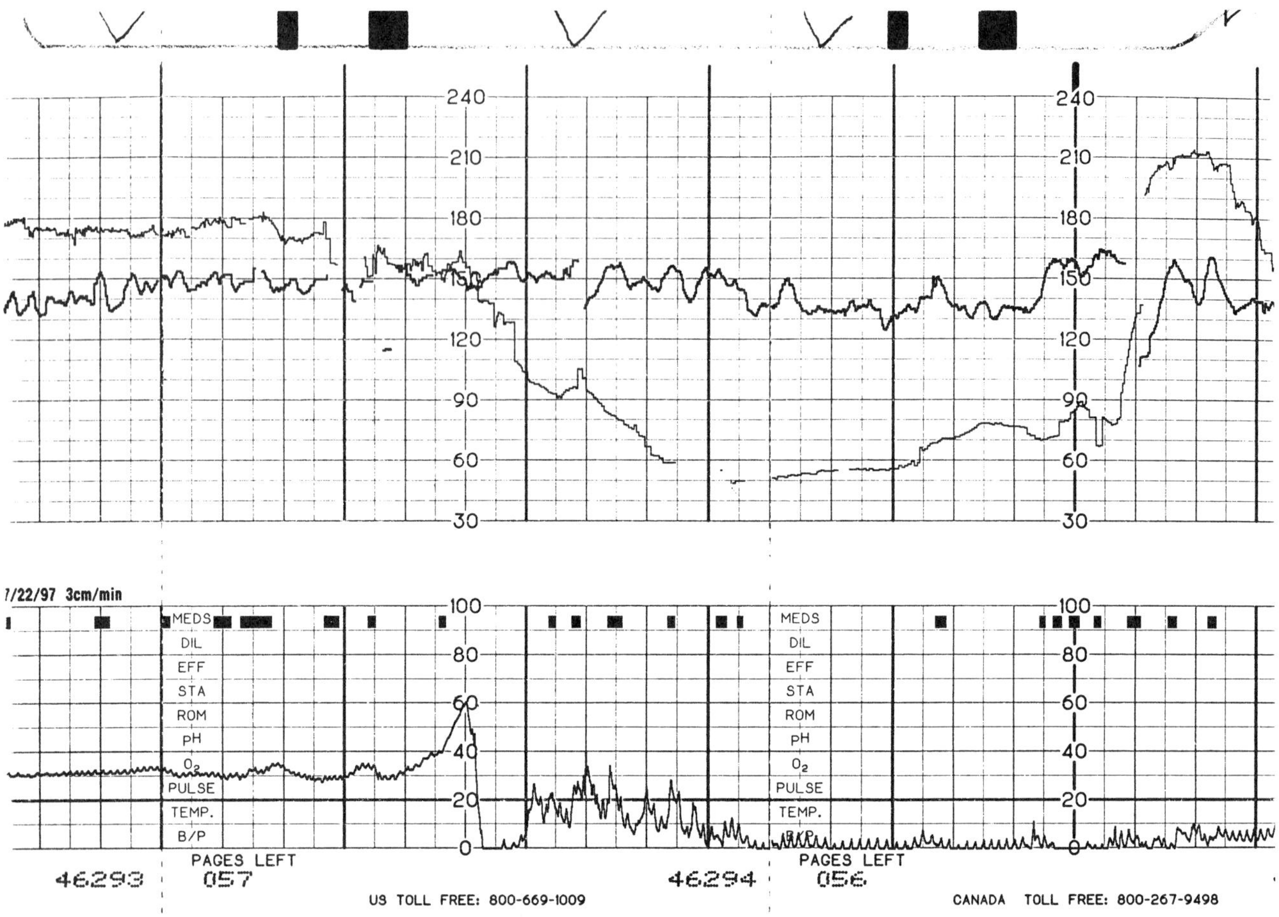

7/22/97 3cm/min

MEDS
DIL
EFF
STA
ROM
pH
O_2
PULSE
TEMP.
B/P

46293 PAGES LEFT 057

US TOLL FREE: 800-669-1009

46294 PAGES LEFT 056

CANADA TOLL FREE: 800-267-9498

A

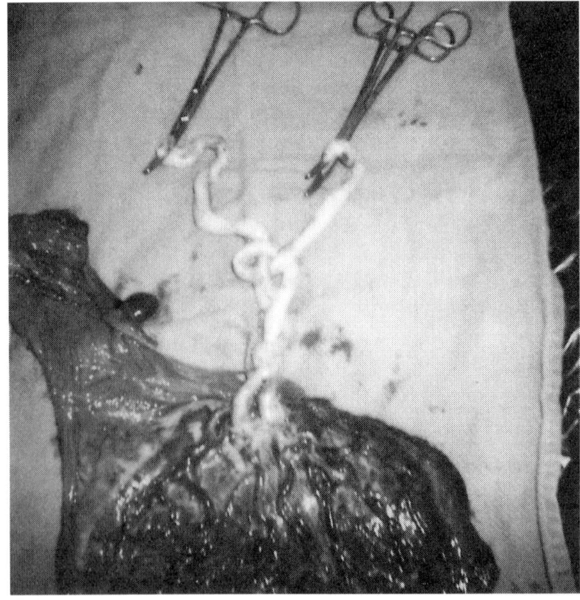

B

FIG. 1. A woman with monoamnionic twins was hospitalized at 33 weeks' gestation. The fetal heart monitor tracing showed a severe deceleration for one twin (**A**). At cesarean delivery a few moments later, there were tangled umbilical cords (**B**).

Ultrasonic imaging is the mainstay of evaluation for twin gestations. Before 10 weeks' gestation, when the chorionic rings are still distinct, chorionicity can reliably be determined. Later in gestation, monochorionic gestation can be ruled out if two placentas are physically separate from one another, if the genders of the twins differ, or if there is a clear "twin peak" sign (Fig. 2) (11). The thickness of the intervening membrane is a clue to chorionicity, but this sign can be misleading, especially later in gestation (12,13). Diagnosis of monoamnionic gestation can be more difficult than it would seem. Often careful scanning will reveal a previously unseen intervening membrane, or the membrane may be so tightly applied to one of the fetuses that it is not distinguishable from the fetal surface with sonography (the "shrink-wrapped" fetus) (14).

Management

Adequate care of twin gestations requires serial sonographic assessment of fetal growth and amniotic fluid volume. Structural fetal anomalies, more common in twin gestations, also may be detected with sonography. Discordancy of fetal growth is variably defined, but marked difference in twin size (greater than 20% to 25%) is associated with increased perinatal mortality (15,16). Smaller than expected size may be due to TTTS (in the donor twin) or, more often, is due to uteroplacental insufficiency or constitutional factors. Abnormalities of amniotic fluid volume are relatively common in twins and are associated with increased perinatal morbidity. Chau et al. (17) described reference ranges for sonographic assessment of amniotic fluid volume in diamnionic twin gestations.

Prematurity

Because prematurity is the greatest threat to twins, successful strategies to prevent preterm birth are needed. Current management, by using preterm labor education, limitation of maternal activity, contraction monitoring, and tocolytic agents is of limited effectiveness. There is some controversy about the ability of glucocorticoids to accelerate lung maturation in twins at increased risk for preterm delivery. Nonetheless, this therapy is reasonable and is widely used (18).

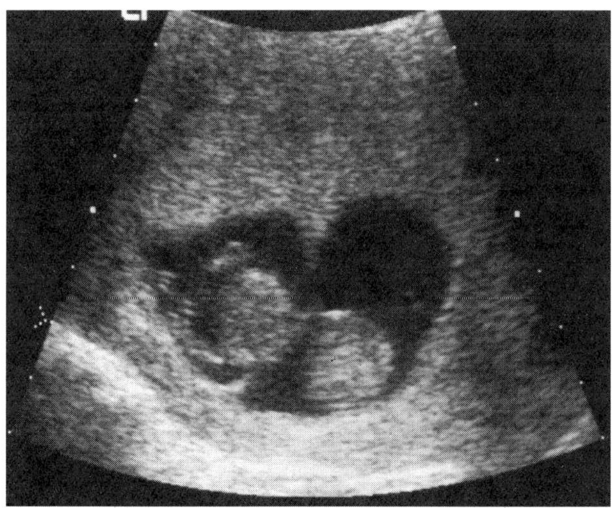

FIG. 2. Twin-peak sign (ultrasound image).

Twin–Twin Transfusion Syndrome

Several therapies are proposed for TTTS. The most widely available is serial amniocentesis from the sac of the recipient twin (19,20). Hydramnios in TTTS can be massive. Up to 5 L of amniotic fluid may be removed during one procedure (21). This approach has resulted in perinatal survival rates of 57% to 65% in recent series (21,22). Significant neonatal and long-term morbidity, mostly prematurity related, is common among survivors (21,23). Two series of patients have undergone intrauterine laser ablation of vascular connections within the shared placenta (24,25). Perinatal survival of 53% has been reported, but fetal loss is common within 24 hours of the procedure (25). The severity and onset of TTTS vary substantially, interfering with facile comparison of therapeutic outcomes between different study populations. The comparative efficacy and safety of treatments for TTTS will remain uncertain until prospective controlled trials are performed. In extreme situations, the donor twin has been aborted by umbilical cord occlusion to salvage the recipient twin (6,26).

MULTIFETAL GESTATIONS

The frequency of pregnancies with three or more fetuses also has increased because of the application of new reproductive technologies (27). Multifetal pregnancies are even more likely to develop all the complications of twin pregnancies; the higher the fetal number, the greater the risk (28,29). The same management strategies applied in twin pregnancies also are used when there are three or more fetuses, except that maternal nutrition is an even greater challenge, and activity restriction and tocolysis are typically started at an earlier gestational age.

To limit the perinatal morbidity and mortality of multifetal pregnancy, particularly when there are four or more fetuses, multifetal reduction procedures are performed at some centers. Reduction of four or more fetuses to twins confers a clear survival advantage and decreases morbidity for the remaining twins (30). There is evidence of improved outcome for the remaining fetuses when triplets are reduced to twins; however, the benefit with triplets is not so clear, and the practice is more controversial than with higher-order gestations (31–34). Twins resulting from multifetal reduction may be at increased risk for some pregnancy complications (preeclampsia, preterm birth, growth restriction, discordant growth) compared with spontaneous twins (35,36). Delivery of multifetal gestations is usually by cesarean section; however, vaginal delivery may be a reasonable option in selected cases (37).

FETAL GROWTH DISORDERS

Small for gestational age (SGA) is a label applied to fetuses with sonographically estimated weights less than the tenth percentile. The diagnosis depends on the accuracy of pregnancy dating and the reference standard used (38). Most fetuses, so designated, are probably constitutionally small and at low risk for perinatal morbidity and mortality. Some fetuses, in contrast, are affected by specific pathology decreasing overall cell number or size. The term intrauterine growth restriction (IUGR) is best reserved for the fetus with a factor or factors interfering with growth (Table 1), as opposed to the constitutionally small, but normal, fetus. In general, the more fetal size deviates from the norm, the more likely there is a pathological cause and the greater the perinatal risk (Fig. 3) (39).

Because the specific diagnosis and prognosis are often in doubt antepartum, obstetricians rely on fetal heart rate monitoring (e.g., nonstress tests) or sonographic assessment (e.g., biophysical profiles) to gain reassurance about fetal well-being and to aid the timing of delivery. Serial sonographic assessment of growth and amniotic fluid volume is essential in management. Doppler flow waveforms from the umbilical artery or other fetal vessels also give prognostic information about perinatal outcome for the small fetus. The finding of absent or reversed diastolic flow in the umbilical artery is a particularly worrisome finding associated with high risk of perinatal mortality (40).

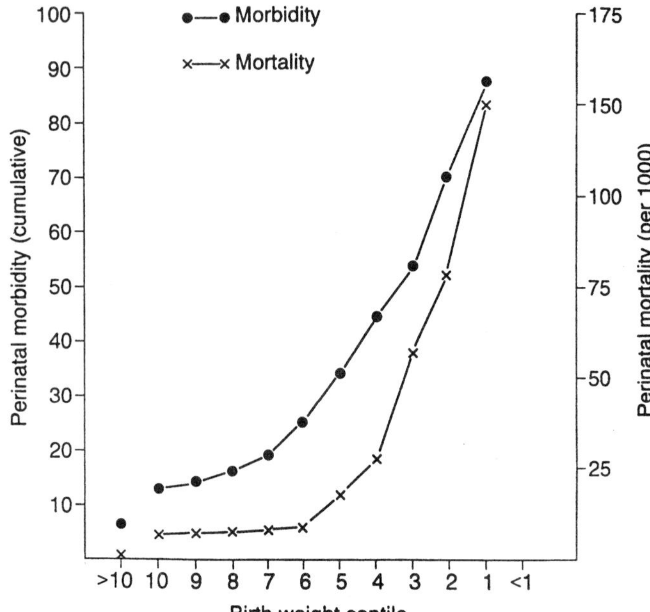

FIG. 3. The relation between birth weight percentile and perinatal morbidity and mortality among fetuses monitored at the University of Manitoba (1987 to 1993). (After ref. 39, with permission.)

TABLE 1. *Some conditions associated with fetal growth restriction*

Maternal disease
Preeclampsia
Chronic hypertension
Diabetic vasculopathy
Collagen vascular disease
Antiphospholipid antibody syndrome
Renal disease
Pulmonary disease
Cyanotic heart disease
Severe malnutrition
Hyperthyroidism
Toxins
Alcohol
Tobacco
Intrauterine infections
Cytomegalovirus
Rubella
Syphilis
Genetic abnormalities
Trisomy (13, 18, 21)
Turner syndrome
Triploidy
Uniparental disomy
Specific syndromes (e.g., Bloom, de Lange)
Fetal structural abnormalities
Abdominal-wall defects
Urinary tract defects
Pancreatic atresia
Multiple gestation

As long as fetal growth continues, and antepartum testing is reassuring, delivery is usually delayed until term or until fetal lung maturity is confirmed by amniotic fluid testing. The fetus that is SGA because of uteroplacental vascular disease may tolerate labor poorly and require cesarean delivery. The fetus also may deteriorate rapidly under conditions of decreased uterine blood flow (i.e., maternal hypotension).

Excessive fetal growth also increases the risk of perinatal morbidity and mortality (41). Large for gestational age (LGA) designates the fetus with sonographically estimated weight greater than the 90th percentile. Macrosomia variably refers to fetuses with birth weight greater than 4,000 or 4,500 grams. Although most LGA fetuses are constitutionally large, maternal diabetes, prolonged gestation, or rare conditions, such as Beckwith–Wiedemann syndrome, predispose to excessive fetal growth. Interestingly, even in nondiabetic pregnancy, there is a positive correlation between relative birth weight and fetal insulin concentration, suggesting an important role for insulin in the modulation of fetal growth (42).

Excessive fetal size increases the risk for abnormal labor, birth trauma, and cesarean section. Currently our ability to decrease this risk is limited. First, sonographic estimation of fetal weight, especially in the large fetus (more than 4,500 g), is frustratingly inaccurate (43). Second, the strategy of labor induction to avoid delivering a larger baby, at least in nondiabetic pregnancy, has not been shown to decrease the likelihood of cesarean section or of shoulder dystocia (44). Third, the routine performance of elective cesarean section based on a sonographic diagnosis of fetal macrosomia is probably a medically unsound approach, except in the presence of maternal diabetes (45,46). Various methods have been proposed to predict shoulder dystocia, one of the more threatening complications associated with excessive fetal growth. All of these methods have low positive predictive value, limiting clinical usefulness. Most clinicians avoid midpelvic operative vaginal deliveries when fetal macrosomia is suspected with a prolonged second stage of labor. This concurrence is associated with a 23% risk of shoulder dystocia (47).

All members of the obstetric team may be urgently needed when shoulder dystocia occurs. For the fetus healthy at the onset of delivery, the obstetrician has about 5 minutes safely to resolve the dystocia. The natural tendency to pull harder on the fetal head must be resisted, as this may injure the fetal brachial plexus. Several standard maneuvers to accomplish delivery are sharp flexion of the maternal hips (the McRobert's maneuver), suprapubic pressure, rotation of the fetus in the pelvis (Woods' or Rubin's maneuvers), or delivery of the posterior fetal arm (48). The anesthesiologist may be asked to support a maternal hip in sharp flexion or to apply firm suprapubic pressure. In rare instances, general anesthesia may be needed to facilitate intravaginal maneuvers or to allow replacement of the fetal head into the uterus, followed by cesarean section (the Zavanelli maneuver) (49).

FETAL DYSRHYTHMIA

Fetal dysrhythmias complicate about 1% to 2% of pregnancies and, fortunately, are often benign and transient (50,51). The most frequent dysrhythmia is repetitive extrasystole, usually of atrial origin, noted with routine fetal heart rate assessment at a prenatal visit. Because of the association between fetal dysrhythmia and structural cardiac defects, a thorough sonographic assessment of fetal cardiac anatomy is warranted in these cases. In the absence of structural defects, the patient may be monitored with periodic assessment of fetal heart rate to rule out development of a sustained tachycardia, although this occurs in only about 1% of cases (52). The mother is advised to avoid caffeine or other substances that may contribute to fetal extrasystoles.

With sustained fetal tachycardia, particularly at rates greater than 230 beats/min, inadequate ventricular filling may lead to fetal hydrops and death (53). The most common fetal tachydysrhythmias are supraventricular tachycardia and atrial flutter, but atrial fibrillation or ventricular tachycardia may occur in utero (51,54). Careful sonographic study of atrial and ventricular activity, by using two-dimensional imaging, M-mode, and pulsed Doppler ultrasonography, allows characterization of the dysrhythmia to guide therapy. In addition, the sonographer looks for evidence of fetal hydrops. A clear indication for intrauterine therapy is sustained fetal tachycardia with hydrops in a pregnancy remote from term. Because lesser degrees of tachycardia may be well tolerated or may resolve spontaneously, the indications for therapy in the absence of hydrops are controversial (51,53). Any coincidental maternal cardiac abnormalities or other conditions that may increase the risk of therapy should be detected and considered in planning management.

Intrauterine therapy of fetal tachyarrhythmias is possible by administering antiarrhythmics to the mother. Maternally administered digitalis has been used to treat fetal tachydysrhythmias since the early 1980s and is generally regarded to be the safest agent available for this purpose (55). Because of increased clearance during pregnancy, higher dosages of digoxin are required (54). Intravenous loading of 1 to 1.5 mg over 24 hours followed by an oral maintenance dose of 0.5 to 0.75 mg per day may be necessary to achieve the desired serum concentration of about 2 ng/mL (56,57). In a series of 35 treated pregnancies, digoxin alone restored sinus rhythm in 55% of nonhydropic fetuses, but in only 8% of hydropic fetuses (56). Flecainide has been used in combination with digoxin or as an alternative first-line agent, especially when there is fetal hydrops, in which case, it appears to be more effective than digoxin alone (56,57). One regimen is to start with 100 mg flecainide three times daily orally and adjust to achieve a serum level of 0.5 to 1 μg/mL (56). Minor increases in serum digoxin concentration may be expected when flecainide is added (54). Although it is widely used, there are some concerns about the safety of flecainide because of one report of a fetal death and the potential for proarrhythmic side effects (57–59).

Refractory fetal tachydysrhythmias associated with fetal decompensation have been treated with amiodarone, a potent iodine-containing antiarrhythmic agent with a relatively high risk of toxicity. Of particular concern is the potential for fetal thyroid dysfunction and, possibly, neurological abnormalities (60,61). Thyroid dysfunction was reported in two of 12 exposed newborns in one series (61). The fetal benefits of therapy must be weighed against the fetal and maternal risks. Anesthetic management for cesarean section in a woman receiving amiodarone is discussed in one report. The authors advocated an epidural block by using lidocaine with epinephrine and fentanyl (62).

Other agents, such as procainamide, quinidine, propranolol, and verapamil, have been used for therapy of fetal tachydysrhythmias. Verapamil has lost favor because it has been implicated in fatal myocardial depression in the neonate and fetus (51,57). A good resource for pharmacologic aspects of transplacental therapy for fetal dysrhythmias is the review by Ito et al. (54). Direct injection of antiarrhythmics (digoxin and adenosine) into the fetal muscle or umbilical vein has been described but is rarely needed (63,64).

Persistent fetal bradycardia, usually associated with complete atrioventricular block, is a less common abnormality, occurring in about 1 in 22,000 live births (65). In about half the cases, complex structural cardiac defects are present, and the perinatal prognosis is poor. In most other cases, there is a maternal antibody (e.g., anti-SSA or anti-SSB) capable of crossing the placenta to injure the fetal cardiac-conduction system (66). The stimulus for maternal antibody production and the mechanism of fetal cardiac injury are unclear (67). Prognosis is related inversely to the ventricular rate and the presence of hydrops (66). Results of pharmacologic therapy in utero have been disappointing. Intrauterine ventricular pacing has been studied in sheep and may be a feasible future therapy (68). A practical issue is how to monitor fetal well-being during labor in cases of fetal atrioventricular block. Various approaches have been described, including sonographic assessment of fetal activity and the atrial heart rate, scalp-blood gas measurement, or intrapartum fetal pulse oximetry (69). At times, cesarean section is used when there is a reasonable chance for viability of the newborn, and intrapartum well-being cannot be assured.

ALLOIMMUNIZATION

Transplacental passage of maternal immunoglobulin G (IgG) antibody allows birth of an infant protected against microbial pathogens in the newborn period. However, antibody directed against fetal tissue antigens can cause fetal disease or death (70). The classic example of such a disorder is red cell alloimmunization. Despite the widespread use of anti-D gamma-globulin to prevent maternal sensitization, anti-D antibody is still the most common cause of alloimmune fetal anemia. Some other antibodies associated with fetal anemia are those directed against other Rhesus antigens (c, C, e, and E), Kell antigens (K and k), Duffy antigens (Fy^a), and Kidd antigens (Jk^a and Jk^b) (71). Fortunately, some common antibodies (e.g., anti-Lewis antibody) are not pathogenic.

Anti-Kell antibody deserves special mention. This antibody can cause fetal anemia at relatively lower titers than other antibodies (72). In addition, when anti-Kell is present, fetal hematocrit is poorly correlated with amniotic fluid bilirubin levels (as measured by the change in optical density at 450 nm) (73). For these reasons, direct umbilical blood sampling is more often required with anti-Kell. Other non-Kell pathogenic antibodies seem to behave similar to anti-D. A flow chart for evaluation of the mother with a positive screen for red cell antibodies is shown in Fig. 4.

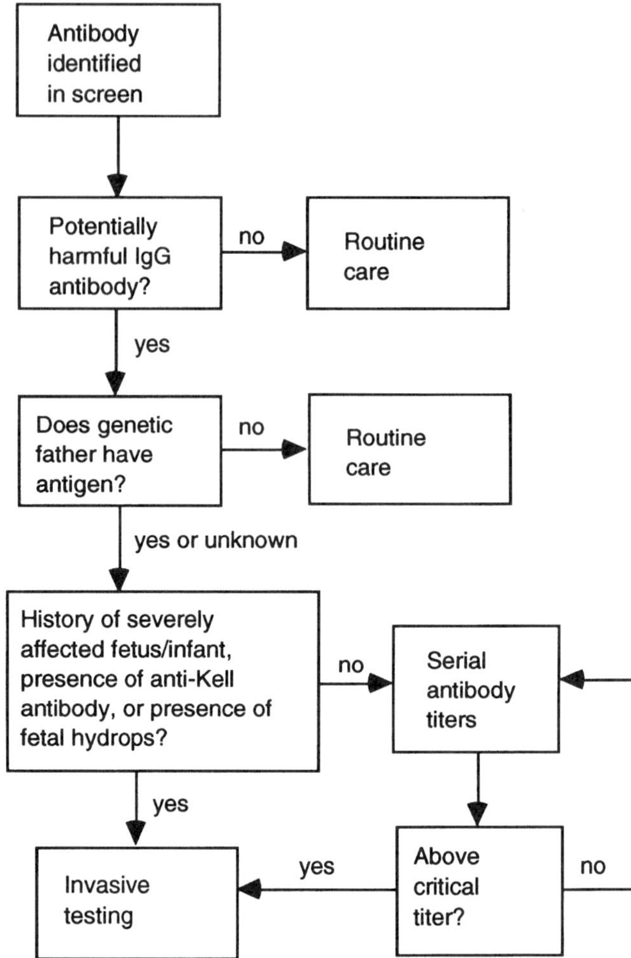

FIG. 4. Evaluation of positive antibody screen.

The outcome for anemic fetuses has improved markedly with the advent of direct fetal transfusion via the umbilical vein, a technique made possible by high-resolution ultrasound imaging. A hypothetical cohort of 100 alloimmunized patients, as presented by Moise (Fig. 5), illustrates current expected outcomes (74). Fetuses requiring intrauterine transfusions who survive the perinatal period appear to have normal long-term development (75).

Fetal hydrops distant from term is a clear indication for intrauterine transfusion. Because the occurrence of hydrops is associated with a less favorable perinatal outcome, a goal of therapy is the prevention of hydrops. The optimal threshold for initiation of intrauterine transfusions is unknown; many centers use a fetal hematocrit cut-off of 30% (74,76,77). Intrauterine transfusions are conceptually straightforward, but technically challenging, and always require meticulous attention to detail. Freshly packed, O-negative, cytomegalovirus (CMV)-negative, irradiated packed red cells spun to a hematocrit of 85% to 90% are transfused to achieve a normal fetal hematocrit (77). The volume required depends on the opening fetal hematocrit and the fetoplacental blood volume, which is

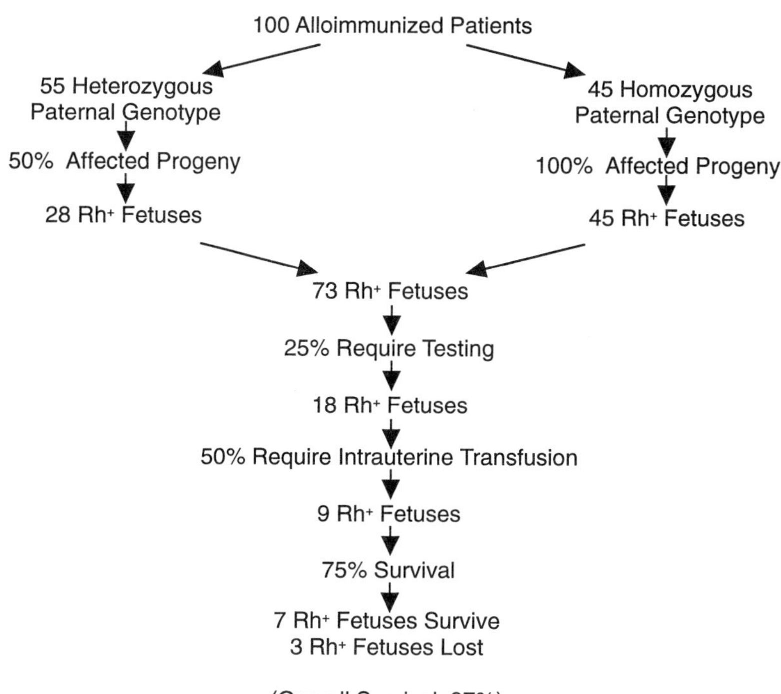

FIG. 5. Expected outcome in 100 patients with red cell alloimmunization.

estimated by using various formulae (78). Especially beyond the threshold of viability (about 24 to 25 weeks' gestation), the anesthesiologist is a critical member of the intrauterine transfusion team. Monitoring the mother's tolerance of the procedure and administering intravenous sedation may improve the ease and success of the transfusion. Depending on the location of the umbilical vein puncture site, fetal administration of muscle relaxants (e.g., pancuronium, 0.1 to 0.3 mg/kg, or vecuronium, 0.1 mg/kg estimated fetal weight) via the umbilical vein may help prevent fetal movement from dislodging the needle (79,80). These agents also can be administered to the fetus intramuscularly by sonographic guidance.

Procedure-related complications during intrauterine transfusions may be dramatic. Major complications include excessive bleeding from the umbilical cord puncture site, cord hematoma, and persistent fetal bradycardia. In the event of a complication, an immediate cesarean section may be needed. The newborn, in this circumstance, will often require intensive volume and ventilatory resuscitation.

Alloimmune thrombocytopenia complicates about 1 of 1,000 pregnancies (81). The most common pathogenic antibody is directed against HPA1 (Pl^{A1}), a platelet glycoprotein antigen absent in about 3% of the population (82). Unlike alloimmune anemia, alloimmune thrombocytopenia is often severe in the first pregnancy. Most cases are referred for evaluation and therapy because of a previously affected sibling (83). The gravest risk is intracranial hemorrhage, which occurs in 10% to 20% of affected fetus/newborns, with 25% to 50% of these occurring antepartum (83). Fetal thrombocytopenia is sometimes severe and of early onset. A case of in utero intracranial hemorrhage at 16 weeks' gestation was reported (84). Antepartum therapies include maternal administration of high-dose intravenous immune globulin (e.g., 1 g/kg/week) with or without glucocorticoids (83–85). In a series of 107 affected fetuses, only one treated fetus had an intracranial hemorrhage (83). Another treatment modality is serial fetal platelet transfusions (84). Umbilical blood sampling is necessary to establish the need for therapy and to monitor response. Initial sampling is often carried out between 20 and 24 weeks' gestation and carries some risk of fetal exsanguination if the platelet count is very low (84,86). Performing immediate intrauterine platelet transfusions if the fetal count is $<50 \times 10^9$/L may help to protect against this complication (86).

As an initial procedure when the father of the baby is heterozygous for a red cell or platelet antigen, or when zygosity is unknown, amniocentesis for amplification of amniocyte DNA can be performed to establish the fetal genotype and the need for further testing. Amniocyte genotyping is available for most pathogenic red cell and platelet antigens (87,88). Single-cell techniques may even be applied to the blastomere for preimplantation diagnosis (89).

FETAL STRUCTURAL ABNORMALITIES

With the widespread use of fetal ultrasound imaging and maternal serum α-fetoprotein testing, many fetal abnormalities are diagnosed before birth. Depending on the parents, antenatal diagnosis allows either pregnancy termination or the time to prepare for the birth of a child with special needs. It also allows the obstetric and pediatric teams to optimize conditions for the transition from intrauterine to extrauterine life. The following abnormalities are relatively common or of special clinical significance for the obstetric team.

Spina Bifida

Spina bifida is the most common of a group of anomalies associated with incomplete closure of the neural tube during embryonic development (Fig. 6). About 80% of lesions are detected prenatally in maternal α-fetoprotein screening programs. Neural tube defects occur in 1 to 2 per 1,000 pregnancies in the United States, with greater frequency in those of northern European extraction than in those of African, Mediterranean, or Asian ethnicity (90). Most lesions are associated with herniation of meninges, a meningocele. In some cases, neural tissue is contained in the hernia sac (i.e., myelomeningocele).

Spina bifida is usually associated with hydrocephalus and posterior fossa anomalies referred to as the Arnold–Chiari, type II malformation. The distorted cranial anatomy is an important clue in the sonographic diagnosis of neural tube defects (91). The range of physical and developmental impairment associated with spina bifida is vast, depending, in part, on the size and location of the lesion. Prenatal sonographic findings are helpful in predicting the degree of functional impairment, but substantial prognostic uncertainty remains (92,93).

The optimal route of delivery for fetuses with spina bifida is highly controversial. Luthy et al. (94) showed that infants exposed to labor had about twice the risk of severe paralysis compared with those delivered by cesarean section without labor. Important confounding variables, including prenatal detection of meningomyelocele and delivery at a tertiary center, which could not be controlled in this retrospective study, may account for some or all of the difference in outcome. Another retrospective study (95) found no benefit to cesarean delivery of the vertex-presenting fetus with meningomyelocele. No randomized clinical trial has been performed to clarify this issue.

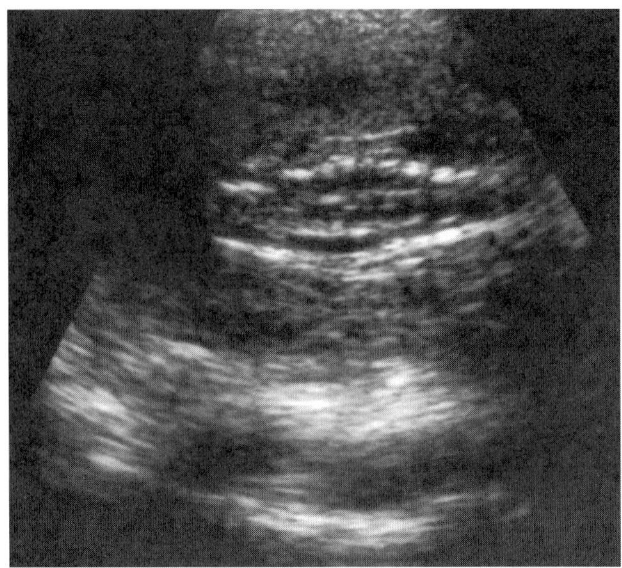

FIG. 6. Spina bifida (ultrasound image).

Hydrocephalus

Dilated fetal cerebral ventricles, unassociated with spina bifida, may be an isolated finding or may be associated with chromosomal or other structural fetal anomalies (Fig. 7). Congenital hydrocephalus, without spina bifida, intracranial tumors, or secondary brain atrophy, is diagnosed in about one child per 1,000 births (96). In boys, isolated dilation of the lateral and third ventricles may be due to X-linked aqueductal stenosis. A thorough sonographic assessment and fetal chromosomal analysis is warranted when hydrocephalus is diagnosed antenatally. Fetal prognosis is largely dependent on the presence of other abnormalities. Prediction of neurological deficit based on the size of the ventricles or the thickness of the cerebral mantle is fraught with uncertainty. However, in general, the more extreme the abnormality, the greater the likelihood of long-term deficit.

Large head size (biparietal diameter greater than 10 cm) associated with progressive hydrocephalus can pose obstetric difficulties. In some cases, labor is induced early, after confirmation of fetal lung maturity by amniocentesis, to allow vaginal delivery before the head is too big. Cesarean section is sometimes necessary and, with extremely large head size, may need to be performed through a vertical uterine incision. In situations with a lethal or dismal prognosis, cephalocentesis to allow a vaginal delivery may be justified. This procedure almost always leads to fetal or neonatal death (97).

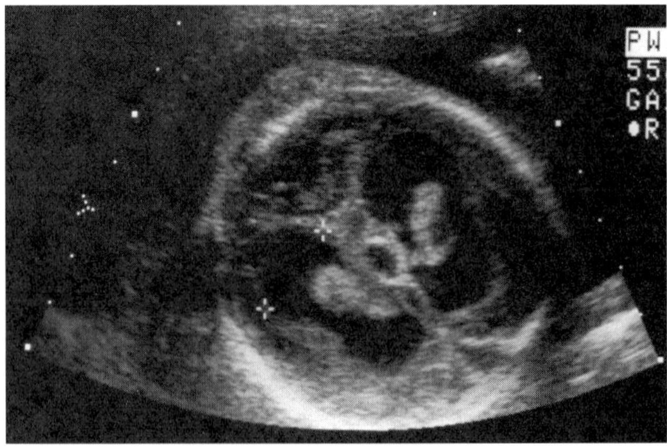

FIG. 7. Hydrocephalus (ultrasound image).

Cardiac Anomalies

A major structural abnormality of the heart affects one in 125 fetuses. Associated noncardiac anomalies are common, and chromosomal abnormalities occur in about 30% of prenatally diagnosed cases (51). The prenatal detection of cardiac anomalies depends on the particular cardiac lesion, the gestational age at assessment, fetal position, maternal habitus, and the thoroughness of sonographic evaluation. Even under the best of circumstances, many cardiac defects are not diagnosed prenatally (98).

Careful diagnosis and planning for delivery can be critical when a fetal cardiac defect is detected. Some lesions (e.g., hypoplastic left heart syndrome) depend on patency of the ductus arteriosus for systemic circulation of oxygenated blood. In these cases, delivery at a tertiary center, with a prostaglandin infusion to maintain ductal patency at hand, may be lifesaving.

Thoracic Anomalies

Noncardiac thoracic anomalies are most often recognized prenatally as masses in the fetal chest, which, depending on size and location, may displace the heart and mediastinum. Any mass of sufficient size presumably can lead to compressive pulmonary hypoplasia.

The differential diagnosis for a thoracic mass includes diaphragmatic hernia (Fig. 8), cystic adenomatoid malformation, and pulmonary sequestration. With the latter two lesions, fetal hydrops may result from hemodynamic alterations and cardiac dysfunction.

The fetal prognosis depends on the presence of associated anomalies or hydrops and the extent to which pulmonary growth and development has been arrested (99). In the presence of fetal hydrops, a preeclamptic state, termed the "mirror syndrome," can threaten the mother and necessitate prompt delivery (100). The newborn with a thoracic mass may seem unaffected at birth or may have profound respiratory insufficiency. Antenatal prediction of newborn pulmonary function is unreliable. Delivery at a site with suitable pediatric and pediatric surgical personnel is critical.

Abdominal Wall Anomalies

Omphalocele and gastroschisis are relatively common fetal anomalies that can be diagnosed prenatally. Gastroschisis is a paramedian, usually right-sided, abdominal wall defect through which free loops of bowel protrude into the amniotic fluid (Fig. 9). Occurring in approximately 1:10,000 births, it is almost always an isolated anomaly with, generally, a good prognosis for repair in the newborn (101). The fetus with gastroschisis is more likely to be SGA and to be delivered preterm (102–105). There appears to be an increased risk of stillbirth and abnormal antepartum fetal testing (106). Dilation of the extra-abdominal fetal bowel loops can sometimes be detected sonographically. This finding is associated with a more complicated and prolonged postsurgical course for the infant, but it remains unproven that an expedited delivery, based on this finding, is beneficial (107,108). The preferred route of delivery with fetal gastroschisis is highly controversial (102,104,105,109–111). Unfortunately, there are no well-controlled studies to help guide obstetric management. At our institution, we favor vaginal delivery unless there is a specific indication for cesarean delivery. Skilled pediatric attendants should be present in the delivery room.

Omphalocele is herniation of abdominal contents within an amnion-covered sac through an umbilical defect. The prevalence of fetal omphalocele is about 2.5 per 10,000 births (112). It is often associated with other

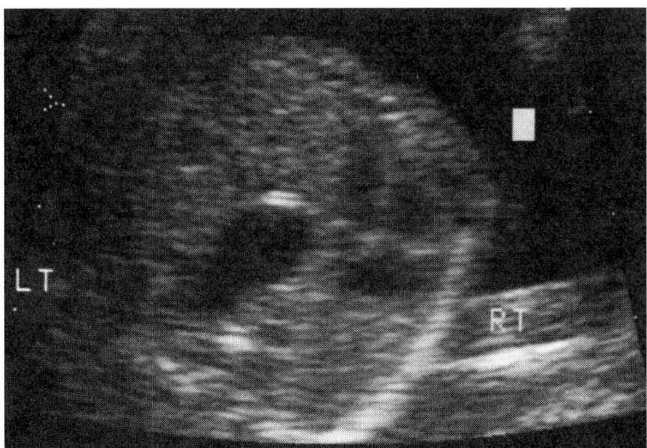

FIG. 8. Diaphragmatic hernia (ultrasound image).

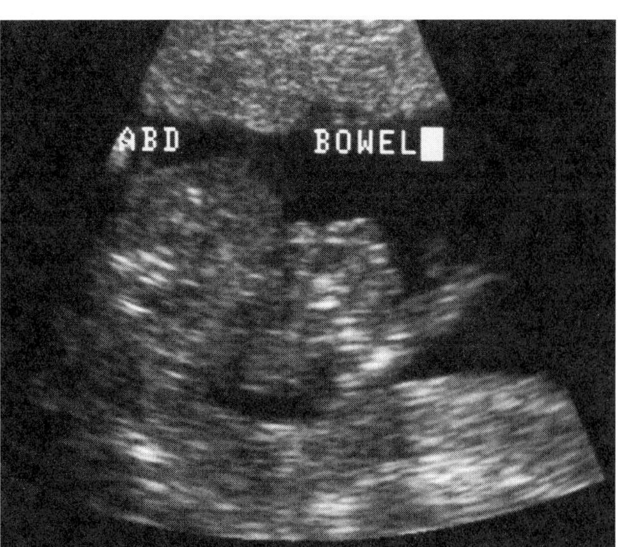

FIG. 9. Gastroschisis (ultrasound image).

anomalies and, in about 30% of cases, there are karyotypic abnormalities, usually trisomy 18 (101,113). Prenatal sonographic findings reported to be associated with karyotypic abnormalities are the presence of other structural abnormalities, absence of liver in the hernia sac, and small hernia size (113). The prognosis with fetal omphalocele depends on the associated anomalies. As with gastroschisis, the fetus with omphalocele is more likely to be SGA, intolerant of labor, and delivered preterm (101). Decision about route of delivery must be individualized. Relevant factors are the size of the defect, prognosis for the newborn, and the presence of other obstetric indications.

Fetal Teratomas

Fetal sacrococcygeal teratomas (occurring in about one in 40,000 pregnancies) are thought to arise from pluripotent cells in the region of Hensen's node near the coccyx and can extend both externally or internally into the pelvis (Fig. 10) (114). They can be quite vascular, behaving like an arteriovenous shunt that can lead to fetal cardiac failure, hydrops, and death (115). Occasionally they are very large and cause soft-tissue dystocia at the time of delivery. In such cases, there is risk of avulsion and hemorrhage. Cesarean delivery is often required to deliver the mass intact safely, particularly if the tumor is greater than 5 cm in diameter (114,116).

Teratomas arising from the fetal neck or oropharynx, fortunately much more rare, can occlude the airway of the newborn at birth (Fig. 11). At a carefully orchestrated delivery, with pediatric and otolaryngologic attendants, the airway can sometimes be secured before delivery of the fetal thorax, a potentially life-saving maneuver (see Chapter 10) (117).

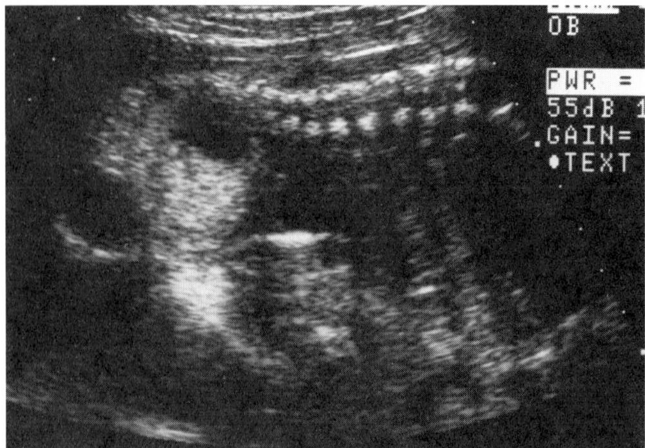

FIG. 10. Sacrococcygeal teratoma (ultrasound image).

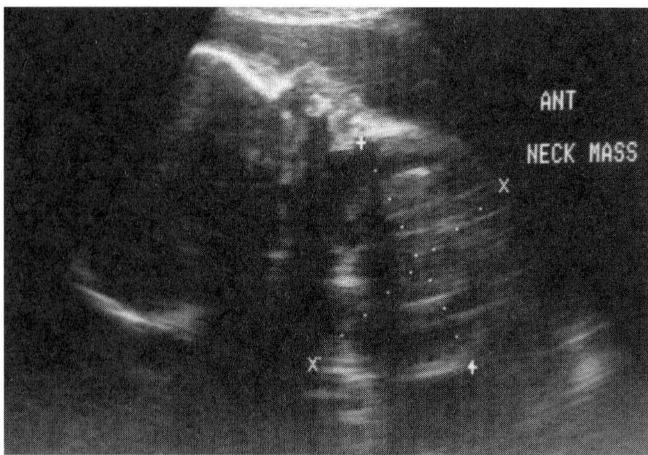

FIG. 11. Anterior neck teratoma (ultrasound image).

CONCLUSION

The fear and anxiety associated with childbirth are heightened for the mother aware of a fetal complication. Especially when referred to the hospital from a distance, she is often accompanied by relatives and friends, all of whom are worried and deprived of sleep. The patient may be less tolerant of pain in this setting. A skilled anesthesiologist, with a calm and comforting manner, can do much to relieve suffering for these pregnant women and their families.

ACKNOWLEDGMENT

We thank Drs. Dorothea Mostello and Diana Gray for their helpful comments regarding this chapter.

REFERENCES

1. Luke B. The changing pattern of multiple births in the U.S.: maternal and infant characteristics. *Obstet Gynecol* 1994;84:101.
2. Newman R, Ellings J. Antepartum management of the multiple gestation: the case for specialized care. *Semin Perinatol* 1995;19:387.
3. Manlon G, Scott K. Contributions of twin pregnancy to perinatal mortality and fetal growth retardation. *Can Med Assoc J* 1978;118:365.
4. Fisk N, Bryan E. Routine prenatal determination of chorionicity in multiple gestation: a plea to the obstetrician. *Br J Obstet Gynaecol* 1993;100:975.
5. Cameron A. The Birmingham twin survey. *Proc R Soc Med* 1968; 61:229.
6. Cincotta R, Fisk N. Current thoughts on twin-twin transfusion syndrome. *Clin Obstet Gynecol* 1997;40:290.
7. Bajoria R, Wigglesworth J, Fisk N. Angioarchitecture of monochorionic placentas in relation to the twin-twin transfusion syndrome. *Am J Obstet Gynecol* 1995;172:856.
8. Schatz F. Eine besondere Art von einseitiger Polyhydramnie mit anderseitiger Oligohydramnie bei eineiigen Zwillingen. *Arch Gynakol* 1882;19:329.
9. Saunders N, Nijders R, Nicolaides K. Therapeutic amniocentesis in twin-twin transfusion syndrome appearing in the second trimester of pregnancy. *Am J Obstet Gynecol* 1992;166:820.
10. Carr S, Aronson M, Coustan D. Survival rates of monoamniotic twins do not decrease after 30 weeks gestation. *Am J Obstet Gynecol* 1990; 163:719.

11. Finberg H. The "twin peak" sign: reliable evidence of dichorionic twinning. *J Ultrasound Med* 1992;11:571.
12. Barss V, Benacerraf B, Frigoletto F. Ultrasonographic determination of chorion type in twin gestation. *Obstet Gynecol* 1985;66:779.
13. Winn H, Gabrielli S, Reece E, et al. Ultrasonographic criteria for the prenatal diagnosis of placental chorionicity in twin gestations. *Am J Obstet Gynecol* 1989;161:1540.
14. Rodis J, Vintzileos A, Campbell W, Deaton J, Fumia F, Nochimson D. Antenatal diagnosis and management of monoamniotic twins. *Am J Obstet Gynecol* 1987;157:1255.
15. O'Brien W, Knuppel R, Scerbo J, et al. Birth weight in twins: an analysis of discordancy and growth retardation. *Obstet Gynecol* 1986;67:483.
16. Crane J, Tomich P, Kopta M. Ultrasonic growth patterns in normal and discordant twins. *Obstet Gynecol* 1980;55:678.
17. Chau A, Kjos S, Kovacs B. Ultrasonographic measurement of amniotic fluid volume in normal diamniotic twin pregnancies. *Am J Obstet Gynecol* 1996;174:1003.
18. NIH Consensus Development Panel. Effect of corticosteroids for fetal maturation on perinatal outcomes. *JAMA* 1995;273:413.
19. Mahony B, Petty C, Nyberg D, Luthy D, Hickok D, Hirsch J. The "stuck twin" phenomenon: ultrasonographic findings, pregnancy outcome and management with serial amniocenteses. *Am J Obstet Gynecol* 1990;163:1513.
20. Elliot J, Urig M, Clewell W. Aggressive therapeutic amniocentesis for treatment of twin-twin transfusion syndrome. *Obstet Gynecol* 1991; 77:537.
21. Trespidi L, Boschetto C, Caravelli E, Villa L, Kustermann A, Nicolini U. Serial amniocenteses in the management of twin-twin transfusion syndrome: when is it valuable? *Fetal Diagn Ther* 1997;12:15.
22. Dickinson J. Severe twin-twin transfusion syndrome: current management concepts. *Aust NZ J Obstet Gynecol* 1995;35:16.
23. Reisner D, Mahony B, Petty C, et al. Stuck twin syndrome: outcome in thirty-seven consecutive cases. *Am J Obstet Gynecol* 1993; 169:991.
24. DeLia J, Kuhlmann R, Harstad T, Cruikshank D. Fetoscopic laser ablation of placental vessels in severe previable twin-twin transfusion syndrome. *Obstet Gynecol* 1995;127:1202.
25. Ville Y, Hyett J, Hecher K, Nicolaides K. Preliminary experience with endoscopic surgery for severe twin-twin transfusion syndrome. *N Engl J Med* 1995;332:224.
26. Wittmann B, Farquharson D, Thomas W, Baldwin V, Wadsworth L. The role of feticide in the management of severe twin transfusion syndrome. *Am J Obstet Gynecol* 1986;155:1023.
27. Callahan T, Hall J, Ettner S, et al. The economic impact of multiple-gestation pregnancies and the contribution of assisted reproduction techniques to their incidence. *N Engl J Med* 1994;331:244.
28. Sassoon D, Castro L, Davis J, Hobel C. Perinatal outcome in triplet versus twin gestations. *Obstet Gynecol* 1990;75:817.
29. Seoud M, Toner J, Druithoff C, Muasher S. Outcome of twin, triplet, and quadruplet in vitro fertilization pregnancies: the Norfolk experience. *Fertil Steril* 1992;57:825.
30. Berkowitz R, Lynch L, Stone J, Alvarez M. The current status of multifetal pregnancy reduction. *Am J Obstet Gynecol* 1996;174:1265.
31. Lipitz S, Reichman B, Uval J, et al. a prospective comparison of the outcome of triplet pregnancies managed expectantly or by multifetal reduction. *Am J Obstet Gynecol* 1994;170:874.
32. Macones G, Schemmer G, Pritts E, Weinblatt V, Wapner R. Multifetal reduction of triplets to twins improves perinatal outcome. *Am J Obstet Gynecol* 1993;169:982.
33. Porreco R, Shannon-Burke M, Hendrix M. Multifetal reduction of triplet and pregnancy outcome. *Obstet Gynecol* 1991;78:335.
34. Boulot P, Hedon B, Pelliccia G, et al. Multifetal pregnancy reduction: a consecutive series of 61 cases. *Br J Obstet Gynecol* 1993;100:63.
35. Groutz A, Yovel I, Amit A, Yaron Y, Azem F, Lessing J. Pregnancy outcome after multifetal pregnancy reduction to twins compared with spontaneously conceived twins. *Hum Reprod* 1996;11:1334.
36. Silver R, Ragin A, Helfand B, Scholl J, Russell T, MacGregor S. Multifetal reduction increases the risk of preterm delivery and growth restriction in twins: a case-control study. *Fertil Steril* 1997;67:30.
37. Houlihan C, Knuppel R. Intrapartum management of multiple gestations. *Clin Perinatol* 1996;23:91.
38. Goldenberg R, Cutter G, Hoffman H, et al. Intrauterine growth retardation: standards for diagnosis. *Am J Obstet Gynecol* 1989;161:271.
39. Manning F. Intrauterine growth retardation: Diagnosis, prognostication, and management based on ultrasound. In: Fleischer A, Manning F, Jeanty P, Romero R, eds. *Sonography in obstetrics and gynecology.* 5th ed. Stamford, CT: Appleton & Lange, 1996:517.
40. Maulik D. Doppler ultrasound velocimetry for fetal surveillance. *Clin Obstet Gynecol* 1995;38:91.
41. Spellacy W, Miller S, Winegar A, Peterson P. Macrosomia: maternal characteristics and infant complications. *Obstet Gynecol* 1985; 66:158.
42. Hoegsberg B, Gruppuso P, Coustan D. Hyperinsulinemia in macrosomic infants of nondiabetic mothers. *Diabetes Care* 1993;16:32.
43. Owaidah M, Ouzounian J, Kjos S. The accuracy of intrapartum ultrasonographic fetal weight estimation in diabetic pregnancies. *Am J Obstet Gynecol* 1997;177:503.
44. Gonen O, Rosen D, Dolfin Z, Tepper R, Markov S, Fejgin M. Induction of labor versus expectant management in macrosomia: a randomized study. *Obstet Gynecol* 1997;89:913.
45. Rouse D, Owen J, Goldenberg R, Cliver S. The effectiveness and costs of elective cesarean delivery for fetal macrosomia diagnosed by ultrasound. *JAMA* 1996;276:1480.
46. Ecker J, Greenberg J, Norwitz E, Nadal A, Repke J. Birth weight as a predictor of brachial plexus injury. *Obstet Gynecol* 1997;89:643.
47. Benedetti T, Gabbe S. Shoulder dystocia: a complication of fetal macrosomia and prolonged second stage of labor with midpelvic delivery. *Obstet Gynecol* 1978;52:526.
48. Morrison J, Sanders J, Magann E, Wiser W. The diagnosis and management of dystocia of the shoulder. *Surg Gynecol Obstet* 1992; 175:515.
49. Sandberg E. The Zavanelli maneuver: a potentially revolutionary method for the resolution of shoulder dystocia. *Am J Obstet Gynecol* 1985;152:479.
50. Fyfe D, Meyer K, Case C. Sonographic assessment of fetal cardiac arrhythmias. *Semin Ultrasound CT MR* 1993;14:286.
51. Simpson L, Gerald R. Diagnosis and treatment of structural fetal cardiac abnormality and dysrhythmia. *Semin Perinatol* 1994;18:215.
52. Kleinman C. Prenatal diagnosis and management of intrauterine arrhythmias. *Fetal Ther* 1986;1:92.
53. Guntheroth W, Cyr D, Shields L, Nghiem H. Rate-based management of fetal supraventricular tachycardia. *J Ultrasound Med* 1996;15:453.
54. Ito S, Magee L, Smallhorn J. Drug therapy for fetal arrhythmias. *Fetal Drug Ther* 1994;21:543.
55. Lingman G, Ohrlander S, Ohlin P. Intrauterine digoxin treatment of fetal paroxysmal tachycardia. *Br J Obstet Gynecol* 1980;87:340.
56. Frohn-Mulder I, Stewart P, Witsenburg M, Den Hollander N, Wladimiroff J, Hess J. The efficacy of flecainide versus digoxin in the management of fetal supraventricular tachycardia. *Prenat Diagn* 1995;15:1297.
57. van Engelen A, Weijtens O, Brenner J, et al. Management outcome and follow-up of fetal tachycardia. *J Am Coll Cardiol* 1994;24:1371.
58. Echt D, Liebson P, Mitchell L, et al. Mortality and morbidity in patients receiving encainide, flecainide or placebo: the Cardiac Arrhythmia Suppression Trial. *N Engl J Med* 1991;324:781.
59. Allan L, Chita K, Sharland G, Maxwell D, Priestley K. Flecainide in the treatment of fetal tachycardias. *Br Heart J* 1991;65:46.
60. De Catte L, De Wolf D, Smitz J, Bougatef A, De Schepper J, Foulon W. Fetal hypothyroidism as a complication of amiodarone treatment for persistent fetal supraventricular tachycardia. *Prenat Diagn* 1994; 14:762.
61. Magee L, Downar E, Sermer M, Boulton B, Allen L, Koren G. Pregnancy outcome after gestational exposure to amiodarone in Canada. *Am J Obstet Gynecol* 1995;172:1307.
62. Fulgencio J, Hamza J. Anaesthesia for caesarean section in a patient receiving high dose amiodarone for fetal supraventricular tachycardia. *Anaesthesia* 1994;49:406.
63. Weiner C, Thompson M. Direct treatment of fetal supraventricular tachycardia after failed transplacental therapy. *Am J Obstet Gynecol* 1988;158:570.
64. Kohl T, Tercanli S, Kececioglu D, Holzgreve W. Direct fetal administration of adenosine for the termination of incessant supraventricular tachycardia. *Obstet Gynecol* 1995;85:873.
65. Ross B. Congenital complete atrioventricular block. *Pediatr Clin North Am* 1990;37:69.
66. Schmidt K, Ulmer H, Silverman N, Kleinman C, Copel J. Perinatal outcome of fetal complete atrioventricular block: a multicenter experience. *J Am Coll Cardiol* 1991;91:1360.
67. Smeenk R. Immunological aspects of congenital atrioventricular block. *PACE Pacing Clin Electrophysiol* 1997;21:2093.

68. Liddicoat J, Klein J, Reddy V, Klautz R, Teitel D, Hanley F. Hemodynamic effects of chronic prenatal ventricular pacing for the treatment of complete atrioventricular block. *Circulation* 1997;96:1025.
69. Dildy G, Loucks C, Clark S. Intrapartum fetal pulse oximetry in the presence of fetal cardiac arrhythmia. *Am J Obstet Gynecol* 1993; 169:1609.
70. Landor M. Maternal-fetal transfer of immunoglobulins. *Ann Allergy Asthma Immunol* 1995;74:279.
71. Weinstein L. Irregular antibodies causing hemolytic disease of the newborn: a continuing problem. *Clin Obstet Gynecol* 1982;25:321.
72. Bowman J, Pollack J, Manning F, Harman C. Maternal Kell blood group alloimmunization. *Obstet Gynecol* 1992;67:285.
73. Vaughan J, Warwick R, Letsky E, Nicolini U, Rodeck C, Fisk N. Erythropoietic suppression in the fetal anemia because of Kell alloimmunization. *Am J Obstet Gynecol* 1994;171:247.
74. Moise K. Changing trends in the management of red blood cell alloimmunization in pregnancy. *Arch Pathol Lab Med* 1994;118:421.
75. Doyle L, Kelley E, Richards A, Ford G, Callanan C. Sensorineural outcome at 2 years for survivors of erythroblastosis treated with fetal intravascular transfusions. *Obstet Gynecol* 1993;81:931.
76. Weiner C, Williamson R, Wenstrom K, et al. Management of fetal hemolytic disease by cordocentesis II. Outcome of treatment. *Am J Obstet Gynecol* 1991;165:1302.
77. Gollin Y, Copel J. Management of the Rh-sensitized mother. *Clin Perinatol* 1995;22:545.
78. Plecas D, Chitkara U, Berkowitz G, Lapinski R, Alvarez M, Berkowitz R. Intrauterine intravascular transfusion for severe erythroblastosis fetalis: how much to transfuse? *Obstet Gynecol* 1990;75:965.
79. Leveque C, Murat I, Toubas F, Poissonnier M-H, Brossard Y, Saint-Maurice C. Fetal neuromuscular blockade with vecuronium bromide: studies during intravascular intrauterine transfusion in isoimmunized pregnancies. *Anesthesiology* 1992;76:642.
80. Ryan G, Morrow R. Fetal blood transfusion. *Fetal Drug Ther* 1994;21: 573.
81. Blanchette V, Chen L, Salomon de Friedberg Z, Hogan V, Trudel E, Decary F. Alloimmunization to the Pl^{A1} platelet antigen: results of a prospective study. *Br J Haematol* 1990;74:209.
82. Levine A, Berkowitz R. Neonatal alloimmune thrombocytopenia. *Semin Perinatol* 1991;15:35.
83. Bussel J, Zabusky M, Berkowitz R, McFarland J. Fetal alloimmune thrombocytopenia. *N Engl J Med* 1997;337:22.
84. Murphy M, Waters A, Doughty H, et al. Antenatal management of fetomaternal alloimmune thrombocytopenia: report of 15 affected pregnancies. *Transfusion Med* 1994;4:281.
85. Bussel J, Berkowitz R, Lynch L, et al. Antenatal management of alloimmune thrombocytopenia with intravenous gamma-globulin: a randomized trial of the addition of low-dose steroid to intravenous gamma-globulin. *Am J Obstet Gynecol* 1996;174:1414.
86. Paidas M, Berkowitz R, Lynch L, et al. Alloimmune thrombocytopenia: fetal and neonatal losses related to cordocentesis. *Am J Obstet Gynecol* 1995;172:475.
87. Bennett P, Le Van Kim C, Colin Y, et al. Prenatal determination of fetal RhD type by DNA amplification. *N Engl J Med* 1993;329:607.
88. McFarland J, Aster R, Bussel J, Gianopoulas J, Derbes R, Newman P. Prenatal diagnosis of neonatal alloimmune thrombocytopenia using allele-specific oligonucleotide probes. *Blood* 1991;78:2276.
89. Van den Veyver I, Chong S, Kristjansson K, Snabes M, Moise K, Hughes M. Molecular analysis of human platelet antigen system 1 antigen on single cells can be applied to preimplantation genetic diagnosis for prevention of alloimmune thrombocytopenia. *Am J Obstet Gynecol* 1994;170:807.
90. Ross H, Elias S. Maternal serum screening for fetal genetic disorder. *Obstet Gynecol Clin North Am* 1997;24:33.
91. Nicolaides K, Campbell S, Gabbe S, Guidetti R. Ultrasound screening for spina bifida: cranial and cerebellar signs. *Lancet* 1986;2:72.
92. Cochrane D, Wilson R, Steinbok P, et al. Prenatal spinal evaluation and functional outcome of patients born with myelomeningocele: information for improved prenatal counseling and outcome prediction. *Fetal Diagn Ther* 1996;11:159.
93. Coniglio S, Anderson S, Ferguson J. Developmental outcomes of children with myelomeningocele: prenatal predictors. *Am J Obstet Gynecol* 1997;177:319.
94. Luthy D, Wardinsky T, Shurtleff D, et al. Cesarean section before the onset of labor and subsequent motor function in infants with meningomyelocele diagnosed antenatally. *N Engl J Med* 1991;324:662.
95. Cochrane D, Aronyk K, Sawatzky B, Wilson D, Steinbok P. The effects of labor and delivery on spinal cord function and ambulation in patients with meningomyelocele. *Childs Nerv Syst* 1991;7:312.
96. Paidas M, Cohen A. Disorders of the central nervous system. *Semin Perinatol* 1994;18:266.
97. Gupta J, Bryce F, Liford R. Management of apparently isolated fetal ventriculomegaly. *Obstet Gynecol Surv* 1994;49:716.
98. Kirk J, Comstock C, Lee W, Smith R, Riggs T, Weinhouse E. Sonographic screening to detect fetal cardiac anomalies: a 5-year experience with 111 abnormal cases. *Obstet Gynecol* 1997;89:227.
99. Sohaey R, Zwiebel W. The fetal thorax: noncardiac chest anomalies. *Semin Ultrasound CT MR* 1996;17:34.
100. Morin L, Crombleholme T, D'Alton M. Prenatal diagnosis and management of fetal thoracic lesions. *Semin Perinatol* 1994;18:228.
101. Paidas M, Crombleholme T, Robertson F. Prenatal diagnosis and management of the fetus with an abdominal wall defect. *Semin Perinatol* 1994;18:196.
102. Sipes S, Weiner C, Sipes D, Grant S, Williamson R. Gastroschisis and omphalocele: does either antenatal diagnosis or route of delivery make a difference in perinatal outcome? *Obstet Gynecol* 1990;76:195.
103. Raynor B, Richards D. Growth retardation in fetuses with gastroschisis. *J Ultrasound Med* 1997;16:13.
104. Moretti M, Khoury A, Rodriquez J, Lobe T, Shaver D, Sibai B. The effect of mode of delivery on the perinatal outcome in fetuses with abdominal wall defects. *Am J Obstet Gynecol* 1990;163:833.
105. Kirk E, Wah R. Obstetric management of the fetus with omphalocele or gastroschisis: a review and report of one hundred twelve cases. *Am J Obstet Gynecol* 1983;146:512.
106. Burge D, Ade-Ajayi N. Adverse outcome after prenatal diagnosis of gastroschisis: the role of fetal monitoring. *J Pediatr Surg* 1997;32:441.
107. Abuhamad A, Mari G, Cortina R, Croitoru D, Evans A. Superior mesenteric artery Doppler velocimetry and ultrasonographic assessment of fetal bowel in gastroschisis: a prospective longitudinal study. *Am J Obstet Gynecol* 1997;176:985.
108. Langer J, Khanna J, Caco C, Dykes E, Nicolaides K. Prenatal diagnosis of gastroschisis: development of objective sonographic criteria for predicting outcome. *Obstet Gynecol* 1993;81:53.
109. Fitzsimmons J, Nyberg D, Cyr D, Hatch E. Perinatal management of gastroschisis. *Obstet Gynecol* 1988;71:910.
110. Lenke R, Hatch E. Fetal gastroschisis: a preliminary report advocating the use of cesarean section. *Obstet Gynecol* 1986;67:395.
111. Pryde P, Bardicef M, Treadwell M, Klein M, Isada N, Evans M. Gastroschisis: can antenatal ultrasound predict infant outcomes? *Obstet Gynecol* 1994;84:505.
112. Calzolari E, Bianchi F, Dolk H, Milan M. Omphalocele and gastroschisis in Europe: a survey of 3 million births 1980-1990. *Am J Med Genet* 1995;58:187.
113. de Veciana M, Major C, Porto M. Prediction of an abnormal karyotype in the fetuses with omphalocele. *Prenat Diagn* 1994;14:487.
114. Gross S, Benzie R, Sermer M, Skidmore M, Wilson S. Sacrococcygeal teratoma: prenatal diagnosis and management. *Am J Obstet Gynecol* 1987;156:393.
115. Bond S, Harrison M, Schmidt K, et al. Death due to high-output cardiac failure in fetal sacrococcygeal teratoma. *J Pediatr Surg* 1990; 25:1287.
116. McCurdy C, Seeds J. Route of delivery of infants with congenital anomalies. *Clin Perinatol* 1993;20:81.
117. Marras T, Poenaru D, Kamal I. Perinatal management of nasopharyngeal teratoma. *J Otolaryngol* 1995;24:310.

PART II

Intraoperative Management

Obstetric Anesthesia, second edition,
edited by Mark C. Norris.
Lippincott Williams & Wilkins, Philadelphia © 1999.

CHAPTER 9

Surgery During Pregnancy

Norman L. Herman

Only for the parturient must an anesthesiologist personally give anesthesia to more than one patient simultaneously. This unique circumstance requires a thorough understanding of the anatomic and physiologic changes associated with pregnancy and the current developmental state and drug sensitivity of the embryo/fetus. As many as 2.2% of pregnant patients undergo surgery during pregnancy (1). This number may be an underestimate, as surgery may be performed before a woman recognizes she is pregnant (2).

GENERAL CONCERNS

Maternal Safety—Physiologic Changes of Pregnancy and How They Relate to Anesthesia

To provide safe anesthesia for the parturient, the anesthesiologist must know and understand not only the physiologic changes that accompany pregnancy (see Chapter 1), but also their timing and anesthetic implications. To that end, this section reiterates some of these adjustments to pregnancy.

Cardiovascular System

Beginning the sixth week of gestation, maternal blood volume expands, increasing by as much as 25% to 40% at term (3). Incremental increases in both plasma volume (50%) and red cell mass (15%) are responsible for this change (Fig. 1) (4). The increase in blood volume has important implications. The unbalanced increase of plasma volume versus red cell mass produces the physiologic anemia of pregnancy. In the face of acute surgical bleeding, the parturient requires transfusion sooner to maintain a hematocrit above 30%, which is needed for optimal fetal oxygenation (5). The rheologic changes that accompany this relative anemia can produce heart murmurs not present in the nongravid state. These murmurs may be indistinguishable from true pathologic conditions (6). Hemodilution also appears to account for a decrease in total plasma protein concentration (7). Fewer plasma proteins increase the free fraction of highly protein-bound drugs. Enhanced drug effect or toxicity at doses normally effective in nonpregnant patients may follow. This reduction in plasma protein concentration also correlates with a decrease in pseudocholinesterase activity (8). Succinylcholine can cause a prolonged neuromuscular blockade (9). Limit the administered dose of succinylcholine (1 to 1.5 mg/kg) and closely monitor neuromuscular blockade with a twitch monitor.

Compression of the great vessels by the gravid uterus when the patient lies supine wreaks havoc on maternal hemodynamics. First, vena caval obstruction and the resultant decrease in venous return from the lower extremities can produce maternal hypotension, tachycardia, pallor, and lightheadedness. This supine hypotension syndrome occurs in up to 10% of pregnant women at term (10), developing as early as 24 to 27 weeks of gestation (3). Even without symptoms of hypotension, 90% of term parturients allowed to lie flat completely obstruct their inferior vena cava (11). Venous blood from the lower body must travel by alternative pathways through the intervertebral venous plexus and azygous veins to reach the superior vena cava. The resulting engorgement of these vessels, particularly the epidural veins, reduces the size of both the subarachnoid and epidural spaces and may contribute to the smaller drug requirements for regional anesthesia in parturients (12). Besides caval compression, the pregnant uterus also can compress the abdominal aorta. Although measured brachial artery pressure remains unchanged, the aortic compression can profoundly decrease both uteroplacental and renal blood flow (13). This occult supine hypotension syndrome can detrimentally affect both mother and fetus (14). For these reasons, second- and

N. L. Herman: Department of Anesthesiology, New York Hospital-Cornell University Medical College, New York, New York 10021.

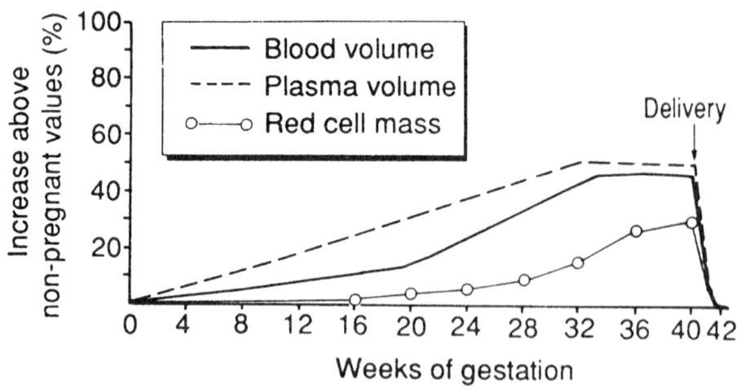

FIG. 1. Increases in blood volume and its constituent components during pregnancy. (From Chamberlain G. ABC of antenatal care. The changing body in pregnancy. *BMJ* 1991; 302:719, with permission.)

third-trimester parturients must avoid the supine position; uterine displacement is essential.

Respiratory System

The progressive upward growth of the pregnant uterus elevates the diaphragm and flares out the lower ribs, decreasing both residual and expiratory reserve volumes and markedly reducing functional residual capacity (FRC) (Fig. 2). These changes begin in the fifth month of gestation and reach a maximal decrease of 20% at term (15–17). In addition, starting at 8 to 12 weeks of gestation, oxygen consumption steadily increases to 20% to 40% above nonpregnant values at term (Fig. 3) (18,19). Because of these two factors, the pregnant patient undergoing surgery risks rapid and severe hypoxemia during periods of apnea (e.g., during rapid-sequence induction and intubation) (20). Pay particular attention to preoxygenation and denitrogenation before induction of general anesthesia. Give supplemental oxygen during regional anesthesia.

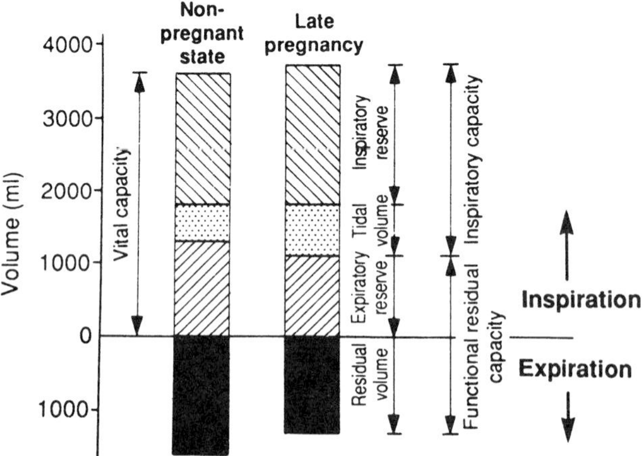

FIG. 2. Changes in inspiratory and expiratory volumes, leading to significant reductions in functional residual capacity (FRC) during pregnancy. (From Chamberlain G. ABC of antenatal care. The changing body in pregnancy. *BMJ* 1991;302: 719, with permission.)

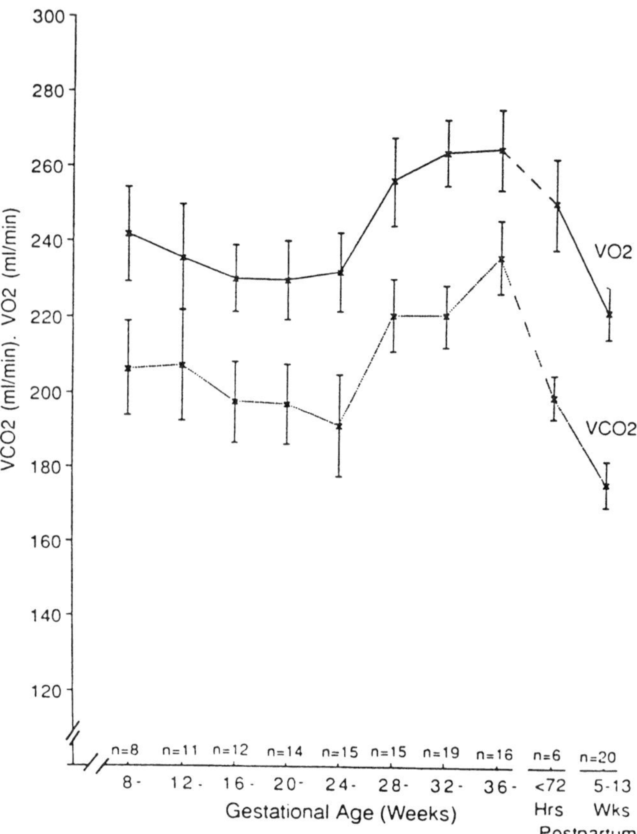

FIG. 3. Pattern of change in oxygen consumption (V_{O_2}) and carbon dioxide production (V_{CO_2}) throughout pregnancy in 20 women. (From ref. 19, with permission.)

Central Nervous System

Pregnancy increases the sensitivity to inhaled anesthetics. The minimal alveolar concentration (MAC) decreases 25% to 40% (21). These changes are well established by 8 to 13 weeks of gestation (22,23). Factors contributing to this reduction may include progesterone, which has a sedating effect (24), and endogenous opioids (25). Use lower concentrations of inhalation agents when performing general anesthesia.

Pregnancy also increases the sensitivity to intravenous agents. The induction dose of thiopental is 18% less than that in nonpregnant controls by weeks 7 to 13 of pregnancy (26). This difference, however, is probably not great enough to justify reducing the dose of thiopental used to induce general anesthesia.

Pregnancy increases the sensitivity to local anesthetics. As early as the first trimester, the extent of sensory blockade after epidural injection of local anesthetics in increased compared with that in nonpregnant women (Fig. 4) (27). Mechanical factors and an increased susceptibility to local anesthetics may play a role. Third-trimester parturients are more sensitive to median nerve block with lidocaine than are nonpregnant controls. These results suggest that pregnancy may directly alter the neural response to these agents (28). However, when

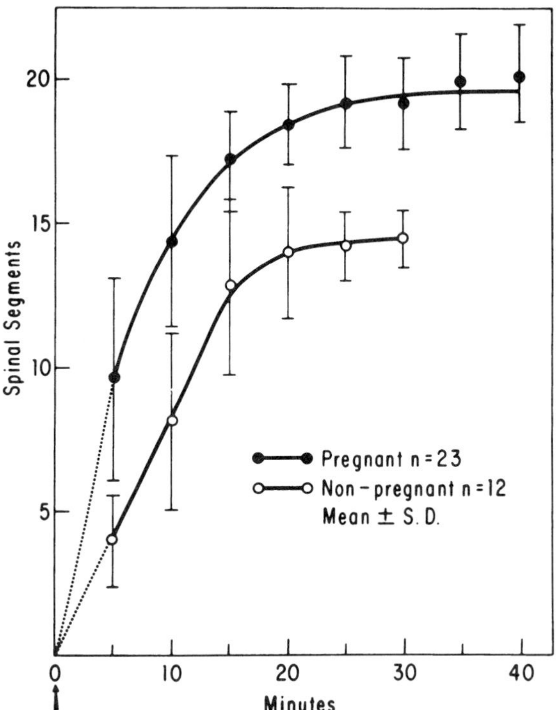

FIG. 4. Pregnancy alters the rate and extent of spread of epidural analgesia. Nonpregnant and first-trimester parturients received comparable doses of epidural local anesthetics. (From ref. 27, with permission.)

rat spinal root axons are directly exposed to bupivacaine, nerves from pregnant animals are less sensitive to local anesthetic blockade than are those from nonpregnant rats (29). Changes in local anesthetic diffusibility through connective tissues or increases in the activity of endogenous analgesic systems might explain the discrepancies between these clinical and laboratory findings. Consider reducing the total dose of local anesthetic for regional anesthesia.

Gastrointestinal System

Several important changes in the gastrointestinal system have implications for the patient undergoing surgery during pregnancy. Placental gastrin release increases the volume and acidity of gastric secretions. It has been a long-held belief that progesterone, by inhibiting smooth-muscle activity, decreases intestinal motility and delays gastric emptying during pregnancy.

There is good evidence for a delay in gastric emptying during labor, but there is little proof of delayed stomach transit before labor. Except for some older reports and investigations in patients scheduled to undergo therapeutic abortion, ethical concerns have prevented resolution of this dilemma by using well-accepted invasive (e.g., nasogastric tube placement) or radiographic (e.g., after barium by using fluoroscopy or radionucleide studies) techniques. Most noninvasive studies consistently failed to show delayed gastric emptying at any time during pregnancy, up to the beginning of labor (30–33). One study, by using paracetamol uptake as an indirect measure of gastric transit, reported decreased gastric emptying beginning as early as 8 to 10 weeks' gestation, which became well manifested by 12 to 14 weeks (34). However, these patients were studied in a supine position (35). When pregnant women are studied sitting, the rate of paracetamol absorption is comparable to that in nonpregnant women (32). Remember, however, that results obtained in these controlled settings may not reflect gastric emptying in parturients with stress, trauma, or pain.

Anatomic displacement of the stomach by the uterus increases intragastric pressure in later pregnancy. Mean barrier pressure (lower esophageal sphincter pressure minus intragastric pressure) decreases (36).

No consensus exists about when during gestation and to what extent the risk of gastric acid aspiration becomes significant. A conservative approach is to give a nonparticulate antacid plus an H_2-receptor antagonist to every patient undergoing surgery during pregnancy (no matter what week of gestation) and do a rapid-sequence induction and intubation with cricoid pressure when providing general anesthesia.

Fetal Safety: Developmental Effect of Anesthetics

The factors that control the passage of anesthetic agents across the blood–brain barrier are the same ones that influence their placental transfer to the embryo/fetus. Virtually all anesthetic agents given to the mother are rapidly shared with the unborn child. The notable exception to this generalization are the neuromuscular blocking drugs, which cross both the blood–brain barrier and placenta with difficulty because they are quaternary ammonium salts (37–40).

This ready drug transfer leads to important questions concerning the safety of these agents in the developing embryo/fetus. Low-molecular-weight compounds [i.e., the vast majority of therapeutic agents (including ***all*** anesthetics)], freely diffuse across the placenta at a rate determined solely by the concentration gradient. This ready transfer raises concerns about developmental effects of maternally administered drugs.

The Food and Drug Administration (FDA) has an established risk-classification system to help physicians weigh risk and benefit when contemplating the use of therapeutic drugs during pregnancy (Federal Register 1980;44:37434) (Table 1). Other sources of information, especially about older, generic drugs, are texts such as *Drug Use in Pregnancy and Lactation* (41) or *Drug: Facts and Comparisons* (42). These texts classify therapeutic drugs on the basis of a thorough review of the current literature. Sometimes the risk category in *Drug Use in Pregnancy and Lactation* differs from that in the package insert [as displayed in the *Physicians' Desk Reference* (43) or *PDR Generics* (44)]. This discrepancy usually

TABLE 1. *FDA fetal-risk categories for therapeutic agents*

Category A:	Controlled studies have shown no risk to the fetus during the first trimester, and later trimesters as well. Risk is remote (e.g., water)
Category B:	Animal studies have demonstrated no fetal risk, but no controlled studies have been performed in humans. Animal studies have shown adverse fetal effects, but these results were not confirmed in controlled human studies. No risk is evident after the first trimester.
Category C:	Either studies have shown fetal risk in animals (teratogenic or embryocidal), but no controlled human studies have been performed, or there are no available data in humans or animals for an agent. Drugs of this class should only be given if benefits outweigh the risks.
Category D:	Confirmed evidence exists for human fetal risk, but benefits are acceptable despite known risk (i.e., life-or-limb situations or serious disease for which no safer drugs exist e.g., diazepam).
Category X:	Agents of this class are contraindicated in pregnant patients for any reason because animal or human studies have displayed teratogenicity or there is evidence of fetal risk from prior human experience. Fetal risk clearly outweighs any clinical benefit of their use in pregnancy (e.g., thalidomide).

Adapted from Federal Register 1980;44:37434–37436, with permission.

occurs because of availability of new information after the manufacturer has presented the data to the FDA for approval.

Changes in Risk Throughout Gestation

Many texts divide the risk of drug administration during pregnancy into problems in early gestation (direct fetal effects, mainly toxicity) and late gestation (maternal effects that indirectly produce fetal injury). Images of the most horrific effects of drugs on embryonic or fetal development easily come to mind: the limb-reducing defects of a child whose mother was treated with thalidomide in early pregnancy or a child with cerebral palsy induced by profound maternal hypoxia or hypotension near birth. Although this demarcation separates the injurious effects of drugs during early and late gestation, drugs can be directly toxic to a fetus after organogenesis, and hypotension and hypoxia can be just as harmful to an embryo.

The early developmental effects of drugs center around teratogenicity. Exposure to a teratogen during gestation can bring about significant changes in the form or function of an infant. Of most concern is exposure during organogenesis, a phase of critical differentiation and development, which occurs between 3 and 8 weeks after conception (45). Because the brain continues to develop even after birth, the duration of central nervous system susceptibility probably extends well beyond the first trimester. Teratogenic effects may be structural anomalies, functional disorders (including behavior), growth retardation, and death. Numerous factors determine whether a given drug exposure will be teratogenic. Timing, dosage, and duration of treatment are most critical. Predicting teratogenicity in humans is complicated by differing species sensitivity. [Thalidomide has no teratogenic effects in rats. Later studies in rabbits found developmental defects similar to those seen in humans (46).] Any agent given in the right dosage at the right time probably can be teratogenic (47). Still, despite conflicting animal data, very few drugs have proven to be teratogenic in humans.

Later in pregnancy, as the fetus grows, its oxygen requirements increase. To meet these demands, many of the physiologic changes of pregnancy aim at increasing maternal blood flow to the enlarging uterus (Fig. 5). Any prolonged disruption of placental oxygen delivery (by either impaired maternal oxygenation or uterine hypoperfusion) can induce fetal asphyxia and its resultant effects (including death). Anesthetic complications that may produce fetal asphyxia include:

- Intubation difficulties with or without gastric acid aspiration,
- Unrecognized esophageal intubation,
- High or complete spinal block during regional anesthesia, and
- Unintended deep inhalational anesthesia.

Induction Agents

Thiopental is teratogenic to chicken embryos when given in doses from 0.2 to 4 mg/egg during the critical phase of development (days 2 to 4) (48). Anomalies included anencephaly, twisted limbs, twisted neck, microphthalmia, everted viscera, cerebral hemorrhage,

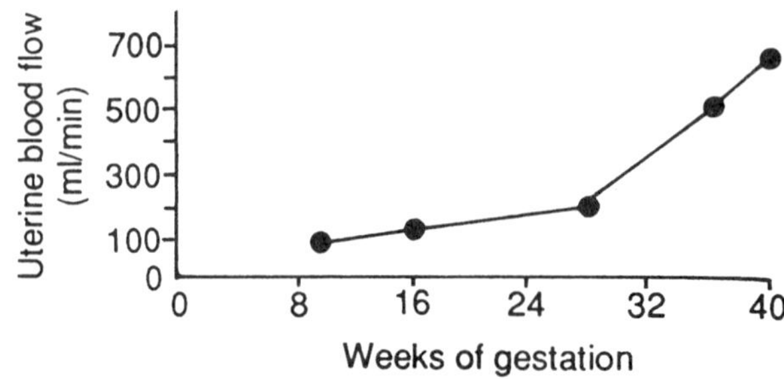

FIG. 5. The elevated metabolic demands of the fetus and placenta require an increasing fraction of cardiac output throughout pregnancy. (From Chamberlain G. ABC of antenatal care. The changing body in pregnancy. *BMJ* 1991;302: 719, with permission.)

and death. Another group noted the growth of aberrant nerve fibers penetrating into the cerebral ventricles and through the cartilage of the presumptive vertebral bodies (49). In mice and rats, up to 100 mg/kg thiopental had no teratogenic effect, although some mice exhibited retarded growth (50,51), but these findings required thiopental doses far in excess of those used clinically. No specific studies directly investigated thiopental teratogenicity or fetal toxicity in humans. Thiopental has been classified as a pregnancy category C agent (44). Its long history of safe administration in pregnant patients justifies its continued use.

Methohexital has been given a category B classification. Reproductive studies in rats and rabbits at 4 and 7 times the recommended human dose, respectively, revealed no teratogenic or embryo/fetal toxic effect (44). Human studies are lacking.

In rats, **ketamine**, 120 mg/kg i.m., had no teratogenic effects when given daily from days 9 to 13 of gestation (52). In contrast, in chick embryos at the stage of greatest organogenesis, ketamine, 400 μg/mL, produced neural tube defects (53). A Russian group found that 40 mg/kg given to rats on gestational days 11, 13, and 15 had "a marked embryolethal action" (route of administration unknown). Doses of between 20 and 40 mg/kg on days 7, 9, and 11 caused internal organ hemorrhage in the embryo (54). No specific reproductive studies have been performed in humans. This agent did not receive pregnancy risk classification by its manufacturer before expiration of its patent, so its risk-assessment category is not noted in *PDR Generics* (44). The pharmaceutical compendium, *Drug: Facts and Comparisons,* has given ketamine a category C rating (42).

In rats, **etomidate** has an embryotoxic effect when administered at 1 and 4 times the normal human dose (44). Doses from 0.3 to 5 mg/kg markedly decreased birth survival in rats and rabbits, although there was no definitive dose–response relation. Stillbirths were also slightly increased at doses between 0.3 and 1.25 mg/kg. Well-controlled studies in pregnant women are absent; therefore, in light of the animal data, etomidate has been given a category C rating by the FDA.

Rats and rabbits given 15 mg/kg of **propofol** (6 times the recommended induction dose in humans) daily throughout pregnancy showed no reproductive effects (44). However, even in the absence of teratogenic action in animals, because developmental effects of propofol in humans are not available, it has been made a pregnancy category B agent.

Inhaled Agents

Potent Agents

Potent inhaled agents are the cornerstone of most general anesthetics. Still, there are no controlled studies of the safety of any of these anesthetics in pregnant surgical patients. Their FDA pregnancy risk classification comes from animal studies.

Halothane is the most studied of the currently available potent agents. Rats exposed to 1 MAC of halothane in 25% O_2 for 12 hours during organogenesis developed skeletal abnormalities (55). In contrast, shorter exposures (1 hour) to about 2 MAC in rats and 3 MAC in rabbits on 5 successive days during different times of development had no effect on pregnancy outcome (56). Long-term exposure to subanesthetic concentrations of halothane resulted in growth retardation but no anomalies (57). In rats, higher doses given either repeatedly or over the long term from preconception through organogenesis caused skeletal abnormalities and embryo/fetal death (58). However, the maternal derangements induced by this regimen, particularly disrupted feeding patterns, hypoventilation, hypoxia (59), and hypothermia (60) themselves have profound effects on development and may have contributed to these findings. At halothane concentrations that did not disturb sleeping and eating, only growth retardation was found. No adequate reproductive studies have been performed in humans. Halothane has been given a pregnancy risk classification of category C (44).

Exposure of mice to **enflurane** (category B) at concentrations of 0.01%, 0.1%, or 1.0% for 4 hours on 6 consecutive days during major organogenesis resulted in an increased incidence of cleft palate (1.9%), fused vertebrae, bent and fused ribs, and renal abnormalities in the highest dose group (61). Subsequent investigations in rats with exposures to 1 MAC (1.68%) of enflurane for 6 hours on 3 succeeding days during organogenesis revealed no teratogenic effect (62). Long-term subanesthetic administration of enflurane to rats before conception (female and male) and through pregnancy was associated with lower birth weights, but no defects (63,64). No controlled studies have been performed in humans.

Studies with **isoflurane** demonstrated treatment-related embryotoxicity in mice at doses 6 times greater than normally used in humans (44). Mazze et al. (65) investigated the effects of lower concentrations of isoflurane in mice. They exposed pregnant mice to either 0.006%, 0.06%, or 0.6% isoflurane for 4 hours daily on days 6 to 15 of gestation (critical period of development). No reproductive effects were noted for the trace (0.006%) and subanesthetic (0.06%) doses. However, 0.6% isoflurane induced significant growth retardation, decreased ossification, and renal abnormalities. They also noted a high incidence of cleft palate (12%). A similar study in rats with 6-hour exposures to 1.05% isoflurane on three successive days during major organogenesis produced no evidence of teratogenic effects (62). No controlled investigations have been done in parturients. Isoflurane has a category C pregnancy risk classification (44).

Rats exposed to 1 MAC-hour/day of **desflurane** through the critical development period to birth had no birth anomalies (43). Because no well-controlled studies have been performed in humans, desflurane has been given a category B classification.

Rats and rabbits exposed to 1 MAC of **sevoflurane** without the use of a CO_2 absorber exhibited no embryotoxic or teratogenic effects (Ultane package insert, sevoflurane volatile liquid for inhalation, 06-9230-R2-Revised June 1995, Abbott Laboratories, North Chicago, IL). Reproductive effects have not been investigated in pregnant patients, making sevoflurane a category B agent. Studies of the reproductive effects of Compound A, formed by the degradation of sevoflurane in the strongly alkaline environment of the CO_2 absorber (soda lime or barium hydroxide lime), have not been done. Maintain at least 3 L/min fresh gas flow when giving sevoflurane to parturients to minimize the inhaled concentration of Compound A.

Nitrous Oxide

Nitrous oxide (N_2O) has been an important anesthetic for many years. It has a long history of apparent safe use for both anesthesia and analgesia in obstetrics. However, in recent years, information about the metabolic effects of N_2O fueled a controversy concerning its use in early pregnancy.

Animal evidence of nitrous oxide teratogenicity is not new. Rat studies showed that exposure to 50% N_2O for 2 to 6 days, or exposure to 70% N_2O for 24 hours during critical phases of early development induced skeletal abnormalities and resorption (abortion) (66,67). Exposing rats to subanesthetic doses of nitrous oxide throughout pregnancy induced resorption, small birth weight, and minor abnormalities of the skeleton (68).

Nitrous oxide impairs deoxyribonucleic acid (DNA) synthesis through its inhibition of methionine synthetase. This enzyme is an important intermediate step in the production of deoxythymidine, a critical component of DNA. N_2O oxidizes the cobalt of the vitamin B_{12} cofactor in the methionine synthetase enzyme complex, which inhibits the conversion of 5-methyl tetrahydrofolate and homocysteine into tetrahydrofolate and methionine (Fig. 6). This effect appears to be the origin of the pernicious anemia-like condition seen in some patients who receive nitrous oxide (69). The most rapidly dividing cells are at greatest risk from this enzyme inhibition. The rapidly growing embryo/fetus may be at risk, particularly during organogenesis. Because nitrous oxide is poorly soluble and readily diffusible, fetal nitrous oxide concentration very rapidly reaches maternal concentration (70). There is evidence of depressed activity of methionine synthetase (71) and DNA content (72) in fetal rats exposed to nitrous oxide. Normally, methionine synthetase is much more active in the embryonic brain, kidney, and liver than later in life (73).

Tetrahydrofolate deficiency from the disruption of methionine synthetase does not fully explain the embryo and fetal toxicity associated with nitrous oxide. Developmental toxicity occurs at doses of nitrous oxide far higher than that required to inhibit methionine synthetase maximally (71). Toxicity is not prevented by administration of folinic acid, as is the case with the pernicious anemia-like syndrome (74). Supplementation with methionine averts the majority of embryo and fetal toxic effects seen with nitrous oxide exposure in the in vitro rat embryo (75). However, the abnormalities induced in rat embryos grown in methionine-deficient growth media are not the same as those seen in nitrous oxide-induced injury (76).

New evidence suggests that the α_1-adrenergic activity of nitrous oxide may be an important aspect of its developmental effects. α_1-Adrenergic antagonists prevent embryo resorption and situs inversus (77). The inference

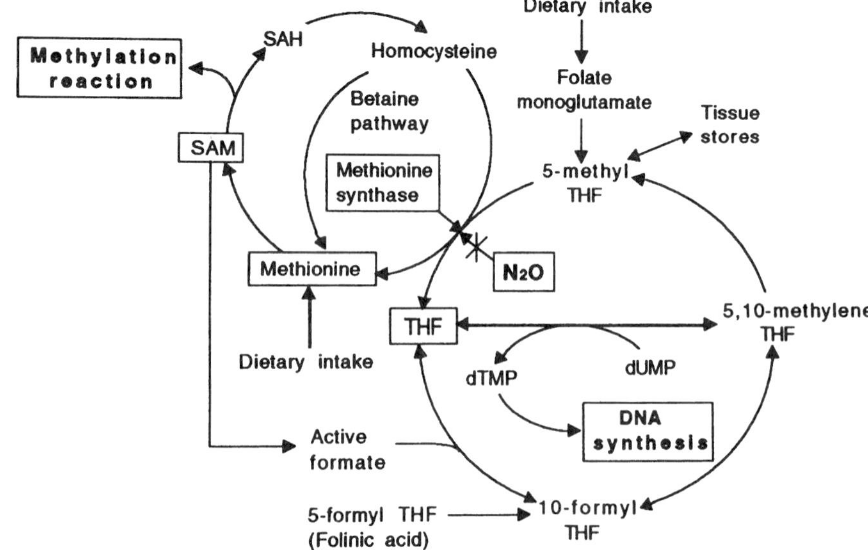

FIG. 6. Metabolic consequences of N_2O inhibition of methionine synthetase. This results in the failure of the conversion of homocysteine into methionine and 5-methyl tetrahydrafolate *(THF)* into THF. Reduced concentrations of THF decrease the available substrate necessary to produce sufficient amounts of 5,10-methylene THF, a one-carbon donor in the conversion of deoxyuridine monophosphate *(dUMP)* to deoxythymidine monophosphate *(dTMP)*, an essential component of DNA. In addition, the decreased quantities of methionine reduce the production of *S*-adenosyl methionine *(SAM)* leading to impaired methylation reactions. *SAH*, *S*-adenosyl homocysteine. (From ref. 59, with permission.)

is that alterations in uteroplacental blood flow may play a role in this nitrous oxide effect. For a more in-depth explanation of the present understanding of the biochemical and molecular biologic effects of nitrous oxide, see the current review by Fujinaga (59).

In light of this evidence of teratogenicity and embryo/fetal toxicity in both intact pregnant rats and cultured rat embryos, some have suggested that nitrous oxide be contraindicated during the first and second trimesters of pregnancy (in other words, be made a category X agent) (78). However, this recommendation involves the direct extrapolation of animal data to humans, a tenuous stretch at best. A 24 hour or longer exposure to nitrous oxide in a rat (or a rat embryo in culture) is not comparable to a pregnant patient undergoing a 1- to 3-hour surgical procedure with a balanced anesthetic technique including nitrous oxide.

Much of the reproductive safety data regarding nitrous oxide in humans comes from epidemiologic studies in female employees in operating rooms and dentist's offices, who could be exposed to trace amounts of this gas for extended periods (79–84). Unfortunately, these types of exposures also are not comparable to those of pregnant patients undergoing surgery with a short-duration nitrous oxide–containing anesthetic.

Studies of embryo/fetal toxicity of nitrous oxide in pregnant patients undergoing surgery are limited. Investigating the etiology of spontaneous abortion after surgery in pregnancy is clouded by multiple potential causes of pregnancy loss, particularly the surgery itself. However, a few of these studies are important to review. Patients undergoing cervical cerclage with general anesthesia including nitrous oxide or conduction block had no difference in the rate of spontaneous abortions (85). In this same study, investigators found no spontaneous abortions in a group of 58 parturients having other surgical procedures under general anesthesia with nitrous oxide. Neither this investigation nor another with an additional 175 patients exposed to nitrous oxide for cervical cerclage (86) revealed any anomalies at birth[1]. A large Swedish registry study provides the most reassuring data about the safety of nitrous oxide in patients having surgery during pregnancy (87). In this study, Mazze and Källén surveyed 720,000 pregnancies between 1973 and 1981. A subset of 5,405 parturients underwent surgery during pregnancy, 2,252 of these in the first trimester and 2,929 under general anesthesia. No significant increase in birth abnormalities was detected in those receiving general anesthesia, 98% of whom received nitrous oxide.

A recent review (59) and the previous edition of this text were reluctant to give nitrous oxide an FDA-type category classification. (Because nitrous oxide is a medical gas, it is not directly regulated by the FDA and is therefore not subject to the pregnancy risk classification requirement and thus never received an official category rating.) These sources instead classified it a category because they believed it could not be precisely defined as either a category C, D, or X agent because of the controversial occupational-exposure data. Clinical data in patients undergoing surgery with nitrous oxide during pregnancy do not support a category X classification. If we exclude the controversial occupational data and consider only patients undergoing surgery with concurrent pregnancy, then a category C would be warranted. Although a conservative approach would be to avoid nitrous oxide, a wealth of clinical data support the safe and continued use of N_2O as part of a balanced anesthetic during all aspects of pregnancy.

Local Anesthetics

Whereas local anesthetics may have direct neurotoxic effects, (88–93), most data suggest that they lack embryo or fetal toxic actions. Procaine, lidocaine, and tetracaine exposure in early chick embryo (53,94) and lidocaine exposure in mice embryo preparations (95) affected neural tube closure. However, no data exist suggesting teratogenicity in intact animals for any local anesthetic. 2-Chloroprocaine and tetracaine are both category C agents because no intact animal studies have been performed, and human data are lacking (44). Bupivacaine also has a C classification because of an increase in fetal and embryo loss in rats and rabbits at 5 to 9 times the maximal clinical dose, although there was no evidence of teratogenicity (44). No controlled studies have assessed the embryo/fetal effects of bupivacaine in humans.

The package insert for lidocaine states that no animal or human studies report adverse embryo or fetal effects, and therefore it has been given a category B classification (44). The chapter on lidocaine in *Drug Use in Pregnancy and Lactation* disagrees with this assessment, giving lidocaine a category C classification (41). These authors cited the neurobehavioral changes (mainly depression) associated with high serum concentrations of lidocaine at birth as one reason for this category change. In addition, they reported the results of the Collaborative Perinatal Project (1959 to 1965), which included 293 first-trimester exposures to lidocaine (96). Although there was no evidence of major or minor malformations with lidocaine, there were some greater than expected increases in respiratory tract anomalies and inguinal hernias. Statistical significance and independent corroboration are lacking.

The recently released local anesthetic ropivacaine lacked teratogenic effects in rats and rabbits at up to 5 times the recommended maximal dose in humans (Naropin package insert, ropivacaine HCl injection, 021683R00, 9/96, Astra USA, Westborough, MA). However, because no definitive controlled studies have been

[1]Editor's note: Remember that cervical cerclage is usually done in the early second trimester, well after organogenesis is complete.

performed in humans, ropivacaine has been classified category B.

SPECIFIC COMMON PROCEDURES

Cervical Cerclage

Definition

Cervical cerclage is the surgical intervention used to prevent second-trimester fetal loss from cervical incompetence. Classically, an obstetrician made a diagnosis of an incompetent cervix after repeated history of painless cervical dilation in the second or early third trimester. Prolapse of the membranes through the cervix or spontaneous rupture of membranes and expulsion of the fetus typically followed. An incompetent cervix seems to result from a weakness of the internal cervical os caused by trauma, congenital factors, or multiple pregnancies. When the fetus attains a critical weight, it overcomes the normal sphincter resistance of the os, and uterine contents begin to extrude. Premature contractions and delivery may follow this mechanical dilatation of the cervix (97).

Making the diagnosis of cervical incompetence is often difficult. Painless cervical dilation of 2 to 4 cm occurs in 24% to 34% of otherwise asymptomatic gravidae who go on to deliver at term. No single pathognomonic physical finding or test confirms a precise diagnosis of an incompetent cervix. It is therefore a diagnosis of exclusion after the obstetrician rules out the other causes of mid-trimester effacement (e.g., preterm labor) (98).

Methods and Types of Cervical Cerclage

Once the diagnosis of an incompetent cervix is made, the goal of therapy is to enhance the resistance of the cervix to effacement and dilatation, and by that, to prevent fetal loss. Vaginal pessary, progesterone therapy, and electrocautery of the cervix have been investigated as treatments with little success. Despite controversy regarding its success, cervical cerclage is the mainstay of therapy for an incompetent cervix (99–101).

The surgical approach for cerclage is either vaginal or transabdominal. Several intravaginal methods have been described since the initial introduction of cerclage in 1950 (102). Shirodkar (103) was first to develop a method of encircling the internal cervical os for reinforcing a weakened cervix.

The Shirodkar procedure involves the incision of the cervix at the level of the internal os, elevating the vaginal mucosa and bladder, and placing a Mersilene 5-mm band (braided dacron) around the cervix. The complex nature of the Shirodkar method makes it difficult during pregnancy and places the urinary tract at risk. Suggestions that this method be avoided in patients with advanced cervical changes, particularly with bulging membranes, notwithstanding (104,105), the Shirodkar technique has been used with success in these parturients (106). A modification of the Shirodkar procedure was described with fewer cervical incisions and a nylon ligature in place of the 5-mm band (107). This modification is equally effective and easier to remove than the original procedure.

The McDonald procedure uses a purse-string suture as high as possible around the exocervix, at approximately the level of the internal os (108). With four to five bites, the suture is placed deeply into the cervix and pulled tightly enough to close the cervical os completely. The McDonald method usually produces less blood loss and trauma to the cervix than the Shirodkar procedure. The McDonald procedure also induces less cervical scarring and a lower incidence of cervical dystocia (scar tissue preventing cervical dilatation) (109).

A far less common procedure is the Würm procedure, which was developed in Australia. This approach uses criss-crossing heavy double-mattress sutures across the cervical opening at the level of the internal os (110). The Würm procedure reportedly can delay delivery until at or near term. It can be used in conjunction with amniocentesis to reduce bulging membranes (111) and as a method for repeated cerclage when either the Shirodkar or McDonald cerclage has failed (112).

The transabdominal cervicoisthmic cerclage is by far the most complex and difficult procedure for the surgical treatment of cervical incompetence (113). It involves the intraabdominal placement of a ligature around the cervix above the cardinal and uterosacral ligaments. It is recommended for patients in whom the cervix is congenitally short, amputated, or scarred from an extensive cone biopsy or unsuccessful prior cerclage, when the fornices are lacerated, or in the presence of subacute cervicitis (114). Because of a high incidence of premature rupture, it is rarely used if the fetal membranes are bulging through a cervix with advanced changes (115,116). Although this technique is effective, with an 85% to 92% rate of fetal salvage (115–117), it has major disadvantages. It requires two abdominal procedures (the cerclage and a subsequent cesarean section). It also has a higher complication rate, related to the high vascularity and proximity of ureters to the surgical site. Although this procedure has received renewed interest recently, it is reserved for women in whom vaginal cerclage has either failed or is impossible.

Cervical cerclage is usually done between weeks 14 and 26 of gestation. Cerclage done between weeks 16 and 19 of gestation has the greatest chance of success (118). Before 14 weeks, pregnancy losses frequently are due to genetic anomalies or imperfect implantation (119). After 26 weeks, cerclage is usually avoided because the survival rates for a fetus of this gestational age are good in an American tertiary neonatal intensive care unit.

Indications and Contraindications for Performing Cerclage

Cervical cerclage is performed to treat cervical incompetence. As mentioned, however, this diagnosis is a difficult one to make. Classically, patients belong in two categories. Either they have a history of repetitive late mid-trimester losses, or they have a partially dilated cervix with intact membranes (120). With the increased use of in vitro fertilization techniques, some obstetricians use cervical cerclage with higher order (more than two) multiple gestations to decrease the dilating stress on the cervix (121,122). Not all studies have found a benefit to this approach (123).

The many reports of improved pregnancy outcome in large series of patients with cerclage have sustained the belief that cervical cerclage prolongs pregnancy. This belief is suspect, however, because most published series are neither controlled and randomized nor do they adequately exclude patients in preterm labor or with previous mid-trimester losses of unknown cause. Cervical cerclage in patients with prior pregnancy losses assumes a high rate of recurrent loss and that any successful pregnancy after cerclage is solely the result of the surgery. This conclusion may be incorrect. Factors predisposing a woman to preterm delivery may resolve spontaneously, independent of treatment (124). Two prospective randomized trials of women with prior preterm pregnancy losses compared cerclage with expectant management. In populations with multiple risks for preterm delivery, cerclage offered no benefit as either a therapy or a prophylaxis for prolonging pregnancy (125,126).

The Medical Research Council/Royal College of Obstetricians and Gynecologists Working Party on Cervical Cerclage issued its final report of a study of 1,292 pregnant women recruited in 12 countries with a history of early delivery or cervical surgery and whose obstetrician was not certain whether or not to perform cerclage during the present pregnancy (99). Each was randomly allocated to receive cerclage or expectant management; 647 received cerclage and 645 did not. There were fewer patients in the cerclage group with delivery before 33 weeks' gestation than in the nontreatment group (13% vs 17%, respectively; $p \leq 0.05$). However, this difference equated to a benefit to one patient in 25 receiving cerclage. The Working Party recommended restricting this surgery to those women with a well-defined diagnosis of an incompetent cervix as the cause of their recurrent losses (e.g., more than three pregnancies ending before 37 weeks' gestation).

A woman with bulging hour-glass membranes protruding through an effaced and dilated cervix requires intervention because a miscarriage is nearly always inevitable. Cerclage in this situation has a poorer prognosis than it does in nonemergency circumstances. Many techniques have been described to reduce the prolapsing membranes before cerclage. Several small series have reported 44% to 100% viable births after emergency cerclage (104,111,112,127). Earlier investigations have reported a dismally low viability rate (13% to 20%) in parturients with prolapsing membranes without subsequent cervical cerclage (104,120,128). Surgical intervention, therefore, appears indicated in this population.

Contraindications to cervical cerclage include (119,129):

- Bleeding,
- Active labor or significant uterine contractions,
- Ruptured membranes (although this is becoming a relative contraindication, as studies have investigated use of cerclage in patients with premature rupture of membranes) (130),
- Cervical dilation greater than 4 cm,
- Intrauterine infection,
- Fetal abnormalities, and
- Abruptio placenta.

Elective Cervical Cerclage

No consensus exists between anesthesiologists and obstetricians as to the choice of anesthesia for vaginal cervical cerclage. The procedure requires adequate analgesia and vaginal-wall relaxation. The surgeon must retract the vagina enough to expose the cervix for surgical manipulation (124). Cerclage has been performed under general (with and without a potent inhalation agent), regional (epidural or spinal), local (a paracervical block or pudendal nerve block), and no anesthesia, all with apparent equal success. The fear that uterine activity might commence with manipulation of the cervix during the procedure has led some to recommend general anesthesia with a potent inhaled agent (97,131) because these afford dose-dependent uterine relaxation (132). However, none of the potent inhalation agents provides uterine relaxation much beyond the end of the anesthetic.

Most anesthesia literature and texts recommend regional block, particularly spinal anesthesia, for cervical cerclage. The small drug dose needed to achieve adequate relaxation and analgesia are the major advantages cited for this technique.

Obstetric texts and reviews of late have been far less committal or dogmatic than they were in the past when many espoused the need for deep general anesthesia for maximal uterine relaxation (97,133,134). Most, if they mention anesthesia at all, suggested that either regional or general anesthesia can be used with success (135–137).

As for any other surgical procedure, the best technique is the one with which the anesthesiologist has the most experience and feels most comfortable. No anesthetic technique is a substitute for diligent intraoperative and postoperative monitoring of uterine activity and use of appropriate tocolytic agents.

Economic concerns have recently crept into the decision-making process for cervical cerclage. Inpatient versus outpatient care after cerclage have been compared. No differences in fetal outcomes or complications have been noted with outpatient care (138,139). Pressures to reduce costs may affect the choice of anesthetic technique if early discharge is planned.

A recent report suggested that bilateral pudendal nerve block provides adequate surgical conditions for McDonald cervical cerclage (140). These authors suggested that pudendal nerve block is a viable option for cerclage and could save significant patient-care dollars by removing the expense of an anesthesiologist and reducing operating room time. The authors of this report described adequate vaginal relaxation and pain relief, even though afferent innervation for the cervix does not transit centrally via the pudendal nerve. They presented patient pain assessments showing no difference between pudendal nerve block and regional anesthesia (epidural and spinal) in relieving the surgical pain of cerclage. However, their pain assessments were not contemporaneous to the surgery, and they converted 10-cm visual-analog pain scale data (a well-validated method of pain assessment) to a 0 to 3 scale (not validated). Success of a pudendal nerve block is subject to operator technique and experience.

Emergency Cerclage

The woman with bulging hour-glass membranes protruding through a dilated cervix raises problems of agreement on anesthetic technique between anesthesiologists and obstetricians. This tenuous circumstance requires emergency reduction of the presenting amniotic sac (with or without fetal presenting parts) and subsequent cervical cerclage. Obstetricians have often recommended general anesthesia for this scenario for two reasons. First, most of those who advocate the use of deep general anesthesia with potent inhalation anesthetics believe it provides uterine relaxation and thereby allows return of the presenting parts to the uterus (97,104,127,134). Second, some fear that the requirement for steep Trendelenberg position to encourage the return of membranes back into the uterine cavity increases the risk of aspiration of stomach contents, although this reason makes little intuitive sense (119).

Numerous recent studies investigating the effectiveness of emergency cerclage have continued to use deep general anesthesia, apparently based solely on tradition (127,141–144). However, spinal and epidural anesthesia have been used effectively in this population without apparent worsening of pregnancy outcomes compared with other studies using general anesthesia (145). When a tocolytic agent is used [e.g., terbutaline (145), ritodrine (142), indomethacin (142), or nitroglycerine (146)], the choice of anesthetic technique makes little difference (147). Another recent report even condemned the use of general anesthesia in patients for emergency cerclage because of the potential for coughing and bucking on intubation and extubation (148).

No randomized study directly investigated the differences in outcome after emergency cerclage under general versus regional anesthesia. Such a study may be as ethically difficult, as is a true randomized prospective trial of the efficacy of cervical cercalge. Growing experience suggests that regional anesthesia is safe and effective for emergency cerclage (Fig. 7). Remember, however, that neuraxial block placed with the patient sitting might

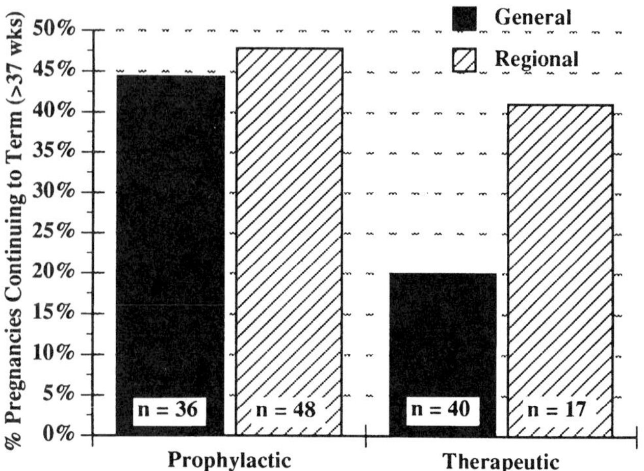

FIG. 7. Success of cervical cerclage after general or regional anesthesia. Prophylactic cerclage was done in women less than 2 cm dilated (n = 84). Therapeutic cerclage was done if the cervix had dilated 2 cm or more (n = 57). Anesthetic technique did not make a statistically significant difference in outcome. (From Engles ED. A retrospective study of regional vs. general anesthesia for cervical cerclage and review of the literature. *Anesthesiology* 1989;71:A888, with permission.)

worsen cervical dilation and membrane bulging and result in rupture of membranes. In addition, consider the interplay between drug baricity and the steep head-down tilt that may be required to reduce the bulging membranes. Last, these are extremely high-risk pregnancies. Membrane rupture at the time of cerclage most likely represents an inevitable outcome, not a shortcoming of anesthetic or obstetric management.

OTHER GYNECOLOGIC SURGERY

Ovarian Surgery

Surgery for ovarian cysts accounts for up to 39% of operations during pregnancy (149). Adnexal masses complicate one in 556 pregnancies (150). About one third are persistent corpus leuteal cysts, and another third are benign cystic teratomas. Of these masses, 2% to 5% are cancerous. A significant number of suspected ovarian masses turn out to be uterine leiomyoma on surgical exploration (151). Indications for the removal of these masses include any suspicion of rupture, torsion, or possible pelvic-outlet obstruction during labor and whenever the mass is larger than 6 to 10 cm (152,153). Magnetic resonance imaging is becoming increasingly useful in defining which masses must be explored and removed (151). Although no detrimental effects have been noted when an ovary with corpus luteum is removed as early as 8 weeks of gestation (154), most experts recommended deferring ovarian surgery at least until weeks 14 to 16 of pregnancy (155). This delay allows the placenta to develop its endocrine function before removing the corpus luteum.

Ectopic Pregnancy

In overall prevalence, implantation outside of the uterus is by far the most important surgical complication of pregnancy. The incidence of ectopic pregnancy has tripled through the 1970s to 1987 to a rate of 16.8 per 1,000 reported pregnancies. Better diagnosis, increased incidence in pelvic inflammatory disease, advanced maternal age, use of intrauterine contraception devices, tubal reanastomosis surgery, and in vitro fertilization techniques may have some role in this alarming increase. In vitro fertilization has introduced a new and unique dimension to ectopic pregnancy, heterotopic pregnancy, in which both tubal and intrauterine pregnancies coexist. The spontaneous occurrence of this situation is extremely rare (1:30,000 pregnancies); however, it complicates 1% to 3% of cases of assisted-reproduction gestations (embryo transfers and ovulation-inducing agents) (156). Ectopic pregnancy is the second leading cause of maternal mortality (157), accounting for 6% to 7% pregnancy-related deaths (158). The risk of dying of an ectopic pregnancy is 10 times greater than that of dying of complications of a term pregnancy.

The significant maternal mortality associated with ectopic pregnancy warrants a high degree of suspicion when a reproductive-age woman has abdominal pain, vaginal bleeding, and a missed period. About 14% of patients with this symptom triad have ectopic pregnancy. Other diagnoses include ovarian cyst, pelvic inflammatory disease, spontaneous abortion, intrauterine pregnancy, and pain of undetermined cause. Even with a positive pregnancy test, only 59% of patients with this triad have ectopic pregnancy (159). Increasingly sensitive pregnancy tests and high-resolution transvaginal ultrasonography have made possible early detection, before rupture and hemorrhage (160). Early diagnosis and improved treatment modalities have dramatically changed the management of ectopic pregnancy.

Traditionally ectopic pregnancy was treated with emergency laparotomy to remove the ruptured fallopian tube. However, with earlier, accurate diagnosis, more than 50% of ectopic pregnancies are unruptured at the time of surgery (161). Earlier diagnosis also has allowed the development of new treatment modalities [e.g., methotrexate (158) and ultrasound-guided transvaginal aspiration (162)].

Laparotomy Versus Laparoscopic Surgery

Until recently, traditional management of both ovarian masses and ectopic pregnancies was exploratory laparotomy. Open exploratory surgery for suspected ruptured ectopic pregnancy or adnexal masses is generally performed through either a laparotomy or minilaparotomy incision. The minilaparotomy incision may limit morbidity and postoperative pain (161). However, laparotomy incision may be needed when extensive abdominal adhesions are anticipated, in a patient in profound hemorrhagic shock, or when the size of an adnexal mass necessitates greater exposure. Although there are suggestions that laparoscopic techniques may replace laparotomy in appropriate situations for removal of adnexal masses [e.g., ovarian cystectomy, oophorectomy (163)], concern about ovarian cancer may require open exploration for proper staging and excision in many cases.

Laparoscopy has become a common nonobstetric gynecologic surgical procedure done during pregnancy (87). Laparoscopy became a tool to diagnose tubal pregnancy before noninvasive tests made early diagnosis possible. Initially laparoscopy was used to confirm the diagnosis of ectopic pregnancy, and treatment by laparotomy or minilaparotomy followed. As operator skills and instruments have improved, progressively more laparoscopic operative procedures are attempted. Advantages of laparoscopic surgery during pregnancy include:

- Reduced pain and limited fetal exposure to postoperative opioids (164),
- Consumption of fewer resources and shorter hospital stay (165),
- A panoramic view of the abdominal contents with minimal uterine manipulation, and
- More rapid return to mobility, reducing incidence of thrombophlebitis (163).

CO_2 Pneumoperitoneum

Whereas the maternal advantages of laparoscopic surgery are clear, its effects on the embryo/fetus are controversial. Laparoscopy requires intraabdominal insufflation of CO_2 to provide adequate exposure. Although anecdotal evidence (163,165–173) suggests that the accompanying increased intraabdominal pressure and maternal hypercarbia are well tolerated by the fetus, more thorough studies are only now being reported.

Hunter et al. (174) studied the fetal effects of CO_2 versus N_2O insufflation for the time required to perform a typical laparoscopic procedure (90 min) in instrumented midterm pregnant ewes. Intraabdominal insufflation with carbon dioxide to 15 mm Hg induced maternal hypercapnia and respiratory acidemia. Fetal pH and pCO_2 followed without delay. In several trials, the fetal pH decreased below 7.2, and pCO_2 increased above 55 mm Hg. Insufflation with N_2O to a similar pressure produced no such changes. In addition, CO_2 insufflation increased the p_aCO_2–end-tidal CO_2 ($ETCO_2$) gradient (normally 15 mm Hg in pregnant sheep). Increasing maternal ventilation improved the fetal acidemia, but capnography gave the mistaken impression of an even greater response because p_aCO_2–$ETCO_2$ gradient became even wider. Fetal tachycardia developed in four fetuses with CO_2 pneumoperitoneum, but only once with N_2O. Fetal central venous pressure (CVP) and intraamniotic pressure responded directly to the changes in intraabdominal pressure with either gas. However, fetal arterial pressure increased 10 to 15 mm Hg with CO_2 insufflation, but not with N_2O. When stepwise increases in CO_2 insufflation pressure were administered at 5-mm Hg intervals up to 25 mm Hg, fetal heart rate (FHR), blood pressure, and p_aCO_2 increased, and fetal pH decreased in a similar stepwise fashion. The greatest aberrations occurred when intraabdominal pressure was more than 15 mm Hg. Fetal p_aO_2 stayed within 4 mm Hg of its starting value throughout.

These authors suggested avoiding CO_2 pneumoperitoneum (174). Instead, they recommended N_2O insufflation or abdominal suspension. Although N_2O can support combustion, it has been safely used for laparoscopy. Whereas suspension devices can lift the abdominal wall away from the abdominal contents, this approach is considered inferior to pneumoperitoneum.

To the anesthesiologist, the authors of this interesting report recommended that maternal respiratory alkalosis be maintained by adjusting ventilator settings. This step is not without its potential problems (see Hyperventilation). Moreover, because they found that the p_aCO_2–$ETCO_2$ gradient worsened with hyperventilation, particularly with increased frequency (probably the result of increased fractional dead-space ventilation), these authors strongly recommended the use of arterial sampling to measure maternal acid–base/p_aCO_2 status directly during insufflation.

This study has its limitations. It included only eight animals. There are differences in implantation and placentation between sheep and humans (174). The placental transfer of both O_2 and CO_2 across the countercurrent multiplier arrangement of maternal–fetal blood flow in the sheep enhances the transfer of both, whereas the concurrent arrangement of the human maternal–fetal interface leads to a simple equilibrium of O_2 and CO_2. This different placental anatomic arrangement in sheep may lead to a far greater increase in fetal CO_2 in response to maternal respiratory acidosis than might be expected in humans. Second, the effect of the acute surgical preparation cannot be excluded from their results. Finally, because of the experimental design, the fetuses could not be followed to delivery. Therefore, the long-term effects of this transient fetal acidemia during the midterm could not be evaluated.

The safety of CO_2 pneumoperitoneum during pregnancy remains unproven. Consider the following when providing anesthesia for laparoscopic surgery:

- Continuously monitor FHR, if possible.
- Limit abdominal insufflation pressure to 15 to 20 mm Hg.
- Increase maternal minute ventilation in response to arising $ETCO_2$
- If signs of fetal compromise develop (i.e., tachycardia or bradycardia), measure maternal blood gas tensions to guide further therapy.
- Consider converting to an open procedure if worrisome FHR changes accompany pneumoperitoneum[2].

NONGYNECOLOGIC SURGERY

Common Operations

Appendectomy

The most common medical problem in the pregnant woman requiring operative intervention is appendicitis, accounting for more than two thirds of all surgery for gastrointestinal disease during pregnancy (175). The incidence of pathologically confirmed appendicitis is between 1:833 (176) and 1:6,600 (175) deliveries. Some suggested that the incidence of appendicitis should be higher during pregnancy because of progesterone-related decreases in gastrointestinal motility. However, the incidence of appendicitis is no different in pregnancy than it is for nonpregnant females of a similar age range (177). The results of a review of several published reports [713 cases (178)] and a large Swedish registry [778 cases (179)] indicate a higher incidence of appendicitis during the second trimester of pregnancy, although some smaller studies with fewer patients found no such difference in incidence among the three trimesters of pregnancy (175).

Diagnosis

The signs and symptoms of acute appendicitis do not easily point the surgeon to the diagnosis. Classic localizing right lower quadrant pain is uncommon after the first trimester, probably the result of the displacement of the appendix upward and laterally by the expanding uterus (Fig. 8). In addition, the gravid uterus isolates the inflamed appendix from the parietal peritoneum, removing the classic peritoneal signs of guarding and rebound, which also may explain the higher incidence of gangrenous and ruptured appendices in later pregnancy (176). The closer to term, the more difficult the symptoms become to unravel. Appendicitis may be mistaken for early labor. Pain may not even be the chief complaint. Patients may be afebrile or with only low-grade temperature elevation. Appendicitis should be considered whenever tenderness is elicited along the right side of the abdomen, particularly with the presence of a positive Adler's sign (fixed right-sided tenderness to palpation when the patient shifts from supine to left lateral position) or Bryan's sign (pain elicited when the pregnant uterus is moved to the right) (177).

[2]Editor's note: Despite the theoretical concerns about CO_2 pneumoperitoneum, the published experience suggests that laparoscopy is safe during pregnancy. This technique will likely see progressively wider use. (Nezhat FR, Tazuke S, Nezhat CS, Seidman DS, Philips DR, Nezhat CR. Laparoscopy during pregnancy: a literature review. *Journal of the Society of Laparoendoscopic Surgeons* 1997;1:17.)

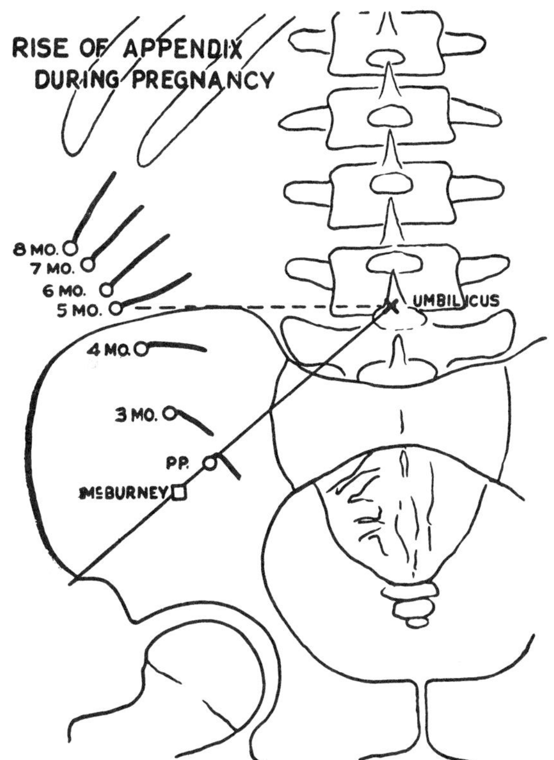

FIG. 8. Changes in position and direction of the appendix during pregnancy. *PP,* prepregnancy; *MO,* months. (From Baer JL, Reis RA, Arens RA. Appendicitis in pregnancy: with changes in position and axis of the normal appendix in pregnancy. *JAMA* 1932;98:1359, with permission.)

Treatment

Appendicitis is a surgical condition. In a classic report in 1908, Babler wrote: ". . . the mortality of appendicitis complicating pregnancy is the mortality of delay" (180). This statement remains true today. Appendiceal rupture complicated 25% of 713 cases of confirmed appendicitis reported in the surgical and obstetric literature since 1960 (178). Among these patients, there were five maternal deaths, yielding a maternal mortality of 2.8% after perforation of the appendix versus 0.7% for all patients with confirmed appendicitis. Fetal mortality was 4.8% in patients with suppurative appendicitis, which increased to 19.4% if this condition progressed to rupture (178) and subsequent fecal peritonitis (181). Delay could mean death; early diagnosis and definitive surgical intervention are key. Pregnancy is not a contraindication to appendectomy, and neither should it be a reason for delay.

The type and location of surgical incision for antepartum appendectomy is determined by the operating surgeon, particularly because the position of the appendix changes over the course of pregnancy (Fig. 8). The most common location is a right midtransverse incision over the site of maximal tenderness (175). However, because other entities are included in the differential diagnosis of abdominal pain during pregnancy, some surgeons will use either a low midline incision or a transverse muscle-cutting incision at the level of the umbilicus to allow optimal abdominal exposure if the appendix is normal.

Anesthesia

Appendectomy during pregnancy has been performed under both regional and general anesthesia. Both provide adequate analgesia and operating conditions. The fear of teratogenicity during embryogenesis (i.e., the first trimester of pregnancy) led some to recommend regional anesthesia during this period (176,177). However, after the first trimester, some recommend general endotracheal anesthesia because it provides better oxygenation, less hypotension, and better abdominal relaxation (177). In reality, both techniques are safe and effective throughout pregnancy. The margin of safety of the majority of anesthetic agents during pregnancy is excellent. The choice of anesthetic technique should be made by the anesthesiologist in consultation with the patient and surgeon.

In a recent report, postoperative pulmonary injury including pulmonary edema and adult respiratory distress syndrome (ARDS) occurred in 18% of parturients undergoing appendectomy (182). Multivariant analysis of the factors common to these cases found an association with intravenous hydration of more than 6 L within the first 46 hours of hospital admission (with surgery usually occurring within the first 24 hours), the use of tocolytic agents, and gestation longer than 20 weeks. These authors suggested use of tocolytic therapy (any agent), only if cervical change has occurred, and judicious intravenous fluid therapy.

Cholecystectomy

A less common, although equally concerning, clinical situation is the pregnant patient with biliary tract disease, either cholelithiasis or acute cholecystitis. Gallbladder disease is the second most common nonobstetric abdominal condition found during pregnancy (183), with as many as one in 1,259 parturients undergoing cholecystectomy (184). Biliary disease has a reported incidence of 0.05% to 0.3% (183,185) during pregnancy. Forty percent of these parturients require surgical intervention (183).

Pregnancy appears to predispose to gallstone formation. Progesterone relaxes gallbladder smooth muscle and decreases its responsiveness to cholecystokinin (186). These physiological changes increase the between-meal and after-meal residual volume within the gallbladder, almost doubling its size (187). In addition, both estrogen and progesterone hypersaturate the bile with cholesterol and alter the character of bile acids (188). The combination of gallbladder stasis and increased bile cholesterol causes sludging (189) and can ultimately lead to stone formation, particularly in multiparous women.

The clinical presentation of a parturient with symptomatic gallbladder disease is much like in the nonpregnant female. Most complain of epigastric or right upper quadrant pain, nausea and vomiting, and intolerance to fatty foods.

Many surgeons advocate conservative management of these patients with intravenous hydration, antibiotics, analgesia, fasting, and nasogastric suction to avoid surgery and the potential for spontaneous abortion or premature labor and delivery (184,185). However, this approach is not without risk. Nutritional problems requiring total parenteral nutrition can develop. Gallbladder disease can progress to gallstone pancreatitis. To avoid these problems, some advocate prompt surgery (188,190). When pancreatitis complicates cholecystitis, maternal mortality, which is negligible for uncomplicated cholecystectomy, increases to 15%, and fetal mortality is 60%.

McKellar et al. (183) reviewed their experience and a number of published series of open cholecystectomy and fetal outcome. They reported a spontaneous abortion rate of 8%. Although this number appears high, it may be an improvement over the risk in patients in whom cholecystectomy is delayed. A comparison between operative and nonoperative management of biliary symptoms during early pregnancy found a 12% rate of fetal wastage in patients managed conservatively versus 14% for those undergoing cholecystectomy (190). Premature labor complicates about 8% of open cholecystectomies (183). The safest time for open cholecystectomy may be during the second trimester, when the risk of abortion and premature labor are lowest.

Indications for cholecystectomy during pregnancy should be individualized to the particular condition and presentation. Surgical intervention is usually indicated when:

- Biliary colic is repetitive or fails to respond to 4 days of conservative therapy,
- Perforation is suspected,
- Significant obstructive jaundice is present,
- Uncontrolled diabetes coexists, or
- Whenever other intraabdominal emergency conditions cannot be ruled out (e.g., perforated peptic ulcer, appendicitis) (191).

Until recently, open cholecystectomy was the technique of choice in parturients. During the last decade, laparoscopic cholecystectomy has become the primary technique for removing the diseased gallbladder in the nonpregnant population. Pregnancy was initially considered an absolute contraindication to laparoscopic cholecystectomy (192). Recently however, there has been a surge of interest in the application of the laparoscopic technique to pregnant patients (165–168,170,173,193,194). Laparoscopic cholecystectomy has been successfully performed during the first (164,165,167–169,195), second (164,165,168,170, 193,194,196), and third trimesters (165,167,173,194). To avoid uterine and fetal trauma during trocar placement, many surgeons use an open Hasson trocar-introduction technique before insufflation (168,193,196), or they place the Veress insufflation needle into an alternative site far from the uterus (169,173).

There are potential advantages to the use of laparoscopy for this procedure. Decreased postoperative pain may decrease opioid analgesic requirements. If intractable premature labor results from the surgery, the smaller surgical incisions might decrease the risk of wound dehiscence with pushing. Patients tend to require less bed rest after laparoscopic gallbladder removal and can therefore decrease their risk of thromboembolism with early ambulation (168).

General anesthesia is the technique of choice for cholecystectomy (open and laparoscopic) (194). Recent case reports described the use of lumbar (to T_8) (197) and thoracic (T_4 to T_{11}) (164) epidural anesthesia for laparoscopic cholecystectomy in parturients at 15 and 19 weeks' gestation. Insufflation of the abdomen was restricted to 10 mm Hg in one patient (164), and an abdominal wall lifting device was used in the other (197). The women were reportedly comfortable and satisfied with their anesthesia. The authors of these reports concluded that epidural anesthesia should be considered when laparoscopic cholecystectomy is indicated in the pregnant patient. If epidural anesthesia for laparoscopic cholecystectomy is contemplated, the anesthesiologist must ensure that the patient is highly motivated for the experience, and the surgeon is agreeable to the use a less than optimal abdominal-expansion method (i.e., significantly reduced degree of pneumoperitoneum or abdominal wall lifters) and a more gentle surgical touch. Regardless of anesthetic technique, questions about the fetal effects of CO_2 pneumoperitoneum remain unanswered (see earlier). Intraoperative FHR monitoring with a transabdominal (if not within the surgical field) or transvaginal ultrasound transducer is recommended. At minimum, preinduction, postinduction, and postsurgical FHR should be assessed if intraoperative monitoring is impossible.

Neurosurgery

Hemorrhage

Intracranial hemorrhage from rupture of an aneurysm or arteriovenous malformation (AVM) is a devastating complication of pregnancy, with a maternal mortality of up to 50% (198). As the obstetric causes of maternal mortality have steadily declined in the past 50 years, nonobstetric causes such as intracranial hemorrhage have become more important reasons for pregnancy-related death. Although rare, occurring in 0.01% to 0.05% of pregnancies (199), intracranial hemorrhage accounts for 4% to 8.5% of maternal deaths (200,201). A recent review of 154 cases of intracranial hemorrhage found that ruptured aneurysm accounted for 77%, whereas AVM made up the other 23%

(202). Fortunately, this incidence is no greater than that in the nonpregnant population; however, there is a strong correlation between hypertension and rupture of aneurysm or AVM (203). The majority of the pregnancy-related intracranial hemorrhages occur antepartum (92%) with only 8% arising after delivery (202).

Early reports of intracranial hemorrhage during pregnancy recommended delaying the repair of the aneurysm or malformation until after delivery to minimize perceived maternal and fetal risks of surgery and anesthesia (204, 205). However, because of the high mortality associated with the 33% to 50% chance of recurrent bleeding during pregnancy, this recommendation has been abandoned. The decision to operate to correct intracranial aneurysms or AVMs should be made based on neurosurgical, not obstetric, indications (199,202). Both the mother and fetus benefit from appropriate repair during pregnancy (202).

Tumors

There is no difference in the incidence of primary intracranial tumors between pregnant and nonpregnant women of similar ages. However, pregnancy may speed the progression and worsen the symptoms of these tumors (206), especially meningiomas, which can have progesterone or estrogen receptors that may accelerate their growth (207,208). The management of intracranial tumors first seen during pregnancy should be tailored to the individual patient (209).

Trauma

Trauma is the number one cause of death in women of childbearing years. The incidence of trauma, particularly head trauma, during pregnancy is no different from that in the nonpregnant population.

Anesthetic Considerations

Management of anesthesia for neurosurgical procedures during pregnancy requires balancing cerebral perfusion and optimal operating conditions with the need to maintain fetal well-being and uterine relaxation. Increased intracranial pressure or the presence of aneurysm or AVM mandates a smooth induction of anesthesia with a controlled intubation. Concerns about full stomach, increased gastric acidity, and high oxygen consumption favor rapid-sequence induction and intubation. Rapid-sequence induction including intravenous lidocaine, fentanyl, β-blockade, or sodium nitroprusside to control responses to laryngoscopy is a reasonable compromise. Controlled hypotension may be lifesaving if the surgeon needs to gain control of a ruptured aneurysm. Sodium nitroprusside has been used effectively in pregnancy (210), but its use requires continuous fetal monitoring to evaluate the effects of maternal hypotension on FHR.

Hyperventilation

Controlled hyperventilation is commonly used in the treatment of increased intracranial pressure. Hypocarbia decreases cerebral blood flow and intracranial blood volume. In the gravid patient, however, hyperventilation may:

- Decrease uterine blood flow,
- Impair placental oxygen transfer by shift of the oxyhemoglobin dissociation curve, and
- Decrease fetal oxygen tension.

Pregnancy itself induces a mild degree of maternal hyperventilation and alkalosis. In late gestation, maternal p_aCO_2 ranges from 26 to 33 mm Hg (211,212) and the pH from 7.40 to 7.47 (213). Additional hyperventilation and hypocarbia accompany pain and anxiety during labor. Fetal tachycardia and decreased umbilical pH have been reported in parturients who hyperventilate to a p_aCO_2 of about 17 mm Hg (214). However, others found no association between maternal hyperventilation and fetal gas values (215). Animal studies reported uterine and sometimes umbilical vasocontriction as a result of maternal hyperventilation. Decreased fetal p_aO_2 and ultimately fetal acidosis follow (216–219).

Most fetuses, however, will tolerate mild to moderate maternal hypocapnia. A recent case report documented successful moderate hyperventilation for aneurysm repair in a parturient. The authors reduced p_aCO_2 to 33 mm Hg (a normal value for a pregnant patient) (220). A target p_aCO_2 of 30 mm Hg is apparently safe (221). Fetal heart rate monitoring may aid in diagnosis of fetal compromise due to excessive maternal hyperventilation.

Cardiac Surgery

The physiologic demands of pregnancy may cause acute decompensation of previously compensated valvular, congenital, or ischemic heart disease. We are thankful that the incidence of heart disease of all types during pregnancy is less than 1%, and severe cardiac dysfunction is very uncommon (222). However, as parturition is pushed to even older ages by advances in fertility and endocrinology, the potential for cardiac disease during pregnancy could increase. When medical management fails, surgery may be the only treatment option. Many advances have been made since the first cardiopulmonary bypass in 1959 and valvotomy during pregnancy in the 1961 (223). Valvular surgery is still the most common cardiac procedure performed during pregnancy. Repair of septal defects and aortic coarctation and coronary bypass are less common (224). Although still uncommon, cardiac surgery has become a safe and effective treatment modality during pregnancy. Fetal survival has increased from 50% (225) to 80% in the modern cardiac operating room (224). Considering the 100% mortality of the fetus if the mother dies or if she undergoes therapeutic abortion to relieve the physiological stress, most experts recommend proceeding with surgery for cardiac and not obstetric indications (225).

The intricate details of anesthetic management of heart surgery during pregnancy are beyond the scope of this chapter. However, some important points are considered. For a more complete discussion, see the recent reviews by Pomini (224) and Strickland (226).

Cardiopulmonary Bypass

Cardiopulmonary bypass is in essence a state of controlled cardiocirculatory shock (224). It places mother, placenta, and fetus at risk by exposing them to a nonphysiologic environment. Some of the deleterious changes include:

- Hypotension,
- Hypothermia,
- Altered coagulation,
- Release of vasoactive factors,
- Rheologic changes in blood,
- Nonpulsatile blood flow, and
- Potential air or particulate emboli (227).

Neither human nor animal controlled studies have examined the effects of cardiopulmonary bypass on the fetus. Pregnant women tolerate cardiopulmonary bypass as well as nonpregnant women of similar age (225,228). This unfortunately is not the case for the embryo/fetus. Bypass, maternal instability, and the emergency circumstances surrounding cardiac surgery probably contribute to this increased fetal mortality.

Cardiopulmonary bypass, which alters the distribution of blood flow, leading to regional inadequacies in tissue perfusion, can have acute affects on uterine blood flow. Because both oxygen consumption and cardiac output increase throughout pregnancy, increased bypass flow rates may be required to maintain fetal well-being (226). Adequate perfusion pressure also is necessary to maintain flow in the low-resistance uteroplacental circulation. Arterial blood pressure decreases precipitately with initiation of bypass. Both hemodilution and release of vasoactive substances contribute to the decreased peripheral vascular resistance (226). Hypotension can decrease placental perfusion. Fetal tachycardia or bradycardia may arise in response to hypoxemia and acidemia.

Fetal bradycardia is especially common during hypothermic cardiopulmonary bypass in parturients (229–235). In one case, umbilical artery Doppler velocimetry demonstrated loss of fetal diastolic flow during bypass with hypothermia. The authors questioned whether hypothermia should be used in pregnant patients (236). Fetal bradycardia responded to an increase in cardiopulmonary pump flow (235). Without some objective means of monitoring the fetus, this deleterious situation can go unnoticed. As oxygen and blood-flow requirements increase even more during the third trimester, these detrimental effects of cardiopulmonary bypass on the fetus may be further accentuated. Some recommended avoiding cardiopulmonary bypass in the third trimester if possible (234).

There is no evidence that any one anesthetic technique is better than another for parturients undergoing cardiopulmonary bypass. Recommendations include (224,226):

- Maintain adequate pump flow and systemic pressure throughout bypass with a cardiac index of 2.0 to 2.7 L/min/m^2 with a mean arterial pressure 60 mm Hg.
- Avoid hypothermia if possible; keep temperature 32°C.
- Monitor FHR.
- Increase pump flow and systemic pressure if fetal bradycardia follows the institution of bypass.
- Minimize the length of bypass.
- Avoid systemic hyperkalemic cardioplegia because of its damaging effects on the fetus and placenta. Retrograde delivery is the method of choice for cardioplegia.

Vasoactive Drugs and Inotropes

Critically ill parturients, particularly those with heart disease, may require hemodynamic support with inotropic or vasoactive agents. These drugs could have profound effects on uterine blood flow. Understanding their actions is important when choosing an agent. (Note: In most cases, human information on the teratogenic effects of these agents is absent, and therefore all of these compounds are classified pregnancy risk category C.)

Epinephrine is a very potent α- and β-adrenoreceptor agonist that produces profound and rapid cardiovascular responses. Epinephrine has an important role in vascular support in cardiac surgery, shock, and for bronchodilatation in acute asthma. However, a classic study in pregnant sheep showed the existence of α-adrenergic receptors in the uterine vascular bed that produce vasocontriction (237). The uterine vessels exhibited no β-adrenergic vasodilatory activity. Epinephrine decreased uterine blood flow in normotensive gravid sheep (238). Bolus administration of epinephrine, 10 and 20 μg, reduced uterine blood flow by 30% to 40% for up to 3 minutes. (Note: This vasoconstrictor action was at normal blood pressures and may not reflect the effect of epinephrine if maternal hypotension exists.) This premise is supported by a case in which fetal bradycardia resolved with an epinephrine infusion in a patient with profound hypotension after being placed on cardiopulmonary bypass (233). Restoration of maternal hemodynamics in this case probably brought about a net increase in uterine blood flow. In addition, in low doses, epinephrine's β-adrenergic agonist action produces uterine relaxation. However, as the plasma concentrations increase, its α-receptor activation predominates, inducing uterine contraction (239).

In the doses typically used to treat hypotensive shock, norepinephrine is a mixed α- and β_1-adrenoreceptor agonist. In gravid sheep, norepinephrine is a potent uterine artery vasoconstrictor, although these effects are minimal at low dose (0.1 to 0.2 μg/kg/min) (240–242). Frequency and intensity of uterine contraction, as well as resting tone, are increased by the α-adrenergic activity of norepinephrine (243). These actions make the use of norepinephrine less than desirable during pregnancy.

Ephedrine is both a direct-acting α- and β-adrenergic agonist and an indirect sympathomimetic (through its enhanced release of norepinephrine from adrenergic nerve terminals). Ephedrine appears to induce systemic vasoconstriction while selectively sparing uterine vessels, thereby enhancing uterine perfusion (244). It continues to be the vasoconstrictor of choice for hypotension in parturients.

Phenylephrine is a selective α_1-adrenergic agonist, which causes marked vaso- and venoconstriction. When blood pressure was increased by 20% with phenylephrine in normotensive gravid ewes, uterine blood flow decreased by 50% (245). In hypotensive healthy term parturients, phenylephrine, 100 μg, restores maternal blood pressure without demonstrable adverse fetal effects (246). Even if phenylephrine produces some uterine vasoconstriction, the restoration of maternal blood pressure outweighs its potential deleterious effects (247). Phenylephrine has been shown to be a safe and efficacious agent for the treatment of hypotension in pregnant patients (246,248). In fact, in circumstances in which increased heart rate and contractility may be poorly tolerated (e.g., in a compromised parturient with severe cardiac disease), ephedrine may not be an optimal drug. Phenylephrine, in conjunction with FHR monitoring, can be carefully titrated to optimal effect without disrupting the delicate balance between myocardial oxygen consumption and delivery (247).

Dopamine, like ephedrine, is both a direct-acting α- and β-adrenergic agonist and an indirect-acting sympathomimetic that stimulates the release of norepinephrine from sympathetic nerve terminals (249). In addition, at low dose (1 to 5 μg/kg/min), it is an agonist at vascular D_1-dopamine receptors, which enhances renal function. This action has been used to induce diuresis in oliguric parturients (250). At higher doses, dopamine increases uterine vascular resistance in a dose-dependent fashion in pregnant sheep and baboons. However, the ultimate effect of dopamine on uterine blood flow is variable. Some studies found that uterine blood flow increased progressively over a range of doses from 5 to 40 μg/kg/min in both normotensive and hypotensive animals (251,252), whereas others reported marked reductions in uterine blood flow, particularly at doses between 20 and 40 μg/kg/min (253–256). In patients with hypotension during spinal anesthesia for cesarean section, dopamine, 2 to 10 μg/kg/min, was as effective as ephedrine in restoring blood pressure (257). Fetal outcome did not differ between dopamine- and ephedrine-treated mothers. Fetal heart rate monitoring is advisable any time a parturient is treated with dopamine.

The synthetic catecholamine dobutamine is a racemic mixture that predominantly activates β_1- and β_2-adrenoreceptors with minimal α-receptor activity [the (–) enantiomer is an α agonist, whereas the (+) enantiomer is an α antagonist] (258). Its net cardiovascular effect is an increase in cardiac output with a concomitant decrease in vascular tone, resulting from stimulation of β_2-adrenergic receptors and reflex withdrawal of sympathetic efferent nerve activity. Dobutamine is ideal for the treatment of cardiac failure associated with increased systemic vascular resistance. This pharmacologic profile suggests dobutamine would be an ideal agent in pregnancy, as it might not increase uterine vascular tone. Unfortunately, in normotensive pregnant ewes, dobutamine induced a dose-dependent reduction in uterine blood flow (particularly at doses between 20 and 40 μg/kg/min), which paralleled a marked increase in heart rate (255). Tachycardia is uncommon in humans treated with dobutamine and may reflect a species-specific phenomenon. In addition, these normotensive animals may not adequately model the patient in cardiogenic shock. The increases in uterine vascular tone with dobutamine were, however, significantly less than those produced by comparable doses of dopamine. Dobutamine may be a better agent in pregnant parturients with heart failure.

Amrinone and milrinone have both inotropic and vasodilatory activity. These two inodilators appear to act by enhancing intracellular cyclic adenosine monophosphate (AMP) concentrations through their selective inhibition of type III phosphodiesterase (259). The newer of these two bipyridines, milrinone, has a shorter half-life and fewer side effects. It also shows greater selectivity for the type III phosphodiesterase, making it the drug of choice in this class (260). Studies in pregnancy are limited. In pregnant baboons, amrinone at clinically useful doses had no effect on uterine blood flow (254). At doses achieving clinically relevant human plasma concentrations, normotensive pregnant ewes treated with milrinone exhibited no significant change in uterine vascular resistance or blood flow (256). With even higher doses, milrinone induced significant increases in uterine blood flow with concomitant decreases in uterine resistance. Whether this change equated to an increase in placental perfusion could not be established. Milrinone could not be detected in fetal plasma at any maternal dose. In a recent case report, amrinone was used in a patient with refractory heart failure at 18 weeks' gestation (261). Cardiac output increased, and total peripheral resistance decreased; however, therapy was stopped because of metabolic acidosis, hypoxemia, and arrhythmias.

Sodium nitroprusside is a potent, short-acting dilator of both arterioles and venules, used to treat severe hypertension. In animals, nitroprusside effectively returned maternal blood pressure to control values after catecholamine-induced hypertension without harming fetal blood flow (241,242,262). It is rapidly metabolized by the endothelium to cyanide (263) and then by the liver to thiocyanate, both toxic compounds. When sodium nitroprusside was administered at very high doses (25 μg/kg/min for 1 hour) to pregnant sheep, more than 60% of the fetuses died (264). However, when infused within the clinically useful dosage range (2.3 μg/kg/min), fetal concentrations remained well below the fetal lethal threshold (242). Sodium nitroprusside effectively controls hypertension associated with severe preeclampsia without evidence of either maternal or fetal toxicity (265). Sodium nitroprusside also can be useful when deliberate hypotension is required, as in intracranial aneurysm clipping (210). Because the low-resistance uteroplacental circulation depends on maternal blood pressure to maintain adequate blood flow, this agent's rapid and potent effect can potentially harm the fetus. This agent should be used only by experienced personnel and only with appropriate maternal and fetal monitoring.

Nitroglycerin is another potent direct-acting vaso- and venodilator. Unlike nitroprusside, it has no apparent toxicity or tachyphylaxis. In normotensive sheep, when nitroglycerin was infused to reduce arterial blood pressure by 30%, uterine blood flow decreased by 40% (266). However, in pregnant ewes with catecholamine-induced hypertension, nitroglycerin infusion returned systemic and pulmonary blood pressure to control levels and increased uterine artery blood flow from 40% to 50% below control to 24% to 30% below control (241,245). Nitroglycerin, 1.5 to 10 μg/kg/min, lacked affect on the circulatory function of the sheep fetus (267). When used as a vasodilator in preeclamptic parturients, nitroglycerin effectively reduced arterial pressure without changes in uterine blood flow, as measured by pulse Doppler velicometry. Pulsatility index (peak systolic velocity – diastolic velocity/mean velocity) within the umbilical artery decreased with this therapy, suggesting a decrease in fetal circulatory resistance (268). Unchanged FHR (and presumably blood pressure) suggests redistribution of fetal blood flow, the ultimate effect of which is unknown. With evidence of comparable efficacy between nitroglycerin and sodium nitroprusside (241), the absence of toxicity and tachyphylaxis with nitroglycerin warrants its choice as the first-line vasodilator for rapid treatment of severe hypertensive crisis.

Other Operations

Ureterolithotomy and Percutaneous Nephrostomy

About one in 1,500 pregnancies is complicated by kidney or urinary tract stones. Even though the risk of renal calculi is no different between pregnant and nonpregnant women, determining the origin of acute abdominal pain in a pregnant woman is a challenge. In addition, stones may predispose a parturient to premature labor (269).

Almost two thirds of urinary tract stones pass spontaneously. Most of the remainder can be managed conservatively and definitive therapy delayed until after pregnancy. However, when persistent obstruction causes declining kidney function, obstruction occurs in a patient with a solitary kidney, pain becomes intractable, infections proximal to the stone become frequent, or colic induces refractory premature labor, intervention may be necessary (269). Conservative therapy involves placing a percutaneous nephrostomy tube or ureteral stents to decompress the kidney. However, these tubes frequently become plugged or infected, requiring frequent manipulation or changes. Frequent instrumentation can increase complications and prompt preterm labor. Although anatomic distortion resulting from pregnancy and risks of radiation to the fetus have restricted definitive stone extraction in the past, recent advances in ureteroscopy have made basket or forceps extraction a more viable option during pregnancy (270). Extracorporeal shock-wave lithotripsy is absolutely contraindicated during pregnancy because of the risk of disrupting developing fetal tissues (269).

When possible, local anesthesia should be used for these procedures (e.g., percutaneous nephrostomy tube placement). However, cystoscopic/ureteroscopic procedures require more than simply local anesthetic. Sedation/analgesia has been used successfully (271) and is recommended by some (270). However, it is advisable only in skilled hands with full monitoring, including fetal, and with minimal sedation to reduce the loss of protective airway reflexes.

Pheochromocytoma

Pheochromocyatoma is a rare tumor that is very uncommon during pregnancy. However, when present, it carries a devastatingly high maternal and fetal mortality. It is a tumor of the sympathetic nervous system that can induce frighteningly high blood pressures, leading to stroke, seizure, and death. If unrecognized before labor, more than 50% of mothers and their children may die (272).

Pheochromocytoma is difficult to differentiate from other diseases of pregnancy, particularly preeclampsia and eclampsia. Because of the increased mortality from missed diagnosis, it should be considered when flushing, sweating, palpitations, anxiety, or faintness accompanies unexplained hypertension (273). Diagnosis rests on the presence of increased levels of catecholamines or their metabolites in blood and urine. Magnetic resonance imaging has been suggested as a powerful tool to assist in localizing the tumor (274).

Preoperative management of pheochromocytoma requires control of the hypercatecholamine state with the α-adrenergic blocker phenoxybenzamine (a pregnancy risk category C agent). This treatment allows restoration of normal vascular tone and intravascular volume. In addition, despite concerns about intrauterine growth retardation and preterm labor, β-blockade, particularly with propranolol, is an important part of blood pressure control in these women (274). If pheochromocytoma is diagnosed before week 24 of gestation, resection proceeds after controlling blood pressure and intravascular volume. After 24 weeks, some advocate delay until maturity of the fetus so that tumor removal can follow cesarean section (272). Intraoperatively, maintain an adequate depth of anesthesia to prevent vascular responses to noxious stimuli. This challenge requires modifying the normal rapid-induction sequence to include opioids, intravenous lidocaine, or a potent agent to blunt hypertensive response to intubation. Intraoperative invasive hemodynamic monitoring is important for prompt recognition and treatment of hypertension before and hypotension after tumor removal (273).

ANESTHETIC CONSIDERATIONS

Maternal Medical Condition

The preoperative assessment of the pregnant patient for nonobstetric surgery should incorporate all the aspects of a routine evaluation for a nonpregnant patient. The anatomic and physiologic changes of pregnancy can strongly influence existing medical conditions. Duration of pregnancy at the time of surgery determines the extent of these physiologic and anatomic influences.

Maternal and Fetal Monitoring

The presence and severity of preexisting maternal disease determine the extent of intraoperative monitoring. An uncomplicated pregnant patient requires the basic monitors recommended in the American Society of Anesthesiologists' Guidelines (Standards for Basic Anesthetic Monitoring, amended October 23, 1996). Pulse oximetry and end-tidal capnography are especially important in these women to help detect hypoxemia and ensure proper endotracheal tube placement. The use of additional monitoring depends on the patient's condition and the surgical procedure to be performed.

Continuous fetal monitoring allows assessment of fetal well-being throughout anesthesia and surgery (275). Fetal heart rate is detectable by transabdominal ultrasound after week 16 of pregnancy (276) and by vaginal ultrasonography even earlier (224). A FHR transducer can easily be positioned and left in place (unless it would interfere with the sterile surgical field) (12). The FHR begins to exhibit fluctuations of six to eight beats/min after weeks 25 to 27 of gestation. These fluctuations, known as beat-to-beat variability, reflect changes in parasympathetic and sympathetic nervous outflows from the fetal medulla. Beat-to-beat variability is a good indicator of fetal well-being (277). The FHR variability is best evaluated by using a fetal scalp electrode, which records well-defined electrocardiographic R-wave potentials for the cardiotachograph to integrate and plot (278). External Doppler transducers have a poor signal-to-noise ratio compared with the fetal scalp electrode and cannot detect subtle changes in beat-to-beat variability. However, because the fetal-scalp electrode is not an option in the majority of surgical cases in pregnant patients, the external transducer must be used. Gross alterations in FHR variability (e.g., loss of beat-to-beat variability) give fairly reliable indications of changes in fetal status. Besides heart-rate variability, changes in baseline FHR are an indication of fetal condition. Moderate degrees of hypoxemia can produce transient to prolonged fetal tachycardia (i.e., FHR more than 160 beats/min) (278). If fetal tachycardia arises intraoperatively, search for maternal hypoxemia, hypovolemia, or any other factors that could interfere with gas exchange at the placental interface (279). Under conditions of profound hypoemxia, acidemia foils the fetus's compensatory efforts by directly depressing cardiac function, resulting in fetal bradycardia (i.e., FHR less than 110 beats/min) (280).

Regional Versus General Anesthesia

Local, regional, and general anesthesia can provide suitable surgical conditions in pregnant women. The ultimate choice of anesthetic should be based on maternal status, extent and anatomic region of the planned surgery, and the expertise of the anesthesiologist (276). Most obstetric anesthesiologists prefer regional anesthesia whenever possible. Regional anesthesia has the following advantages:

- Reduces the risk of maternal aspiration, as long as supplemental sedation is kept to a minimum,
- Decreases fetal drug exposure, particularly if a subarachnoid block is used,
- Uses local anesthesias, which unlike inhalational agents, are not known teratogens (12), and
- Allows the use of intrathecal or epidural opioids for intraoperative and postoperative pain relief.

From this list of regional anesthesia advantages, the reader should not infer that general anesthesia is unsuitable. In many circumstances, regional and local anesthesia are not options. A carefully performed general anesthetic presents no greater maternal risk than does either local or regional anesthesia.

Premature Labor

Parturients undergoing anesthesia and surgery are at significant risk for premature labor and spontaneous abortion (1,281,282). During the second trimester, the risk of spontaneous abortion is fivefold greater than that in matched controls (283). Whether this increased risk of abortion results from the surgery or the anesthesia remains unknown (282,284). No matter the cause of premature labor after surgery, these data point to the need for postoperative uterine monitoring and aggressive tocolytic management if contractions are associated with cervical change (285).

ANESTHETIC TECHNIQUE

A preoperative visit is vital to the anesthetic management of the pregnant surgical patient. The anesthesiologist can allay the woman's concerns and fears and reduce her apprehension by discussing the anesthetic plan and answering her questions. As with any other patient group, a reassuring preoperative visit can reduce the need for premedication (286).

Aspiration prophylaxis is an important consideration for any gravid patient undergoing surgery. Increased gastric acidity with pregnancy warrants conservative gastrointestinal prophylaxis for all parturients. Give an H_2-receptor antagonist (cimetadine, famotidine, nizatidine, or ranitidine) the night before and the morning of surgery to reduce gastric acid secretion (both acidity and volume). A nonparticulate antacid (0.3 *M* sodium citrate, 30 mL) 15 to 30 minutes before induction will increase the pH of any existing gastric contents. Metoclopramide, 10 mg orally or intravenously, will reduce gastric volume by enhancing emptying in this patient population (287) and could be a part of an overall aspiration-prophylaxis regimen. However, metoclopramide may induce maternal tachycardia (288), particularly in response to surgical stress (289).

To avoid aortocaval compression, no woman at more than 25 weeks of gestation should be transported to or placed on the operating room table supine. If FHR and uterine-contraction monitoring are feasible (greater than 17 weeks' gestation) and not within the surgical field, place external transducers before induction. If fetal monitoring is impossible and an intravaginal probe is not available, then assess FHR before and after induction of anesthesia and then again at the end of surgery. Because the reading and interpretation of continuous FHR and uterine-contraction patterns are not part of the day-to-day job of an anesthesiologist, close consultation with an obstetrician may be necessary if unusual changes occur intraoperatively.

To avoid hypotension, infuse at least 1 L of balanced salt solution before inducing either spinal or epidural anesthesia. Be prepared to administer more fluid if hypotension does arise. If blood pressure decreases more than 15% below the preanesthetic level or the patient exhibits symptoms of cerebral hypoperfusion (e.g., nausea, vomiting, altered level of consciousness), give ephedrine, 5 to 10 mg intravenously.

For general anesthesia remember the following:

- Carefully denitrogenate the patient by using 100% oxygen by mask before induction to reduce the risk of maternal and fetal hypoxemia.
- Even with adequate gastric acid prophylaxis therapy, do a rapid-sequence induction and intubation with a cuffed endotracheal tube and cricoid pressure. Oral or nasogastric suctioning after intubation may help minimize the possibility of periopertive passive aspiration.
- Aspiration is as great a problem on extubation as on intubation. Delay extubation. Look for objective signs of intact airway reflexes and motor strength (e.g., adequate tidal volumes, train-of-four without a decrement, tetany at 50 Hz without a fade, head lift for 5 seconds).
- Proper ventilation is very important during general anesthesia in the parturient. Mechanical hyperventilation markedly reduces uterine blood flow (218). To avoid this risk, monitor end-tidal capnography closely, and sample arterial blood gases, if necessary, to maintain p_aCO_2 within normal pregnancy limits (30 to 35mm Hg). Remember, pregnancy decreases the arterial to end-tidal CO_2 gradient. End-tidal CO_2 approximates p_aCO_2 (Fig. 9) (290).

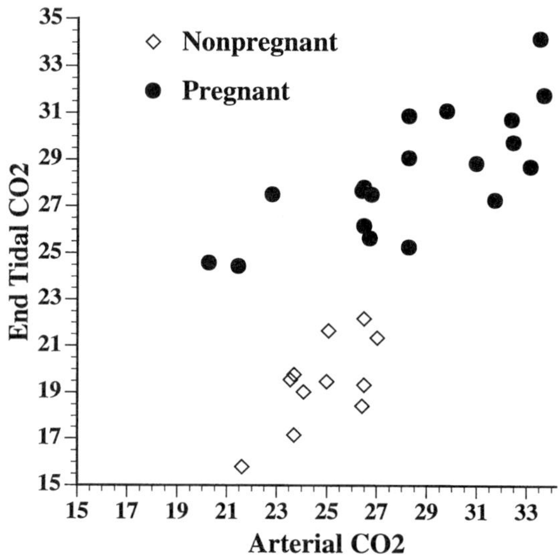

FIG. 9. End-tidal to arterial CO_2 gradient during general endotracheal anesthesia in pregnant and nonpregnant patients. (From ref. 290, with permission.)

REFERENCES

1. Brodsky JB, Cohen EN, Brown BW Jr, Wu ML, Whitcher C. Surgery during pregnancy and fetal outcome. *Am J Obstet Gynecol* 1980;138:1165.
2. Manley S, de Kelaita G, Joseph NJ, Salem MR, Heyman HJ. Preoperative pregnancy testing in ambulatory surgery: incidence and impact of positive results. *Anesthesiology* 1995;83:690.
3. Lees MM, Taylor SH, Scott DB, Kerr MG. A study of cardiac output at rest throughout pregnancy. *J Obstet Gynaecol Br Commonw* 1967;74:319.
4. Lund CJ, Donovan JC. Blood volume during pregnancy: significance of plasma and red cell volumes. *Am J Obstet Gynecol* 1967;98:393.
5. Martin C, Varner MW. Physiologic changes in pregnancy: surgical implications. *Clin Obstet Gynecol* 1994;37:241.
6. Cutforth R, MacDonald CB. Heart sounds and murmurs in pregnancy. *Am Heart J* 1966;71:741.
7. Song CS, Merkatz IR, Rifkind AB, Gillette PN, Kappas A. The influence of pregnancy and oral contraceptive steroids on the concentration of plasma proteins: studies with a quantitative immunodiffusion method. *Am J Obstet Gynecol* 1970;108:227.

8. Leighton BL, Cheek TG, Gross JB, et al. Succinylcholine pharmacodynamics in peripartum patients. *Anesthesiology* 1986;64:202.
9. Weissman DB, Ehrenwerth J. Prolonged neuromuscular blockade in a parturient associated with succinylcholine. *Anesth Analg* 1983;62:444.
10. Howard BK, Goodson JH, Mengert WF. Supine hypotensive syndrome in late pregnancy. *Obstet Gynecol* 1953;1:371.
11. Kerr MG, Scott DB, Samuel E. Studies of the inferior vena cava in late pregnancy. *BMJ* 1964;1:532.
12. Pedersen H, Finster M. Anesthetic risk in the pregnant surgical patient. *Anesthesiology* 1979;51:439.
13. Bieniarz J, Crottogini JJ, Curuchet E, et al. Aortocaval compression by the uterus in late human pregnancy. II. An arteriographic study. *Am J Obstet Gynecol* 1968;100:203.
14. McMorland GH. Cardiovascular and respiratory changes in late pregnancy. In: Datta S, ed. *Common problems in obstetric anesthesia.* 2nd ed. St. Louis: Mosby, 1995:1.
15. Cugell DW, Frank NR, Gaensler EA, Badger TL. Pulmonary function in pregnancy. I. Serial observations in normal women. *Am Rev Tuberc* 1953;67:568.
16. Prowse CM, Gaensler EA. Respiratory and acid-base changes during pregnancy. *Anesthesiology* 1965;26:381.
17. Alaily AB, Carrol KB. Pulmonary ventilation in pregnancy. *Br J Obstet Gynaecol* 1978;85:518.
18. Pernoll ML, Metcalfe J, Schlenker TL, Welch JE, Matsumoto JA. Oxygen consumption at rest and during exercise in pregnancy. *Respir Physiol* 1975;25:285.
19. Rees GB, Pipkin FB, Symonds EM, Patrick JM. A longitudinal study of respiratory changes in normal human pregnancy with cross-sectional data on subjects with pregnancy-induced hypertension. *Am J Obstet Gynecol* 1990;162:826.
20. Archer GW Jr, Marx GF. Arterial oxygen tension during apnoea in parturient women. *Br J Anaesth* 1974;46:358.
21. Palahniuk RJ, Shnider SM, Eger EI II. Pregnancy decreases the requirement for inhaled anesthetic agents. *Anesthesiology* 1974;41:82.
22. Gin T, Chan MTV. Decreased minimum alveolar concentration of isoflurane in pregnant humans. *Anesthesiology* 1994;81:829.
23. Chan MTV, Mainland P, Gin T. Minimum alveolar concentration of halothane and enflurane are decreased in early pregnancy. *Anesthesiology* 1996;85:782.
24. Merryman W, Boiman R, Barnes L, Rothchild I. Progesterone "anesthesia" in human subjects [Letter]. *J Clin Endocrinol Metab* 1954; 14:1567.
25. Lyrenäs S, Nyberg F, Lindberg B, Terenius L. Cerebrospinal fluid activity of dynorphin-converting enzyme at term pregnancy. *Obstet Gynecol* 1988;72:54.
26. Gin T, Mainland P, Chan MTV, Short TG. Decreased thiopental requirements in early pregnancy. *Anesthesiology* 1997;86:73.
27. Fagraeus L, Urban BJ, Bromage PR. Spread of epidural analgesia in early pregnancy. *Anesthesiology* 1983;58:184.
28. Butterworth JF IV, Walker FO, Lysak SZ. Pregnancy increases median nerve susceptibility to lidocaine. *Anesthesiology* 1990;72:962.
29. Dietz FB, Jaffe RA. Pregnancy does not increase susceptibility to bupivacaine in spinal root axons. *Anesthesiology* 1997;87:610.
30. Hunt JN, Murray FA. Gastric function in pregnancy. *J Obstet Gynaecol Br Emp* 1958;65:78.
31. O'Sullivan GM, Sutton AJ, Thompson SA, Carrie LE, Bullingham RE. Noninvasive measurement of gastric emptying in obstetric patients. *Anesth Analg* 1987;66:505.
32. Macfie AG, Magides AD, Richmond MN, Reilly CS. Gastric emptying in pregnancy. *Br J Anaesth* 1991;67:54.
33. Carp H, Jayaram A, Stoll M. Ultrasound examination of the stomach contents of parturients. *Anesth Analg* 1992;74:683.
34. Simpson KH, Stakes AF, Miller M. Pregnancy delays paracetamol absorption and gastric emptying in patients undergoing surgery. *Br J Anaesth* 1988;60:24.
35. O'Sullivan G. Gastric emptying during pregnancy and the puerperium. *Int J Obstet Anesth* 1993;2:216.
36. Brock-Utne JG, Dow TGB, Dimopoulos GE, Welman S, Downing JW, Moshal MG. Gastric and lower oesophageal sphincter (los) pressures in early pregnancy. *Br J Anaesth* 1981;53:381.
37. Moya F, Kvisselgaard N. The placental transmission of succinylcholine. *Anesthesiology* 1961;22:1.
38. Abouleish E, Wingard LB Jr, de la Vega S, Uy N. Pancuronium in caesarean section and its placental transfer. *Br J Anaesth* 1980; 52:531.
39. Demetriou M, Depoix J-P, Diakite B, Fromentin M, Duvaldestin P. Placental transfer of Org NC 45 in women undergoing caesarean section. *Br J Anaesth* 1982;54:643.
40. Shearer ES, Fahy LT, O'Sullivan EP, Hunter JM. Transplacental distribution of atracurium, laudanosine and monoquaternary alcohol during elective caesarean section. *Br J Anaesth* 1991;66:551.
41. Briggs GG, Freeman RK, Yaffee SJ. *Drugs in pregnancy and lactation: a reference guide to fetal and neonatal risk.* 4th ed. Baltimore: Williams & Wilkins, 1994.
42. Kastrup EK, Hebel SK, eds. *Drugs: facts and comparisons.* St. Louis: Facts and Comparisons, 1997.
43. Arky R, ed. *Physicians' desk reference.* 52nd ed. Montvale, NJ: Medical Economics Company, 1998.
44. Gray M, Noueihed LA, eds. *PDR Generics.* 3rd ed. Montvale, NJ: Medical Economics Company, 1997.
45. Moore KL, ed. *The developing human: clinically oriented embryology.* 3rd ed. Philadelphia: WB Saunders, 1982.
46. Tuchmann-Duplessis H. Selection of animal species for teratological drug testing. In: Neubert D, Merker H-J, Kwasigroch TE, eds. *Methods in prenatal toxicity: evaluation of embryotoxic effects in experimental animals.* Stuttgart: Georg Thieme Publishers, 1977:25.
47. Shepard TH. Human teratogens: how can we sort them out? *Ann N Y Acad Sci* 1986;477:105.
48. Novitt AD, Gilani SH. Abnormal embryogenesis induced by thiopental. *J Clin Pharmacol* 1979;19:697.
49. Ojeda JL. Aberrant nerve fibres in embryos treated with thiopental. *Experientia* 1969;25:516.
50. Persaud TVN. Tierexperimentelle untersuchungen zur frage der teratogenen wirkung von barbituraten. *Acta Biol Med Ger* 1965;14:89.
51. Tanimura T, Owaki Y, Nishimura H. Effect of administration of thiopental sodium to pregnant mice upon the development of their offspring. *Okajimas Folia Anat Jpn* 1967;43:219.
52. el-Karim AHB, Benny R. Embryotoxic and teratogenic action of ketamine hydrochloride in rats. *Ain Shavis Med J* 1976;27:459.
53. Lee H, Nagele RG. Neural tube defects caused by local anesthetics in early chick embryos. *Teratology* 1985;31:119.
54. Bandazhevskii II, Shimanovich AI. The characteristics of the embryotoxic action of kalipsol (English trans.). *Farmakol Toksikol* 1991;54:58.
55. Basford AB, Fink BR. The teratogenicity of halothane in the rat. *Anesthesiology* 1968;29:1167.
56. Kennedy GL Jr, Smith SH, Keplinger ML, Calandra JC. Reproductive and teratologic studies with halothane. *Toxicol Appl Pharmacol* 1976; 35:467.
57. Lansdown ABG, Pope WDB, Halsey MJ, Bateman PE. Analysis of fetal development in rats following maternal exposure to subanesthetic concentrations of halothane. *Teratology* 1976;13:299.
58. Wharton RS, Wilson AI, Mazze RI, Baden JM, Rice SA. Fetal morphology in mice exposed to halothane. *Anesthesiology* 1979;51:532.
59. Fujinaga M. Anesthetics. In: Kavlock RJ, Daston GP, eds. *Drug toxicity in embryonic development II: advances in understanding mechanisms of birth defects: mechanistic understanding of human developmental toxicants.* Berlin: Springer, 1997:295.
60. Smoak IW, Sadler TW. Hypothermia: teratogenic and protective effects on the development of mouse embryos in vitro. *Teratology* 1991;43:635.
61. Wharton RS, Mazze RI, Wilson AI. Reproduction and fetal development in mice chronically exposed to enflurane. *Anesthesiology* 1981; 54:505.
62. Mazze RI, Fujinaga M, Rice SA, Harris SB, Baden JM. Reproductive and teratogenic effects of nitrous oxide, halothane, isoflurane, and enflurane in Sprague-Dawley rats. *Anesthesiology* 1986;64:339.
63. Strout CD, Nahrwold ML, Taylor MD, Zagon IS. Effects of subanesthetic concentrations of enflurane on rat pregnancy and early development. *Environ Health Perspect* 1977;21:211.
64. Halsey MJ, Green CJ, Monk SJ, Doré C, Knight JF, Luff NP. Maternal and paternal chronic exposure to enflurane and halothane: fetal and histological changes in the rat. *Br J Anaesth* 1981;53:203.
65. Mazze RI, Wilson AI, Rice SA, Baden JM. Fetal development in mice exposed to isoflurane. *Teratology* 1985;32:339.
66. Fink BR, Shepard TH, Blandau RJ. Teratogenic activity of nitrous oxide. *Nature* 1967;214:146.

67. Shepard TH, Fink BR. Teratogenic activity of nitrous oxide in rats. In: Fink BR, ed. *Toxicity of anesthetics*. Baltimore: Williams & Wilkins, 1968:308.
68. Vieira E, Cleaton-Jones P, Austin JC, Moyes DG, Shaw R. Effects of low concentrations of nitrous oxide on rat fetuses. *Anesth Analg* 1980; 59:175.
69. Chanarin I. Cobalamins and nitrous oxide: a review. *J Clin Pathol* 1980;33:909.
70. Marx GF, Joshi CW, Orkin LR. Placental transmission of nitrous oxide. *Anesthesiology* 1970;32:429.
71. Baden JM, Serra M, Mazze RI. Inhibition of fetal methionine synthase by nitrous oxide. *Br J Anaesth* 1984;56:523.
72. Hansen DK, Billings RE. Effects of nitrous oxide on macromolecular content and DNA synthesis in rat embryos. *J Pharmacol Exp Ther* 1986;238:985.
73. Gaull GE, von Berg W, Räihä NCR, Sturman JA. Development of methyltransferase activity of human fetal tissues. *Pediatr Res* 1973; 7:527.
74. Mazze RI, Fujinaga M, Baden JM. Halothane prevents nitrous oxide teratogenicity in Sprague-Dawley rats; folinic acid does not. *Teratology* 1988;38:121.
75. Fujinaga M, Baden JM. Methionine prevents nitrous oxide-induced teratogenicity in rat embryos grown in culture. *Anesthesiology* 1994; 81:184.
76. Baden JM, Fujinaga M. Effects of nitrous oxide on day 9 rat embryos grown in culture. *Br J Anaesth* 1991;66:500.
77. Fujinaga M, Baden JM, Suto A, Myatt JK, Mazze RI. Preventive effects of phenoxybenzamine on nitrous oxide-induced reproductive toxicity in Sprague-Dawley rats. *Teratology* 1991;43:151.
78. Nunn JF, Chanarin I. Nitrous oxide inactivates methionine synthetase. In: Eger EI, ed. *Nitrous oxide/N_2O*. New York: Elsevier, 1985:211.
79. Cohen EN, Bellville JW Brown BW Jr. Anesthesia, pregnancy, and miscarriage: a study of operating room nurses and anesthetists. *Anesthesiology* 1971;35:343.
80. Spence AA, Cohen EN, Brown BW Jr., Knill-Jones RP, Himmelberger DU. Occupational hazards for operating room-based physicians: analysis of data from the United States and the United Kingdom. *JAMA* 1977;238:955.
81. Cohen EN, Gift HC, Brown BW, et al. Occupational disease in dentistry and chronic exposure to trace anesthetic gases. *J Am Dent Assoc* 1980;101:21.
82. Ericson HA, Källén AJB. Hospitalization for miscarriage and delivery outcome among Swedish nurses working in operating rooms 1973-1978. *Anesth Analg* 1985;64:981.
83. Hemminki K, Kyyrönen P, Lindbohm M-L. Spontaneous abortions and malformations in the offspring of nurses exposed to anaesthetic gases, cytostatic drugs, and other potential hazards in hospitals, based on registered information of outcome. *J Epidemiol Community Health* 1985;39:141.
84. Spence AA. Environmental pollution by inhalation anaesthetics. *Br J Anaesth* 1987;59:96.
85. Crawford JS, Lewis M. Nitrous oxide in early human pregnancy. *Anaesthesia* 1986;41:900.
86. Aldridge LM, Tunstall ME. Nitrous oxide and the fetus: a review and the results of a retrospective study of 175 cases of anaesthesia for insertion of Shirodkar suture. *Br J Anaesth* 1986;58:1348.
87. Mazze RI, Källén B. Reproductive outcome after anesthesia and operation during pregnancy: a registry study of 5405 cases. *Am J Obstet Gynecol* 1989;161:1178.
88. Ready LB, Plumer MH, Haschke RH, Austin E, Sumi SM. Neurotoxicity of intrathecal local anesthetics in rabbits. *Anesthesiology* 1985; 63:364.
89. Myers RR, Kalichman MW, Reisner LS, Powell HC. Neurotoxicity of local anesthetics: altered perineurial permeability, edema, and nerve fiber injury. *Anesthesiology* 1986;64:29.
90. Kalichman MW, Powell HC, Myers RR. Pathology of local anesthetic-induced nerve injury. *Acta Neuropathol (Berl)* 1988;75:583.
91. Kalichman MW, Powell HC, Myers RR. Quantitative histologic analysis of local anesthetic-induced injury to rat sciatic nerve. *J Pharmacol Exp Ther* 1989;250:406.
92. Kalichman MW, Moorhouse DF, Powell HC, Myers RR. Relative neural toxicity of local anesthetics. *J Neuropathol Exp Neurol* 1993;52:234.
93. de Jong RH. Last round for a "heavyweight"? [Editorial]. *Anesth Analg* 1994;78:3.
94. Lee H, Bush KT, Nagele RG. Time-lapse photographic study of neural tube closure defects caused by xylocaine in the chick. *Teratology* 1988;37:263.
95. O'Shea KS, Kaufman MH. Neural tube closure defects following in vitro exposure of mouse embryos to xylocaine. *J Exp Zool* 1980; 214:235.
96. Heinonen OP, Slone D, Shapiro S. *Birth defects and drugs in pregnancy.* Littleton, MA: Publishing Sciences Group, 1977.
97. McDonald IA. Cervical cerclage. *Clin Obstet Gynaecol* 1980;7:461.
98. Lidegaard O. Cervical incompetence and cerclage in Denmark 1980-1990: a register based epidemiological survey. *Acta Obstet Gynecol Scand* 1994;73:35.
99. MRC/RCOG Working Party on Cervical Cerclage. Final report of the Medical Research Council/Royal College of Obstetricians and Gynaecologists multicentre randomized trial of cervical cerclage. *Br J Obstet Gynaecol* 1993;100:516.
100. Ayhan A, Mercan R, Tuncer ZS, Tuncer R, Kiniçi HA. Postconceptional cervical cerclage. *Int J Gynecol Obstet* 1993;42:243.
101. Golan A, Wolman I, Arieli S, Barnan R, Sagi J, David MP. Cervical cerclage for the incompetent cervical os: improving the fetal salvage rate. *J Reprod Med* 1995;40:367.
102. Lash AF, Lash SR. Habitual abortion: the incompetent internal os of the cervix. *Am J Obstet Gynecol* 1950;59:68.
103. Shirodkar VN. A method of operative treatment for habitual abortions in the second trimester of pregnancy. *Antiseptic* 1955;52:299.
104. Olatunbosun OA, Dyck F. Cervical cerclage operation for a dilated cervix. *Obstet Gynecol* 1981;57:166.
105. Goodlin RC. Surgical treatment of patients with hour glass shaped or ruptured membranes prior to the twenty-fifth week of gestation. *Surg Gynecol Obstet* 1987;165:410.
106. Novy MJ, Haymond J, Nichols M. Shirodkar cerclage in a multifactorial approach to the patient with advanced cervical changes. *Am J Obstet Gynecol* 1990;162:1412.
107. Caspi E, Schneider DF, Mor Z, Langer R, Weinraub Z, Bukovsky I. Cervical internal os cerclage: description of a new technique and comparison with Shirodkar operation. *Am J Perinatol* 1990;7:347.
108. McDonald IA. Suture of the cervix for inevitable miscarriage. *J Obstet Gynaecol Br Emp* 1957;64:346.
109. Weissman A, Jakobi P, Zahi S, Zimmer EZ. The effect of cervical cerclage on the course of labor. *Obstet Gynecol* 1990;76:168.
110. Hefner JD, Patow WE, Ludwig JM Jr. A new surgical procedure for the correction of incompetent cervix during pregnancy: the Wurm procedure. *Obstet Gynecol* 1961;18:616.
111. Goodlin RC. Cervical incompetence, hourglass membranes, and amniocentesis. *Obstet Gynecol* 1979;54:748.
112. McGahan JP, Hanson F. Prolapsing amniotic membranes: detection, sonographic appearance, and management. *J Perinatol* 1987;7:204.
113. Benson RC, Durfee RB. Transabdominal cervicouterine cerclage during pregnancy for the treatment of cervical incompetence. *Obstet Gynecol* 1965;25:145.
114. Cammarano CL, Herron MA, Parer JT. Validity of indications for transabdominal cervicoisthmic cerclage for cervical incompetence. *Am J Obstet Gynecol* 1995;172:1871.
115. Novy MJ. Transabdominal cervicoisthmic cerclage: a reappraisal 25 years after its introduction. *Am J Obstet Gynecol* 1991;164:1635.
116. van Dongen PWJ, Nijhuis JG. Transabdominal cerclage. *Eur J Obstet Gynecol Reprod Biol* 1991;41:97.
117. Gibb DMF, Salaria DA. Transabdominal cervicoisthmic cerclage in the management of recurrent second trimester miscarriage and preterm delivery. *Br J Obstet Gynaecol* 1995;102:802.
118. Seppälä M, Vara P. Cervical cerclage in the treatment of incompetent cervix: a retrospective analysis of the indications and results of 164 operations. *Acta Obstet Gynecol Scand* 1970;49:343.
119. Harger JH. Cervical cerclage: patient selection, morbidity, and success rates. *Clin Perinatol* 1983;10:321.
120. Stromme WB, Wagner RM, Reed SC. Surgical management of the incompetent cervix. *Obstet Gynecol* 1960;15:635.
121. Goldman GA, Dicker D, Peleg D, Goldman JA. Is elective cerclage justified in the management of triplet and quadruplet pregnancy? *Aust N Z J Obstet Gynaecol* 1989;29:9.
122. Flynn A, Scott F, Birrell W, Evans N. Delayed-interval delivery in a quadruplet pregnancy: the use of transperineal ultrasound and cervical cerclage. *Aust N Z J Obstet Gynaecol* 1995;35:280.
123. Mordel N, Zajicek G, Benshushan A, Schenker JG, Laufer N,

Sadovsky E. Elective suture of uterine cervix in triplets. *Am J Perinatol* 1993;10:14.

124. Ayers JWT. Cervical incompetence: diagnosis and management of preterm effacement. In: Dilts PV Jr, Sciarra JJ, eds. *Gynecology and obstetrics.* Philadelphia: JB Lippincott, 1989:1.
125. Rush RW, Isaacs S, McPherson K, Jones L, Chalmers I, Grant A. A randomized controlled trial of cervical cerclage in women at high risk of spontaneous preterm delivery. *Br J Obstet Gynaecol* 1984; 91:724.
126. Lazar P, Gueguen S, Dreyfus J, Renaud R, Pontonnier G, Papiernik E. Multicentered controlled trial of cervical cerclage in women at moderate risk of preterm delivery. *Br J Obstet Gynaecol* 1984;91:731.
127. Scheerer LJ, Lam F, Bartolucci L, Katz M. A new technique for reduction of prolapsed fetal membranes for emergency cervical cerclage. *Obstet Gynecol* 1989;74:408.
128. Lauersen NH, Fuchs F. Experience with Shirodkar's operation and postoperative alcohol treatment. *Acta Obstet Gynecol Scand* 1973; 52:77.
129. Cousins L. Cervical incompetence, 1980: a time for reappraisal. *Clin Obstet Gynecol* 1980;23:467.
130. Kurzel RB, Ott H Jr. Cerclage, tocolysis and antibiotics for premature rupture of the membranes in previable twins. a case report. *J Reprod Med* 1992;37:289.
131. Weingold AB, Palmer JI, Stone ML. Cervical incompetency: a therapeutic enigma. *Fertil Steril* 1968;19:244.
132. Munson ES, Embro WJ. Enflurane, isoflurane, and halothane and isolated human uterine muscle. *Anesthesiology* 1977;46:11.
133. Coutifaris B, Coutifaris C. Management of the incompetent uterine cervix: a modified technique. In: Hafez ESE, ed. *Spontaneous abortion.* Lancaster: MTP Press, 1984:337.
134. McDonald IA. Cervical incompetence as a cause of spontaneous abortion. In: Bennett MJ, Edmonds DK, eds. *Spontaneous and recurrent abortion.* Oxford: Blackwell Scientific Publications, 1987:168.
135. Harger JH. Comparison of success and morbidity in cervical cerclage procedures. *Obstet Gynecol* 1980;56:543.
136. Shortle B, Jewelewicz R. *Clinical aspects of cervical incompetence.* Chicago: Yearbook Medical Publishers, 1989.
137. Fox R, James M, Tuohy J, Wardle P. Transvaginal ultrasound in the management of women with suspected cervical incompetence. *Br J Obstet Gynaecol* 1996;103:921.
138. Wetchler BV, Brick J. Safety of outpatient cerclage. *J Reprod Med* 1990;35:243.
139. Golan A, Wolman I, Barnan R, Niv D, David MP. Outpatient versus inpatient cervical cerclage. *J Reprod Med* 1994;39:788.
140. McCulloch B, Bergen S, Pielet B, Keller J, Elrad H. McDonald cerclage under pudendal nerve block. *Am J Obstet Gynecol* 1993;168:499.
141. Charles D, Glover DD. Incompetent cervical os. In: Cibils LA, ed. *Surgical disease in pregnancy.* New York: Springer-Verlag, 1990:1.
142. MacDougall J, Siddle N. Emergency cervical cerclage. *Br J Obstet Gynaecol* 1991;98:1234.
143. Lipitz S, Libshitz A, Oelsner G, et al. Outcome of second-trimester, emergency cervical cerclage in patients with no history of cervical incompetence. *Am J Perinatol* 1996;13:419.
144. Schorr SJ, Morales WJ. Obstetric management of incompetent cervix and bulging fetal membranes. *J Reprod Med* 1996;41:235.
145. Higuchi M, Hirano H, Maki M. Emergency cervical cerclage using a metreurynter in patients with bulging membranes. *Acta Obstet Gynecol Scand* 1992;71:34.
146. Cousins LM, Pue A. Nitroglycerin facilitates therapeutic cerclage placement. *J Perinatol* 1996;16:127.
147. Aarts JM, Brons JTJ, Bruinse HW. Emergency cerclage: a review. *Obstet Gynecol Surv* 1995;50:459.
148. Barth WH Jr. Cervical incompetence and cerclage: unresolved controversies. *Clin Obstet Gynecol* 1994;37:831.
149. Levine W, Diamond B. Surgical procedures during pregnancy. *Am J Obstet Gynecol* 1961;81:1046.
150. Hopkins MP, Duchon MA. Adnexal surgery in pregnancy. *J Reprod Med* 1986;31:1035.
151. Curtis M, Hopkins MP, Zarlingo T, Martino C, Graciansky-Lengyl M, Jenison EL. Magnetic resonance imaging to avoid laparotomy in pregnancy. *Obstet Gynecol* 1993;82:833.
152. Thornton JG, Wells M. Ovarian cysts in pregnancy: does ultrasound make traditional management inappropriate? *Obstet Gynecol* 1987; 69:717.
153. Hess LW, Peaceman A, O'Brien WF, Winkel CA, Cruikshank DP, Morrison JC. Adnexal mass occurring with intrauterine pregnancy: report of fifty-four patients requiring laparotomy for definitive management. *Am J Obstet Gynecol* 1988;158:1029.
154. Bryan WMJ. Surgical emergencies in pregnancies and the puerperium. *Am J Obstet Gynecol* 1955;70:1204.
155. Struyk APHB, Treffers PE. Ovarian tumors in pregnancy. *Acta Obstet Gynecol Scand* 1984;63:421.
156. Rojansky N, Schenker JG. Heterotopic pregnancy and assisted reproduction: an update. *J Assist Reprod Genet* 1996;13:594.
157. Atrash HK, Friede A, Hogue CJR. Ectopic pregnancy mortality in the United States, 1970-1983. *Obstet Gynecol* 1987;70:817.
158. Jehle D, Krause R, Braen GR. Ectopic pregnancy. *Emerg Med Clin North Am* 1994;12:55.
159. Gonzalez FA, Waxman M. Ectopic pregnancy: a prospective study on differential diagnosis. *Diagn Gynecol Obstet* 1981;3:101.
160. Nager CW, Murphy AA. Ectopic pregnancy. *Clin Obstet Gynecol* 1991;34:403.
161. Loffer FD. Surgical settings and incisions for the management of ectopic pregnancies. *J Reprod Med* 1986;31:94.
162. Feichtinger W, Kemeter P. Conservative treatment of ectopic pregnancy by transvaginal aspiration under sonographic control and methotrexate injection [Letter]. *Lancet* 1987;1:381.
163. Nezhat F, Nezhat C, Silfen SL, Fehnel SH. Laparoscopic ovarian cystectomy during pregnancy. *J Laparoendosc Surg* 1991;1:161.
164. Costantino GN, Vincent GJ, Mukalian GG, Kliefoth WL Jr. Laparoscopic cholecystectomy in pregnancy. *J Laparoendosc Surg* 1994; 4:161.
165. Lemaire BMD, van Erp WFM. Laparoscopic surgery during pregnancy. *Surg Endosc* 1997;11:15.
166. Cristalli B, Cayol A, Izard V, Levardon M. Benefit of operative laparoscopy for ovarian tumors suspected of benignity. *J Laparoendosc Surg* 1992;2:69.
167. Elerding SC. Laparoscopic cholecystectomy in pregnancy. *Am J Surg* 1993;165:625.
168. Hart RO, Tamadon A, Fitzgibbons RJ Jr, Fleming A. Open laparoscopic cholecystectomy in pregnancy. *Surg Laparosc Endosc* 1993; 3:13.
169. Chandra M, Shapiro SJ, Gordon LA. Laparoscopic cholecystectomy in the first trimester of pregnancy. *Surg Laparosc Endosc* 1994;4:68.
170. Lanzafame RJ. Laparoscopic cholecystectomy during pregnancy. *Surgery* 1995;118:627.
171. Posta CG. Laparoscopic surgery in pregnancy: report on two cases. *J Laparoendosc Surg* 1995;5:203.
172. Curet MJ, Allen D, Josloff RK, et al. Laparoscopy during pregnancy. *Arch Surg* 1996;131:546.
173. Eichenberg BJ, Vanderlinden J, Miguel C, et al. Laparoscopic cholecystectomy in the third trimester of pregnancy. *Am Surg* 1996; 62:874.
174. Hunter JG, Swanstrom L, Thornburg K. Carbon dioxide pneumoperitoneum induces fetal acidosis in a pregnant ewe model. *Surg Endosc* 1995;9:272.
175. Babaknia A, Parsa H, Woodruff JD. Appendicitis during pregnancy. *Obstet Gynecol* 1977;50:40.
176. Weingold AB. Appendicitis in pregnancy. *Clin Obstet Gynecol* 1983; 26:801.
177. Moawad AH. Acute appendicitis during pregnancy. In: Cibils LA, ed. *Surgical disease in pregnancy.* New York: Springer-Verlag, 1990:105.
178. Mahmoodian S. Appendicitis complicating pregnancy. *South Med J* 1992;85:19.
179. Mazze RI, Källén B. Appendectomy during pregnancy: a Swedish registry study of 778 cases. *Obstet Gynecol* 1991;77:835.
180. Babler EA. Perforative appendicitis complicating pregnancy. *JAMA* 1908;51:1310.
181. Calì V, Pepe G, Pepe F, Panella P, Ingegneros L. Fecal peritonitis in pregnancy. *Clin Exp Obstet Gynecol* 1987;14:68.
182. de Veciana M, Towers CV, Major CA, Lien JM, Toohey JS. Pulmonary injury associated with appendicitis in pregnancy: who is at risk? *Am J Obstet Gynecol* 1994;171:1008.
183. McKellar DP, Anderson CT, Boynton CJ, Peoples JB. Cholecystectomy during pregnancy without fetal loss. *Surg Gynecol Obstet* 1992;174:465.
184. Hill LM, Johnson CE, Lee RA. Cholecystectomy in pregnancy. *Obstet Gynecol* 1975;46:291.

185. Printen KJ, Ott RA. Cholecystectomy during pregnancy. *Am Surg* 1978;44:432.
186. Scott LD. Gallstone disease and pancreatitis in pregnancy. *Gastroenterol Clin North Am* 1992;21:803.
187. Braverman DZ, Johnson ML, Kern F Jr. Effects of pregnancy and contraceptive steroids on gallbladder function. *N Engl J Med* 1980;302:362.
188. Davis A, Katz VL, Cox R. Gallbladder disease in pregnancy. *J Reprod Med* 1995;40:759.
189. Maringhini A, Marceno MP, Lanzarone F, et al. Sludge and stones in gallbladder after pregnancy. prevalence and risk factors. *J Hepatol* 1987;5:218.
190. Dixon NP, Faddis DM, Silberman H. Aggressive management of cholecystitis during pregnancy. *Am J Surg* 1987;154:292.
191. Simon JA. Biliary tract disease and related surgical disorders during pregnancy. *Clin Obstet Gynecol* 1983;26:810.
192. Gadacz TR, Talamini MA. Traditional versus laparoscopic cholecystectomy. *Am J Surg* 1991;161:336.
193. Comitalo JB, Lynch D. Laparoscopic cholecystectomy in the pregnant patient. *Surg Laparosc Endosc* 1994;4:268.
194. Steinbrook RA, Brooks DC, Datta S. Laparoscopic cholecystectomy during pregnancy: review of anesthetic management, surgical considerations. *Surg Endosc* 1996;10:511.
195. Weber AM, Bloom GP, Allan TR, Curry SL. Laparoscopic cholecystectomy during pregnancy. *Obstet Gynecol* 1991;78:958.
196. Schorr RT. Laparoscopic cholecystectomy and pregnancy. *J Laparoendosc Surg* 1993;3:291.
197. Edelman DS. Alternative laparoscopic technique for cholecystectomy during pregnancy. *Surg Endosc* 1994;8:794.
198. Barrett JM, Van Hooydonk JE, Boehm FH. Pregnancy-related rupture of arterial aneurysms. *Obstet Gynecol Surv* 1982;37:557.
199. Minielly R, Yuzpe AA, Drake CG. Subarachnoid hemorrhage secondary to ruptured cerebral aneurysm in pregnancy. *Obstet Gynecol* 1979;53:64.
200. Kaunitz AM, Hughes JM, Grimes DA, Smith JC, Rochat RW, Kafrissen ME. Causes of maternal mortality in the United States. *Obstet Gynecol* 1985;65:605.
201. Rochat RW, Koonin LM, Atrash HK, Jewett JF. Maternal mortality in the United States: report from the maternal mortality collaborative. *Obstet Gynecol* 1988;72:91.
202. Dias MS, Sekhar LN. Intracranial hemorrhage from aneurysms and arteriovenous malformations during pregnancy and the puerperium. *Neurosurgery* 1990;27:855.
203. Simolke GA, Cox SM, Cunningham FG. Cerebrovascular accidents complicating pregnancy and the puerperium. *Obstet Gynecol* 1991; 78:37.
204. Rhoads EE. Congenital aneurysms of the circle of Willis associated with pregnancy. *Am J Obstet Gynecol* 1947;54:533.
205. De Carle DW. Pregnancy and cerebrovascular complications. *West J Surg Obstet Gyecol* 1949;57:181.
206. Wan WL, Geller JL, Feldon SE, Sadun AA. Visual loss caused by rapidly progressive intracranial meningiomas during pregnancy. *Ophthalmology* 1990;97:18.
207. Donnell MS, Meyer GA, Donegan WL. Estrogen-receptor protein in intracranial meningiomas. *J Neurosurg* 1979;50:499.
208. Pliskow S, Herbst SJ, Saiontz HA, Cove H, Ackerman RT. Intracranial meningioma with positive progesterone receptors: a case report. *J Reprod Med* 1995;40:154.
209. Isla A, Alvarez F, Gonzalez A, García-Grande A, Perez-Alvarez M, García-Blazquez M. Brain tumor and pregnancy. *Obstet Gynecol* 1997; 89:19.
210. Rigg D, McDonogh A. Use of sodium nitroprusside for deliberate hypotension during pregnancy. *Br J Anaesth* 1981;53:985.
211. Cohen AV, Schulman H, Romney SL. Maternal acid-base metabolism in normal human parturition. *Am J Obstet Gynecol* 1970;107:933.
212. Lim VS, Katz AI, Lindheimer MD. Acid-base regulation in pregnancy. *Am J Physiol* 1976;231:1764.
213. Huch R. Maternal hyperventilation and the fetus. *J Perinat Med* 1986;14:3.
214. Müller G, Huber JC, Salzer H, Reinold E. Maternal hyperventilation as a possible cause of fetal tachycardia sub partu: a clinical and experimental study. *Gynecol Obstet Invest* 1984;17:270.
215. Lumley J, Renou P, Newman W, Wood C. Hyperventilation in obstetrics. *Am J Obstet Gynecol* 1969;103:847.
216. Motoyama EK, Rivard G, Acheson F, Cook CD. Adverse effect of maternal hyperventilation on the foetus. *Lancet* 1966;1:286.
217. Leduc B. The effect of hyperventilation on maternal placental blood flow in pregnant rabbits. *J Physiol (Lond)* 1972;225:339.
218. Levinson G, Shnider SM, de Lorimier AA, Steffenson JL. Effects of maternal hyperventilation on uterine blood flow and fetal oxygenation and acid-base status. *Anesthesiology* 1974;40:340.
219. Oakes GK, Walker AM, Ehrenkranz RA, Cefalo RC, Chez RA. Uteroplacental blood flow during hyperthermia with and without respiratory alkalosis. *J Appl Physiol* 1976;41:197.
220. van Buul BJA, Nijhuis JG, Slappendel R, Lerou JGC, Bakker-Niezen SH. General anesthesia for surgical repair of intracranial aneurysm in pregnancy: effects on fetal heart rate. *Am J Perinatol* 1993;10:183.
221. Bray RS, Lynch R, Grossman RG, Foreman D. Management of neurosurgical problems in pregnancy. *Clin Perinatol* 1987;14:243.
222. de Swiet M. Heart disease in pregnancy. In: de Swiet M, ed. *Medical disorders in obstetric practice.* 3rd ed. Oxford: Blackwell Science, 1995:143.
223. Sullivan HJ. Valvular heart surgery during pregnancy. *Surg Clin North Am* 1995;75:59.
224. Pomini F, Mercogliano D, Cavalletti C, Caruso A, Pomini P. Cardiopulmonary bypass in pregnancy. *Ann Thorac Surg* 1996;61:259.
225. Zitnik RS, Brandenburg RO, Sheldon R, Wallace RB. Pregnancy and open-heart surgery. *Circulation* 1969;39:I-257.
226. Strickland RA, Oliver WC Jr, Chantigian RC, Ney JA, Danielson GK. Anesthesia, cardiopulmonary bypass, and the pregnant patient. *Mayo Clin Proc* 1991;66:411.
227. Chambers CE, Clark SL. Cardiac surgery during pregnancy. *Clin Obstet Gynecol* 1994;37:316.
228. Becker RM. Intracardiac surgery in pregnant women. *Ann Thorac Surg* 1983;36:453.
229. Koh KS, Friesen RM, Livingstone RA, Peddle LJ. Fetal monitoring during maternal cardiac surgery with cardiopulmonary bypass. *Can Med Assoc J* 1975;112:1102.
230. Trimakas AP, Maxwell KD, Berkay S, Gardner TJ, Achuff SC. Fetal monitoring during cardiopulmonary bypass for removal of a left atrial myxoma during pregnancy. *Johns Hopkins Med J* 1979;144:156.
231. Levy DL, Warriner RA III, Burgess GE III. Fetal response to cardiopulmonary bypass. *Obstet Gynecol* 1980;56:112.
232. Bahary CM, Ninio A, Gorodesky IG, Neri A. Tococardiography in pregnancy during extracorporeal bypass for mitral valve replacement. *Isr J Med Sci* 1980;16:395.
233. Lamb MP, Ross K, Johnstone AM, Manners JM. Fetal heart monitoring during open heart surgery: two case reports. *Br J Obstet Gynaecol* 1981;88:669.
234. Eilen B, Kaiser IH, Becker RM, Cohen MN. Aortic valve replacement in the third trimester of pregnancy: case report and review of the literature. *Obstet Gynecol* 1981;57:119.
235. Bernal JM, Miralles PJ. Cardiac surgery with cardiopulmonary bypass during pregnancy. *Obstet Gynecol Surv* 1986;41:1.
236. Goldstein I, Jakobi P, Gutterman E, Milo S. Umbilical artery flow velocity during maternal cardiopulmonary bypass. *Ann Thorac Surg* 1995;60:1116.
237. Greiss FC Jr, Pick JR Jr. The uterine vascular bed: adrenergic receptors. *Obstet Gynecol* 1964;23:209.
238. Hood DD, Dewan DM, James FM III. Maternal and fetal effects of epinephrine in gravid ewes. *Anesthesiology* 1986;64:610.
239. Kaiser IH, Harris JS. The effect of adrenalin on the pregnant human uterus. *Am J Obstet Gynecol* 1950;59:775.
240. Greiss FC Jr, Van Wilkes D. Effects of sympathominetic drugs and angiotensin on the uterine vascular bed. *Obstet Gynecol* 1964;23:925.
241. Wheeler AS, James FM III, Meis PJ, et al. Effects of nitroglycerin and nitroprusside on the uterine vasculature of gravid ewes. *Anesthesiology* 1980;52:390.
242. Ellis SC, Wheeler AS, James FM III, et al. Fetal and maternal effects of sodium nitroprusside used to counteract hypertension in gravid ewes. *Am J Obstet Gynecol* 1982;143:766.
243. Cibils LA, Pose SV, Zuspan FP. Effect of 1-norepinephrine infusion on uterine contractility and the cardiovascular system. *Am J Obstet Gynecol* 1962;84:307.
244. Tong C, Eisenach JC. The vascular mechanism of ephedrine's beneficial effect on uterine perfusion during pregnancy. *Anesthesiology* 1992;76:792.
245. Craft JB Jr, Co EG, Yonekura ML, Gilman RM. Nitroglycerin therapy for phenylephrine-induced hypertension in pregnant ewes. *Anesth Analg* 1980;59:494.

246. Ramanathan S, Grant GJ. Vasopressor therapy for hypotension due to epidural anesthesia for cesarean section. *Acta Anaesthesiol Scand* 1988;32:559.
247. Johnson MD, Saltzman DH. Cardiac disease. In: Datta S, ed. *Anesthesia and obstetric management of high risk pregnancy.* 2nd ed. St. Louis: Mosby, 1996:200.
248. Thomas DG, Robson SC, Redfern N, Hughes D, Boys RJ. Randomized trial of bolus phenylephrine or ephedrine for maintenance of arterial pressure during spinal anaesthesia for caesarean section. *Br J Anaesth* 1996;76:61.
249. Hoffman BB, Lefkowitz RJ. Catecholamines, sympathomimetic drugs, and adrenergic receptor antagonists. In: Hardman JG, Limbird LE, Molinoff PB, Ruddon RW, Gilman AG, eds. *Goodman & Gilman's the pharmacological basis of therapeutics.* 9th ed. New York: McGraw-Hill, 1996:199.
250. Kirshon B, Lee W, Mauer MB, Cotton DB. Effects of low-dose dopamine therapy in the oliguric patient with preeclampsia. *Am J Obstet Gynecol* 1988;159:604.
251. Blanchard K, Dandavino A, Nuwayhid B, Brinkman CR III, Assali NS. Systemic and uterine hemodynamic responses to dopamine in pregnant and nonpregnant sheep. *Am J Obstet Gynecol* 1978;130:669.
252. Cabalum T, Zugaib M, Lieb S, Nuwayhid B, Brinkman CR III, Assali NS. Effect of dopamine on hypotension induced by spinal anesthesia. *Am J Obstet Gynecol* 1979;133:630.
253. Rolbin SH, Levinson G, Shnider SM, Biehl DR, Wright RG. Dopamine treatment of spinal hypotension decreases uterine blood flow in the pregnant ewe. *Anesthesiology* 1979;51:37.
254. Fishburne JI Jr, Dormer KJ, Payne GG, Gill PS, Ashrafzadeh AR, Rossavik IK. Effects of amrinone and dopamine on uterine blood flow and vascular responses in the gravid baboon. *Am J Obstet Gynecol* 1988;158:829.
255. Fishburne JI, Meis PJ, Urban RB, et al. Vascular and uterine responses to dobutamine and dopamine in the gravid ewe. *Am J Obstet Gynecol* 1980;137:944.
256. Santos AC, Baumann AL, Wlody D, Pedersen H, Morishima HO, Finster M. The maternal and fetal effects of milrinone and dopamine in normotensive pregnant ewes. *Am J Obstet Gynecol* 1992;166:257.
257. Clark RB, Brunner JA III. Dopamine for the treatment of spinal hypotension during cesarean section. *Anesthesiology* 1980;53:514.
258. Ruffolo RR Jr, Yaden EL. Vascular effects of the stereoisomers of dobutamine. *J Pharmacol Exp Ther* 1983;224:46.
259. Geraci SA. Pharmacologic approach in patients with heart failure. In: Chernow B, ed. *The pharmacologic approach to the critically ill patient.* 3rd ed. Baltimore: Williams & Wilkins, 1994:80.
260. Kelly RA, Smith TW. Pharmacological treatment of heart failure. In: Hardman JG, Limbird LE, Molinoff PB, Ruddon RW, Gilman AG, eds. *Goodman & Gilman's the pharmacological basis of therapeutics.* 9th ed. New York: McGraw-Hill, 1996:809.
261. Jelsema RD, Bhatia RK, Ganguly S. Use of intravenous amrinone in the short-term management of refractory heart failure in pregnancy. *Obstet Gynecol* 1991;78:935.
262. Ring G, Krames E, Shnider SM, Wallis KL, Levinson G. Comparison of nitroprusside and hydralazine in hypertensive pregnant ewes. *Obstet Gynecol* 1977;50:598.
263. Bates JN, Baker MT, Guerra R Jr, Harrison DG. Nitric oxide generation from nitroprusside by vascular tissue: evidence that reduction of the nitroprusside anion and cyanide loss are required. *Biochem Pharmacol* 1991;42[Suppl]:S157.
264. Naulty J, Cefalo RC, Lewis PE. Fetal toxicity of nitroprusside in the pregnant ewe. *Am J Obstet Gynecol* 1981;139:708.
265. Stempel JE, O'Grady JP, Morton MJ, Johnson KA. Use of sodium nitroprusside in complications of gestational hypertension. *Obstet Gynecol* 1982;60:533.
266. de Rosayro M, Nahrwold ML, Hill AB, Tait AR, Busch MDT, Kirsh MM. Plasma levels and cardiovascular effect of nitroglycerin in pregnant sheep. *Can Anaesth Soc J* 1980;27:560.
267. Bootstaylor BS, Roman C, Parer JT, Heymann MA. Fetal and maternal hemodynamic and metabolic effects of maternal nitroglycerin infusions in sheep. *Am J Obstet Gynecol* 1997;176:644.
268. Grunewald C, Kublickas M, Carlström K, Lunell N-O, Nisell H. Effects of nitroglycerin on the uterine and umbilical circulation in severe preeclampsia. *Obstet Gynecol* 1995;86:600.
269. Kroovand RL. Stones in pregnancy and in children [Editorial]. *J Urol* 1992;148:1076.
270. Ulvik NM, Bakke A, Hisaeter PÅ. Ureteroscopy in pregnancy. *J Urol* 1995;154:1660.
271. Rittenberg MH, Bagley DH. Ureteroscopic diagnosis and treatment of urinary calculi during pregnancy. *Urology* 1988;32:427.
272. Schenker JG, Granat M. Phaeochromocytoma and pregnancy: an updated appraisal. *Aust N Z J Obstet Gynaecol* 1982;22:1.
273. Mitchell SZ, Freilich JD, Brant D, Flynn M. Anesthetic management of pheochromocytoma resection during pregnancy. *Anesth Analg* 1987;66:478.
274. Harper MA, Murnaghan GA, Kennedy L, Hadden DR, Atkinson AB. Phaeochromocytoma in pregnancy: five cases and a review of the literature. *Br J Obstet Gynaecol* 1989;96:594.
275. Liu PL, Warren TM, Ostheimer GW, Weiss JB, Liu LMP. Foetal monitoring in parturients undergoing surgery unrelated to pregnancy. *Can Anaesth Soc J* 1985;32:525.
276. Steinberg ES, Santos AC. Surgical anesthesia during pregnancy. *Int Anesthesiol Clin* 1990;28:58.
277. Paul RH, Suidan AK, Yeh S-Y, Schifrin BS, Hon EH. Clinical fetal monitoring. VII. the evaluation and significance of intrapartum baseline FHR variability. *Am J Obstet Gynecol* 1975;123:206.
278. Petrie RH. Effect of drugs and anesthetics on the fetal heart rate. *Semin Perinatol* 1978;2:147.
279. Ramanathan S. Anesthesia in nonobstetric situations. In: *Obstetric anesthesia.* Philadelphia: Lea & Febiger, 1988:296.
280. Harris AP. Fetal physiology. In: Chestnut DH, ed. *Obstetric anesthesia: principles and practice.* St. Louis: Mosby, 1994:76.
281. Shnider SM, Webster GM. Maternal and fetal hazards of surgery during pregnancy. *Am J Obstet Gynecol* 1965;92:891.
282. Duncan PG, Pope WDB, Cohen MM, Greer N. Fetal risk of anesthesia and surgery during pregnancy. *Anesthesiology* 1986;64:790.
283. Harger JH, Caritis SN. Preterm cervical dilation. In: Queenan JT, ed. *Managing OB/GYN emergencies.* 2nd ed. Oradell, NJ: Medical Economics Books, 1983:56.
284. Brodsky JB. Anesthesia and the pregnant patient. *Reg Anesth* 1984;9:119.
285. Leicht CH. Anesthesia for the pregnant patient undergoing nonobstetric surgery. *Anesthesiol Clin North Am* 1990;8:131.
286. Egbert LD, Battit GE, Turndorf H, Beecher HK. The value of the preoperative visit by an anesthetist: a study of doctor patient rapport. *JAMA* 1963;185:553.
287. Wyner J, Cohen SE. Gastric volume in early pregnancy: effect of metoclopramide. *Anesthesiology* 1982;57:209.
288. Bevacqua BK. Supraventricular tachycardia associated with postpartum metoclopramide administration. *Anesthesiology* 1988;68:124.
289. Eisenach JC, Dewan DM. Metoclopramide exaggerates stress-induced tachycardia in pregnant sheep. *Anesth Analg* 1996;82:607.
290. Shankar KB, Moseley H, Kumar Y, Vemula V. Arterial to end tidal carbon dioxide tension difference during caesarean section anaesthesia. *Anaesthesia* 1986;41:698.

Obstetric Anesthesia, second edition,
edited by Mark C. Norris.
Lippincott Williams & Wilkins, Philadelphia © 1999.

CHAPTER 10

Anesthesia for Fetal Surgery

Steven T. Fogel and Jacob C. Langer

In the past three decades, our ability to detect fetal abnormalities has grown remarkably. Therapeutic modalities have paralleled these diagnostic advances and transformed the fetus from passive bystander to patient. During the 1960s, amniocentesis made possible the cytogenetic and biochemical analyses that are commonplace today (1–3). Liley (4) is credited with the first direct treatment of the fetus for hemolytic disease. Subsequently, outcomes improved with the development of percutaneous techniques (5). Finally, the refinement of ultrasound, coupled with the discovery of biochemical markers for congenital anomalies, provided strong impetus for the development of medical and surgical fetal therapies (Table 1) (6–11).

PRINCIPLES OF FETAL SURGERY

Fetal surgery involves both mother and fetus. Surgical techniques are continually being refined, with only a few centers actively investigating methods and outcome. The complexity of open fetal surgery (fetal surgery performed via hysterotomy) and the initial lack of guidelines for this therapy led to the formation of the International Fetal Medicine and Surgery Society in 1982, which proposed the following general criteria for fetal surgery (12):

- The fetus should be a singleton with no concomitant anomalies, as determined by level II ultrasound and amniocentesis for karyotype, α-fetoprotein, and viral cultures.
- The family should be fully counseled about the risks and benefits and should agree to treatment.
- A multidisciplinary team, including a perinatologist, an ultrasonographer, a pediatric surgeon, and a neonatologist must be actively involved in patient care.
- There must be access to a level III high-risk obstetric unit and intensive care nursery.
- Availability of bioethical and psychological consultation must be present.

Successful fetal surgery requires proper patient selection and intensive perioperative monitoring. Although potentially life saving, fetal surgery has not been uniformly successful (13–15). In 1994, further criteria were developed, aiming to improve maternal and neonatal outcomes after fetal surgery (16):

- Reliable diagnosis,
- The natural history and pathophysiology of the lesion understood,
- Animal models show that appropriately timed fetal intervention reverses the pathophysiology and significantly improves survival,
- A predictably poor prognosis without fetal intervention, and
- Low maternal risk.

Anesthetic techniques must be appropriate for both mother and fetus. Attenuation of the stress response to surgery in the fetus is especially important (15). Adequate operating conditions require a flaccid uterus and an immobile fetus. Both mother and fetus must be monitored. Finally, intensive postoperative monitoring of both mother and fetus must pay particular attention to the prevention of preterm labor (16–19).

INDICATIONS FOR FETAL SURGERY AND TREATMENT MODALITIES

The great majority of fetal defects are neither amenable to surgical therapy nor meet the criteria for fetal surgery. Many defects are best treated after delivery (20). However, some conditions may be successfully treated in utero by either minimally invasive or open techniques (Table 2) (21).

S.T. Fogel: Department of Anesthesiology, Washington University School of Medicine, St. Louis, Missouri 63110.
J.C. Langer: Department of Surgery, Division of Pediatric Surgery, Washington University School of Medicine, St. Louis, Missouri 63110.

TABLE 1. *First reports of fetal operations*

Year	Physician	Procedure	Outcome
1963	Liley AW	Intrauterine transfusion of fetus for erythroblastosis fetalis	Alive (after 4 wk of follow-up study)
1981	Clewell WH	Ventriculoamionitic shunt for hydrocephalus	Alive (4 mo at publication)
1982	Golbus MS	Hydronephrosis decompressed by vesicoamniotic shunt	Alive (1 yr at publication)
1982	Harrison MR	Hydronephrosis decompressed by open bilateral ureterostomies	Alive (after 4 yr of follow-up)
1987	Clark SL	Thoracoamniotic shunt of cystic adenomatoid malformation	Alive (14 mo at publication)
1988	Rodeck C	Pleuroamniotic shunt for fetal hydrothorax	Delivery with pulmonary distress
1989	Harrison MR	Open resection of sacrococcygeal teratoma	Death; pulmonary distress, delivery at 26-weeks' gestation after premature rupture of membranes
1990	Harrison MR	Open repair of diaphragmatic hernia	Alive (8 mo at publication)
1990	Adzick NS	Open resection of cystic adenomatoid malformation	Alive (5 mo at publication)
1990	De Lia JE (11)	Fetoscopic laser occlusion of placental vessels for severe twin–twin transfusion	4 of 6 infants alive at time of publication
1994	Quintero RA (10)	Fetoscopic umbilical cord ligation of acardiac twin	Normal twin alive at time of publication (3 mo of age)

Modified from ref. 8, with permission.

TABLE 2. *Malformations that may benefit from in utero treatment*

Condition	Recommended treatment
Life-threatening defects	
Urinary obstruction (urethral valves)	Percutaneous catheter Fetoscopic vesicostomy Open vesicostomy
Cystic adenomatoid malformation	Open pulmonary lobectomy Percutaneous thoracoamniotic shunt
Diaphragmatic hernia	Open repair Bowel exteriorization Temporary tracheal occlusion
Sacrococcygeal teratoma	Resection of tumor Fetoscopic vascular occlusion
Twin–twin transfusion syndrome	Open fetectomy Fetoscopic obliteration of placental vessels
Aqueductal stenosis	Ventriculoamniotic shunt Open ventriculoperitoneal shunt[a]
Complete heart block	Percutaneous pacemaker Open pacemaker
Pulmonary–aortic obstruction	Percutaneous valvuloplasty Open valvuloplasty[a]
Tracheal atresia–stenosis–obstruction by tumor	Fetoscopic tracheostomy[a]
Nonlethal defects	
Myelomeningocele	Fetoscopic coverage Open repair
Cleft lip and palate	Fetoscopic repair[a] Open repair[a]
Metabolic–cellular defects	Fetal stem cell transplant or gene therapy with fetal stem cells (autologous–allogenic)
Stem cell–enzyme defects	
Predictable organ failure	Induce tolerance for postnatal organ transplant[a]

[a]Procedure not yet performed in humans.
Modified from ref. 21, with permission.

Congenital Diaphragmatic Hernia

Congenital diaphragmatic hernia (CDH) occurs when a posterolateral defect in the developing diaphragm allows incomplete separation of the chest and abdominal cavities. The pleuroperitoneal canal fails to close by the time the bowel returns to the abdomen at 8 to 10 weeks' gestation (Fig. 1) (22). This abnormality is corrected by removing the bowel from the chest and closing the diaphragmatic defect (23,24). Neonatal mortality is high because of pulmonary hypoplasia and pulmonary hypertension resulting from pulmonary arteriolar hyperplasia (25–27). In addition, hypoplasia of the left ventricle and interventricular septum was documented in both humans and fetal lambs with CDH (28). Correction of CDH in utero reverses these abnormalities (29).

CDH occurs in approximately 1:3,000 to 1:5,000 live births (30,31). The mortality is close to 60% (32). Risk factors for poor neonatal outcome include (14,33–43):

- Detection of CDH before 25 weeks' gestation,
- Cardiac ventricular disproportion,
- Low lung area-to-head circumference ratio,
- Large distended stomach in chest,
- Large volume of liver in chest, and
- Polyhydramnios.

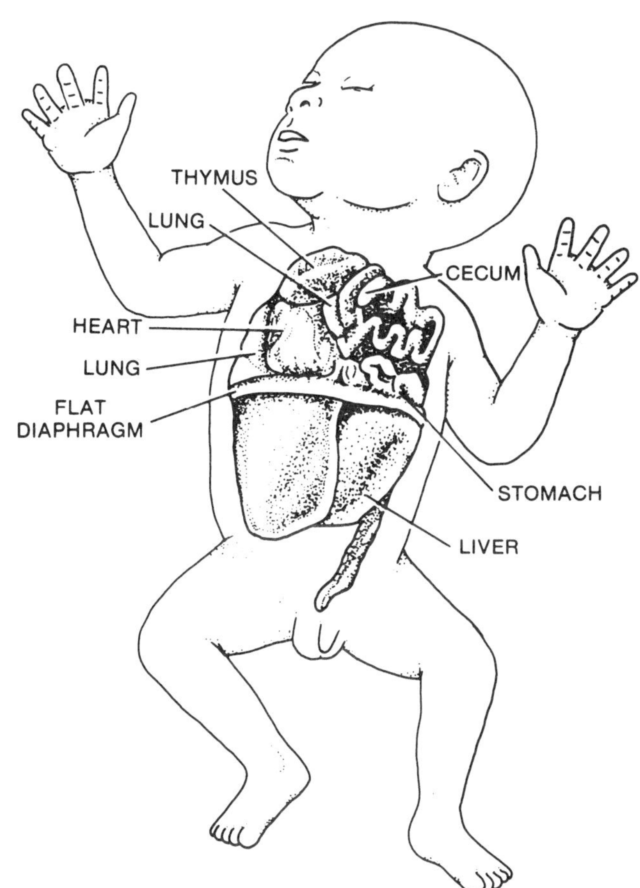

FIG. 1. Neonate with diaphragmatic hernia. (From ref. 22, with permission.)

In animals, in utero correction of CDH prevents mortality (44–46). In fetal lambs, the effects of CDH can be mimicked by placing an inflatable balloon in the chest cavity. Deflating the balloon then simulates correction of CDH. Deflating the intrathoracic balloon midway in gestation improves survival in these lambs compared with control lambs in which the balloon remains inflated (45,46). Diaphragmatic hernia also can be surgically created and then repaired in fetal lambs (47,48). Surgical correction in fetal lambs prevents both the pulmonary hypoplasia and pulmonary vascular abnormalities associated with CDH (49). These observations provide a physiologic rationale for in utero repair of CDH (Fig. 2).

Despite these promising animal results, correction of CDH by open fetal surgery in humans has had limited success (14,33,41,50). Definitive in utero repair may be complicated and hazardous to the fetus. Technical problems have resulted in a high mortality for a subgroup of fetuses in whom the liver has herniated into the chest (51). Although the results of open fetal repair for fetuses without liver in the chest have been encouraging, they are no better than the natural history of the same subgroup of untreated patients. For these reasons, complete repair of CDH in utero has largely been abandoned. (N.S. Adzick, personal communication, 1998.)

An alternative approach to the problem of CDH involves fetal tracheal ligation. Temporary occlusion of the fetal trachea results in increased fetal lung growth in animal models of fetal pulmonary hypoplasia (52–55). The reasons for this effect are unclear. Alterations in fetal lung expansion may have a potent and rapid impact on pulmonary DNA synthesis. Subsequent changes in growth-factor gene expression may stimulate pulmonary development (56). In humans, successful open fetal tracheal clip application, followed by postnatal definitive surgical correction of CDH, has been reported (57,58). (A.W. Flake, personal communication, 1995.) In fetal sheep, tracheal clips have been successfully placed by using less invasive endoscopic techniques, and a number of human fetuses have now undergone this procedure (58,59). Further refinements will no doubt have a significant impact on the management of the fetus with CDH (Fig. 3).

Obstructive Uropathy

Fetal urinary obstruction can lead to abnormalities of the face, abdominal wall, and musculoskeletal system (Potter's syndrome), renal dysplasia, and hydronephrosis. With complete or nearly complete obstruction, oligohydramnios or anhydramnios may lead to pulmonary hypoplasia and an associated high mortality (Fig. 4) (60). In the fetal lamb, urethral obstruction produces hydronephrosis, renal dysplasia, and pulmonary hypoplasia. In utero vesicostomy reverses these effects by restoring urine excretion and amniotic fluid volume (61,62). In a similar animal model, early mid-trimester ureteral

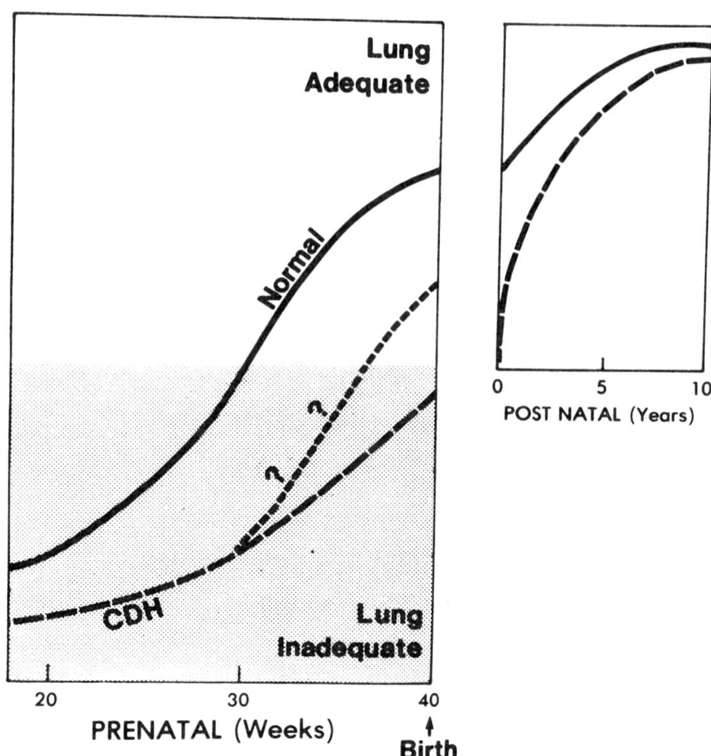

FIG. 2. Pathophysiologic rationale for correction of congenital diaphragmatic hernia (CDH) in utero. Human lung growth and development versus time plotted on an arbitrary scale. CDH limits lung growth and development during the prenatal and postnatal periods. In utero correction of CDH may allow improved growth and development in the fetus (dotted line). (From ref. 46, with permission.)

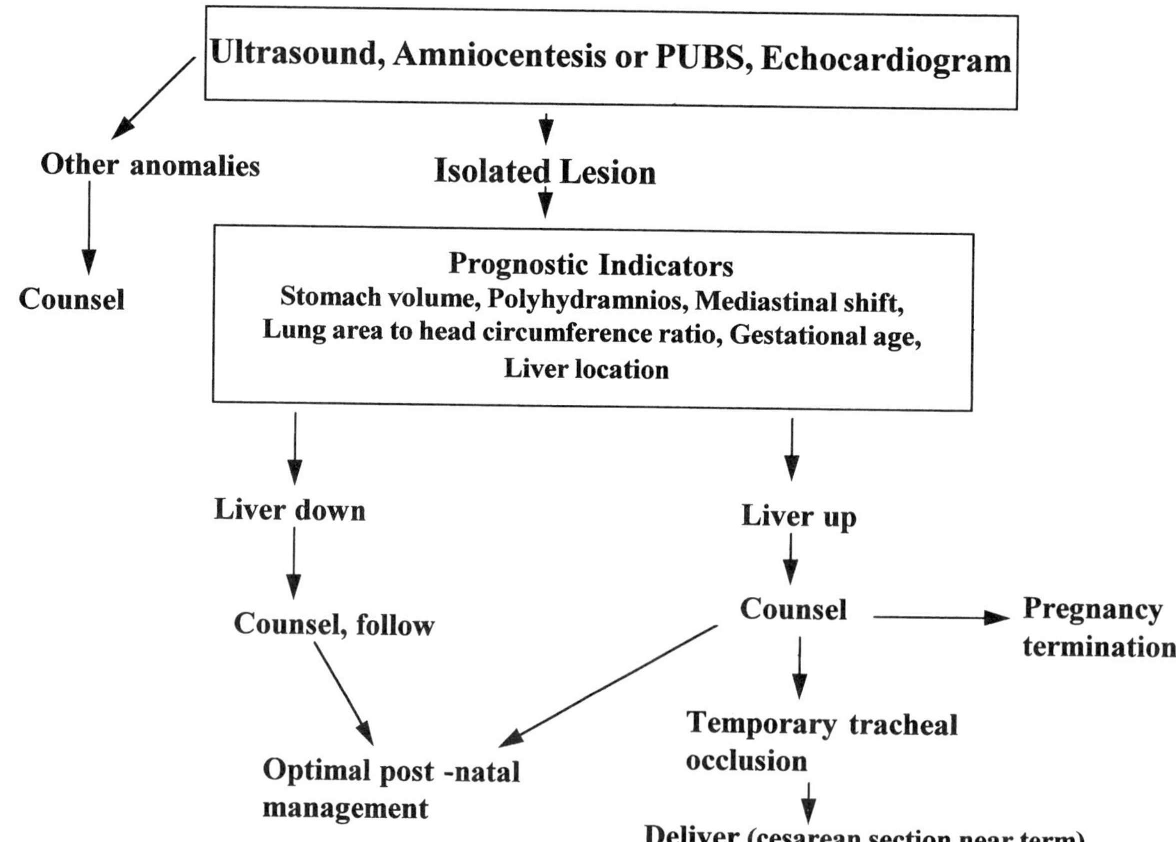

FIG. 3. Algorithm for managing fetus with congenital diaphragmatic hernia (CDH). (Modified from ref. 51, with permission.)

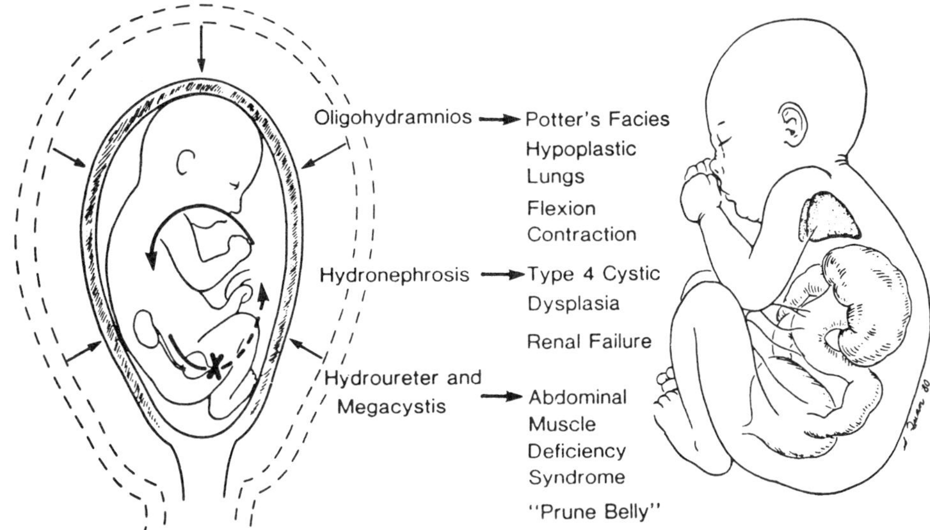

FIG. 4. Consequences of fetal urethral blockage. Obstruction causes hydroureter, megacystis, and hydronephrosis. Blockage of fetal urinary excretion alters normal amniotic fluid dynamics and produces oligohydramnios. (From Bond SJ, Harrison MR. Obstructive uropathy—when to intervene. *Contemp Obstet Gynecol* (Special Issue) 1987:65, with permission.)

obstruction produces renal dysplasia, and in utero decompression prevents renal injury in a time-dependent fashion (63,64).

A treatment algorithm, based on the results of serial sonographic examinations, allows selection of appropriate candidates for in utero intervention (Fig. 5) (51). This algorithm relies on the ability of the sonographic appearance of the fetal kidneys, fetal urine electrolytes, and fetal urine β_2-microglobulin concentration to predict postnatal renal function (51). When present, sonographically detected cortical cysts are diagnostic of renal dysplasia. However, ultrasonography often fails to detect cortical cysts in cases of renal dysplasia (65,66). Normal fetal urine is hypotonic. A fetal urine sodium of less than 70 mEq/L is a good predictor of postnatal renal function. Fetal urine β_2-microglobulin concentration less than 2 mg/L also predicts normal postnatal renal function (66). Serial analyses of fetal urine (Fig. 6) improves the ability to predict survival and normal renal function (60).

In fetuses with urinary tract obstruction, oligohydramnios, and immature lungs, several surgical options are available. The bladder can be decompressed in utero by percutaneous ultrasound-guided vesicoamniotic shunt placement, which often successfully reconstitutes amniotic fluid volume and prevents pulmonary hypoplasia. Open fetal surgery with vesicostomy or bilateral nephrostomy also has been reported, but is no better than shunting (Fig. 7) (21,67,68). Experience treating fetuses with obstructive uropathy suggests that selection criteria are sufficient to avoid inappropriate intervention (21). It is unclear, however, whether intervention in humans alters the course of renal dysplasia or improves renal functional development (51).

Sacrococcygeal Teratoma

Sacrococcygeal teratoma (SCT) is a rare congenital tumor. Although most affected fetuses can be treated postnatally, intrauterine mortality can occur as a result of high-output cardiac failure and fetal hydrops. Arteriovenous shunts within the enlarging tumor are thought to cause fetal cardiac failure, and Doppler ultrasound measurements have documented the high-output physiology of SCT (8,69). Mortality is inversely related to fetal age at diagnosis, and the development of hydrops is almost universally fatal (8,70). When hydrops develops before lung maturity, open fetal surgery may be considered. In human fetuses, removal of the tumor in utero has reversed fetal cardiac dilation, scalp edema, ascites, and pleural effusions (71). In several recent cases, fetal surgery for SCT resulted in a viable infant (72) (M.R. Harrison, N.S. Adzick, personal communication, 1998). For SCT with hydrops after 30 weeks, preterm delivery and postnatal surgical excision are recommended.

Congenital Cystic Adenomatous Malformation of the Lung

Congenital cystic adenomatous malformation of the lung (CCAM) is a benign developmental lesion that usually is first seen in infancy. CCAM may be diagnosed prenatally, and in some cases may be associated with fetal hydrops. In this subgroup of fetuses, the large cystic lung mass produces a marked mediastinal shift, fetal ascites, pleural and pericardial effusions, and scalp edema (51,73). Hydrops in these fetuses probably

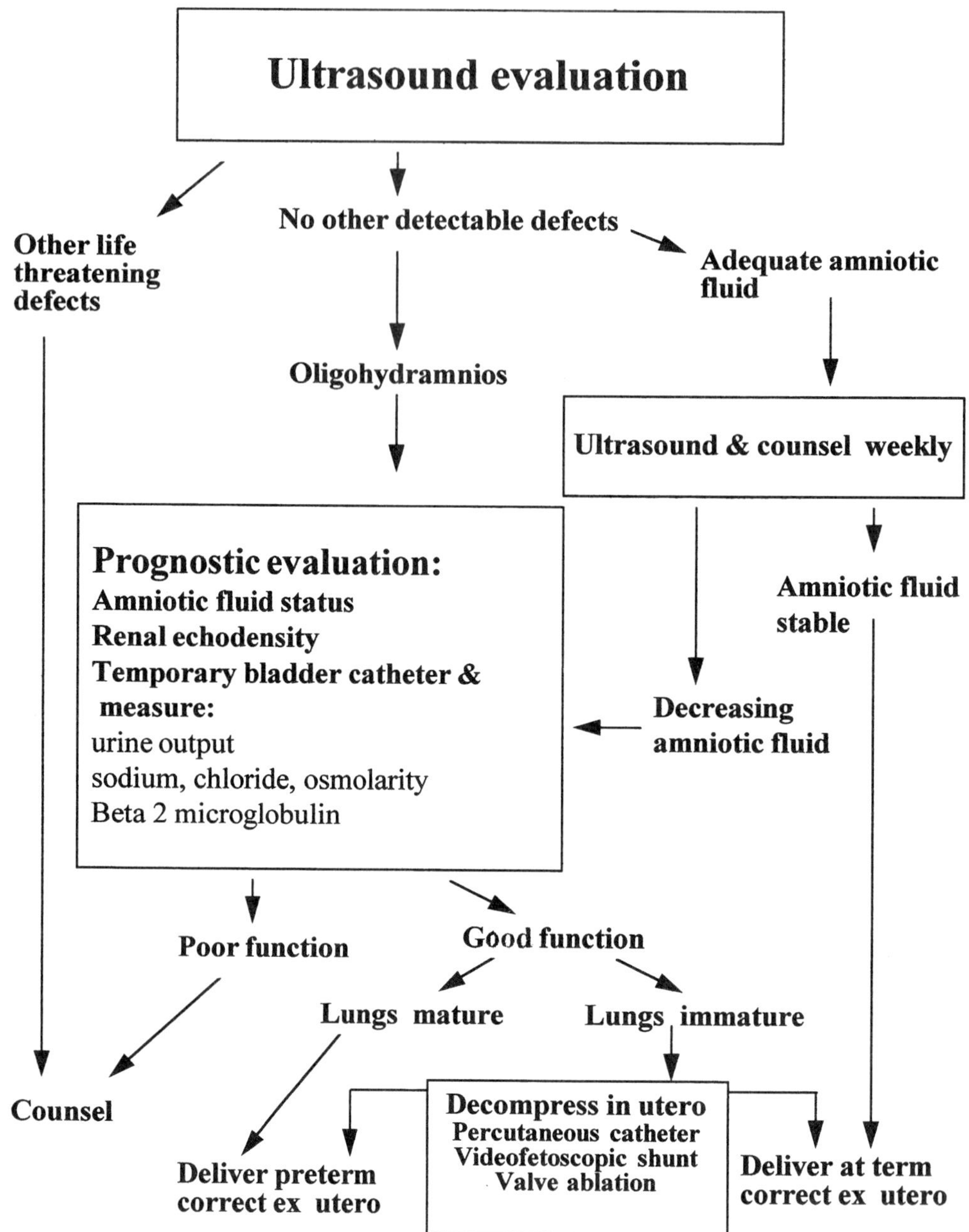

FIG. 5. Algorithm for managing a fetus with bilateral hydronephrosis. (Modified from ref. 51, with permission.)

results from obstruction of cardiac venous return and central venous hypertension (74). Resection of fetal lung is technically feasible and stimulates compensatory lung growth in sheep (51). Although both open fetal surgery and thoracoamniotic shunts have been performed successfully in human fetuses with CCAM, many lesions will resolve spontaneously (51,75–77). Fetal intervention should be reserved for hydropic fetuses who are too immature to undergo preterm delivery and postnatal therapy (see Fig. 7).

Hydrocephalus

Fetal hydrocephalus and ventriculomegaly were the focus of intense study in the 1980s because of the ease of diagnosis with ultrasonography and a desire to avoid neurological disability (78). The natural history and associated pathology were examined in an effort to select appropriate candidates for fetal therapy (79). This task proved difficult. Infants with associated anomalies, which preoperative screening frequently failed to detect,

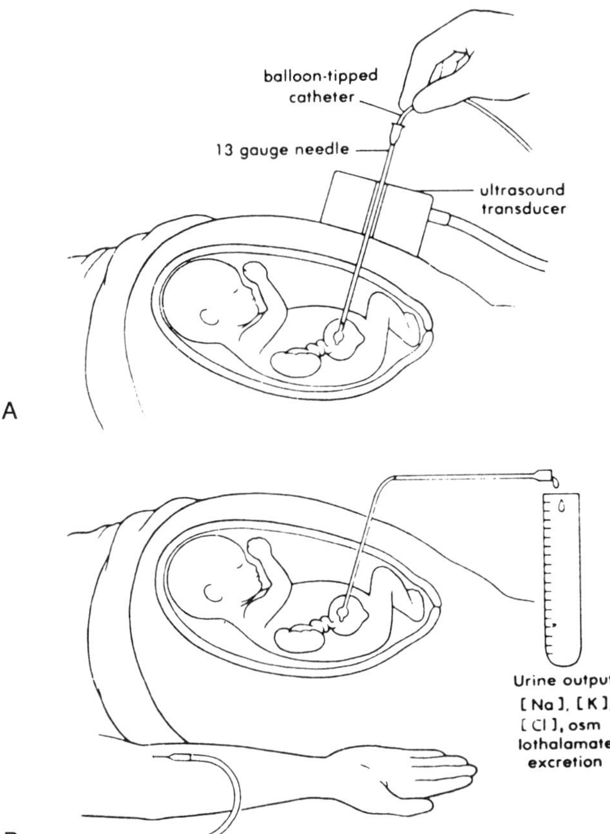

FIG. 6. Technique for diagnostic urinary catheterization. **A:** A catheter is placed into the fetal bladder under ultrasound guidance. **B:** Sample of fetal urine is collected for laboratory analysis. (From Glick PL, Harrison MR, Golbus MS. Management of the fetus with congenital hydronephrosis II: Prognostic criteria and selection for treatment. *J Pediatr Surg* 1985;20:376, with permission.)

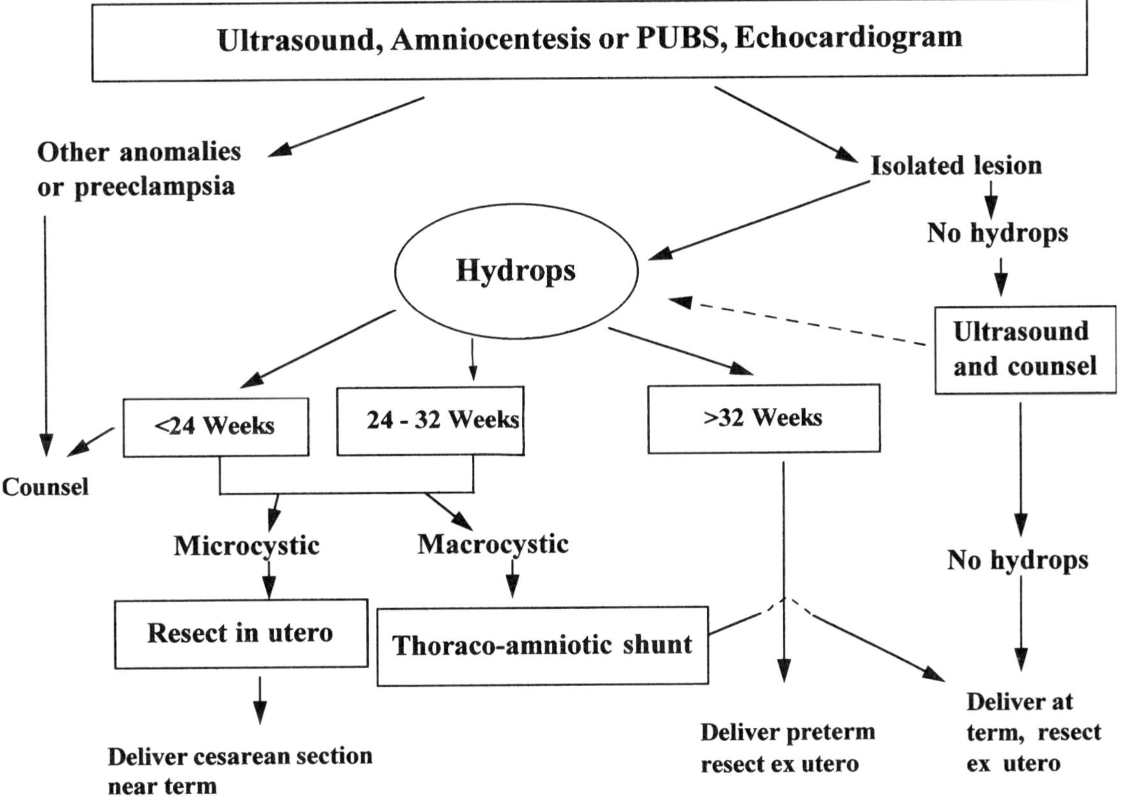

FIG. 7. Algorithm for managing a fetus with cystic adenomatoid malformation of the lung. (Modified from ref. 51, with permission.)

had a uniformly poor outcome regardless of treatment. As of 1990, 44 cases of in utero shunting for ventriculomegaly had been reported. Whereas overall survival rate was higher for the shunted than conventionally managed infants, shunting procedures did not improve neurological function (80). Because of the overall poor neurological prognosis and inability to identify clearly fetuses who may benefit, there has been a moratorium on in utero treatment for obstructive hydrocephalus (80,81). Some authors, however, believe that shunting procedures may be useful in the future, because techniques and selection criteria may improve with experience and further study (8,13).

Nonlethal Conditions

While the previously mentioned procedures have been performed for lethal or potentially lethal conditions, fetal surgery also has been advocated for nonlethal conditions. One reason for this interest is the prospect of scarless surgery.

Cleft Lip

Wound healing in the fetus differs from that in the adult. Simple fetal wounds heal without scarring early in gestation, and become more adult-like in the third trimester (82,83). The reasons for this difference are complex and are currently under intensive study (84–86). This phenomenon has significant implications for fetal surgery, particularly for functional defects such as cleft lip. Endoscopic repair of cleft lip without scar formation has been done in fetal lambs (87). Human application of this approach awaits improvements in maternal safety and the control of preterm labor.

Myelomeningocele

Myelomeningocele can be detected antenatally with α-fetoprotein screening and ultrasonography. Neonates born with this condition can have marked neurological impairment. Although neurological injury may be an inherent outcome of the defect, studies in fetal lambs suggest that direct exposure of the spinal cord to the intrauterine environment may be responsible. In utero correction, using a latissimus dorsi flap, prevents the associated neurological impairment in the fetal lamb. Once appropriate selection criteria have been developed, fetal myelomeningocele repair by using either an open or fetoscopic approach, may prove useful in humans (21,88–90).

Hematopoietic Stem Cell Transplantation

Contemporary technology makes possible the prenatal detection of a number of congenital metabolic and hematologic disorders (91). In utero hematopoietic stem cell transplantation could be curative, while avoiding some of the problems encountered with postnatal bone marrow transplants (limited donor availability, graft rejection, graft-vs-host disease, and fetal deterioration before transplantation). The preimmune fetus (fewer than 15 weeks of gestation) will not reject transplanted cells, and the myeloablation and immune suppression often needed for postnatal transplants are unnecessary. In addition, in utero transplantation may allow early treatment and avoid injury from the underlying disease (Table 3).

Although not insurmountable, there are difficulties with these procedures (see Table 3). Inherent risks are associated with the techniques of diagnosis early in gestation (chorionic villus sampling, amniocentesis) and the interventional treatment of a very small fetus. The degree of engraftment or chimerism achieved may not be sufficient to cure some diseases. The treatment of some enzymatic deficiencies may require that only a small number of transplanted cells survive. For other disorders, such as hemoglobinopathies, the degree of engraftment needed for a cure might be impossible. Inducing tolerance in utero for subsequent postnatal booster injections, however, may be a solution to this problem (21).

Hematopoietic stem cell transplants in both fetal sheep and fetal monkeys have yielded donor cell lines in neonates without evidence of graph-vs-host disease (92,93). In humans, successful in utero hematopoietic stem cell transplants at 12 to 28 weeks' gestation, by using fetal liver stem cells, either cured or considerably improved the neonatal condition of fetuses with immunodeficiency disease or thalassemia major (94,95). Successful treatment of X-linked severe combined immunodeficiency disease with in utero transplantation of paternal bone marrow also has been reported (96).

Other Anomalies

In utero treatment of other abnormalities and defects is actively being investigated. In utero fetal cardiac bypass for the repair of congenital heart defects was reported in animals (97–101). The feasibility of in utero intracranial and spinal surgery was investigated, and attempts at in utero organ transplants were reported (102–104). With further development and refinement of in utero surgical techniques, fetal surgery is likely to become used for an ever-increasing list of indications.

TABLE 3. *Hematopoietic stem cell transplantation for genetic disease*

Age of recipient	Advantages	Disadvantages
Preimmune fetus (<15wks)	No rejection of graft Marrow empty and primed to receive hematopoietic cells No ablation or immunosuppression Treatment is before disease causes irreversible damage	Risks of fetal diagnosis and treatment Partial engraftment (chimerism) may not "cure" disease
Immunocompetent neonate (up to adult)	Complete replacement of marrow likely to cure disease	Rejection of donor HSC[a] Requires marrow ablation/immunosuppression Requires marrow ablation to "make room" for donor HSC Damage from disease that occurs before treatment
Source of donor hematopoietic stem cells		
Preimmune fetal liver (<15wks)	No graft-vs-host disease T-cell depletion not necessary Increased proliferative capacity Increased homing capacity	Abortion issues Contamination (bacterial/viral) Number of cells limited
Adult marrow-blood; neonatal cord blood	Living related transplant possible Repeated transplant from same donor possible Large number of cells	Graft-vs-host disease T-cell depletion necessary T-cell depletion hinders engraftment

[a]Human stem cell.
From ref. 21, with permission.

SURGICAL CONSIDERATIONS

The fetus can be approached either percutaneously, endoscopically, or by open techniques (i.e., hysterotomy).

Percutaneous Procedures

The most common percutaneous intrauterine procedure is amniocentesis, which is usually performed for genetic diagnosis and for determining fetal lung maturity. Most often, the procedure is done with small-diameter needles and local or no anesthesia. Other percutaneous procedures include fetal blood sampling, fetal skin sampling, fetal liver biopsy, and muscle biopsy (91). Therapeutic percutaneous procedures include fetal blood transfusion, which is widely performed for fetuses severely affected by isoimmunization.

Percutaneously placed vesicoamniotic shunts allowed in utero decompression of fetal bladder-outlet obstruction (Fig. 8). These procedures can be complicated by blocked or dislodged catheters, and recatheterization is sometimes needed (105,106). Needle drainage of fetal fluid collections [e.g., fetal lung cysts (107)] can be performed percutaneously and repeated if necessary. Although minimally invasive, percutaneous procedures require expert ultrasound guidance, a cooperative patient, and optimal fetal positioning.

Endoscopic Procedures

Although fetal endoscopy has been used for many years as a diagnostic tool (91), several groups recently developed techniques for minimally invasive intrauterine fetal surgery. The problems of access, intrauterine environment, and postoperative amniotic fluid leak have been addressed in sheep and primate models (108–112). The ideal operative medium has yet to be determined. While CO_2 has been used as an intrauterine operative medium (87,110,113), it is associated with acidosis in the fetal lamb (112,114).

Human experience has now been reported by using fetoscopy for umbilical cord ligation of an acardiac twin (11), vessel ablation for twin–twin transfusion syndrome (10,115), antegrade ablation of posterior urethral valves (116), tracheal occlusion for CDH (58), and fetal repair of myelomeningocele (Fig. 9) (117). In general, for fetoscopic procedures in humans, a liquid medium is preferred, and small endoscopes and instruments that can pass through a needle are used. For more complex procedures requiring larger instruments, maternal laparotomy is performed, and the uterus is approached directly. Full-thickness purse-string sutures are placed under ultrasound guidance to avoid amniotic fluid leak after the trocar is removed (59,87,110,111,113, 118,119).

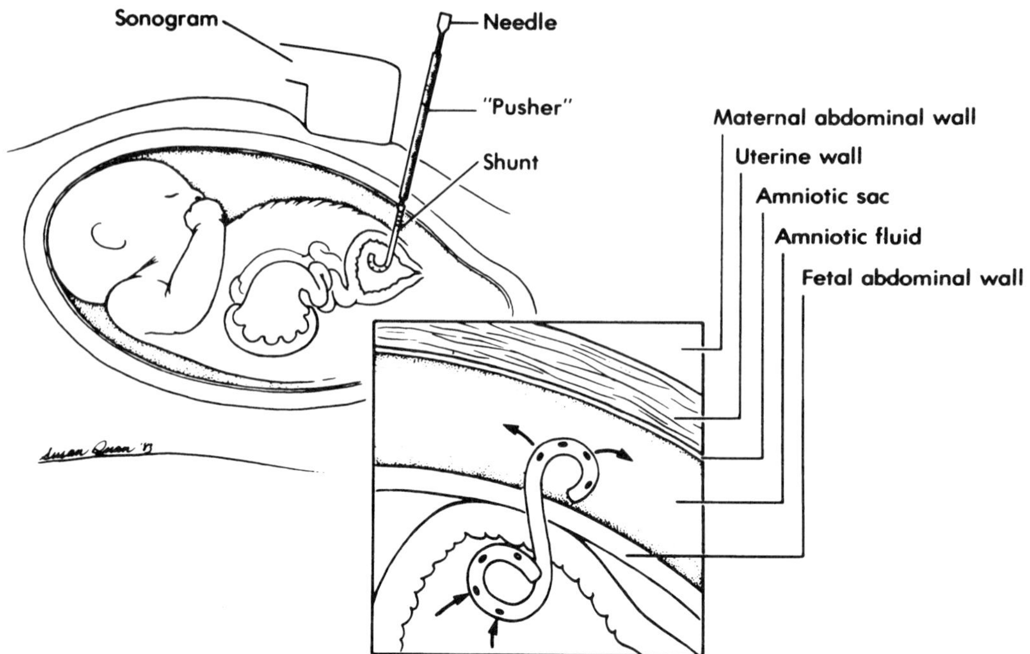

FIG. 8. Technique for placement of Harrison double-pigtailed catheter into the fetal bladder under ultrasound guidance. (From ref. 105, with permission.)

Open Fetal Surgery

Only a few centers are performing open fetal surgery in humans. The experimental nature of these complex procedures and the requirements for intensive intraoperative and postoperative care have limited their widespread use.

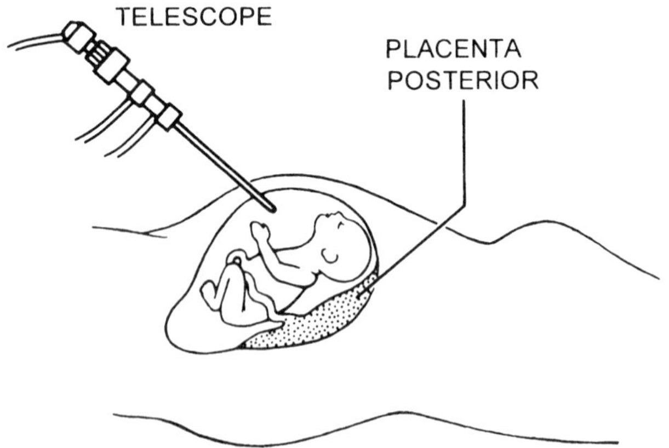

FIG. 9. Fetoscopy in the human. The fetoscope is placed directly through the anterior portion of the uterus. (From ref. 58, with permission.)

Preoperative ultrasound examination determines the intrauterine position of the fetus and placenta. The fetus is approached via maternal laparotomy, and the uterus is brought into the operative field (Fig. 10). A sterile ultrasound probe is used to locate the placenta (71). The hysterotomy is planned as far away from the placenta as possible, while keeping the fetal anatomy of interest accessible. A variety of approaches, including posterior uterine incisions, are used (71). Amniotic fluid is withdrawn, and a uterine incision is made with a device that maintains hemostasis at the uterine edges with absorbable staples (120). When the uterine cavity is entered, the fetus is exposed and the area to be operated on is brought into the field. In some cases, such as fetal tracheal ligation procedures for CDH, the fetus may remain in situ, whereas in others, such as SCT, a portion must be delivered from the uterine cavity (71,121) (A.W. Flake, personal communication, 1995.) During the operative procedure, warm saline is circulated through the uterine cavity to maintain fetal temperature and uterine distention. After completion of the operative procedure, the operated-on fetal part is returned, and the uterine incision is closed with three layers of sutures and fibrin glue (see Fig. 10) (21,121).

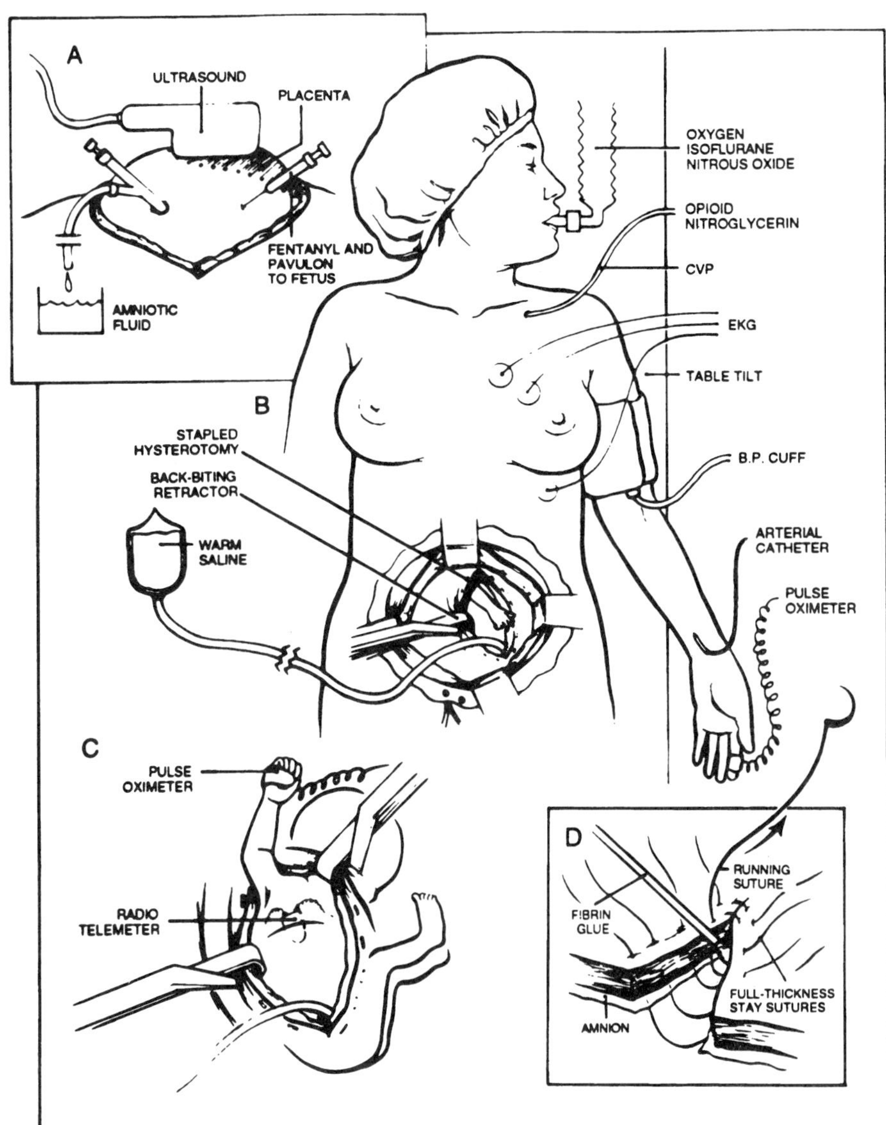

FIG. 10. Fetal surgery techniques. **A:** The uterus is exposed through a maternal laparotomy, and ultrasonography is performed. **B:** The uterus is opened with a cutting/stapling device that provides hemostasis and seals the membranes. **C:** The fetal part of interest is exposed. **D:** After fetal repair, the uterine incision is closed with absorbable sutures and fibrin glue. Amniotic fluid is restored with warm lactated Ringer's solution. (From ref. 21, with permission.)

ANESTHETIC CONSIDERATIONS

Maternal Anesthesia

Anesthesia for fetal surgery requires the simultaneous administration and monitoring of anesthesia to both mother and fetus. Anesthetic considerations applicable to anesthesia during pregnancy for nonobstetric surgery are pertinent to our discussion. Although these issues are covered elsewhere (see Chapter 9), several general principles are worth noting. The key physiologic changes of pregnancy to remember include:

- Increased cardiac output,
- Increased blood volume,
- Increased O_2 consumption,
- Increased minute ventilation,
- Decreased functional residual capacity,
- Increased sensitivity to anesthetics [decreased minimum alveolar concentration (MAC)],
- Prolonged gastric emptying,
- Increased gastric acid production, and
- Decreased lower esophageal sphincter competence (122–126).

Uterine blood flow is determined by the gradient between mean arterial pressure and venous pressure and is inversely proportional to uterine arterial resistance. During pregnancy, there is no uterine artery autoregulation, and the uterine vasculature is near maximally dilated (122,127). Consequently, uteroplacental blood flow can be decreased by:

- Decreased uterine artery pressure,
- Increased uterine venous pressure,
- Increased myometrial pressure, or
- Uterine artery vasoconstriction resulting from either increased levels of endogenous catecholamines or exogenous vasopressors.

Any of these changes can ultimately lead to fetal acidosis (128–130). In addition, maternal respiratory alkalosis or maternal acidosis from any cause can be associated with fetal acidosis (131,132). Finally, consider the potential teratogenic effects of the anesthetics used.

Fetal Anesthesia

An unanesthetized fetus will respond with changes in heart rate and hormonal output when subjected to surgery (133). An older fetus with normal acid–base status will show heart-rate increases when subjected to loud noises or scalp stimulation (122). Both the preterm and term neonate mount a stress response to surgical stimulation with increases in fetal catecholamine concentrations and changes in aldosterone, corticosterone, pyruvate, and blood glucose. Not only can anesthesia suppress these responses in neonates, but the type of anesthesia also can have an impact on clinical outcome (134–137). In addition, recent studies have shown that the human fetus responds to hepatic vein transfusion with increases in cortisol and β-endorphins (138). Giving the fetus fentanyl ameliorates this response (139). Finally, there is anatomic and physiological evidence that the fetus can feel pain. By 22 weeks' gestation, myelination of nerve tracts in the spinal cord and brain stem is present. By 28 to 30 weeks, cortical evoked potentials can be elicited (Fig. 11) (140).

The goals of fetal anesthesia therefore are similar to those for that of the newborn:

- Providing analgesia,
- Rendering the patient immobile, and
- Maintaining cardiovascular homeostasis.

The issue of providing amnesia is unresolved.

Although not ideal, halogenated inhalational agents approach these goals. It is fortuitous that the fetal MAC of anesthetic is less than MAC for adults. In fetal sheep, halothane MAC is 0.33%. In adult sheep, it is 0.69% (141). At maternal MAC, the fetal blood concentration of anesthetic agent is equivalent to a calculated end-tidal concentration of 0.54% (141). The lower MAC for the fetus may be related to increased progesterone concentrations. As progesterone concentration decreases in neona-

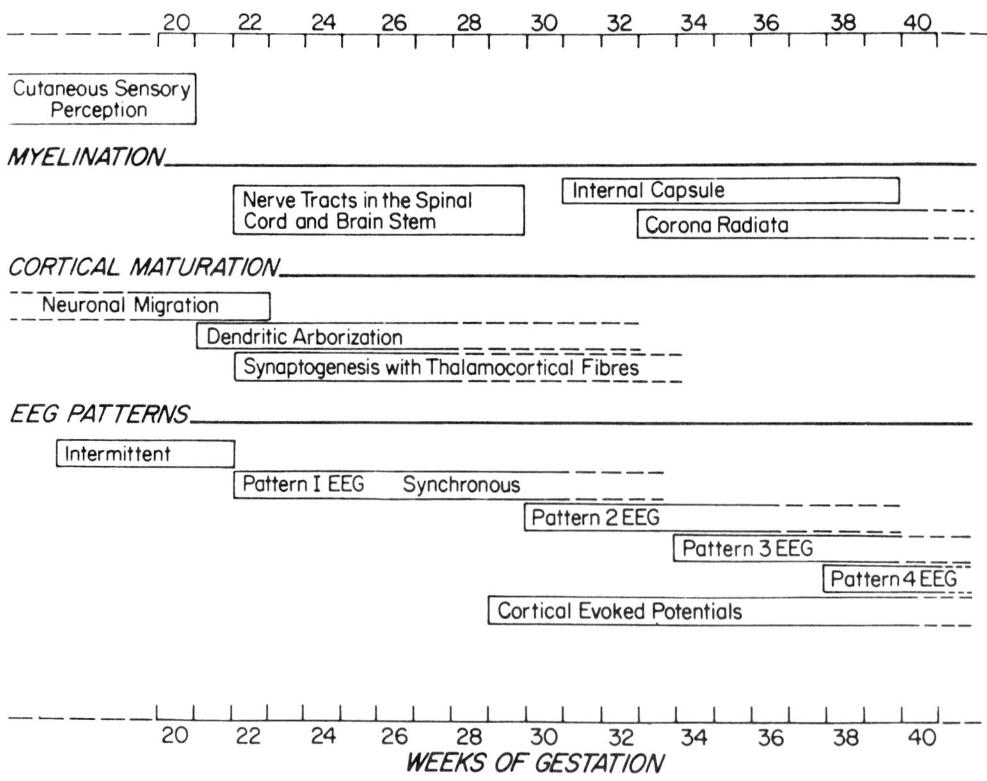

FIG. 11. Schematic diagram of the development of cutaneous sensory perception. (From ref. 140, with permission.)

tal sheep, halothane MAC increases (141). Halothane administered maternally quickly reaches the fetus. While fetal halothane concentration remains below maternal concentration, a steady state occurs by 24 minutes (Fig. 12) (142). The maternal–fetal pharmacokinetics of isoflurane resemble those of halothane (Fig. 13) (143). In sheep, the calculated fetal MAC for isoflurane is 0.34% (Table 4) (141,144).

Although maternal administration of volatile anesthetics provides fetal anesthesia, cardiovascular and acid–base changes can still occur. In healthy sheep, uteroplacental blood flow, fetal acid–base status, and fetal O_2 saturation remain stable with maternal administration of 1.0 and 1.5 MAC of halothane or isoflurane. Two MAC of either agent causes these parameters to deteriorate, primarily because of maternal cardiovascular depression (145). Biehl et al. (146) found that maternal administration of 1.5% halothane (2.0 MAC) decreased fetal mean arterial pressure by 27% but did not alter blood flow to vital organs, cardiac output, oxygenation, or acid–base status in the fetus. Unlike the earlier investigators, who measured end-tidal halothane concentration, Biehl et al. measured maternal blood halothane concentration instead. Thus the effective concentration of halothane in this study was slightly more than one MAC (142,146).

In the stressed (asphyxiated) fetus, 15-minute exposure to 1.0% to 1.5% (1.5 to 2.0 MAC) halothane did not cause further fetal deterioration (147,148). During longer fetal operations (up to 1 hour), potent anesthetics are associated with decreased fetal cardiac output and placental blood flow and increased total vascular resistance. Placental vascular resistance increases out of proportion to fetal systemic vascular resistance. The resulting shunting of blood away from the placental circulation depresses respiratory gas exchange, increases p_aCO_2, and produces fetal acidosis (149). In the isolated fetal lamb heart, even low doses of halothane adversely affect both diastolic and systolic cardiac function (150).

From the fetal perspective, isoflurane has no clear advantage over halothane. Biehl et al. (143) administered 2.0% isoflurane to maternal sheep. After approximately 90 minutes, fetal pH, base excess, and cardiac index decreased significantly (143). This deterioration in fetal acid–base status may have been the result of excessive isoflurane. MAC for isoflurane is 0.86% and 0.34% for maternal and fetal sheep, respectively (144). After 90 minutes of maternal 2.0% isoflurane, fetal blood concentration was almost 0.8%, more than twice the fetal MAC. Maternal blood isoflurane concentration, however, was 0.98%, just slightly greater than 1 MAC. Administration of isoflurane 2.0% for shorter periods (i.e., up to 30 minutes) produces neither fetal acidosis nor a decrease in cardiac output (144). Thus the fetal effects of potent anes-

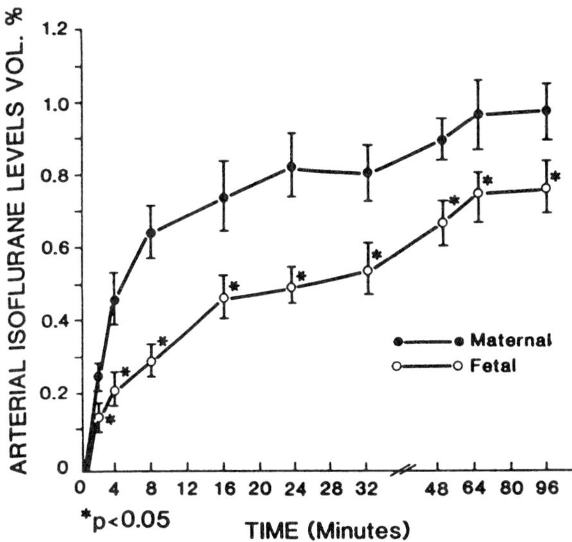

FIG. 13. Maternal and fetal arterial isoflurane concentration during administration of isoflurane at an inspired concentration of 2.0% for 96 minutes (n = 8; mean ± SEM). (From ref. 143, with permission.)

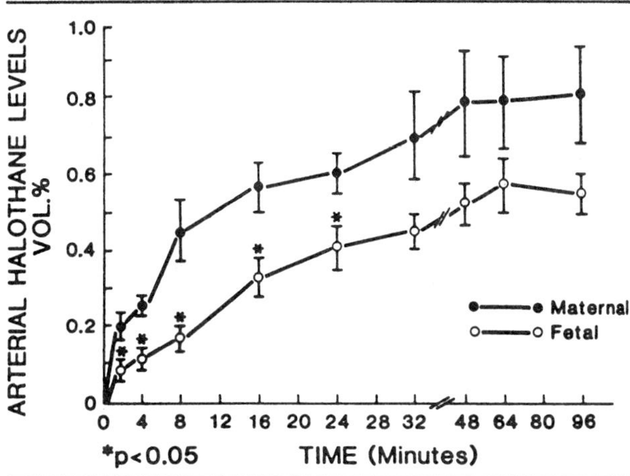

FIG. 12. Maternal and fetal arterial halothane concentration during administration of halothane at an inspired concentration of 1.5% for 96 minutes (n = 6; mean ± SEM). (From ref. 142, with permission.)

TABLE 4. *Maternal and fetal MAC for halothane and isoflurane in the sheep model*

Agent	Maternal	Fetal
Halothane	0.69%	0.33%
Isoflurane	0.86%	0.34%

MAC, minimum alveolar concentration.
From refs. 141 and 144.

thetics depend on the dose and duration of anesthesia as well as the presence of fetal stress and maternal hemodynamics. A short duration of anesthesia (less than 60 minutes) and a low to moderate inspired concentration of potent agent (1 to 1.5 MAC) seem to be reasonably well tolerated.

Other anesthetics and techniques have been examined. In sheep, fetal spinal anesthesia blocks the stress response to surgery (151). One study compared fetal cervical subarachnoid block with 2 mg/kg tetracaine administered via a small hysterotomy with intramuscular ketamine, 25 mg/kg. Maternal anesthesia was provided with a continuous intravenous infusion of ketamine that did not produce fetal anesthesia. Surgical manipulation consisted of exposure of the fetus and placement of venous and arterial lines. After 90 minutes of exposure, the fetal lambs in the spinal-anesthesia group had significantly higher cardiac outputs, and higher brain, total body, and placental blood flows than did those in the ketamine group. In addition, cardiac output in the spinal-anesthesia group approximated that found in unstressed, long-term instrumented fetal sheep. These results suggest that fetal spinal anesthesia may allow stress-free surgery in the fetus. Both technical difficulties and fetal safety issues pose significant obstacles to the use of spinal anesthesia in human fetuses.

The fetal effects of propofol also have been examined. In fetal sheep, maternal propofol infusion, at dosages ranging from 150 to 450 μg/kg/min, did not adversely affect uterine blood flow, fetal mean arterial pressure, heart rate, or base excess (152). Fetal heart rate variability decreased as propofol dosage increased. Although the fetuses were not subjected to exposure or manipulation, the decreased fetal heart rate variability suggested the presence of fetal anesthesia.

Finally, in humans, fentanyl and vecuronium were given directly to the fetus during open surgery (153). Unfortunately, there are no published reports comparing anesthetic techniques for fetal surgery in humans. Nevertheless, some conclusions can be drawn from the available data. Maternally administered volatile inhalational anesthesia may harm the fetus if duration and inspired concentration are excessive. Total spinal anesthesia is not currently technically feasible in humans, and propofol has not been sufficiently studied. Although the use of fentanyl and vecuronium for fetal surgery has not been examined to the same extent as volatile anesthetics, outcome data in human neonates undergoing cardiac surgery have shown an opioid-based anesthetic regimen to be superior to a light inhalational–opioid anesthetic regimen (137). Extrapolating these data to the human fetus suggests that direct fetal administration of opioid and muscle relaxant may be the most appropriate anesthetic currently available for fetal surgery.

Uterine Relaxation and Prevention of Preterm Labor

In addition to adequate maternal and fetal anesthesia, open uterine procedures require profound tocolysis (19,33). This end can be accomplished with a potent volatile anesthetic. Halothane, isoflurane, and enflurane produce dose-dependent uterine relaxation (154,155). In nonhuman primates, 1.5 MAC isoflurane provides satisfactory uterine relaxation for open fetal surgery [Fogel ST, Langer JC, Ball RH, Paul MJ, Downey JC, Talcott M. Anesthesia for fetal surgery in the rhesus monkey (unpublished data)]. Similar concentrations of inhalational agents have been reported to produce satisfactory uterine relaxation in many cases of open fetal surgery in humans (156–158). Additional uterine relaxation may be supplied by supplemental tocolytics such as terbutaline, nitroglycerin, magnesium sulfate, or temporary increases in the concentration of volatile agent. Indomethacin, a nonsteroidal antiinflammatory agent with potent tocolytic effects, is often administered preoperatively to provide additional intraoperative and postoperative tocolysis (10,17,18,153,158) (C.B. Cauldwell, A.W. Flake, personal communication, 1995). Using 1.5 MAC potent agent also usually provides fetal anesthesia and a motionless operative field. Maternal isoflurane (1.5 MAC) consistently provided satisfactory fetal anesthesia for tracheal occlusion procedures in the rhesus monkey. In humans, Gaiser et al. (158) were similarly able to induce fetal anesthesia and uterine relaxation with maximal maternal end-tidal isoflurane concentrations of 1.69% ± 0.07% (mean ± SEM). They used magnesium sulfate to provide additional intraoperative tocolysis (158).

Remember, animal studies reported fetal acidosis after 60 to 90 minutes of maternal end-tidal concentrations of slightly more than 1 MAC isoflurane (143). None of the investigators experienced in human or primate open fetal surgery studied fetal acid–base changes associated with maternal inhalational anesthesia. We monitored fetal status with intraoperative ultrasound measurement of fetal heart rate, whereas Gaiser et al. (158) used fetal pulse oximetry. In both studies the fetuses clinically appeared to tolerate the procedures well. Other groups used lower doses of potent agents (less than 1 MAC) plus N_2O and opioids. Uterine relaxation was maintained with a nitroglycerin infusion (153) (C.B. Cauldwell, A.W. Flake, personal communication, 1995).

Postoperative premature labor is the single most important source of fetal loss in open surgery (99,159). The incidence of coordinated uterine contractions, which often lead to preterm labor (type I contractions), is directly related to the degree of uterine manipulation and myometrial trespass (Fig. 14) (62). The development and application of minimally invasive surgical techniques is therefore appealing.

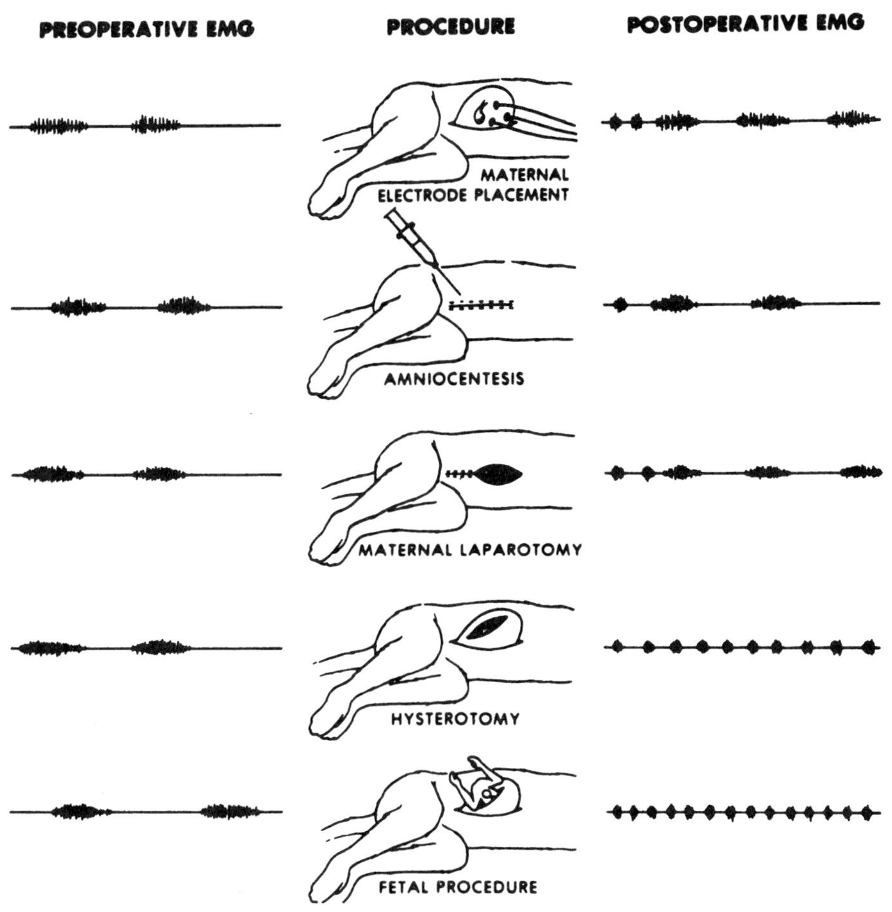

FIG. 14. Postoperative electromyogram (EMG) after procedures in the pregnant rhesus monkey. (From Nakayama DK, Harrison MR, Seron-Ferre M, Villa RL. Fetal surgery in the primate II. Uterine electromyographic response to operative procedures and pharmacologic agents. *J Pediatr Surg* 1984;19:333, with permission.)

CLINICAL RECOMMENDATIONS

Percutaneous Procedures

Percutaneous procedures are not uncommon. Amniocentesis is widely used for diagnostic purposes and usually requires only local anesthesia (7). More extensive percutaneous procedures such as percutaneous umbilical blood sampling (PUBS) and intrauterine transfusions frequently require an immobile fetus as well as maternal comfort (160–162). Although regional or general anesthesia can be administered safely, many of these procedures can be done with local infiltration with or without maternal sedation.

Preoperative Evaluation and Management

Emergency cesarean section may be necessary in patients undergoing percutaneous fetal procedures. These women require the usual preoperative evaluation. In addition, note the current gestational age, which may determine the type of intervention for a sudden fetal complication. Most of these women will not require preoperative anxiolysis. An explanation of planned events should be sufficient. In the rare event that preoperative anxiolytics are necessary, use a short-acting benzodiazepine such as midazolam, and titrate to effect. Immediately before the procedure give a clear, nonparticulate antacid.

Monitoring

Use routine monitors for the mother. Assess mental status and respiratory rate frequently when maternal sedation is required. Monitor the fetus with intraoperative ultrasound, paying particular attention to fetal heart rate, fetal positioning, instrumentation, and fetal movement.

Induction and Maintenance

Position the patient with left uterine displacement and give oxygen. Titrate any maternal sedatives or analgesics as needed. As when providing analgesia and sedation for nonpregnant patients, we and others prefer short-acting agents (i.e., midazolam, propofol, and fentanyl) (163).

When needed, fetal immobility can be provided by direct fetal intramuscular or intravenous injection of nondepolarizing neuromuscular blockers. Although the use of pancuronium has been reported, we have had good success with vecuronium and more recently *cis*-atracurium (161,164,165).

Postoperative Management

Allow patients who have received sedatives or analgesics to recover in a postanesthesia-care unit setting. Monitor fetal status with continuous electronic heart rate monitoring and tocodynometry. Watch for preterm labor, rupture of membranes, or placental abruption. Parenteral analgesics are rarely needed after percutaneous procedures.

Open Uterine Procedures

Open uterine procedures (Table 5) may be complex and require careful advanced planning. They will require multidisciplinary involvement of surgeon, perinatologist, neonatologist, anesthesiologist, and specialized nursing support. As in many complex cases, success depends on meticulous preparation.

Preoperative Evaluation and Management

Preoperative evaluation and management is very similar to that for patients undergoing percutaneous procedures. Be sure that these parturients have adequate cardiopulmonary reserves to tolerate extensive tocolytic therapy. Blood loss may be significant. Be prepared for blood and fluid replacement. Some fetal anomalies may lead to polyhydramnios, increasing the risk of maternal regurgitation and aspiration. In addition:

- Determine gestational age and whether the fetus will be delivered as an emergency in the event of intraoperative deterioration.
- Determine the nature of the fetal lesion and the planned procedure.
- Determine the location of the placenta and the planned site of the uterine incision.
- Determine the obstetric condition of the patient, presence or absence of uterine activity, and cervical dilatation.
- Determine the presence of associated obstetric conditions such as pregnancy-induced hypertension, gestational diabetes, placenta previa, prior preterm labor, or uterine anomalies.
- Because blood loss can be considerable, check a preoperative hematocrit.
- Obtain electrocardiogram (ECG) and chest radiograph if there is an indication of maternal cardiopulmonary compromise.
- Assure that at least 2 units of packed red blood cells are available.
- If intraoperative fetal blood transfusion is anticipated, determine the availability of O-negative, cytomegalovirus-negative, irradiated blood.
- Keep the patient NPO (nil per os) for at least 6 to 8 hours preoperatively, but keep her well hydrated. Begin maintenance intravenous fluids the night before surgery with a large-bore i.v.

TABLE 5. *Suggested anesthetic technique for open fetal surgery*

Preoperative preparation
- Indomethacin, 50 mg, rectally at HS and on call to OR
- Epidural catheter for postop pain management[a]
- Nonparticulate clear antacid, 30 mL p.o.

Monitors
- Maternal
  - ECG
  - Pulse oximeter
  - Direct arterial pressure
  - Central venous pressure
  - Peripheral nerve stimulator
  - Temperature
- Fetal[b]
  - Intraoperative ultrasound
  - Implantable telemetric temperature, heart rate, intraamniotic pressure monitor
  - Pulse oximetery

Intraoperative management
- Induction
  - Left uterine displacement
  - Rapid-sequence induction (opioid, sodium thiopental, succinylcholine) and intubation
- Maintenance
  - Maternal
    - Isoflurane at <1 MAC
    - N_2O, 50%
    - Opioid
    - Vecuronium for muscle relaxation
    - Maintain CVP at 10–12 mm Hg
    - Maintain MAP >65 mm Hg
  - Fetal
    - Fentanyl, 25–50 µg/kg i.m.
    - Vecuronium or pancuronium, 0.1–0.2 mg/kg i.m.

Intraoperative tocolysis
- Nitroglycerin infusion ≤20 µg/kg/min
- Additional tocolysis as needed
  - Terbutaline boluses i.v., 0.25 mg
  - Brief increases in inspired isoflurane
  - $MgSO_4$, 4 gm bolus, 1–2 gm/h infusion

Emergence Anticipate extubation

Postoperative care
- Continue tocolysis
  - Nitroglycerin
  - Magnesium sulfate
  - Terbutaline, ritodrine
  - Indomethancin
  - Calcium channel blockers
- Continue invasive monitoring
  - Arterial blood pressure
  - CVP or PAWP
- Monitor fluid balance
  - Foley catheter
- Monitor uterine activity and fetal well-being
  - Tocodynometer
  - External fetal heart-rate monitor
  - Repeated fetal ultrasound examination

HS, bedtime; MAC, minimum alveolar concentration; CVP, central venous pressure; MAP, mean arterial pressure; PAWP, pulmonary artery wedge pressure.

[a]Optional.

[b]For some procedures (e.g., tracheal ligation for CDH performed in situ), monitoring via intraoperative ultrasound may be sufficient.

- Counsel the patient about anticipated events including the need for invasive central and arterial monitoring and possible postoperative intubation.
- Discuss with the patient plans for postoperative pain management via either continuous lumbar epidural catheter or intravenous patient-controlled analgesia.
- Give the patient indomethacin, 50 mg per rectum, the night before surgery.
- On the morning of surgery, give indomethacin, 100 mg per rectum.
- Anticipate more than the usual degree of preoperative anxiety. Consider intravenous midazolam on the morning of surgery.
- If planning continuous lumbar epidural analgesia for postoperative pain management, insert the catheter.
- Give 30 mL of a nonparticulate antacid before transporting the patient to the operating room.

Monitoring

Use all standard maternal monitors (ECG, pulse oximetry, noninvasive blood pressure, end-tidal CO_2 and temperature). Intraoperative β-mimetic tocolytics can decrease maternal blood pressure. Rapid infusion of large fluid volumes may be needed. For this reason, intraarterial blood pressure monitoring and a central venous pressure (CVP) catheter may be appropriate. Use a Foley catheter to monitor urine output.

Monitor fetal heart rate with intraoperative ultrasound. Other techniques of fetal monitoring include the use of modified ECG electrodes, fetal pulse oximetry, and implantable telemetric devices capable of measuring fetal ECG, heart rate, temperature, and intrauterine pressure (19,33,166) (C.B. Cauldwell, A.W. Flake, personal communication, 1995).

Postoperatively, plan to continue to monitor maternal intraarterial pressure, CVP, and uterine activity. Monitor fetal status with an external heart rate monitor and intermittent ultrasound examinations.

Induction and Maintenance

Position the patient with left uterine displacement (Fig. 10). Use a rapid-sequence induction. Facilitate intubation with either succinylcholine or rocuronium. Maintain anesthesia with low-dose isoflurane (less than 1 MAC) and 50% N_2O in oxygen. Provide supplemental analgesia with opioids as needed. Provide fetal anesthesia and paralysis with fentanyl, 25 to 50 μg, and pancuronium or vecuronium, 0.1 to 0.3 mg, given intramuscularly via a transuterine approach. Maintain uterine tocolysis with a continuous controlled infusion of nitroglycerin in doses of up to 20 μg/kg/min. Nitroglycerin lacks deleterious cardiovascular effects in fetal sheep and may be preferable to high doses of isoflurane (167). If needed, provide additional tocolysis with intravenous terbutaline, 0.25 mg, magnesium sulfate (4-g bolus over 30 minutes followed by 1 to 2 g/h), or brief increases in the inhaled isoflurane concentration. Use intravenous fluids (keep CVP 10 to 12 mm Hg) and ephedrine to maintain maternal mean arterial pressure near 65 mm Hg (153) (C.B. Cauldwell, A.W. Flake, personal communication, 1995). If using magnesium sulfate, remember that it can prolong and intensify nondepolarizing neuromuscular blockade.

An alternative anesthetic uses higher doses of isoflurane for maintenance (158). Give isoflurane in oxygen to end-tidal concentration of approximately 1.5 MAC. Gaiser et al. (159) reported that maximal end-tidal isoflurane levels of 1.69% ± 0.07% (mean ± SEM) usually provided sufficient maternal and fetal anesthesia. Limit supplemental opioids to maximize tolerable isoflurane concentration. Maintain tocolysis with isoflurane and supplemental magnesium sulfate if required.

Plan to extubate the patient at the end of the procedure. Minimize coughing and straining on the endotracheal tube at the time of extubation with intravenous lidocaine or supplemental opioids.

Postoperative Care

Open fetal surgery is associated with a number of postoperative complications. Allow patients to recover in an intensive-care unit setting. Premature labor remains a constant threat (19,168,169). Continue tocolytics. Use β-mimetics, magnesium sulfate, indomethacin, or calcium channel blockers (for a more detailed discussion of tocolytic therapy, see Chapter 34) (8). Nitric oxide donors such as nitroglycerin also have yielded encouraging results (16,153,170). The limiting factor in the use of tocolytics is the large volume of fluid needed to maintain hemodynamic stability and the consequent threat of pulmonary edema (16).

Pulmonary edema associated with tocolysis may not be the simple result of fluid overload and elevated pulmonary artery occlusion pressures (PAOP). In a recent case of pulmonary edema after open fetal surgery, DiFrederico (171) suggested a causative role for low oncotic pressure and increased capillary permeability. PAOP was only 13 mm Hg. There was no evidence of ventricular dysfunction. Plasma protein concentration was 3.95 mg/dL (normal pregnant range, 5.5 to 7.5 mg/dL). In addition, the ratio of protein in alveolar fluid and plasma was 0.99, suggesting increased pulmonary capillary permeability (171).

Observe these women closely for the development of pulmonary edema. Continue CVP or PAOP monitoring into the postoperative period. Monitor fluid balance closely and follow electrolytes and arterial blood gases as indicated. If magnesium sulfate is used for tocolysis, follow serum magnesium concentration. If using β-mimetics, also follow glucose. Continue antibiotics for several days (C.B. Cauldwell, A.W. Flake, personal communication, 1995).

Uterine rupture is an additional threat, and although this complication has not been reported in humans, it has been seen in the nonhuman primate (172). Monitor uterine contractions and fetal well-being with tocodynometry and repeated fetal ultrasound and echocardiography. Once uterine activity has subsided, wean the patient to either oral tocolytic therapy with terbutaline or ritodrine, or parenteral terbutaline via an implantable pump (16).

Amniotic fluid leaks and subsequent oligohydramnios also have been reported after open fetal surgery (168). Evaluate these patients frequently for this complication.

Finally, because open fetal surgery frequently involves a uterine incision placed over the fundus, these women are no longer candidates for a trial of labor (16).

Fetoscopic Procedures

Reducing the degree of uterine intrusion by using fetoscopic surgery should decrease the risk of preterm labor. Indeed, van der Wildt et al. (173) observed a distinct absence of uterine activity 24 hours postoperatively in rhesus monkeys after intrauterine endoscopic surgical access. In sheep, endoscopic fetal surgery did not alter uterine artery blood flow or uteroplacental oxygen delivery, whereas hysterotomy decreased oxygen delivery to near-critical values (174).

Fetoscopic procedures have been successfully performed in humans for a variety of indications (10,11,58, 115–117). Surgical techniques have included both percutaneous approaches to the fetus (11,115,116) and maternal laparotomy with a transuterine approach (Fig. 15) (10,58). Most have been performed under general anesthesia. The anesthetic goals for fetoscopic surgery are the same as for open fetal surgery: maternal and fetal anesthesia, fetal immobility, and tocolysis. The perioperative management of patients for fetoscopic surgery are therefore the same as for open fetal surgery (see earlier). Myometrial trespass is usually less for fetoscopic procedures than for open fetal surgery. Potent volatile anesthetics may therefore provide sufficient intraoperative uterine tocolysis and fetal anesthesia. Consider direct fetal administration of nondepolarizing muscle relaxants to assure fetal immobility. Use small boluses of nitroglycerin, 50 to 200 μg i.v., or terbutaline, 250 μg i.v., if needed for tocolysis. Administer indomethacin preoperatively, but consider reserving supplemental tocolytic infusions for the more complex procedures and for the postoperative period. Postoperative magnesium sulfate has proven successful (58,175) (R.R. Gaiser, personal communication, 1998; A.W. Flake, personal communication, 1998). Patients who have undergone fetoscopic procedures may not require subsequent cesarean delivery because only small incisions have been

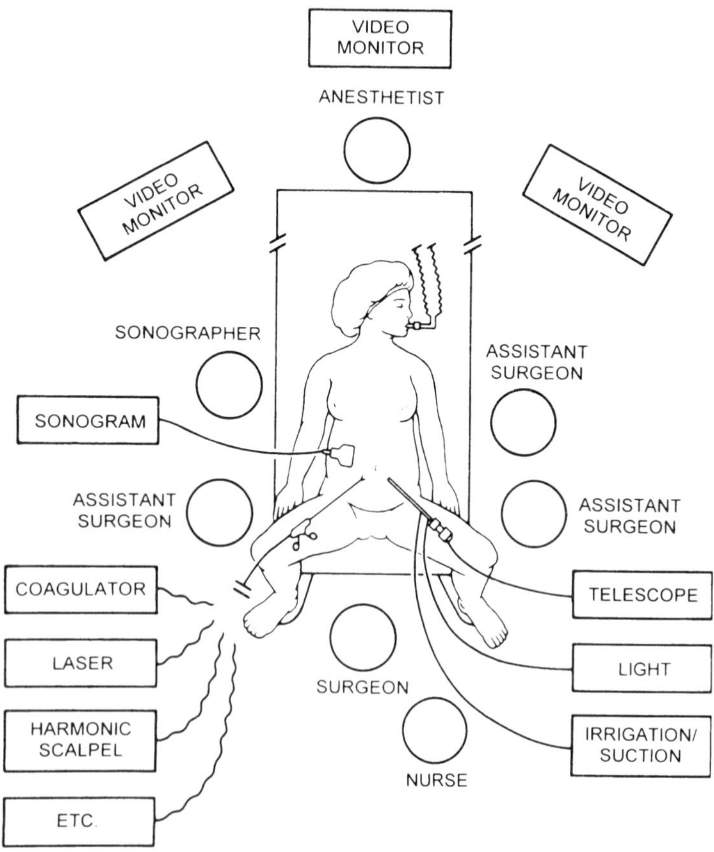

FIG. 15. Operating room set up for fetoscopic surgery in the human. General anesthesia is used, and the uterus is approached via a laparotomy. Fetoscopic instruments are then placed directly through the uterus. (From ref. 58, with permission.)

made in the uterus (R.R. Gaiser, personal communication, 1998). Keep in mind, however, that endoscopic fetal operations have the potential of turning into open uterine procedures.

Perinatal Operations While on Placental Support

Perinatologists and anesthesiologists are, on rare occasion, presented with the problem of delivering a fetus with a known lesion obstructing the upper airway (156,176). The application of anesthetic techniques for intrauterine fetal operations has shown promise in managing this rare but difficult problem.

The management of prenatally diagnosed neck masses and upper airway lesions has been described in the literature and referred to as OOPS (operation on placental support) or the EXIT (ex utero intrapartum treatment) (57,177). Delivery is usually managed via cesarean section. The uterine incision is made in a manner similar to open uterine surgery. Uterine relaxation and fetal anesthesia are obtained, and a surgical airway is established in the neonate, while oxygenation is maintained via continued placental function. Once an intact airway is established, the neonate is delivered.

The largest series to date (eight cases) was reported by Mychaliska et al. (57) with few maternal or fetal complications. They suggested the following anesthetic technique:

- Evaluate and prepare the patient as for open fetal surgery (see earlier).
- Place the patient in left lateral uterine tilt, and perform a rapid-sequence induction of general anesthesia.
- Maintain anesthesia with high-dose inhalational agent (isoflurane, 2% to 3% in oxygen). Provide muscle relaxation with vecuronium and monitor with a peripheral nerve stimulator.

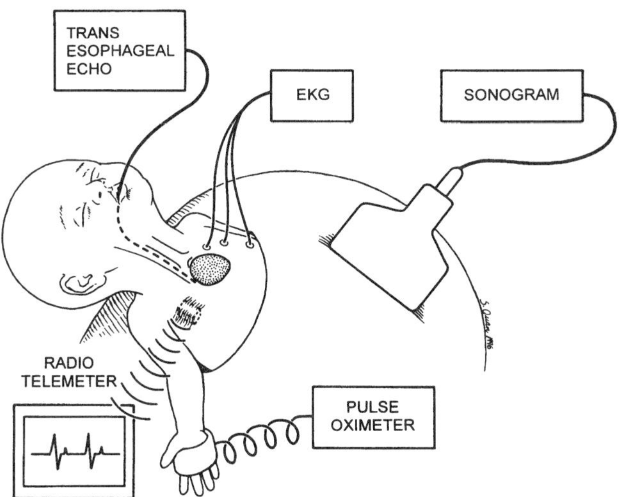

FIG. 16. Fetal monitoring options during an ex utero intrapartum treatment (EXIT) procedure. (From ref. 57, with permission.)

- If high-dose isoflurane does not achieve sufficient uterine relaxation, add small i.v. boluses of terbutaline, 250 μg, or nitroglycerin, 50 to 100 μg. Treat hypotension with fluids and ephedrine.
- If needed, give vecuronium, 0.1 mg/kg, intramuscularly to the fetus for immobility.
- Monitor the fetus with ultrasound and or pulse oximetry (Fig. 16).
- Once an airway has been established (this step may take 60 minutes or more), and the neonate delivered, add pitocin to the intravenous fluids, and change the anesthetic to a low-dose isoflurane/opioid/nitrous oxide technique.
- Allow the patient to recover in a postanesthesia recovery unit, and watch for postpartum bleeding and uterine atony.

MATERNAL AND FETAL OUTCOME

Open fetal surgery is currently performed primarily for life-threatening fetal conditions based on the premise that, absent intervention, the fetus or neonate would die. Although it is ultimately the parent's decision to proceed, maternal risks must be acceptable (see Table 6).

Although maternal deaths directly related to open fetal surgery have not been reported, significant maternal morbidity can occur (21,51). At the Fetal Treatment Center, University of California, San Francisco, reported blood

TABLE 6. *Maternal outcome with open fetal surgery*[a]

	Median	Range
Maternal age (yr)	26	18–43
Gestational age of fetus (wk)	25.0	17–28
Operative time, total (min)	127.4	69–182
Operative time, fetal repair (min)	34	10–92
Blood loss (mL)	455	150–1,400
Interval to delivery (wk)	4.0	1–15
Gestational age at delivery (wk)	28.0	22–36
Complications		
Preterm labor	50	
Transfusion	6	
Pulmonary edema	4	
Amniotic fluid leak		
Intraperitoneal	2	
Transvaginal	5	
Subsequent pregnancy history		
Term cesarean delivery, healthy baby	24[b]	
Pregnant (at time of publication)	1	
History of infertility	9	
Not attempted not desired, too early, etc.	18	
Subsequent uterine disruptions	2	

[a]University of California, San Francisco, Fetal Treatment Center; 50 cases through 1994.
[b]Two women had two subsequent pregnancies each.
Modified from ref. 21, with permission.

loss has ranged from 150 to 1,400 mL, with a median of 455 mL. Six of 50 patients required blood transfusion (21). Virtually all patients developed preterm labor. Pulmonary edema is a common complication of tocolysis in these women (21).

Maternal mirror syndrome, also known as Ballantyne syndrome, is a complication of fetal hydrops. Patients have high-output cardiac failure and findings consistent with preeclampsia. The mechanism is unclear but appears to be related to fetal or placental hydrops (178,179). It is not believed to be the result of the operative procedure itself and is most commonly seen in situations in which fetal surgery is being done because of fetal hydrops (8). Correction of fetal hydrops is not uniformly followed by regression of maternal symptoms. Termination of the pregnancy may be required (16,178,180).

The uterine incisions typically made for open fetal surgery can place the patient at risk for subsequent scar dehiscence. No patient thus far has experienced uterine wound disruptions postoperatively, but two had a dehiscence of the uterine wound in a subsequent pregnancy. Both patients did well with satisfactory neonatal outcome (21,51). A final consideration is the potential impact of open fetal surgery on future fertility. Fetal surgery trials in the nonhuman primate model have shown no decrease in fertility relative to colony controls as long as nonabsorbable sutures or clips were not left in the uterus (181). Similarly, there appears to be no negative impact on fertility in humans (21).

Fetal outcome varies considerably and depends on the initial lesion. Results for open fetal surgery for CDH have not been encouraging. Of 14 patients undergoing open fetal surgery for correction of CDH, five died intraoperatively. Of the remaining nine, there were only four survivors (16). A less complicated approach with the use of temporary fetal tracheal occlusion may prove more promising. In distinct contrast, however, are the results obtained for CCAM. Harrison reported a series of nine patients undergoing open uterine surgery for CCAM with five survivors, all of whom had normal postnatal growth and development (16,21). Fetal outcome after less invasive percutaneous procedures, such as those used to treat urinary obstruction, also has been encouraging (21,78).

Neurological outcome also is of considerable interest. Of 33 infants born after open fetal surgery, seven had significant central nervous system (CNS) abnormalities (182). The remaining 26 appeared neurologically normal (as determined by postmortem examination in the 12 nonsurviving patients, or by imaging or clinical evaluation in the 14 survivors). Periventricular hemorrhage, intraventricular hemorrhage, and periventricular leukomalacia were the major abnormalities identified. All seven abnormal fetuses had been treated for CDH. Although the overall incidence of CNS abnormalities (21%) was similar to gestationally matched premature neonates, the authors thought that these injuries were the result of sudden changes in fetal cerebral blood flow. They speculated that such changes in fetal cerebral hemodynamics may have been due to either maternal hypoxia or maternally administered tocolytic drugs. Fetal outcome, however, can be expected to improve with further refinements in surgical technique and perioperative care.

SUMMARY

Fetal surgery offers the opportunity to improve markedly the lives of children with previously untreatable disorders. Whereas many procedures are still investigational, improvements in surgical technique and perioperative care are likely to bring many interventional procedures into widespread use. A multidisciplinary approach to the fetus as a surgical patient and meticulous attention to detail will be required of all personnel involved to achieve consistently successful outcomes. The provision of stress-free fetal anesthesia, appropriate fetal monitoring, and continuous attention to maternal welfare from the time of admission to well into the postoperative period will be the primary responsibilities of the anesthesiologist.

REFERENCES

1. Steele MW, Breg WR. Chromosome analysis of human amniotic fluid cells. *Lancet* 1966;1:383.
2. Nadler HL. Antenatal detection of hereditary disorders. *Pediatrics* 1968;42:912.
3. Nadler HL, Berbie AB. Role of amniocentesis in the intrauterine detection of genetic disorders. *N Engl J Med* 1970;282:596.
4. Liley AW. Intrauterine transfusion of foetus in hemolytic disease. *Br Med J* 1963;2:1107.
5. Liggins GC. Fetal transfusion by the impaling technique. *Obstet Gynecol* 1966;27:323.
6. Cunningham FG, MacDonald PC, Gant NF, et al. *Williams obstetrics*. Stamford, CT: Appleton & Lange, 1997:1023.
7. Cunningham FG, MacDonald PC, Gant NF, et al. *Williams obstetrics*. Stamford, CT: Appleton & Lange, 1997:919.
8. Langham MR, Rieger KM. Advances in fetal surgery. *Surg Ann* 1994; 26:193.
9. Quintero RA, Puder KS, Cotton DB. Embryoscopy and fetoscopy. *Obstet Gynecol Clin North Am* 1993;20:563.
10. De Lia JE, Cruikshank DP, Keye WR Jr. Fetoscopic neodymium:YAG laser occlusion of placental vessels in severe twin-twin transfusion syndrome. *Obstet Gynecol* 1990;75:1046.
11. Quintero RA, Reich H, Puder KS, et al. Brief report: umbilical-cord ligation of an acardiac twin by fetoscopy at 19 weeks of gestation. *N Engl J Med* 1994;330:469.
12. Harrison MR, Filly RA, Golbus M, et al. Fetal treatment. *N Engl J Med* 1982;307:1651.
13. Nakayama DK, Harrison MR, Chinn DH, et al. Prenatal diagnosis and natural history of the fetus with a congenital diaphragmatic hernia: initial clinical experience. *J Pediatr Surg* 1985;20:118.
14. Harrison MR, Adzick NS, Flake AW, et al. Correction of congenital diaphragmatic hernia in utero: VI. Hard-earned lessons. *J Pediatr Surg* 1993;28:1411.
15. Ford WDA. Fetal intervention for congenital diaphragmatic hernia. *Fetal Diagn Ther* 1994;9:398.
16. Sullivan KM, Adzick NS. Fetal surgery. *Clin Obstetr Gynecol* 1994; 37:355.
17. Rosen M. Anesthesia and monitoring for fetal intervention. In: Harrison MR, Golbus MS, Filly RA, eds. *The unborn patient: prenatal diagnosis and treatment*. Philadelphia: WB Saunders, 1990:172.
18. Scheerer LJ, Katz M. Tocolysis for fetal intervention. In: Harrison MR, Golbus MS, Filly RA, eds. *The unborn patient: prenatal diagnosis and treatment*. Philadelphia: WB Saunders, 1990:82.

19. Harrison MR, Anderson J, Rosen MA, Ross NA, Hendrickx AG. Fetal surgery in the primate I. Anesthetic, surgical, and tocolytic management to maximize fetal-neonatal survival. *J Pediatr Surg* 1982;17:115.
20. Harrison MR, Golbus MS, Filly RA. Management of the fetus with a correctable congenital defect. *JAMA* 1981;246:774.
21. Harrison MR. Fetal surgery. *Am J Obstet Gynecol* 1996;174:1255.
22. Harrison MR. The fetus with a diaphragmatic hernia: pathophysiology, natural history, and surgical treatment. In: Harrison MR, Golbus MS, Filly RA, eds. *The unborn patient: prenatal diagnosis and treatment*. Philadelphia: WB Saunders, 1991:295.
23. Harrison MR, de Lorimier AA. Congenital diaphragmatic hernia. *Surg Clin North Am* 1981;61:1023.
24. Harrison MR, Bjordal RI, Landmark F, Knutrud O. Congenital diaphragmatic hernia: the hidden mortality. *J Pediatr Surg* 1979;13:227.
25. Inselman LS, Mellins RB. Growth and development of the lung. *Pediatrics* 1981;98:1.
26. Levin DL. Morphologic analysis of the pulmonary vascular bed in congenital left sided diaphragmatic hernia. *J Pediatr* 1978;92:805.
27. Reid L. The lung: its growth and remodeling in health and disease. *Am J Roentgenol* 1977;129:777.
28. Allan LD, Irish MS, Glick PL. The fetal heart in diaphragmatic hernia. *Clin Perinatol* 1996;23:795.
29. Karamanoukian HL, O'Toole SJ, Rossman JR, Sharma A, Azizkhan RG, Glick PL. Fetal surgical interventions and the development of the heart in congenital diaphragmatic hernia. *J Surg Res* 1996;65:5.
30. Harrison MR, Bjordal RI, Langmark F, Knutrud O. Congenital diaphragmatic hernia: the hidden mortality. *J Pediatr Surg* 1978;13:227.
31. Brandsma AE, Tenbrinck R, Ijsselstijn H, et al. Congenital diaphragmatic hernia: new models, new ideas. *Pediatr Surg Int* 1995;10:10.
32. Harrison MR, Adzick NS, Estes JM, Howell LJ. A prospective study of the outcome for fetuses with diaphragmatic hernia. *JAMA* 1994;271:382.
33. Harrison MR, Langer JC, Adzick NS, et al. Correction of congenital diaphragmatic hernia in utero. V: Initial clinical experience. *J Pediatr Surg* 1990;25:47.
34. Adzick NS, Vacanti JP, Lillehei CW, O'Rourke PP, Crone RK, Wilson JM. Fetal diaphragmatic hernia: ultrasound diagnosis and clinical outcome in 38 cases. *J Pediatr Surg* 1989;24:654.
35. Sharland KG, Lockhart SM, Heward AJ, Allan LD. Prognosis in fetal diaphragmatic hernia. *Am J Obstet Gynecol* 1992;166:9.
36. Burge DM, Atwell JD, Freeman NV. Could the stomach site help predict outcome in babies with left sided congenital diaphragmatic hernia diagnosed antenatally? *J Pediatr Surg* 1989;24:567.
37. Goodfellow T, Hyde I, Burge DM, Greeman NV. Congenital diaphragmatic hernia: the prognostic significance of the site of the stomach. *Br J Radiol* 1987;60:993.
38. Crawford DC, Wright VM, Drake DP, Allan LD. Fetal diaphragmatic hernia: the value of fetal echocardiography in the prediction of postnatal outcome. *Br J Radiol* 1989;96:705.
39. Crawford DC, Drake DP, Kwaitkowski DK, Chapman MG, Allan LD. Prenatal diagnosis of reversible cardiac hypoplasia associated with congenital diaphragmatic hernia: implications for postnatal management. *J Clin Ultrasound* 1986;14:718.
40. Kamata S, Hasegawa T, Ishikawa S, et al. Prenatal diagnosis of congenital diaphragmatic hernia and perinatal care: assessment of lung hypoplasia. *Early Hum Dev* 1992;29:375.
41. Harrison MR, Adzick NS, Flake AW, Jennings RW. The CDH two-step: a dance of necessity. *J Pediatr Surg* 1993;28:813.
42. Dommergues M, Louis-Sylvestre C, Mandelbrot L, et al. Congenital diaphragmatic hernia: can prenatal ultrasonography predict outcome? *Am J Obstetr Gynecol* 1996;174:1377.
43. Metkus AP, Filly RA, Stringer MD, Harrison MR, Adzick NS. Sonographic predictors of survival in fetal diaphragmatic hernia. *J Pediatr Surg* 1996;31:148.
44. Haller JAJ, Signer RD, Gollader ES, Inon AE, Harrington DD, Shermeta DW. Pulmonary and ductal hemodynamics in studies of simulated diaphragmatic hernia of fetal and newborn lambs. *J Pediatr Surg* 1976;11:675.
45. Harrison MR, Jester JA, Ross NA. Correction of congenital diaphragmatic hernia in utero. I. The model: intrathoracic balloon produces fatal pulmonary hypoplasia. *Surgery* 1980;88:174.
46. Harrison MR, Bressack MD, Churg AM, de Lorimier AA. Correction of congenital diaphragmatic hernia in utero. II. Simulated correction permits fetal lung growth with survival at birth. *Surgery* 1980;88:260.
47. Harrison MR, Ross NA, de Lorimier AA. Correction of congenital diaphragmatic hernia in utero. III. Development of a successful surgical technique using abdominoplasty to avoid compromise of umbilical blood flow. *J Pediatr Surg* 1981;16:934.
48. Soper RT, Pringle KC, Scofield JC. Creation and repair of diaphragmatic hernia in the fetal lamb: technique and survival. *J Pediatr Surg* 1984;19:33.
49. Adzick NS, Outwater KM, Harrison MR, et al. Correction of congenital diaphragmatic hernia in utero. IV. An early gestational fetal lamb model for pulmonary vascular morphometric analysis. *J Pediatr Surg* 1985;20:673.
50. Harrison MR, Adzick NS, Longaker MT, et al. Successful repair in utero of a fetal diaphragmatic hernia after removal of herniated viscera from the left thorax. *N Engl J Med* 1990;322:1582.
51. Harrison MR, Flake AW. Fetal surgery. *Ann Rev Med* 1995;46:67.
52. Wilson JW, DiFiore JW, Peters CA. Experimental fetal tracheal ligation prevents the pulmonary hyperplasia associated with fetal nephrectomy: possible application for congenital diaphragmatic hernia. *J Pediatr Surg* 1993;28:1433.
53. Luks FI, Gilchrist BF, Jackson BT, Piasecki GJ. Endoscopic tracheal obstruction with expanding device in a fetal lamb model: preliminary considerations. *Fetal Diagn Ther* 1996;11:67.
54. DiFiore JW, Wilson JM. Lung liquid, fetal lung growth, and congenital diaphragmatic hernia. *Pediatr Surg Int* 1995;10:2.
55. Bealer JF, Skarsgard ED, Hedrick MH, et al. The PLUG odyssey: adventures in experimental fetal tracheal occlusion. *J Pediatr Surg* 1995;30:361.
56. Hooper SB, Han VK, Harding R. Changes in lung expansion alter pulmonary DNA synthesis and IGF-II gene expression in fetal sheep. *Am J Physiol* 1993;265:L403.
57. Mychaliska GB, Bealer JF, Graf JL, Rosen MA, Adzick NS, Harrison MR. Operating on placental support: the ex utero intrapartum treatment procedure. *J Pediatr Surg* 1997;32:227.
58. VanderWall KJ, Skarsgard ED, Filly RA, Eckert J, Harrison MR. Fetendo-clip: a fetal endoscopic tracheal clip procedure in a human fetus. *J Pediatr Surg* 1997;32:970.
59. VanderWall KJ, Bruch SW, Meuli M, et al. Fetal endoscopic (Fetendo) tracheal clip. *J Pediatr Surg* 1996;31:1101.
60. Johnson MP, Bukowski TP, Reitleman C, Isada ND, Pryde PG, Evans MI. In utero surgical treatment of fetal obstructive uropathy: a new comprehensive approach to identify appropriate candidates for vesicoamniotic shunt therapy. *Am J Obstet Gynecol* 1994;170:1770.
61. Harrison MR, Ross N, Noall R, de Lorimier AA. Correction of congenital hydronephrosis in utero I. The model: fetal urethral obstruction produces hydronephrosis and pulmonary hypoplasia in fetal lambs. *J Pediatr Surg* 1983;18:247.
62. Harrison MR, Nakayama DK, Noall R, de Lorimier AA. Correction of congenital hydronephrosis in utero II: decompression reverses the effects of obstruction on the fetal lung and urinary tract. *J Pediatr Surg* 1982;17:965.
63. Glick PL, Harrison MR, Noall RA, Villa RL. Correction of congenital hydronephrosis in utero III. Early mid-trimester ureteral obstruction produces renal dysplasia. *J Pediatr Surg* 1983;18:681.
64. Glick PL, Harrison MR, Adzick NS, Noall RA, Villa RL. Correction of congenital hydronephrosis in utero IV: in utero decompression prevents renal dysplasia. *J Pediatr Surg* 1984;19:649.
65. Mahony BS, Filly RA, Callen PW, et al. Sonographic evaluation of fetal renal dysplasia. *Radiology* 1984;152:143.
66. Crombleholme TM, Harrison MR, Golbus M, et al. Fetal intervention in obstructive uropathy: prognostic indicators and efficacy of intervention. *Am J Obstet Gynecol* 1990;162:1239.
67. Crombleholme TM, Harrison MR, Langer JC, et al. Early experience with open fetal surgery for congenital hydronephrosis. *J Pediatr Surg* 1988;23:1114.
68. Harrison MR, Golbus M, Filly RA, et al. Fetal hydronephrosis: selection and surgical repair. *J Pediatr Surg* 1987;22:556.
69. Schmidt KG, Silverman NH, Harrison MR, Callen PW. High-output cardiac failure in fetuses with large sacrococcygeal teratoma: diagnosis by echocardiography and Doppler ultrasound. *J Pediatr* 1989;114:1023.
70. Bond SJ, Harrison MR, Schmidt KG, et al. Death due to high-output cardiac failure in fetal sacrococcygeal teratoma. *J Pediatr Surg* 1990;25:1287.
71. Langer JC, Harrison MR, Schmidt KG, et al. Fetal hydrops and death from sacrococcygeal teratoma: rationale for fetal surgery. *Am J Obstet Gynecol* 1989;160:1145.

72. Bullard KM, Harrison MR. Before the horse is out of the barn- fetal surgery for hydrops. *Semin Perinatol* 1995;19:462.
73. Adzick NS, Harrison MR, Glick PL, et al. Fetal cystic adenomatoid malformation: prenatal diagnosis and natural history. *J Pediatr Surg* 1985;20:483.
74. Rice HE, Estes JM, Hedrick MH, Bealer JF, Harrison MR, Adzick NS. Congenital cystic adenomatoid malformation: a sheep model of fetal hydrops. *J Pediatr Surg* 1994;29:692.
75. Adzick NS, Harrison MR, Flake AW, Howell LJ, Golbus MS, Filly RA. Fetal surgery for cystic adenomatoid malformation of the lung. *J Pediatr Surg* 1993;28:806.
76. MacGillivray TE, Harrison MR, Goldstein RB, Adzick NS. Disappearing fetal lung lesions. *J Pediatr Surg* 1993;28:1321.
77. Miller JA, Corteville JE, Langer JC. Congenital cystic adenomatoid malformation in the fetus-natural history and predictors of outcome. *J Pediatr Surg* 1996;31:805.
78. Evans MI, Drugan A, Manning FA, Harrison MR. Fetal surgery in the 1990s. *Am J Dis Child* 1989;143:1431.
79. Hudgins R, Edwards MSB. The fetus with a CNS malformation: natural history and management. In: Harrison MR, Golbus MS, Filly RA, eds. *The unborn patient: prenatal diagnosis and treatment*. Philadelphia: WB Saunders, 1991:437.
80. Manning FA, Harrison MR, Rodeck CH. Special Report. Catheter shunts for fetal hydronephrosis and hydrocephalus: report of the International Fetal Surgery Registry. *N Engl J Med* 1986;315:336.
81. Clewell WH. The fetus with ventriculomegaly: selection and treatment. In: Harrison MR, Golbus MS, Filly RA, eds. *The unborn patient: prenatal diagnosis and treatment*. Philadelphia: WB Saunders, 1991:444.
82. Longaker MT, Kaban LB. Experimental craniofacial abnormalities. In: Harrison MR, Golbus MS, Filly RA, eds. *The unborn patient: prenatal diagnosis and treatment*. Philadelphia: WB Saunders, 1991:590.
83. Dixon JB. Inflammation in the foetal and neonatal rat: the local reactions to skin burns. *J Pathol Bacteriol* 1960;80:73.
84. Sullivan KM, Lorenz HP, Meuli M, Lin RY, Adzick NS. A model of scarless human fetal wound repair is deficient in transforming growth factor beta. *J Pediatr Surg* 1995;30:198.
85. Estes JM, Adzick NS, Harrison MR, Longaker MT, Stern R. Hyaluronate metabolism undergoes an ontogenic transition during fetal development: implications for scar-free wound healing. *J Pediatr Surg* 1993;28:1227.
86. Martin P. Mechanisms of wound healing in the embryo and fetus. *Curr Topics Dev Biol* 1996;32:175.
87. Estes JM, Whitby DJ, Lorenz HP, et al. Endoscopic creation and repair of fetal cleft lip. *Plast Reconstr Surg* 1992;90:743.
88. Meuli-Simmen C, Meuli M, Hutchins GM, et al. Fetal reconstructive surgery: experimental use of the latissimus dorsi flap to correct myelomeningocele in utero. *Plast Reconstr Surg* 1995;96:1007.
89. Meuli M, Meuli-Simmen C, Yingling CD, et al. Creation of myelomeningocele in utero: a model of functional damage from spinal cord exposure in fetal sheep. *J Pediatr Surg* 1995;30:1028.
90. Meuli M, Meuli-Simmen C, Hutchins GM, et al. In utero surgery rescues neurological function at birth in sheep with spina bifida. *Nature Med* 1995;1:342.
91. Simpson JL, Elias S. Prenatal diagnosis of genetic disorders. In: Creasy RK, Resnik R, eds. *Maternal fetal medicine: principles and practice*. Philadelphia: WB Saunders, 1994:61.
92. Flake AW, Harrison MR, Adzick NS, Zanjani ED. Transplantation of fetal hematopoietic stem cells in utero: the creation of hematopoietic chimeras. *Science* 1986;233:776.
93. Harrison MR, Slotnick RN, Crombleholme TM, Golbus MS, Tarantal AF, Zanjani ED. In-utero transplantation of fetal liver haemopoietic stem cells in monkeys. *Lancet* 1989;2:1425.
94. Touraine JL, Raudrant D, Rebaud A, et al. In utero transplantation of stem cells in humans: immunological aspects and clinical follow-up of patients. *Bone Marrow Transplant* 1992;9[Suppl 1]:121.
95. Raudrant D, Touraine JL, Rebaud A. In utero transplantation of stem cells in humans: technical aspects and clinical experience during pregnancy. *Bone Marrow Transplant* 1992;9[Suppl 1]:98.
96. Flake AW, Roncarolo MG, Puck JM, et al. Treatment of X-linked severe combined immunodeficiency by in utero transplantation of paternal bone marrow. *N Engl J Med* 1996;335:1806.
97. Fishman NH, Hof RB, Rudolph AM, Heymann MA. Models of congenital heart disease in fetal lambs. *Circulation* 1978;58:354.
98. Bical O, Gallix P, Toussaint M, et al. Intrauterine versus postnatal repair of created pulmonary artery stenosis in the lamb: morphologic comparison. *J Thorac Cardiovasc Surg* 1990;99:685.
99. Harrison MR, Adzick NS. The fetus as a patient: surgical considerations. *Ann Surg* 1991;213:279.
100. Reddy VM, Liddicoat JR, Klein JR, McElhinney DB, Wampler RK, Hanley, FL. Fetal cardiac bypass using an in-line axial flow pump to minimize extracorporeal surface and avoid priming volume. *Ann Thorac Surg* 1996;62:393.
101. Reddy VM, Liddicoat JR, Klein JR, Wampler RK, Hanley FL. Long-term outcome after fetal cardiac bypass: fetal survival to full term and organ abnormalities. *J Thorac Cardiovasc Surg* 1996;111:536.
102. Brodner RA, Markowitz RS, Lantner HJ. Feasibility of intracranial surgery in the primate fetus: model and surgical principles. *J Neurosurg* 1987;66:276.
103. Albright L. Techniques of spinal cord surgery in fetal rats. *Neurosurgery* 1987;20:240.
104. Niederhuber JE, Shermeta D, Turcotte JG, Gikas PW. Kidney transplantation in the fetal lamb: technique and histopathology of rejection. *Transplantation* 1971;12:161.
105. Harrison MR, Filly RA. The fetus with obstructive uropathy: pathophysiology, natural history, selection, and treatment. In: Harrison MR, Golbus MS, Filly RA, eds. *The unborn patient: prenatal diagnosis and treatment*. Philadelphia: WB Saunders, 1991:328.
106. Appleman Z, Golbus MS. The management of fetal urinary tract obstruction. *Clin Obstet Gynecol* 1986;29:483.
107. Brown MF, Lewis D, Brouillette RM, Hilman B, Brown EG. Successful prenatal management of hydrops, caused by congenital cystic adenomatoid malformation, using serial aspirations. *J Pediatr Surg* 1995;30:1098.
108. Skarsgard ED, Meuli M, VanderWall KJ, Bealer JF, Adzick NS, Harrison MR. Fetal endoscopic tracheal occlusion (Fetendo-PLUG) for congenital diaphragmatic hernia. *J Pediatr Surg* 1996;31:1335.
109. Skarsgard ED, Bealer JF, Meuli M, Adzick NS, Harrison MR. Fetal endoscopic (Fetendo) surgery: the relationship between insufflating pressure and the fetoplacental circulation. *J Pediatr Surg* 1995;30:1165.
110. Estes JM, MacGillivray TE, Hedrick MH, Adzick NS, Harrison MR. Fetoscopic surgery for the treatment of congenital anomalies. *J Pediatr Surg* 1992;27:950.
111. Crombleholme TM, Dirkes K, Whitney TM, Alman B, Garmel S, Connelly RJ. Amniotic band syndrome in fetal lambs: fetoscopic release and morphometric outcome. *J Pediatr Surg* 1995;30:974.
112. Pelletier GJ, Srinathan SK, Langer JC. Effects of intraamniotic helium, carbon dioxide, and water on fetal lambs. *J Pediatr Surg* 1995;30:1155.
113. Estes JM, Szabo Z, Harrison MR. Techniques for in utero endoscopic surgery: a new approach for fetal intervention. *Surg Endosc* 1992;6:215.
114. Luks FI, Deprest JA, Marcus M, et al. Carbon dioxide pneumoamnios causes acidosis in the fetal lamb. *Fetal Diagn Ther* 1994;9:105.
115. Ville Y, Hyett J, Hecher K, Nicolaides K. Preliminary experience with endoscopic laser surgery for severe twin-twin transfusion syndrome. *N Engl J Med* 1995;332:224.
116. Quintero RA, Hume R, Smith C, et al. Percutaneous fetal cystoscopy and endoscopic fulguration of posterior urethral valves [Comments]. *Am J Obstet Gynecol* 1995;172:206.
117. Bruner JP, Tulipan NE, Richards WO. Endoscopic coverage of fetal open myelomeningocele in utero [Letter]. *Am J Obstet Gynecol* 1997;176:256.
118. Luks FI, Deprest JA, Vandenberghe K, Brosens IA, Lerut T. A model for fetal surgery through intrauterine endoscopy. *J Pediatr Surg* 1994;29:1007.
119. Hedrick MH, Jennings RW, MacGillivray TE, et al. Endoscopic catheterization of placental vessels for chronic fetal vascular access. *Surg Forum* 1992;43:504.
120. Bond SJ, Harrison MR, Slotnick RN, Anderson J, Flake AW, Adzick NS. Cesarean delivery and hysterotomy using an absorbable stapling device. *Obstet Gynecol* 1989;74:25.
121. Harrison MR, Longaker MT. Maternal risk and the development of fetal surgery. In: Harrison MR, Golbus MS, Filly RA, eds. *The unborn patient: prenatal diagnosis and treatment*. Philadelphia: WB Saunders, 1991:189.
122. Cunningham FG, MacDonald PC, Gant NF, et al. *Williams obstetrics*. Stamford, CT: Appleton & Lange, 1997:191.

123. Davison JS, Davison MC, Hay DM. Gastric emptying time in late pregnancy and labor. *J Obstet Gynecol Br Commonw* 1970;77:37.
124. Pernoll ML, Betcalfe J, Schlenker TL, Welch E, Matsumoto JA. Oxygen consumption at rest and during exercise in pregnancy. *Respir Physiol* 1975;25:285.
125. Palahniuk RJ, Shnider SM, Eger EI. Pregnancy decreases the requirement of inhaled anesthetic agents. *Anesthesiology* 1974;41:82.
126. Attia RR, Ebeid AM, Fischer JE, Goudsouzian NG. Maternal fetal and placental gastrin communications. *Anaesthesia* 1982;37:18.
127. Thaler I, Mansor D, Itskovitz J, et al. Changes in uterine blood flow during human pregnancy. *Am J Obstet Gynecol* 1990;162:121.
128. Adamson K, Jueller-Heubach E, Myers RE. Production of fetal asphyxia in the rhesus monkey by administration of catecholamines to the mother. *Am J Obstet Gynecol* 1971;109:248.
129. Ralston DH, Shnider SM, de Lorimier AA. Effects of equipotent ephedrine, metaraminol, mephentermine and methoxamine on uterine blood flow in the pregnant ewe. *Anesthesiology* 1974;40:354.
130. Shnider SM, Wright RG, Levinson G, et al. Uterine blood flow and plasma norepinephrine changes during maternal stress in the pregnant ewe. *Anesthesiology* 1979;50:542.
131. Motoyama EK, Rivard G, Acheson F, Cook CD. The effect of changes in maternal pH and P_{CO_2} on the P_{O_2} of fetal lambs. *Anesthesiology* 1967;28:891.
132. Levinson G, Shnider SM, de Lorimier AA, Steffenson JL. Effects of maternal hyperventilation on uterine blood flow and fetal oxygenation and acid-base status. *Anesthesiology* 1974;40:340.
133. Rose JC, MacDonald AA, Heymann MA, Rudolph AM. Developmental aspects of the pituitary-adrenal axis response to hemorrhagic stress in lamb fetuses in utero. *J Clin Invest* 1978;61:42.
134. Anand KJ, Brown MJ, Bloom SR, Aynsley-Green A. Studies on the hormonal regulation of fuel metabolism in the human newborn infant undergoing anaesthesia and surgery. *Hormone Res* 1985;22:115.
135. Anand KJ, Brown MJ, Causon RC, Christofides ND, Bloom SR, Aynsley-Green A. Can the human neonate mount an endocrine and metabolic response to surgery? *J Pediatr Surg* 1985;20:41.
136. Anand KJ, Sippell WG, Aynsley-Green A. Randomized trial of fentanyl anaesthesia in preterm babies undergoing surgery: effects on the stress response. *Lancet* 1987;1:62.
137. Anand KJ, Hickey PR. Halothane-morphine compared with high-dose sufentanil for anesthesia and postoperative analgesia in neonatal cardiac surgery [Comments]. *N Engl J Med* 1992;326:1.
138. Giannakoulopoulos X, Sepulveda W, Kourtis P, Glover V, Fisk NM. Fetal plasma cortisol and beta-endorphin response to intrauterine needling. *Lancet* 1994;344:77.
139. Fisk NM. Report to the International Fetal Medicine and Surgery Society May, 1997.
140. Anand KJ, Hickey PR. Pain and its effects in the human neonate and fetus. *N Engl J Med* 1987;317:1321.
141. Gregory GA, Wade JG, Beihle DR, Ong BY, Sitar DS. Fetal anesthetic requirement (MAC) for halothane. *Anesth Analg* 1983;62:9.
142. Biehl DR, Cote J, Wade JG, Gregory GA, Sitar D. Uptake of halothane by the foetal lamb in utero. *Can Anaesth Soc J* 1983;30:24.
143. Biehl DR, Yarnell R, Wade JG, Sitar D. The uptake of isoflurane by the foetal lamb in utero: effect on regional blood flow. *Can Anaesth Soc J* 1983;30:581.
144. Bachman CR, Biehl DR, Sitar D, Cumming M, Pucci W. Isoflurane potency and cardiovascular effects during short exposures in the foetal lamb. *Can Anaesth Soc J* 1986;33:41.
145. Palahniuk RJ, Shnider SM. Maternal and fetal cardiovascular and acid-base changes during halothane and isoflurane anesthesia in the pregnant ewe. *Anesthesiology* 1974;41:462.
146. Biehl DR, Tweed AW, Cote J, Wade JG, Sitar D. Effect of halothane on cardiac output and regional flow in the fetal lamb in utero. *Anesth Analg* 1983;62:489.
147. Yarnell R, Biehl DR, Tweed AW, Gregory GA, Sitar D. The effect of halothane anaesthesia on the asphyxiated foetal lamb in utero. *Can Anaesth Soc J* 1983;30:474.
148. Cheek DBC, Hughes SD, Dailey PA, et al. Effect of halothane on regional cerebral blood flow and cerebral metabolic oxygen consumption in the fetal lamb in utero. *Anesthesiology* 1987;67:361.
149. Sabik JF, Assad RS, Hanley FL. Halothane as an anesthetic for fetal surgery. *J Pediatr Surg* 1993;28:542.
150. Davis DA, Speziali G, Wagerle CL, Heckman JL, Russo RA. Effects of halothane on the immature lamb heart. *Ann Thorac Surg* 1995;59:695.
151. Fenton KN, Heinemann MK, Kickey PR, Hanley FL. The stress response during fetal surgery is blocked by total spinal anesthesia. *Surg Forum* 1992;43:631.
152. Alon E, Ball RH, Gillie MH, Parer JT, Rosen MA, Shnider SM. Effects of propofol and thiopental on maternal and fetal cardiovascular and acid-base variables in the pregnant ewe. *Anesthesiology* 1993;78:562.
153. Cauldwell CB, Rosen MA, Harrison MR. The use of nitroglycerin for uterine relaxation during fetal surgery [Abstract]. *Anesthesiology* 1995;83:A929.
154. Munson ES, Embro WJ. Enflurane, isoflurane, and halothane and isolated human uterine muscle. *Anesthesiology* 1977;46:11.
155. Calvello DC, Abadir AR, Chaudhry MR, Doss NW. Isoflurane effect on isolated non-pregnant human myomtrium. *Proceedings Western Pharmacology Society* 1987;30:179.
156. Norris MC, Joseph J, Leighton BL. Anesthesia for perinatal surgery. *Am J Perinatol* 1989;6:39.
157. Johnson MD, Birnbach DJ, Burchman C, Greene MF, Datta S, Ostheimer GW. Fetal surgery and general anesthesia: a case report and review. *J Clin Anesth* 1989;1:363.
158. Gaiser RR, Cheek TG, Kurth CD, Jackson GM, Adzick NS. Perioperative management of the parturient presenting for fetal surgery [Abstract]. *Soc Obstet Anesth Perinatol* 1997;60.
159. Adzick NS, Harrison MR. Fetal surgical therapy. *Lancet* 1994;343:897.
160. Reece EA, Copel JA, Scioscia AL, Grannum PA, DeGennaro N, Hobbins JC. Diagnostic fetal umbilical blood sampling in the management of isoimmunization. *Am J Obstet Gynecol* 1988;159:1057.
161. Copel JA, Grannum PA, Harrison D, Hobbins JC. The use of intravenous pancuronium bromide to produce fetal paralysis during intravascular transfusion. *Am J Obstet Gynecol* 1988;158:170.
162. Sacher RA, Falchuk SC. Percutaneous umbilical blood sampling. *Crit Rev Clin Lab Sci* 1990;28:19.
163. Spielman FJ, Seeds JW, Corke BC. Anaesthesia for fetal surgery. *Anaesthesia* 1984;39:756.
164. Seeds JW, Corke BC, Spielman FJ. Prevention of fetal movement during invasive procedures with pancuronium bromide. *Am J Obstet Gynecol* 1986;155:818.
165. Moise KJ Jr, Carpenter RJ Jr, Deter RL, Kirshon B, Diaz SF. The use of fetal neuromuscular blockade during intrauterine procedures. *Am J Obstet Gynecol* 1987;157:874.
166. Jennings RW, Adzick NS, Longaker MT, Lorenz HP, Harrison MR. Radiotelemetric fetal monitoring during and after open fetal operation. *Surg Gynecol Obstet* 1993;176:59.
167. de Rosayro M, Nahrwold ML, Hill AB, Tait AR, Busch MD, Kirsh MM. Plasma levels and cardiovascular effect of nitroglycerin in pregnant sheep. *Can Anaesth Soc J* 1980;27:560.
168. Longaker MT, Adzick NS, Harrison MR. Update on the status of fetal surgery. *Surg Ann* 1991;23:53.
169. Harrison MR. Fetal surgery. *Am J Obstet Gynecol* 1996;174:1255.
170. Harrison MR. Nitric oxide and preterm labor. *Fetal Treat Center Newsl* 1994;4.
171. DiFederico EM, Harrison M, Matthay MA. Pulmonary edema in a woman following fetal surgery. *Chest* 1996;109:1114.
172. Flake AW, Harrison MR, Adzick NS. Intrauterine intervention: fetal surgery in the nonhuman primate. In: Bruns YW, Kuehl TTJ, eds. *Nonhuman primates in perinatal research*. New York: John Wiley, 1988:245.
173. van der Wildt B, Luks FI, Steegers EAP, Deprest JA, Peers KHE. Absence of electrical uterine activity after endoscopic access for fetal surgery in the rhesus monkey. *Eur J Obstet Gynecol Reprod Biol* 1995;58:213.
174. Luks FI, Peers KHE, Deprest JA, Lerut TE, Vandenberghe K. The effect of open and endoscopic fetal surgery on uteroplacental oxygen delivery in the sheep. *J Pediatr Surg* 1996;31:310.
175. Crombleholme TM, VanderWall KJ. Fetendo-clip: a fetal endoscopic tracheal clip procedure in a human fetus. *J Pediatr Surg* 1997;32:972.
176. Langer JC, Tabb T, Thompson P, Paes BA, Caco CC. Management of prenatally diagnosed tracheal obstruction: access to the airway in utero prior to delivery. *Fetal Diagn Ther* 1992;7:12.
177. Skarsgard ED, Chitkara U, Krane EJ, Riley ET, Halamek LP, Dedo HH. The OOPS procedure (operation on placental support): in utero airway management of the fetus with prenatally diagnosed tracheal obstruction. *J Pediatr Surg* 1996;31:826.
178. Longaker MT, Golbus MS, Filly RA, Rosen MA, Chang SW, Harrison MR. Maternal outcome after open fetal surgery. *JAMA* 1991;265:737.

179. van Selm M, Kanhai HH, Gravenhorst JB. Maternal hydrops syndrome: a review. *Obstet Gynecol Surv* 1991;46:785.
180. Bock B, Riess R, Wunsch PH, Feige A. [Prenatal diagnosis of a sacrococcygeal teratoma with hydrops fetalis and placental hypertrophy consequences for the further course of pregnancy]. [German]. *Geburtshilfe Frauenheilkd* 1990;50:647.
181. Adzick NS, Harrison MR, Glick PL, et al. Fetal surgery in the primate III: maternal outcome after fetal surgery. *J Pediatr Surg* 1986;21:477.
182. Bealer JF, Raisanen J, Skarsgard ED, et al. The incidence and spectrum of neurological injury after open fetal surgery. *J Pediatr Surg* 1995;30:1150.

Obstetric Anesthesia, second edition,
edited by Mark C. Norris.
Lippincott Williams & Wilkins, Philadelphia © 1999.

CHAPTER 11

Obstetric Management of Labor

Linda Chan and Ji-Bin Liu

EVENTS BEFORE PARTURITION

Definitions

The average duration of pregnancy in humans is 280 days (40 weeks) from the first day of the last menstrual period, or 267 days after ovulation. A fetus reaches term at 40 ± 2 weeks, and is viable at 500 grams and mature at 2,500 grams. Labor at 40 ± 2 weeks is labor at term. Preterm labor is labor between 20 and 37 completed weeks of pregnancy. A fetus born before 20 completed weeks of pregnancy is an abortus.

Preparatory Events

Before labor begins, several physiologic phenomena commonly occur. These events serve to ready the fetus and uterus for the onset of true labor (1).

Lightening

Lightening is a subjective sensation felt by the mother as the baby settles into the brim of the pelvis. The abdominal shape changes. The fundal region flattens, while the lower abdomen, just above the pubic bone, bulges. The uterus now compresses the bladder, inciting urinary frequency. In primigravid women, lightening (or engagement) commonly occurs 2 to 3 weeks before the onset of labor. Further descent of the fetus does not occur until late in labor. In most multigravid women, lightening does not take place until early labor.

L. Chan: Division of Maternal-Fetal Medicine, Department of Obstetrics, Gynecology and Reproductive Science, Temple University School of Medicine, Philadelphia, Pennsylvania 19140.

J.-B. Liu: Division of Diagnostic Ultrasound, Department of Radiology, Thomas Jefferson University, Philadelphia, Pennsylvania 19107.

Cervical Ripening, Effacement, and Bloody Show

Before the onset of parturition, the cervix frequently softens and becomes increasingly flexible, a process called "ripening." The softening of the cervix results from:

- An increase in its water content caused by an increase in the relative amount of various glycosaminoglycans that have the capacity to retain water, and
- Collagen lysis and rearrangement of the collagen fibers.

With cervical ripening, effacement ("thinning" or "obliteration") of the cervix occurs as it is taken up into the lower uterine segment. Because of cervical effacement, the mucous plug (which often is blood-tinged) filling the cervical canal may break free. Labor usually begins several hours to a few days after this "bloody show." The average length of the unripe, uneffaced cervix is 2.5 cm. During labor, the cervix gradually thins until it is completely retracted and the cervicovaginal angle completely disappears (100% effaced) (Fig. 1).

False Labor

During the later part of pregnancy, the uterus undergoes irregular, sporadic, brief contractions that produce neither progressive effacement and dilatation of the cervix, nor descent of the presenting part. These contractions, so-called "false labor" or "Braxton Hicks" contractions, may serve a physiologic role in preparing the uterus and cervix for true labor. Braxton Hicks contractions are often confined to the lower abdomen and groin and do not usually involve all the myometrium. The contractions of true labor usually originate in the fundal region and spread over the entire uterus and through to the lower back. False labor can be rhythmic and of mild intensity. However, these contractions may be painful and prevent the patient from sleeping and resting. The hazards of false labor include maternal physical and mental exhaustion, apprehension, and premature intervention by the obstetri-

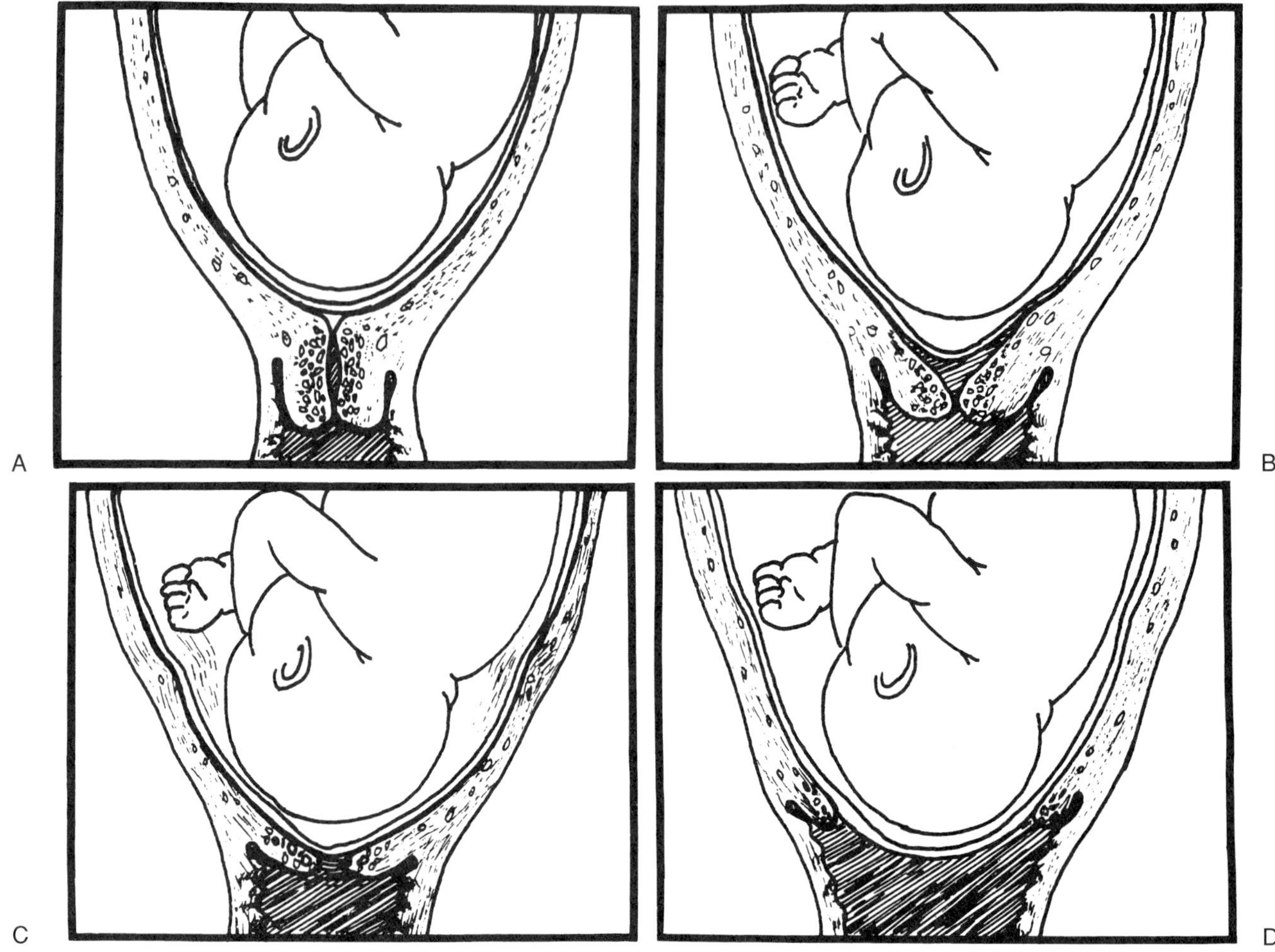

FIG. 1. Progression of cervical effacement and dilation. **A:** 0% effacement, closed cervix. **B:** 50% effacement, closed cervix. **C:** 100% effacement, 2- to 3-cm cervical dilation. **D:** 100% effacement, 9-cm cervical dilation.

cian. The treatment for false labor is sedation and rest. When Braxton Hicks contractions occur before 37 completed weeks of pregnancy, it is important to distinguish them from true preterm labor.

INITIATION OF PARTURITION

The exact mechanism of the initiation and progression of labor in humans is not entirely clear. Two schools of thought argue whether the fetus or the extrafetal tissues of the conceptus are the origins of the chain of events that begins parturition. A communication system exists between fetus and mother. It has two functional arms:

- the fetal–placental–maternal endocrine arm, and
- the fetal–decidual paracrine arm.

Regardless of whether the chain begins within or outside the fetus, the signal is translated into the activation of the maternal myometrium and labor (2).

The uterine muscle cells undergo hypertrophy and hyperplasia up to week 20 of gestation. Then distention and stretching of muscle fibers predominates. Throughout most of gestation, the uterus rests in a somewhat quiescent state. Progressive increases in myometrial contractions antecede parturition. Possibly labor begins when the myometrial fibers have stretched to their maximum (i.e., pregnancy at term, polyhydramnios, multiple gestations).

Chemical Mediators

Oxytocin, an octapeptide hormone made by the posterior pituitary gland, induces uterine contractions and, during lactation, causes milk "let-down." It was once thought to play a key role in the onset of labor. As parturition nears, the uterus becomes maximally sensitive to oxytocin as oxytocin-receptor concentrations increase. However, an increase in circulating oxytocin concentration is difficult to prove, questioning the importance of oxytocin in the initiation of labor. Still, the increase in oxytocin-receptor density may allow the myometrium to react to a small increase in circulating oxytocin. This change in the uterine sensitivity to endogenous oxytocin may plan an adjuvant role in the initiation of parturition (3,4). Oxytocin stimulates endometrial/decidual prostaglandin synthesis. In addition, prostaglandins make the myometrium more sensitive to oxytocin. Possibly oxytocin plays a role in labor initiation in conjunction with prostaglandins (3).

The decidua vera of pregnancy is macrophage-like and may play a role in the initiation and maintenance of labor. Its activation results in an outpouring of prostaglandins ($PGF_{2\alpha}$ and PGE_2), arachidonic acid, platelet-activating factor, and selected cytokines including interleukin-1. These factors, alone or in concert, can facilitate labor. Bacterial endotoxins or immunologic mechanisms may stimulate the decidua to synthesize and release these compounds. The decidua vera may link infection in pregnancy with the onset of labor. The prevention of decidual activation may ensure myometrial quiescence and the maintenance of pregnancy (1,2,5).

The fetal membranes, the amnion and chorion laeve, also may serve a pivotal role in the initiation of parturition. They are rich in arachidonic acid, the substrate for prostaglandin synthesis. The amnion and chorion laeve produce almost exclusively PGE_2, a potent uterotropin (serving to prepare the uterus for labor) that accumulates in the amniotic fluid. Early in labor, the amniotic fluid concentration of PGE_2, probably amnionic in origin, increases. As labor progresses, amniotic fluid $PGF_{2\alpha}$, preferentially synthesized by the decidua, and its metabolite, PGFM, increase (1,6).

Progesterone and estrogen play only minor roles in the initiation of parturition in humans. The reduction of maternal plasma progesterone concentration before labor commonly seen in sheep and other animal species does not play a role in the onset of labor in humans. Estrogen serves only a permissive function in parturition. Prolonged gestation or dysfunctional labor occasionally correlates with hypoestrogenism (fetal anencephaly, fetal adrenal hypoplasia, and placental sulfatase deficiency) (7).

Onset of Labor

Labor is characterized by regular, painful, progressive uterine contractions that cause dilation and effacement of the cervix, with descent of the presenting fetal part. The result is the delivery of the fetus and placenta through the birth canal.

The mechanism of labor comprises various movements of the fetus to enable its head to adapt to the bony maternal pelvic canal through which the fetus must pass during the birth process. Familiarity with the shape and size of the various types of pelves facilitates the understanding of normal and abnormal mechanisms of labor.

THE FEMALE PELVIS

Anatomy

The true pelvis is the only bony canal through which the fetus must pass during its birth. This passageway lies beneath the pelvic brim, or linea terminalis. The pelvis is divided into four imaginary planes to allow description of the location of the fetus (Figs. 2 and 3). These planes are:

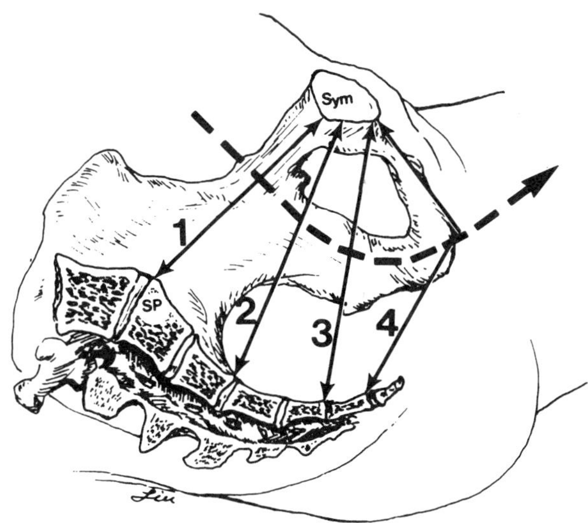

FIG. 2. Sagittal section of an adult female pelvis. 1, Plane of pelvic inlet; 2, plane of greatest dimensions; 3, plane of mid-pelvis (least pelvic dimensions); 4, plane of pelvic outlet.

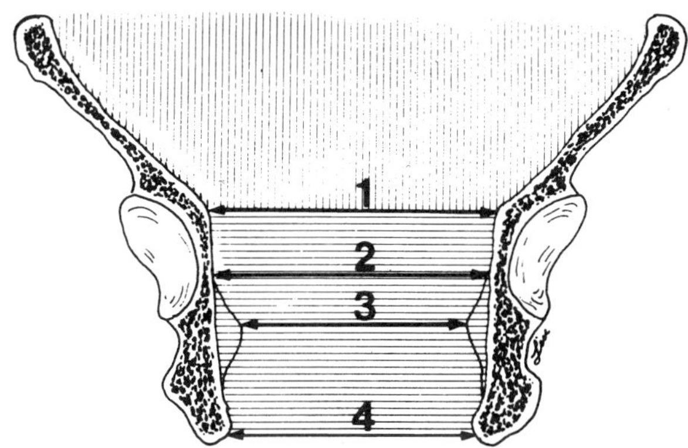

FIG. 3. Coronal section of an adult female pelvis. 1, Plane of pelvic inlet; 2, plane of greatest dimensions; 3, plane of mid-pelvis (least pelvic dimensions); 4, plane of pelvic outlet.

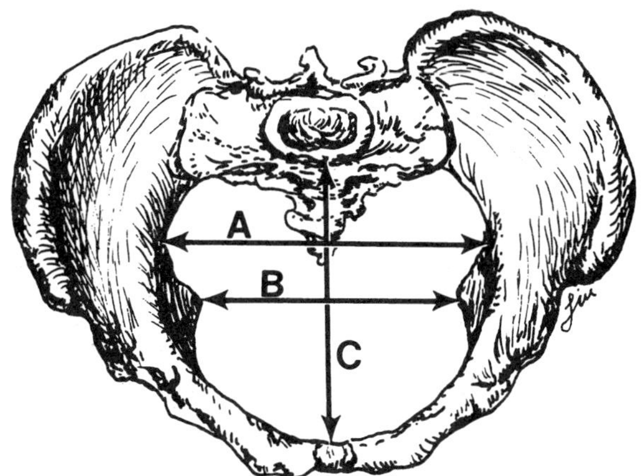

FIG. 4. Anteroposterior view of the female pelvis. *A,* Transverse diameter of pelvic inlet (13.5 cm). *B,* Interspinous diameter of the mid-pelvis (10 cm). *C,* Anteroposterior diameter of the inlet, or the obstetrical conjugate (10.5 cm).

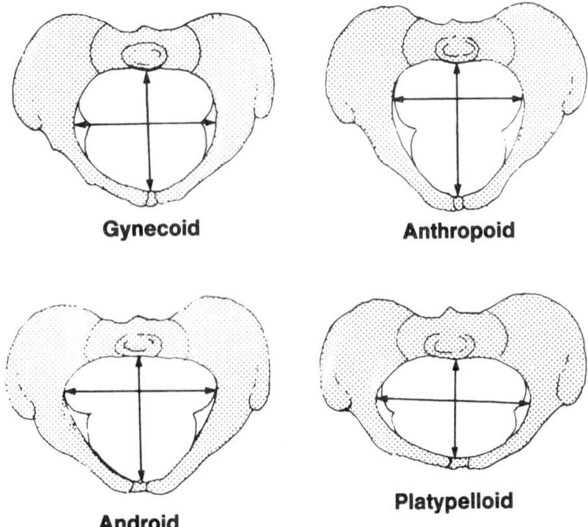

FIG. 5. The Caldwell and Moloy classification of the four pure types of pelvis.

- The plane of pelvic inlet,
- The plane of greatest dimensions,
- The plane of the mid-pelvis (least pelvic dimensions), and
- The plane of pelvic outlet.

The typical adult female pelvic inlet has an anteroposterior diameter of 10.5 cm (the obstetric conjugate) and a transverse diameter of 13.5 cm. The plane of least pelvic dimensions in the mid-pelvis has an anteroposterior diameter of 12 cm and a transverse or interspinous diameter (between the ischial spines) of greater than 10 cm (Fig. 4). This mid-pelvis plane is the most important because it has the least room; it is here where the arrest of labor progress often occurs. The plane of greatest dimensions lacks obstetric significance. If the areas of the pelvic inlet and mid-pelvis are adequate, the pelvic outlet will usually pose no problem to labor and delivery of the fetus (8,9).

Classification

According to Caldwell and Moloy (10), there are four pure types of pelves. They are named based on the shape of the inlet, with mention of the nonconforming outlet. The four basic types of pelves are gynecoid, android, anthropoid, and platypelloid (Fig. 5). Many pelves are mixed, with characteristics of more than one basic type. The gynecoid pelvis is the normal female pelvis with a round or transverse oval inlet. It is the most common type of pelvis, occurring in almost 50% of women. Approximately 20% of women have an android pelvis; a male-type pelvis with a heart- or wedge-shaped inlet. The extreme form of android pelvis is frequently associated with obstructed labor and difficult deliveries. The anthropoid pelvis has a long anteroposterior oval inlet. Twenty five percent of women, commonly non-white, have this type of pelvis. The platypelloid pelvis, seen in only 3% to 5% of women, is flat with a flat transverse oval inlet. Labor in women with the platypelloid-type pelvis often ends with cesarean birth (9,10).

CHARACTERISTICS OF THE FETUS

Fetal Presentations

Presentation, or lie, is the relation of the long axis of the fetus to the long axis of the mother. It is the pole of the fetus that occupies the lower portion of the uterus. The fetal lie may be either longitudinal or transverse. With a longitudinal lie, the presenting part is either the head (cephalic) or the breech. With a transverse lie, the shoulder presents. Oblique lie is in between the longitudinal and transverse presentations.

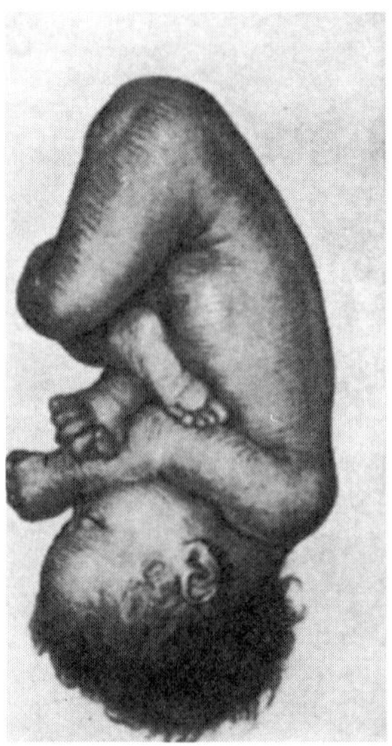
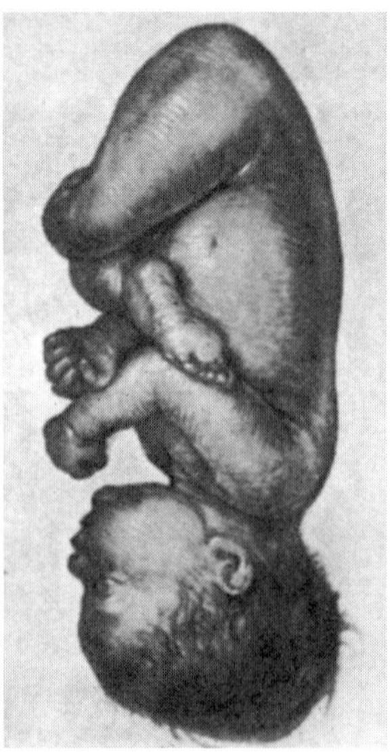
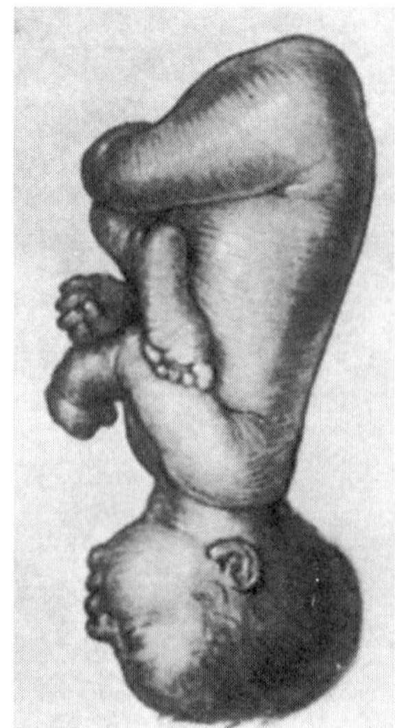
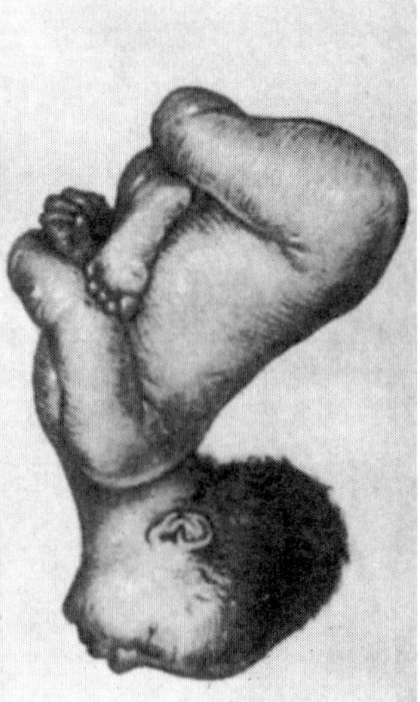

FIG. 6. Differences in attitude of fetus in vertex, sinciput, brow, and face presentations. (From ref. 1, with permission.)

Cephalic presentations are classified according to the relation of the head to the body of the fetus (fetal attitude or habitus). Depending on the degree of flexion or extension of the fetal head, the occiput (vertex), face, mentum (chin), sinciput (large fontanelle), or brow may present (Fig. 6). Sinciput and brow presentations are considered intermediate conditions. They usually convert spontaneously to vertex or face presentations during labor.

Breech presentations are classified according to the flexion or extension of the thighs and knees (Fig. 7). If both thighs and knees are flexed, it is a complete breech. If the thighs are flexed with both knees extended, it is a frank breech. A single-footling breech has one leg extended at the thigh and knee, with the foot as the presenting part. The other leg is flexed at the thigh with either flexion or extension of the knee. A double-footling

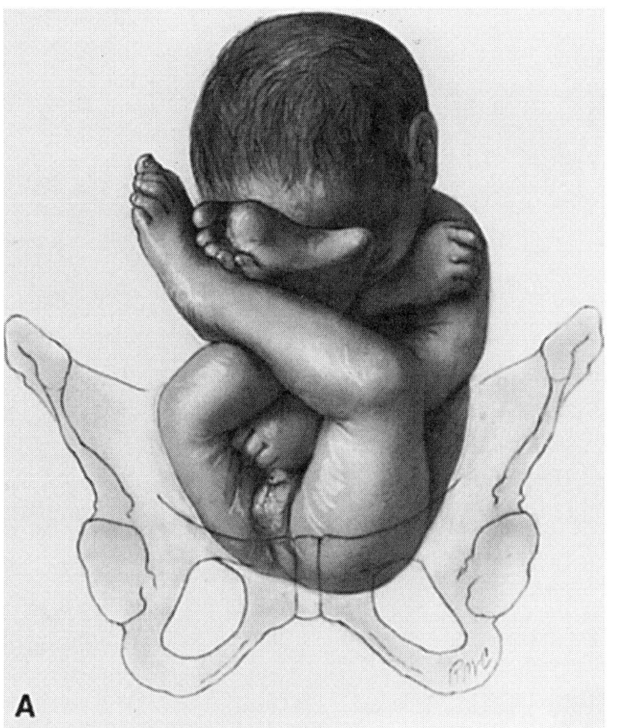

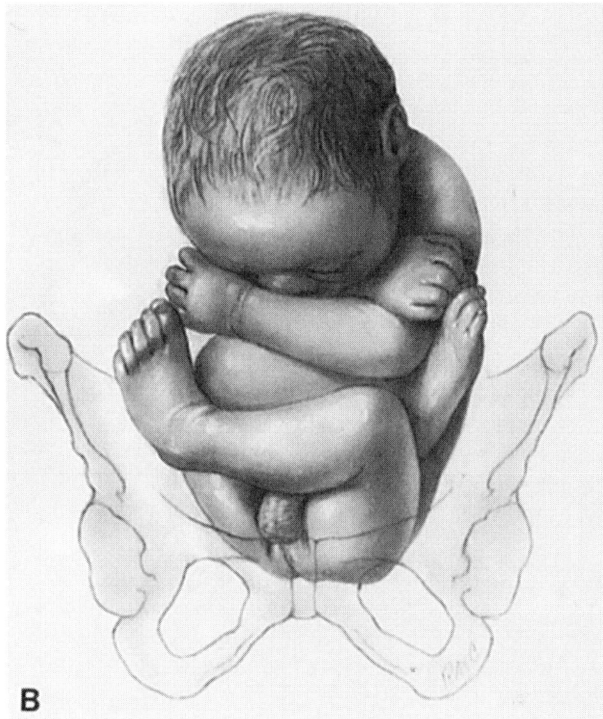

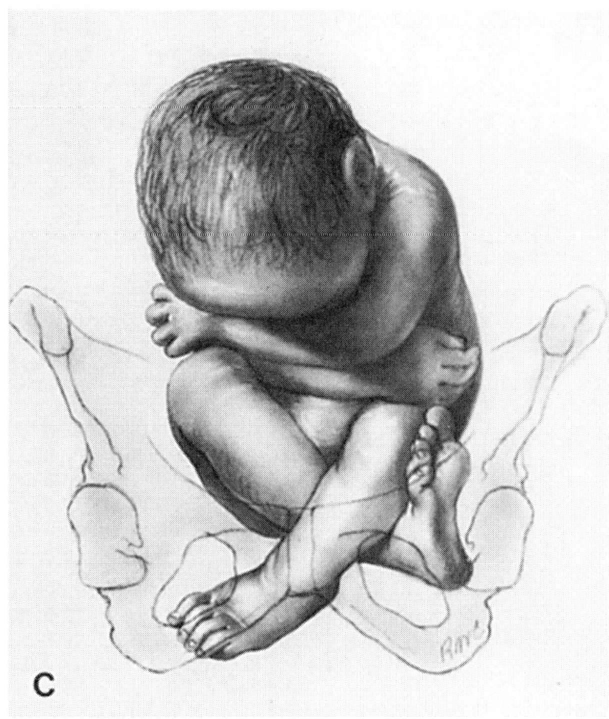

FIG. 7. A: Frank breech presentation. **B:** Complete breech presentation. **C:** Incomplete, or footling, breech presentation. (From ref. 1, with permission.)

breech has both legs extended at the thigh and knee, and both feet presenting.

Fetal Head

The fetal head is important from the obstetric viewpoint because it is the largest and the least compressible part of the fetus. In the cephalic presentation, the head must change its shape (molding) to adapt to the maternal pelvis. The force of uterine contractions, the resistance of the bony pelvis, and the loose connections between the bones of the fetal skull combine to mold the fetal head to the shape of the pelvis.

The anterior fontanelle (bregma) is the diamond-shaped junction of the parietal and frontal bones. The posterior fontanelle is the triangular junction of the two parietal bones and the occipital bone (Figs. 8 and 9). These landmarks and suture lines can be felt during a pelvic examination to confirm fetal position during labor. The average dimensions of the fetal head diameters are listed in Table 1. Figure 10 shows some examples of fetal positions in the vertex presentation.

In prolonged labor, a caput succedaneum (edematous scalp swelling) may form in the portion of the fetal scalp immediately over the cervical os before complete cervical dilatation. Caput succedaneum can prevent the examiner from differentiating sutures and fontanelles.

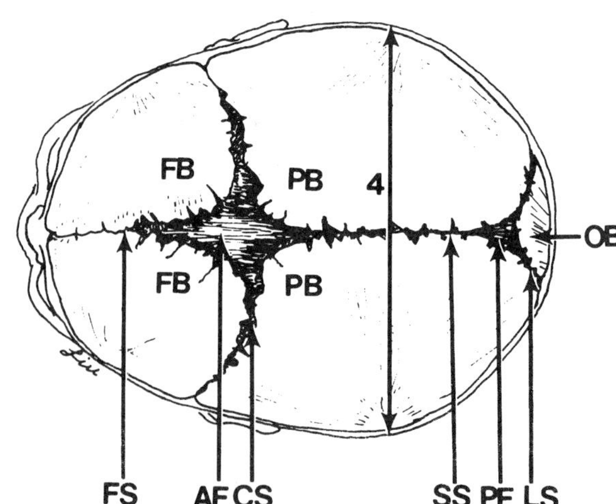

FIG. 9. Common landmarks, suture lines, and diameter of the fetal head. *FS*, frontal suture; *FB*, frontal bone; *AF*, anterior fontanelle; *CS*, coronal suture; *PB*, parietal bone; *Line 4*, biparietal diameter; *SS*, sagittal suture; *PF*, posterior fontanelle; *LS*, lambdoid suture; *OB*, occipital bone.

Diagnosis of Fetal Presentation and Position

The diagnosis of fetal presentation and position is made by abdominal palpation, pelvic examination, and auscultation of the location of the fetal heart. Ultrasonography helps to confirm fetal position in cases in which the physical examination may be difficult (i.e., oligohydramnios or polyhydramnios, abnormal fetal lie, preterm pregnancies). In addition, sonography is valuable in placental localization, especially in cases with abnormal vaginal bleeding.

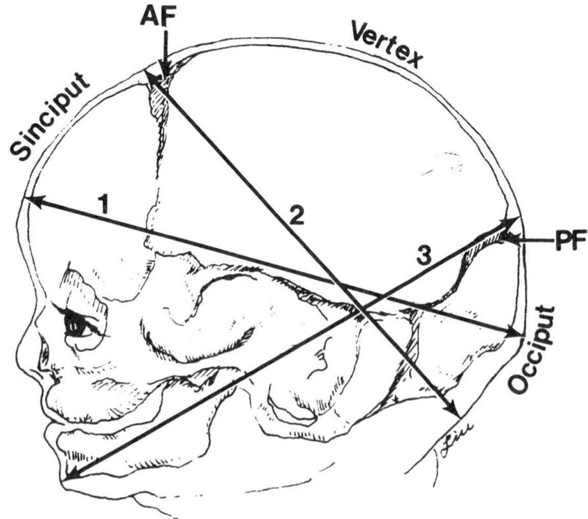

FIG. 8. Common diameters of the fetal head. *AF*, anterior fontanelle; *PF*, posterior fontanelle; *Line 1*, occipitofrontal diameter; *Line 2*, suboccipitobregmatic diameter; *Line 3*, occipitomental diameter.

Fetal Station and Engagement

Station is the distance from the fetal presenting part to an imaginary line drawn between the maternal ischial spines. The leading bony portion of the fetal head (not the caput succedaneum) is used to estimate station in a cephalic presentation. In the breech presentation, the buttocks at the bitrochanteric diameter are used. By convention, station zero is when the presenting part is at the level of the ischial spines. Two systems exist for the

TABLE 1. *Common fetal head diameters*

Diameter	Average dimension (cm)	Comment
Occipitofrontal	11.0–11.5	Presents in military attitude
Bipareital	9.5	The greatest transverse diameter
Bitemporal	8.0	The shortest transverse diameter
Occipitomental	12.5–13.5	The longest anteroposterior diameter; brow presentation
Suboccipitobregmatic	9.5	The anteroposterior diameter that present in well-flexed head

Adapted from Cunningham FG, MacDonald PC, Grant NF. The morphological and functional development of the fetus. In: Cunningham FG, MacDonald PC, Gant NF, eds. *Williams obstetrics.* 18th ed. Connecticut: Appleton & Lange, 1987:87, with permission.

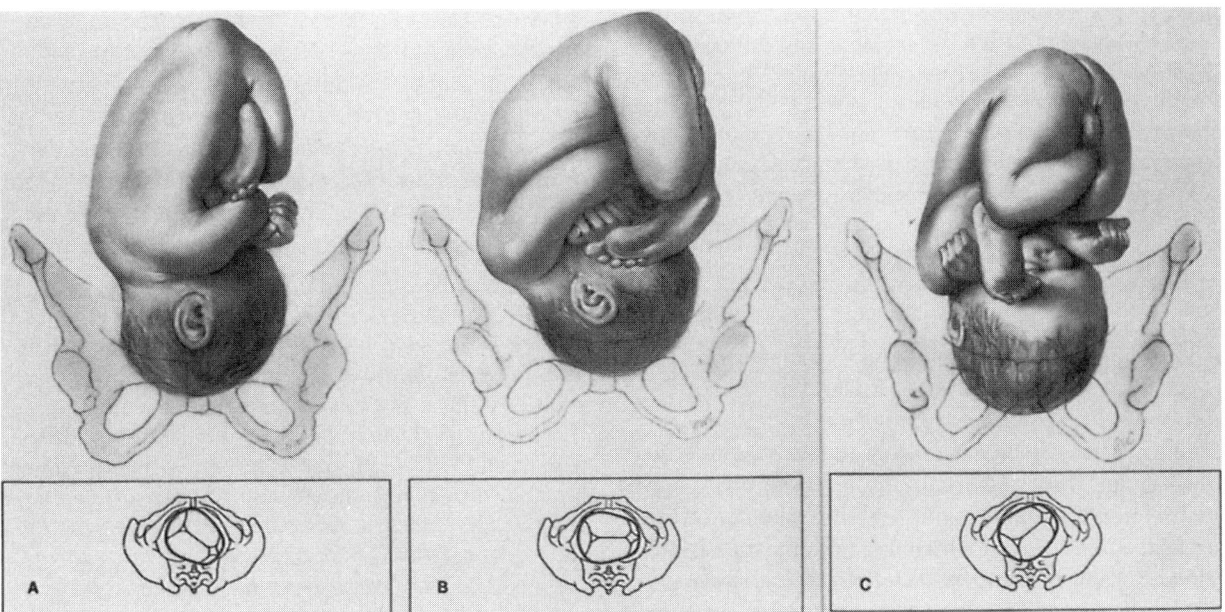

FIG. 10. Vertex presentation. **A:** Right occipitoanterior position. **B:** Right occipital transverse position. **C:** Right occipitoposterior position. (From ref. 1, with permission.)

designation of fetal stations, the three-level and the five-level classifications. In the three-level system, the long axis of the birth canal is divided into thirds from the pelvic inlet to the ischial spines and again divided into thirds from the ischial spines to the pelvic outlet. When the presenting part is above the ischial spines, the station is designated with a minus sign (stations −1, −2, −3). When the presenting part is below the ischial spines, a plus sign is given (stations +1, +2, +3). In the five-level system, the station of the fetal head is estimated in centimeters away from the ischial spines. The fetus traverses the pelvis from about −5 station at the true pelvic inlet to +5 station at the outlet (bulging perineum). In Fig. 3, line 1 represents −5 station, line 3 represents 0 station, and line 4 represents +5 station as the presenting part descends through the pelvis (11,12).

In the vertex presentation, engagement occurs when the fetal biparietal diameter passes the plane of the pelvic inlet, and the leading bony portion of the head is at or below the ischial spines (Fig. 11). Most heads engage in the occiput transverse position and deliver in the occiput anterior position. Engagement in the transverse position is common in gynecoid, android, and platypelloid pelves, whereas oblique engagement is more frequent in the anthropoid-type pelvis.

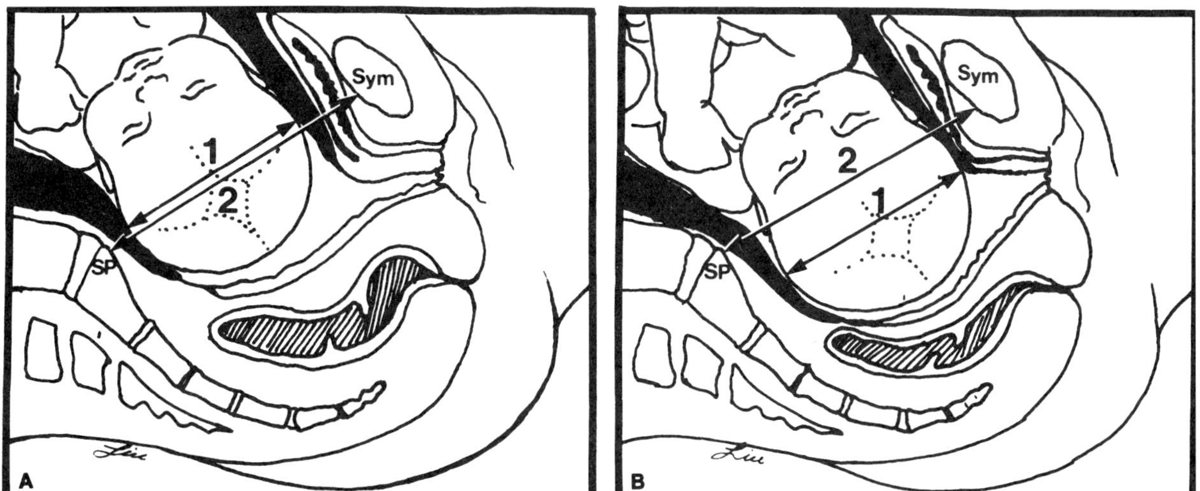

FIG. 11. A: Unengaged fetal head in the maternal pelvis. **B:** Engaged fetal head in the maternal pelvis. (Line 1, biparietal diameter; line 2, pelvic inlet.)

STAGES OF LABOR

There are four stages of labor. The first stage of labor begins with the onset of true labor and ends with the complete dilation of the cervix (10 cm). The average duration of the first stage of labor is 8 hours in the primigravida (or nullipara) and 5 hours in the multipara (range, 6 to 18 hours and 2 to 10 hours, respectively). The second stage of labor extends from full dilation of the cervix to the birth of the fetus. The average duration of the second stage is 50 minutes in the nullipara and 20 minutes in the multipara (range, 30 minutes to 3 hours and 5 to 30 minutes, respectively). The third stage of labor begins with the birth of the fetus and ends with the complete expulsion or extraction of the placenta. The third stage is usually complete within 30 minutes of the delivery of the fetus for both primipara and multipara. The fourth stage begins with the delivery of the placenta and ends at approximately 1 hour postpartum when the parturient is stabilized (11,12).

The major difficulty in diagnosing labor is differentiating it from false labor. Unlike true labor, false labor is not accompanied by progressive cervical change or descent of the presenting fetal part.

First Stage of Labor

The first stage of labor must overcome cervical resistance. It is divided into latent and active phases. Early cervical effacement and softening may occur before true labor, yet during the first stage of labor, the entire cervical length retracts into the lower uterine segment as the cervix progressively dilates.

The latent phase of labor is the time between the onset of regular uterine contractions and the beginning of the active phase (appreciable cervical effacement and more rapid cervical dilation). The duration of the latent phase varies. It can be differentiated from the active phase of labor with certainty only in retrospect. The average latent phase in nulliparas lasts 6.4 hours with a standard deviation of 5.1 hours. By 20 hours, 95% of patients will complete the latent phase of labor. The latent phase is prolonged when it exceeds 20 hours in the nullipara and 14 hours in the multipara. The latent phase usually ends at 3- to 4-cm cervical dilation (12,13). During the latent phase, contractions produce mild to moderate discomfort and may be irregular and infrequent. Eventually a regular pattern of painful contractions begins.

The active phase of labor usually begins when the cervix reaches 3- to 4-cm dilation. The active phase of labor is subdivided into an acceleration phase, the phase of maximal slope, and the deceleration phase. The existence of a deceleration phase is not universally accepted. Its occurrence may be an artifact in clinical observation (i.e., not an actual slowing in cervical dilation, but the cervix being retracted cephalad around the fetal presenting part). When cervical dilation is plotted against time, the curve typically takes on a sigmoid shape (Fig. 12). The fetal presenting part begins to descend in earnest during the phase of maximal slope. Descent then continues at its maximal rate through the second stage of labor. Most nulliparae have a maximal slope of cervical dilation in the active phase of more than 1.2 cm/h and a maximal slope of descent of 1.0 cm/h. In multiparae, the maximal rates of cervical dilation and descent are 1.5 cm/h and 2.0 cm/h in the phase of maximal slope and the deceleration phase, respectively (12,13).

Friedman (12) separated labor into three functional divisions. The first is the preparatory division. Here, there are

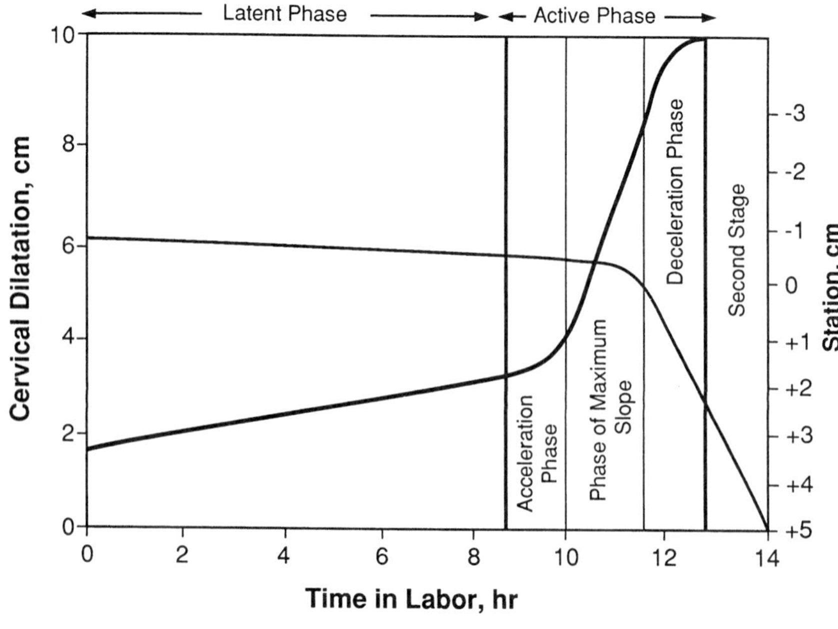

FIG. 12. Composite of cervical dilatation and fetal descent curves illustrating their interrelation and their component phases. (From ref. 12, with permission.)

changes in the ground substance and connective tissues in the cervix and possibly the uterus. The preparatory division includes the latent and the acceleration phases and is presumed to be sensitive to sedation and analgesia. The second division is the dilatational division. It occurs during the phase of maximal slope in the active phase of labor. This division is predominantly involved with rapid cervical dilation and is usually not affected by sedation or analgesia. The third division is the pelvic division. It begins with the deceleration phase and continues through the second stage of labor simultaneous with the phase of maximal slope of descent. It is during the pelvic division of labor that the cardinal movements of the delivery of the fetus take place (please refer to "Delivery of the Fetus") (1).

MANAGEMENT OF NORMAL LABOR

First and Second Stages of Labor

Patient Evaluation, Preparation, and the Administration of Fluids

Maternal vital signs such as temperature, blood pressure, pulse, and respiratory rate are evaluated and recorded. Vital signs should be checked as clinically indicated, but at least every 1 to 2 hours during the first and more frequently during the second stage of labor. Blood for hemoglobin and hematocrit, a blood group, rhesus type, and antibody screen is drawn on admission. This blood may be later cross-matched if needed for transfusion in case of obstetric hemorrhage and emergencies. Additionally, a voided urine specimen should be examined for protein and glucose.

Obstetrics experts no longer advocate the routine use of enema and perineal preparation (pubic and vulvar shaving). An enema may help minimize fecal contamination during labor and delivery in patients who are constipated or have large amounts of palpable stool. Enema should not be used to stimulate labor.

Because gastric emptying slows during labor, the patient should take nothing by mouth with the onset of labor. This precaution will, we hope, lessen the risk of aspiration pneumonitis, especially if general anesthesia is required for an unforeseen emergency delivery.

An intravenous catheter with infusion of crystalloid solution should be established in active labor to prevent dehydration. Any patient needing analgesia for relief of labor pain especially requires intravenous access. A large-bore (16- or 18-gauge) intravenous catheter should be used; these women may require transfusion for obstetric hemorrhage or need other medical treatments. Oxytocin, to facilitate uterine contraction before or after delivery, also may be given intravenously.

A careful record of fluid intake and urine output is necessary for the laboring patient. Oxytocin has considerable antidiuretic activity. Conduction analgesia can obliterate the urge to void. The bladder should be catheterized and emptied if the patient has difficulty voiding and the bladder is distended.

Diagnosis of Ruptured Membranes and Amniotomy

Spontaneous rupture of the amniotic membranes may occur at any time before (premature rupture of membranes) or during labor. The obstetrician may choose to rupture membranes artificially (amniotomy) during labor. Amniotomy may shorten the duration of labor slightly but increases the risk of chorioamnionitis if labor is prolonged. If the presenting part is not engaged, the umbilical cord may prolapse or become compressed between the presenting part and the pelvis after amniotomy. Immediately after rupture of the membranes, a vaginal examination should be done to evaluate cervical dilation and to detect prolapse of the umbilical cord. Amniotomy is not routinely needed unless internal monitoring is indicated. At the time of ruptured membranes, the volume of amniotic fluid and the presence or absence of meconium are noted (11).

Vaginal Examinations and Evaluation of Labor Progress

The obstetrician should determine fetal presentation and position on admission to the labor suite by abdominal and vaginal examination. If the patient has vaginal bleeding, the possibility of placenta previa or abruption must be eliminated before vaginal examination. At this time, station, cervical dilatation, and effacement also should be evaluated and recorded.

The vaginal examinations should be kept to a minimum and done under aseptic conditions to minimize bacterial contamination and decrease the risk of intrauterine infection. This precaution is especially important during the latent phase or after the membranes rupture. Once in the active phase of labor, cervical examination approximately every 2 hours helps monitor the progress of labor. If the patient reports severe rectal pressure and the urge to push, vaginal examination will decide whether full cervical dilatation and fetal descent has occurred (i.e., imminent delivery of the fetus). If a significant fetal heart-rate deceleration occurs, prompt vaginal examination is needed to rule out a prolapsed umbilical cord.

At the beginning of the second stage, the parturient usually has a desire to bear down with each contraction. It is important to instruct the patient not to bear down before complete cervical dilation.

Uterine Activity

Uterine contractility defines the power or adequacy of labor. The frequency and duration of uterine contractions may be palpated by an examiner or quantified by an external tocodynamometer. However, a pressure catheter in the amniotic cavity (intrauterine pressure catheter) is the only accurate way to measure the intensity or strength of uterine contractions. The use of an intrauterine pressure catheter is recommended during oxytocin augmentation of labor or in patients undergoing a trial of labor after a previous cesarean delivery.

An effective uterine contraction reaches an intensity of 40 to 60 mm Hg. Uterine contractions of an intensity less than 25 mm Hg are ineffective and rarely produce cervical dilatation. In adequate labor, an average of three uterine contractions occurs every 10 minutes. Uterine work is measured in Montevideo units. This number represents the sum of the peak amplitude of all contractions within a 10-minute period. Adequate labors may have between 95 and 395 Montevideo units. Failure to progress or arrest of labor in the active phase is diagnosed when there are at least 200 Montevideo units per 10 minutes for at least 2 hours without cervical change (13).

Maternal Position

During the first stage of labor, the parturient may ambulate, sit, or recline if intermittent monitoring confirms fetal well-being. In patients lying in bed, the lateral recumbent position, instead of the supine position, avoids aortocaval compression and helps assure adequate uteroplacental perfusion. To avoid prolapse of the umbilical cord, patients with ruptured membranes and an unengaged presenting fetal part should not ambulate. During the second stage, the mother may assume any comfortable position that allows effective bearing down.

Intrapartum Fetal Heart-Rate Monitoring

During labor, the fetal heart rate may be counted intermittently with a fetal stethoscope or a Doppler ultrasonic device. Alternatively, continuous electronic monitoring of the fetal heart rate and uterine contractions may be used. Retrospective studies suggested that continuous electronic fetal monitoring detected fetal asphyxia in labor (14) and decreased the frequency of intrapartum stillbirth (15). However, seven randomized controlled studies of low- and high-risk pregnancies did not confirm this finding. Perinatal mortality does not differ between those women monitored with auscultation and those monitored with electronic fetal monitoring (16–20). One recent study found a significant reduction in perinatal deaths due to asphyxia with intrapartum electronic fetal heart-rate monitoring (21). Most studies, however, found only a significant increase in operative vaginal and abdominal deliveries in women receiving intrapartum continuous electronic fetal monitoring.

For low-risk patients, the American College of Obstetricians and Gynecologists and the American Academy of Pediatrics have recommended intermittent auscultation of the fetal heart every 30 minutes during the active phase of the first stage of labor, and at least every 15 minutes during the second stage. For higher risk patients, they recommend listening every 15 minutes during active labor and every 5 minutes in the second stage of labor. Intermittent auscultation of the fetal heart requires a 1:1 nurse/patient ratio. It is done during a uterine contraction and for 30 seconds afterward. When using continuous electronic monitoring, the tracings should be evaluated at the same time intervals as recommended for intermittent auscultation (22).

Delivery of the Fetus

During labor in an occiput presentation, the baby undergoes a series of movements to adapt to the irregular shape of the maternal pelvic canal. These movements, the so-called cardinal movements of labor, are:

- Engagement,
- Descent,
- Flexion,
- Internal rotation,
- Extension,
- External rotation, and
- Expulsion.

In a typical occipitoanterior labor, the head delivers by extension over the perineum, followed by external rotation (or restitution) back to the transverse or anterior position. The anterior shoulder then delivers under the symphysis pubis, followed by the posterior shoulder over the perineal body. The rest of body follows quickly after the delivery of the posterior shoulder. Figure 13 illustrates the cardinal movements of labor and delivery in the left occiput anterior position.

The mechanism of labor in most occipitoposterior presentations is similar to that of the occipitoanterior presentation, except that the head has to rotate 135 degrees to the anterior before extension. Deviation from the normal mechanism of labor may occur if:

- The head does not completely rotate, resulting in transverse arrest, or
- If ineffective contractions, large fetus, or inadequate flexion of the head lead to persistent occiput posterior position.

Forceps Delivery

Obstetric forceps are used for traction and rotation of the fetal head to hasten delivery of the fetus electively, or for fetal or maternal indications (Table 2). Forceps applications are classified as outlet, low, or mid, depending on the station (by using the five-level or centimeter system) and position of the fetal head (Table 3). Mid-forceps deliveries are reserved for sudden severe fetal or maternal compromise. Simultaneous preparation for cesarean delivery must

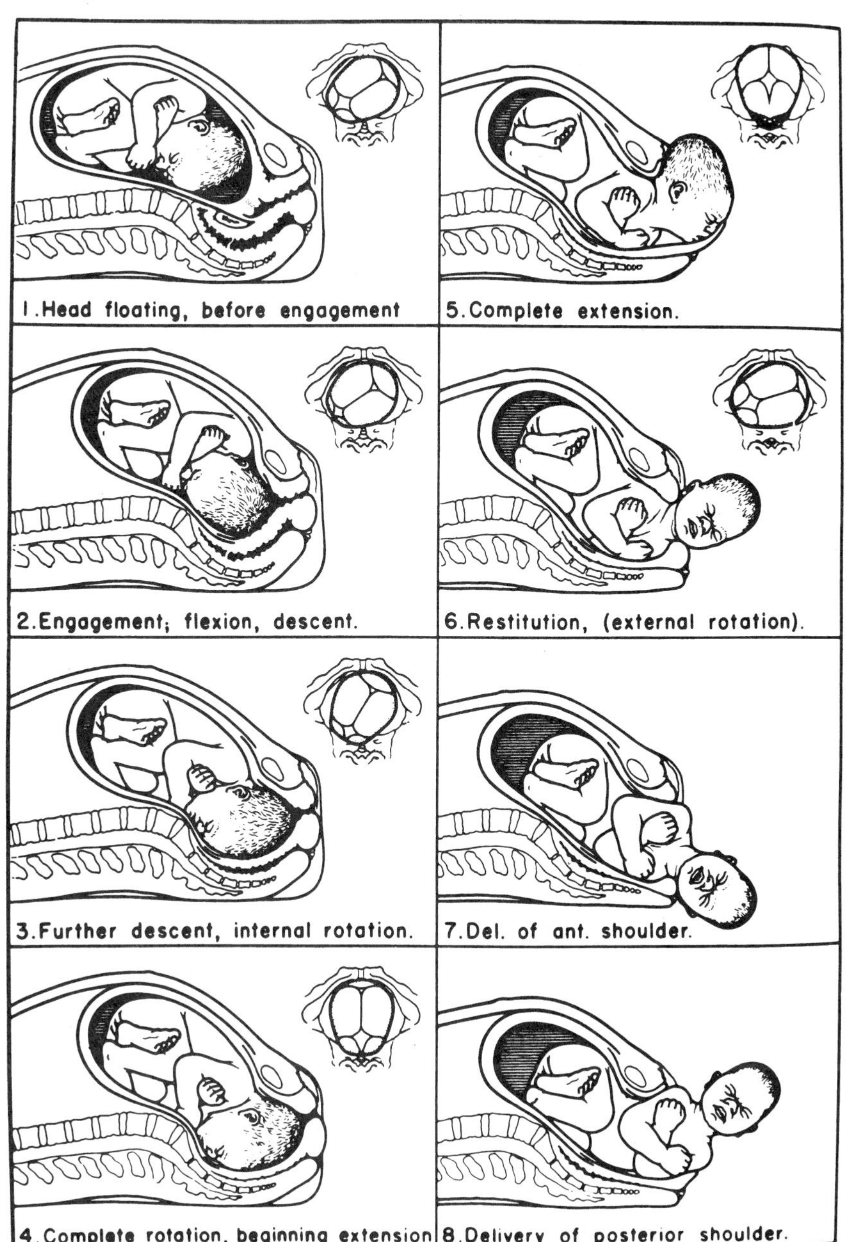

FIG. 13. Cardinal movements in the mechanism of labor and delivery, left occiput anterior position. (From ref. 1, with permission.)

begin if forceps delivery fails. High forceps (unengaged fetal head) and difficult mid-forceps deliveries have no place in modern obstetrics because of the associated maternal and fetal morbidity and mortality.

Episiotomy

Episiotomy can be done as the head is crowning or distending the vulva and perineum to prevent perineal lacerations during delivery of the fetus. Episiotomy is routinely cut during forceps or vacuum delivery. It may be a midline incision, from the fourchette to middle of the perineum before the rectum, or it may be a mediolateral incision from the fourchette into the perineum approximately 45 degrees laterally and away from the rectum. Median episiotomy offers less blood loss, ease of repair, and less pain. The disadvantage of the median episiotomy is the risk of extension through the anal sphincter and into the rectum. The mediolateral episiotomy rarely extends through the anal sphincter and into the rectum. Disadvantages of the mediolateral episiotomy include greater blood loss, more difficult repair, more painful, and occasionally, dyspareunia.

Theoretically, episiotomy prevents pelvic relaxation and the possible long-term consequences of childbirth, such as cystocele, urinary incontinence, rectocele, and the prolapse of the uterus. However, some argue against the use of routine prophylactic episiotomy because, by

TABLE 2. *Indications for obstetric forceps delivery shortening the second stage by outlet forceps*

	Definition
Prolonged second stage	
Nulliparous	3 h with regional anesthesia 2 h without regional anesthesia
Multiparous	2 h with regional anesthesia 1 h without regional anesthesia
Fetal indications	
Nonreassuring fetal heart-rate pattern	
Failure to deliver spontaneously after an appropriately managed second stage	
Fetal malposition (deflexion and asynclitism)	
Maternal indications	
Need to avoid voluntary expulsive effort	
Exhaustion	
Lack of cooperation	
Excessive analgesia	

Adapted from American College of Obstetricians and Gynecologists. *Operative vaginal delivery.* ACOG technical bulletin 196. Washington, DC: ACOG, August 1994, with permission.

the time the episiotomy is done, damage to the pelvic musculature has already occurred (23). Nonetheless, episiotomy is indicated if the perineum is not adequately stretched and lacerations are anticipated, or when additional vaginal space is needed for operative delivery or for breech extractions.

A straight incision from an episiotomy is usually easier to repair than ragged lacerations. By definition, a first-degree perineal laceration involves only the vaginal mucosa or perineal skin. A second-degree laceration involves the submucosal tissue with or without damage to the perineal body. A third-degree laceration involves an extension into the body of the anal sphincter, and a fourth-degree laceration involves damage through the rectal mucosa.

TABLE 3. *Definitions of obstetric forceps according to station and rotation*

Outlet forceps
Fetal scalp visible at the introitus without separating the labia
Fetal skull reached the pelvic floor
Fetal head is at or on the perineum
Sagittal suture in the following positions
Anterior-posterior diameter
Right or left occiput anterior
Right or left occiput posterior
Rotation cannot exceed 45 degrees
Low forceps
Leading point of the fetal skull is at station +2 or more and not on the pelvic floor
Rotation ≤45°
Rotation ≥45°
Midforceps
Fetal head is engaged
Station above +2
High forceps
Not included in classification

Adapted from American College of Obstetricians and Gynecologists. *Operative vaginal operative delivery.* ACOG committee opinion 196. Washington, DC: ACOG, August 1994, with permission.

Complications of inadequate repair of an episiotomy or perineal lacerations include infection, urinary retention, hematomas, and occasionally, hemorrhagic shock. A digital rectal examination, done after repair of the episiotomy or lacerations, ensures intact anal sphincter and rectum and should detect any sutures penetrating the rectal mucosa.

Analgesia

The method of pain control may affect the progress of labor. The preparatory division of labor (latent and acceleration phases) is purported to be sensitive to sedation and analgesia. The dilatational division of labor (phase of maximal slope) is not. The duration of the second stage also may vary with the type of analgesia.

The Third and Fourth Stages of Labor

Separation of the placenta generally occurs within 10 minutes of the end of the second stage. Signs of placental separation include:

- A sudden gush of blood from the vagina,
- Lengthening of the umbilical cord, and
- The uterus becoming firm and globular with the fundal portion rising up in the abdomen.

No traction should be applied to the umbilical cord until the placenta has separated. Forceful traction may invert the uterus, producing life-threatening hemorrhage and shock (11).

After its delivery, the placenta should be immediately inspected to assure its complete removal. If there is a torn vessel on the chorionic membrane or if there is a missing cotyledon, the uterus must be immediately explored for the removal of retained placental fragments. Retained placenta may incite immediate or delayed postpartum hemorrhage. The perineum, cervix, vagina, sphincter ani, and rectum should be examined for injuries and surgical repair done if needed.

The uterus contracts dramatically after the delivery of the fetus and the placenta. Myometrial contractions that occlude the open, bleeding sinuses provide the primary mechanism of cessation of uterine bleeding from the placental implantation site. Bimanual uterine massage can facilitate this process. Alternatively, when the placenta completely delivers, 10 to 20 units of oxytocin can be added to the intravenous infusion (at a rate of approximately 200 mU/min). Ergot derivatives such as methergine or ergotrate (0.2 mg, i.m.) may be given instead of oxytocin immediately postpartum. Avoid ergot derivatives in hypertensive parturients. These compounds can increase blood pressure themselves. The intramuscular route yields fewer hypertensive side effects.

Postpartum hemorrhage is defined as blood loss in excess of 500 mL during the first 24 hours after delivery. In the presence of excessive bleeding or if the placenta has not delivered after 30 minutes in the third stage, manual removal of the placenta under appropriate anesthesia will shorten the third stage and can limit blood loss.

The hour immediately after delivery is the fourth stage of labor. It is during this time that postpartum hemorrhage most commonly occurs. Vital signs and uterine blood loss should be monitored closely. Complaints of severe pelvic pain suggest significant pelvic or perineal trauma. The principal causes of postpartum hemorrhage are uterine atony, trauma to the genital tract, and retained placenta (Table 4).

TABLE 4. *Predisposing factors and causes of obstetrical hemorrhage*

Trauma to the genital tract
Large episiotomy, including extensions
Perineal, cervical, or vaginal lacerations
Uterine rupture
Bleeding from placental implantation site
Hypotonic myometrium/uterine atony
Halogenated hydrocarbon anesthetics
Conduction analgesia
Poorly perfused uterus
Hemorrhage
Hypotension
Overdistended uterus
Large fetus
Multiple gestation
Hydramnios
Exhausted uterus
Prolonged labor
Rapid or precipitate labor
Oxytocin induction or augmentation of labor
High parity
Previous history of uterine atony
Chorioamnionitis
Retained placental tissue
Avulsed cotyledon
Succenturiate or accessory lobe
Abnormally adherent placenta
Placenta accreta, increta, or percreta
Coagulation defects

Adapted from Cunningham FG, MacDonald PC, Grant NF. Obstetrical hemorrhage. In: Cunningham FG, MacDonald PC, Gant NF, eds. *Williams obstetrics.* 18th ed. Connecticut: Appleton & Lange, 1989:695, with permission.

The treatment of uterine atony includes bimanual uterine massage and the administration of oxytocin or ergot derivatives. Intramuscular injection of the 15-methyl derivative of PGF_{2a} at 15- to 30-minute intervals may help if the uterus does not respond to other physical and pharmacotherapy. If retained placental fragments are suspected, manual removal, manual exploration, and possibly curettage of the uterus may be necessary. The genital tract should be carefully inspected and any lacerations repaired. A blood sample can be drawn immediately for the observation of clot formation within 5 minutes to rule out clinical hypofibrinogenemia. In addition, blood tests (hemoglobin/hematocrit, platelet count, fibrinogen, fibrin-split products, prothrombin time, and partial thromboplastin time) may diagnose consumptive coagulopathy. Placenta accreta, increta, or percreta should be considered a differential diagnosis in cases of postpartum hemorrhage unresponsive to conventional therapy. In cases in which conventional therapy fails, a laparotomy is indicated for possible bilateral hypogastric artery ligation or hysterectomy as a life-saving procedure. The uterus generally should not be packed during the treatment of postpartum hemorrhage because it might mask excessive accumulation of blood behind the packing.

MANAGEMENT OF ABNORMAL LABOR

Dystocia

Three main factors influence the course of labor:

- The powers (uterine contractions),
- The passage (bony pelvis and maternal soft tissues), and
- The passenger (size and position of the fetus) (13).

The gradual descent or change in station of the presenting part in the pelvis determines the progress of labor. Determining the correct fetal station is important for the evaluation of labor progress. Molding, asynclitism (lateral flexion), deflexion, and caput succedaneum can lead to erroneous diagnosis of station because the head may feel lower than it is.

Dystocia, difficult labor or childbirth, may be caused by:

- Abnormal or inadequate uterine contractions (uterine dysfunction),
- Abnormalities of the maternal pelvic architecture or size, or
- Abnormalities in fetal size, presentation, or development.

Any of these factors may occur alone or in combination with others. For example, uterine dysfunction often accompanies a contracted pelvis.

Table 5 lists the definitions, diagnostic criteria, and treatment of the major labor disorders (24). Figure 14

TABLE 5. *Major disorders of labor*

Phase of labor	Nullipara	Multipara	Treatment
Latent phase			
Prolonged latent phase	>20 h	>14 h	Rest or oxytocin
Active phase protraction disorders			
Protracted dilatation	<1.2 cm/h	<1.5 cm/h	Oxytocin for inadequate contractions
Protracted descent	<1.0 cm/h	<2.0 cm/h	
Active phase arrest disorders			
Secondary arrest of dilatation	>2 h	>2 h	Oxytocin or forceps/vacuum delivery or cesarean section
Arrest of descent	>1 h	>1 h	
Prolonged deceleration phase	>3 h	>1 h	
Second stage			
Failure to descend	No descent after complete dilatation	No descent after complete dilatation	Oxytocin or cesarean section

Modified from Friedman EA. Dysfunctional labor. In: Cohen WR, Friedman EA, eds. *Management of labor.* 1st ed. Maryland: Aspen Publishers, 1983:11, with permission.

illustrates some examples of the major labor aberrations (25). Active-phase arrest cannot be diagnosed until the latent phase has been completed (cervical dilation of at least 3 to 4 cm) and adequate uterine contractions have been documented (at least 200 Montevideo units every 10 minutes for 2 hours) (13). If using oxytocin to augment labor, the obstetrician should have a timetable in mind for the evaluation of labor progress. If cephalopelvic disproportion (i.e., the fetus is large relative to the maternal bony pelvis) is suspected by the abnormal progress of labor, the initiation or continuation of oxytocin stimulation is contraindicated, and a cesarean section is indicated.

Shoulder Dystocia

Shoulder dystocia occurs if, after delivery of the fetal head, the delivery of the shoulders (and therefore the rest of the fetal body) arrests. Serious fetal consequences of shoulder dystocia are fractured humerus or clavicle, Erb's palsy caused by brachial nerve damage, severe fetal asphyxia, possible neurological damage, and death. Maternal consequences of shoulder dystocia are postpartum hemorrhage because of uterine atony or genital tract trauma and infection.

If shoulder dystocia is suspected antepartum or intrapartum, a cesarean section is a reasonable and indicated alternative. However, the prediction of fetal shoulder dystocia by history and sonographic estimation of fetal biometry and weight is imprecise, and unexpected cases will always occur. The term "large for gestational age" applies to infants whose birth weight is above the 90th percentile. The term "macrosomia" applies to fetuses with estimated fetal weights of more than 4,500 g. Fetal macrosomia with the fetal abdominal circumference larger the fetal head circumference is a major predisposing factor for shoulder dystocia. The fetal abdomen also may be enlarged because of fetal ascites, enlarged liver or kidneys, or marked bladder distention. Maternal obesity, previous macrosomic infant, diabetes mellitus, and postterm pregnancy also correlate with fetal macrosomia. However, the prognostic usefulness of labor abnormalities to identify patients at high risk for shoulder dystocia and birth injury is debatable. Dysfunctional labor, such as

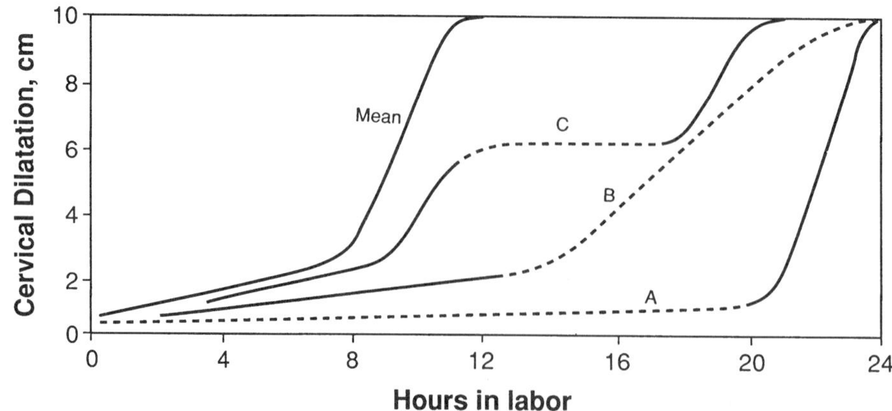

FIG. 14. The major labor aberrations shown in comparison with the mean cervical dilatation–time curve for nulliparas. *A,* Prolonged latent phase. *B,* Protracted active-phase dilatation (primary dysfunctional labor). *C,* Secondary arrest of dilatation. (From ref. 25, with permission.)

arrest and protraction disorders, prolonged second stage, and instrumental delivery have been reported to increase the risk of shoulder dystocia, especially when the fetus is strongly suspected to be macrosomic (26,27).

The management of shoulder dystocia requires the presence of a physician experienced in maneuvers to deliver the fetal shoulders, adequate anesthesia, and a neonatal team for the resuscitation of the newborn (28). If vaginal delivery fails, the Zavanelli maneuver, pushing the fetal head back into the vagina and delivering the fetus by cesarean section, may be tried (29).

Abnormal Intrapartum Fetal Monitoring

Fetal intolerance to labor or nonreassuring fetal status in labor occurs in 1% to 2% of most obstetric populations. Electronic fetal monitoring (EFM) can prove a useful screening test for fetal acidosis. A normal fetal heart-rate pattern (120 to 160 beats/min, short-term variability greater than 6 beats/min, normal long-term variability, acceleration with fetal movements, and absence of decelerations) is highly predictive of a nonacidotic fetus and normal outcome. Yet an abnormal or nonreassuring EFM test has poor specificity for detecting fetal compromise and little positive predictive value for subsequent neonatal morbidity or mortality (30). Some examples of nonreassuring fetal heart-rate patterns are:

- Repetitive variable decelerations,
- Severe bradycardia,
- Decelerations,
- Prolonged deceleration,
- Unexplained tachycardia and loss of baseline variability, and
- Sinusoidal pattern.

In the presence of nonreassuring intrapartum fetal heart-rate patterns, other tests may help evaluate fetal well-being and the safety of continued labor (22).

Intrapartum Assessment of Fetal Well-Being

Some of the available modalities for the intrapartum evaluation include fetal scalp-blood sampling, fetal scalp stimulation, and vibroacoustic stimulation. In a healthy baby, the fetal heart rate should accelerate at least 15 beats above the baseline after fetal scalp stimulation via digital pelvic examination, scalp puncture during fetal blood sampling (31,32), or with transabdominal vibroacoustic stimulation via an artificial larynx (33). A reactive fetal heart-rate response after these stimulations correlates with a nonacidotic fetus. In those fetuses with a non-reactive fetal heart response, acidosis is present in approximately 50% (31).

Obtaining fetal blood for blood gas analysis via fetal scalp-blood sampling (Fig. 15) confirms fetal acid–base status in the presence of nonreassuring fetal heart-rate patterns. Fetal scalp-blood sampling requires ruptured membranes and sufficient cervical dilation for the application of the endoscope to the presenting fetal part. The scalp is punctured with a 2-mm blade, and fetal blood is collected in a heparinized capillary tube for blood gas analysis. Some contraindications to fetal scalp-blood sampling are maternal hemophilia carrier status with fetal status unknown, maternal acquired immunodeficiency syndrome, and active maternal genital infections (34,35).

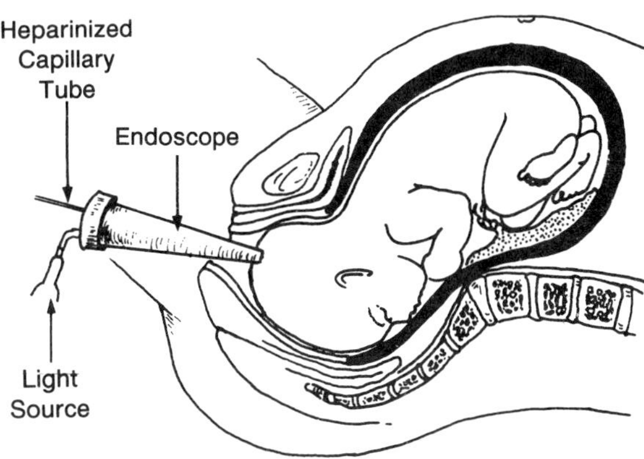

FIG. 15. Fetal scalp-blood sampling in labor.

Fetal scalp-blood pH of 7.25 is normal. Repeated blood sampling depends on the fetal heart-rate pattern and progress of labor. Fetal pH between 7.20 and 7.25 is equivocal or suggestive of fetal metabolic compromise. In this setting, the procedure should be repeated in 20 to 30 minutes to detect a possible downward trend. Traditionally, fetal scalp pH less than 7.20 was considered abnormal, suggestive of fetal acidemia and mandating rapid intervention. However, most newborns with a scalp pH less than 7.20 near delivery have normal Apgar scores and are vigorous at birth without any neurological consequences. Recently some investigators advocated a lower threshold to define significant fetal acidemia. An umbilical arterial pH of 7.10 is within 2 standard deviations of the mean and can be a normal finding in 5% of newborns. A more realistic criterion of pathologic fetal acidemia is an umbilical arterial pH less than 7.00 with a metabolic acidosis and neurological sequelae. However, even with this low critical value, most newborns with umbilical arterial pH of less than 7.00 at birth will be neurologically normal (35). The American College of Obstetricians and Gynecologists recommended that the term birth "asphyxia" be reserved for damaging acidemia, hypoxia, and metabolic acidosis with all of the following findings:

- Profound metabolic or mixed acidemia (umbilical arterial or venous pH less than 7.00), if obtained,
- Persistent Apgar score of 0 to 3 for longer than 5 minutes, and
- Evidence of neonatal neurological sequelae and multisystem organ dysfunction (36).

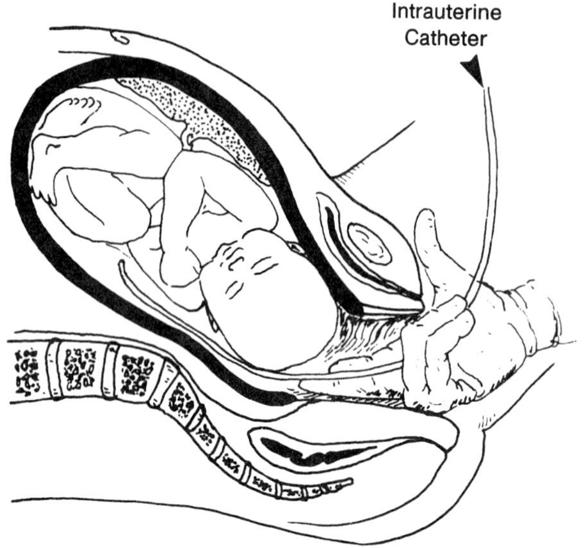

FIG. 16. Application of an intrauterine water pressure catheter (IUPC). Amnioinfusion is performed with infusion of saline solution into the amniotic cavity via the IUPC.

Intrapartum Resuscitation

Nonreassuring fetal heart-rate patterns during labor require prompt action. Maximize uteroplacental perfusion by repositioning the mother to the lateral position. Improve placental intervillous space perfusion and correct maternal hypotension with rapid infusion of intravenous fluids. Oxygen by face mask at 8 to 10 L/min may improve fetal oxygenation. Intrauterine infusion of saline (amnioinfusion) may diminish recurrent fetal variable decelerations. Amnioinfusion of saline probably works by reducing umbilical cord compression by expanding the intrauterine fluid volume (Fig. 16) (37,38). If these measures fail to improve the nonreassuring fetal heart-rate pattern, expedient delivery, either vaginally or abdominally via a cesarean section, is indicated (34).

Uterine activity should be assessed when abnormal fetal heart-rate patterns occur. Uterine hyperactivity or hyperstimulation should be ruled out. If oxytocin is being used, it should be stopped. Some investigators advocate the use of tocolytic agents, such as magnesium sulfate or β-mimetics, to relax the uterus to resolve or temporize the abnormal heart-rate pattern. This treatment allows time for in utero fetal resuscitation (improvement in the fetal metabolic status) while awaiting continued progress in labor or expedient delivery (39–41). Assessment of umbilical cord gases for acid–base status at birth is important in further diagnosis and prompt treatment of the neonate (35).

INDUCTION AND AUGMENTATION OF LABOR

Induction of labor is the initiation of labor by artificial means. Both medical (oxytocin or prostaglandins) and surgical (amniotomy) approaches are used. Augmentation of labor is the artificial stimulation, with oxytocic agents, of a spontaneous labor.

Labor is usually induced by combined amniotomy and oxytocin. Uterine contractions produced by oxytocin help apply the presenting part to the lower uterine segment. A well-applied presenting fetal part reduces the likelihood of prolapsed umbilical cord when the membranes are later ruptured. Amniotomy might increase uterine sensitivity and facilitate the progress of labor by reducing uterine volume. In patients with a favorable cervix, labor usually starts within 12 hours of amniotomy. However, the loss of amniotic fluid increases the risk of cord compression and consequent fetal intolerance to labor.

The Bishop score, which evaluates the station of the fetal head and the status of the cervix (Table 6), can help predict the likelihood of successful induction of labor in multiparous patients (42). This score ranges from 0 to 13. A score of at least nine (a "ripened" or "favorable" cervix) suggests a very good chance of successful induction and vaginal delivery. A score below five (an "unripe" or "unfavorable" cervix) indicates a poor chance of success.

Indications and Contraindications

An obstetrician may decide to induce or augment labor for many reasons (43). Elective induction of labor, induction for convenience alone, risks iatrogenic prematurity, uterine hyperstimulation causing abnormal fetal heart rate and fetal hypoxia, or failed induction requiring cesarean section. Assessing fetal maturity (Table 7) before elective induction of labor is important to decide the timing of induction (44).

Therapeutic induction of labor may be needed for medical or obstetric reasons. Labor may be induced before term if the continuation of the pregnancy presents significant risks to the mother or fetus (Table 8). If an overlarge fetus is mature, labor may be induced close to term to prevent the complications of macrosomia (shoulder dystocia, cesarean section).

Some contraindications to induction of labor include:

- Absolute cephalopelvic disproportion (i.e., contracted pelvis),

TABLE 6. *Bishop scoring system*

	0	1	2	3
Cervix				
Dilatation (cm)	0	1–2	3–4	≥5
Effacement (%)	0–30	40–50	60–70	≥80
Position	Posterior	Mid	Anterior	
Consistency	Firm	Medium	Soft	
Fetal head				
Station	−3	−2	−1/0	+1/+2

Adapted from ref. 42, with permission.

TABLE 7. *Fetal maturity assessment before delivery*

Documentation of one of the following (no amniocentesis required)
- Documented fetal heart tones for
  - 20 weeks by nonelectronic fetoscope, or
  - 30 weeks by Doppler
- 36 weeks have elapsed since a positive serum or urine human chorionic gonadotropin pregnancy test was found (performed by a reliable laboratory)
- Ultrasound measurement of the crown–rump length, obtained at 6–11 weeks, supports a gestational age ≥39 weeks
- Ultrasound examination at 12–20 weeks confirms the gestational age of ≥39 weeks determined by clinical history and physical examination

These criteria are not intended to preclude the use of menstrual dating. If any one of these criteria confirms gestational age determined from menstrual dates in a patient with normal menstrual cycles and no immediately antecedent use of contraceptives, it is appropriate to schedule delivery at ≥39 weeks by the menstrual dates. Ultrasound may be considered confirmatory of menstrual dates if there is gestational age agreement within 1 week by crown–rump measurement obtained at 6–11 weeks or within 10 days by the average of multiple measurements at 12–20 weeks.

Awaiting the onset of spontaneous labor is another option.

Adapted from ref. 44, with permission.

TABLE 8. *Indications for induction of labor*

Maternal
- Premature rupture of membranes
- Preeclampsia/eclampsia
- Cardiac disease
- Renal disease
- Pulmonary disease
- Chorioamnionitis
- Maternal medical problems (diabetes, malignancy, etc.)
- History of rapid labor (distance from hospital)

Fetal
- Intrauterine growth restriction
- Premature rupture of membranes
- Nonreassuring antepartum surveillance (abnormal biophysical profile, or contraction stress test)
- Postdate pregnancy
- Intrauterine fetal demise
- Hemolytic disease of the newborn (Rh isoimmunization, Kell sensitization, etc.)

Adapted from ref. 43, with permission.

- Previous uterine surgery that involved the full thickness of the uterus (i.e., classic cesarean section, myomectomy, or uterine reconstruction for congenital anomalies),
- Placenta previa or vasa previa,
- Invasive cervical carcinoma, and
- Certain abnormal positions or presentations (i.e., transverse lie, funic or umbilical cord presentation).

Some of these contraindications may not apply in certain clinical situations (i.e., a dead fetus).

Augmentation of labor is indicated when labor is abnormal in the presence of inadequate uterine contractions (Table 5). Contraindications to augmentation of labor are similar to those for induction of labor. Intrauterine pressure should be directly measured when augmenting labor, especially in a patient with previous low transverse cesarean section, to avoid hyperstimulation and possible uterine rupture.

Oxytocin

In the United States, oxytocin is approved for the purpose of induction and augmentation of labor. The uterine response to oxytocin varies with gestational age. The uterus is maximally sensitive to oxytocin close to term. It is somewhat unresponsive at the beginning of gestation and after parturition. As the sensitivity of the uterus changes, so does the oxytocin-receptor concentration in the myometrium (3,4).

Although oxytocin has been used intravenously, intramuscularly, and transbuccally, the intravenous route is the only one used in pregnant women. Oxytocin has a half-life of 3 to 5 minutes. Plasma concentration stabilizes 40 to 60 minutes after beginning the infusion. The physiologic effects of oxytocin will abate within 30 minutes of stopping the infusion.

A maximal infusion rate of 2 to 8 mU of oxytocin per minute should provide adequate augmentation of labor at term (45). Induction of labor usually requires more oxytocin than does augmentation of labor. Oxytocin may be infused at an initial rate of 0.5 to 1 mU/min. This rate is then increased every 40 to 60 minutes in increments of 1 to 2 mU/min (46). Other experts advocated initial infusion rate of 1 to 2 mU/min, increasing every 15 minutes in 1-mU/min increments (47). Oxytocin must be stopped in the presence of uterine hypertonus (a resting tone more than 20 mm Hg between contractions) or fetal intolerance to labor (abnormal fetal heart-rate pattern or "fetal distress") (22,43).

The major complications from the use of oxytocin are:

- Uterine hyperstimulation causing fetal intolerance to labor,
- Tetanic contractions leading to rupture of the uterus, and
- Possible water intoxication due to an intrinsic antidiuretic effect associated with high doses (more than 40 mU/min) of oxytocin (11).

Prolonged oxytocin infusion also may induce myometrial resistance to its effect. After delivery, uterine atony and hemorrhage may follow.

Prostaglandins

Prostaglandins play a role in the initiation of labor and cause cervical ripening. The Food and Drug Administration (FDA) approved prostaglandin E_2 (PGE_2), 20 mg, for use as an abortifacient in mid-trimester pregnancies. Currently, the PGE_2 derivative, dinoprostone, is the only prostaglandin approved by the FDA for cervical ripening and labor induction. This preparation is expensive and its cost is further increased because many women require two or more doses to achieve adequate cervical ripening (48,49). For continued uterine stimulation, oxytocin infusion can begin 4 hours after the last dose of prostaglandin. Oxytocin given with PGE_2 can cause uterine hyperstimulation (50,51).

Misoprostol

Cervical ripening is of fundamental importance to the successful induction of labor, but the optimal regimen for cervical ripening and labor induction remains unclear. Recently a PGE_1 analog, misoprostol, received attention as a potential cervical-ripening agent. This medication is inexpensive, easy to store, and stable at room temperature. Misoprostol is currently marketed in the United States for the prevention and treatment of peptic ulcers. Several recent randomized controlled trials of vaginal misoprostol and dinoprostone found misoprostol to be an effective agent for cervical ripening and labor induction. Most investigators found a significant reduction in the rate of cesarean delivery, as well as shorter duration of labor and reduced need for oxytocin augmentation with misoprostol (48,52–54). In addition, there is a low incidence of maternal side effects. However, one investigator (48) found that nonreassuring fetal heart-monitoring patterns associated with hyperstimulation were significantly more frequent in women treated with misoprostol compared with dinoprostone. There also was one report of uterine rupture in a 34-year-old multipara 5 hours after the administration of a second 25-mg dose of intravaginal misoprostol (55). A meta-analysis of the eight randomized controlled trials in the literature (56) confirmed reports that women who received misoprostol had a significantly lower overall cesarean rate and a higher incidence of vaginal delivery. Although misoprostol was associated with a higher incidence of uterine tachysystole, the risk of hyperstimulation and adverse perinatal outcome were not increased.

The optimal dose of intravaginal misoprostol for cervical ripening and labor induction has yet to be determined. Most investigators used 25 to 50 mg of misoprostol intravaginally every 3 to 6 hours. Wing et al. (49,57) recently published two studies assessing the safety and efficacy of intravaginal misoprostol for cervical ripening and labor induction. Both studies compared intravaginal misoprostol with intracervical dinoprostone. The 25-mg dose was as effective as the 50-mg dose in achieving a successful induction with fewer complications. These same investigators found that women with a 6-hour dosing schedule had longer intervals to delivery, more frequently required oxytocin augmentation, and had more failed inductions than patients with 3-hour dosing. One group (58) compared oral misoprostol (50 mg every 4 hours) with intracervical or vaginal prostaglandins. They reported that oral misoprostol was an effective and safe induction agent with minimal gastrointestinal side effects. Other investigators (59) compared vaginal versus oral misoprostol (100 mg every 3 hours) for induction of labor and found that the vaginal route of administration achieved a higher success rate in a shorter time with a lower dose. Significant differences in the pharmacokinetics of orally and vaginally administered misoprostol have been reported. Zienman et al. (60) reported that the systemic bioavailability of vaginally administered misoprostol is three times higher than that of orally administered misoprostol. Peak plasma concentrations are reached more slowly with vaginal administration but are sustained for longer periods, suggesting that longer dosage intervals may be appropriate with vaginal administration. These preliminary data suggest that misoprostol therapy is both efficacious and safe, although additional studies are needed to determine the optimal dose, route, and frequency of administration.

ACTIVE MANAGEMENT OF LABOR

There is widespread concern about the use of cesarean section in the United States. Cesarean delivery is associated with increased maternal morbidity and mortality and is more expensive than vaginal delivery. The active management of labor has been proposed as a strategy to lower the incidence of cesarean section for dystocia, although it was designed to prevent prolonged labor. Active management of labor was first described in Dublin, Ireland, in the 1960s (61,62). However, the first trial in the United States was reported by Boylan in 1991 (63), who found no significant change in forceps use or length of labor but a halving of the cesarean section rate.

Active management of labor is organized into two components (64). The first is the organizational component, which attempts to ensure consistent, appropriate care through the provision of prenatal education classes, midwife labor attendants, and peer review of all cesarean sections. The second approach is the medical component. Patients are encouraged not to come to the hospital until contractions are both regular and painful. According to the Dublin protocol, labor is diagnosed by the quality of the contractions in conjunction with at least one of the following: complete cervical effacement, rupture of membranes, or bloody show, versus cervical dilatation (61,62).

If membranes are still intact, amniotomy is performed soon after the diagnosis of labor. The most noticeable difference between the active management of labor and traditional labor-management protocols is the manner in which oxytocin is used for labor augmentation. If at any time the patient fails to dilate at least 1 cm/hour in the first stage of labor or the presenting part does not descend for an hour in the second stage of labor, augmentation with oxytocin is initiated. Infusion is started at 6 mU/min and increased at 6 mU/min every 15 minutes until a frequency of seven contractions per 15 minutes is achieved or a maximal rate of 40 mU/min is reached. If delivery does not occur within 12 hours of the onset of labor, a cesarean section is performed (61,62).

In the United States, the first randomized trial of active management of labor with concurrent controls was reported in 1992. Lopez-Zeno et al. (65) found a 26% reduction in cesarean section and a mean decrease in the length of labor of almost 2 hours. In addition, maternal infectious morbidity was halved. Frigoletto et al. (66) reported conflicting results in a second randomized trial. Here, the length of labor was shortened by more than 2 hours, and the risk of maternal febrile illness was reduced by 40%, but the incidence of cesarean section did not change. Both trials reported no differences between actively managed patients and controls in the incidence of low Apgar scores, birth injuries, neonatal deaths, seizures, or admissions to the neonatal intensive care unit. More recently, Glantz and McNanley (67) performed a meta-analysis of the published literature regarding the active management of labor. They found a 34% reduction in the rate of cesarean section delivery for dystocia in nulliparas without an increase in adverse neonatal outcomes.

There appear sufficient data to indicate that active labor-management programs can be instituted without deleterious effects on neonatal outcome. Although not uniformly successful, active management of labor may be one way to reduce the rate of operative delivery.

PRETERM LABOR

Definitions

The onset of labor is preterm or premature when it occurs before 37 completed weeks of gestation. Low birth weight is a fetal weight of less than 2,500 g. Very low birth weight is a fetal weight of less than 1,500 g, and extremely low birth weight is birth weight less than 1,000 g. A fetus born weighing less than 500 g, or less than 20 weeks, is an abortus.

Epidemiology and Neonatal Outcome of Preterm Birth

Neonatal survival and long-term cognitive, motor, or neurological function depend on birth weight as a reflection of gestational age. With the advances in neonatal intensive care medicine, the developmental outcome for the group of infants with birth weight more than 1,000 g is approaching the expected outcome for term neonate. For the very immature infants (birth weight less than 1,000 g), the risk of abnormal developmental outcome (cerebral palsy, blindness, bronchopulmonary dysplasia, sensorineural deficiencies, and developmental delay) remains significant (68). In most cases of preterm labor, the cause is unknown (Table 9). Fifty percent of preterm births have no identifiable risk factors (69).

In the United States, preterm delivery occurs in approximately 10% of all births. Prematurity is the leading cause of perinatal, neonatal, and infant mortality and morbidity. Pharmacologic inhibition of preterm labor has not convincingly reduced the rate of preterm birth or neonatal death. Once the decision is made to treat preterm labor, the goal is to reduce the frequency of uterine contractions and arrest cervical change.

TABLE 9. *Common causes of preterm labor*

Maternal causes
Genital tract colonization and infection (group B streptococci, *N. gonorrhoea,* gardenerella vaginitis, etc.)
Abdominal surgery
Preeclampsia/eclampsia
Diabetic ketoacidosis
Pyelonephritis
Appendicitis
Thyroid storm
Systemic illness
Maternal smoking or cocaine use
Prepregnancy weight <45 kg
Fetal causes
Fetal demise
Fetal anomalies
Uterine placental causes
Overdistended uterus
Multiple gestations
Polyhydramnios
Abnormal placentation
Placenta previa
Abruptio placentae
Second trimester bleeding
Chorioamnionitis
Premature rupture of membranes
Uterine or cervical anomalies
Cervical incompetence
Other
No prenatal care
Previous second trimester abortion
Prior preterm delivery
Low socioeconomic status
Nonwhite race
Maternal age <18 or >40 years
Single parent

Adapted from ref. 69, with permission.

Indications and Contraindications for the Use of Labor-Inhibiting (Tocolytic) Agents

Prerequisites for use of a labor-inhibiting (tocolytic) agent include:

- Presence of regular uterine contractions with documented cervical change (effacement or dilation),
- A gestational age at which treatment will benefit the fetus, and
- The absence of medical or obstetric contraindications to the inhibition of labor or the tocolytic agent.

As with term labor, early differentiation between true and false preterm labor is difficult. Ideally, preterm labor is diagnosed by the presence of regular uterine contractions that produce progressive cervical dilatation or effacement after 20 but before 37 weeks of gestation. The success of tocolysis diminishes when advanced cervical dilatation or effacement have occurred. Most fetal mortality and serious morbidity occur before 34 weeks' gestation. The fetus most likely to benefit from labor inhibition is probably at a gestational age of less than 32 to 34 weeks. Corticosteroids should be considered for all women between 24 and 34 weeks' gestation at risk for preterm delivery for the purpose of induction of fetal lung maturity (70). The upper gestational age limit for labor inhibition is individually determined. Tocolysis also may be of some value to prevent delivery during maternal transport to an appropriate medical facility (69).

Treatment of Preterm Labor

Treatment of premature labor includes bed rest, mild sedation, hydration, and the use of tocolytic agents.

Infection

Subclinical chorioamnionitis with bacterial colonization decreases the effectiveness of tocolysis (71). Bacterial vaginosis increases the risk of spontaneous preterm birth (75) and low-birth-weight infants (76). Antibiotics may prolong pregnancy when included in the treatment of idiopathic preterm labor (72–74). Treatment of bacterial vaginosis with metronidazole or erythromycin may reduce the risk of spontaneous preterm birth (77–79). In addition to treating specific genital tract pathogens, it is important to follow current guidelines for the administration of intrapartum group B streptococcus (GBS) prophylaxis when preterm birth or prolonged membrane rupture is anticipated (80).

Other predictors of preterm birth and perinatal infection include the presence of fetal fibronectin and a short cervix (75,81).

Fetal Fibronectin

Fetal fibronectin is an extracellular matrix protein found in the fetal membranes, decidua, and amniotic fluid. It is normally present in cervicovaginal fluid before week 20 of gestation but infrequently thereafter. Its presence after 20 weeks' gestation indicates evidence of pathologic changes at the interface of fetal and maternal tissues. The production of fetal fibronectin is stimulated by bacteria and inflammatory mediators.

Fetal fibronectin has been gaining popularity as a diagnostic test for preterm labor, although its use as a screening test remains investigational. In a multicenter trial of women with suspected preterm labor, the detection of fetal fibronectin in cervicovaginal secretions identified a population of women at high risk for preterm delivery (82).

An enzyme immunoassay kit has recently been approved by the FDA for use in symptomatic patients to diagnose preterm labor. The Committee on Obstetric Practice of the American College of Obstetricians and Gynecologists recommends the following criteria be met for its use:

- Amniotic membranes are intact,
- Cervical dilatation is minimal (less than 3 cm), and
- Sampling no earlier than 24 weeks, 0 days, and no later than 34 weeks, 6 days of gestation (83).

Tocolytic Agents for the Treatment of Preterm Labor

Ritodrine is the only drug approved by the FDA for the use as a tocolytic agent in the treatment of preterm labor. However, other drugs have also been used for tocolysis. The β-adrenergic agonists, ritodrine and terbutaline, in addition to magnesium sulfate, are the most commonly used first-line intravenous tocolytic agents in the United States. (Some physicians prefer subcutaneous terbutaline instead of the intravenous agents as the initial tocolytic drug.)

Once uterine contractions have stopped for 12 to 24 hours, tocolysis is commonly maintained until 35 to 37 weeks of gestation with an oral agent such as ritodrine or terbutaline. Oral magnesium produces subtherapeutic increases in the serum magnesium concentration and may not be clinically effective as a tocolytic maintenance agent. In addition, oral magnesium is a potent cathartic (69,82).

Tocolytic agents are titrated until uterine contractions stop. Once labor is inhibited, infusion usually continues for 12 to 24 hours. All tocolytic agents have significant maternal hemodynamic and metabolic effects (Table 10). These drugs should be stopped if significant maternal side effects, especially pulmonary edema, occur. The pulmonary edema is multifactorial; it is associated with fluid overload, chorioamnionitis, use of steroids, prolonged tocolytic therapy, and multiple gestations. The toxic effects of magnesium such as cardiac arrest and respiratory paralysis are rarely seen below a serum concentration of 10 mg/dL (69,84). Table 11 lists contraindications to tocolysis for preterm labor.

In a few medical centers, indomethacin has been used with good clinical outcome as the first-line tocolytic agent in the short-term treatment of selected cases of

TABLE 10. *Potential complications of tocolytic agents*

β-Adrenergic agents
Hyperglycemia
Hypokalemia
Hypotension
Pulmonary edema
Cardiac insufficiency
Arrhythmias
Myocardial ischemia
Maternal death
Magnesium sulfate
Pulmonary edema
Respiratory depression[a]
Cardiac arrest[a]
Maternal tetany[a]
Profound muscular paralysis[a]
Profound hypotension[a]
Indomethacin
Hepatitis[b]
Renal failure[b]
Gastrointestinal bleeding[b]
Nifedipine
Transient hypotension

[a]Effect is rare; seen with toxic levels.
[b]Effect is rare; associated with chronic use.
Adapted from ref. 69, with permission.

preterm labor. An initial dose of 50 to 100 mg can be given orally or as a rectal suppository and followed by 25 mg every 4 to 6 hours for 24 to 48 hours. The major limitation of indomethacin is closure of the fetal ductus arteriosus. This drug should be avoided after 34 weeks of gestation, when this fetal risk is greatest. In addition, oligohydramnios may occur with its prolonged use. The contraindications to use are a history of gastric ulcer, renal disease, and known bleeding disorders (69,84,85).

The calcium channel blocking agents have been investigated for their safety and efficacy in the treatment of preterm labor. There have now been several small prospective, randomized clinical trials of nifedipine versus other tocolytic agents for the treatment of preterm labor (86–91). These studies suggested that nifedipine is at least as effective for tocolysis as ritodrine, terbutaline, or magnesium sulfate in the prevention of preterm delivery. In addition, although animal studies raised concerns about the fetal safety of calcium channel blockers, there is no evidence that nifedipine compromises the fetus in human clinical trials. As a result, these agents are gaining popularity as second-line tocolytics when other agents fail.

The antihypertensive diazoxide is an effective tocolytic agent and has been used with success in some clinical studies. However, its potent vasodilating effects and its early misuse have limited its use in obstetrics (92). Preliminary data on atosiban, an oxytocin antagonist, also has been promising (93). Studies on the efficacy and safety of using multiple agents for labor inhibition are limited and conflicting (69,94). Combination tocolytic therapy may be reserved for the selected high-risk patients for whom conventional single-agent therapy failed, but only after careful consideration of the mechanisms and side effects of each agent. A recent meta-analysis of controlled randomized trials found no benefit to oral tocolytic maintenance therapy (95).

TABLE 11. *Contraindications to tocolysis for preterm labor*

General contraindications
Acute fetal distress (except intrauterine resuscitation)
Chorioamnionitis
Eclampsia or severe preeclampsia
Fetal demise (singleton)
Fetal maturity
Maternal hemodynamic instability
Contraindications for specific tocolytic agents
β-Mimetic agents
Maternal cardiac rhythm disturbance or other cardiac disease
Poorly controlled diabetes, thyrotoxicosis, or hypertension
Magnesium sulfate
Hypocalcemia
Myasthenia gravis
Renal failure

Adapted from ref. 69, with permission.

Acceleration of Fetal Pulmonary Maturation

In an attempt to decrease the frequency of severe respiratory distress syndrome, various antenatal treatments have tried to speed the maturation of the fetal lungs. When given between 24 and 34 weeks' gestation, maternal administration of glucocorticoids (betamethasone or dexamethasone) appears to reduce the incidence of neonatal respiratory distress syndrome, intraventricular hemorrhage, and mortality (70).

Thyrotropin-releasing hormone (TRH) also has been used in combination with corticosteroids to accelerate fetal lung maturation. In initial clinical trials, TRH therapy was associated with a reduced incidence of respiratory distress syndrome and chronic lung disease. However, two large multicenter studies (ACTOBAT and the North American TRH Trial) found that antenatal TRH and corticosteroids did not improve outcome in preterm infants (96,97).

Several preliminary clinical studies reported that either of the two active forms of the thyroid hormone, thyroxin (T_4) or triiodothyronine (T_3) alone accelerate fetal lung maturity (98,99). Adamsons et al. (100) and Romaquera et al. (101) reported an increase in the amniotic fluid lecithin-to-sphingomyelin (L/S) ratio in premature fetuses after intraamniotic T_4 injection. Barkai et al. (102) reported similar findings by using a fluorescence polarization assay to quantify amniotic fluid surfactant. Animal data support the maturational effect of T_3 on fetal lung development (103). Current clinical trials are evaluating the safety and efficacy of antenatal thyroxine and corticosteroids for the reduction of complications of prematurity.

Preterm Rupture of the Membranes

Premature rupture of membranes is rupture any time before the onset of labor, regardless of the duration of gestation at the time of rupture. Preterm rupture is rupture of membranes before 37 weeks of gestation. Although premature rupture of the membranes may occur at any stage of pregnancy, its incidence increases as term approaches. Premature rupture of membranes complicates approximately 10% of pregnancies. Preterm rupture of membranes happens in at least 30% of preterm deliveries. The time between rupture of the membranes and the onset of labor is inversely proportional to the gestational age at which rupture of membranes occurs. In preterm patients, labor occurs in 50% of women within 24 hours of ruptured membranes. At term, labor begins within 24 hours of membrane rupture in 90% of patients.

The cause of premature rupture of membranes is unknown, but it is associated with premature delivery, maternal sepsis, and increased perinatal morbidity and mortality. Factors associated with premature rupture of membranes include hydramnios, multiple gestation, chorioamnionitis, incompetent cervix, abruptio placentae, and amniocentesis. Guinn et al. (104) found that black race, multiparity, a history of abortion or preterm birth, advanced cervical dilatation, and positive amniotic fluid markers also were associated with premature rupture of membranes in women with preterm labor.

It is important to diagnose ruptured membranes promptly to allow appropriate management. Vaginal fluid should be examined for group B streptococcus, chlamydia, and gonococcus. The presence of bacterial vaginosis should be sought. Standard practices should be applied regarding group B streptococcal intrapartum prophylaxis with either penicillin or ampicillin (69,80). In addition, the L/S ratio and the presence of PG (phosphatidyl glycerol), or other markers of fetal lung maturity, should be evaluated (44).

If insufficient amniotic fluid is available from the vaginal pool for complete evaluation, amniocentesis may help clarify the pulmonary maturity status of the fetus. Amniotic fluid obtained via amniocentesis also should be sent for Gram stain and cultures. Instillation of indigo carmine dye into the amniotic cavity before withdrawal of the amniocentesis needle may clarify questionable cases of rupture of the membranes.

The obstetric management of premature rupture of membranes is controversial. If membranes break after 36 weeks, or before 36 weeks with documented fetal lung maturity, delivery is recommended. If there are no signs of infection, it is reasonable to wait 12 to 24 hours for the onset of spontaneous labor. In the presence of chorioamnionitis at any gestational age, antibiotic therapy and prompt delivery are recommended. Chorioamnionitis in preterm rupture of membranes increases the risk of neonatal respiratory distress, intraventricular hemorrhage, sepsis, low 1-minute Apgar score, and mortality.

In the management of preterm rupture of membranes, current consensus is to use glucocorticoids for the acceleration of fetal lung maturity in gestational ages between 24 and 32 to 34 weeks in cases without clinical evidence of chorioamnionitis (70). Recent clinical trials support the use of antimicrobial therapy in the expectant management of preterm premature rupture of the membranes by demonstrating prolongation of pregnancy and a reduction in maternal and infant infectious morbidities (105–107).

REFERENCES

1. Cunningham FG, MacDonald PC, Gant NF. Parturition: biomolecular and physiological processes. In: Cunningham FG, MacDonald PC, Gant NF, eds. *Williams obstetrics.* 19th ed. Connecticut: Appleton & Lange, 1993:297.
2. Casey ML, MacDonald PC. Decidual activation: the role of prostaglandins in labor. In: McNellis D, Challis JRG, MacDonald PC, Nathanielsz PW, Roberts JM, eds. *The onset of labor: cellular and integrative mechanisms: reproductive and perinatal medicine.* Vol 9. Ithaca, NY: Perinatology Press, 1988:141.
3. Soloff MS. The role of oxytocin in the initiation of labor, and oxytocin-prostaglandin interactions. In: McNellis D, Challis JRG, MacDonald PC, Nathanielsz PW, Roberts JM, eds. *The onset of labor: cellular and integrative mechanisms: reproductive and perinatal medicine.* Vol 9. Ithaca, NY: Perinatology Press, 1988:87.
4. Soloff MS. Oxytocin receptors and mechanism of oxytocin action. In: Amico JA, Robinson AG, eds. *Oxytocin clinical and laboratory studies. Excerpta medica ICS 666.* New York: Elsevier Science Publishing Company, 1985:259.
5. Casey ML,MacDonald PC. Biomolecular processes in the initiation of parturition: decidual activation. *Clin Obstet Gynecol* 1988;31:533.
6. Mitchell MD. Sources of eicosanoids within the uterus during pregnancy. In: McNellis D, Challis JRG, MacDonald PC, Nathanielsz PW, Roberts JM, eds. *The onset of labor: cellular and integrative mechanisms: reproductive and perinatal medicine.* Vol 9. Ithaca, NY: Perinatology Press, 1988:165.
7. Challis JRG. Steroid production by the fetal membranes in relation to the onset of parturition. In: McNellis D, Challis JRG, MacDonald PC, Nathanielsz PW, Roberts JM, eds. *The onset of labor: cellular and integrative mechanisms: reproductive and perinatal medicine.* Vol 9. Ithaca, NY: Perinatology Press, 1988:233.
8. Oxorn H, Foote WR. Obstetric pelvis. In: Oxorn H, ed. *Human labor and birth.* 4th ed. New York: Appleton-Century-Crofts, 1980:22.
9. Cunningham FG, MacDonald PC, Gant NF. The normal pelvis. In: Cunningham FG, MacDonald PC, Gant NF, eds. *Williams obstetrics.* 19th ed. Connecticut: Appleton & Lange, 1993:283.
10. Steer CM, Moloy HC. General morphology of the pelvis. In: Steer CM, ed. *Moloy's evaluation of the pelvis in obstetrics.* 3rd ed. New York: Plenium Medical Book Company, 1975:1.
11. Cunningham FG, MacDonald PC, Gant NF. Conduct of normal labor and delivery. In: Cunningham FG, MacDonald PC, Gant NF, eds. *Williams obstetrics.* 19th ed. Connecticut: Appleton & Lange, 1993:371.
12. Friedman EA. Normal and dysfunctional labor. In: Cohen WR, Acker DB, Friedman EA, eds. *Management of labor.* 2nd ed. Rockville, MD: Aspen, 1989:1.
13. American College of Obstetricians and Gynecologists. *Dystocia and the augmentation of labor.* ACOG technical bulletin 218. Washington, DC: ACOG, December 1995.
14. Beard RW. The detection of fetal asphyxia in labor. *Pediatrics* 1974;53(2):157.
15. Paul RH, Huey JR Jr, Yaeger CF. Clinical fetal monitoring: Its effects on cesarean section rate and perinatal mortality: five-year trends. *Postgrad Med* 1977;61(4):160.

16. Wood C, Renou P, Oats J, Farrell E, Beischer N, Anderson I. A controlled trial of fetal heart rate monitoring in a low-risk obstetric population. *Am J Obstet Gynecol* 1981;141:527.
17. Leveno KJ, Cunningham FG, Nelson S, et al. A prospective comparison of selective and universal electronic fetal monitoring in 34,995 pregnancies. *N Engl J Med* 1986;315:615.
18. Luthy DA, Shy KK, vanBelle G, et al. A randomized trial of electronic fetal heart monitoring in premature labor. *Obstet Gynecol* 1987;69:687.
19. MacDonald D, Grant A, Sheriden-Pereira M, Boylan P, Chalmers I. The Dublin randomized controlled trial of intrapartum fetal heart rate monitoring. *Am J Obstet Gynecol* 1985;152:524.
20. Renou P, Chang A, Anderson I, Wood C. Controlled trial of fetal intensive care. *Am J Obstet Gynecol* 1976;126:470.
21. Vintzileo AM, Antsaklis A, Varvarigos I, Papas C, Sofatzis I, Montgomery JT. A randomized trial of intrapartum electronic fetal heart rate monitoring versus intermittent auscultation. *Obstet Gynecol* 1993;81:899.
22. American College of Obstetricians and Gynecologists. *Fetal heart rate patterns:* monitoring, *interpretation, and management.* ACOG technical bulletin 207. Washington, DC: ACOG, July 1995.
23. Thacker SB, Banta HD. Benefits and risks of episiotomy: an interpretative review of the English language literature, 1860-1980. *Obstet Gynecol Surv* 1983;38:322.
24. Friedman EA. Dysfunctional labor. In: Cohen WR, Friedman EA, eds. *Management of labor.* 1st ed. Maryland: University Park Press, 1983:11.
25. Friedman EA. Chapter 57. Dysfunctional labor. In: Greenhill JP, ed. *Obstetrics.* 13th ed. Philadelphia: WB Saunders, 1965:831.
26. American College of Obstetricians and Gynecologists. *Fetal macrosomia.* ACOG technical bulletin 159. Washington DC: ACOG, September 1991.
27. Cohen WR. The pelvic division of labor. In: Cohen WR, Acker DB, Friedman EA, eds. *Management of labor.* 2nd ed. Rockville, MD: Aspen Publishers, 1989:19.
28. Cunningham FG, MacDonald PC, Gant NF. Dystocia due to abnormalities in presentation, position, or development of the fetus. In: Cunningham FG, MacDonald PC, Gant NF, eds. *Williams obstetrics.* 19th ed. Connecticut: Appleton & Lange, 1993:493.
29. Sandberg EC. The Zavanelli maneuver: a potentially revolutionary method for the resolution of shoulder dystocia. *Am J Obstet Gynecol* 1985;152:479.
30. Smith CV. Fetal distress. In: Phelan JP, Clark SL, eds. *Cesarean delivery.* New York: Elsevier Science Publishing, 1988:70.
31. Clark SL, Gimovsky ML, Miller FC. The scalp stimulation test: a clinical alternative to fetal scalp blood sampling. *Am J Obstet Gynecol* 1984;148:274.
32. Clark SL, Gimovsky, Miller FC. Fetal heart rate response to scalp blood sampling. *Am J Obstet Gynecol* 1982;144:706.
33. Smith CV, Nguyen HN, Phelan JP, Paul RH. Intrapartum assessment of fetal well-being: a comparison of fetal acoustic stimulation with acid-base determinations. *Am J Obstet Gynecol* 1986;155:726.
34. Cohen WR, Schifrin BS. Clinical management of fetal hypoxemia. In: Cohen WR, Acker DB, Friedman EA, eds. *Management of labor.* 2nd ed. Rockville, MD: Aspen Publishers, 1989:283.
35. American College of Obstetricians and Gynecologists. *Umbilical artery blood acid-base analysis.* ACOG technical bulletin 216. Washington, DC: ACOG, November 1995.
36. American College of Obstetricians and Gynecologists. *Inappropriate use of the terms fetal distress and birth asphyxia.* ACOG committee opinion 197. Washington, DC: ACOG, February 1998.
37. Owen J, Henson BV, Hauth JC. A prospective randomized study of saline solution amnioinfusion. *Am J Obstet Gynecol* 1990;162:1146.
38. Haubrich KL. Amnioinfusion: a technique for the relief of variable deceleration. *J Obstet Gynecol Neonatal Nurs* 1990;19:299.
39. Lipshitz J. Use of a β_2-sympathomimetic drug as a temporizing measure in the treatment of acute fetal distress. *Am J Obstet Gynecol* 1977;129:31.
40. Burke MS, Porreco RP, Day D, et al. Intrauterine resuscitation with tocolysis. An alternate month clinical trial. *J Perinat* 1989;9:296.
41. Shekarloo A, Mendez-Bauer C, Cook V, Freese U. Terbutaline (intravenous bolus) for the treatment of acute intrapartum fetal distress. *Am J Obstet Gynecol* 1989;160:615.
42. Bishop EN. Pelvic scoring for elective induction. *Obstet Gynecol* 1964;24:266.
43. American College of Obstetricians and Gynecologists. *Induction of labor.* ACOG technical bulletin 217. Washington, DC: ACOG, December 1995.
44. American College of Obstetricians and Gynecologists. *Assessment of fetal lung maturity.* ACOG educational bulletin 230. Washington, DC: ACOG, November 1996.
45. Seitchik J, Castillo M. Oxytocin augmentation of dysfunctional labor. I. Clinical data. *Am J Obstet Gynecol* 1982;144:899.
46. Seitchik J, Castillo M. Oxytocin augmentation of dysfunctional labor. II. Uterine activity data. *Am J Obstet Gynecol* 1983;145:529.
47. Hauth JC, Hankins GDV, Gilstrap LC, Strickland DM, Vance P. Uterine contraction pressures with oxytocin induction/augmentation. *Obstet Gynecol* 1986;68:305.
48. Buser D, Mora G, Arias F. A randomized comparison between misoprostol and dinoprostone for cervical ripening and labor induction in patients with unfavorable cervices. *Obstet Gynecol* 1997;89:581.
49. Wing DA, Ortiz-Omphroy G, Paul RH. A comparison of intermittent vaginal administration of misoprostol with continuous dinoprostone for cervical ripening and labor induction. *Am J Obstet Gynecol* 1997;177:612.
50. Brindley BA, Sokol RJ. Induction and augmentation of labor: basis and methods for current practice. *Obstet Gynecol Surv* 1988;43:730.
51. Rayburn WF. Prostaglandin E2 gel for cervical ripening and induction of labor: critical analysis. *Am J Obstet Gynecol* 1989;160:529.
52. Wing DA, Randall A, Jones MM, Goodwin TM, Paul RH. Misoprostol: an effective agent for cervical ripening and labor induction. *Am J Obstet Gynecol* 1995;172:1811.
53. Varaklis K, Gumina R, Stubblefield PG. Randomized controlled trial of vaginal misoprostol and intracervical prostaglandin E2 gel for induction of labor at term. *Obstet Gynecol* 1995;86:541.
54. Mundle WR, Young DC. Vaginal misoprostol for induction of labor: A randomized controlled trial. *Obstet Gynecol* 1996;88:521.
55. Bennett BB. Uterine rupture during induction of labor at term with intravaginal misoprostol. *Obstet Gynecol* 1997;89:832.
56. Sanchez-Ramos L, Kaunitz AM, Wears RL, Delke I, Gaudier FL. Misoprostol for cervical ripening and labor induction: a meta-analysis. *Obstet Gynecol* 1997;89:663.
57. Wing DA, Paul RH. A comparison of differing dosing regimens of vaginally administered misoprostol for preinduction cervical ripening and labor induction. *Am J Obstet Gynecol* 1996;175:158.
58. Windrim R, Bennett K, Mundle W, Young DC. Oral administration of misoprostol for labor induction: A randomized controlled trial. *Obstet Gynecol* 1997;89:392.
59. Toppozada MK, Anwar MYM, Hassan HA, El-Gazaerly WS. Oral or vaginal misoprostol for induction of labor. *Int J Gynecol Obstet* 1997;56:135.
60. Zieman M, Fong SK, Benowitz NL, Banskter D, Darney PD. Absorption kinetics of misoprostol with oral or vaginal administration. *Obstet Gynecol* 1997;90:88.
61. O'Driscoll K, Jackson RJA, Gallagher JT. Prevention of prolonged labor. *Br Med J* 1969;2:477.
62. O'Driscoll K, Jackson RJA, Gallagher JT. Active management of labour and cephalopelvic disproportion. *J Obstet Gynaecol Br Commonw* 1970;77:385.
63. Boylan P, Frankowski R, Roundtree R, Selwyn B, Parrish K. Effect of active management of labor on the incidence of cesarean section for dystocia in nulliparas. *Am J Perinat* 1991;8:373.
64. Peaceman AM, Socol ML. Active management of labor. *Am J Obstet Gynecol* 1996;175:363.
65. Lopez-Zeno JA, Peaceman AM, Adashek JA, Socol ML. A controlled trial of a program for the active management of labor. *N Engl J Med* 1992;326:450.
66. Frigoletto FD, Lieberman E, Lang JM, et al. A clinical trial of active management of labor. *N Engl J Med* 1995;333:745.
67. Glantz JC, McNanley TJ. Active management of labor: a meta-analysis of cesarean delivery rates for dystocia in nulliparas. *Obstet Gynecol Surv* 1997;52:497.
68. Escobedo MB. Follow-up of prematurely born infants. *Clin Obstet Gynecol* 1988;31:662.
69. American College of Obstetricians and Gynecologists. *Preterm labor.* ACOG technical bulletin 206, Washington DC: ACOG, June 1995.
70. Effects of corticosteroids for fetal maturation on perinatal outcomes: NIH Consensus Statement. *Am J Obstet Gynecol* 1995;173:246.

71. Roberto R, Mazor M. Infection and preterm labor. *Clin Obstet Gynecol* 1988;31:553.
72. McGregor JA, French JI, Reller LB, Todd JK, Makowski EL. Adjunctive erythromycin treatment for idiopathic preterm labor: results of a randomized, double-blinded, placebo-controlled trial. *Am J Obstet Gynecol* 1986;154:98.
73. Morales WJ, Angel JL, O'Brien WF, Knuppel RA, Finazzo M. A randomized study of antibiotic therapy in idiopathic preterm labor. *Obstet Gynecol* 1988;72:829.
74. Newton ER, Dinsmoor MJ, Gibbs RS. A randomized, blinded, placebo-controlled trial of antibiotics in idiopathic preterm labor. *Obstet Gynecol* 1989;74:562.
75. Goldenberg RL, Ians JD, Mercer BM, et al. The preterm prediction study: the value of new vs standard risk factors in predicting early and all spontaneous preterm births: NICHD MFMU Network. *Am J Public Health* 1998;88:233.
76. Hillier SL, Nugent RP, Eschenbach DA, et al. Association between bacterial vaginosis and preterm delivery of a low-birth-weight infant: the vaginal infections and prematurity study group. *N Engl J Med* 1995;333:1737.
77. McDonald HM, O'Loughlin JA, Vigneswaran R, et al. Impact of birth in women with bacterial vaginosis flora (gardnerella vaginosis): A randomized, placebo controlled trial. *Br J Obstet Gynecol* 1997;104:1391.
78. Steele RW. Reduced incidence of preterm delivery with metronidazole and erythromycin in women with bacterial vaginosis. *Clin Pediatr* 1996;35:378.
79. Hauth JC, Goldenberg RL, Andrew WW, DuBard MB, Copper RL. Reduced incidence of preterm delivery with metronidazole and erythromycin in women with bacterial vaginosis. *N Engl J Med* 1995; 333:1732.
80. Mercer BM, Lewis R. Preterm labor and preterm premature rupture of the membranes: diagnosis and management. *Infect Dis Clin North Am* 1997;11:177.
81. Goldenberg RL, Thom E, Moawad AH, Johnson F, Roberts J, Caritis SN. The preterm prediction study: Fetal fibronectin, bacterial vaginosis and peripartum infection: NICHD Maternal Fetal Medicine Units Network. *Obstet Gynecol* 1996;87:656.
82. Lockwood CJ, Senyei AE, Dische MR, et al. Fetal fibronectin in cervical and vaginal secretions as a predictor of preterm delivery. *N Engl J Med* 1991;325:669.
83. American College of Obstetricians and Gynecologists. *Fetal fibronectin preterm labor risk test.* ACOG committee opinion 187. Washington, DC: ACOG, 1997.
84. Caritis SN, Darby MJ, Chan L. Pharmacologic treatment of preterm labor. *Clin Obstet Gynecol* 1988;31(3):635.
85. Niebyl JR, Witter FR. Neonatal outcome after indomethacin treatment for preterm labor. *Am J Obstet Gynecol* 1986;155:747.
86. Ferguson JE, Dyson DC, Shultz T, Stevenson DK. A comparison of tocolysis with nifedipine or ritodrine: analysis of efficacy and maternal, fetal and neonatal outcome. *Am J Obstet Gynecol* 1990:163:105.
87. Bracero LA, Leikin E, Kirshenbaum N, Tejani N. comparison of nifedipine and ritodrine for the treatment of preterm labor. *Am J Perinat* 1991;8:365.
88. Kupferminc M,. Lessing JB, Yaron Y, Peyser MR. Nifedipine versus ritodrine for suppression of preterm labour. *Br J Obstet Gynaecol* 1993;100:1090.
89. Smith CS, Woodland MB. Clinical comparison of oral nifedipine and subcutaneous terbutaline for initial tocolysis. *Am J Perinat* 1993;10:280.
90. Glock JL, Morales WJ. Efficacy and safety of nifedipine versus magnesium sulfate in the management of preterm labor: a randomized study. *Am J Obstet Gynecol* 1993;169:960.
91. Pirhonen JP, Erkkola RU, Ekblad UU, Nyman L. Single dose of nifedipine in normotensive pregnancy: nifedipine concentrations, hemodynamic responses, and uterine and fetal flow velocity waveforms. *Obstet Gynecol* 1990;76:807.
92. Adamsons K, Wallach RC. Diazoxide and calcium antagonists in preterm labor. In: Fuchs FF, Stubblefield PG, eds. *Preterm birth: causes, prevention, and management.* New York: Macmillan, 1984: 249.
93. Goodwin TM, Paul R, Silver H, et al. The effect of the oxytocin antagonist atosiban on preterm uterine activity in the human. *Am J Obstet Gynecol* 1994;170:474.
94. Hatagandi S, Nathanielsz P, Knupzel R, Lake M. The tocolytic interaction between atosiban and terbutaline: Society of Perinatal Obstetricians. *Am J Obstet Gynecol* 1995;172:256.
95. Macones GA, Berlin M, Berlin J. Efficacy of oral beta-agonist maintenance therapy in preterm labor: a meta-analysis. *Obstet Gynecol* 1995;85:313.
96. Crowther CA, Hiller JE, Haslam RR, Robinson JS, ACTOBAT Study Group. Australian collaborative trial of antenatal thyrotropin-releasing hormone (ACTOBAT) for prevention of neonatal respiratory disease. *Lancet* 1995;345:877.
97. Ballard RA, Ballard PL, Canaan A, et al. The North American trial of antenatal thyrotropin releasing hormone (TRH) for the prevention of lung disease in the preterm infants. *N Engl J Med* 1998;338:493.
98. Mashiach S, Barkai G, Sack J, et al. The effect of intraamniotic thyroxine administration on fetal lung maturity in man. *J Perinat Med* 1979;7:161.
99. Schreyer P, Caspi E, Letko Y, Ron-El R, Pinto N, Zeidman JL. Intraamniotic triiodothyronine instillation for prevention of respiratory distress syndrome in pregnancies complicated by hypertension. *J Perinat Med* 1982;10:27.
100. Adamsons K, Romaquera J, Wallach RC. Acceleration of fetal maturation by intra-amniotic administration of thyroxine. *J Perinat Med* 1984:12:21.
101. Romaquera J, Zorrilla C, Vega ADL, et al. Responsiveness of L-S ratio of the amniotic fluid to intra-amniotic administration of thyroxine. *Acta Obstet Gynecol Scand* 1990;69:119.
102. Barkai G, Reichman B, Lusky A, et al. The effect of thyroxine and corticosteroids upon amniotic fluid fluorescence polarization: A randomized controlled study. *J Perinat Med* 1992;20:459.
103. Chan L, Miller TF, Yuxin J, et al. Antenatal triiodothyronine improves neonatal pulmonary function in preterm lambs. *J Soc Gynecol Invest* 1998;5(3):122.
104. Guinn DA, Goldenbery RL, Hauth JC, Andrews WW, Thom E, Romero R. Risk factors for the development of preterm premature rupture of membranes. *Am J Obstet Gynecol* 1995;173:1310.
105. Mercer BM, Arheart KL. Antimicrobial therapy in expectant management of preterm premature rupture of the membranes. *Lancet* 1995; 346:1271.
106. Gibbs RS, Eschenbach DA. Use of antibiotics to prevent preterm birth. *Am J Obstet Gynecol* 1997;177:375.
107. Lovett SM, Weiss JD, Diogo MJ, Williams PT, Garite JJ. A prospective, double-blind, randomized controlled clinical trial of ampicillin-sulbactam for preterm premature rupture of membranes in women receiving antenatal corticosteroid therapy. *Am J Obstet Gynecol* 1997;176:1030.

Obstetric Anesthesia, second edition,
edited by Mark C. Norris.
Lippincott Williams & Wilkins, Philadelphia © 1999.

CHAPTER 12

Mechanisms of Labor Pain

Gabriela Rocha Lauretti

Cinema scenes of women clutching at bedposts and emitting blood-curdling screams, plus discussion with those who have given birth, are among the sources of the nullipara's expectations about labor pain (1). Many approaches may relieve this pain, but most can impair episodic memory of the vivid and emotional moment that is childbirth.

LABOR PAIN AS A MODEL OF ACUTE PAIN

Labor is a well-authenticated model of acute pain (2). The afferent uterine roots are T_{11} to T_{12} (3). Labor pain involves the T_{10} to L_1 or L_3 spinal segments (Fig. 1) (4,5), and the second to fourth sacral segments, which innervate the cervix, vagina, and perineum (4). During labor, pain is felt in the dermatomes supplied by the spinal cord segments that receive input from the uterus, cervix, pelvis, and perineum. In the absence of therapeutic intervention, these painful stimuli cause spinal sensitization, activating adjacent segments, extending the field of pain.

Stages of Labor

Labor is characterized by painful, progressive uterine contractions that cause dilatation and effacement of the cervix. Descent and delivery of the fetus and placenta through the birth canal follow. There are four stages of labor. The first stage, which must overcome cervical resistance, is further divided into latent and active phases. The latent phase usually ends at 3- to 4-cm cervical dilation. The active phase ends with the complete dilation of the cervix (10 cm). During the second stage of labor, descent continues at its maximal rate. The fetus undergoes a series of movements to adapt to the maternal pelvic canal and is finally born. Episiotomy is often done at the end of the second stage, although by this time, damage to the pelvic musculature has already occurred (6). The third stage of labor begins with the birth of the fetus and ends with complete expulsion or extraction of the placenta. The fourth stage ends 1 hour postpartum.

First and Second Stages of Labor

Pain of the first stage of labor results from uterine contractions that cause effacement of the cervicovaginal angle and dilatation, distention, stretching, and tearing of the cervix and perineum. The force of uterine contractions against the closed or dilating cervix and perineum places pressure on nerve endings that lie among the muscle fibers of the body and fundus of the uterus (7,8) and induces inflammatory changes within uterine muscle (7). Other sources of pain can be contraction of an ischemic myometrium and cervix (9), and vasoconstriction resulting from sympathetic hyperactivity (10). Peripheral tissue injury and uterine contractions enhance the responsiveness of both the peripheral and central nervous systems (sensitization). Peripheral sensitization reduces the firing threshold of nociceptor afferent peripheral nerve terminals. Central sensitization produces an activity-dependent increase in the excitability of spinal neurons. The resulting pain is felt between the umbilicus and pubes, across the back at the level of the top of the sacrum (Fig. 2) (11), and is a summation of:

- Acute deep and superficial somatic pain from the pelvic joints, vagina, and perineum,
- Acute visceral pain from the uterus and cervix, and
- Pain referred to skin and muscle of the abdominal wall and the back.

During the second stage of labor, the nociceptive stimulation from the fully dilated cervix decreases, but the presenting part of the fetus distends pain-sensitive struc-

G. R. Lauretti: Department of Surgery, Orthopedics, and Traumatology, Faculty of Medicine of Ribeirão Preto, University of São Paulo, São Paulo 14049, Brazil.

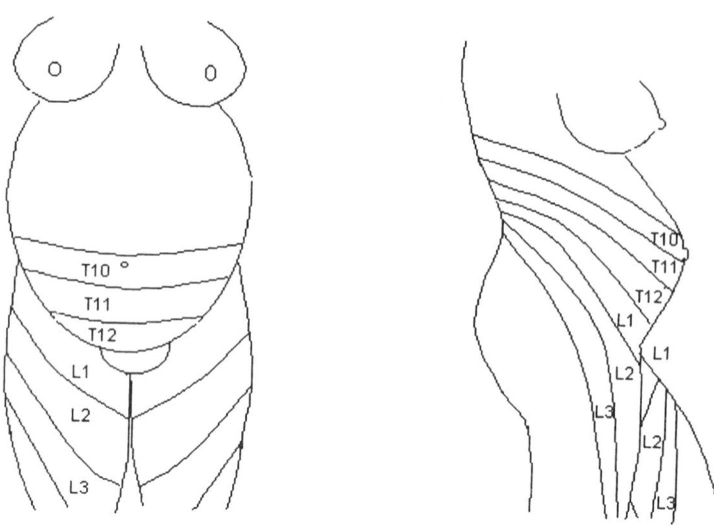

FIG. 1. Labor pain involves T_{10} to L_3 spinal segments and the second to fourth sacral segments (not shown). Some patients develop aching, burning pain in the legs, probably reflecting L_1 to L_3 and S_2 dermatome involvement, and representing areas of referral pain.

tures in the pelvis and perineum, adding to the ongoing pain. Progressively greater distention stretches and tears fascia and subcutaneous tissue of the vagina and adjacent structures (urethra, bladder, fascia and muscle of the pelvic cavity, peritoneum, and uterine ligaments) (8). Some patients also report aching, burning, or cramping in the thighs or legs, probably reflecting secondary hyperalgesia involving the L_1 to L_3 and S_2 dermatomes (Fig. 1).

Acute tissue destruction, such as occurs during labor, induces both primary and secondary hyperalgesia. Primary hyperalgesia occurs at the site of injury and results from sensitization of peripheral sensory receptors of A_δ and C fibers. Central sensitization has only a small role in primary hyperalgesia.

In contrast, secondary hyperalgesia, which occurs distant from the site of injury, is mediated by central sensiti-

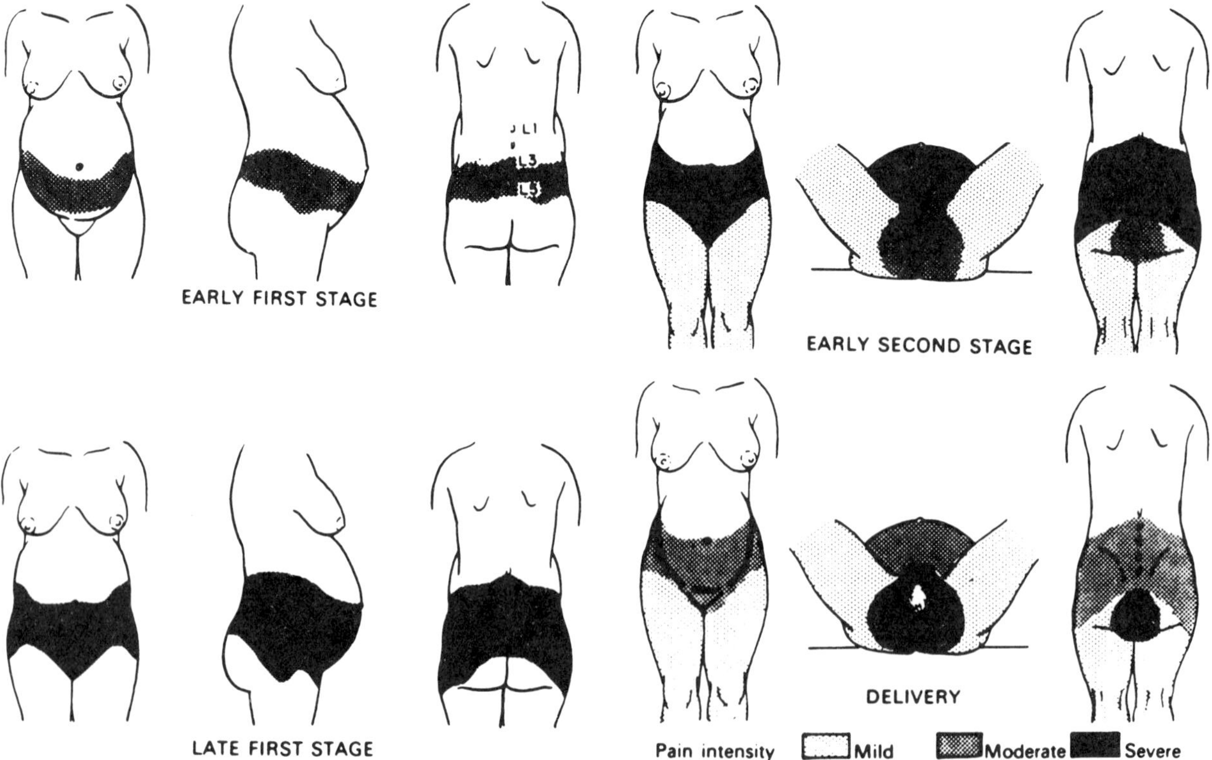

FIG. 2. Surface distribution of pain throughout labor. The location and intensity of pain varies with the progress of labor. (From ref. 11, with permission.)

zation (12), enabling Aβ fiber activation to produce pain. Secondary hyperalgesia can be modulated by:

- Opioids and acetylcholine,
- *N*-methyl-D-aspartate (NMDA) antagonists (13),
- Substance P antagonists,
- Antiinflammatories with a central site of action [i.e., diclofenac (14) or dipyrone (15)],
- Neuraxial local anesthetics (16), and
- Nitric oxide (17).

Repeated C-fiber input (18) or central summation of C and A_δ nociceptive activity (19) facilitates nerve activity within the dorsal horn and induces central sensitization. This enhanced responsiveness of dorsal horn neurons, also called "wind up," is due partly to the interaction of three mediators released by the C-fiber terminals:

- Glutamate, which acts on 9-amino-3-hydroxy-5-methyl-isoxazole (AMPA) and NMDA receptors,
- Substance P, which acts on neurokinin-1 receptors, and
- Neurokinin A, which acts on neurokinin-2 receptors and appears to play a major role in acute nociception (20).

Glutamate stimulation of the NMDA receptor allows Ca^{2+} to enter the cell. Ca^{2+} interacts with second messengers, activating additional AMPA receptors, enhancing the response to subsequent glutamate activation (21). Central sensitization then alters the spatial extent, responsiveness, and threshold of the receptive fields of the dorsal horn neurons (22). NMDA antagonists (i.e., ketamine) can block central hypersensitive states. Opioids, like morphine, bind to presynaptic inhibitory opioid receptors on C-fiber terminals and can delay or block wind-up by reducing or stopping C-fiber input into the dorsal horn nociceptive neurons (23).

Sometimes itching occurs within the field of pain. Pain and itch have much in common. Both are transmitted by unmyelinated sensory afferent nerve fibers (C fibers) with perhaps a contribution from thinly myelinated ones (A_δ fibers). Itch, like pain, is abolished by anterolateral cordotomy (24). Both itch and pain can occur in areas of secondary hyperalgesia (25,26). Despite these similarities, differential effects of noxious counterstimuli on itch and pain show that itch is not merely subclinical pain (27).

Third and Fourth Stages of Labor

Pain during the third and fourth stages of labor reflects the noxious stimuli that have previously accompanied fetal descent and the separation of the placenta. The central and peripheral hyperalgesic state present by delivery normally diminishes as the damaged visceral and somatic tissue recuperates. Mechanical hyperalgesia (conducted by Aβ fibers) may persist for several days after the incision or cutting of tissue (28), such as the episiotomy.

Pain Pathways

Afferent Pain Pathways

The quality of pain depends on the tissue innervated. Tissue injury and inflammation activates somatic or visceral peripheral afferent nociceptors by releasing many chemicals including:

- Bradykinin,
- Histamine,
- Eicosanoids,
- Substance P,
- 5-Hydroxytryptamine (5-HT),
- Adenosine triphosphate,
- Hydrogen ion,
- Noradrenaline,
- Nerve growth factor, and
- Opioid peptides (29).

Noxious stimulation induces release of substance P peripherally from C fibers (30) and into the cerebrospinal fluid (CSF) from central C-fiber projections (31). Parturients have lower plasma substance P concentrations than do nonpregnant women. This difference is not related to hemodilution. It also is unrelated to the presence of acute pain, as both laboring patients and those awaiting elective cesarean section have similar decreases in substance P plasma concentrations (32). This difference may be unrelated to pain processing, as both substance P and calcitonin gene-related peptide, another neuromodulator, also may regulate myometrial contractility (33).

Superficial and Deep Somatic Pain Pathways

Dilation, distention, and stretching of the muscles, pelvic joints, and vagina during labor produces somatic pain. Deep somatic pain follows activation of nociceptors in muscle, nerves (34), or joints. Cutaneous activation of nociceptors produces superficial somatic pain (Fig. 3).

Nociceptive information is conveyed from the periphery to the central nervous system (CNS) via myelinated (A_δ) and unmyelinated (C) primary afferent fibers. These nerves have average conduction velocities of 15 m/sec and less than 1 m/sec, respectively. They subserve different aspects of pain. A_δ fibers are the major peripheral source of information on the more discriminative or epicritic/phasic aspects of pain. This pain, known as first pain, is well localized, sharp, and pricking in nature and provides early warning of tissue damage. A_δ fibers respond most strongly to noxious heat and pressure and less strongly to chemical stimulation (35). C fibers have been implicated in protopathic/tonic pain perception, often described as dull, burning, or aching. This pain is known as second pain and is preferentially attenuated by opioids (36). Nociceptors, associated with the free nerve endings of C fibers, are most strongly activated by chem-

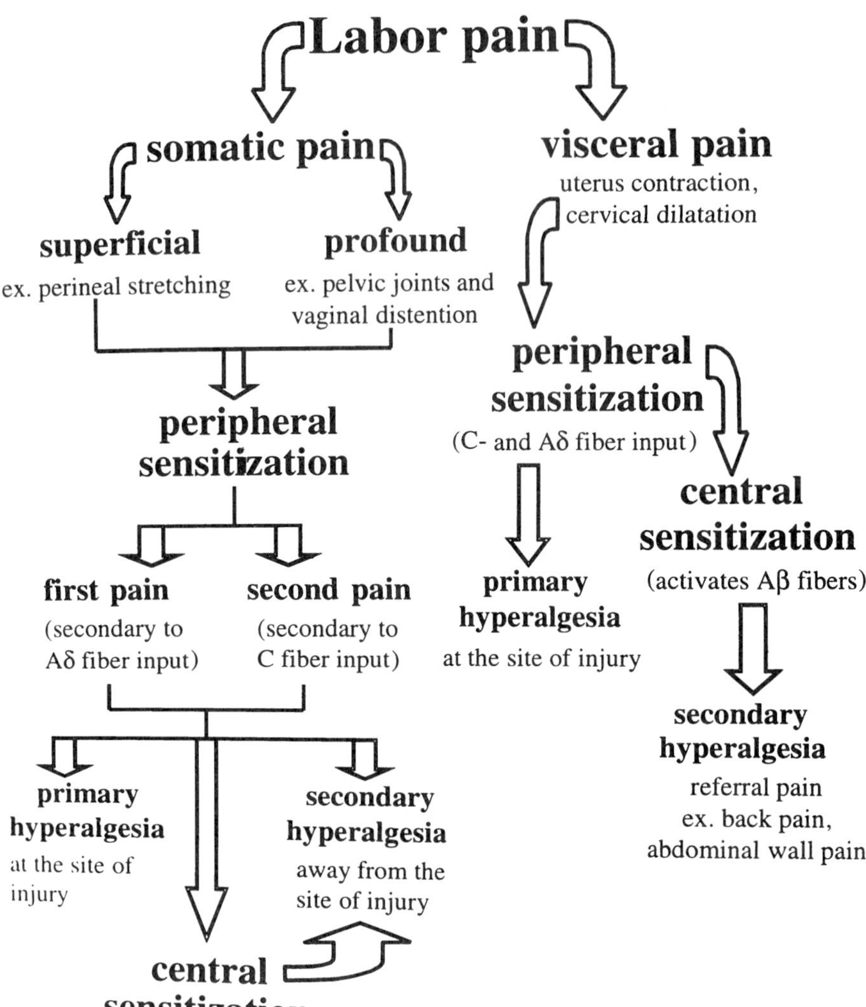

FIG. 3. Untreated labor pain results in acute somatic and visceral pain that will lead to peripheral and central sensitization.

ical mediators. Central sensitization from a noxious stimulus, such as incisional pain, also can activate other nerve fibers, such as the large, low-threshold mechanoreceptive Aβ-primary sensory neurons, which are not usually involved in pain (28).

Nociceptors are polymodal: they respond to thermal, mechanical, and chemical noxious (or painful) stimuli. Under normal circumstances, most are inactive and unresponsive ("silent" or "sleeping"). Silent nociceptors have been described in joint structures and cutaneous and visceral nerves (37,38). Inflammation can sensitize these nociceptors (38,39). They develop spontaneous discharges and become more responsive to peripheral stimulation.

Inflammatory mediators, released in damaged tissue, sensitize nociceptors by activating second-messenger systems (38–40). Afferent nociceptors have pharmacologic receptors on their surface membranes for:

- Opioids,
- γ-Aminobutyric acid (GABA) [benzodiazepines applied spinally were more efficient for somatic than for visceral pain (41)],
- Bradykinin,
- Histamine,
- Serotonin,
- Capsaicin (42), and
- Excitatory amino acids (43).

After peripheral injury, many afferent fibers also express newly formed adrenoreceptors (44,45).

After leaving the periphery, the afferent nerve fibers accompany the sympathetic nerves, passing to the uterine plexus, then to the inferior, middle, and superior hypogastric plexus, and finally to the aortic plexus of the celiac plexus. The nociceptive afferents then travel to the lumbar sympathetic chain and run cephalad with the lower thoracic sympathetic nerves. They leave the sympathetic chain through the rami communicantes associated with the T_{10}, T_{11}, T_{12}, and L_1 (occasionally L_2 and L_3) spinal nerves (Fig. 4). The cell bodies of these afferent fibers lie within the dorsal root ganglia. The afferent fibers pass through the posterior spinal nerve roots and make synaptic contact in the dorsal horn of the spinal gray matter, at:

- Lamina I,
- Laminae II and III (substantia gelatinosa),
- Laminae IV to VI (nucleus proprius) (46), and in the ventral horn, at
- Laminae VII and VIII (47), and
- Lamina X (48).

Visceral Pain Pathways

Visceral pain from labor starts during the later part of pregnancy as the uterus begins irregular, sporadic contractions known as false labor or Braxton Hicks contractions. Uterine visceral pain during false labor can be treated with rest and the peripheral anticholinergic *N*-butyl scopolamine. Whether this compound's analgesic action comes from blockade of nicotinic receptors in sympathetic ganglia or a direct muscarinic antispasmodic effect on the viscera is unclear (49). The onset of labor is characterized by regular, active, painful uterine contractions, which decrease in intensity after birth but continue beyond the fourth stage of labor (see Fig. 3).

Acute pain after visceral injury is often intense, vaguely localized, referred to distant regions of the body (referred pain), and accompanied by powerful motor and autonomic reactions, including spasms of the abdominal musculature and increased sympathetic outflow (50). The area of referral is segmental and superficial (muscle or skin) and corresponds to the spinal segments that innervate the involved viscera. Stimulation of visceral nerves at low intensities produces a vague feeling of fullness and nausea. Higher intensities cause a sensation of pain (51).

The viscera are innervated by vagal and spinal afferent pathways comprising thinly myelinated A_δ fibers and unmyelinated C fibers. Silent nociceptors also have been described in visceral nerves (37,38). These nociceptors are found in mucosal, muscle, and serosal layers of viscera and exhibit chemosensitivity, thermosensitivity, and mechanosensitivity. Spinal visceral nerve cell bodies are located in dorsal root ganglia. On their route to the spinal cord, these nerves typically pass through or near prevertebral ganglia (where they can give off collateral axons to autonomic ganglion cell bodies) and paravertebral ganglia. Visceral afferent nerve fibers display a consistent pattern of central termination throughout the spinal cord. Areas of projection include laminae I and V, but not the intermediate dorsal horn. Visceral afferent nerve fibers reach the dorsal horn via Lissauer's tract and join medial and lateral bundles of fine fibers that run along the edges of the dorsal horn (Figs. 5 and 6) (52). Somatic neurons are located mainly in laminae II, III, and IV of the dorsal horn, whereas viscera–somatic neurons are located in laminae I, V, and in the ventral horn (53).

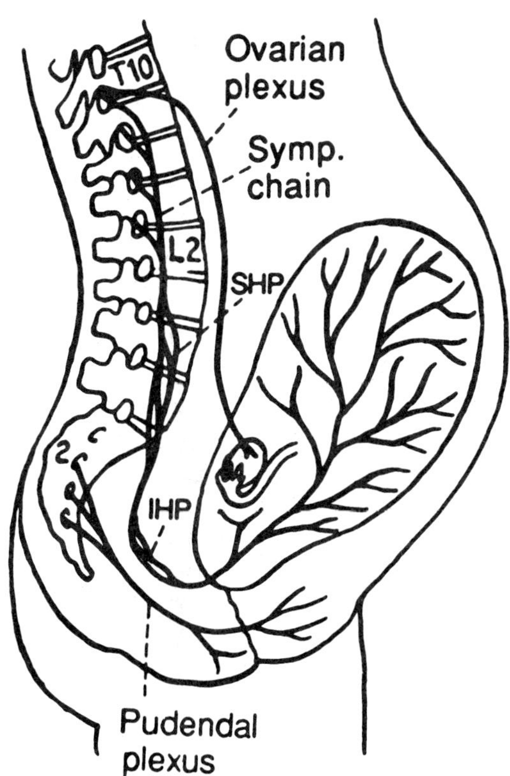

FIG. 4. Peripheral nociceptive pathways involved in the pain of parturition. The uterus, including the cervix and lower uterine segments, is supplied by afferents that accompany sympathetic nerves through the inferior hypogastric plexus (SHP), to the lumbar and lower thoracic sympathetic chain. Then they enter the spinal cord at T_{10}, T_{11}, T_{12}, and L_1. (From ref. 8, with permission.)

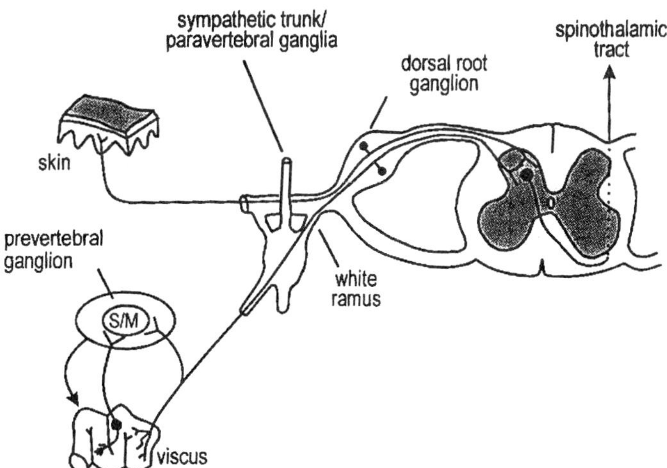

FIG. 5. Anatomic organization of visceral afferent fibers and convergence of cutaneous and visceral afferent inputs in the spinal dorsal horn. *S* and *M*, secretory and motor functions, respectively, of postganglionic neurons; not illustrated are the efferent inputs to the prevertebral ganglion. (From ref. 52, with permission.)

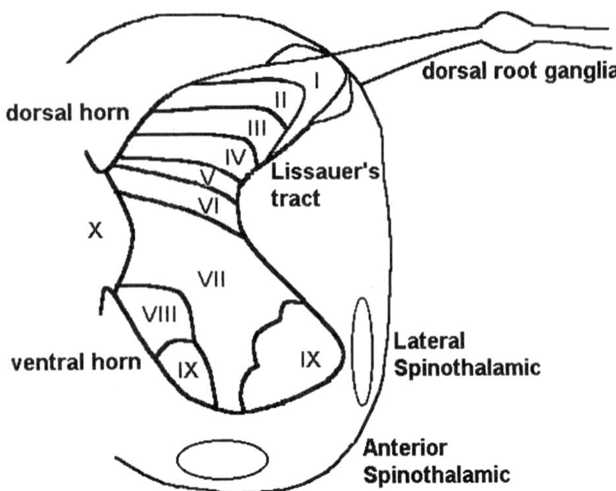

FIG. 6. Spinal laminae and tracts. (From Figs. 5 and 6, ref. 52, with permission.) Somatic neurons are mainly located in laminae II, III, and IV of the dorsal horn, whereas viscera–somatic neurons are located in laminae I, V, and in the ventral horn. Visceral afferent nerve fibers reach the dorsal horn via Lissauer's tract.

The viscera are sparsely innervated, and many C fibers respond to stimuli from more than one organ. Spinal visceral afferents compose only 2% to 10% of the total spinal afferent nerve fibers. Conversely, somatic tissue is more richly innervated. Consequently, visceral pain is vague and poorly localized, whereas somatic input is promptly localized. Some compensation for the low number of visceral afferents is provided by the significantly greater rostrocaudal intraspinal spread of visceral afferent nerve terminals. Finally, the spinal neurons on which visceral afferents terminate typically receive convergent cutaneous and deep input.

Most mechanosensitive afferents innervate muscle, but two populations of mechanosensitive afferents innervate viscera: 70% to 80% of fibers have a low response threshold, and 20% to 30% have high threshold. The uterus is innervated by a population of afferent fibers that do not begin to respond until the distending stimulus intensity is in the range of pressures associated with pain. Whether these afferents are nociceptors is currently a matter of debate.

Opioid receptors also play a role in activating sympathetic and parasympathetic low-threshold visceral nerves (54). Spinal μ-opioid (55), κ-opioid (56), and α_2-adrenergic receptors (55) are involved in visceral and somatic antinociception. Although animal data suggest a synergistic interaction between μ-opioid and α_2-adrenergic sites (55), data from parturients after cesarean section suggest only an additive interaction (57).

Visceral afferents undergo peripheral and central sensitization, which produces visceral hyperalgesia, felt mainly as discomfort and pain associated with visceral disorders. Sensitization of afferent visceral fibers increases afferent neural input to the spinal cord and alters sensation. Spinal cord release of neurotransmitters, including glutamate and peptides, such as substance P, follows activation of silent nociceptors. These compounds alter the excitability of spinal neurons. Thus visceral hyperalgesia produces central sensitization by a mechanism similar to cutaneous models. Nerve growth factor also may have a role in the peripheral and central sensitization (58).

Visceral inflammation enhances the effect of opioids (3 times for morphine and 1.9 times for fentanyl) at peripheral, but not central, receptors. Intestinal inflammation sensitizes μ, but not κ-opioid receptors (59). It is currently unknown whether a similar phenomenon occurs in the uterus.

Spinal Pain Modulation

Peripheral nociceptive afferents terminate in an ordered way in the dorsal horn of the spinal cord. The thinly myelinated A_δ fibers end in laminae I and V. The unmyelinated C fibers enter outer lamina I and lamina II. These high-threshold sensory fibers activate a large number of second-order interneurons within the dorsal horn (60). There are functionally two main groups of dorsal horn cells:

- The "nociceptive-specific," and
- The "multireceptive" (also called "wide dynamic range" or "convergent").

The former respond solely to noxious stimuli, whereas the latter also are activated by innocuous stimuli (61). Interneuronal networks in the spinal gray matter modulate nociceptive information and transmit it to neurons that project to the brain. While certain stimuli sensitize these projection neurons and increase nociceptive transmission, other inputs produce inhibition. The balance between the excitatory and inhibitory processes is the basis of the gate theory of pain transmission (62).

Apparently the progressive stretching of the uterine muscle fibers during pregnancy from fetal growth does not sensitize visceral afferents or cause visceral central sensitization, which would decrease sensitivity to anesthetics or analgesics. Conversely, during pregnancy, there is an increased susceptibility to local anesthetic neural blockade (63). There is a high prevalence of back pain (49%) during pregnancy (64). Back pain during labor is associated with cervical dilation (L_1 and L_2 roots) (65), whereas the progressive uterine muscle fibers stretching from the fetal growth during pregnancy (T_{11} and T_{12} roots) might play a role in patients who complain of back pain during pregnancy.

Spinal Neurotransmitters and Neuromodulators

The spinal neurotransmitters come from afferent nerve fibers, intrinsic neurons, and descending fibers. These transmitters include (Fig. 7):

- Excitatory amino acids, particularly glutamate,
- Neuropeptides, such as substance P,
- Calcitonin gene-related peptide,
- Vasoactive intestinal polypeptide (66),
- Prostaglandins,
- Dopamine,
- Serotonin,
- GABA,
- Catecholamines,
- Somatostatin,
- Acetylcholine,
- Histamine,
- Nitric oxide, and
- Others (67–69).

As with peripheral nociceptors, sensitization of dorsal horn nociceptive neurons is the result of activation of second-messenger systems. Particular signal-transduction cascades involved include the protein kinase C system (70,71) and probably other pathways (51). In addition, noxious stimulation evokes expression of c-Fos from dorsal horn spinal cord neurons (72). The protein c-Fos is a nuclear product encoded by the immediate-early gene c-*fos* and is an indicator of a noxious stimulus. The μ-opioid agonists and several antiinflammatories reduce noxious stimulus–evoked c-Fos expression in the spinal cord (73–75).

Inhibitory neurotransmitters in the nociceptive circuits of the dorsal horn include:

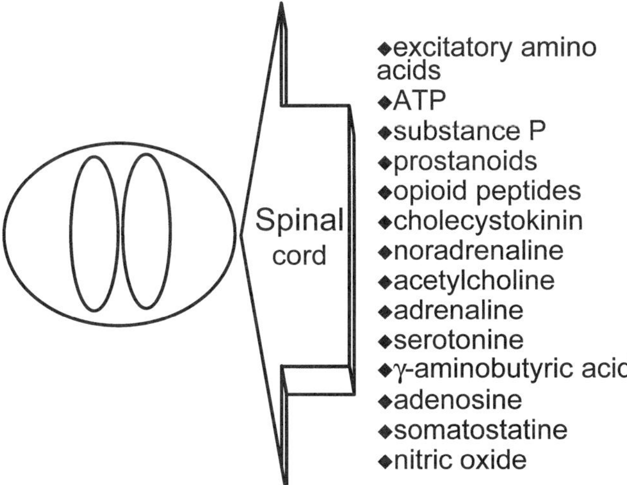

FIG. 7. Spinal neurotransmitters and neuromodulators involved in pain processing.

- Opioid agonists,
- Enkephalins,
- GABA,
- Glycine, and
- Noradrenaline.

The analgesia produced by spinal opioids comes from binding to specific opioid receptors located on the primary afferents and second-order neurons. Opioid binding inhibits nociceptive transmission to the thalamus and cortex. There are μ, δ-, and κ-opioid receptors in the substantia gelatinosa (laminae II and III) and nucleus proprius (laminae IV, V, and VI) of the dorsal horn (76). Spinal opioids also decrease the release of substance P and calcitonin gene-related peptide (77), and block N-type voltage-dependent Ca^{2+} channels (78). In addition, stimulation of both spinal and supraspinal opioid-sensitive sites may be essential for the production of analgesia by spinally administered opioids (79,80). Morphine produces analgesia by binding at supraspinal μ_1 receptors and the spinal μ_2 receptors. Respiratory depression is secondary to binding at supraspinal μ_2 receptors (79). Another important mechanism by which opioids produce analgesia is activation of neurons in the mid-brain and medulla with descending inhibitory projections to the spinal cord dorsal horn (81). NMDA receptors in the rostral ventromedial medulla modulate the transmission of opioid pain-inhibitory signals from the periaqueductal gray matter (82).

The $GABA_A$ and $GABA_B$ receptor subtypes have both pre- and postsynaptic inhibitory actions. Glycine acts postsynaptically to inhibit nociceptive transmission (83,84). Norepinephrine diminishes substance P release from primary A_δ and C afferents (85) and reduces response of dorsal horn neurons to noxious stimuli (86). It also modulates pain by stimulating acetylcholine release by binding to α_2-adrenoreceptors on spinal cholinergic interneurons (87). Centrally, presynaptic α_2 activation may exacerbate pain, but postsynaptic α_2 and α_1 binding sites may be involved in inhibitory descending pain pathways that relay to the nucleus proprius (laminae IV, V, and VI of the medulla).

Ascending Pain Pathways

After processing in the dorsal horn, nociceptor input travels directly, or via brainstem relay nuclei, to the thalamus and then into the cortex, where the conscious sensation of pain is generated. Simultaneously, output from the dorsal horn activates flexor motor neurons in the ventral horn, generating the withdrawal reflex. Both the sensation of physiologic pain and the flexion withdrawal reflex occur together (88).

Nociceptive projection neurons in the spinal cord transmit information to a number of regions of the brainstem and diencephalon, including:

- Thalamus,
- Periaqueductal gray matter,
- Parabrachial region,
- Bulbar reticular formation,
- Limbic structures in the hypothalamus,
- Amygdaloid nucleus,
- Septal nucleus, and
- Cortex and other sites (51).

These projection neurons travel in the spinothalamic, spinomesencephalic, spinoreticular, and spinolimbic (66) tracts, which lie in the anterolateral quadrant of the spinal cord. Pathways in the dorsal quadrant include the spinocervicothalamic and postsynaptic dorsal column tracts.

A large fraction of spinothalamic and spinomesencephalic tract cells are concentrated in the lumbar and sacral laminae I, IV to VI, and X (46). Some spinothalamic neurons respond to stimulation of receptors in muscle (89), joints (90), or viscera (91,92). A visceral nociceptive pathway exists in the dorsal column (93–95). Spinothalamic neurons with a dominant input from viscera or muscle are situated in segments just rostral and caudal to segments containing spinothalamic tract cells with a dominant cutaneous input from the distal part of an extremity (96).

Uterine and vaginal distention induces nociceptive activity in neurons of the dorsal column nuclei (97). These responses may be triggered by unmyelinated primary afferent fibers that ascend in the dorsal column directly to the dorsal column nuclei (98,99). Alternatively, they could be mediated through the postsynaptic dorsal column pathway (100) and cells of the gracile nucleus (93,94). This visceral information is relayed together with cutaneous epicritic (i.e., somatic pain conducted by A_δ fibers) information in the medial lemniscus to the thalamus. Most neurons (85%) in the ventral posterior lateral nucleus of the thalamus respond to both cutaneous and visceral stimuli (101,102). Although the cutaneous input is somatotopic, the visceral input is not viscerotopic (102).

Descending Pain Pathways

The sensation of pain is subject not only to modulation during its ascending transmission from the periphery through the medulla to the cortex, but also to segmental modulation and descending control from higher centers (Fig. 8). This control is manifested via pathways that originate at the level of the cortex, the thalamus, and the brainstem [the periaqueductal gray, the raphe nuclei (raphe dorsal nucleus and raphe magnus), and locus coeruleus and subcoeruleus complex]. Other structures involved include limbic structures, the Kölliker–Fuse nuclei, and several nuclei of the bulbar reticular formation. Descending inhibition from the thalamus is in part mediated via relay stations in the brainstem. Projections

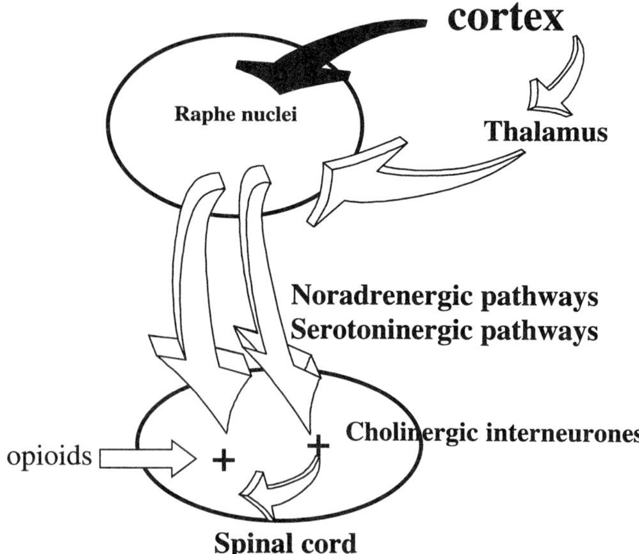

FIG. 8. The descending control of pain is manifested via pathways that originate at the level of the cortex, the thalamus, and the brainstem. Descending noradrenergic pain pathways would activate chroninergic spinal interneurones to inhibit pain transmission. (From ref. 87, with permission.)

of the spinomesencephalic tract to the periaqueductal gray matter could activate the descending analgesia system that arises from the periaqueductal gray matter. Most of the connections of the periaqueductal gray to the spinal cord are indirect (51,103).

The main neurotransmitter systems implicated in descending pain control are (61,71,87):

- Serotonin ($5\text{-}HT_{1A}$ and $5\text{-}HT_3$ receptors),
- α_2-adrenoreceptors,
- $GABA_A$ receptors,
- Glycine receptors,
- Acetylcholine receptors, and
- Opioid receptors.

Whether $GABA_A$ and glycine are released from long descending axons from the rostral ventromedial medulla (104) or from inhibitory interneurons in the spinal cord is unclear (51). In addition to catecholaminergic modulation, dopaminergic inhibition of nociceptive dorsal horn cells has been reported (105).

FACTORS INFLUENCING THE SEVERITY OF LABOR PAIN

Pain is a subjective phenomenon commonly characterized as a multidimensional experience, varying in quality and intensity. Pain-intensity scales can be used clinically to guide the provision of analgesia and to quantify pain. They consist of a line with two opposites that can be numeric (varying from 0, "no pain at all," to 10 cm, "worst possible pain"), or categoric (varying from "no pain" to "worst possible pain") (Fig. 9). Pain-descriptor questionnaires such as the McGill Pain Questionnaire (106) assess both the quality and intensity of pain. It consists of 20 sets of words describing sensory, affective, evaluative, and miscellaneous dimensions of the experience of pain (Fig. 10).

The severity of labor pain varies widely (Fig. 11: pain scores from the McGill Pain Questionnaire), with many factors influencing its severity.

Neurohumoral Changes

Neurohumoral changes occurring in pregnancy may modify the responses to pain (107). Pregnancy is associated with an increased nociceptive tolerance related to increased plasma β-endorphin concentrations. The opioid antagonist naltrexone reverses this effect (107). Lower plasma substance P concentration also may contribute to the altered pain tolerance in pregnancy (108,109). In addition, progesterone (110) modifies deactivation of substance P by an endopeptidase (111). Clinically, pregnant women need approximately 30% less local anesthetics for epidural analgesia than do nonpregnant women (112). Although some of this effect may be related to increased sensitivity to local anesthetics (see later), some also may be related to changes in pain tolerance associated with pregnancy.

Pregnancy also is associated with an increased sensitivity to both regional and general anesthetics (113,114). This altered susceptibility may be due to:

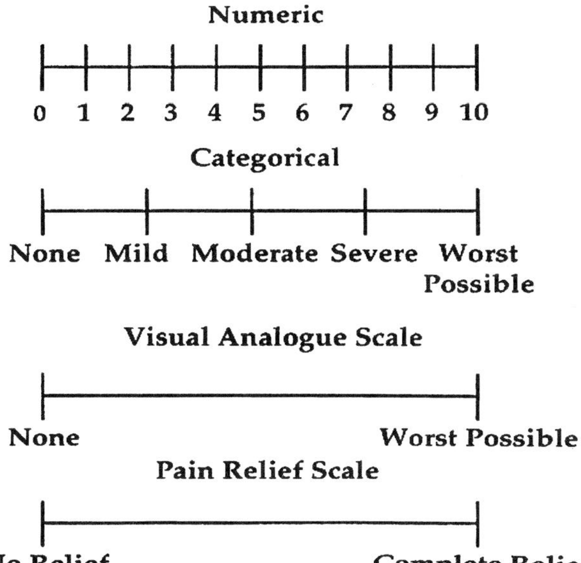

FIG. 9. Pain Intensity Scales. (From Ferrante FM. *ASA Guidelines for Cancer Pain Management.* ASRA Notebook, 1996 Annual Meeting, 423, with permission.)

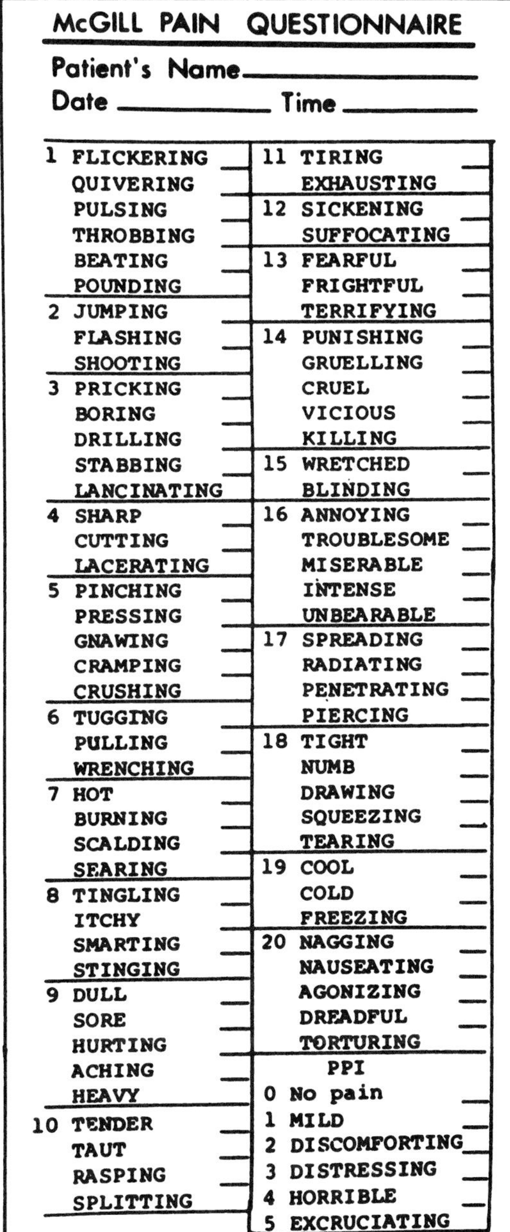

McGILL PAIN QUESTIONNAIRE

Patient's Name ____________
Date ________ Time ________

1 FLICKERING, QUIVERING, PULSING, THROBBING, BEATING, POUNDING	11 TIRING, EXHAUSTING
2 JUMPING, FLASHING, SHOOTING	12 SICKENING, SUFFOCATING
3 PRICKING, BORING, DRILLING, STABBING, LANCINATING	13 FEARFUL, FRIGHTFUL, TERRIFYING
4 SHARP, CUTTING, LACERATING	14 PUNISHING, GRUELLING, CRUEL, VICIOUS, KILLING
5 PINCHING, PRESSING, GNAWING, CRAMPING, CRUSHING	15 WRETCHED, BLINDING
6 TUGGING, PULLING, WRENCHING	16 ANNOYING, TROUBLESOME, MISERABLE, INTENSE, UNBEARABLE
7 HOT, BURNING, SCALDING, SEARING	17 SPREADING, RADIATING, PENETRATING, PIERCING
8 TINGLING, ITCHY, SMARTING, STINGING	18 TIGHT, NUMB, DRAWING, SQUEEZING, TEARING
9 DULL, SORE, HURTING, ACHING, HEAVY	19 COOL, COLD, FREEZING
10 TENDER, TAUT, RASPING, SPLITTING	20 NAGGING, NAUSEATING, AGONIZING, DREADFUL, TORTURING
	PPI: 0 No pain, 1 MILD, 2 DISCOMFORTING, 3 DISTRESSING, 4 HORRIBLE, 5 EXCRUCIATING

FIG. 10. McGill Pain Questionnaire. Categories of pain sensory, 1 to 10; affective, 11 to 15; evaluative, 16; and miscellaneous, 17 to 20. Rank value for each word based on position of word category. Sum of rank values = pain-rating index (PRI). Index of present pain intensity (PPI) is based on scale of 0 to 5. (From ref. 135, with permission.)

- A direct effect of progesterone on membrane excitability,
- Indirect actions of neurotransmitters,
- Increased permeability of the neural sheath,
- Potentiation of the analgesic effect of endogenous opioids (116), or

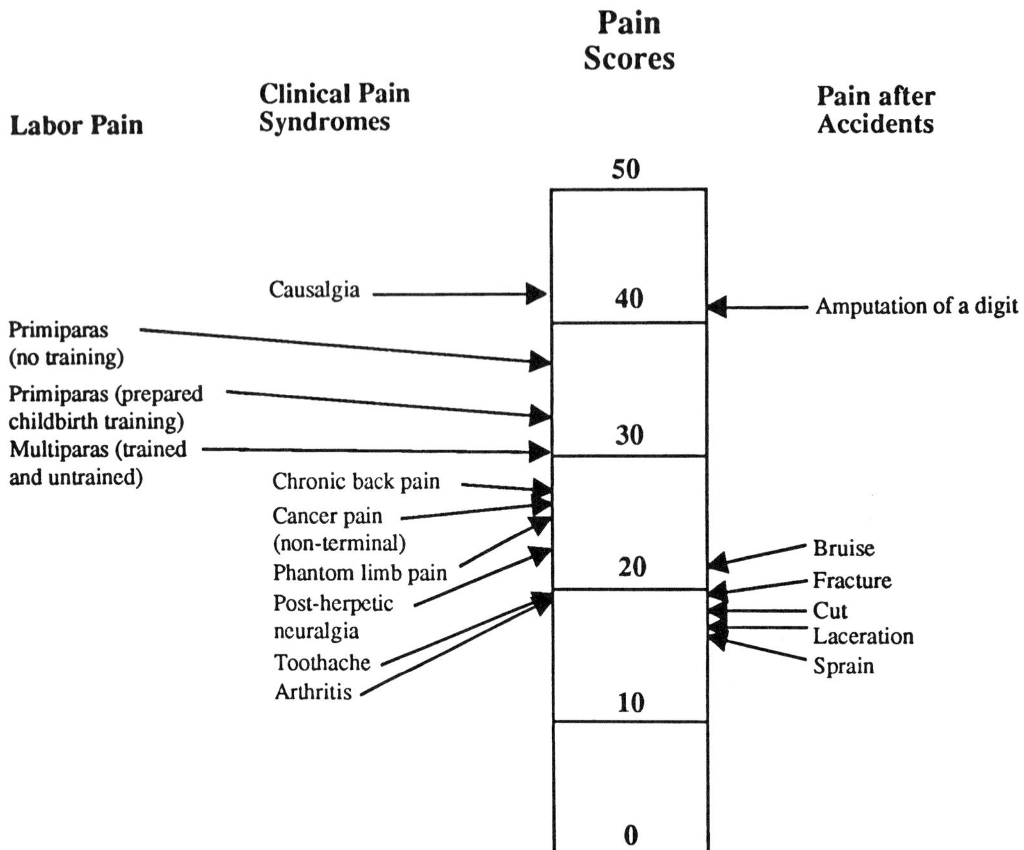

FIG. 11. Pain scores derived from the McGill Pain Questionnaire. The graph compares the severity of labor pain with pain recorded in the emergency room after a variety of accidents. In addition, the graph depicts pain intensity as reported in pain clinics for several clinical pain syndromes. (From ref. 119, with permission.)

- Pharmacokinetic and pharmacodynamic differences between pregnant and nonpregnant women.

While studies in humans find that pregnancy is associated with increased susceptibility to local anesthetic blockade (113), some controversy surrounds this issue (115). C fibers from ventral and dorsal nerve root axons of pregnant rats are less sensitive to local anesthetics than are those from nonpregnant rats (115).

Related to central sensitization, the hormonal changes of pregnancy may influence pain neuropeptides in the spinal cord. The increase in pain threshold is likely to be maximal toward the end of gestation, possibly related to opioid activity in the spinal cord (117). Both somatic and visceral antinociceptive effects of epidural lidocaine are potentiated in near-term pregnant rats (63). However, smaller doses of epidural lidocaine are more effective for visceral than for somatic pain (63). Whether the increased endogenous opioid reduces the noxious stimuli-evoked c-Fos expression at the spinal cord, as observed in animals (118), has not been investigated.

Obstetric Factors

Labor is less painful in multigravidae than primigravidae (see Fig. 11) (119). Women having their first labor complain of more intense pain, have longer labors, and consume more analgesics than do multiparous patients (120). The frequency of contractions and cervical dilatation predict pain for primigravid women, but only the amount of cervical dilatation predicts pain in multiparae (121). Regardless of parity, untreated parturients report the highest pain scores at 8- to 10-cm cervical dilatation. Advanced cervical dilation requires an increased concentration of epidural bupivacaine for analgesia (122). Histories of severe menstrual and low-back pain also correlate with pain scores in labor (123), whereas the roles of fetal position (124) and oxytocin (125) are controversial.

Physical and Chemical Factors

Both physical and chemical factors may alter a patient's response to epidural labor analgesia. Pregnancy alters the distribution of local anesthetics within the spinal canal and enhances the sensitivity of nerves to local anesthetic blockade. Reduced thoracic kyphosis and caudad position of the apex of the lumbar lordosis may help enhance cephalad spread of spinal analgesia in late pregnancy (116). In addition, Bromage et al. (112) and Gin et al. (114) found increased spread of spinal and epidural blockade in early pregnancy. These changes are unlikely to be related to changes in posture, but instead may be related to enhanced neural sensitivity (63).

Independent of pregnancy, cephalad spread of analgesia may be reduced in patients with history of extradural anesthesia because of local aseptic inflammatory changes, and these inflammatory changes are unrelated to the number of previous epidurals. Inflammatory changes observed include proliferation of connective tissue, adhesions between the dura mater and the ligamentum flavum, granulations, and irregularities of the extradural spaces (126). However, other authors showed no differences in success rate of subsequent epidural anesthetics (127).

CSF pH is higher in the second and third trimesters of gestation (7.33 to 7.34) compared with that in nonpregnant patients (7.30). Higher pH increases the amount of local anesthetic in the nonionized base form, which should enhance the rate of diffusion across the nerve sheath and nerve membrane, contributing to faster onset of block in pregnant patients (128). However, clinical studies showed that pregnancy-induced changes in acid–base state of CSF (CSF pH, pCO_2, HCO_3^-) have little effect on the spread of spinal anesthesia (128).

Demographic Variables

There are marked differences in pain beliefs among different cultures (129). Each patient has a unique background, personality, religion, previous experience, and expectation, all of which can influence the pain experience. For example, American women expected labor to be more painful than Dutch women (130), and Catholic women reported less pain during active labor than either Protestant or nonreligious parturients (131).

Aging impairs pain perception (132). Although both A_δ and C fibers are clearly affected, preferential loss of myelinated fibers occurs with aging (133). Vibrotactile sensitivity, which is subserved by $A\beta$ fibers, seems to provide the earliest detectable evidence of age-related disturbance of sensory function (134). In agreement, older women have less painful labors than younger women (135).

Anxiety

Untrained primigravidae reported more severe labor pain than those attending childbirth classes (see Fig. 11) (119). Neurons from the spinothalamic tract that project to the central lateral nucleus in the median thalamus have large receptive fields and may have a role in the motivational–affective aspects of pain (136) rather than in sensory discrimination (51). Motivational–affective circuits can mimic pain states, most notably in patients with anxiety (i.e., an untrained primigravida).

Although the available data suggest that a prepared mother will be less anxious and cope better with labor pain, the mechanism of anxiety's impact on pain is controversial. Anxiety shows a strong correlation with visual-analog scale (VAS) ratings of pain and unpleasantness. The higher the levels of anxiety, the higher the VAS scores of pain and unpleasantness (132). In addition, anxiety and stress induce release of epinephrine, which may sensitize or directly activate peripheral nociceptors. Cholecystokinin (CCK) also may play a role in anxiety and the transmission of nociceptive information (137). Selective CCK_A or CCK_B antagonists may potentiate morphine analgesia (138).

Conversely, anxiety also may release endogenous opioids, and there are strong suggestions that anxiety can inhibit pain perception, not directly, but by diverting attention from the painful stimulus (139). Anxiety focused on pain may increase pain, whereas anxiety focused on other sources may reduce pain.

Placebo Responders

The placebo phenomenon has not been studied in labor. Placebo analgesia is a situation in which the administration of a substance known to be nonanalgesic, such as saline solution, produces analgesia in a believer. It is mediated by endogenous opiates (μ- and δ-, but not κ-receptors) (140,141), is antagonized by naloxone (142), and there may be a role for cholecystokinin in placebo responders (143).

ANALGESIA AND LABOR

Little is known of the effects of epidural analgesia on the progress of labor, method of delivery, and neonate. In the second stage of labor, there is evidence that epidural analgesia attenuates endogenous oxytocin production (Ferguson's reflex) (144) and reduces uterine contractility (145). It is assumed that the motor block associated with epidural analgesia reduces maternal effort during pushing and causes relaxation of the pelvic floor, which predisposes to malrotation of the fetal head. In the first-stage labor, epidural analgesia does not reduce uterine contractility, but may slow cervical dilatation (146). Intravenous atropine, 250 μg, increases maternal cervical dilatation during the active phase of the first stage in women receiving epidural analgesia (G.R.F. Silva, personal communication, 1997).

Fluid infused before regional analgesia transiently decreases uterine activity. A liter of normal saline decreases uterine activity for 10 to 20 minutes (147). The rapid volume expansion may cause a sudden release of the atrial natriuretic peptide (ANP) or have a direct mechanical effect on the uterine vasculature, producing local release of endothelial vasoactive peptides (147). ANP is directly secreted by the atrium. It causes vasodilatation, natriuresis and diuresis, and inhibits the secretion and action of angiotensin II and noradrenaline (148). It is also a potent inhibitor of the uterine contractility (149). Plasma concentration of ANP increases slightly during pregnancy and further with volume loading. Intravenous infusion of 250 mL of dextran 40 in laboring patients increased plasma concentration of ANP by 172% (150).

IMPLICATIONS

Pain can be therapeutically approached at the supraspinal, spinal, and peripheral levels. Supraspinal structures such as the ventral posterior lateral nucleus or the spinal dorsal column nuclei could be specifically stimulated to produce labor analgesia. Peripherally, the observation that most nociceptors are normally "silent" or "sleeping" but become sensitized by inflammation suggests that blocking peripheral sensitization or the respective spinal field can minimize pain. Central sensitization requires that temporal or spatial summation of postsynaptic excitatory potentials exceeds the action-potential threshold of the cell. The receptive field of a dorsal horn neuron is divided into the firing zone and the subliminal zone, which surrounds the former and does not respond to the initial repetitive stimuli (151). In this subliminal zone, an increase in excitability can convert a previously subthreshold stimulus to a suprathreshold stimulus and generate a hyperexcitable state. This phenomenon can be reduced or avoided by preadministration of various agents, such as opioids, local anesthetics, nonsteroidal antiinflammatory drugs, clonidine, nitric oxide or ketamine (preemptive analgesia) (152–154). However enticing the concept of preemptive analgesia may be, its role in the routine management of labor pain is limited, as pain has already occurred and sensitization changes are already established by the time the parturient seeks medical assistance. Unfortunately, postinjury analgesia has a much-diminished effect on an established state of hyperexcitability. Low doses of morphine prevent central sensitization, but once it is established, high doses are necessary to suppress it (155).

An alternative approach to labor analgesia should involve searching for a synergistic combination of drugs that would enhance pre- and postsynaptic inhibition of dorsal horn nociceptive circuits. The ideal method of analgesia would relieve pain before and during tissue injury and last until complete tissue healing occurs. Intrathecal, but not epidural, local anesthetics inhibit temporal summation of repeated electric stimuli (156,157). These data may provide a rationale for the use of combined spinal/epidural or continuous spinal techniques in laboring women.

RATIONALE FOR PAIN RELIEF

The pain of labor serves no useful purpose. Women neither want nor need to experience labor pain. Unfortunately, some still believe that the experience of labor pain enhances a parturient's birth experience. Others fear that adequate analgesia will impair the progress of labor, and many anesthesiologists are unwilling to commit the time and resources needed to offer effective labor analgesia to women who request it.

Although the severity of labor pain may decrease with subsequent pregnancies, its characteristics remain constant (1). The semantic memory of this pain is deeply imbedded in our culture. This memory will remain even without constant reinforcement that occurs when an individual parturient suffers. By using our growing understanding of pain processing and the mechanisms of analgesia, anesthesiologists can strive to provide safe, effective labor analgesia that does not adversely effect the progress or outcome of labor (158).

REFERENCES

1. Niven CA, Brodie EE. Memory for labor pain: context and quality. *Pain* 1995;64:387.
2. Melzak R. Labour pain as a model of acute pain. *Pain* 1993;53:117.
3. Cleland JGP. Paravertebral anaesthesia in obstetrics. *Surg Gynecol Obstet* 1933;57:51.
4. Head H. On disturbances of sensation with special reference to the pain of the visceral disease. *Brain* 1983;16:1.
5. Mackenzie J. *Symptoms and their interpretation.* New York: Paul B Hoeber, 1912.
6. Thacker SB, Banta HD. Benefits and risks of episiotomy: an interpretative review of the English language literature, 1860-1980. *Obstet Gynecol Surv* 1983;38:322.
7. Reynolds SRM. *Physiology of the uterus.* 2nd ed. New York: Paul B Hoeber, 1949.
8. Bonica JJ. *The management of pain.* 2nd ed. Philadelphia: Lea & Febiger, 1990:1326.
9. Moir C. The nature of the pain of labor. *J Obstet Gynecol* 1939;46:409.
10. Dick-Read G. *Childbirth without fear.* New York: Harper, 1953.
11. Bonica JJ. *Obstetric analgesia and anesthesia.* 2nd ed. Seattle: University of Washington Press, 1980:46.
12. Cervero F, Meyer RA, Campbell JN. A psychophysical study of secondary hyperalgesia: evidence for increased pain to input from nociceptors. *Pain* 1994;58:21.
13. Choe H, Choi Y-S, Kim Y-H, et al. Epidural morphine plus ketamine for upper abdominal surgery: improved analgesia from preincisional versus postincisional administration. *Anesth Analg* 1997;84:560.
14. Jurna I, Sohree B, Bock R. Intrathecal injection of acetylsalicylic acid, salicylic acid and indomethacin depresses C fibre-evoked activity in the rat thalamus and spinal cord. *Pain* 1992;49:249.
15. Akman H, Aksu F, Gaveltekin I, et al. A possible central antinociceptive effect of dipyrone in mice. *Pharmacology* 1996;53:71.
16. Nagy I, Woolf C. Lignocaine selectively reduces C fibre-evoked neuronal activity in rat spinal cord in vitro by decreasing *N*-methyl-D-aspartate and neurokinin receptor-mediated post-synaptic depolarizations; implications for the development of novel centrally acting analgesics. *Pain* 1996;64:59.
17. Meller ST, Gebhart GF. Nitric oxide (NO) and nociceptive processing in the spinal cord. *Pain* 1993;52:127.
18. MacMahon SB, Lewin GR, Wall PD. Central hyperexcitability triggered by noxious inputs. *Curr Opin Neurobiol* 1993;3:602.
19. Andersen OK, Jensen LM, Brennum J, Arendt-Nielsen L. Evidence for central summation of C and A_δ nociceptive activity in man. *Pain* 1994;59:273.
20. Nagy I, Maggi CA, Dray A, Woolf CJ, Urban L. The role of neu-

rokinin and *N*-methyl-D-aspartate receptors in synaptic transmission from capsaicin sensitive primary afferents in the rat spinal cord in vitro. *Neuroscience* 1993;52:1029.
21. Pockett S. Spinal cord synaptic plasticity and chronic pain. *Anesth Analg* 1995;80:173.
22. Cook AJ, Woolf CJ, Wall PD, McMahon SB. Dynamic receptive field plasticity in the rat spinal cord dorsal horn following C-primary afferent inputs. *Nature* 1987;325:151.
23. Yamamoto T, Yaksh TL. Studies on the spinal interactions of morphine and the NMDA receptor antagonists MK-801 on the hyperesthesia observed in a rat model of sciatic mononeuropathy. *Neurosci Lett* 1992;135:67.
24. Nathan PW. Touch and surgical division of the anterior quadrant of the spinal cord. *J Neurol Neurosurg Psychiatry* 1990;53:935.
25. Simone DA, Alreja M, Lamotte RH. Psychophysical studies of the itch sensation and itchy skin (allokinesis) produced by intracutaneous injection of histamine. *Somatosens Mot Res* 1991;8:271.
26. LaMotte RH, Shain CN, Simone DA, Tsai EFP. Neurogenic hyperalgesia: psychological studies of underlying mechanisms. *J Neurophysiol* 1991;41:509.
27. Ward L, Wright E, McMahon SB. A comparison of the effects of noxious and innocuous counterstimuli on experimentally induced itch and pain. *Pain* 1996;64:129.
28. Brenann TJ, Vandermeulen EP, Gebhart GF. Characterization of a rat model of incisional pain. *Pain* 1996;64:493.
29. Pleuvry BJ, Lauretti GR. Biochemical aspects of chronic pain and its relationship to treatment. *Pharmacol Ther* 1996;71:313.
30. Marshall KW, Chui B, Inman RD. Substance P and arthritis: analysis of plasma and synovial fluid levels. *Arthritis Rheum* 1990;33:87.
31. Basbaum A. Mechanisms of substance P-mediated nociception and opioid-mediated nociception. In: Stanley T, Ashburn M, eds. *Anesthesiology and pain management*. Dordrecht: Kluwer Academic, 1994:1.
32. Dalby PL, Ramanathan S, Rudy TE, Roy L, Amenta JS, Aber A. Plasma and saliva substance P levels: the effects of acute pain in pregnant and non-pregnant women. *Pain* 1997;69:263.
33. Traurig HH, Papka RE, Shew RL. Substance P and related peptides associated with the afferent and autonomic innervation of the uterus. *Ann N Y Acad Sci* 1991;632:304.
34. Terebjrk HE, Ochoa JL, Schady W. Referred pain from intraneural stimulation of muscle fascicles in the median nerve. *Pain* 1984;18:145.
35. Rang HP, Bevans SJ, Dray A. Chemical activation of nociceptive peripheral neurones. *Br Med Bull* 1991;47:534.
36. Yeomans DC, Cooper BY, Vierck CJ Jr. Effects of systemic morphine on responses of primates to first or second pain sensations. *Pain* 1996;66:253.
37. Handwerker HO, Kilo S, Reeh PW. Unresponsive afferent nerve fibres in the sural nerve of the rat. *J Physiol* 1991;435:229.
38. Davis KD, Meyer RA, Campbell JN. Chemosensitivity and sensitization of nociceptive afferents that innervate the hairy skin of the monkey. *J Neurophysiol* 1993;69:1071.
39. Birrell GJ, McQueen DS, Iggo A, Grubb BD. Prostanoid-induced potentiation of the excitatory and sensitizing effects of bradykinin on articular mechanonociceptors in the rat ankle joint. *Neuroscience* 1993;54:537.
40. Schepelmann K, Messlinger K, Schmidt RF. The effects of phorbol ester on slowly conducting afferents of the cat's knee joint. *Exp Brain Res* 1993;92:391.
41. Goodchild CS, Noble DJ. The effects of intrathecal midazolam on sympathetic nervous system reflexes in man: a pilot study. *Br J Clin Pharmacol* 1987;23:279.
42. Dray A. Chemical activation and sensitization of nociceptors. In: Besson JM, Guilbaud G, Ollat H, eds. *Peripheral neurons in nociception: physio-pharmacological aspects*. Paris: John Libbey Eurotext, 1994:49.
43. Lawand NB, Westlund KN, Willis WD. The effects of excitatory amino acids (EAAs) on the discharge of articular sensory receptors in rats. *Neuroscience* 1996;22:1369.
44. Bossut DF, Perl ER. Effects of nerve injury on sympathetic excitation of Aδ mechanical nociceptors. *J Neurophysiol* 1995;73:1721.
45. Xie J, Yoon YW, Yom SS, Chung JM. Norepinephrine rekindles mechanical allodynia in sympathectomized neuropathic rat. *Analgesia* 1995;1:107.
46. Apkarian AV, Hodge CJ. Primate spinothalamic pathways: I. A quantitative study of the cells of origin of the dorso lateral and ventral spinothalamic pathway. *J Comp Neurol* 1989;288:447.
47. Kevetter GA, Haber LH, Yezierski RP, Chung JM, Martin RF, Willis WD. Cells of origin of the spinoreticular tract in the monkey. *J Comp Neurol* 1982;207:61.
48. Willis WD, Kenshalo DR, Leonard RB. The cells of origin of the primate spinothalamic tract. *J Comp Neurol* 1979;188:543.
49. Lauretti GR, Lima ICPR. Intrathecal neostigmine effects on somatic and visceral pain: improvement by association with a peripheral anticholinergic. *Anesth Analg* 1996;82:617.
50. Cervero F, Meyer RA, Campbell JN. Prickle and pain in normal and hyperalgesic skin: evidence that low threshold mechanoreceptors are responsible for the pain of secondary hyperalgesia. *Soc Neurosci Abstr* 1991;17:293.
51. Willis WD, Westlund KN. Neuroanatomy of the pain system and of the pathways that modulate pain. *J Clin Neurophysiol* 1997;14:2.
52. Gebhart GF. Visceral pain: from basic science to patients. Annual Meeting, American Society of Regional Anesthesia, 1996:157.
53. MacMahon SB. Mechanisms of sympathetic pain. *Br Med Bull* 1991;47:584.
54. Balkowiek A, Kukula K, Szulczyk P. Influence of morphine on the activity of low-threshold visceral mechanoreceptors in cats with acute pericarditis. *Pain* 1994;59:251.
55. Harada Y, Nishioka K, Kitahata LM, Kishikawa K, Collins JG. Visceral antinociceptive effects of spinal clonidine combined with morphine, (D-Pen2, D-Pen5) enkephalin, or U50,488H. *Anesthesiology* 1995;83:344.
56. Danzebrink RM, Green AS, Gebhart GF. Spinal mu and delta, but not kappa, opioid-receptor agonists attenuate responses to noxious colorectal distension in the rat. *Pain* 1995;63:49.
57. Eisenach JC, D'Angelo R, Taylor C, Hood DD. An isoholographic study of epidural clonidine and fentanyl after cesarean section. *Anesthesiology* 1994;79:285.
58. MacMahon SB, Dmitrieva N, Koltzenburg M. Visceral pain. *Br J Anaesth* 1995;75:132.
59. Pol O, Sanchez B, Puig MM. Peripheral effects of opioids in a model of intestinal inflammation in mice. *Pharmacology* 1996;53:340.
60. Woolf CJ. Somatic pain: pathogenesis and prevention. *Br J Anaesth* 1995;75:169.
61. Stamford JA. Descending control of pain. *Br J Anaesth* 1995;75:217.
62. Melzak R, Wall PD. Pain mechanisms: a new theory. *Science* 1965; 150:971.
63. Kaneko M, Saito Y, Kirihara Y, Kosaka Y. Pregnancy enhances the antinociceptive effects of extradural lignocaine in the rat. *Br J Anaesth* 1994;72:657.
64. Ostgaard HC, Andersson GBJ, Karlsson K. Prevalence of back pain in pregnancy. *Spine* 1991;16:549.
65. MacEvilly M, Buggy D. Back pain and pregnancy: a review. *Pain* 1996;64:405.
66. Willis WD, Coggeshall RE. *Sensory mechanisms of the spinal cord.* 2nd ed. New York: Plenum Press, 1991.
67. Dickenson AH. Spinal cord pharmacology of pain. *Br J Anaesth* 1995; 75:193.
68. Lauretti GR. Uso de fármacos no analégsicos por via espinal. *Rev Soc Espan Dolor* 1997;4:421.
69. Krukowski J, Hood DD, Eisenach JC. Intrathecal neostigmine for post-cesarean section analgesia: dose-response. *Anesth Analg* 1997; 84:1269.
70. Palecek J, Paleckova PM, Dougherty PM, Willis WD. The effect of phorbol esters on the responses of primate spinothalamic neurons to mechanical and thermal stimuli. *J Neurophysiol* 1994;71:529.
71. Lin Q, Peng YB, Willis WD. Possible role of protein kinase C in the sensitization of primate spinothalamic tract neurons. *J Neurosci* 1996;16:3026.
72. Zieglgänsberger W, Tölle TR. The pharmacology of pain signaling. *Curr Opin Neurobiol* 1993;3:611.
73. Presley RW, Menétrey D, Levine JD, Basbaum AI. Systemic morphine suppresses noxious stimulus-evoked fos protein-like immunoreactivity in the rat spinal cord. *J Neurosci* 1990;10:323.
74. Honoré P, Buritova J, Besson JM. Carrageenan-evoked c-*fos* expression in rat lumbar spinal cord: the effects of indomethacin. *Eur J Pharmacol* 1995;272:249.
75. Buritova J, Honoré P, Besson JM. Enhanced effects of co-administered dexamethasone and diclofenac on inflammatory pain processing and associated spinal cord c-*fos* expression in the rat. *Pain* 1996; 64:559.
76. Willetts J, Balster RL, Leander JD. The behavioral pharmacology of

NMDA receptor antagonists. *Trends in Pharmacology Sciences,* Special Report, Elsevier Science Publ., Amsterdam, 1991;62.
77. Takano M, Takano Y, Yaksh TL. Release of calcitonin gene-related peptide (CGRP), substance P (SP), and vasoactive intestinal polypeptide (VIP) from rat spinal cord: modulation by α_2 agonists. *Peptides* 1993;14:371.
78. Schroeder JE, Fishbach PS, Zheng D, McCleskey EW. Activation of μ opioid receptors inhibits transient high- and low-threshold Ca^{++} currents, but spares a sustained current. *Neuron* 1991;6:13.
79. Pasternack GW. Pharmacological mechanisms of opioid analgesics. *Clin Neuropharmacol* 1993;16:1.
80. Ferouz F, Norris MC, Arkoosh VA, Leighton BL, Boxer LM, Corba RJ. Baricity, needle direction and intrathecal sufentanil labor analgesia. *Anesthesiology* 1997;86:592.
81. Hields HL, Heinricher MM, Mason P. Neurotransmitter in nociceptive modulatory circuits. *Ann Rev Neurosci* 1991;14:219.
82. Spinella M, Cooper ML, Bodnar R. Excitatory animo acid antagonists in the ventromedial medulla inhibit mesencephalic morphine analgesia in rats. *Pain* 1996;64:545.
83. Carlton SM, Westlund KN, Zhang D, Willis WD. GABA-immunoreactive terminals synapse on primate spinothalamic tract cells. *J Comp Neurol* 1992;322:528.
84. Curtis DR, Lacey G. GABA-B receptor-mediated spinal inhibition. *Neuroreport* 1994;5:540.
85. Kuraishi Y, Hirota N, Sato Y, Kaneko S, Satoh M, Takagi H. Noradrenergic inhibition of the release of substance P from the primary afferents in the rat spinal dorsal horn. *Brain Res* 1985;359:177.
86. Headley PM, Duggan AW, Griersmith BT. Selective reduction by noradrenaline and 5-hydroxytryptamine of nociceptive responses of cat dorsal horn neurones. *Brain Res* 1978;145:185.
87. Bouaziz H, Chuanyao T, Yoon Y, Hood DD, Eisenach JC. Intravenous opioids stimulate norepinephrine and acetylcholine release in spinal cord dorsal horn. *Anesthesiology* 1996;84:143.
88. Willer JC. Comparative study of perceived pain and nociceptive flexion reflex in man. *Pain* 1979;3:69.
89. Foreman RD, Schmidt RF, Willis WD. Effects of mechanical and chemical stimulation of fine muscle afferents upon primate spinothalamic tract cells. *J Physiol* 1979;286:215.
90. Dougherty PM, Sluka KA, Sorkin LS, Westlund KN, Willis WD. Neural changes in acute arthritis in monkeys. I. Parallel enhancement of responses of spinothalamic tract neurons. *Brain Res Rev* 1992; 17:1.
91. Ammons WS. Primate spinothalamic cell responses to ureteral occlusion. *Brain Res* 1989;496:124.
92. Ammons WS. Electrophysiological characteristics of primate spinothalamic neurons with renal and somatic inputs. *J Neurophysiol* 1989; 60:1121.
93. Al-Chaer ED, Lawand NB, Westlund KN, Willis WD. Visceral nociceptive input into the ventral posterolateral nucleus of the thalamus: a new function for the dorsal column pathway. *J Neurophysiol* 1996; 76:2661.
94. Al-Chaer ED, Lawand NB, Westlund KN, Willis WD. Pelvic visceral input into the nucleus gracilis is largely mediated by the postsynaptic dorsal column pathway. *J Neurophysiol* 1996;76:2675.
95. Hishberg RM, Al-Chaer ED, Lawand NB, Westlund KN, Willis WD. Is there a pathway in the posterior funiculus that signals visceral pain? *Pain* 1996;67:291.
96. Hoobs SF, Chandler MJ, Bolser DC, Foreman RD. Segmental organization of visceral and somatic input onto C3-T6 spinothalamic tract cells of the monkey. *J Neurophysiol* 1992;68:1575.
97. Berkley KJ, Hubscher CH. Are there separate central nervous system pathways for touch and pain? *Nature Med* 1995;1:766.
98. Patterson JT, Coggeshall RE, Lee WT, Chung K. Long ascending unmyelinated primary afferent axons in the rat dorsal column: immunohistochemical localizations. *Neurosci Lett* 1990;108:6.
99. Conti F, De Biasi S, Giuffrida R, Rustioni A. Substance P-containing projections in the dorsal columns of rats and cats. *Neuroscience* 1990;34:607.
100. Noble R, Riddell JS. Cutaneous excitatory and inhibitory input to neurones of the postsynaptic dorsal column system in the cat. *J Physiol* 1988;396:497.
101. Chandler MJ, Hobbs SF, Fu QG, Kenshalo DR, Blair RW, Foreman RD. Responses of neurons in the ventroposterolateral nucleus of primate thalamus to urinary bladder distension. *Brain Res* 1992;571:26.
102. Brüggemann J, Shi T, Apkarian AV. Squirrel monkey lateral thalamus. II. Viscerosomatic convergent representation of urinary bladder, colon, and esophagus. *J Neurosci* 1994;14:6796.
103. Cameron AA, Khan IA, Westlund KN, Willis WD. The efferent projections of the periaqueductal gray in the rat: a *Phaseolus vulgaris* leucoagglutination study. II. Descending projections. *J Comp Neurol* 1995;351:585.
104. Antal M, Petko M, Polgar E, Heizmann CW, Storm-Mathisen J. Direct evidence of an extensive GABAergic innervation of the spinal cord dorsal by fibres descending fron the restro ventro-medial medulla. *Neuroscience* 1996;73:509.
105. Barasi S, Bem-Steri MM, Clatworthy AL, et al. Dopamine-receptor-mediated spinal antinociception in the normal and haloperidol pretreated rat: effects of sulpiride and SCH23390. *Br J Pharmacol* 1987; 90:15.
106. Melzack R. The McGill Pain Questionnaire: major properties and scoring methods. *Pain* 1975;1:277.
107. Iwasaki H, Collins JG, Saito Y, Kerman-Hinds A. Naloxone-sensitive pregnancy-induced changes in behavioral responses to colorectal distension: pregnancy-induced analgesia to visceral stimulation. *Anesthesiology* 1991;74:927.
108. Mouton SM, Kambam JM, Naukum RB, Blanks SC, Sastry BPR. Substance P levels are decreased in pregnancy. *Anesthesiology* 1991; 75:A842.
109. Dalby PL, Ramathan S, Rudy TE, Roy L, Amenta JS, Aber A. Plasma and saliva substance P levels: the effects of acute pain in pregnant and non-pregnant women. *Pain* 1997;69:263.
110. Jayaram AM, Carp HP. Progesterone-mediated potentiation of spinal sufentanil in rats. *Anesth Analg* 1993;76:745.
111. Casey ML, Smith JW, Nagai K, Hersh LB, MacDonald PC. Progesterone-regulated cyclic modulation of membrane metalloendopeptidase (enkephalinase) in human endometrium. *J Biol Chem* 1991;266: 23041.
112. Bromage PR. Spread of analgesic solutions in the epidural space and their site of action: a statistical study. *Br J Anaesth* 1962;34:161.
113. Butterworth JF, Walker FO, Lysak SZ. Pregnancy increases median nerve susceptibility to lidocaine. *Anesthesiology* 1990;72:962.
114. Gin T, Mainland P, Chan MTV, Short TG. Decreased thiopental requirements in early pregnancy. *Anesthesiology* 1997;86:73.
115. Deitz FB, Jaffe A. Pregnancy does not increase susceptibility to bupivacaine in spinal root axons. *Anesthesiology* 1997;87:610.
116. Hirabayashi Y, Shimizu R, Saitoh K, Fukuda H. Cerebrospinal fluid progesterone in pregnant women. *Br J Anaesth* 1995;75:683.
117. Whipple B, Josimovich JB, Kamisaruk BR. Sensory thresholds during the antepartum, intrapartum, and postpartum periods. *Int J Nurs Stud* 1990;27:213.
118. Tölle TR, Schadrack J, Castro-Lopes JM, Evan G, Roques BP, Zieglgansberger W. Effects of Kelatorphan and morphine before and after noxious stimulation on immediate-early gene expression in rat spinal cord neurons. *Pain* 1994;56:103.
119. Bonica JJ. After Melzak R: the myths of painless childbirth (The John Bonica Lecture). *Pain* 1984;19:231.
120. Gaston-Johansson F, Fridh G, Turner-Norvell K. Progression of labor pain in primiparas and multiparas. *Nurs Res* 1988;37:86.
121. Lowe N. Parity and pain during parturition. *J Obstet Gynecol Neonatal Nurs* 1987;September/October 1987;5:340.
122. Capogna G, Celleno D, Lyons G, Fusco P. Minimum local analgesic concentration of extradural bupivacaine increases with progression of labour. *Br J Anaesth* 1998;80:11.
123. Melzak R, Belonger E. Labour pain: correlations with menstrual pain and acute low back pain before and during pregnancy. *Pain* 1989;36:225.
124. Wuichick M, Bakal D, Lipshitz J. The clinical significance of pain and cognitive activity in latent labor. *Obstet Gynecol* 1989;73:35.
125. Onur E, Ercal T, Karslioglu I. Prolactin and cortisol levels during spontaneous and oxytocin-induced labour and the effect of meperidine. *Arch Gynecol Obstet* 1989;244:227.
126. Igarashi T, Hirabayashi Y, Shimizu R, et al. Inflammatory changes after extradural anaesthesia may affect the spread of local anaesthetic within the extradural space. *Br J Anaesth* 1996;77:347.
127. Blanche R, Eisenach JC, Dewan DM. Previous wet tap does not reduce success rate of labor epidural analgesia. *Anesth Analg* 1994; 79:291.
128. Hirabayashi Y, Shimizu R, Fukuda H, Igarashi T. Acid-base state of

cerebrospinal fluid during pregnancy and its effect on spread of spinal anaesthesia. *Br J Anaesth* 1996;77:352.
129. Thomas VJ, Rose FD. Ethnic differences in the experience of pain. *Soc Sci Med* 1991;32:1063.
130. Senden IPM, Wetering MD, Eskes TKAB, Brerkens PB, Laube DW, Pitkin RM. Labor pain: a comparison of parturients in a Dutch and an American teaching hospital. *Obstet Gynecol* 1988;71:541.
131. Wuitchick M, Hesson K, Bakal D. Perinatal predictors of pain and distress during labor. *Birth* 1990;17:186.
132. Chakour MC, Gibson SJ, Bradbeer M, Helme RD. The effect of age on Aδ- and C-fibre thermal pain perception. *Pain* 1996;64:143.
133. Ochoa J, Mair WGP. The normal sural nerve in man. II. Changes in the axons and Schwann cells due to aging. *Acta Neuropathol* 1969;13:217.
134. Katzman R, Rowe JW. *Principles of geriatric neurology.* Philadelphia: Davis, 1992:281.
135. Melzak R, Kinch R, Dobkin P, Lebrun M, Taenzer P. Severity of labour pain: influence of physical as well as psychologic variables. *Can Med Assoc J* 1984;130:579.
136. Ammons WS, Girardot MN, Foreman RD. T2-T5 spinothalamic neurons projecting to medial thalamus with viscerosomatic input. *J Neurophysiol* 1985;54:73.
137. Woodruff GN, Hughes J. Cholecystokinin antagonists. *Annu Rev Pharmacol Toxicol* 1991;31:469.
138. Singh L, Oles RJ, Field MJ, Atwal P, Wooddruff GN, Hunter JC. Effect of CCK receptor antagonists on the antinociceptive, reinforcing and gut motility properties of morphine. *Br J Pharmacol* 1996;118:1317.
139. Janssen AS, Arntz A. Anxiety and pain: attentional and endorphinergic influences. *Pain* 1996;66:145.
140. Lord JAH, Waterfield AA, Hughes J, Kosterlitz HW. Endogenous opioid peptides: multiple agonists and receptors. *Nature* 1977;267:495.
141. Lavigne GJ, Hargreaves KM, Schmidt EA, Dionne RA. Proglumide potentiates morphine analgesia for acute postsurgical pain. *Clin Pharmacol Ther* 1989;45:666.
142. Levine JD, Gordon NC, Fields HL. The mechanism of placebo analgesia. *Lancet* 1978;2:654.
143. Benedetti F. The opposite effects of the opiate antagonist naloxone and the cholecystokinin antagonist proglumide on placebo analgesia. *Pain* 1996;64:535.
144. Goodfellow CF, Hull MGR, Swaab DF, Dogterom J, Buijs RM. Oxytocin deficiency at delivery with epidural analgesia. *Br J Obstet Gynecol* 1983;90:214.
145. Bates RG, Helm CW, Duncan A, Edmonds DK. Uterine activity in the second stage of labour and the effect of epidural analgesia. *Br J Obstet Gynecol* 1985;92:1246.
146. Newton ER, Schroeder BC, Knape KG, Bennett BL. Epidural analgesia and uterine function. *Obstet Gynecol* 1995;85:749.
147. Cheek TG, Samuels P, Miller F, Tobin M, Gutsche BB. Normal saline iv load decreases uterine activity in active labour. *Br J Anaesth* 1996;77:632.
148. Genest J, Cantin M. Atrial natriuretic factor. *Circulation* 1987;75:118.
149. Beck T, Ottesen B, Fahrenkrung J. The effect of gallanin, CGRP and ANP on spontaneous smooth muscle activity of rat uterus. *Peptides* 1988;9:497.
150. Eledjam JJ, Thomas H, Macheboeuf M, Baudin G, Ferrer JM, D'Athis F. Influence of vascular loading on the secretion of the atrial natriuretic factor during epidural analgesia for labor. *Anesthesiology* 1989;71:A876.
151. Woolf CJ, King AE. Physiology and morphology of multireceptive neurons with C-afferent fibre inputs in the deep dorsal horn of the rat lumbar spinal cord. *J Neurophysiol* 1987;58:460.
152. Coderre TJ, Katz J, Vaccarino AL, Melzak R. Contribution of central neuroplasticity to pathological pain review of clinical and experimental evidence. *Pain* 1993;53:259.
153. Lauretti GR, Azevedo VMS. Intravenous ketamine or fentanyl prolongs postoperative analgesia after intrathecal neostigmine. *Anesth Analg* 1996;83:766.
154. Woolf CJ, Chong M-S. Preemptive analgesia: treating postoperative pain by preventing the establishment of central sensitization. *Anesth Analg* 1993;77:1.
155. Woolf CJ, Wall PD. Morphine-sensitive and morphine-insensitive actions of C-fibre input on the rat spinal cord. *Neurosci Lett* 1986;64:221.
156. Curatolo M, Pelersen-Felix S, Arendt-Nielsen L, Fischer M, Zbinder AM. Temporal summation during extradural anaesthesia. *Br J Anaesth* 1995;75:634.
157. Curatolo M, Petersen-Felix S, Arendt-Nielsen L, Zbinder AM. Spinal anesthesia inhibits central temporal summation. *Br J Anaesth* 1997;78:88.
158. Chestnut DH, McGrath JM, Vincent RD Jr, et al. Does early administration of epidural analgesia affect obstetric outcome in nulliparous women who are in spontaneous labor? *Anesthesiology* 1994;80:1201.

Obstetric Anesthesia, second edition,
edited by Mark C. Norris.
Lippincott Williams & Wilkins, Philadelphia © 1999.

CHAPTER 13

Alternatives to Conduction Analgesia

H. Jane Huffnagle and Suzanne Lynne Huffnagle

NONPHARMACOLOGIC PAIN RELIEF

When the anesthetic effects of ether and chloroform were discovered in the mid-1800s, the British clergy argued that human intervention in the miracle of birth was a sin against the will of God. Once Queen Victoria used "blessed chloroform" during her eighth confinement, the practice of limiting labor pain gained wider acceptance (1–3). As labor analgesia became more widely practiced, maternal and infant morbidity and mortality fell. Many attributed this improved outcome to the absence of pain that permitted the obstetrician to work unhindered in difficult labors.

Viewed historically, childbirth has undergone several incarnations:

- A providentially appointed occasion to suffer,
- A ritualized event in the female community,
- A highly charged emotional and physical brush with death, and
- A pathology requiring medical intervention.

Concern for maternal–fetal safety and the desire for a satisfactory birth experience have fostered an "antianesthesia" atmosphere in some obstetric suites. Some claim that "intervention" is unnecessary in the "natural" process of parturition. To them, the use of anesthesia represents patient failure and risks disastrous fetal outcome. This sentiment has led some patients and obstetricians to seek alternative methods of labor pain relief. These options include:

- Prepared childbirth, encompassing techniques of Grantly Dick-Read, Lamaze's psychoprophylaxis, and Leboyer's childbirth without violence,
- Hypnosis,
- Acupuncture,
- Transcutaneous electrical nerve stimulation (TENS), and
- Biofeedback.

Some women also consider nonhospital and often nonmedical delivery (home delivery) options. Laboring women may use these techniques alone or in combination. None precludes the use of other analgesic medications. These methods avoid exogenous drugs; however, most leave the parturient with considerable pain. The birth experience may still be unsatisfactory (or at least very painful).

Prepared Childbirth

Natural Childbirth: The Dick-Read Method

During the past few decades, women in the United States have increasingly elected to have a "natural" childbirth. American culture defines natural childbirth in a variety of ways (4). Some consider it the absence of analgesics during the first stage of labor. Others deem it the absence of monitoring, episiotomies, and all analgesic, anesthetic, and oxytocic medications.

Grantly Dick-Read coined the term *natural childbirth.* He suggested that labor pain arose from socially induced expectations about parturition. He asserted that childbirth is not an inherently painful process. "There is no physiologic function in the body which gives rise to pain in the normal course of health" (5). He outlined the "fear-tension-pain syndrome." In this syndrome, fear incites tension in the circular muscle fibers of the lower part of the uterus. This tension produces pain perception. To eliminate labor pain, Dick-Read advocated correcting the faulty expectations regarding parturition and the use of progressive muscle relaxation. He also introduced breathing exercises, advocating deep breathing during early stages of labor, more rapid breathing during contractions

H. J. Huffnagle and S. L. Huffnagle: Department of Anesthesiology, Thomas Jefferson University Hospital, Philadelphia, Pennsylvania 19107.

toward the end of the first stage, panting during a contraction if bearing down was undesirable, and breath-holding during the process of bearing down (5,6). This method of natural childbirth does have its limitations; even Dick-Read admitted that normal labor could involve some pain.

Psychoprophylaxis

A second major theory of childbirth preparation was developed in the Soviet Union in 1954 by A. Nikolayev. The technique, known as psychoprophylaxis, was presented to Western scientists by Velvovsky (6,7) who, like Dick-Read, postulated that labor was not an inherently painful experience. If a multipara felt pain, she was having "conditioned reflex labor pain." Cortical pain came from neural impulses arising in labor and experienced as painful because of disruption of excitatory–inhibitory processes in the cortex and subcortex. Psychoprophylaxis would prevent excitatory–inhibitory imbalance through:

- Deep breathing during each contraction,
- Stroking of sections of the abdomen combined with deep breathing, and
- Pressure applied to "pain-prevention points" along the small of the back and the medial surface of the anterior superior ilia (8).

Lamaze

A French obstetrician, Fernand Lamaze (Fig. 1), became acquainted with the teaching of Velvovsky in 1951 while touring Russia. Upon returning to France, he began using the techniques, with some of his own variations (9). First, he added rapid breathing during the second stage of labor, and panting during crowning and delivery. Second, he advocated the use of controlled neuromuscular relaxation during labor, which "economizes on oxygen and reduces the production of waste products." He deleted the use of stroking, pain-prevention points, and timing of contractions from Velvovsky's technique (2).

The Lamaze method is the most popular approach to prepared childbirth in the United States, although it is often modified with parts of the Dick-Read method. Differences in preparatory techniques reflect variance in trainers, treatment settings, and theoretical orientations (7). Most programs however, include three distinct components:

- Information about normal anatomy and physiology of pregnancy, labor, and delivery,
- Relaxation training, and
- Breathing techniques that usually follow variations of the format outlined by Dick-Read.

To these three components, many instructors add husband participation. The husband takes an active role in

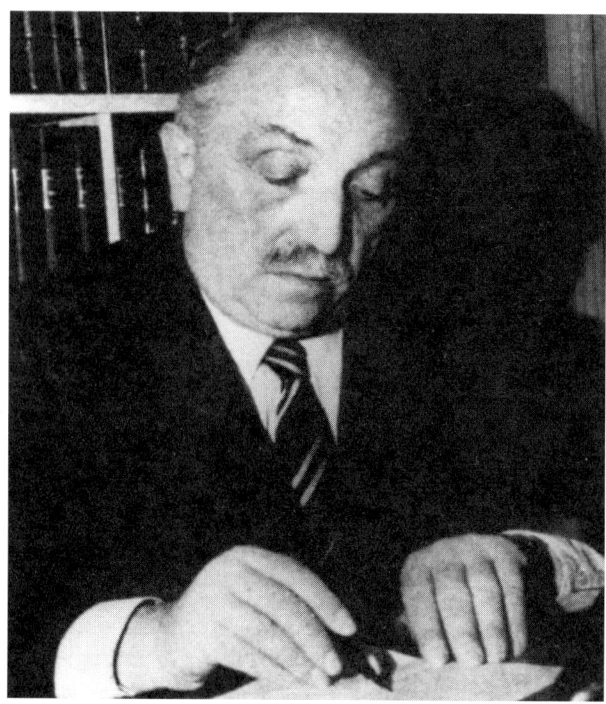

FIG. 1. Fernand Lamaze. (Photo courtesy of Richard Clark, M.D., and Patrick Sim [ASA Library].)

timing contractions, delivering reminders about the use of breathing techniques, and providing support.

Natural childbirth techniques do provide some degree of pain relief. In one study, primiparas who had completed antepartum Lamaze training were given narcotics less frequently during labor, received conduction anesthesia less often, and had a higher frequency of spontaneous vaginal deliveries compared to "matched" controls (Table 1) (8). Melzak and colleagues (10) report that primiparas who had prepared childbirth training reported lower pain scores than those with no training. However, 81% of the prepared childbirth patients still requested epidural anesthesia. Relaxation training is the most therapeutically active component of the Lamaze regimen (11). Lamaze classes teach women breathing, pushing, and relaxation techniques. They hope to instill in mothers the confidence to use these techniques to successfully manage labor (12). Self-evaluation of performance during labor is one of the most important components of the childbirth experience (12).

Bradley

The second most popular form of childbirth education in the United States originates from the work during the 1940s of Robert Bradley, M.D., who believed that women could be taught to cope with labor pain as animals did. He introduced husbands into the labor room and argued against the "meddlesome interference

TABLE 1. *Effect of Lamaze preparation on labor pain and obstetric outcome in primiparous women*

	Lamaze group	Control group	*p* Value
Number of patients	129	129	NS
Oxytocin induction or augmentation (n)	17	20	NS
Mean duration, first stage of labor (h ± SD)	8.98 ± 4.91	8.83 ± 4.34	NS
Mean duration, second stage of labor (min ± SD)	51.0 ± 35.4	56.9 ± 37.8	NS
Spontaneous vaginal delivery (%)	62.8	36.4	<0.001
Low forceps (%)	24.8	53.5	<0.001
Mid forceps (%)	6.2	5.4	NS
Cesarean section (%)	6.2	4.7	NS
No analgesia, first stage of labor (n)	36	9	<0.001
Narcotics	84	109	<0.001
Epidural or caudal	18	52	<0.001
Pudendal block	83	59	<0.001

Data from ref. 8.

with nature's instinctual conduct and plans" and the "terrible indignities of drugs" (13–15). Today, proponents of the Bradley method continue to emphasize unmedicated childbirth, arguing that with the proper preparation and a supportive coach, 9 of 10 women can give birth without medication (16).

Duola

Reassurance and support are important aspects of natural childbirth regimens. A "duola," or supportive lay companion, significantly improves labor outcome. One study examined the effects of a duola on the length of labor and mother–infant interaction in healthy Guatemalan primigravidae (17). Women were initially assigned to a duola or no companion on a random basis. Control women had a significantly higher rate of subsequent perinatal problems (i.e., cesarean section or meconium staining). The authors had to admit 103 mothers to the control group and 33 to the duola group to get 20 uncomplicated deliveries in each group. In the final sample, women having a duola delivered 8.8 hours after admission to the hospital compared to 19.3 hours for those laboring alone. Mothers who had a duola present during labor were awake more after delivery and stroked, smiled at, and talked to their babies more than the control mothers. This same group repeated their study in a hospital in the United States and obtained similar results (18). These observations suggest that constant human support during labor may offer substantial benefits. Lower maternal anxiety and, hence, decreased catecholamine concentrations may be their etiology.

Leboyer

The French obstetrician Frederick Leboyer developed the concept of "childbirth without violence" (19). He believed that noise, bright lights, and other stimulation associated with a traditional delivery caused psychological trauma to the newborn. He advocated delivery in semidarkness, with minimal noise to avoid disturbing the neonate. Immediately after delivery, the baby is lifted onto the mother's abdomen. When the umbilical cord stops pulsating, the baby is lowered into a warm bath. Leboyer's methods have met with considerable controversy. Among the objections:

- Subdued lighting may hinder assessment of the baby's condition and color.
- Hypothermia may develop while the baby is on the mother's abdomen or in the bath.
- Placing the baby on the mother's abdomen, which is higher than the placenta, until the cord stops pulsating can allow a serious loss of blood from baby to placenta.
- Placental transfusion to neonate can result in volume overload, increased hematocrit and blood viscosity, and pulmonary hypertension (20–22).

Henschel (23) addressed some of these concerns by comparing the Leboyer technique to conventional delivery. That study reported the following results:

- Hypothermia did not occur in babies who had skin-to-skin contact with their mother at birth.
- Immersion in the water bath had no adverse effects.
- No baby suffered from treatable jaundice.
- No baby suffered from anemia due to delayed clamping of the cord.
- The quiet and subdued lighting did not interfere with communication or observation of the mother's or baby's condition.

The Leboyer babies cried considerably less, and the mothers' memories of the birth experience were always positive. But, one randomized clinical trial found that the Leboyer method offered no infant or maternal advantage over a gentle, conventional delivery (24).

Nelle et al. (20–22) addressed the placental transfusion issues. Blood transfusion from the placenta to the neonate occurs when the umbilical cord clamping is delayed for more than 5 seconds after delivery and the neonate is at or below the level of the placenta. Up to 35 mL/kg of blood flows to the neonate (25–28). Even with Leboyer deliveries, when the baby is placed on the mother's abdomen, higher than the level of the placenta, there still can be a marked transfusion of placental blood (20). Blood volume may increase rapidly by 50%. Although most infants respond with compensatory vasodilation, some may suffer marked volume overload (21). Plasma extravasates and the resulting hemoconcentration may increase the hematocrit (up to 67%) and the blood viscosity (50%). Even in the absence of clinical signs, this increase in hematocrit may produce pulmonary hypertension lasting several days (22). The amount of placental transfusion during Leboyer deliveries varies. Infants who receive a full placental transfusion of 35 mL/kg are in a state of acute vascular distension and at high risk of cardiac failure, and respiratory and central nervous system problems (29). However, a placental transfusion of 20 mL/kg may be optimal for oxygen transport. Infants delivered according to the Leboyer method should be examined carefully for signs and symptoms of hyperviscosity (21).

Although these various methods of prepared childbirth training may decrease maternal anxiety and pain, many women will still request additional analgesia. Childbirth classes should include reliable information about anesthetic options. Regional anesthesia can be a reasonable compromise that minimizes pain and stress but still allows participation of the mother and father in the birth of their infant.

Hypnosis

Hypnosis has long been used to lessen or relieve the pain of labor and delivery, and it has advantages over other forms of pain relief:

- Hypnosis does not obtund airway reflexes, impair the sensorium, or produce hypoventilation (30).
- It produces neither hypotension nor decreased uteroplacental perfusion.
- It does not cause itching or nausea and vomiting.
- It does not depress the neonate (31).

One study has suggested that hypnosis significantly shortened the first stage of labor (32). Others, however, have found the opposite effect (33). Moya and James (31) reported better acid–base status after birth using hypnosis compared to general anesthesia. Also, infants recover more rapidly from birth asphyxia with hypnosis compared to either general or regional anesthesia (31). A psychologist has described her experience with Lamaze and hypnosis for labor pain relief. She preferred hypnosis, feeling that Lamaze requires much more effort and causes anxiety in anticipation of contractions. She suggests that women can easily learn hypnosis during pregnancy and use it successfully in labor (34). Maternity nurses or labor coaches could help with simple "deepening techniques," eliminating the need for constant physician attendance.

Harmon et al. (35) studied the benefits of hypnotic analgesia as an adjunct to childbirth education in 60 nulliparous women. Hypnotic training significantly raised the pain threshold in susceptible parturients (Figs. 2A and 2B). Women who used hypnosis had a shorter first stage of labor, used less medication, and had more frequent spontaneous deliveries than controls (Table 2). Their infants had higher Apgar scores. Highly susceptible, hypnotically treated women had lower depression scores after birth as well. Superior outcomes in the hypnosis group may result from reduced pain perception as

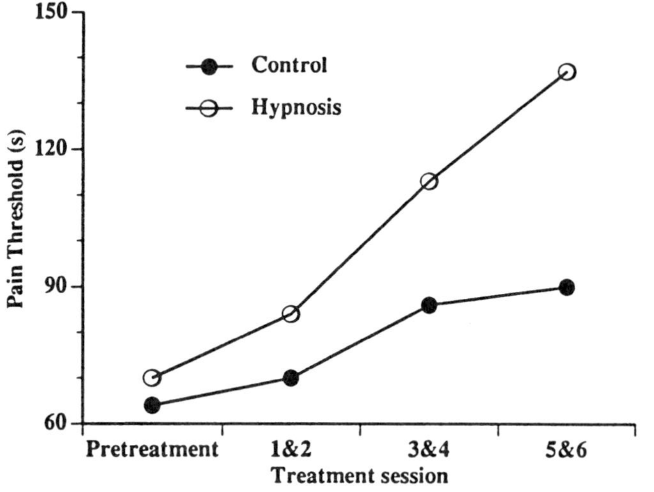

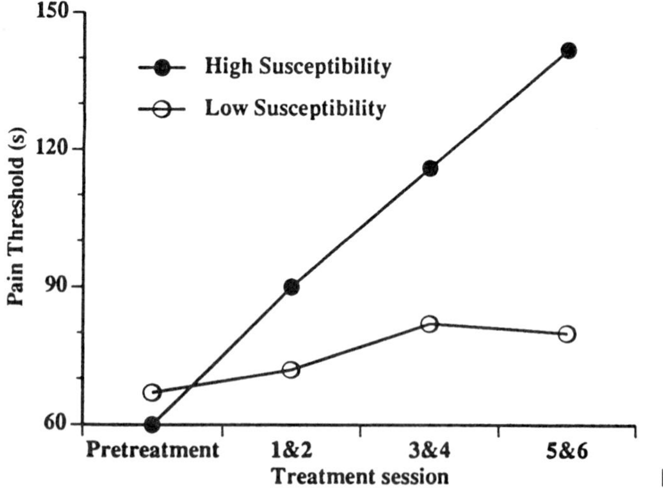

FIG. 2. A: Mean pain threshold for hypnosis and control subjects for tourniquet-induced ischemia. **B:** Mean pain threshold for subjects with high or low susceptibility to hypnosis for tourniquet-induced ischemia. (After ref. 35.)

TABLE 2. *Obstetric outcomes in primiparous women using hypnotic analgesia and skill mastery combined with childbirth education*

	Hypnosis	Control
Stage 1 (min)	78.9 ± 55.3[a]	247.9 ± 141.5
Stage 2 (min)	46.5 ± 27.0	63.5 ± 26.0
Spontaneous delivery	87%[a]	60%
Tranquilizer use	13%[a]	53%
Narcotic use	7%[a]	53%
Oxytocics	33%[a]	93%

[a] $p < 0.01$ vs control. All women listened to childbirth education tapes. Women in the hypnosis group also received instruction and practiced hypnotic induction. Women in both groups were initially determined to have "high susceptibility" to hypnosis.

Data from ref. 35.

well as a higher tolerance to pain (35). Study subjects were highly motivated volunteers, willing to try hypnosis. They participated in twice the typical amount of childbirth training.

Women interested in hypnoanalgesia can be evaluated for suggestibility by using the eye roll test (36). Preparation before labor consists of a series of conditioning sessions about 30 minutes in length. With each session, a greater degree of trance is obtained. One technique consists of an induction involving a counting down from 10 to 0 while descending a flight of stairs. The trance is deepened by imagining peaceful scenes, suggestions of arm levitation, glove anesthesia, and finally abdominal anesthesia (35).

Oster (37) presents a model of psychological preparation that appears to be superior to Lamaze. It uses the following elements:

- An opportunity for the mother to tailor the protocol to her needs and includes husband or "coach" participation in the training,
- Utilization of a "parts model" for the hypnotic induction, deepening, and imagery,
- Incorporation of "hypnotic reversal," dissociation, time distortion, and cognitive reframing, and
- Continued application of the hypnotic procedure after delivery and into the recovery period.

Following delivery, for which they had been specifically prepared, the women in this study reported they also were able to use their hypnosis skills as needed in other medical or dental situations (37).

Hypnosis, however, is not for everyone. Of any random group, only 25% are easily hypnotized (30). Reported complications range from acute anxiety to frank psychosis. Wahl (30) lists seven strong contraindications to hypnosis:

- Evidence of psychosis,
- Evidence of latent, unconscious homosexuality,
- Evidence of a strong unconscious wish to regress,
- History of psychoneurotic hysterical conversion reactions,
- Evidence of strong fear or ambivalence regarding birth or motherhood,
- Hyperemesis gravidarum during the first trimester, and
- Nightmares in the last trimester.

In addition to relieving the pain of labor, hypnosis has been used successfully as an adjunct to the medical treatment of premature labor (38) and in the treatment of acute pregnancy-associated hypertension (39). Although hypnosis may offer advantages over conventional methods of labor analgesia, it will not be effective with everyone and should be used only in carefully selected patients.

Acupuncture

Chinese acupuncture is based upon a belief that chi (qi) energy runs along 12 meridians (channels). There are two forms of energy, yin and yang, which must be in balance; imbalance causes disease and pain. Balance can be regained by inserting needles into acupuncture points, which lie on the meridians, and gently vibrating them. Traditionally, vibrations were generated by hand, but today electrical stimuli are more common (40).

Acupuncture has been used to help control labor pain in China and the Far East for many years. However, even in China, acupuncture produces surgical analgesia in only 60% to 70% of patients (41). It is least effective for pain in the lower part of the body (42). Its success depends on patient selection and motivation, as well as deeply embedded cultural conditioning. Acupuncture can produce a state of hypoalgesia that varies with a given patient's pain threshold. It does not provide complete pain relief. This hypoalgesic state may be mediated by endogenous opioids (endorphins) (43,44).

Abouleish and Depp (45) studied electroacupuncture (the needles are electrically vibrated continuously after insertion) in 12 laboring women. Needles were inserted at selected points depending upon whether the patient was in stage 1 or stage 2 of labor (Fig. 3). The angle, depth, or site of insertion was changed until "Teh-Chi" (warmth, numbness, or tightness at the site of insertion, sometimes radiating along the corresponding meridian) was obtained. The needles were then vibrated at a frequency of 5 to 10 cycles/s. The output from the machine was increased until the patient felt the needles vibrating but no associated discomfort. Four women received no pain relief. Seven reported a 66% reduction of pain. None was completely free of pain. Ten of the 12 required regional anesthesia for delivery; one delivered under acupuncture alone. Another group used only three acupuncture points,

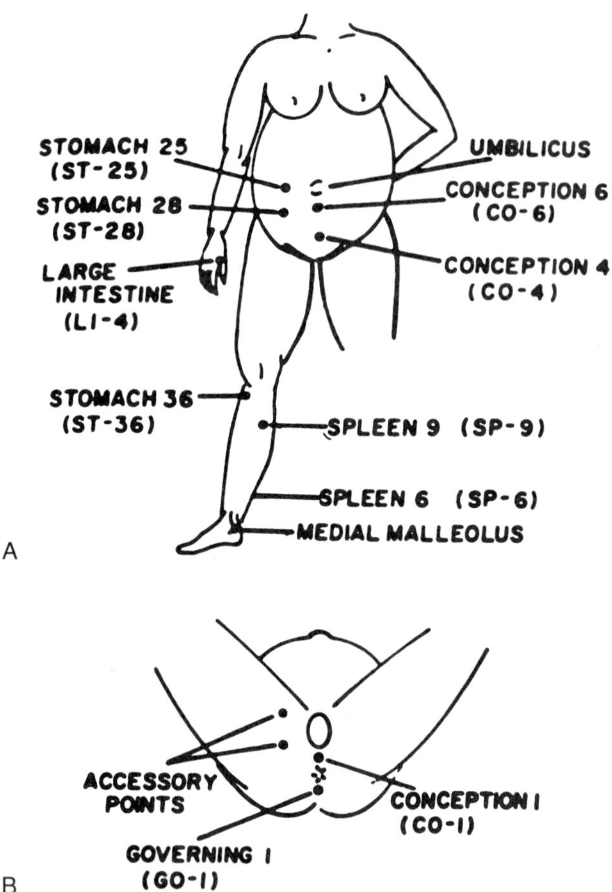

FIG. 3. Acupuncture meridians for pain relief during first stage **(A)** and second stage **(B)** of labor. (Reprinted from ref. 45, with permission.)

all located on one leg (46). Of 85 patients in the acupuncture group, 37 required additional analgesia; however, the first stage of labor was 2.5 hours shorter for primigravidae in the acupuncture group compared with the control group.

In a third study, patients used acupuncture repeatedly in the month before delivery (47). Acupuncture did not improve the women's overall experience of labor and delivery. Still, 95% of the women in the acupuncture group stated that they would request this treatment before a future delivery. Women who received acupuncture felt more in control of their labor and delivery (46).

Acupuncture analgesia is incomplete, unpredictable, inconsistent, and time consuming. Needles may become dislodged, patients' movements are restricted, and electroacupuncture can interfere with electronic monitoring of mother and fetus (45).

Transcutaneous Electrical Nerve Stimulation

Over the past decade, TENS techniques have been developed for chronic pain of various etiologies. Electricity has been used in medicine since A.D. 46, when Scribonius Largus, a Roman physician, used the torpedo fish for the treatment of headache and gout. The shock from the ray stimulated the area and relieved the pain (48). The use of TENS in modern medicine derives from the gate-control theory of pain (49). Accordingly, cells in the posterior horn of the spinal gray matter have a gating function. Activity in low-threshold, large afferent fibers (not conducting pain) closes the gate to the pain pathways. The pain experienced is controlled by the balance between the activity in the low-threshold, large afferent fibers, which have no pain function, and that in the afferent pain fibers (50). TENS is thought to work by a combination of increasing the release of endogenous opiates and "closing the pain gate" (40).

Dilation of the cervix and contraction of the uterus produce most of the pain of the first stage of labor. Visceral fibers of nerve roots T_{10} to L_1 carry this information to the central nervous system. Distention of the pelvic outlet and perineum, and pressure on and stretching of other structures incite pain during the transitional and second stages of labor. This pain travels mostly in somatic fibers of the sacral plexus (51).

The TENS stimulator is a dual-output device. Each output can be varied in both amplitude and rate. The amplitude varies from 0 to 220 V, and frequency ranges from 40 to 150 Hz (52). Two pairs of silicon electrodes are placed paravertebrally at the T_{10} to L_1 and S_2 to S_4 spinal levels (Fig. 4). The amplitude and frequency at the upper level is adjusted until the patient is aware of a tingling or tickling sensation. This stimulation is maintained continuously as background through labor. The amplitude and frequency at the lower level are set higher than the upper. The lower-level electrodes are stimulated from the beginning until 30 seconds after each contraction (52,53). As labor progresses, the frequency and amplitude of stimulation are varied to achieve the best results.

Usually, TENS provides some relief of pain during the first stage of labor. It is less effective in the second stage

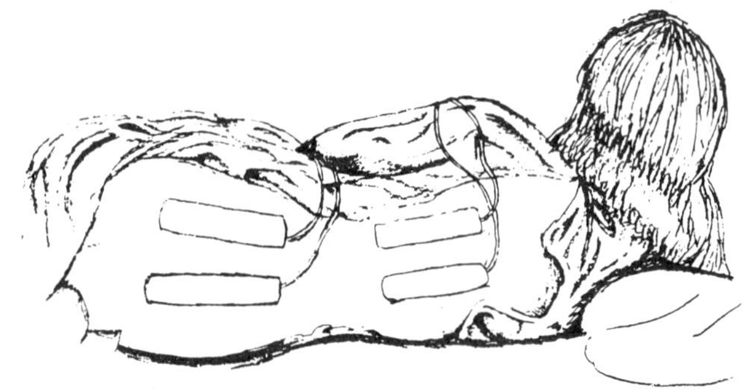

FIG. 4. Transcutaneous electrical nerve stimulation (TENS) electrode placement. The wires connect to a nerve stimulator.

(48,52–54). Some patients find TENS especially helpful with "back labor" (51,53). Augustinsson et al. (55) reported that 44% of 147 laboring women treated with TENS considered the pain relief good or very good, 44% reported moderate pain relief, and 12% felt that it had no effect. Over 70% of parturients find TENS helpful enough to request it for a subsequent labor (48,56). Kemp (40) suggests that placing TENS over acupuncture points would be more efficient than the present placement. TENS decreases the need for narcotic analgesics and may shorten the first stage of labor (48,50). A few cases of TENS interfering with fetal heart monitoring have been reported (50,56,57). The electrical stimulation from the TENS unit causes artifact on the cardiotocograph, which may produce a distorted reading. The TENS unit can be turned off momentarily to obtain a reading, or a filter that suppresses TENS interference can be applied (57).

TENS has certain advantages over other forms of labor analgesia. It is safe, noninvasive, instantly reversible, and can easily be administered by a trained midwife. Although TENS appears to be of minimal benefit in the second stage of labor, it can compliment conventional methods of analgesia (54).

Biofeedback

Biofeedback has been used for more than a decade to help patients cope with chronic pain (58). It has recently been investigated for use during labor and delivery. St. James-Roberts and associates (59) studied two methods of biofeedback training: the autonomic or skin conductance level (SCL) method, and the voluntary-muscle relaxation or electromyographic (EMG) method. In the SCL method, electrodes are placed on the patient's second and third fingers of the left hand, and she wears an earphone. SCL is detected by the electrodes and is indicated to the patient by a series of clicks heard through the earphones. An increase in SCL, heard as an increase in the rate of clicks, indicates increased arousal (Fig. 5). For the EMG method, electrodes are applied 5 cm apart in the mid-line of the abdomen. The ground electrode is placed above the umbilicus and the two active electrodes are placed below (see Fig. 5). The patient also wears an earphone. As with the SCL method, increased EMG activity (decreased relaxation) is indicated by a faster rate of clicks through the earphones. By reducing tension of voluntary muscles, biofeedback may reduce some of the perineal trauma associated with delivery. Second, by concentration and focusing on relaxation, the woman may be distracted from her pain. Muscle relaxation also may reduce perineal trauma and enhance descending modulatory pain pathways (58).

The EMG method seems to the more effective (59). Biofeedback seems more effective in early than active labor. However, women using EMG biofeedback report lower levels of pain both by visual analog scale and by verbal descriptor scale than controls. In one study, women in the biofeedback group labored 2 hours less than the control group and used 30% fewer medications (58).

Biofeedback is easily taught. Instruction can be given in group format, usually in four to six weekly training sessions followed by daily practice at home. However, patients should receive this training before labor.

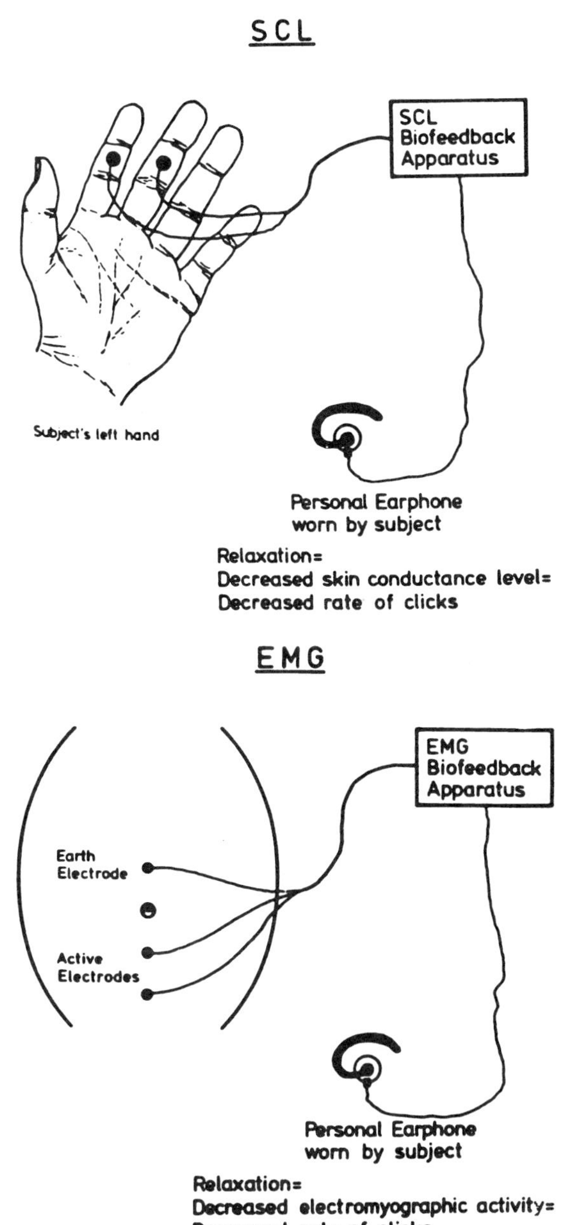

FIG. 5. Biofeedback electrode placement: skin conductance level *(SCL)* and electromyographic *(EMG)* methods. (Reprinted from ref. 59, with permission.)

SYSTEMIC ANALGESICS IN OBSTETRICS

Systemic drugs have been used to decrease pain in labor since 1847. Although spinal or epidural analgesia are the most effective methods of analgesia in labor, the use of systemic medications is still very common for several reasons:

- They are simple to administer and do not require anesthesia personnel.
- They require minimal monitoring.
- They have a low incidence of complications.
- Neuraxial analgesia may not be available in all hospital settings.
- Regional analgesia may be contraindicated in certain conditions.
- Some women fear regional analgesia.

Systemic medications do have their disadvantages, however:

- They seldom provide complete analgesia.
- They cause sedation and possibly respiratory depression in parturients and neonates.
- They delay gastric emptying parturients and may precipitate nausea/vomiting.
- They have been associated with adverse fetal and neonatal effects (loss of beat-to-beat variability, neonatal neurobehavioral changes).

Opioid Analgesics

Parenteral opioids may be given by intermittent bolus or by patient-controlled analgesia (PCA). Intermittent bolus doses can be given either by subcutaneous (s.c.), intramuscular (i.m.), or intravenous (i.v.) injection. The route and timing of administration influence maternal uptake and placental transfer. The s.c. and i.m. injections are simple, but painful. The resultant analgesia is delayed in onset and variable in quality and duration. The i.v. injection provides more uniform quality and onset, so drugs are easier to titrate. PCA is associated with:

- Better pain relief with lower drug doses,
- Less risk of maternal respiratory depression,
- Less placental transfer of drug,
- Less nausea/vomiting, and
- Greater patient satisfaction (60,61).

Smaller, more frequent dosing produces more stable plasma drug concentrations and more consistent analgesia. The intermittent and intensifying episodes of pain that occur during labor unfortunately limit the efficacy of i.v. PCA (62).

Morphine

Morphine, a phananthrene derivative, is the most important alkaloid of opium. It binds in a stereo-specific manner to saturable sites (ν receptors) in the brain, spinal cord, and other tissues (63). The usual doses for maternal analgesia are 2 to 5 mg i.v. or 5 to 10 mg i.m. Onset is 3 to 5 minutes after intravenous or 20 to 40 minutes after intramuscular injection. Morphine is metabolized in the liver to morphine-3-glucuronide and then excreted by the kidneys (64). Morphine rapidly crosses the placenta and the blood–brain barrier of the immature fetus (65). Maternal morphine decreases fetal heart rate (FHR) variability and also may lower baseline FHR (66). Neonates are very susceptible to the respiratory depressant effects of morphine. They are more sensitive to morphine than meperidine, possibly due to a greater permeability of the infant brain to morphine (67). This sometimes profound newborn respiratory depression and excessive maternal sedation have caused morphine to fall into disfavor as a labor analgesic. However, because of the short maternal elimination half-life, Gerdin et al. (64) suggest its use as an analgesic in labor be reevaluated.

Meperidine

Meperidine is a narcotic analgesic qualitatively similar to morphine. A 60- to 80-mg i.v. dose is approximately equianalgesic with 10 mg of morphine (63). Because of its potency and lipophilicity (which speed onset), meperidine is one of the most widely used opioids for labor analgesia. Doses range from 25 to 50 mg i.v. or 50 to 100 mg i.m. every 2 to 4 hours. Onset is within 5 minutes after i.v. and 45 minutes after i.m. injection. Meperidine is usually given with a phenothiazine because it can cause significant nausea and vomiting. After i.v. injection, maternal plasma meperidine concentration peaks within 1 minute and remains detectable throughout labor. A 50-mg dose of i.v. meperidine appears in fetal blood within 90 seconds and equilibrates between maternal and fetal compartments in 6 minutes (68). Its half-life is about 2.5 hours in the mother (69) and 18 to 23 hours in the neonate (70).

Meperidine is metabolized in the liver to three compounds: meperidic acid, normeperidic acid, and the pharmacologically active normeperidine. Normeperidine is first detectable in maternal plasma 10 minutes after injection. Plasma concentration rises rapidly for 20 minutes and then continues to increase slowly throughout labor (69). Normeperidine readily crosses the placenta and its half-life in the neonate is about 60 hours (60). Neonatal concentrations may be further increased by its own metabolism of placentally transferred meperidine.

Maternal meperidine has been associated with neonatal depression. The incidence of neonatal depression is related to the time between injection and delivery, the quantity of drug administered, and the rate of maternal metabolism (71). Maximal neonatal depression occurs 2 to 3 hours after maternal injection (72,73). When the drug is given within 1 hour of birth, neonatal depression is rare.

The variable neonatal response to maternal meperidine correlates with the drug's fetal kinetics. In the first 2 hours, fetal tissue uptake limits plasma meperidine concentrations. After 3 hours, the fetus is clearing the drug from its tissues (74). In addition, normeperidine is a potent respiratory depressant, and this compound, rather than meperidine, may be responsible for neonatal depression (71). Others argue that neonatal depression is related, not to normeperidine, but to the amount of unmetabolized meperidine passing from mother to fetus (73,74). Even if normeperidine is not the main culprit after a single maternal dose of meperidine, it may become clinically important following multiple doses. Multiple maternal doses of meperidine create a continuous diffusion gradient from mother to fetus, maximizing fetal exposure to both meperidine and normeperidine. Both compounds accumulate in fetal tissues (75,76). Pharmacologically, the best time to be born following maternal meperidine is within 1 hour, or more than 4 hours, after a single, small i.v. dose (76). Both meperidine and normeperidine may produce subtle changes in neonatal neurobehavior (77–80).

Maternal meperidine administration can diminish FHR variability for up to 1 hour. Long-term variability is impaired more than short-term variability (81). Maternal meperidine also decreases the frequency and duration of fetal movements. This effect is maximal in the first 20 minutes after injection (82). These two issues may cause confusion when trying to assess the fetal state (81).

Finally, although traditional teaching states that meperidine decreases uterine contractility and slows latent labor, the opposite may be true. Animal studies report increased frequency (83,84) and amplitude (84) of uterine contractions after meperidine administration. Women who receive meperidine for analgesia appear to have shorter labors than those who receive morphine (85). Devoe et al. (86) conclude that meperidine does not stop true labor and is often associated with an increase in uterine contractility. Elimination of pain or awareness of pain will decrease adrenal medullary release of epinephrine, a known inhibitor of uterine activity, and should lead to increased uterine activity. Meperidine's ability to stimulate cervical proteases may accelerate cervical effacement and distention (87).

Fentanyl

Fentanyl is a very lipid-soluble and highly protein-bound drug, which is about 100 times as potent as morphine and about 750 times as potent as meperidine (63). Its onset is almost immediate when given intravenously and 7 to 8 minutes following i.m. injection. Maximal analgesia and respiratory depression may not occur immediately. Analgesia usually persists 30 to 60 minutes after a single i.v. dose of up to 100 μg and 1 to 2 hours after i.m. injection. As with all opioid analgesics, the respiratory depressant effects may outlast analgesia (63). Because of its rapid onset, short duration, absent active metabolites, and low emetic activity, fentanyl appears attractive for use in laboring patients.

Fentanyl rapidly crosses the placenta. In sheep, fentanyl can be detected in fetal blood within 1 minute of maternal i.v. injection. Peak fetal blood concentrations occur at 5 minutes (Fig. 6). Fentanyl had no deleterious effects on maternal cardiovascular function or uterine blood flow (88). In monkeys, maternal administration of fentanyl within 10 minutes of delivery did not produce any detectable neonatal impairment (89). In laboring women, fentanyl produced temporary mild analgesia but failed to completely eradicate uterine contraction pain, especially in late labor (90). FHR variability decreased for 30 minutes, but maternal fentanyl did not impair newborn respiratory function, Apgar scores, or neurological and adaptive capabilities. In an unblinded comparison, meperidine caused more maternal nausea, vomiting, and sedation, and neonatal respiratory depression than fentanyl (91).

Nalbuphine

Nalbuphine is a synthetic opioid agonist–antagonist of the phenanthrene series, chemically related to both the opioid analgesic oxymorphone and the narcotic antagonist naloxone (Table 3) (63,92,93). Nalbuphine's analgesic potency is equivalent to morphine on a milligram basis. The usual dose is 10 to 20 mg every 4 to 6

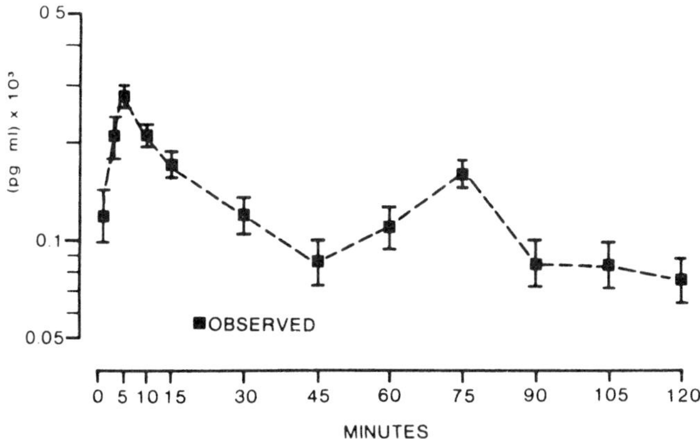

FIG. 6. Mean plasma concentration of fentanyl in fetal arterial blood after a maternal bolus injection of 50, 75, or 100 μg. Each point represents the mean blood concentration of all three doses ± SEM when normalized to the 50-μg dose. There was a minimum of 24 determinations at each time period. (Reprinted from ref. 88, with permission.)

TABLE 3. *Structures of opioids and opioid antagonists chemically related to morphine*

Nonproprietary name	Chemical radicals and positions[a] 3	6	17	Other changes[b]
Morphine	—OH	—OH	$—CH_3$	—
Heroin	$—OCOCH_3$	$—OCOCH_3$	$—CH_3$	—
Hydromorphone	—OH	=O	$—CH_3$	(1)
Oxymorphone	—OH	=O	$—CH_3$	(1), (2)
Levorphanol	—OH	—H	$—CH_3$	(1), (3)
Levallorphan	—OH	—H	$—CH_2CH{=}CH_2$	(1), (3)
Codeine	$—OCH_3$	—OH	$—CH_3$	—
Hydrocodone	$—OCH_3$	=O	$—CH_3$	(1)
Oxycodone	$—OCH_3$	=O	$—CH_3$	(1), (2)
Nalmefene	—OH	$—CH_2$	$—CH_2$—◁	(1), (2)
Nalorphine	—OH	—OH	$—CH_2CH{=}CH_2$	—
Naloxone	—OH	=O	$—CH_2CH{=}CH_2$	(1), (2)
Naltrexone	—OH	=O	$—CH_2$—◁	(1), (2)
Buprenorphine	—OH	$—OCH_3$	$—CH_2$—◁	(1), (2), (4)
Butorphanol	—OH	—H	$—CH_2$—◇	(2), (3)
Nalbuphine	—OH	—OH	$—CH_2$—◇	(1), (2)

[a]The number 3, 6, and 17 refer to positions in the morphine molecule, as shown above.
[b]Other changes in the morphine molecule are as follows:
(1) Single instead of double bond between C_7 and C_8.
(2) OH added to C_{14}.
(3) No oxygen between C_4 and C_5.
(4) *Endo*etheno bridge between C_6 and C_{14}; 1-hydroxy-1,2,2-trimethylpropyl substitution on C_7.

hours. Onset occurs within 2 to 3 minutes of i.v. administration, and in less than 15 minutes after s.c. or i.m. injection. The plasma half-life is 5 hours and, in clinical studies, the duration of analgesic activity ranges from 3 to 6 hours (63). Like morphine and other opioids, nalbuphine is a respiratory depressant. However, unlike pure opioid agonist drugs, nalbuphine-induced respiratory depression peaks after a dose of 10 to 20 mg. Larger or repeated doses of drug do not depress respiratory drive any further (92,94). Although repeated doses of nalbuphine can produce prolonged analgesia without cumulative effects on respiration, larger doses do not increase the intensity of pain relief. One author reported that nalbuphine provides adequate maternal analgesia in labor without apparent adverse maternal, fetal, or newborn side effects (92). Nalbuphine delivered by PCA may produce better pain relief than meperidine in primiparous patients in the first stage of labor (95). But others see no advantage of nalbuphine over meperidine for pain relief in labor (93). In one study, infants whose mothers were given nalbuphine had significantly lower 2- to 4-hour neurobehavioral scores than infants whose mothers were given meperidine, possibly due to easier placental transfer (93).

Butorphanol

Butorphanol is a synthetically derived opioid agonist–antagonist of the phenanthrene series (Table 3). In man, the analgesic potency of butorphanol appears to be five to eight times that of morphine and 30 to 50 times that of meperidine on a per milligram basis (96,97). The usual dose in labor is 1 to 2 mg i.v. or i.m. every 3 to 4 hours. Onset of analgesia is within a few minutes after i.v. injection and 10 to 15 minutes after i.m. injection. Peak analgesic activity occurs in 30 to 60 minutes (63). The analgesic dose of butorphanol (2 mg) depresses respiration to a similar degree as equivalent analgesic doses of morphine (10 mg) or meperidine (70 mg). However, doubling the dose (4 mg) does not produce appreciably greater depression. This ceiling effect on respiration is of particular interest for treating pain of labor where respiratory depression is especially contraindicated (97).

Several studies have compared the analgesia of butorphanol with meperidine in labor (97–99). Butorphanol provides similar or significantly more analgesia than meperidine at 30 minutes and 1 hour after administration based on pain intensity and pain relief scores (97,98). Fetal effects (Apgar scores, time to sustained respiration, umbilical venous pH, FHR, neonatal neurobehavioral scores) also are similar (98,99). Maternal side effects, although infrequent, were more commonly reported after meperidine (99).

Butorphanol also has been compared with fentanyl for labor analgesia. Both drugs were equally safe and without effect on active labor, but butorphanol provided better initial analgesia than fentanyl with fewer patient requests for more medication (100).

Pentazocine

Pentazocine is a member of the benzazocine series (also known as the benzomorphan series). It has both agonist and weak antagonist properties. A 30-mg dose of pentazocine is usually as effective an analgesic as morphine (10 mg) or meperidine (75 to 100 mg). Analgesia and sedation usually occur within 15 to 20 minutes of an i.m. injection and 2 to 3 minutes after i.v. administration. Pentazocine weakly antagonizes the analgesic effects of morphine and meperidine, and partially reverses the cardiovascular, respiratory, and behavioral depression induced by the latter. It has about 1/50th the antagonistic activity of another agonist–antagonist, nalorphine. The plasma half-life of pentazocine is 2 to 3 hours (63). Most commonly, a single i.m. 30-mg dose is administered during labor. An i.v. 20-mg dose has given adequate pain relief to some laboring patients. This dose may be repeated two to three times at 2- to 3-hour intervals as needed (63). Respiratory depression can be seen with pentazocine but with a ceiling at 40 to 60 mg. Side effects from pentazocine differ somewhat from those opioids. The most commonly reported is sedation, followed by sweating, and dizziness or lightheadedness. Nausea occurs, but vomiting is less common than with morphine. Psychotomimetic effects such as anxiety, nightmares, weird thoughts, fear of impending death, and hallucinations have been reported. These are seen with increasing frequency when doses approach and exceed 60 mg (101). These psychotomimetic effects have limited pentazocine's use in obstetrics.

Nonnarcotic Analgesics/Tranquilizers

Phenothiazines

Phenothiazines are sometimes combined with opioids in labor. They provide sedation and decrease the potential for opioid-induced nausea and vomiting. Rapid placental transfer may decrease FHR beat-to-beat variability. Neonatal effects have not been extensively studied, but neonatal depression is rare (102). Chlorpromazine, promazine, and prochlorperazine may cause maternal hypotension via α-adrenergic blockade.

Promethazine (Phenergan) is the most commonly used phenothiazine. In early labor, promethazine 50 mg provides sedation and anxiolysis. In active labor, 25 to 75 mg may be given i.m. or i.v. with an appropriately reduced dose of any desired opioid analgesic (usually meperidine). This drug combination can be repeated once or twice at 4-hour intervals. The maximum total recommended dose of promethazine during labor is 100 mg in 24 hours (63). Promethazine also is a mild respiratory stimulant and may counteract opioid respiratory depression.

Hydroxyzine

Hydroxyzine (Vistaril) is an antihistamine that provides sedation and prevents maternal nausea and vomiting. It is usually used in combination with a reduced dose of an opioid (hydroxyzine potentiates the action of opioids and barbiturates) (63). The usual dose in labor is 25 to 50 mg i.m. (i.v. injection is very irritating to the veins). Hydroxyzine does not appear to cause neonatal respiratory depression (103,104).

Scopolamine

In the past, the anticholinergic scopolamine was used for amnesia and sedation in laboring women. It is not a respiratory depressant. In combination with an opioid, scopolamine produces "twilight sleep." A high incidence of agitation and excitement has reduced its use to virtually zero (105). In addition, scopolamine crosses the placenta, increases the FHR, and obliterates beat-to-beat variability (106). This effect may be reversed by maternal physostigmine (107).

Barbiturates

Barbiturates (pentobarbital, secobarbital, amobarbital) are hypnotics, not analgesics. These medications can cause maternal sedation and anxiolysis. They are most commonly used as sedative hypnotics during early latent labor, when delivery is remote. Barbiturates may increase the perception of pain when given without an opioid (108). The most commonly used barbiturates are pentobarbital 100 to 200 mg and secobarbital 100 mg. Both drugs are given by mouth or i.m. All barbiturates are lipid soluble and readily cross the placenta. When administration is limited to early labor, a single dose of barbiturate rarely results in neonatal depression (60). However, the addition of secobarbital to meperidine for labor analgesia increases not only the incidence of neonatal depression but also the time before birth in which the infant is at risk of opioid-induced depression (72). Barbiturates also may be used to help a patient to sleep who is in false labor (105).

Ketamine

Ketamine is a phencyclidine derivative that, when given i.m. or i.v., induces a dissociative state of intense analgesia with or without amnesia. One mg/kg i.v. produces unconsciousness. Ketamine stimulates the sympathetic nervous system and can exacerbate hypertension in preeclamptic patients. Intravenous ketamine has a rapid onset and a short duration. Bolus injection of 10 to 20 mg can provide analgesia for vaginal delivery. This dose can be repeated every 2 to 5 minutes, but should not exceed 1 mg/kg in 30 minutes (60) or a total dose of 100 mg (109).

No significant maternal or newborn complications have been reported with this low dose (109). Larger doses of ketamine (1.5 to 2.0 mg/kg) have been associated with maternal laryngospasm, increased uterine tone, low Apgar scores, and neonatal depression (110).

Nonsteroidal Antiinflammatory Drugs

Ketorolac is a member of the pyrrolo-pyrrole group of nonsteroidal antiinflammatory drugs. It inhibits the synthesis of prostaglandins by inhibiting the enzyme prostaglandin synthetase. Ketorolac has no known effect on opiate receptors (63). Ketorolac is not recommended in obstetric analgesia because it may suppress uterine contractions and cross the placenta, causing closure of the fetal ductus arteriosus (63). Therefore, few data are available on the use of ketorolac in labor. Walker et al. (111) compared ketorolac 10 mg with meperidine 50 to 100 mg in laboring women. Ketorolac provided less pain relief than either dose of meperidine, but all three were relatively ineffective. Ketorolac produced less maternal sedation and fetal depression. Ketorolac crosses the placenta. The fetal:maternal plasma ratio is low compared with other analgesics used to treat labor pain (112). The authors feel that prostaglandin synthetase inhibitors "may have a subsidiary role in the management of labour pain."

Benzodiazepines

Benzodiazepines act primarily by binding to specific postsynaptic receptors in the central nervous system. They increase the efficacy or availability of the inhibitory amino acid, glycine. They also increase the effect of γ amino butyric acid (GABA), an inhibitory neurotransmitter. These effects provide anxiolysis, sedation, and muscle relaxation. Benzodiazepines have never been used extensively in obstetric patients because of significant side effects.

Diazepam, both alone and as an adjunct to opioids, was first used in obstetrics in 1964 (108). It provided maternal sedation and decreased anxiety, apprehension, and fear. Diazepam readily crosses the placenta and may accumulate in the fetus. Fetal blood concentration may exceed maternal concentration (113,114). Diazepam has a long maternal half-life (24 to 48 hours). It is metabolized in the liver to the active metabolites desmethyldiazepam and oxazepam, whose half-lives are greater than 50 hours.

Hypotonicity and hypoactivity are characteristic of diazepam-exposed neonates. Low Apgar scores, apneic spells, reluctance to feed, and impaired temperature regulation and metabolic responses to cold stress also are seen with larger doses (108,115–117). Diazepam can displace bilirubin from albumin-binding sites, increasing the risk of kernicterus (105). Finally, there may be a significant reduction in the mother's recall of labor and delivery due to diazepam's amnestic effect.

Unlike diazepam, midazolam is water soluble and is rapidly metabolized to minimally active compounds, which limits its duration. It is two to five times as potent as diazepam due to a greater affinity for the benzodiazepine receptor (108,118). Midazolam, given before cesarean section, rapidly crosses the placenta. The umbilical vein:maternal vein ratio is approximately 0.65, and the neonatal elimination half-life is 6.3 hours (60,119). Neonates exposed to induction doses of midazolam have a high incidence of respiratory depression and may have decreased temperature and tone (120,121). Midazolam, like diazepam, is a potent amnestic and may reduce maternal recall of labor and delivery (122). Some suggest delaying maternal midazolam until after pediatric ministrations to the neonate are completed and the mother has seen the child (123,124), or limiting its use to special indications (125).

Inhalational Analgesia

Although uncommon in the United States, inhalational analgesia is still an acceptable form of labor pain relief. In 1981, none of the surveyed hospitals in the United States used intermittent inhalational analgesia for labor, and only 6% used inhalational agents for vaginal delivery (126,127). Inhalational analgesia is used frequently in Europe and Canada if regional analgesia is unavailable. Nitrous oxide remains the agent of choice. In Great Britain, it may be administered even by unsupervised midwives (128).

Inhalational analgesia does not usually provide complete relief of severe labor pain, but it can provide substantial analgesia and a cooperative mother.

Nitrous Oxide

Joseph Priestley identified nitrous oxide in 1772, and Stanislav Klikovicz introduced it into obstetrics in 1880. It was first used to treat hyperemesis gravidarum, then to help ease the pain of labor (129). Throughout the world, nitrous oxide continues to be a commonly used inhalational labor analgesic (128).

Nitrous oxide does not completely eliminate the pain of contractions but reportedly provides satisfactory labor analgesia in about 50% of parturients using a concentration of 50% or greater (130). A recent study, however, has questioned the efficacy of nitrous oxide as a labor analgesic. Pain scores did not differ between parturients who breathed either 50% nitrous oxide in oxygen or compressed air (128). Upon completion of the study, the women were given the choice of continuing to use N_2O for labor analgesia or not. Most chose to continue using N_2O.

To maximize the concentration of nitrous oxide in the blood and brain, the parturient must hold a mask and begin inhaling the gas as soon as she feels a contraction. A nitrous oxide/oxygen blender or a premixed 1:1 cylinder limits the delivered concentration of nitrous oxide. Even these devices must be checked frequently to prevent unintentional administration of high concentrations of nitrous oxide and hypoxic gas mixtures. One may improve the analgesic efficacy of nitrous oxide by administering the mixture continuously via a nasal cannula in addition to inhaling it during contractions (131).

In addition to its limited efficacy, nitrous oxide has other deficiencies. Multiple studies have reported pollution of the labor suite with nitrous oxide concentrations above 25 ppm (132–134). Nitrous oxide, in high concentrations, reduces methionine synthase activity, which may interfere with the synthesis of deoxythymidine and deoxyribonucleic acid. This decrease produces megaloblastic bone marrow changes and neurological abnormalities (134). Although controversial, unscavenged nitrous oxide may increase the risk of spontaneous abortion, infertility, and other health problems among exposed health care workers (135).

Inadequate pain relief in parturients using nitrous oxide for labor analgesia places them at risk for hypoxemia. Pain-mediated hyperventilation may result in maternal hypoxia and neonatal acidosis. Alkalemia shifts the oxyhemoglobin dissociation curve to the left, impairing the release of oxygen to both maternal tissues and fetal blood (136). Maternal hypocapnia also may lead to vasoconstriction of the umbilical and uteroplacental vasculature.

Diffusion hypoxemia also may result from administration of nitrous oxide for labor analgesia (137–140). Active hyperventilation during maternal contractions causes a rapid uptake and distribution of nitrous oxide. After a contraction, parturients breathe room air. Nitrous oxide diffuses outward, lowering the alveolar partial pressure of oxygen, producing maternal hypoxemia (136). The combined use of nitrous oxide and the respiratory depressant meperidine further increases the risk of maternal hypoxemia (138,139). However, one study reported that parturients breathing 50% nitrous oxide and oxygen intermittently had higher oxygen saturations after a contraction than women breathing compressed air (128).

Nitrous oxide does not interfere with uterine activity (129), but it does directly depress the myocardium in both animals and humans (141,142). In animals, inhalation of nitrous oxide produces sympathetic stimulation, which may increase peripheral resistance. Depressed myocardial activity plus increased vascular resistance may decrease uterine perfusion (143). Despite these theoretical concerns, a recent study found no changes in maternal blood pressure and heart rate, or uterine artery pressure associated with nitrous oxide (144). Nitrous oxide did decrease the pulsatility index in both maternal and fetal cerebral vessels, indicating increased cerebral blood flow. Although neither mother nor fetus suffered any clinically detectable adverse effects, the authors suggested that the decreased pulsatility index and increased cerebral blood flow could predispose a preterm fetus to cerebral hemorrhage from cerebral hyperemia in the presence of immature cerebral autoregulation (144).

In the neonate, nitrous oxide is eliminated via the lings within a few minutes of birth. There is very little metabolism, and nitrous oxide lacks effect on neonatal respirations or neurobehavioral function (131,140).

Potent Halogenated Agents

All potent halogenated agents produce dose-related relaxation of uterine smooth muscle (145). At 0.5 minimum alveolar concentration (MAC), halothane, enflurane, or isoflurane diminish spontaneous uterine activity, but the uterine muscle still responds to oxytocin (146). Greater concentrations decrease the uterine contractile response to oxytocin (146,147).

Methoxyflurane

Methoxyflurane was a popular inhaled agent for labor analgesia in the late 1960s and early to mid-1970s. It provided better pain relief, less restlessness, and had a less pungent odor than trichloroethylene (130). Methoxyflurane was a better labor analgesic than 50% nitrous oxide in oxygen, but parturients seemed drowsier (130). The potential for nephrotoxicity after long exposure sharply limited the use of methoxyflurane. However, there are no reports of this complication in parturients.

Enflurane

Intermittent enflurane inhalation was introduced after a study demonstrated its superiority over 50% nitrous oxide for relieving labor pain. Parturients appeared to be more drowsy with enflurane, but no mother became unresponsive to verbal stimulus (148). Abboud et al. (149) also studied enflurane during the second stage of labor and found that mothers and anesthesiologists rated enflurane and nitrous oxide similarly for pain relief. But obstetricians rated enflurane superior to nitrous oxide. Estimated blood loss, Apgar scores, as well as umbilical cord blood gas and acid–base measurements were similar for the two groups. Oxygenation was slightly better in the enflurane group as higher concentrations of oxygen can be given than with nitrous oxide. Biochemical tests did not detect maternal or fetal renal dysfunction. Intermittent enflurane inhalation did not increase maternal inorganic fluoride concentrations at 24 hours after birth, and umbilical cord fluoride concentrations were only minimally elevated. Enflurane does not adversely affect neonatal neurobehavioral scores at 24 hours after delivery (140).

Isoflurane

Isoflurane has a low blood:gas solubility and produces anesthesia rapidly without significant accumulation (150). These properties make it a good inhalational agent for labor analgesia (150). Isoflurane provides satisfactory labor analgesia with no adverse effects on maternal or fetal renal function, newborn Apgar scores, or neonatal neurobehavioral scores (151). Maternal amnesia is rarer than with enflurane (149,151). Parturients using isoflurane or enflurane experienced mild drowsiness and commented on the pungent odor of both agents (148,150).

Desflurane

Desflurane has a blood:gas solubility coefficient (0.42) similar to that of nitrous oxide and a MAC of between 6% and 7.25% (152). Like isoflurane, it provides labor analgesia and then dissipates rapidly. A recent study demonstrated its effectiveness in providing analgesia in the second stage of labor without affecting Apgar scores, neonatal acid–base and blood gas data, and neurobehavioral scores. Biochemical tests found no signs of maternal renal dysfunction. Nine of 40 parturients using desflurane were amnestic for delivery. Breath-holding also can occur (153).

Sevoflurane

Sevoflurane, another new inhalational agent, has been studied in elective cesarean birth (154). No published studies using sevoflurane for labor analgesia exist to date. Sevoflurane has a low blood:gas partition coefficient of 0.69 and a MAC of about 2% (155,156). These characteristics make it a good inhalational agent for labor analgesia. In addition, sevoflurane is less pungent than other agents. The use of sevoflurane for elective cesarean section results in similar maternal hemodynamics, uterine tone, maternal awakening times, and neonatal outcome and neurobehavioral scores as isoflurane (154). However, parturients complained of some mild coughing and pharyngitis postoperatively. Although sevoflurane was associated with increased serum fluoride ion concentrations, there were no cases of maternal renal dysfunction.

PERIPHERAL NERVE BLOCKS

Although lumbar epidural analgesia provides excellent pain relief for labor in most parturients, it is not always available. Epidural block is contraindicated in some parturients and rejected by others. Alternatives include:

- Paracervical, lumbar sympathetic, and sterile water blocks for the pain of the first stage of labor,
- Pudendal block for the second stage, and
- Ilioinguinal block for postcesarean section pain.

During the first stage of labor, dilation of the cervix and distention of the lower uterine segment and upper vagina stimulate small unmyelinated nerve fibers. These afferent visceral nerve impulses coalesce in the paracervical plexus, enter the sympathetic chain at L_2 to L_3, and then join the somatic nerves of the spinal cord at T_{10} to L_1 (see Chapter 12) (157,158). Afferent information travels to the cerebral cortex and is experienced as pain. Peripheral nerve blocks attempt to interrupt these neural impulses before they reach the central nervous system.

With the exception of the water block, peripheral nerve blocks use local anesthetics. Because of the ever present risk of systemic toxicity of these drugs, intravenous access and readily available resuscitation equipment and drugs are necessities before attempting these techniques.

Paracervical Block

Paracervical block was first reported in 1926, and the first description of this technique in the North American literature was in 1945 (158). This block stops afferent nerve transmission at the paracervical or Frankenhauser's plexus, which lies lateral and posterior to the junction of the uterus and cervix, at the base of the broad ligament (158). Local anesthetic solution bathes the parametrial tissues, blocking nerve transmission and alleviating pain during the first stage of labor (159).

Technique

Paracervical block is usually done with the parturient in the lithotomy position with left uterine displacement (160). The optimal time for paracervical block is during the acceleration phase of labor (159). Doing the block after the cervix is dilated 8 cm greatly increases the risk of injecting local anesthetic into the fetal head. Paracervical block is not as effective late in labor because it does not relieve second-stage pain (158). Usually, a 12- to 14-cm, 22-gauge needle with a guide is used. The needle guide prevents injury to the birth canal and fetus, and it precisely defines the depth of local anesthetic injection. The most popular guides are the Kobak needle and guide and the Iowa trumpet (Fig. 7) (158). The index and middle fingers of the right hand introduce the needle guide into the lateral fornix of the cervix for the right side of the pelvis and vice versa for the left side. This maneuver helps divert the needle laterally into Frankenhauser's plexus and lowers the risk of intrafetal or intramyometrial injection (Fig. 8)

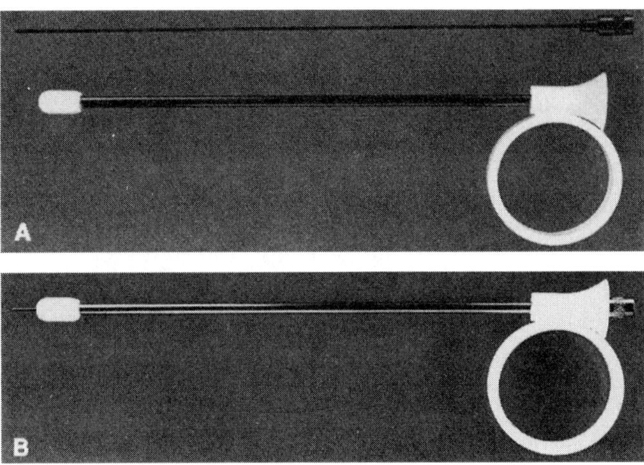

FIG. 7. A: Needle guide and needle for paracervical and pudendal block. **B:** Note that the guide prevents needle from passing deeply into tissues.

(158,161). Excessive pressure during needle placement will decrease the distance to the uterine vessels.

After the needle is placed in the paracervical area and gentle aspiration has ruled out intravascular location, increments of local anesthetic are injected slowly. Limiting the depth of injection to no more than 3 mm will deposit local anesthetic paracervically just below the epithelium, allowing slow diffusion into the loose intervascular connective tissue (162). Superficial injection limits the risk of depositing drug directly into the paracervical venous plexus (162). After drug injection, the parturient assumes the left lateral position, and her heart rate, blood pressure, and the FHR are monitored for at least 30 minutes (161).

The precise site of drug injection varies. Originally, two 10-mL injections were made at the 3 and 9 o'clock cervical positions (159,163). Others recommended placing the needle further from the uterine vessels and injecting the local anesthetic at 4 and 8 o'clock (159,163). Still others advocate 3- to 5-mL injections at four sites around the cervix (4, 5, 7, and 8 o'clock) to further decrease the chance of injecting a large amount of local anesthetic near a vessel (158). Reportedly, there are fewer paracervical block failures when the anesthetic is injected at four points instead of two (164). Another author injects small volumes (3 mL) at six different sites, stating that the onset of pain relief is faster and the analgesic effect is more consistent (165). Radiologic studies show that local anesthetic spreads uniformly regardless of injection site(s) (163).

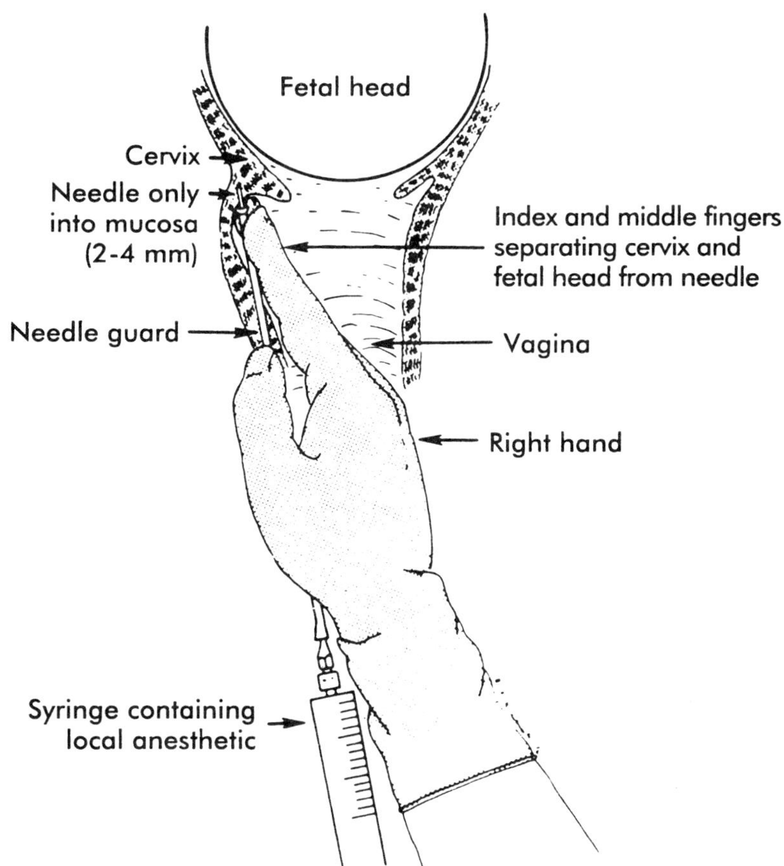

FIG. 8. Paracervical nerve block. Direct the needle through the vagina and into the lateral fornix of the cervix. (Reprinted from ref. 161, with permission.)

Some recommend a 10- to 15-minute delay before blocking the other side of the cervix (164), but a more recent study found no increase in complications when injecting the contralateral side immediately (166). Most now recommend waiting approximately two maternal contractions, or 5 minutes, before injecting the contralateral side (158,159). Uterine displacement and patient selection are more important in preventing problems while performing the block (166).

Pain relief after paracervical block usually begins within 5 minutes. Success depends on operator experience and timing (159). Complete relief develops in 62% to 80% of parturients, partial relief in 10% to 25%, and no relief in 5% to 13% (157,159,167,168). The block can be repeated in 30 minutes if the parturient is still uncomfortable (157).

The duration of pain relief depends on the anesthetic used and the parturient's cervical dilation (Table 4) (157–159,168,169). Epinephrine prolongs the duration of lidocaine and 2-chloroprocaine but not bupivacaine or mepivacaine (159,169). Phenylephrine increases the duration of mepivacaine but not lidocaine (159). Epinephrine may cause fetal hypoxemia by inducing uterine artery vasoconstriction or prolong the first stage of labor by decreasing uterine activity (159,161,169).

Paracervical block may be repeated, but most obstetricians do not exceed a total of four blocks (159). Tafeen et al. (170) describe placement of a paracervical catheter for continuous analgesia. This technique is complicated and the catheter often becomes dislodged. It is rarely used.

Choice of Local Anesthetic

Most proponents of paracervical blocks advocate small volumes of dilute solutions of local anesthetic (158–160). There is no need to inject more than 10 mL of local anesthetic on each side.

The choice of local anesthetic remains controversial. Aminoesters, particularly 2-chloroprocaine, are popular because of rapid metabolism and low toxicity. Some investigators report lower rates of postblock fetal bradycardia with 2-chloroprocaine than with lidocaine (161, 171,172). Only traces of 2-chloroprocaine persist in fetal blood at delivery, in contrast to significant amounts of unmetabolized lidocaine (171). The major disadvantage of 2-chloroprocaine is its short duration (Table 4).

TABLE 4. *Duration of pain relief after paracervical block*

Drug	Duration
Lidocaine, 1%	45–90 min
Chloroprocaine, 2%	30–45 min
Mepivacaine, 1%	45–90 min
Prilocaine, 1%	60–90 min
Bupivacaine, 0.25%	90–120 min

Amide local anesthetics are metabolized in the liver. The immature fetal liver clears these drugs slowly, and unmetabolized drug may be found in significant concentrations in the fetus (171). Mostly, amide local anesthetics leave the fetal circulation by diffusion through the placenta to maternal blood. Unmetabolized mepivacaine has been blamed for perinatal death following paracervical block (173). Prilocaine, which undergoes significant extrahepatic metabolism, may be less likely to produce fetal bradycardia (10.9%) than lidocaine (22.1%) or mepivacaine (21.9%) (174). However, prilocaine may produce methemoglobinemia in the infant following a single paracervical block (174). Lidocaine is associated with increased beat-to-beat variability in the FHR following paracervical block, but no change in maternal and fetal acid–base status (175).

Bupivacaine is not yet approved for paracervical block in the United States, although several studies demonstrate its safety (168,169,176,177). Analgesia lasts about 2 hours, and the reported incidence of fetal bradycardia is low (2.0%) (168,169). Paracervical block with 0.25% bupivacaine is not associated with any neonatal neurobehavioral changes (177). But, a review of 50 cases of perinatal death associated with paracervical block found that bupivacaine was the local anesthetic used in over half (178).

Effect on Labor

Paracervical block probably has no significant effect on the progress of labor. Individual responses vary greatly. In aggregate, only small, variable changes in uterine activity occur after block (170,171,175,176,179,180). Although the rate of cervical dilation may increase slightly after block, this effect most likely represents the normal progress of labor (176).

Maternal Complications

Maternal complications of the paracervical block are uncommon. Anaphylaxis is very rare (159). Pain and maternal fright can trigger neurogenic syncope. Most other complications stem from either error in technique or infection.

Systemic toxic reactions are due to intravascular injection or overdose of local anesthetic. This complication usually presents as central nervous system irritability with symptoms of palpitations, metallic taste, tinnitus, dysarthria, drowsiness, confusion, and convulsions. These symptoms are usually transient, but occasionally hypotension and cardiovascular collapse are seen.

Hematoma of the broad ligament due to laceration of uterine vessels and superficial laceration of the vagina from the tip of the needle can occur (159,161). Inadvertent sciatic nerve block may result while performing a paracervical block. This results in sensory disturbances of the lower extremities (usually unilateral), which resolve with resolution of the block (159).

Postpartum parametritis and subgluteal and retropsoal abscesses have been reported after paracervical block (159,181). Subgluteal and retropsoal infection can spread laterally to the hip joint, resulting in severe pain, limitation of motion, and fever. These symptoms may occur a few hours to several days after the block. Treatment consists of antibiotics for gram-negative and anaerobic organisms. Large abscesses require surgical debridement (181).

The incidence of neuropathy following paracervical block is 1:2,000. This syndrome begins with severe buttock pain radiating down the posterior surface of the ipsilateral leg. As pain worsens, the patient cannot walk. The onset of neuropathy ranges from 12 hours to 10 days after block. Symptoms may worsen over 1 to 10 days, followed by progressive improvement and complete recovery. Most likely, the injury results from direct trauma to the sacral plexus or to hematoma formation around the plexus. A palpable sacroiliac mass without fever is suggestive. Treatment consists of analgesics and early assisted ambulation (182).

Fetal Complications

The most common and serious complication of the paracervical block is fetal bradycardia. The reported incidence is 2% to 70% (158,160). This variable rate relates to different definitions of bradycardia, methods of fetal monitoring, drug dosages, local anesthetics, and patient selection (158). Bradycardia begins 2 to 10 minutes after injection and usually resolves within 20 minutes (183). It is more common in parturients with preexisting nonreassuring FHR tracings (184).

The etiology of fetal bradycardia after paracervical block is unclear. There at least four theories.

Reflex Bradycardia

Manipulation of the fetal head, uterus, or the uterine blood vessels during performance of the block may cause reflex fetal bradycardia (159,160). Reflex bradycardia is thought to be harmless and usually resolves promptly.

Direct Fetal Central Nervous System and Myocardial Depression

Paracervical block requires injection of large amounts of local anesthetic close to the uteroplacental circulation. Local anesthetic rapidly crosses the placenta and may have a direct toxic effect on the fetal central nervous system and myocardium (161,166,176, 185,186). Fetuses with bradycardia after paracervical block have higher plasma concentrations of mepivacaine than their mothers (185,187). Possibly, local anesthetic reaches the fetus by a more direct route than maternal systemic absorption, i.e., diffusion across the uterine arteries, producing higher concentrations of drug in placental intervillous blood. Fetal acidosis would worsen this effect through ion trapping (160,185, 188). However, other reports find that fetal local anesthetic concentrations are consistently lower than maternal concentrations (175,184,185). Freeman et al. (183) injected 300 mg of mepivacaine directly into the fetal scalp of two anencephalic fetuses. The QRS complex widened and the PR interval lengthened, but no bradycardia developed (183). In contrast, neither QRS complex nor PR interval is prolonged during bradycardia from paracervical block in normal fetuses (183). Thus, fetal hypoxemia, not direct myocardial depression, is most likely responsible for bradycardia after paracervical block.

Increased Uterine Activity

Increased uterine activity decreases utereoplacental perfusion. The resultant fetal hypoxemia can produce bradycardia. Direct injection of bupivacaine into the uterine arteries of gravid ewes increases uterine tone (180). Lidocaine intermediately increases uterine tone, whereas 2-chloroprocaine has no effect (180). Other authors also report an increase in uterine activity after paracervical block (166,183). Conversely, Read and Miller (176) and Jenssen (179) noted no increase and even a slight decrease in uterine activity following paracervical block. They only observed one brief episode of fetal bradycardia following paracervical block.

Uterine Artery Vasoconstriction

Currently available evidence strongly supports the existence of local anesthetic-induced vasoconstriction that significantly decreases uterine blood flow (189–191). In vitro, local anesthetics have a direct, nonadrenergic, vasoconstrictive effect (Fig. 9) (189,190). Others have reported significant decreases in uterine blood flow at local anesthetic concentrations comparable to those occurring during paracervical blockade (179,190,191,192). Decreased uterine blood flow produces fetal hypoxemia, which causes sinoatrial node suppression and narrow QRS complex fetal bradycardia (183). LeFevre (184) found a fivefold increase in fetal bradycardia after paracervical block in parturients with evidence of preexisting

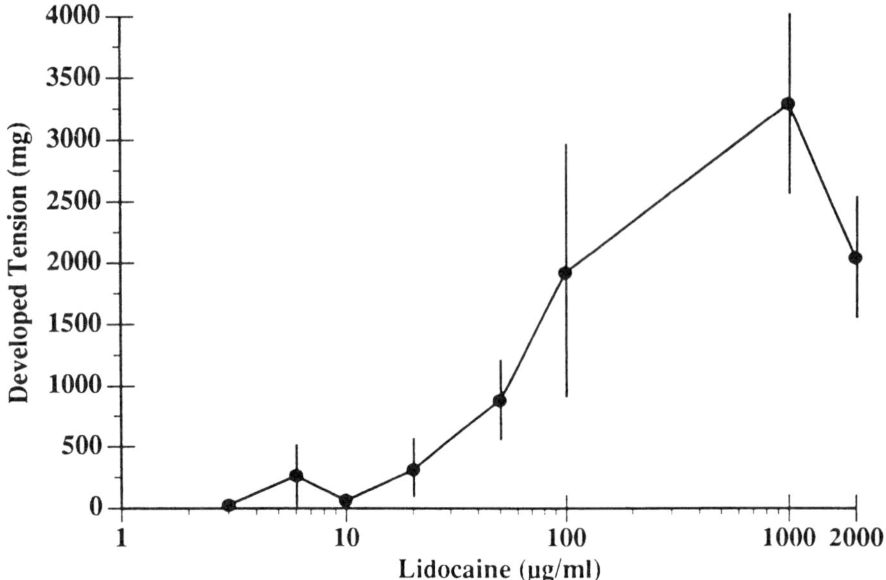

FIG. 9. Dose–response curve of pregnant human uterine artery to lidocaine (n = 9). (Reprinted from ref. 189, with permission.)

uteroplacental insufficiency. Using transcutaneous electrode monitoring, Baxi et al. (193) demonstrated a decrease in pO_2 in ten fetuses after paracervical block. They attributed this change to a decrease in fetal perfusion secondary to uterine artery vasoconstriction. This seemed to be independent of advancing labor and variations due to uterine contractions. Most of their patients had increases in mean uterine activity during the first 60 minutes following paracervical block; only one had a period of decreased uterine activity.

The significance of fetal bradycardia varies. The fetus develops a transient metabolic acidosis only when bradycardia lasts longer than 10 minutes (183). The fetus needs time in utero to recover from the effects of bradycardia. Apgar scores are better in fetuses delivered more than 30 minutes after a bradycardic episode (188). Shnider et al. (187) found depressed 1-minute Apgar scores in fetuses experiencing bradycardia, but all had normal scores by 5 minutes. Meperidine analgesia is more commonly associated with fetal distress (umbilical artery pH $\leq$ 7.15 and a 1-minute Apgar score $\leq$ 7) than paracervical block (194). Neurobehavioral testing on neonates exposed to the paracervical block did not reveal significant long-term effects compared to unmedicated controls (177).

If bradycardia occurs, treatment aims at optimizing uteroplacental perfusion. Maintain uterine displacement, assure adequate maternal blood pressure, and give supplemental oxygen (161). Avoid immediate delivery to allow time for intrauterine resuscitation (158). If bradycardia persists longer than 10 minutes, fetal scalp pH sampling may help determine the need for rapid delivery (160). Bradycardia lasting longer than 45 minutes results in severe fetal hypoxemia and intrauterine death (173). Postnatal exchange transfusion may be used to treat local anesthetic toxicity if immediate delivery is unavoidable (161).

Summary

Although epidural analgesia for labor is very popular in academic obstetrical practices, community use of the paracervical block is significant. In 1989, two thirds of laboring parturients in a community hospital in Minnesota received a paracervical block (167).

Most experts agree on following recommendations concerning paracervical block for labor analgesia:

- Avoid this block in parturients with preterm or stressed fetuses, or those with suspected uteroplacental insufficiency.
- Avoid the block in complicated deliveries such as breech or multiple gestations.
- Do not place the block when the cervix is more than 8 cm dilated.
- Maintain uterine displacement during and after placement of the block.
- Limit the depth of injection to 3 mm. Aspirate frequently.
- After injecting the local anesthetic on one side, wait 5 to 10 minutes and observe FHR before injecting the other side.
- Use small volumes (10 mL on each side) of dilute local anesthetic without epinephrine.
- Monitor the FHR continuously after the block.
- Have resuscitative equipment available.

Lumbar Sympathetic Block

Dellepiane and Badino first described the use of lumbar sympathetic blocks in parturients in 1927 and Cleland introduced this procedure in the United States in 1933 (157,160,195). Cleland (195) showed that lower uterine and cervical afferent sensory fibers join the sympathetic chain at L_2 to L_3 (195). Paravertebral lumbar sympathetic block interrupts the transmission of pain impulses from the cervix and lower uterine segment at the sympathetic chain before the nerves enter the spinal cord (157,160).

The uterus, cervix, vagina, and supporting structures have a dual innervation from the sympathetic and parasympathetic nervous systems (196). During labor, both are activated and balance each other. Parasympathetic efferent impulses activate longitudinal uterine musculature. Contracting circular muscular structures, which are innervated by sympathetic efferent fibers, resist the longitudinal contraction. Distention, tension, and pulling of cervix and lower uterine segment during labor produce painful impulses, which are conducted centrally by the sympathetic nerves (196). Lumbar sympathetic block provides adequate analgesia during the first stage of labor, but does not relieve pain during the second stage (157,196). It is particularly useful in the parturient with previous back surgery in whom epidural anesthesia can be difficult or impossible, or in the parturient who refuses lumbar epidural analgesia (160,197).

Technique

The parturient sits to provide maximal flexion of the spine, facilitating identification of the spinous process of L_2 (Fig. 10A) (157,196,197). After sterile preparation, make a skin wheal of local anesthetic 5 to 8 cm laterally from the mid-point of the L_2 spinous process on each side of the back (196–199). Contact the transverse process of L_2 (Fig. 10B–10D) by introducing a 10-cm, 22-gauge needle at a 20-degree angle cephalad. While placing this needle, inject local anesthetic along the anticipated tract to ensure patient comfort (198). Then withdraw the needle to the skin and redirect it to pass below the transverse process. With the needle directed medially, advance approximately 4.5 cm to contact the vertebral body. Again, inject a small amount of local anesthetic (198). Attempt to "walk off" the ver-

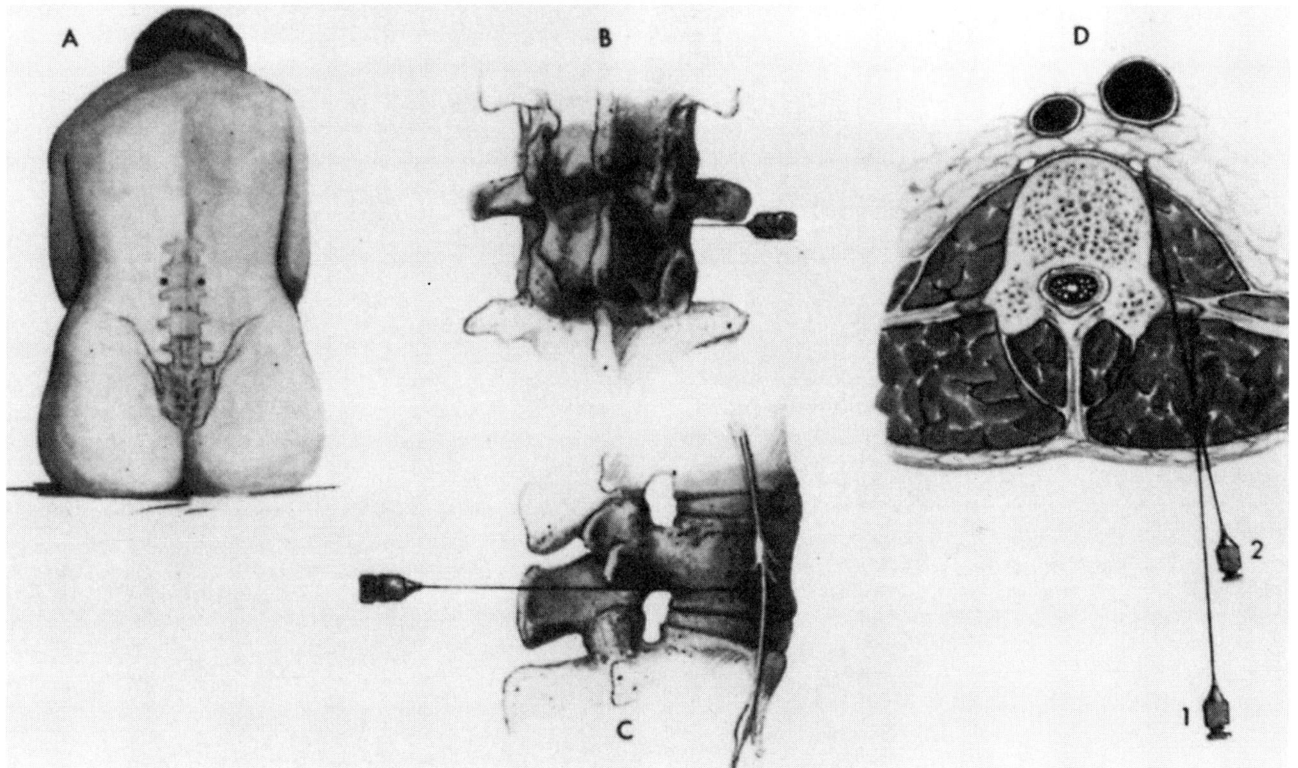

FIG. 10. Technique of lumbar sympathetic block. **A:** Patient in the sitting position with spine flexed. Note that the two skin wheals are opposite the mid-portion of the spinous process of the second lumbar vertebra. **B:** Enlarged posterior view of the vertebral column with details of these landmarks. **C:** Side view showing relation of needles to the bones. **D:** Cross-section showing two of the steps used in inserting the needle. (Reprinted from ref. 157, with permission.)

tebral body by redirecting the needle laterally 5 to 10 degrees. The needle will then be located anterolateral to the vertebral body, at the medial attachment of the psoas muscle (Fig. 10D) (157,160). A loss of resistance syringe may then be used to determine when the needle is beyond the psoas muscle fascia. There is resistance to injection of air in the muscle, but a "pop" may be felt and resistance is lost when the needle advances through the psoas fascia and into the area of the lumbar sympathetic trunk (198). Aspirate frequently while injecting local anesthetic in two 5-mL aliquots to avoid an intravascular injection (the inferior vena cava lies on the right side and the aorta on the left) (160,198). The needle also is close to the subarachnoid and epidural spaces. Question the patient to elicit signs of spinal or epidural blockade. Repeat the procedure on the opposite side.

A disadvantage of lumbar sympathetic block is its finite duration, which varies with the choice of local anesthetic. Lidocaine 1% without epinephrine provides pain relief for 60 to 90 minutes; lidocaine with epinephrine provides pain relief for approximately 120 minutes (156). Tetracaine 0.5% lasts up to 4 hours (197). Meguiar and Wheeler (197) used 20 mL of bupivacaine 0.5% with epinephrine 1:200,000 for bilateral lumbar sympathetic blocks and obtained good analgesia in 38 of 40 parturients. Most patients delivered before regression of the block, but 12 required a second procedure. The mean duration of the analgesia was 283 minutes. Reich (196) described a technique of passing catheters through the needle used for the block to allow repeated injections without repeating the whole procedure (Fig. 11) (196).

Effect on Labor

Lumbar sympathetic blocks do not interfere with the progress of labor (157). Some evidence suggests they may accelerate labor (196–200). In one study, 5 to 15 minutes of uterine hypertonus followed lumbar sympathetic block in 20 of 39 patients (200). This hypertonus was due to increased frequency of contractions. The other 19 patients had no change in labor pattern. Lumbar sympathetic block converted an abnormal uterine contractile pattern to a normal one in 14 of 19 patients. Others reported rapid progression of labor after block, with an average time of 158 minutes from block to complete cervical dilation (197,199). Because no motor block develops, this technique does not affect the second stage of labor (199).

Maternal Complications

The most common side effect of lumbar sympathetic block is hypotension, which occurs 15% to 20% of the time (157,196,197). Local anesthetic spreads to the celiac and splanchnic plexi, producing splanchnic vasodilation and hypotension (157). A smaller volume of drug may

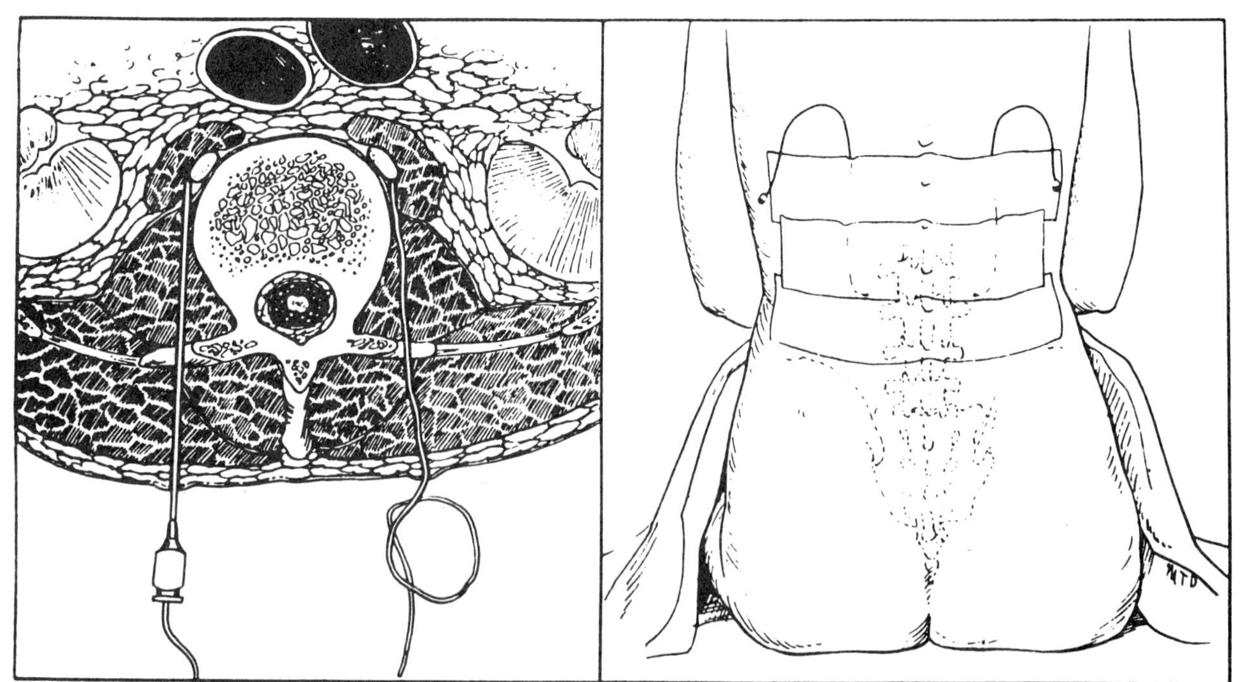

FIG. 11. Technique of continuous lumbar sympathetic block. **A:** After placing the needle in proper position, pass a catheter to just beyond its tip, then remove the needle. **B:** The catheters are then secured in place. (Reprinted from ref. 157, with permission.)

decrease the magnitude of the hemodynamic changes. Administrating a 500-mL bolus of fluid may help offset this hypotension (197).

Other complications include systemic toxicity with seizures and injection into an intervertebral foramen resulting in subarachnoid or epidural block (157,196–198). In an early review of 1,200 patients, 3 experienced convulsions, 4 had minor systemic symptoms, 2 had subarachnoid injections, and 5 had epidural injection with sensory blockade up to T_6 (157). Rarely, parturients may suffer retroperitoneal hemorrhage (157,197). Other complications associated with this block include: parasthesia and pain on injection (198), motor paralysis of the lower extremities possibly due to anterior spinal artery ischemia (201,202), transient lower extremity motor block from local anesthetic spread to the genitofemoral nerve (198), total spinal anesthesia (203), postdural puncture headache (204), Horner's syndrome (205), and intralymphatic injection with possible lymphocele formation (206).

Fetal Complications

There are no direct fetal complications reported with lumbar sympathetic block (157). The fetus may suffer from significant maternal hypotension. Use caution if contemplating this block in situations of fetal distress and uteroplacental insufficiency (197). Increased uterine activity after the block also could affect the fetus, resulting in possible fetal bradycardia (200). However, there are no reports of fetal asphyxia related to uterine tetany.

Summary

Lumbar sympathetic block is used infrequently in labor and delivery. It is technically difficult to place and parturients are more uncomfortable during placement than they are during induction of epidural analgesia (197). This technique provides a finite duration of analgesia unless one places catheters (196). A pudendal or caudal block is commonly used in addition to the lumbar sympathetic block to relieve pain during the second stage of labor (157,195,197,199). Lumbar sympathetic block does not produce motor blockade and may speed labor (196,197,199,200). Consider lumbar sympathetic block in patients who cannot have a lumbar epidural because of back problems or other contraindications (160).

Sterile Water Block

About one third of laboring women experience continuous low back pain during labor, and others feel the pain of contractions primarily in the back (207). Low back pain in labor is more common with an occipitoposterior presentation of the fetus (208).

Pain impulses from the posterior part of the cervix and uterus are transmitted to the spinal cord segments T_{11} to L_1 and cutaneous branches from these segments supply the skin over the low back area (209). Pain originating in the cervix can be localized to the back through these cutaneous nerves (208). A number of analgesic techniques may relieve this pain, including transcutaneous nerve stimulation, application of a local anesthetic agent to the skin via a direct compress, and intradermal or subcutaneous infiltration of the skin with local anesthetic (208,210).

Intradermally injected hypotonic sterile water causes local irritation and stimulates the surrounding tissues, inducing analgesia (208). This analgesia may originate in the mid-brain centers or be caused by gate control at the spinal level (208). This hyperstimulation of the skin area can affect perception of visceral pain. The mechanism of referred pain is reversed to produce referred analgesia.

Intradermal injection of small amounts of sterile water has been reported to successfully treat ureteral colic (211). Trolle et al. (208) evaluated intradermal injection of sterile water or saline in laboring parturients complaining of severe low back pain. The injections were made with 0.1 mL intradermally at four different spots in the low back area, approximately corresponding to the borders of the sacrum (Fig. 12). Analgesia occurred in 2 minutes. Women given sterile water blocks reported

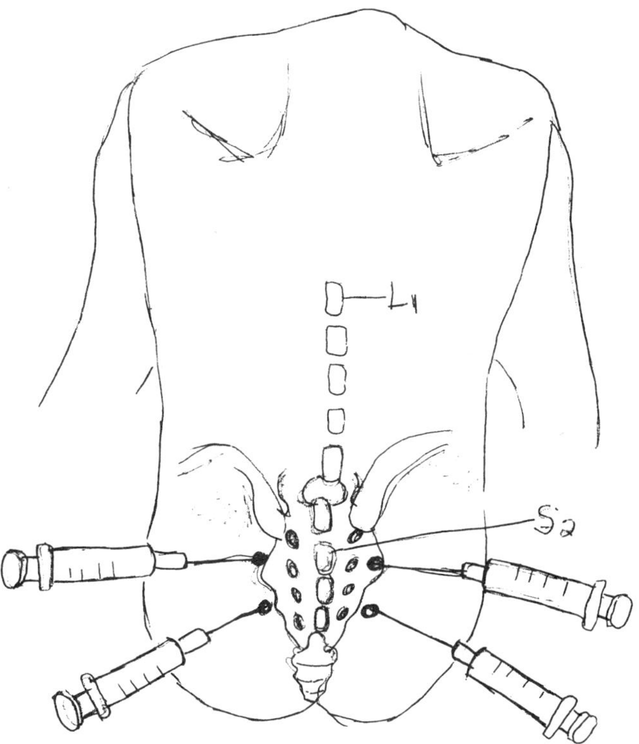

FIG. 12. Sterile water block injection sites corresponding to the boarders of the sacrum.

better analgesia than the women given sterile saline blocks. Epidural and paracervical blocks were not available to these women. They were offered pethidine or nitrous oxide in oxygen and pudendal block for delivery.

Trigger Point Injections

Chronic low back pain is common. In the general population, the leading cause is myofascial pain (212). A myofascial trigger point is a hyperirritable locus within a taut band of skeletal muscle or fascia (213). An acute muscle strain disrupts the sarcoplasmic reticulum, releasing calcium and causing a sustained or repeated contraction. Tissue ischemia results, producing adenosine triphoshate depletion, failure of myosin release from actin, and release of nociceptor sensitizing substances (214). Myofascial pain may be acute, or a result of chronic muscle fatigue. The pain is steady, deep and aching, and can be exacerbated with strenuous activity. During pregnancy, low back pain is a common complaint. The parturient probably experiences myofascial pain during gestation as well as during labor.

Tsen and Camann (215) used trigger point injections to treat a parturient with myofascial pain in her right lower back despite epidural local anesthetic injection. They used two injections of 6 mL of 0.25% bupivacaine with good results. They caution that when using continuous lumbar epidural analgesia and trigger point injections in the parturient, one must be aware of the total amount of local anesthetic used to avoid cumulative toxicity.

Pudendal Block

Mueller described the pudendal nerve block in 1908, but it was not until 1916 that King published the first American article on the subject (157). Klink described the technique of perineal pudendal nerve block in 1953, and Kohl reported the now more commonly used technique of transvaginal block in 1954 (157). Distention of the lower vagina, vulva, and perineum produces pain at the end of the first stage and during the second stage of labor (157,158). The pudendal nerve is the major source of sensation in this area. This nerve is the largest branch of the pudendal plexus and carries somatic fibers from the anterior divisions of the second, third, and fourth sacral nerves. It also provides the motor innervation of the perineal muscles (157,158,160).

The pudendal nerve travels through the lower part of the greater sciatic foramen and enters the gluteal region. The nerve then passes posterior to the ischial spine and continues into the lesser sciatic foramen. It enters Alcock's canal, where it lies along the lateral border of the ischiorectal fossa. The pudendal nerve then divides into the perineal nerve, the dorsal nerve to the clitoris, and the inferior hemorrhoidal nerve (Fig. 13) (158). The success of this block requires blocking the nerve after the formation of the anterior divisions of S_2, S_3, and S_4 but before the division into the three terminal branches. The pudendal nerve is located posterior to the ischial spine. It is blocked here between the sacrotuberous and sacrospinous ligaments (157,158,160). This block pro-

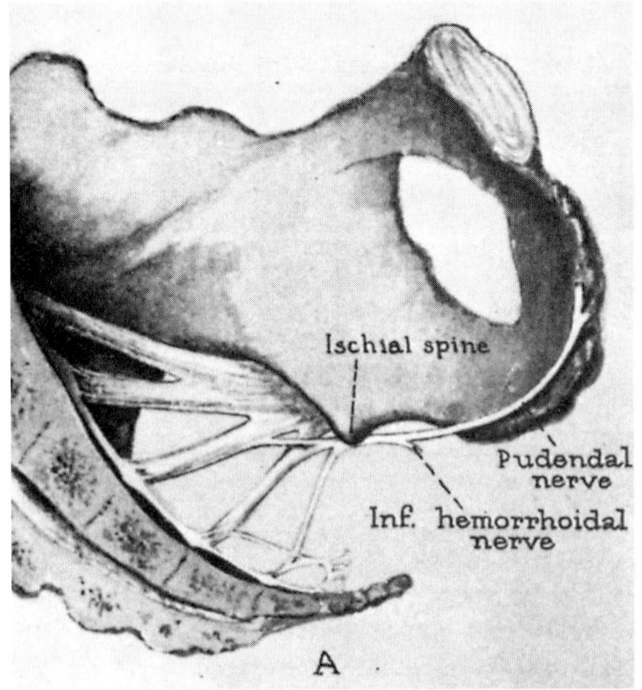

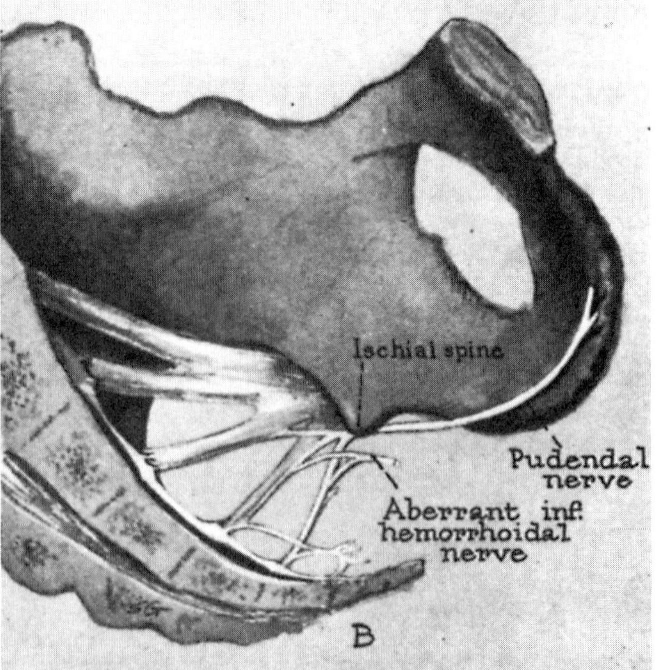

FIG. 13. Origin and course of the pudendal nerve in relation to the bones of the pelvis. Note particularly its relation to the ischial spine. (Reprinted from ref. 157, with permission.)

vides pain relief during the second stage of labor. It also provides analgesia for low forceps delivery and repair of vaginal and perineal lacerations (157,158).

Technique

The pudendal nerve block is most commonly performed transvaginally, but it also may be done through the perineum. The obstetrician uses an Iowa trumpet or Kobak needle and guide to protect the vaginal mucosa and the fetal presenting part (157,160,162). The parturient places herself in the lithotomy position. For the transvaginal technique, hold the needle between the middle and index fingers of the right hand to block the right pudendal nerve and palpate the ischial spine. The left hand holds the needle for the left side. The sacrospinous ligament lies 1 cm medial and posterior to the ischial spine (158). Direct the needle through the sacrospinous ligament to a depth of about 1 cm. One may use a loss of resistance syringe, applying constant pressure to it, while piercing the sacrospinous ligament. There is a sudden loss of resistance as the needle goes through the ligament into the area of the pudendal nerve (Fig. 14) (157). Aspirate for blood and inject 10 mL of local anesthetic on each side. Abouleish (161) describes an alternative method of injecting 7 mL of local anesthetic in the location described and an additional 3 mL of drug 1 cm distal to the ischial spine to block any aberrant nerve branches. Analgesia begins in 2 to 10 minutes and lasts 20 to 60 minutes depending upon the local anesthetic used (158).

Choice of Local Anesthetic

Pudendal block involves injection of local anesthetic into well-perfused tissue. The parturient rapidly absorbs

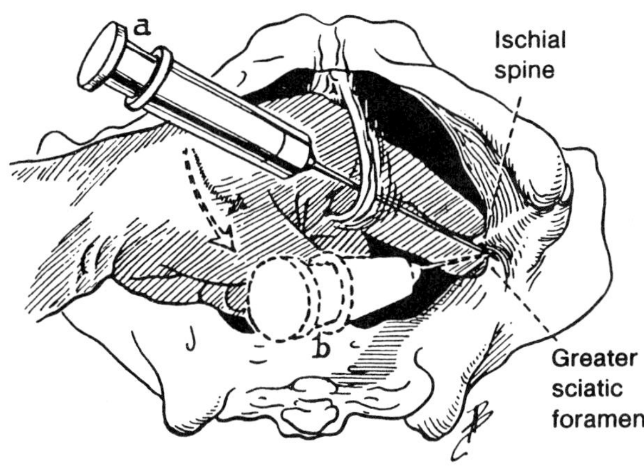

FIG. 14. Transvaginal pudendal block. *a,* The position of the syringe directed downward and laterally to pierce the vagina just below the projection of the ischial spine. *b,* The redirection of the needle to make it parallel with the longitudinal axis of the mother is indicated by the *arrows.* (Reprinted from ref. 227, with permission.)

this drug (216). In addition, most fetuses deliver shortly after the block and lack the benefits of placental clearance if exposed to large amounts of local anesthetic. Lidocaine 1% appears in maternal and fetal blood within 5 minutes of the block, with peak concentrations appearing within 10 to 20 minutes (216). The addition of epinephrine prolongs the block and lowers the maternal and fetal blood concentrations of lidocaine. Matenal lidocaine concentrations are lower than those reported after epidural blockade with the same dose of drug. Some obstetricians favor 2-chloroprocaine because of its rapid onset and metabolism. These properties decrease the likelihood of fetal or maternal systemic toxicity. 2-Chloroprocaine has a short duration, but the block may be repeated (160).

Mepivacaine 1%, with and without epinephrine, is safe for pudendal block (217). In one study, the addition of epinephrine prolonged the time to delivery.

Merkow et al. (218) compared bupivacaine 0.5%, 2-chloroprocaine 3%, and mepivacaine 1% for pudendal block and found no significant differences in most neonatal neurobehavioral responses. Neonatal response to pinprick with mepivacaine at 4 hours was better than with the other local anesthetics.

Regardless of local anesthetic, use dilute drug solutions for pudendal nerve block to limit maternal absorption and decrease the risk of maternal or fetal systemic toxicity if repeat blocks are necessary (160).

Effect on Labor

Obstetricians in the United States commonly perform pudendal nerve block immediately before delivery. Many believe that perineal analgesia prolongs the second stage of labor (160). By eliminating the urge to bear down, pudendal block may impair the parturient's ability to push. One study compared obstetric outcome in 24 parturients who received pudendal block at complete cervical dilation and 24 parturients who did not receive pudendal block (216). Pudendal block slightly prolonged the second stage of labor; the addition of epinephrine prolonged it even further. The incidence of instrumental deliveries did not increase.

Pudendal block appears to have little effect on uterine activity (157,216). Epinephrine appears to intensify any transient effects of this block on uterine activity (216).

Maternal Complications

The most frequent complication of this block is failure to provide adequate analgesia for delivery because of performing the block too late (157,158). As with other regional blocks, the patient may experience symptoms of systemic local anesthetic toxicity from intravascular injection, rapid absorption, or administration of a large amount of drug (158). Retroperitoneal hematoma from vascular injury to the internal pudendal artery also can occur (219). Temperature elevation in a parturient with a decreasing hematocrit heralds an infected retroperitoneal hematoma. Treatment includes broad spectrum antibiotics and blood replacement, if necessary. Retropsoal or subgluteal abscesses have been reported for pudendal as well as paracervical blocks (216,219).

Fetal Complications

Serious fetal complications secondary to pudendal block are extremely rare. One must limit the dose of drug injected to avoid fetal toxicity (158).

Summary

Pudendal block provides analgesia during the second stage of labor and for delivery. It is useful in patients who do not have a functioning epidural catheter. This technique also is used for operative vaginal deliveries (vacuum or low outlet forceps). Vaginal and perineal damage may be repaired using pudendal block. This block is not adequate for repair of deep vaginal or cervical lacerations. It is not effective for mid-forceps deliveries or intrauterine manipulations (158).

Ilioinguinal Nerve Block

Three nerves, the iliohypogastric, the ilioinguinal, and the genitofemoral, supply the inguinal area. They originate from the lumbar plexus (220). The iliohypogastric nerve (from L_1) gives off an anterior cutaneous branch, which runs in a ventrocaudal direction. It lies between the transversus and internal oblique muscles and reaches the lower part of the anterior abdominal wall two finger breadths medial to the anterior superior iliac spine. It supplies the skin immediately above the inguinal ligament. The ilioinguinal nerve (from L_1) runs parallel to and below the iliohypogastric nerve. It exits through the superficial inguinal ring and gives off branches to the surrounding skin and to the labia majora. The genitofemoral nerve (from L_1 and L_2) divides on the anterior aspect of the psoas muscle above the inguinal ligament, into the genital and the femoral branches. The genital branch supplies the labia majora, and the femoral branch supplies the skin over the upper part of the femoral triangle (Fig. 15) (220).

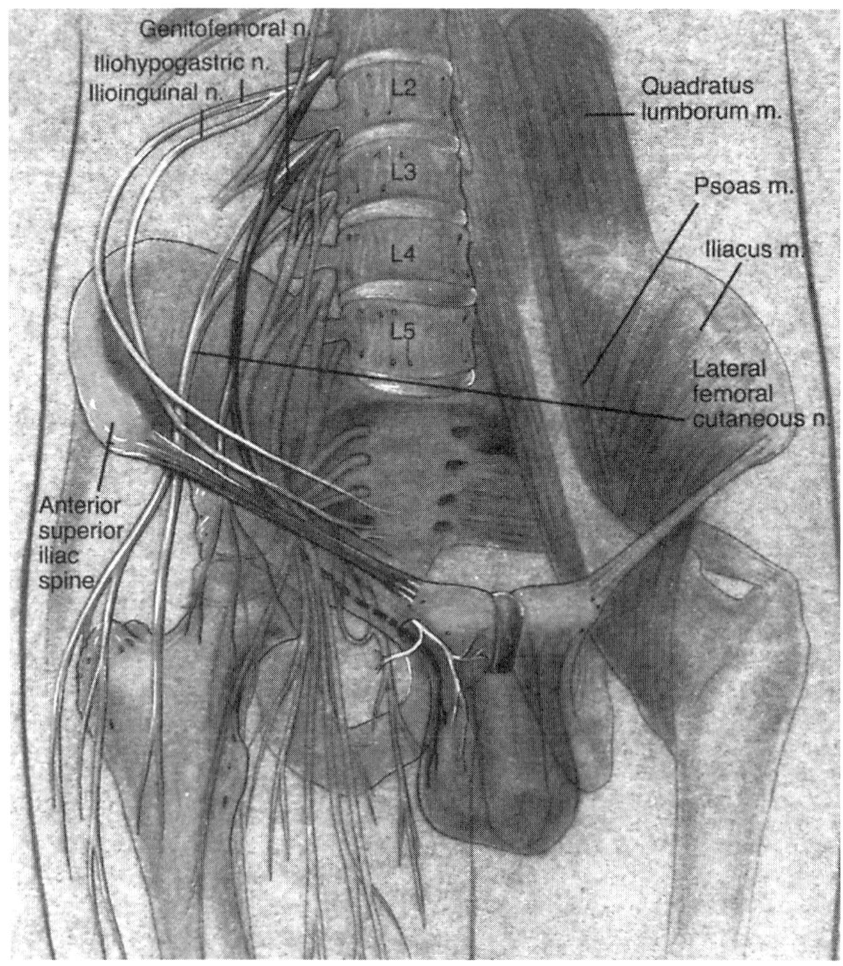

FIG. 15. Inguinal anatomy. (Reprinted from ref. 225, with permission.)

The Pfannenstiel incision, performed for a cesarean section, also lies within the L_1 dermatome (Fig. 16). Blocking the ilioinguinal and the iliohypogastric nerves bilaterally should provide analgesia following this incision (221). Ilioinguinal nerve block does not, however, abolish postcesarean section pain arising from visceral structures (221). Women who receive ilioinguinal nerve block after cesarean section under general anesthesia report lower pain scores than those who do not (221). The women who do not receive the block use more opioids in the first 24 hours than the blocked women; however, all have some pain postoperatively. In a recent retrospective study, unblocked patients used twice as much MSO_4 postoperatively as blocked patients (222). Both bilateral ilioinguinal nerve block and local wound infiltration provide analgesia after cesarean section. These blocks produce similar pain scores (223).

Huffnagle et al. (224) also studied the effects of ilioinguinal nerve block for postoperative pain relief following spinal anesthesia for elective cesarean section. One group had blocks placed before surgical incision, one group had blocks placed at the end of the procedure, and one group did not have nerve blocks. Patient satisfaction and postoperative morphine usage did not differ among the groups. Patients in the group receiving ilioinguinal nerve blocks at the end of the procedure occasionally reported more pain than those in either of the other two groups. These authors concluded that there is no benefit to ilioinguinal nerve blocks either before or after cesarean section in patients receiving spinal anesthesia. Ilioinguinal nerve block alone is not sufficient to block the somatic and visceral components of postcesarean delivery pain.

Technique

Stand to one side of the supine patient and locate the anterior superior iliac spine. At a point two finger breadths medial to the anterior superior iliac spine, inject local anesthetic into the muscles in front of the pelvic bone using a short beveled needle (Fig. 17) (220). Then, pierce the aponeurosis of the external oblique muscle and inject local anesthetic solution in two directions, caudal and mediocaudal (one feels a slight "pop" when the needle pierces the aponeurosis) (Fig. 18). Finally, inject local anesthetic subcutaneously in a caudal direction toward the inguinal fold and mediocaudally as far as the mid-

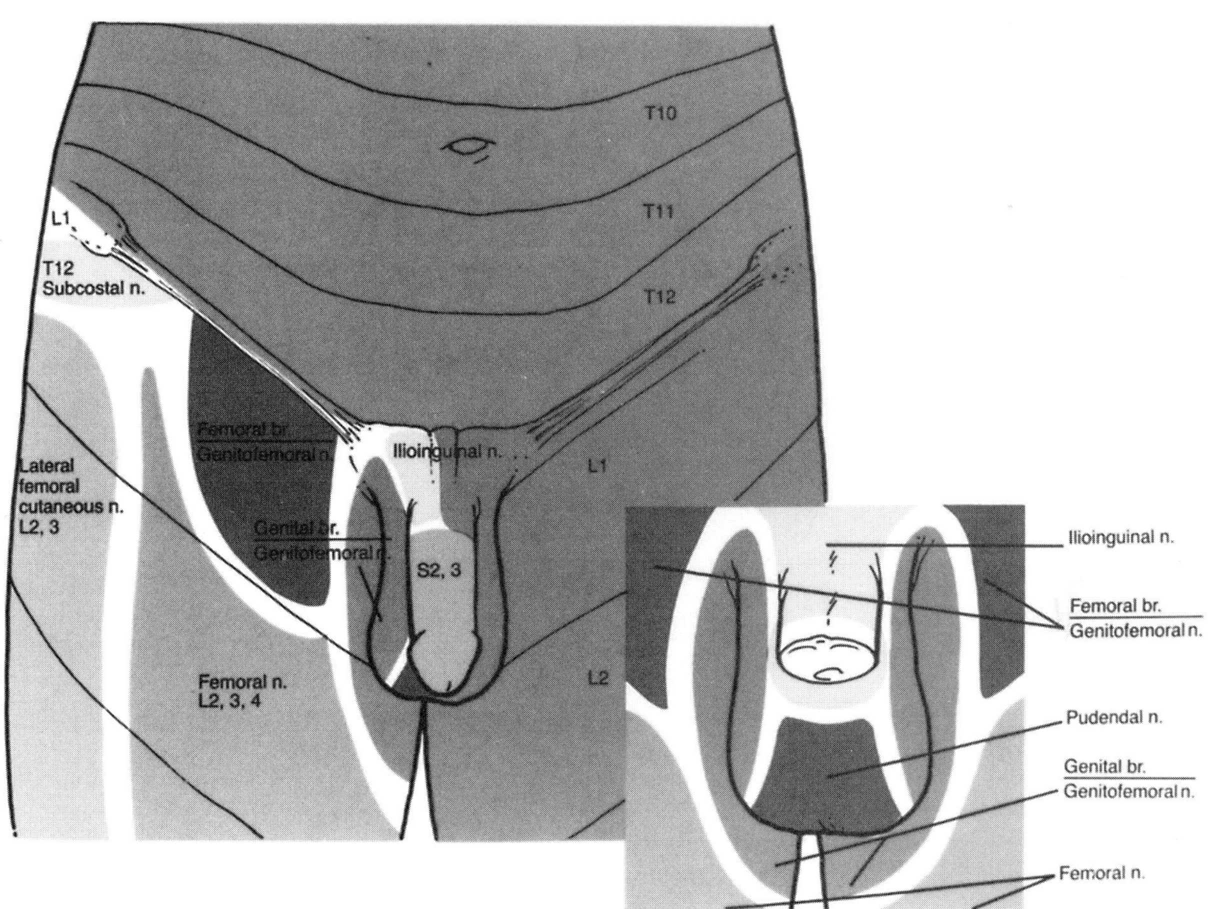

FIG. 16. The dermatomal sensory distribution in the inguinal area. (Reprinted from ref. 225, with permission.)

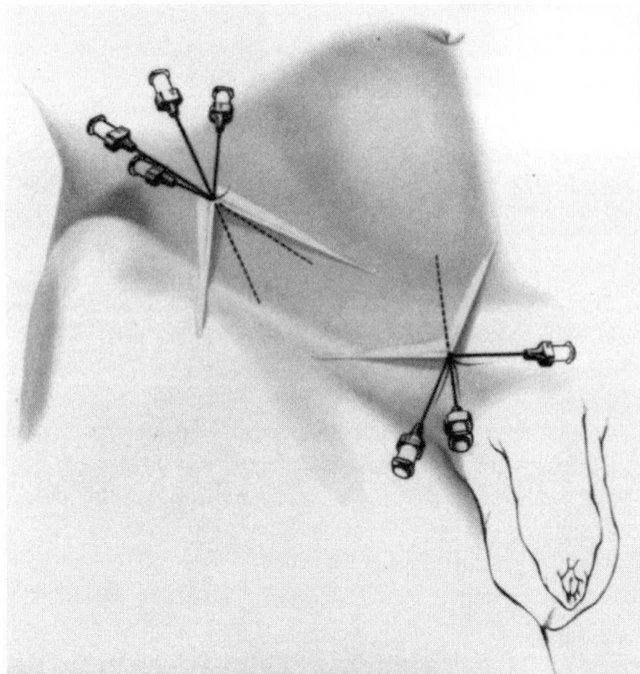

FIG. 17. Position of the needle for ilioinguinal nerve block in a male patient. (Reprinted from ref. 220, with permission.)

line. Repeat the procedure on the opposite side. From a second point, proximal to the pubic tubercle, inject local anesthetic extraperitoneally along the superior margin of the pubic bone, within the aponeurosis of the external oblique muscle, and about 5 cm cranially (Fig. 17). Also inject subcutaneously in a fanwise manner, laterally as far as the inguinal fold and mediocranially as far as the midline (220).

Alternatively, start 3 cm medial and inferior to the anterosuperior iliac spine, raise a skin wheal, and insert an 8-cm, 22-gauge needle in the cephalolateral direction to contact the inner surface of the ilium (Fig. 19, needle 1). Inject local anesthetic while withdrawing the needle through the layers of the abdominal wall. Then, reinsert the needle at a steeper angle to penetrate all three abdominal muscles (Fig. 19, needle 2) and inject the same way. Create a subcutaneous field block by injecting from the initial skin wheal to the umbilicus, and from the umbilicus to the pubis (Fig. 20). Repeat this procedure on the opposite side with the exception of the subcutaneous injection from the umbilicus to the pubis (225).

Choice of Local Anesthetic

Von Bahr used prilocaine 0.5% with epinephrine for ilioinguinal nerve block for inguinal herniorrhaphy in males using the first technique described (220). He used a total of 50 to 90 mL of local anesthetic depending upon the size of the patient. Studies describing ilioinguinal block for postcesarean section pain utilize bupivacaine 0.5%, 10 mL on each side (221–224).

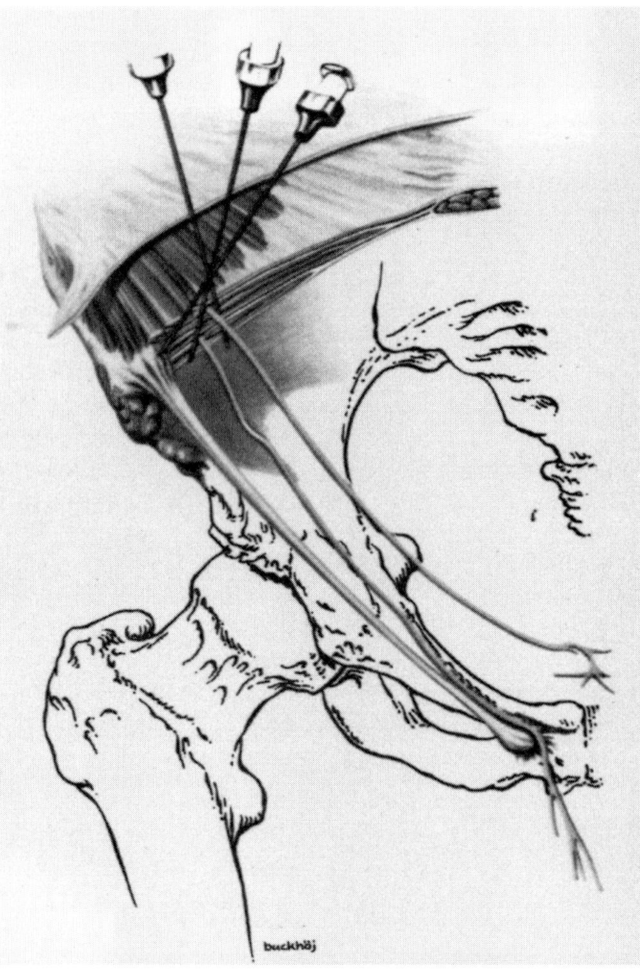

FIG. 18. Ilioinguinal nerve block. Note the needle pierces the aponeurosis of the external oblique muscle. Inject local anesthetic solution in two directions, caudal and mediocaudal. (Reprinted from ref. 220, with permission.)

Maternal Complications

It is moderately difficult to place ilioinguinal block in patients before cesarean delivery because the gravid uterus markedly distorts the anatomy in the area of the block (220,224). One author quotes a 50% failure rate of the block placed before cesarean section (224).

Other complications include possible infection, hematoma formation, and systemic toxic reaction from overdose of local anesthetic or intravascular injection. Local anesthetic may track medially and collect around the femoral nerve, resulting in transient femoral nerve palsy (226).

Fetal Complications

No fetal complications have been reported when ilioinguinal nerve block is placed before cesarean section. Remember to maintain uterine displacement while placing the block.

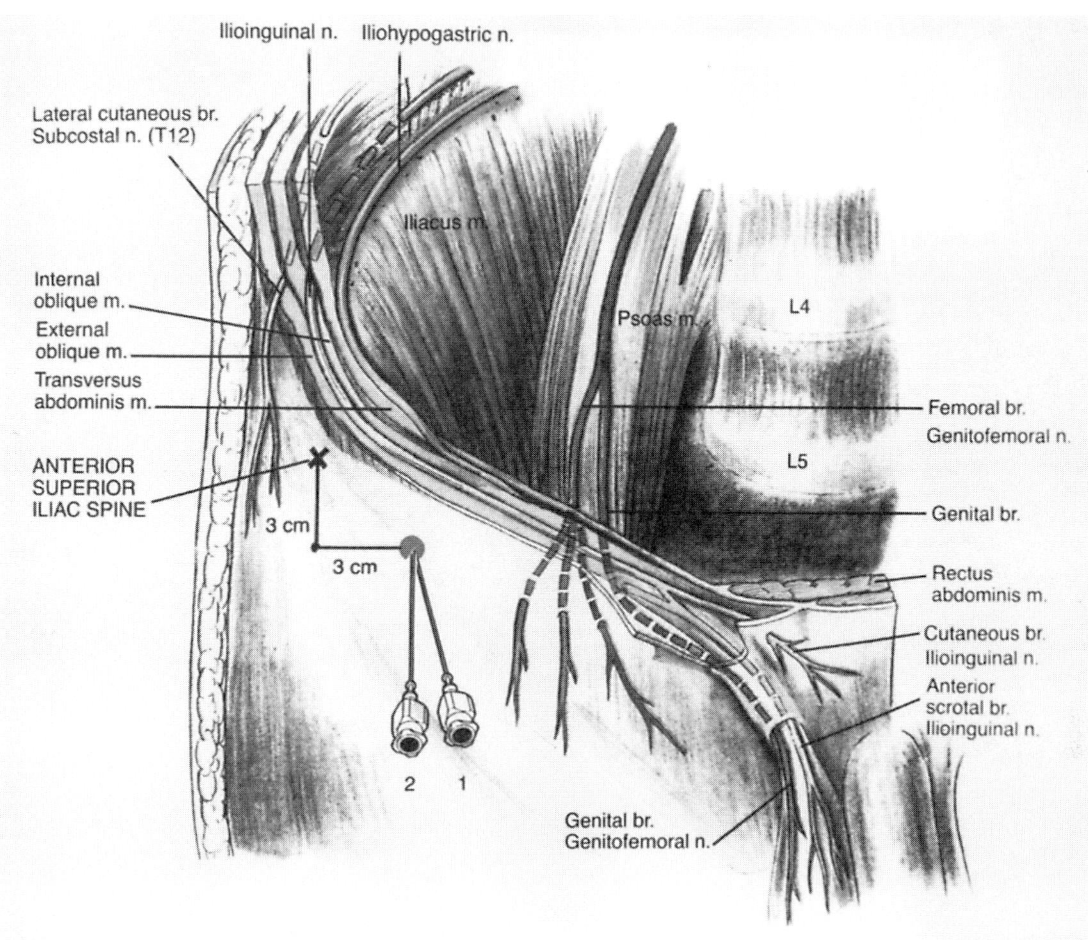

FIG. 19. Ilioinguinal nerve block. Start 3 cm medial and inferior to the anterior superior iliac spine. (Reprinted from ref. 225, with permission.)

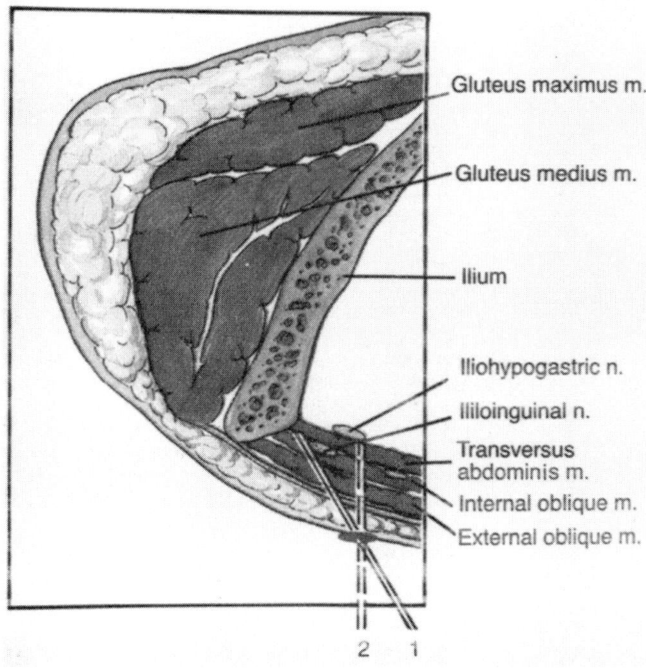

FIG. 20. Ilioinguinal nerve block. Raise a skin wheal in the cephalolateral direction contacting the ileum (needle 1). Reinsert the needle at a steeper angle to penetrate all three abdominal muscles (needle 2). (Reprinted from ref. 225, with permission.)

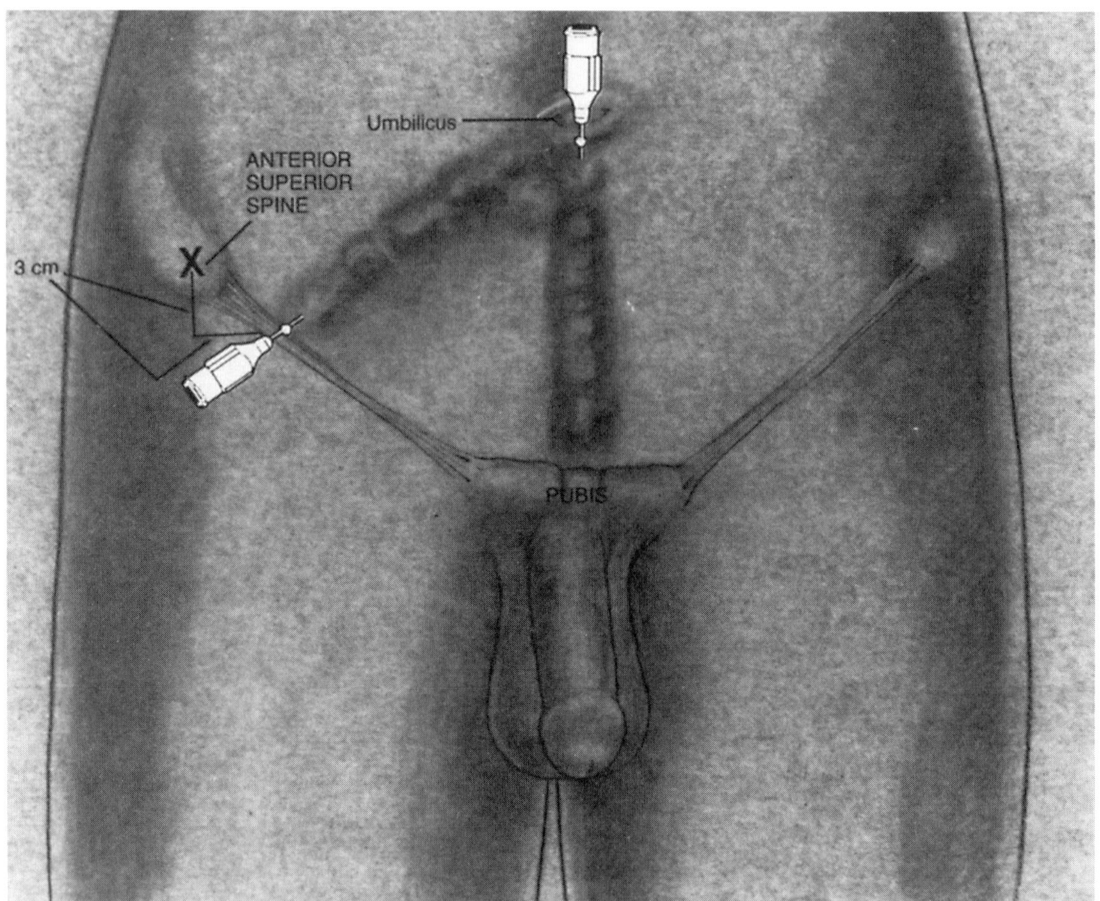

FIG. 21. Ilioinguinal nerve block. Create a subcutaneous field by injecting from the initial skin wheal to the umbilicus and from the umbilicus to the pubis. (Reprinted from ref. 225, with permission.)

Summary

Ilioinguinal nerve block alone following general anesthesia for cesarean delivery may alleviate some incisional pain (Fig. 21) (221). But, it is unclear if this block offers any advantage over local infiltration of the incision (223). It does not appear to offer any benefit for postcesarean section pain relief after spinal anesthesia (224).

CONCLUSIONS

This chapter has explored various nonpharmacologic methods of pain relief and coping available to the parturient as well as some common systemic medications, inhalational analgesic techniques, and peripheral nerve blocks used as alternatives to neuraxial analgesia. Not all methods are suitable for every patient. Some may still leave the mother with considerable pain. Neuraxial techniques remain the most reliable, effective methods of maternal pain relief.

REFERENCES

1. Crafter H. Pain-free labor. *Nurs Times* 1989;85:66.
2. Pitcock CDH, Clark RB. From Fanny to Fernand: the development of consumerism in pain control during the birth process. *Am J Obstet Gynecol* 1992;167:581.
3. Weintraub S. *Queen Victoria: an intimate biography*. New York: EP Dutton, 1987:224.
4. Stanton ME. The myth of "natural" childbirth. *J Nurse-Midwife* 1979; 24:25.
5. Dick-Read G. *Childbirth without fear,* 2nd ed. New York: Harper and Row, 1959.
6. Beck NC, Geden EA, Brouder GT. Preparation for labor: a historical perspective [Review]. *Psychosom Med* 1979;41:243.
7. Beck NC, Hall D. Natural childbirth—a review and analysis. *Obstet Gynecol* 1978;52:371.
8. Scott JR, Rose NB. Effects of psychoprophylaxis (Lamaze preparation) on labor and delivery in primaparas. *N Engl J Med* 1976;294:1205.
9. Lamaze F. *Painless childbirth.* London: Burke, 1958. LB Celestin, translator.
10. Melzak R, Taenzer P, Feldman P, Kinch R. Labor is still painful after prepared childbirth training. *Can Med Assoc J* 1981;125:357.
11. Geden E, Beck N, Brouder G, Glaisler J, Pohlman S. Self-report and psychophysiological effects of Lamaze preparation: an analogue of labor pain. *Res Nurs Health* 1985;8:155.
12. Mackey MC. Women's evaluation of their childbirth performance. *Maternal-Child Nursing J* 1995;23:57.
13. Bradley RA. *Husband-coached childbirth,* 4th ed. New York: Bantam Books, 1996.
14. Bradley RA. *Husband-coached childbirth,* 3rd ed. New York: Harper and Row, 1981.
15. Monto MA. Lamaze and Bradley childbirth classes: contrasting perspectives toward the medical model of birth. *Birth* 1996;23:193.
16. Rosegg S, Rosegg P. *Natural childbirth the Bradley way.* New York: EP Dutton, 1984.

17. Sosa R, Kennell J, Klaus M, Robertson S, Urrulia J. The effects of a supportive companion on perinatal problems, length of labor, and mother-infant interaction. *N Engl J Med* 1980;303:587.
18. Kennell J, Klaus M, McGrath S, Robertson S, Hinkley C. Continuous support during labor in a U.S. Hospital. *JAMA* 1991;265:2197.
19. LeBoyer F. *Birth without violence.* New York: Alfred A. Knopf, 1975.
20. Nelle M, Zilow EP, Kraus M, Bastert G, Linderkamp O. The effect of LeBoyer delivery on blood viscosity and other hemorheologic parameters in term neonates. *Am J Obstet Gynecol* 1993;169:189.
21. Nelle M, Zilow EP, Bastert G, Linderkamp O. Effect of LeBoyer childbirth on cardiac output, cerebral and gastrointestinal blood flow velocities in full-term neonates. *Am J Perinatol* 1995;12:212.
22. Nelle M, Kraus M, Bastert G, Linderkamp O. Effects of LeBoyer childbirth on left- and right systolic time intervals in healthy term neonates. *J Perinat Med* 1996;24:513.
23. Henschel D. LeBoyer versus conventional care. *Nurs Mirror* 1982; September:38.
24. Nelson MN, Enkin NW, Saigal S, Bennett KJ, Milner R, Sackett DL. A randomized clinical trial of the LeBoyer approach to childbirth. *N Engl J Med* 1980;302:655.
25. Oh W, Blankenship W, Lind J. Further study of neonatal blood volume in relation to placental transfusion. *Ann Paediatr* 1966;207:147.
26. Yao AC, Lind J. Effect of gravity on placental transfusion. *Lancet* 1969;2:505.
27. Linderkamp O. Placental transfusion: determinants and effects. *Clin Perinatol* 1982;9:559.
28. Linderkamp O, Nelle M, Kraus M, Zilow EP. The effect of early and late cord-clamping on blood viscosity and other hemorheological parameters in full-term neonates. *Acta Paediatr* 1992;81:745.
29. Saigal S, Usher RH. Symptomatic neonatal polycythemia. *Biol Neonate* 1977;32:62.
30. Wahl CW. Contraindications and limitations of hypnosis in obstetric analgesia. *Am J Obstet Gynecol* 1962;84:1869.
31. Moya F, James LS. Medical hypnosis for obstetrics. *JAMA* 960;174:2026.
32. Davidson JA. An assessment of the value of hypnosis in pregnancy and labour. *Br Med J* 1962;95:1.
33. Freeman RM, Macaulay AJ, Eve L, Chamberlain GV, Bhat AV. Randomized trial of self hypnosis for analgesia in labour. *Br Med J* 1986; 292:657.
34. Weishaar BB. A comparison of Lamaze and hypnosis in the management of labor. *Am J Clin Hypn* 1986;28:214.
35. Harmon TM, Hynan MT, Tyre TE. Improved obstetric outcomes using hypnotic analgesia and skill mastery combined with childbirth education. *J Consult Clin Psychol* 1990;58:525.
36. Spiegel H. An eye-roll test for hypnotizability. *Am J Clin Hypn* 1972; 15:25.
37. Oster MI. Psychological preparation for labor and delivery using hypnosis. *Am J Clin Hypn* 1994;37:12.
38. Omer H. A hypnotic relaxation technique for the treatment of premature labor. *Am J Clin Hypn* 1987;29:206.
39. Smith C. Acute pregnancy-associated hypertension treated with hypnosis: a case report. *Am J Clin Hypn* 1989;31:209.
40. Kemp T. The use of transcutaneous electrical nerve stimulation on acupuncture points in labour. *Midwives* 1996;109:318.
41. Palahniuk RJ, Shnider SM, Wu SW. Acupuncture analgesia in obstetrics. *ASA Sci Abstr* 1973;49.
42. McIntyre JWR. Observations on the practice of anesthesia in the People's Republic of China. *Anesth Analg* 1974;53:107.
43. Sjolund B, Teranius L, Erickson MBE. Increased cerebrospinal fluid levels of endorphins after electroacupuncture. *Acta Physiol Scand* 1977;100:382.
44. Moir DD, ed. Pain relief in labour. In: *A handbook for midwives,* 5th ed. New York: Churchill Livingstone 1986:21.
45. Abouleish E, Depp R. Acupuncture in obstetrics. *Anesth Analg* 1975; 54:83.
46. Skelton IF, Flowerden MW. Acupuncture and labor—a summary of results. *Midwives Chronical Nursing Notes* 1988;May:134.
47. Lyrenas S, Lutsch H, Hetta J, Nyberg F, Willdeck-Lundh G, Lindberg B. Acupuncture before delivery: effect on pain perception and the need for analgesics. *Gynecol Obstet Invest* 1990;29:118.
48. Miller-Jones CMH. Transcutaneous nerve stimulation in labour (forum). *Anaesthesia* 1980;35:372.
49. Melzack R, Wall PD. Pain mechanism: a new theory. *Science* 1965; 150:972.
50. Bundsen P, Peterson LE, Selstam U. Pain relief in labor by transcutaneous electrical nerve stimulation—a prospective matched study. *Acta Obstet Gynecol Scand* 1981;60:459.
51. Bonica JJ. The nature of pain of parturition. *Clin Obstet Gynecol* 1975;2:516.
52. Stewart P. Transcutaneous nerve stimulation as a method of analgesia in labour. *Anaesthesia* 1979;34:361.
53. Robson J. Transcutaneous nerve stimulation for pain relief in labour (forum). *Anaesthesia* 1979;34:357.
54. Lee ENC, Chung IWY, Lee JYL, Lam PNY, Chin RKH. The role of transcutaneous electrical nerve stimulation in management of labour in obstetric patients. *Asia-Oceanis J Obstet Gynaecol* 1990;16:247.
55. Augustinsson LE, Bohlin P, Bundsen P, et al. Pain relief during delivery by transcutaneous electrical nerve stimulation. *Pain* 1977;4:59.
56. Hughes SC, Dailey PA, Partridge C. Transcutaneous electrical nerve stimulation for labor analgesia. *Anesth Analg* 1988;67:599.
57. Bundsen P, Erickson K. Pain relief in labor by transcutaneous electrical nerve stimulation safety aspects. *Acta Obstet Gynecol Scand* 1982; 61:1.
58. Duchene P. Effects of biofeedback on childbirth pain. *J Pain Symptom Manage* 1989;4:117.
59. St. James-Roberts I, Hutchinson C, Haran F, Chamberlain G. Biofeedback as an aid to childbirth. *Br J Obstet Gynaecol* 1983;90:56.
60. Wakefield ML. Systemic analgesia: opioids, ketamine, and inhalational agents. In: Chestnut DH, ed. *Obstetric anesthesia principles and practice.* St. Louis: Mosby-Year Book, Inc., 1994;13:340.
61. Podlas J, Breland BD. Patient-controlled analgesia with nalbuphine during labor. *Obstet Gynecol* 1987;70:202.
62. McIntosh DG, Rayburn WF. Patient-controlled analgesia in obstetrics and gynecology. *Obstet Gynecol* 78;1991:1129.
63. *Physicians' desk reference.* Montvale, NJ: Medical Economics Company, 1996.
64. Gerdin E, Salmonson T, Lindberg B, Rane A. Maternal kinetics of morphine during labour. *J Perinat Med* 1990;18:479.
65. Gerdin E, Rane A, Lindberg B. Transplacental transfer of morphine in man. *J Perinat Med* 1990;18:305.
66. Grimwade J, Walker D, Wood C. Morphine and the fetal heart rate. *Br Med J* 1971;7:373.
67. Way WL, Costley EC, Way EL. Respiratory sensitivity of the newborn infant to meperidine and morphine. *Clin Pharm Ther* 1965;6:454.
68. Shnider SM, Way EL, Lord MJ. Rate of appearance and disappearance of meperidine in fetal blood after administration of narcotic to the mother. *Anesthesiology* 1966;27:227.
69. Kuhnert BR, Kuhnert PM, Tu ASL, Lin DCK, Foltz RL. Meperidine and normeperidine levels following meperidine administration during labor I. Mother. *Am J Obstet Gynecol* 1979;133:904.
70. Caldwell J, Wakile LA, Notarianni LJ, et al. Maternal and neonatal disposition of pethidine in childbirth—a study using quantitative gas chromatography-mass spectrometry. *Life Sci* 1978;22:589.
71. Morrison JC, Whybrew WD, Rosser SI, Bucovaz ET, Wiser WL, Fish SA. Metabolites of meperidine in the fetal and maternal serum. *Am J Obstet Gynecol* 1976;126:997.
72. Shnider SM, Moya F. Effects of meperidine on the newborn infant. *Am J Obstet Gynecol* 1964;89:1009.
73. Belfrage P, Boréus LO, Hartvig P, Irestedt L, Raabe N. Neonatal depression after obstetrical analgesia with pethidine. The role of the injection-delivery time interval and of the plasma concentrations of pethidine and norpethidine. *Acta Obstet Gynecol Scand* 1981;60:43.
74. Kuhnert BR, Kuhnert PM, Tu ASL, Lin DCK. Meperidine and normeperidine levels following meperidine administration during labor. II. Fetus and neonate. *Am J Obstet Gynecol* 1979;133:909.
75. Kuhnert BR, Philipson EH, Kuhnert PM, Syracuse CD. Disposition of meperidine and normeperidine following multiple doses during labor. I. Mother. *Am J Obstet Gynecol* 1985;51:406.
76. Kuhnert BR, Kuhnert PM, Philipson EH, Syracuse CD. Disposition of meperidine and normeperidine following multiple doses during labor. II. Fetus and neonate. *Am J Obstet Gynecol* 1985;151:410.
77. Hodgkinson R, Bhatt M, Wang CN. Double-blind comparison of the neurobehaviour of neonates following the administration of different doses of meperidine to the mother. *Can Anaesth Soc J* 1978;25:405.
78. Belsey EM, Rosenblatt DB, Lieberman BA, et al. The influence of maternal analgesia on neonatal behaviour: I. Pethidine. *Br J Obstet Gynaeol* 1981;88:398.
79. Kuhnert BR, Linn PL, Kennard MJ, Kuhnert PM. Effects of low doses of meperidine on neonatal behavior. *Anesth Analg* 1985;64:335.

80. Golub MS, Donald JM. Effect of intrapartum meperidine on behavior of 3- to 12-month-old infant Rhesus monkeys. *Biol Neonate* 1995;67: 140.
81. Kariniemi V, Ämmälä P. Effects of intramuscular pethidine on fetal heart rate variability during labour. *Br J Obstet Gynaecol* 1981;88:718.
82. Zimmer EZ, Divon MY, Vadasz A. Influence of meperidine on fetal movements and heart rate beat-to-beat variability in the active phase of labor. *Am J Perinatol* 1988;5:197.
83. Fazackerley J, Pleuvry BJ. Stimulant action of pethidine on the pregnant rat uterus in-vitro. *J Pharm Pharmacol* 1987;39:491.
84. Sivalingam T, Pleuvry BJ. Actions of morphine, pethidine and pentazocine on the oestrus and pregnant rat uterus in vitro. *Br J Anaesth* 1985;57:430.
85. Campbell C, Phillips OC, Frazer TM. Analgesia during labour: a comparison of pentobarbital, meperidine and morphine. *Obstet Gynaecol* 1961;17:714.
86. DeVoe SJ, DeVoe K, Rigsby WC, McDaniels BA. Effect of meperidine on uterine contractility. *Am J Obstet Gynecol* 1969;105:1004.
87. Milwidsky A, Finci-Yeheskel Z, Mayer M. Direct stimulation of urokinase, plasmin, and collagenase by meperidine: a possible mechanism for the ability of meperidine to enhance cervical effacement and dilation. *Am J Perinatol* 1993;10:130.
88. Craft JB, Coaldrake LA, Bolan JC, et al. Placental passage and uterine effects of fentanyl. *Anesth Analg* 1983;62:894.
89. Eisele JH, Wright R, Rogge P. Newborn and maternal fentanyl levels at cesarean section. *Anesth Analg* 1982;61:179.
90. Rayburn W, Rathke A, Leuschen P, Chleborad J, Weidner W. Fentanyl citrate analgesia during labor. *Am J Obstet Gynecol* 1989;161:202.
91. Rayburn WF, Smith CV, Parriott JE, Woods RE. Randomized comparison of meperidine and fentanyl during labor. *Obstet Gynecol* 1989; 74:604.
92. Wilson SJ, Errick JK, Balkon J. Pharmacokinetics of nalbuphine during parturition. *Am J Obstet Gynecol* 1986;155:340.
93. Wilson CM, McClean E, Moore J, Dundee JW. A double-blind comparison of intramuscular pethidine and nalbuphine in labour. *Anaesthesia* 1986;41:1207.
94. Romagnili A, Keats AS. Ceiling effect for respiratory depression by nalbuphine. *Clin Pharmacol Ther* 1980;27:478.
95. Frank M, McAteer EJ, Cattermole R, Loughnan B, Stafford LB, Hitchcock AM. Nalbuphine for obstetric analgesia. *Anaesthesia* 1987; 42:697.
96. DelPizzo A. A double-blind study of the effects of butorphanol compared with morphine in balanced anaesthesia. *Can Anaesth Soc J* 1978;25:392.
97. Quillgan EJ, Keegan KA, Donahue MJ. Double-blind comparison of intravenously injected butorphanol and meperidine in parturients. *Int J Gynaecol Obstet* 1980;18:363.
98. Maduska AL, Hajghassemali M. A double-blind comparison of butorphanol and meperidine in labour: maternal pain relief and effect on the newborn. *Can Anaesth Soc J* 1978;25:398.
99. Hodgkinson R, Huff RW, Hayashi R, Husain F. Double-blind comparison of maternal analgesia and neonatal neurobehaviour following intravenous butorphanol and meperidine. *J Int Med Res* 1979;7:224.
100. Atkinson BD, Truitt LJ, Rayburn WF, Turnbull GL, Christensin HD, Wlodaver A. Double-blind comparison of intravenous butorphanol (Stadol) and fentanyl (Sublimaze) for analgesia during labor. *Am J Obstet Gynecol* 1994;171:993.
101. Jaffe JH, Martin WP. Opioids with mixed actions: partial agonists. In: Gilman AG, Rall TW, Nies AS, Taylor P, eds. *Pharmacological basis of therapeutics,* 8th ed. New York: Pergamon Press, 1990;15:510.
102. McQuitty FM. Relief of pain in labour. A controlled double-blind trial comparing pethidine and various phenothiazine derivatives. *J Obstet Gynaecol Br Cmnwlth* 1967;74:925.
103. Brelje MC, Garcia-Bunuel R. Meperidine-hydroxyzine in obstetric analgesia. *Obstet Gynecol* 1966;27:350.
104. Zsigmond EK, Patterson RL. Double-blind evaluation of hydroxyzine hydrochloride in obstetric anesthesia. *Anesth Analg* 1967;46:275.
105. Clark RB, Seifen AB. Systemic medication during labor and delivery. *Obstet Gynecol Ann* 1983;12:165.
106. Boehm FH, Growdon JH. The effect of scopolamine on fetal heart rate baseline variability. *Am J Obstet Gynecol* 1974;120:1099.
107. Boehm FH, Ehilmez A, Smith BE. Physostigmine's effect on the diminished fetal heart rate variability caused by scopolamine, meperidine, and propiomazine. *J Perinat Med* 1977;5:214.
108. Coalson DW, Glosten B. Alternatives to epidural analgesia. *Sem Perinatol* 1991;15:375.
109. Akamatsu TJ, Bonica JJ, Rehmet R, Eng M, Ueland K. Experiences with the use of ketamine for parturition: I. Primary anesthetic for vaginal delivery. *Anesth Analg* 1974;53:284.
110. Little B, Chang T, Chucot L, et al. Study of ketamine as an obstetric anesthetic agent. *Am J Obstet Gynecol* 1972;113:247.
111. Walker JJ, Johnston J, Fairlie F, Lloyd J, Bullingham R. A comparative study of intramuscular ketorolac and pethidine in labour pain. *Eur J Obstet Gynecol Reprod Biol* 1992;46:87.
112. Walker JJ, Johnstone J, Lloyd J, Rocha CL. The transfer of ketorolac tromethamine from maternal to foetal blood. *Eur J Clin Pharmacol* 1988;34:509.
113. Dawes JA. The distribution and action of drugs on the fetus in utero. *Br J Anaesth* 1973;45:766.
114. Desilva JAF, D'Anconte L, Kaplan J. The determination of blood levels and the placental transfer of diazepam in humans. *Curr Ther Res* 1964;6:121.
115. Cree JE, Meyer J, Hailey KM. Diazepam in labour: its metabolism and effects on the clinical condition and thermogenesis of the newborn. *Br Med J* 1973;3:251.
116. McAllister CB. Placental transfer and neonatal effects of diazepam when administered to women just before delivery. *Br J Anaesth* 1980; 52:423.
117. Owen JR, Irani SF, Blair AW. Effect of diazepam administered to mothers during labour on temperature regulation of the neonate. *Arch Dis Child* 1972;47:107.
118. Bramwell S. Systemic medications for labor analgesia. In: Norris MC, ed. *Obstetric anesthesia.* Philadelphia: JB Lippincott, 1993:281.
119. Bach V, Carl P, Ravlo O, et al. A randomized comparison between midazolam and thiopental for elective cesarean section anesthesia: III. Placental transfer and elimination in neonates. *Anesth Analg* 1989;68:238.
120. Bland BAR, Lawes EG, Duncan PW, et al. Comparison of midazolam and thiopental for rapid sequence anesthetic induction for elective cesarean section. *Anesth Analg* 1987;66:1165.
121. Ravel O, Carl P, Crawford ME, et al. A randomized comparison between midazolam and thiopental for elective cesarean section anesthesia: II. Neonate. *Anesth Analg* 1989;68:234.
122. Camann W, Cohen MB, Ostheimer GW. Is midazolam desirable for sedation in parturients? *Anesthesiology* 1986;65:441.
123. Heyman HJ, Salem MR. Is midazolam desirable for sedation in parturients—reply. *Anesthesiology* 1987;66:577.
124. Ginsberg FB, Bell SN. Midazolam in obstetric anesthesia—a reply. *Anesthesiology* 1988;68:296.
125. Seidman SF, Marx GF. Midazolam in obstetric anesthesia. *Anesthesiology* 1987;67:443.
126. Gibbs CP. Obstetric anesthesia: a national survey. *Anesthesiology* 1986;65:298.
127. Hawkins JL, Gibbs CP, Orleans M, Martin-Salvaj G, Beaty B. Obstetric anesthesia work force survey, 1981 versus 1992. *Anesthesiology* 1997;87:135.
128. Carstoniu MA, Levytam S, Norman P, Daley D, Katz J, Sandler AN. Nitrous oxide in early labor. *Anesthesiology* 1994;80:30.
129. Marx GF, Katsnelson T. The introduction of nitrous oxide analgesia into obstetrics. *Obstet Gynecol* 1992;80:715.
130. Rosen, M. Recent advances in pain relief in childbirth: inhalation and systemic analgesia. *Br J Anaesth* 1971;43:837.
131. Brownridge P. Treatment options for the relief of pain during childbirth. *Drugs* 1991;41:69.
132. Bernow J, Bjrdal J, Wiklund KE. Pollution of delivery ward air by nitrous oxide. Effects of various modes of room ventilation, excess and close scavenging. *Acta Anaesthesiol Scand* 1984;28:119.
133. Munley AJ, Railton R, Gray WM, Carter KB. Exposure of midwives to nitrous oxide in four hospitals. *Br Med J* 1986;293:1063.
134. Mills GH, Singh D, Longan M, O'Sullivan J, Caunt JA. Nitrous oxide exposure on the labour ward. *Int J Obstet Anesth* 1996;5:160.
135. Cheek TG, Gutsche BB. Comment. *Surv Anesth* 1987;31:276.
136. Deckardt R, Fembacker PM, Schneider KTM, Graeff H. Maternal arterial oxygen saturation during labor and delivery: pain-dependent alterations and effects on the newborn. *Obstet Gynecol* 1987;70:21.
137. Lin DM, Reisner LS, Benumof J. Hypoxemia occurs intermittently and significantly with nitrous oxide labor analgesia. *Anesth Analg* 1989;68:S167(abst).

138. Norman PH, Kavanagh B, Daley MD. Nitrous oxide analgesia in labour. *Anesth Analg* 1992;74:S222(abst).
139. Reed PN, Coloquhoun AD, Hanning CD. Maternal oxygenation during normal labour. *Br J Anaesth* 1989;62:316.
140. Stefani SJ, Hughes SC, Shnider SM, et al. Neonatal neurobehavioral effects of inhalation analgesia for vaginal delivery. *Anesthesiology* 1982;56:351.
141. Rudgren B, Dottori O, Nordström G, Seeman T. Hemodynamic effects in dogs of nitrous oxide-meperidine and meperidine, respectively, in comparison with nitrous oxide. *Acta Anaesthesiol Scand* 1990;34:585.
142. Eriksen S, Johannsen G, Frost N. Effects of nitrous oxide on systolic time interval. *Acta Anaesth Scand* 1980;24:74.
143. Westling F, Milsom I, Zetterström H, Ekström-Jodal B. Effects of nitrous oxide/oxygen inhalation on the maternal circulation during vaginal delivery. *Acta Anaesthesiol Scand* 1992;36:175.
144. Polvi HJ, Pirhonen JP, Efkkola RU. Nitrous oxide inhalation: effects on maternal and fetal circulations at term. *Obstet Gynecol* 1996; 87:1045.
145. Munson ES, Embro WJ. Enflurane, isoflurane, and halothane and isolated human uterine muscle. *Anesthesiology* 1977;46:11.
146. Marx GF, Kim YI, Lin CC, Halevy S, Schulman H. Postpartum uterine pressures under halothane or enflurane anesthesia. *Obstet Gynecol* 1978;51:695.
147. Abadir AR, Humayun SG, Calvello D, Gintautas J. Effects of isoflurane and oxytocin on gravid human uterus in vitro. *Anesth Analg* 1987;66:S1(abst).
148. McGuinness C, Rosen M. Enflurane as an analgesic in labour. *Anaesthesia* 1984;39:24.
149. Abboud TK, Shnider SM, Wright RG, et al. Enflurane analgesia in obstetrics. *Anesth Analg* 1981;60:133.
150. McLeod DD, Ramayya GP, Tunstall ME. Self-administered isoflurane in labour. *Anaesthesia* 1985;40:424.
151. Abboud TK, Gangolly J, Mosaad P, Crowell D. Isoflurane in obstetrics. *Anesth Analg* 1989;68:388.
152. Rampil IJ, Zwass M, Lockhart S, et al. MAC of 1653 in surgical patients. *Anesthesiology* 1989;71:A269(abst).
153. Abboud TK, Swart F, Qhu J, Donovan MM, DaSilva P, Yakal K. Desflurane analgesia for vaginal delivery. *Acta Anaesthesiol Scand* 1995; 39:259.
154. Gambling DR, Sharma SK, White PF, Van Beveren T, Bala AS, Gouldson R. Use of sevoflurane during elective cesarean birth: a comparison with isoflurane and spinal anesthesia. *Anesth Analg* 1995;81:90.
155. Katoh T, Kazuyuki I. The minimum alveolar concentration (MAC) of sevoflurane in humans. *Anesthesiology* 1987;66:301.
156. Eger EI. New inhaled anesthetics. *Anesthesiology* 1994;80:906.
157. Bonica JJ. *Principles and practice of obstetrical anesthesia.* Philadelphia: FA Davis, 1967:487.
158. King JC, Sherline DM. Paracervical and pudendal block. *Clin Obstet Gynecol* 1981;24:587.
159. Thiery M, Vroman S. Paracervical block analgesia during labor. *Am J Obstet Gynecol* 1972;113:988.
160. Chestnut DH. *Alternative regional anesthetic techniques: paracervical block, lumbar sympathetic block, pudendal block, and perineal infiltration.* St. Louis: Mosby-Year Book, Inc., 1994:420.
161. Abouleish E. *Paracervical block.* In: Abouleish E. Pain control in obstetrics. Philadelphia: JB Lippincott, 1977:342.
162. Jgerhorn M. Paracervical block in obstetrics. An improved injection method. *Acta Obstet Gynecol Scand* 1975;54:9.
163. Kobak AJ, Sadove MS, Mazeros WT. Anatomic studies of transvaginal regional anesthesia. *Obstet Gynecol* 1962;19:302.
164. Saloheimo AM. Paracervical block anesthesia in labor. *Acta Obstet Gynecol Scand* 1968;47[Suppl 5]:3.
165. Ranney B. Paracervical block for first-stage pain in primigravidas. *Obstet Gynecol* 1966;27:757.
166. Van Dorsten JP, Miller FC, Yeh S. Spacing the injection interval with paracervical block: a randomized study. *Obstet Gynecol* 1981;58:696.
167. Day TW. Community use of paracervical block in labor. *J Fam Pract* 1989;28:545.
168. Ranta P, Jouppila P, Spalding M, Kangas-Saarela T, Jouppila R. Paracervical block—a viable alternative for labor pain relief? *Acta Obstet Gynecol Scand* 1995;74:122.
169. Nesheim B. Which local anesthetic is best suited for paracervical blocks? *Acta Obstet Gynecol Scand* 1983;62:261.
170. Tafeen CH, Freedman HL, Harris H. A system of continuous paracervical block anesthesia. *Am J Obstet Gynecol* 1966;94:854.
171. Weiss RR, Halevy S, Almonte RO, Gundersen K, Hinsvark ON, O'Brien JE. Comparison of lidocaine and 2-chloroprocaine in paracervical block: clinical effects and drug concentrations in mother and child. *Anesth Analg* 1983;62:168.
172. Philipson EH, Kuhnert BR, Syracuse CB, Reese AL, Rosen MG. Intrapartum paracervical block anesthesia with 2-chloroprocaine. *Am J Obstet Gynecol* 1983;146:16.
173. Rosefsky JB, Petersiel ME. Perinatal deaths associated with mepivacaine paracervical block anesthesia in labor. *N Engl J Med* 1968;27: 530.
174. Shnider SM, Gildea J. Paracervical block anesthesia in obstetrics. *Am J Obstet Gynecol* 1973;16:320.
175. Miller FC, Quesnel G, Petrie RH, Paul RH, Hon EH. The effects of paracervical block on uterine activity and beat-to-beat variability of the fetal heart rate. *Am J Obstet Gynecol* 1978;130:284.
176. Read JA, Miller FC. The bupivacaine paracervical block in labor and its effect on quantitative uterine activity. *Obstet Gynecol* 1979;53: 166.
177. Saarela-Kangas T, Jouppila R, Puolakka J, Jouppila P, Hollmn A, Puukka M. The effect of bupivacaine paracervical block on the neurobehavioural responses of newborn infants. *Acta Anaesthesiol Scand* 1988;32:566.
178. Teramo K. Effects of obstetrical paracervical blockade on the fetus. *Acta Obstet Gynecol Scand [Suppl]* 1971;16:1.
179. Jenssen H. The effect of paracervical block on cervical dilatation and uterine activity. *Acta Obstet Gynecol Scand* 1973;52:13.
180. Fishburne JI, Greiss FC, Hopkinson R, Rhyne AL. Responses of the gravid uterine vasculature to arterial levels of local anesthetic agents. *Am J Obstet Gynecol* 1979;133:753.
181. Hibbard LT, Snyder EN, McVann RM. Subgluteal and retropsoal infection in obstetric practice. *Obstet Gynecol* 1972;39:137.
182. Gaylord TG, Pearson JW. Neuropathy following paracervical block in the obstetric patient. *Obstet Gynecol* 1982;60:521.
183. Freeman RK, Gutierrez NA, Ray ML, Stovall D, Paul RH, Hon EH. Fetal cardiac response to paracervical block anesthesia. Part I. *Am J Obstet Gynecol* 1972;113:583.
184. LeFevre ML. Fetal heart rate pattern and postparacervical fetal bradycardia. *Obstet Gynecol* 1984;64:343.
185. Gordon HR. Fetal bradycardia after paracervical block. *N Engl J Med* 1968;279:910.
186. Asling JH, Shnider SM, Margolis AJ, Wilkinson GL, Way EL. Paracervical block anesthesia on obstetrics. *Am J Obstet Gynecol* 1970; 107:626.
187. Shnider SM, Asling JH, Holl JW, Margolis AJ. Paracervical block anesthesia in obstetrics. *Am J Obstet Gynecol* 1970;107:619.
188. Teramo K. Studies on foetal acid-base values after paracervical blockade during labour. *Acta Obstet Gynecol Scand [Suppl]* 1969; 48:80.
189. Gibbs CP, Noel SC. Response of arterial segments from gravid human uterus to multiple concentrations of lignocaine. *Br J Anaesth* 1977; 49:409.
190. Cibils LA. Response of human uterine arteries to local anesthetics. *Am J Obstet Gynecol* 1976;126:202.
191. Greiss FC, Still JG, Anderson SG. Effects of local anesthetic agents on the uterine vasculatures and myometrium. *Am J Obstet Gynecol* 1976;124:889.
192. Van Dorsten JP, Miller FC. Fetal heart rate changes after accidental intrauterine lidocaine. *Obstet Gynecol* 1981;57:257.
193. Baxi LV, Petrie RH, James LS. Human fetal oxygenation following paracervical block. *Am J Obstet Gynecol* 1979;135:1109.
194. Jensen F, Qvist I, Brocks V, Secher NJ, Westergaard LG. Submucous paracervical blockade compared with intramuscular meperidine as analgesia during labor: a double-blind study. *Obstet Gynecol* 1984; 64:724.
195. Cleland JGP. Paravertebral anaesthesia in obstetrics. *Surg Gynecol Obstet* 1933;57:51.
196. Reich AM. Paravertebral lumbar sympathetic block in labor. *Am J Obstet Gynecol* 1951;61:1263.
197. Meguiar RV, Wheeler AS. Lumbar sympathetic block with bupivacaine: analgesia for labor. *Anesth Analg* 1978;57:486.
198. Brown DL. *Regional anesthesia and analgesia.* Philadelphia: WB Saunders, 1996:369.

199. Jarvis SM. Paravertebral sympathetic nerve block, a method for the safe and painless conduct of labor. *Am J Obstet Gynecol* 1944;47:335.
200. Hunter CA. Uterine motility studies during labor. *Am J Obstet Gynecol* 1963;85:681.
201. Parris WC, Kirshner HS. Motor paralysis of the lower extremities following lumbar sympathetic block. *Anesthesiology* 1993;78:981.
202. Nagaro T, Arai T. Anterior spinal artery syndrome (comment)? *Anesthesiology* 1993;79:1156.
203. Gay GR, Evans JA. Total spinal anesthesia following lumbar paravertebral block: a potentially lethal complication. *Anesth Analg* 1971; 50:344.
204. Artuso JD, Stevens RA, Lineberry PJ. Post dural puncture headache after lumbar sympathetic block: a report of two cases. *Reg Anesth* 1991;16:288.
205. Wills MH, Korbon GA, Arasi R. Horner's syndrome resulting from a lumbar sympathetic block. *Anesthesiology* 1988;68:613.
206. Haynsworth RF, Noe CE, Raymond Fassy L. Intralymphatic injection: another complication of lumbar sympathetic block. *Anesthesiology* 1994;80:460.
207. Melzack R, Schaffelberg D. Low-back pain during labor. *Am J Obstet Gynecol* 1987;156:901.
208. Trolle B, Møller M, Kronborg H, Thomsen S. The effect of sterile water blocks on low back labor pain. *Am J Obstet Gynecol* 1991;164:1277.
209. Bonica JJ. Peripheral mechanisms and pathways of parturition pain. *Br J Anaesth* 1979;51:3S.
210. Ulmsten U, Sandahl B, Lunden C, Andersson KE. Treatment of labor pain with locally applied ketocaine. *Acta Obstet Gynecol Scand* 1980; 59:209.
211. Bengtsson J, Worning AM, Gertz J. Pain due to urolithiasis treated by intracutaneous injection of sterile water. *Ugreskr Laeger* 1981; 143:3463.
212. Raj PP. *Practical management of pain.* Chicago: Year Book Medical Publishers, 1986:569.
213. Wall PD, Melzack R. *Textbook of pain,* 3rd ed. London: Churchill Livingstone, 1994:5110.
214. Travell JG, Simons DG. *Myofascial pain and dysfunction: the trigger point manual*. Baltimore: Williams & Wilkins, 1983.
215. Tsen SC, Camann WR. Trigger point injections for myofascial pain during epidural analgesia for labor. *Reg Anesth* 1997;22:466.
216. Zador G, Lindmark G, Nilsson BA. Pudendal block in normal vaginal deliveries. *Acta Obstet Gynecol Scand [Suppl]* 1974;34:51.
217. Schierup L, Schmidt JF, Jensen T, Rye BAO. Pudendal block in vaginal deliveries. *Acta Obstet Gynecol Scand* 1988;67:195.
218. Merkow AJ, McGuinness GA, Erenberg A, Kennedy RL. The neonatal neurobehavioral effects of bupivacaine, mepivacaine, and 2-chloroprocaine used for pudendal block. *Anesthesiology* 1980;52:309.
219. Kurzel RB, Au AH. Retroperitoneal hematoma as a complication of pudendal block. Diagnosis made by computed tomography. *Westein Journal of Medicine* 1996;164:523.
220. Eriksson E. *Illustrated handbook in local anesthesia.* London: Lloyd-Luke, 1979:52.
221. Bunting P, McConachie I. Ilioinguinal nerve blockade for analgesia after caesarean section. *Br J Anaesth* 1988;61:773.
222. Bell ED, Greengrass R, Spahn T, Penning DH. Iliohypogastric and ilioinguinal peripheral nerve blocks reduce postoperative morphine requirements after cesarean section. *Anesthesiology* 1997;87:A869.
223. Ganta R, Samra SK, Maddineni VR, Furness G. Comparison of the effectiveness of bilateral ilioinguinal nerve block and wound infiltration for postoperative analgesia after caesarean section. *Br J Anaesth* 1994;72:229.
224. Huffnagle HJ, Norris MC, Leighton BL, Arkoosh VA. Ilioinguinal iliohypogastric nerve blocks—before or after cesarean delivery under spinal anesthesia? *Anesth Analg* 1996;82:8.
225. Brown DL. *Atlas of regional anesthesia.* Philadelphia: WB Saunders, 1992:236.
226. Derrick JL, Aun CST. Transient femoral nerve palsy after ilioinguinal block [Letter]. *Anaesth Intens Care* 1996;24:115.
227. Kobak AJ, Evans FE, Johnson GR. Transvaginal pudendal nerve block. A simple procedure for effective anesthesia in operative delivery. *Am J Obstet Gynecol* 1956;71:981.

Obstetric Anesthesia, second edition,
edited by Mark C. Norris.
Lippincott Williams & Wilkins, Philadelphia © 1999.

CHAPTER 14

Anatomy of the Epidural Space

Quinn Hogan

Regional anesthesia for labor and cesarean section requires appropriate patient selection, choice of agents, management of side effects, and avoidance of complications. In addition to this complex sequence of decisions, the obstetric anesthetist also must achieve a basic technologic goal—successful delivery of anesthetics into the epidural or subarachnoid space. Proper placement of neuraxial needles and catheters is an exercise in applied anatomy and requires a clear mental image of locations and relations of various structures.

This chapter describes anatomic features in progression from outside inward. Three aspects of spinal anatomy emerge as recurring themes. First, it is evident that many published accounts of the soft tissues of the vertebral canal are inaccurate. This shortcoming probably results from several reasons:

- Study of preserved and distorted material,
- Examination by methods that create artifact such as epiduroscopy or radiologic imaging after contrast injection,
- The inherent challenges of scrutinizing frail tissues hidden within very sturdy walls, and
- The imagination of medical illustrators.

Second, variability is part of nature, and anatomic features display expected interindividual differences. Finally, it is impossible to know too much anatomy. The images we carry in our minds of the objects a needle strikes, the location of the catheter tip, or the pattern of solution spread are the basis upon which we plan redirection of the needle or speculate on the cause of unexpected anesthetic distribution. Text and images are an imperfect means of instruction in anatomy. Frequent examination of a skeleton is helpful in mastering the intricate topography of the vertebrae. Dissection is invaluable in gaining an appreciation of actual anatomy and can usually be arranged at medical schools, refresher courses, or in the autopsy lab.

Q. Hogan: Department of Anesthesiology, Medical College of Wisconsin, Milwaukee, Wisconsin 53226.

SURFACE LANDMARKS

The extent of blockade associated with both spinal and epidural anesthesia depends on vertebral level of injection. In the absence of imaging, determination of the site of needle insertion requires inferring vertebral level from palpable bony landmarks. Data show a disappointing success rate of less than 50% in accurately predicting vertebral level of insertion (1–3). Lumbar levels of puncture are typically used in obstetrics, and Tuffier's line, or the line between the iliac crests, is the most common reference (Fig. 1). The utility of this method is compromised in part by variations in the amount of subcutaneous fat, resulting in a more rostral apparent site in obese patients. In addition, the level of the iliac crests is widely variable (Fig. 2). The line between them crosses the vertebral column with a maximal incidence at the L_{4-5} disc (perhaps higher on

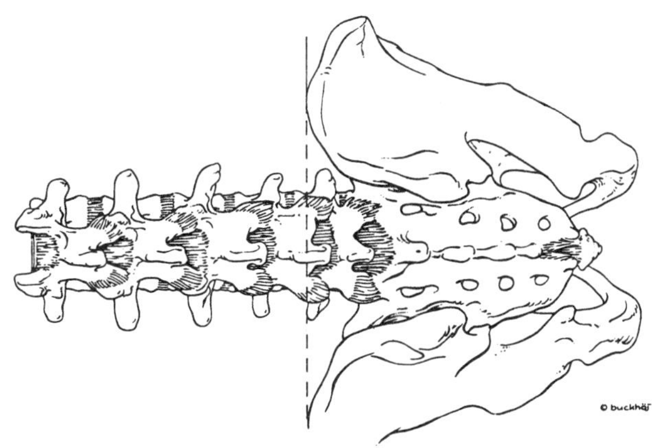

FIG. 1. The most common reference for level of insertion of lumbar epidural or spinal needles is the line between the iliac crests, or Tuffier's line. (Reproduced from ref. 51, with permission.)

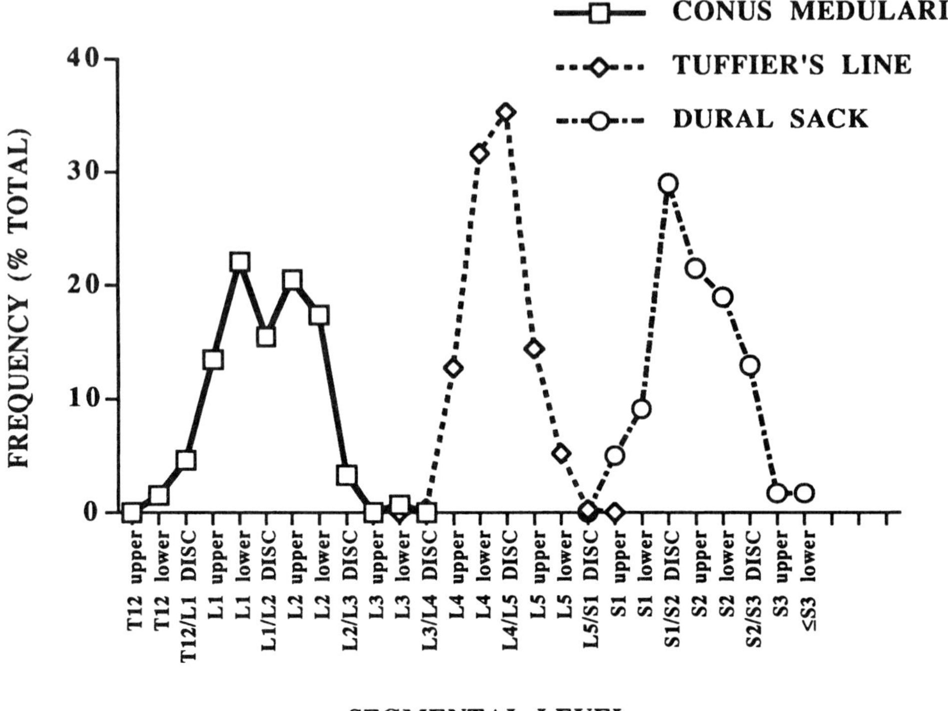

FIG. 2. Anatomic features show interindividual variation in a normal distribution. The level at which the line between the iliac crests (Tuffier's line) crosses the vertebral column is most often the L_{4-5} disc but may be as high as the L_{3-4} disc and as low as the L_5–S_1 disc. The caudal tip of the dural sac and the end of the spinal cord (the conus medularis) show similar variability.

average in men than women), but the range is from as low as the L_5–S_1 disc to as high as the L_{3-4} disc (4).

Identification of the mid-line may be difficult when palpation of spinous processes is impeded by abundant subcutaneous tissue. Symmetry and a mid-line skin crease may be helpful in locating the mid-line in a sitting patient, provided the subject is positioned squarely on the bed and there is no deformity. In the lateral position, visible landmarks are not useful and palpation may be deceptive, because the apparent location of the vertebral column can be more dependent than the location at which the mid-line structures are ultimately found. Use of a small-gauge needle to contact the spinous process may be necessary to establish the bony mid-line. A 2-inch, 22-gauge needle can be used to locate bony structures while anesthetizing superficial tissues. In the obese subject, a 22-gauge spinal needle might be necessary as a finder needle to locate the spinous processes. A mid-line tuft of hair or dimple is a superficial indication of a possible partial spinal bifida. In this setting, a normal epidural space may not exist, and the nerve roots cannot be assumed to be free in the cerebrospinal fluid (CSF).

Although the sacral hiatus is widely patent in children, this anatomic region is particularly unpredictable in adulthood. Palpation often fails to identify the sacral crurae on either side of the hiatus. Fusion of the posterior roof of the sacral vertebral canal is typically complete down to the S_5 level, where the sacral hiatus remains open. However, an entire lack of any posterior bony roof or virtually complete closure or the sacral vertebral canal are found in about 8% of subjects (5). In 5% of adult sacral bones, the anterior–posterior diameter of the canal at the hiatus is 2 mm or less.

POSTERIOR LIGAMENTS

The supraspinous ligament joins the tips of the spinous processes and may be felt as a heavy band in the mid-line in thin individuals (Fig. 3). In the lower lumbar region, it thins and vanishes (6) to allow greater flexion there. The interspinous ligament is a narrow mid-line web between the spinous processes with fibers running in a posterocranial direction. Slit-like cavities filled with fat may develop in this ligament and result in a loss of resistance to the advancement of the needle and to injection, creating the false impression of having entered the epidural space. The ligament is so narrow that a slightly oblique needle may pass out of the side of the ligament, which also may be perceived as epidural entry (Fig. 4). Because the supraspinous and interspinous ligaments are composed largely of fibrous collagen, a needle passing through them generates a characteristic snapping sensation as the fibers are severed.

At its anterior margin, the interspinous ligament blends into the ligamentum flavum. Unlike the more superficial ligaments, the ligamentum flavum is 80% elastin, which gives it a characteristic yellow color. It has a dense homogenous texture, which is readily appreciated as a needle passes through it. Tension in the ligamentum

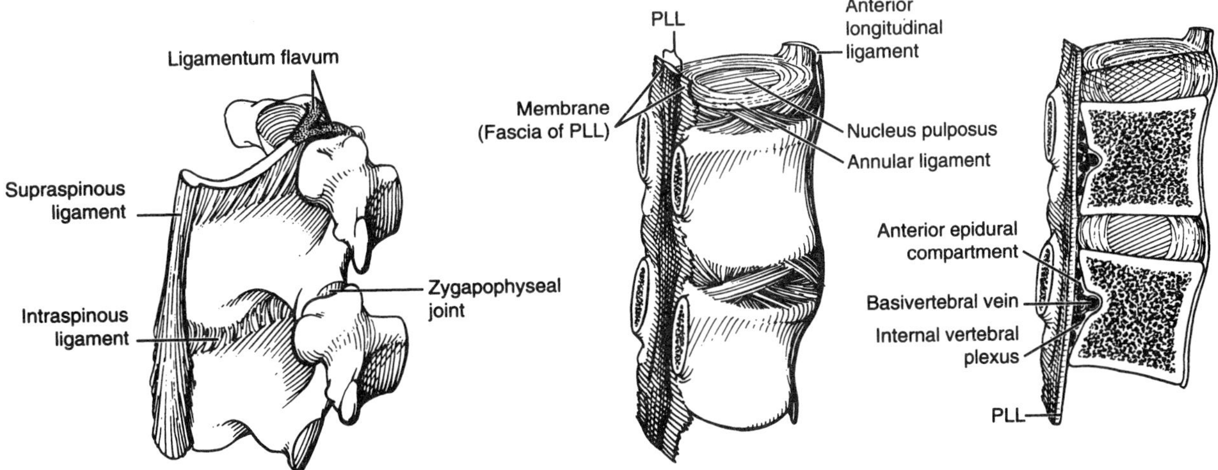

FIG. 3. Ligaments of the lumbar vertebral column. The supraspinous ligament joins the tips of the spinous processes, and the interspinous ligaments form a web between them. The posterior longitudinal ligament *(PLL)* runs behind the vertebral bodies joining the discs and extends laterally as a membrane, whereas the broad anterior longitudinal ligament reinforces the front of the column. Veins occupy the area anterior to the PLL. The annular ligament surrounds the nucleus pulposus of the intervertebral disc. (Reproduced from ref. 52, with permission.)

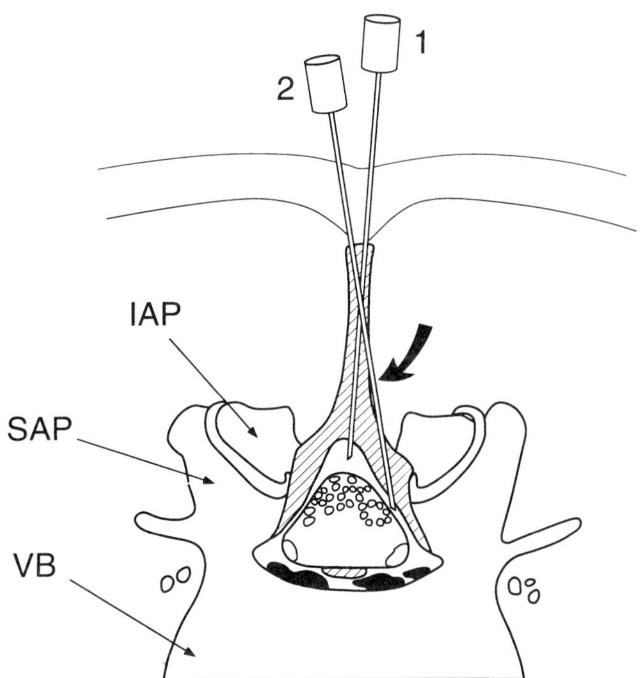

FIG. 4. A needle inserted exactly in the mid-line will travel in the interspinous ligament and then into the ligamentum flavum (shown together as *cross-hatched* in this drawing). The epidural space is thickest from posterior to anterior (between the ligamentum flavum and dura) in the mid-line. A needle inserted slightly at an angle (in this image, about 13 degrees from the sagittal plane) may exit the interspinous ligament *(arrow)* before reaching the ligamentum flavum, creating the impression of a loss of resistance. Also, when not in the mid-line, a needle will encounter the ligamentum flavum at a greater depth and will travel a longer course through the ligamentum flavum before reaching the epidural space. Finally, the thickness of the epidural space decreases away from the mid-line so that the dura is encountered immediately upon piercing the ligamentum flavum. (Traced from cryomicrotome data as in Fig. 10; the caudal tip of a spinous process evident in Fig. 10 is eliminated in this drawing to represent the plane of the needle course.)

flavum is evident as it retracts to half its length when cut. It spans from the anterior surface of the rostral lamina of an adjacent pair of vertebrae to the posterior aspect of the lower lamina. The right and left halves meet at an angle of less than 90 degrees, and a gap may be present in the mid-line (7). The lateral edges of the ligamenta flava wrap anteriorly around the medial margin of the facet joints, reinforcing the joint capsule. Bone, which may occasionally impede the passage of spinal and epidural needles, may grow into the margins of the ligamentum flavum, even in young patients (8,9).

The thickness of the ligamentum flavum typically is reported as between 2 and 5 mm (10,11). This dimension is not, however, a useful parameter in judging the placement of an epidural needle. If it passes through the mid-line slit between the right and left halves, the needle may occasionally enter the epidural space without engaging the ligamentum flavum. Furthermore, because the ligament is not in a coronal plane but rather is steeply angled and the needle will not engage it at right angles, the pathway through the ligamentum flavum may be substantially longer (Fig. 4).

VERTEBRAL BONES

The lumbar vertebral column often has more or less than five vertebrae. The L_5 vertebra is fused to S_1 in 6.2% of normal subjects, and the S_1 vertebra shows incomplete fusion to S_2 in 5.3% (12). Developmental defects in a lumbar vertebral arch occur in 3.9% of subjects. In the paramedian approach to the epidural space, the posterior bony elements are contacted first as a reference point, so absent bone could result in uncertain needle placement.

The lumbar vertebral bones (Fig. 5) are complicated structures that can best be appreciated as elements encir-

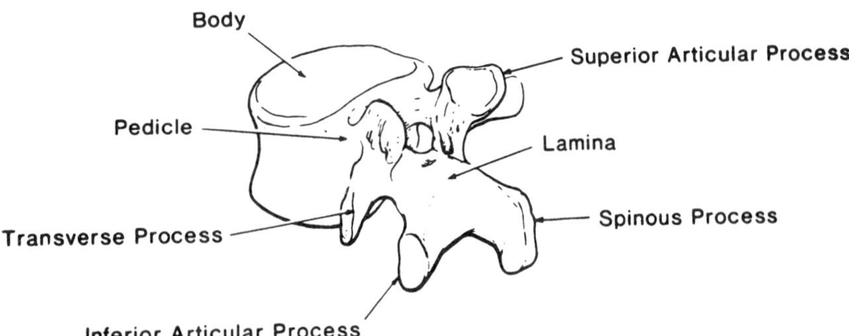

FIG. 5. Components of a lumbar vertebra.

cling the central vertebral canal, combined with processes extending from them. Anterior to the vertebral canal, the vertebral body is the largest part of the vertebral bone and carries a large part of the load supporting the body. It is markedly wider at the endplates than in the middle, resulting in an hourglass shape. They articulate with adjacent vertebral bodies by the intervertebral discs and are further joined by the heavy anterior longitudinal ligament in the front and the band of posterior longitudinal ligament behind.

The pedicles arise from the posterior aspect of the vertebral bodies and form the lateral walls of the vertebral canal. The plate-like laminae close the circle and form the posterior boundary of the vertebral canal. The transverse processes extend laterally from the junction of the pedicle and lamina, and the spinous process extends from the mid-line fusion of the laminae but may not remain in the mid-line as it extends posteriorly. Superior and inferior articular processes attach to either side of the lateral laminae and, with their corresponding members from the adjacent vertebra, form the zygapophyseal (facet) joints.

During mid-line epidural and spinal needle placement, the gap between the spinous processes must be identified.

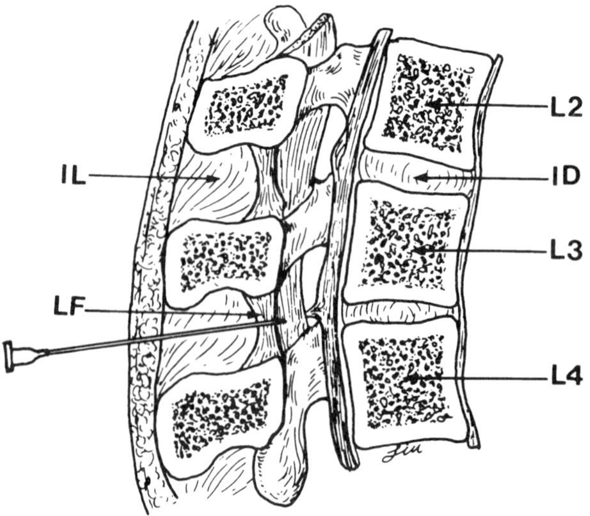

FIG. 6. Sagittal view of the course of an epidural needle into the epidural space.

The inferior edge of the spinous processes are somewhat concave downward (Fig. 6). The space between the interspinous processes lies at an angle of about 63 to 83 degrees from the axial plane (13), so the clearest path for a needle is slightly rostral in angle from a starting point closer to the lower spinous process than the upper one. Flexion of the spine widens the space between the spinous processes. Loss of disc height may narrow or obliterate the space between spinous processes as well as diminish the interlaminar gap through which the needle must ultimately pass (14). The lamina is the bone most commonly encountered by the needle, which usually indicates a need for a more rostral needle direction. Arthritic changes can lead to expansion of the zygapophyseal joints, which may then encroach upon the needle path, but these impediments are not characteristic of patients in the obstetric age range. By far the most common anatomic error in needle placement is mistaken identification of the mid-line.

EPIDURAL SPACE

The epidural space is the area inside the vertebral canal but outside the dural sac. Nature has provided the spinal cord and nerve roots with a sturdy but flexible surrounding wall. The padding and lubricating effects of the fat and membranes in the epidural space provide free motion of the dural sac within the walls of the vertebral canal.

Artists depictions of epidural anatomy typically show a space of uniform width completely encircling the dura. However, in its undisturbed state as revealed by cryomicrotome sections (Figs. 7–11) (7) and in vivo imaging, the lumbar vertebral canal is mostly filled by the dural sac. The epidural space is empty (a "potential space") in large areas where dura contacts the bone and ligament of the vertebral canal wall. Rather than being spread out in a uniform layer, epidural contents are contained in a series of metamerically and circumferentially discontinuous compartments separated by zones where the dura contacts the canal wall (Fig. 12). Inferior to the L_4–L_5 disc and in the sacral canal, the dural sac tapers to a smaller diameter and does not fill the canal as completely, so there is a proportionate increase in the abundance of epidural fat (Fig. 11). The variability of sacral

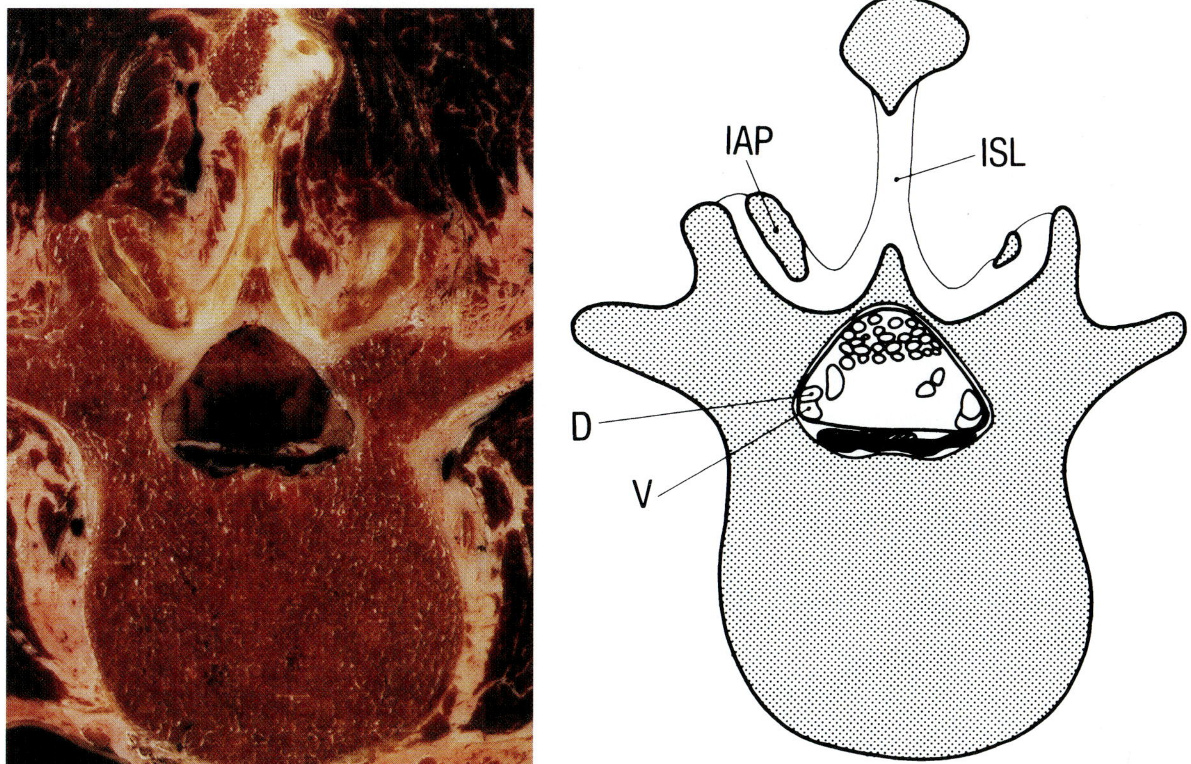

FIG. 7. Axial cryomicrotome sections through the lumbar vertebrae of a single subject at four different levels. This figure is at the level of the pedicles of the third lumbar vertebra. Cortical bone is white and medullary bone is red. *D*, dorsal root ganglion; *IAP*, inferior articular process; *ISL*, intraspinous ligament; *V*, ventral root. Posterior is at the top of the image.

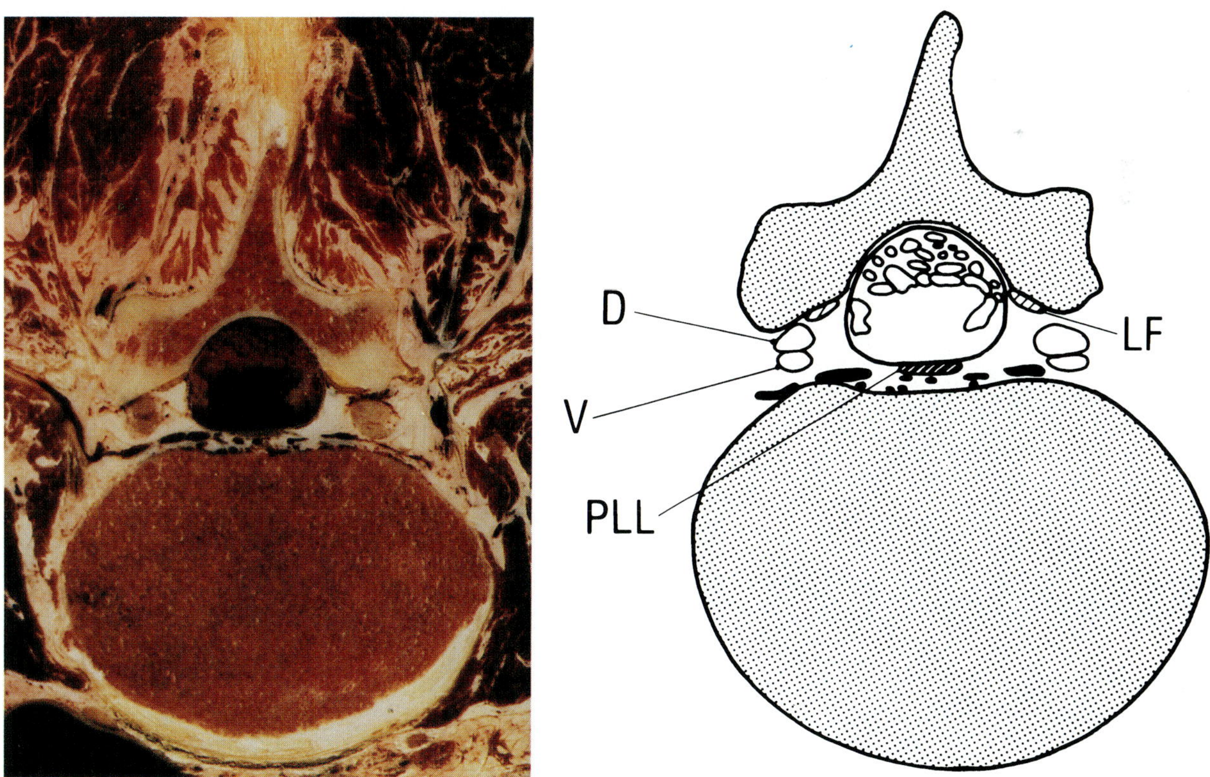

FIG. 8. Axial cryomicrotome sections through the lumbar vertebrae of a single subject at four different levels. This figure is at a more caudal level through the L_3–L_4 intervertebral foramen. Cortical bone is white and medullary bone is red. *D*, dorsal root ganglion; *LF*, ligamentum flavum; *PLL*, posterior longitudinal ligament; *V*, ventral root. Posterior is at the top of the image.

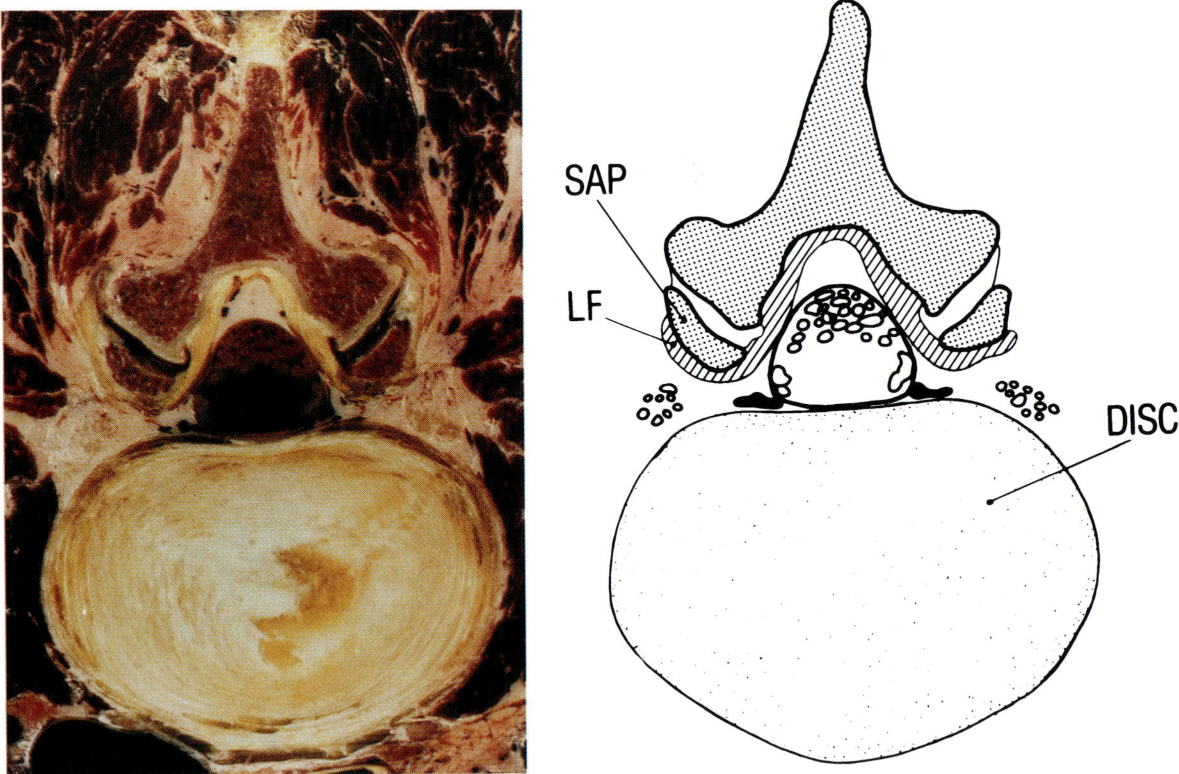

FIG. 9. Axial cryomicrotome sections through the lumbar vertebrae of a single subject at four different levels. This figure is at a somewhat more caudal level through the L_3–L_4 disc. Cortical bone is white and medullary bone is red. *LF*, ligamentum flavum; *SAP*, superior articular process. Posterior is at the top of the image.

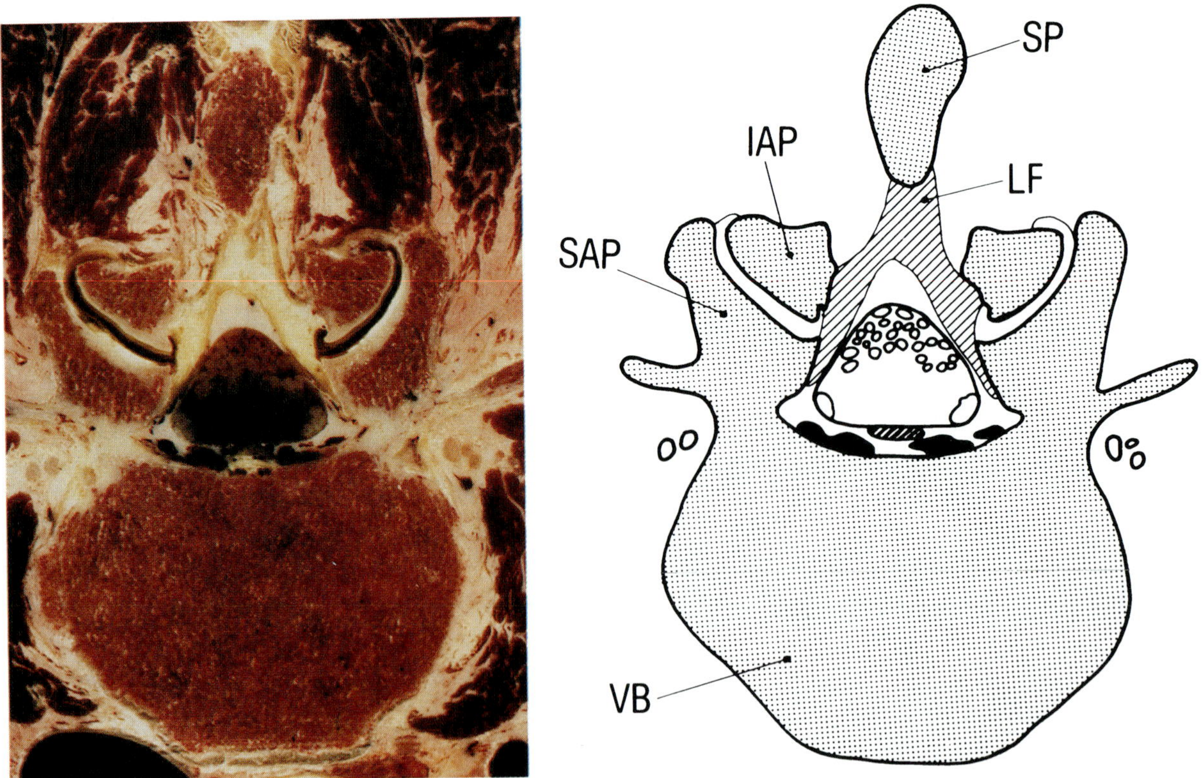

FIG. 10. Axial cryomicrotome sections through the lumbar vertebrae of a single subject at four different levels. This figure is through the vertebral body and pedicles of L_4. Cortical bone is white and medullary bone is red. *IAP*, inferior articular process; *LF*, ligamentum flavum; *SAP*, superior articular process; *SP*, spinous process; *VB*, vertebral body. Posterior is at the top of the image.

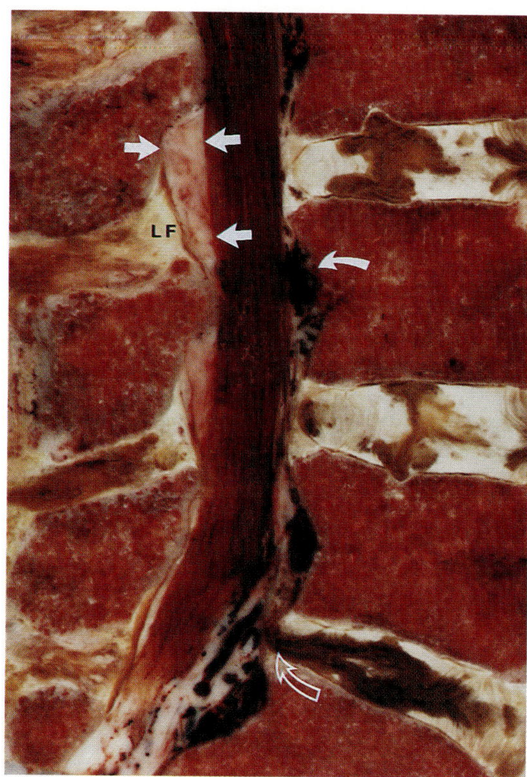

FIG. 11. Mid-line sagittal cryomicrotome section through the vertebral column at the levels L_3–S_1. Anterior is to the right. *Outlined arrow*, herniated nucleus pulposus at the L_5–S_1 disc; *straight arrows*, posterior epidural fat; *solid curved arrow*, anterior epidural veins.

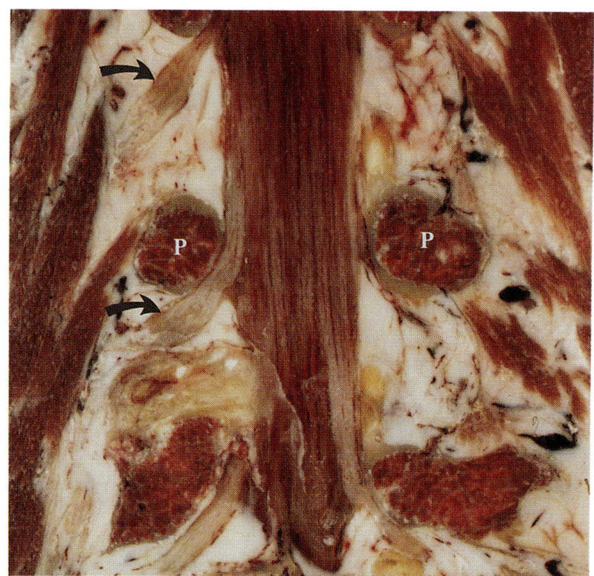

FIG. 13. Coronal cryomicrotome section through the pedicles and intervertebral foramina of L_3 (just visible at the top of the image), L_4, and L_5. The plane is slightly oblique so that the nerve roots and dorsal root ganglia *(arrow)* are evident on the *left* but not the *right*, and yellow-appearing ligamentum flavum is evident where the plane of section leaves the foramen and catches the more posterior ligamentum flavum. The lateral boundary of the spinal canal has more window (intervertebral foramina) than wall (pedicles) so the spinal canal is in free communication with the retroperitoneal space through foramina filled with fat and nerve roots.

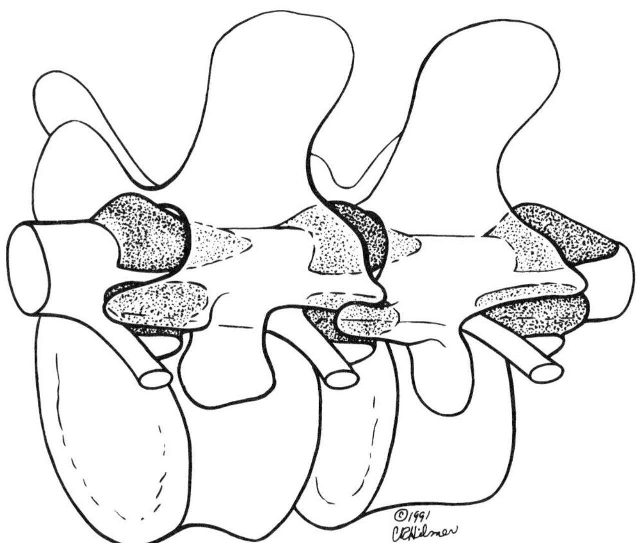

FIG. 12. Drawing of the distribution of the contents of the epidural space. The *stippled areas* represent posterior (toward the top of the image) and lateral epidural compartments, separated by areas in which the dura contacts the canal wall and there are no contents. The anterior epidural space is not shown.

anatomy is reflected in the highly unpredictable sacral canal volume, which may vary in adults from 12 to 65 mL (15).

Posterior Epidural Space

The area of most interest to anesthesiologists is the posterior compartment of the epidural space into which needles are inserted. It is filled by a fat pad that is triangular in axial section, confined between the dura and ligamenta flava. Longitudinally the fat extends slightly under the caudal-most portion of the lamina above. For the most part, this fat is not adherent to adjacent structures, which allows movement of the dura within the canal during spinal flexion. This lack of adhesion also permits catheters or fluid to pass between the surfaces of the fat, canal wall, and dura, and allows air or solution entry during loss of resistance technique as the needle tip first advances from ligamentum flavum into the vertebral canal.

The distance a needle must travel from the skin to reach the vertebral canal has been measured by noting the length of needle inserted when loss of resistance is first observed (16–24) and by ultrasound (25,26) or magnetic resonance (13) examination. These studies show that the depth at which the epidural space is encountered is not easily predicted in any particular subject. Although the average depth is about 4.5 to 5.5 cm, the wide range, from 3 to 9 cm, precludes the use of the published data to guide needle insertion. The depth is slightly greater at L_1–L_2 than at L_3–L_4, and depth is somewhat related to weight, but the correlation is not very strong. Part of the variability is due to natural differences between individuals, but a second factor is due to the geometry of the posterior epidural compartment. The epidural space is closest to the skin at the posterior apex of the triangular area under the ligamentum flavum. Near the mid-line, a needle may pass through the ligamentum flavum perhaps 1 cm less deep than off the mid-line near the facet joint where the ligamentum flavum is less superficial (Fig. 4).

The posterior epidural fat pad is attached along its posterior mid-line by a vascular pedicle that enters through the gap between the right and left ligamenta flava. This mesentery-like attachment and the accompanying fat pad may be seen as a mid-line filling defect in radiologic contrast studies and as an incomplete "membrane" during epiduroscopy. Claims of a mid-line fibrous septum are not confirmed by cryomicrotome (7) or histologic (27) examinations, which show no fibrous elements in the epidural space. In fact, the epidural fat is unique in the body in having virtually no fibrous content (28,29). Asymmetric development of cutaneous anesthesia after epidural local anesthetic injection is often attributed to the hypothetical median septum, but a technical error of needle or catheter insertion is the usual correct explanation because reinsertion in these cases results in complete block (30).

As in the pleural cavity and joint spaces elsewhere in the body, the rigid enclosure of the posterior epidural space allows the tissues to generate a subatmospheric tissue fluid pressure (31), due to the usual action of lymphatics and the balance of osmotic and hydrostatic forces across the capillary endothelium (Starling forces). This, and deformation of fat and dura as the needle advances further, produces the force that aspirates a hanging drop into the needle hub as the tip enters the compartment.

Segmental nerves, vessels, and fat fill the lateral epidural compartment that forms just medial to each intervertebral foramen. The pedicles are an incomplete lateral wall for the vertebral canal (Fig. 13). Except in advanced degenerative disease, the intervertebral foramina are widely open and allow the free egress of solution injected within the vertebral canal. Because of the extent to which the lateral epidural wall is incomplete and the lack of a rigid barrier in the intervertebral foramina, the pressure in the epidural space closely reflects intraabdominal pressure. Increased abdominal pressure, such as during a cough or pregnancy, is readily transmitted to the epidural space (32), which can be expected to press structures together under greater force, resulting in more extensive spread of injected solution injected between the structures. This mechanism probably contributes to the greater spread of epidural anesthesia in pregnant subjects. There is no reason to believe that veins passing through the intervertebral foramina in some way play a special role in conducting pressure changes from the abdomen to the vertebral canal. However, epidural veins may enlarge if the vena cava is obstructed, causing diversion of venous flow. This effect also may alter the distribution of injected solution.

Anterior Epidural Space

The anterior epidural compartment is separated from the rest of the vertebral canal by a fine membrane that stretches laterally from the posterior longitudinal ligament. The anterior space is almost entirely filled by a nearly confluent internal vertebral plexus, from which the mid-line basivertebral vein originates as it penetrates into the vertebral body. In most subjects, this is the only epidural site with large veins and is the most common place where epidural catheters encounter veins. Catheters passed 3 cm or more into the epidural space are, therefore, more likely to encounter veins, often with a perceptible sudden yield ("pop"). If a more cephalad needle angle is used, as is done with thoracic epidural catheterization or during a paramedian approach, the catheter is less apt to advance anteriorly where the majority of large epidural veins exist.

Clinical Correlations

The behavior of solutions and catheters within the epidural space can be explained by anatomic findings. As a needle tip traverses the ligamentum flavum, injected air or saline enters the plane between the nonadherent posterior fat pad and vertebral canal wall. This is the loss of resistance noted when the syringe plunger suddenly yields to pressure exerted during needle advancement. Less commonly, the needle might pass into the substance of the posterior fat pad, making catheter passage difficult. Solution or air injected into the epidural space readily distributes between the surfaces of the various structures and encircles the dura, with only an occasional and limited impediment in the posterior mid-line where the dura may adhere to the lamina or fat.

The distance that a needle must travel after entering the epidural space within the ligamentum flavum before penetrating the dura is typically about 7 mm (20,22,24,33), but the range is from 2 mm to as much as 2.5 cm. This measurement in part reflects indentation of the dura by the needle, because larger needles require greater advance-

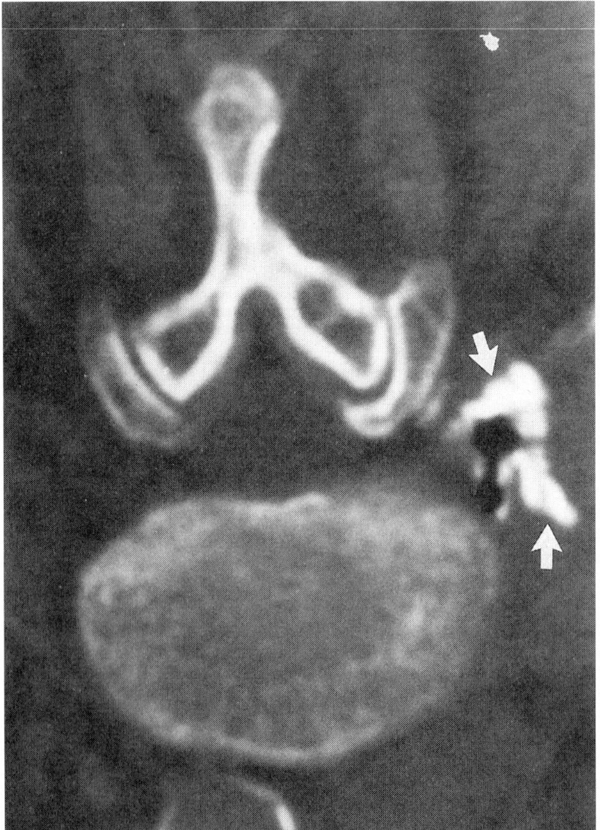

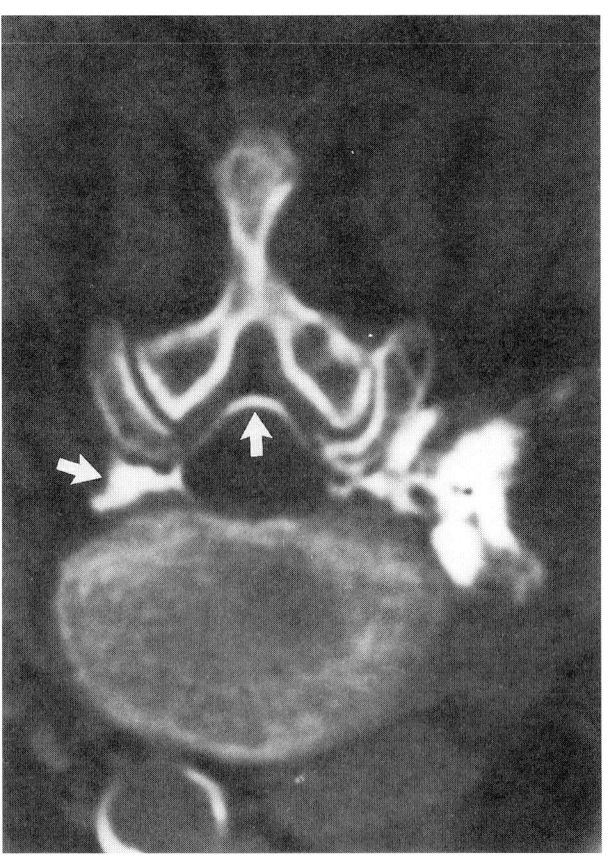

FIG. 14. Axial computerized tomography images of contrast injection through a lumbar epidural catheter that provided good postoperative analgesia. Injection of 4 mL of solution **(A)** distributes only in the area of the catheter tip beyond the intervertebral foramen *(arrows)*, but injection of an additional 10 mL **(B)** encircles the dural sac and even exits the contralateral foramen *(arrows)*. Small amounts of air appear black.

ment to reach CSF (20). Magnetic resonance imaging measurements show a range of 4 to 9 mm (13). In clinical practice, there is great variability in this dimension, because the posterior epidural compartment has a complex shape (Fig. 12) and the anterior–posterior dimension will depend on exactly where the space is traversed. If the needle enters the spinal canal away from the mid-line, it may encounter the dura with no further advancement because the posterior epidural fat pad thins toward its lateral margin (Fig. 4). The largest lumbar space is at the L_3–L_4 level (Fig. 11). As a catheter is passed through the needle, there may be a brief resistance to advancement as the tip impinges upon the dura.

Observations by computerized tomography show that a catheter tip inserted 3 cm into the vertebral canal after a mid-line skin puncture most commonly travels to a site in the lateral epidural space, but injected solution still surrounds the dura circumferentially. Uneven distribution of injected fluid is typically evident only with small volumes (e.g., 4 mL) and, in these cases, larger volumes (e.g., 10 mL) consistently show uniform distribution. This effect is consistent with clinical observations that incomplete blockade can usually be remedied by additional injection (34). Even when the catheter tip lies exterior to the intervertebral foramen in the paravertebral space, distribution of the injectate is preferentially back into the vertebral canal (Fig. 14). The muscular confines of the perivertebral space cause high pressures to develop with injection, whereas the adjacent spinal canal has a maximum pressure equal to the CSF pressure (about 15 cm H_20) and accepts flow by displacing CSF.

MENINGES AND CEREBROSPINAL FLUID

The goal of needle placement for spinal anesthesia is to place the tip through the dural and arachnoid membranes and within the CSF of the subarachnoid space. The spinal dura mater is a connective tissue sac that extends from the skull, where its fusion with the foramen magnum terminates the epidural space, to its caudal terminus at about the S_2 level (Fig. 2). Other attachments are weak, except fibrous slips to the posterior longitudinal ligament, particularly in the lumbar region (35), and anchoring of the dural nerve root sleeves to the epineural tissue in the intervertebral foramen.

Dura Mater

A posterior fold, termed the plica dorsalis medianalis, has been observed when epidural injectate (air or solution) compresses the dural sac. Scattered attachments tether the dura to the posterior epidural fat and lamina forming the fold as adjacent dura is pressed inward. In the undisturbed state, however, the dura is circular or oval in axial section (7). The thickest portion of the dura is in the posterior mid-line (36), where it is tough enough to prevent puncture by epidural catheters (37). Cases have been noted in which CSF can be aspirated from previously normal functioning catheters or in which massive spinal anesthesia resulted from injection of an epidural dose after previous doses performed normally. These reports are almost certainly not due to migration of the epidural catheter tip through intact dura.

Dura is composed of lamellae made up predominantly of collagen and some elastin elements, separated by clefts filled with ground substance (38), which account for dural permeability (39). Because there are no rigid elements, the dural sac is freely compressible. Valsalva's maneuver dramatically and immediately collapses the lumbar and thoracic dural sac, displacing CSF rostrally (40–43). By this mechanism, coughing after spinal anesthetic injection may produce a greater than expected anesthetic distribution. Increased abdominal pressure, such as with obesity and pregnancy, is freely transmitted

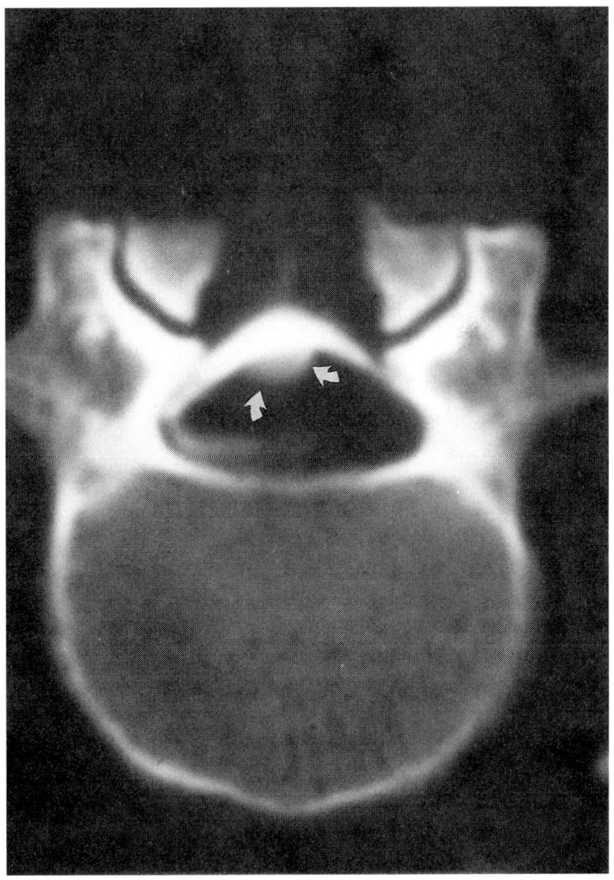

FIG. 15. Solution may accumulate in the subdural space between the dura and arachnoid membranes *(arrows)* without evidence of excessive anesthesia. Rupture of a bleb such as is shown, for instance, during an epidural top-off injection, would release a collection of local anesthetic into the subarachnoid space, resulting in sudden extensive block and the appearance of catheter migration.

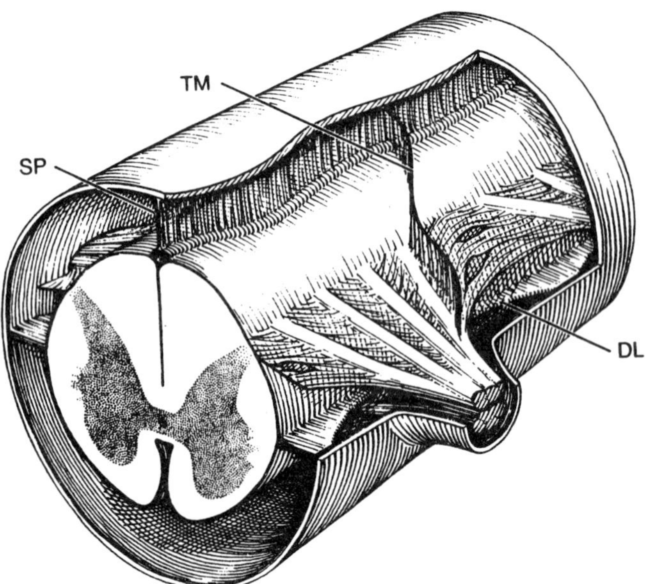

FIG. 16. The posterior subarachnoid space is subdivided by membranous partitions. The septum posticum *(SP)* runs down the mid-line and gives off transverse membranes *(TM)*, which span to the posterior roots, which are themselves enmeshed in a membrane. The dentate ligaments *(DL)* attach the cord to the lateral dura. (Reproduced from ref. 52, with permission.)

to the epidural space through the intervertebral foramina, which compresses the dural sac and results in decreased CSF volume (44). Decreased dilution of anesthetic then causes greater anesthetic effect. Longitudinal oscillation of CSF with the heartbeat is accentuated with elevated abdominal pressure and may contribute to greater anesthetic spread of spinal anesthesia during pregnancy.

Arachnoid Mater

Arachnoid mater is a thin membrane within the dura that encloses the subarachnoid space and the CSF, and forms a physiologically active barrier (45). The arachnoid layer is only loosely attached to the inner aspect of the dura and may recede from an advancing needle, making clean puncture uncertain. During myelography, injections of contrast intended for the subarachnoid space commonly flow in part into the subdural space between the dura and arachnoid, demonstrating the potential for partial subdural injection after subarachnoid needle placement. Local anesthetic injected during spinal anesthesia will have a much diminished effect if placed in the subdural space, whereas epidural doses may produce extensive, sometimes unilateral, anesthesia when injected subdurally. It is possible that an epidural catheter placed in the subdural space (or perhaps with some of the holes of a multiholed catheter in the subdural space) will produce a bleb of loculated anesthetic (Fig. 15), which will only break free into the CSF after repeated dosing. This event will create the appearance of catheter migration, because initial aspiration is negative for CSF, and the first or second anesthetic dose may have minimal or expected performance.

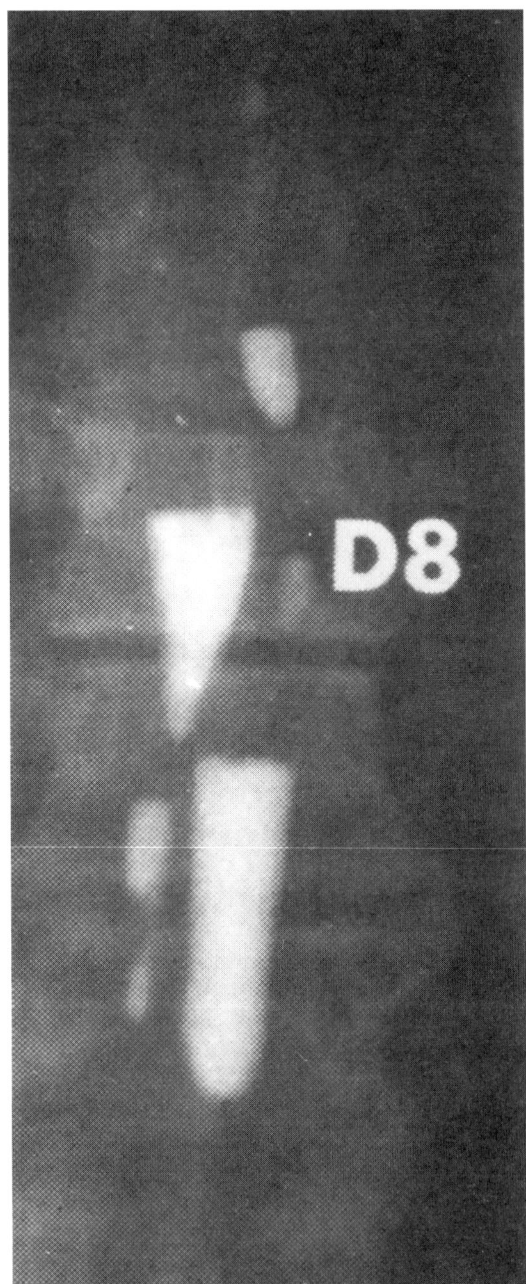

FIG. 17. Subarachnoid cysts, shown highlighted by hyperbaric contrast in an upright subject, are most common at thoracic levels but may be a cause for failed spinal anesthesia. (Reproduced from ref. 41, with permission.)

Subarachnoid Space

In contrast to the anterior subarachnoid space, which is empty of structures, the posterior subarachnoid space is crowded with membranous elements (Fig. 16) (46–48). A mesh of trabeculae spans the space from arachnoid to join the pia mater, the meningeal layer that envelops the surface of the cord and nerve roots. Denticulate ligaments extend laterally from the sides of the cord to suspend it within the dural sac. A fenestrated partition, the subarachnoid septum or septum posticum, extends from the posterior mid-line of the cord to the inner aspect of the arachnoid in most subjects at the cervical and thoracic levels and often at lumbar levels (47). The degree to which it affects distribution of anesthetic solutions is unknown. An additional problem for the anesthetist is the occurrence of cysts within the subarachnoid space (Fig. 17). These saccular dilatations of the septum posticum are present in 45% (49) to 84% (50) of normal subjects. Injection into them is a potential cause of inadequate spinal anesthesia because local anesthetic will not distribute into the CSF.

REFERENCES

1. Sjögren P, Gefke K, Banning A, Parslov M, Olsen LBO. Lumbar epidurography and epidural analgesia in cancer patients. *Pain* 1989; 36:305.
2. Gielen MJ, Slappendel R, Merx JL. Asymmetric onset of sympathetic blockade in epidural anesthesia shows no relation to epidural catheter position. *Acta Anaesth Scand* 1991;35:81.
3. Van Gessel EF, Forster A, Gamulin Z. Continuous spinal anesthesia: where do spinal catheters go? *Anesth Analg* 1993;76:1004.
4. Hogan Q. Tuffier's line: the normal distribution of anatomic parameters. *Anesth Analg* 1993;78:194.
5. Norenberg A, Johanson DC, Gravenstein JS. Racial differences in sacral structure in caudal anesthesia. *Anesthesiology* 1979;50:549.
6. Heylings JA. Supraspinous and intraspinous ligaments of the human lumbar spine. *J Anat* 1978;125:127.
7. Hogan Q. Lumbar epidural anatomy: a new look by cryomicrotome section. *Anesthesiology* 1991;75:767.
8. Williams DM, Gabrielsen TO, Latack JT. Ossification in the caudal attachments of the ligamentum flavum. *Radiology* 1982;145:693.
9. Williams DM, Gabrielsen TO, Latack JT, Martel W, Knake JE. Ossification in the cephalic attachment of the ligamentum flavum. *Radiology* 1984;150:423.
10. Zarzur E. Anatomic studies of the human lumbar ligamentum flavum. *Anesth Analg* 1984;63:499.
11. Parkin IG, Harrison GR. The topographical anatomy of the lumbar epidural space. *J Anat* 1985;141:211.
12. Willis TA. An analysis of vertebral anomalies. *Am J Surg* 1929;6:163.
13. Westbrook JL, Renowden SA, Carrie LES. Study of the anatomy of the extradural region using magnetic resonance imaging. *Br J Anaesth* 1993;71:495.
14. Hogan QH. Epidural anatomy examined by cryomicrotome section: influence of age, level and disease. *Reg Anesth* 1996;21:395.
15. Trotter M. Variations of the sacral canal: their significance in the administration of caudal analgesia. *Anesth Analg* 1947;26:192.
16. Palmer SK, Abram SE, Maitra AM, von Colditz JH. Distance from the skin to the lumbar epidural space in an obstetric population. *Anesth Analg* 1983;62:944.
17. Rosenberg H, Keykhak MM. Distance to the epidural space in nonobstetric patients. *Anesth Analg* 1984;63:538.
18. Harrison GR, Clowes NWB. The depth of the lumbar epidural space from the skin. *Anaesthesia* 1985;40:685.
19. Meiklejohn BH. Distance from skin to the lumbar epidural space in an obstetric population. *Reg Anesth* 1990;15:134.
20. Holloway TE, Telford RJ. Observations on deliberate dural puncture with a Touhy needle: depth measurements. *Anaesthesia* 1991;46:722.
21. Sutton DN, Linter SPK. Depth of extradural space and dural puncture. *Anaesthesia* 1991;46:97.
22. Bevacqua BK, Haas T, Brand F. A clinical measure of the posterior epidural space depth. *Reg Anesth* 1996;21:456.
23. Segal S, Beach M, Eappen S. A multivariate model to predict the distance from skin to the epidural space in an obstetric population. *Reg Anesth* 1996;21:451.
24. Hoffmann VLH, Vercauteren MP, Buczkowoski PW, Vanspringel GLJ. A new combined spinal-epidural apparatus: measurement of the distance to the epidural and subarachnoid spaces. *Anaesthesia* 1997;52:350.
25. Cork RC, Kryc JJ, Vaughan RW. Ultrasonic localization of the lumbar epidural space. *Anesthesiology* 1980;52:513.
26. Currie JM. Measuring of the depth to the extradural space using ultrasound. *Br J Anaesth* 1984;56:345.
27. Hogan Q, Lynch K, Lacitis I. Histologic features of epidural soft tissue and its relation to the dura and canal wall. *Reg Anesth* 1991;8(S):54.
28. Ramsey HJ. Fat in the epidural space of young and adult cats. *Am J Anat* 1959;104:345.
29. Ramsey HJ. Comparative morphology of fat in the epidural space. *Am J Anat* 1959;105:219.
30. Asato F, Hirikawa N, Oda M, et al. A median epidural septum is not a common cause of unilateral epidural blockade. *Anesth Analg* 1990; 71:427.
31. Guyton AC, Granger HJ, Taylor AE. Interstitial fluid pressure. *Physiol Rev* 1971;51:527.
32. Shah JL. Influence of cerebrospinal fluid on epidural pressure. *Anaesthesia* 1981;36:627.
33. Nickalls RWD, Kokri MS. The width of the epidural space in obstetric patients. *Anaesthesia* 1986;41:432.
34. Caseby NG. Epidural analgesia for the surgical induction of labour. *Br J Anaesth* 1974;46:747.
35. Blikra G. Intradural herniated lumbar disc. *J Neurosurg* 1969;31:676.
36. Cheng PA. The anatomical and clinical aspects of epidural anesthesia. *Anesth Analg* 1963;42:398.
37. Hardy PAJ. Can epidural catheters penetrate dura mater? An anatomic study. *Anaesthesia* 1986;41:1145.
38. Fink BR, Walker S. Orientation of fibers in human dorsal lumbar dura mater in relation to lumbar puncture. *Anesth Analg* 1989;69:768.
39. Bernards C, Hill H. Morphine and alfentanil permeability through the spinal dura, arachnoid and pia mater of dogs and monkeys. *Anesthesiology* 1990;73:1214.
40. Reitan H. On movements of fluid inside the cerebro-spinal space. *Acta Radiol* 1941;22:762.
41. Scott WG, Furlow LT. Myelography with pantopaque and a new technique for its removal. *Radiology* 1944;43:241.
42. Epstein BS. The effect of increased interspinal pressure on the movement of iodized oil within the spinal canal. *AJR* 1944;52:196.
43. Martins BS, Wiley JK, Myers PW. Dynamics of the cerebrospinal fluid and the spinal dura mater. *J Neurol Neurosurg Psychiat* 1972; 35:468.
44. Hogan QH, Prost R, Kulier A, Taylor ML, Liu S, Mark L. Magnetic resonance imaging of cerebrospinal fluid volume and the influence of body habitus and abdominal pressure. *Anesthesiology* 1996;84:1341.
45. Shanthaveerappa TR, Bourne GH. The perineural epithelium, a metabolically active, continuous, protoplasmic cell barrier surrounding peripheral nerve fasciculi. *J Anat* 1962;96:527.
46. Jirout J. *Pneumomyelography.* 2nd ed. Springfield: CC Thomas, 1969:27.
47. DiChiro G, Timins EL. Supine myelography and the septum posticum. *Radiology* 1974;111:319.
48. Nauta HJW, Dolan E, Yasaargil MG. Microsurgical anatomy of spinal subarachnoid space. *Surg Neurol* 1983;19:431.
49. Teng P, Papatheodorou C. Spinal arachnoid diverticula. *Br J Radiol* 1966;39:249.
50. Teng P, Rudner N. Multiple arachnoid diverticula. *AMA Arch Neurol* 1960;2:348.
51. Covino BG, Scott DB. Handbook of epidural anaesthesia and analgesia. Orlando: Grune & Stratton, 1985.
52. Hogan QH. A reexamination of anatomy in regional anesthesia. In: Brown D, ed: *Regional anesthesia.* Philadelphia: WB Saunders, 1996:50.

Obstetric Anesthesia, second edition,
edited by Mark C. Norris.
Lippincott Williams & Wilkins, Philadelphia © 1999.

CHAPTER 15

Neuraxial Analgesia for Labor

Part I: Techniques

Richard N. Wissler and Mark C. Norris

Both epidural and combined spinal–epidural (CSE) techniques can be used to provide effective labor analgesia. Both approaches begin by placing a needle in the epidural space. With a sound knowledge of anatomy and careful teaching, this procedure can be easy. Still, controversy surrounds many aspects of the techniques of epidural and CSE labor analgesia. This chapter will review many of these controversies and try to provide useful information to help the reader with this cardinal task.

ANATOMY

Bones and Ligaments

A thorough understanding of the anatomy of the lumbar epidural region (see Chapter 14) is essential to the successful performance of either technique. The epidural space lies deep to the vertebral laminae and the ligamenta flava. The lateral outer boundaries of the epidural space are composed of vertebral pedicles, intervertebral foraminae, and lateral extensions of the ligament flava. The vertebral bodies and intervertebral discs, covered by the posterior longitudinal ligament, comprise the anterior outer boundary of the epidural space (1). The posterior longitudinal ligament is named in relation to the vertebral bodies, although it lies anterior to the other structures within the vertebral canal. The inner boundary of the epidural space is the dura mater, a viscoelastic membrane containing 13% elastin and 54% collagen (2–4). Nonpregnant cadaveric lumbar dura is uniformly 0.25 to 0.28 mm thick (5). Because of its intrinsic physical properties and the in vivo core of cerebrospinal fluid (CSF) connected to an intracranial reservoir, the dura resists puncture by blunt or conical-shaped needles.

A posterior mid-line or median approach to the epidural space passes sequentially through the supraspinous and interspinous ligaments and the ligamenta flava before reaching the epidural space. In contrast, a paramedian approach traverses the paraspinal soft tissues and the ligamenta flava before entering the epidural space.

The lumbar epidural space consists of posterior, lateral, and anterior segmented compartments (6–10). These compartments are continuous and repeat at each lumbar vertebral level. The anterior and posterior epidural compartments are connected at each lumbar vertebral level by two lateral compartments. At most lumbar levels, the anterior epidural space is small. A prominent mid-line attachment between the dura and the posterior longitudinal ligament limits fluid passage across the anterior mid-line.

The posterior epidural compartment is the target for the needle and catheter during placement of a lumbar epidural block. In the sagittal plane, this compartment has a "saw-tooth" appearance (Fig. 1). This pattern is due to the close apposition of the vertebral laminae to the dura mater, with severe anteroposterior narrowing of the posterior epidural space at each lumbar vertebral level. The narrowed portion of the posterior epidural space is not a significant barrier to the passage of fluid or catheter (11). Therefore, the anesthetic significance of the narrowed portion is primarily related to epidural space depth. The hindmost border of each posterior lumbar epidural compartment is curved (Fig. 1). Therefore, the mid-line depth of each posterior epidural compartment varies from one lamina to the next. Each is deepest near its cephalad end (6,7,9).

R. N. Wissler: Departments of Anesthesiology and Obstetrics & Gynecology, University of Rochester School of Medicine and Dentistry, Rochester, New York 14642.

M. C. Norris: Department of Anesthesiology, Washington University School of Medicine, St. Louis, Missouri 63110-1083.

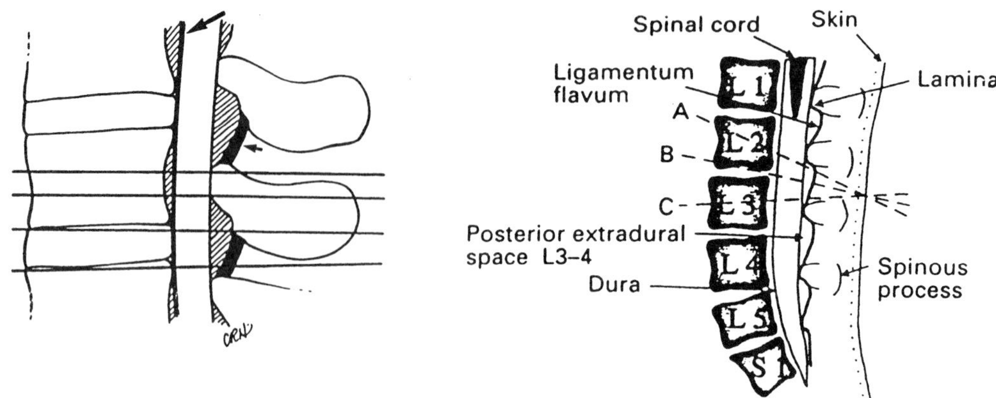

FIG. 1. Segmentation of the lumbar epidural space. Sagittal plane diagrams illustrate the variable depth of the posterior lumbar epidural space at each vertebral level. (Reproduced from refs. 6 and 9, with permission.)

The ligamenta flava are 3.5 to 5.0 mm thick and form the interlaminar posterior outer border or roof of the epidural space. A controversy exists about the mid-line continuity of the ligamenta flava. A mid-line gap containing a vascular pedicle for the posterior epidural fat may separate the right and left portions of ligamenta flava (1,6,12). Other evidence suggests that the ligamenta flava are continuous in the posterior mid-line (13,14). If a mid-line gap exists, a true mid-line technique may enter the epidural space without encountering the ligamenta flava.

Distances

The posterior epidural compartment has a saw-tooth shape on sagittal section and a triangular shape on cross-section (Fig. 2) (6,7,9,10,12,14,25). Thus, the depth of the lumbar posterior epidural space varies along both longitudinal and transverse axes. As a result, the distance from skin to ligamenta flava to dura mater varies for both patient and technical reasons. Among these factors are:

- Size of the patient,
- Angle of epidural needle,
- Lateral offset of insertion site from the mid-line (Fig. 2), and
- Relative intervertebral position (Fig. 1, Table 1).

The mean distance from skin to lumbar posterior epidural space in parturients is 4.4 to 5.3 cm (Fig. 3) (15–19,22,59). The distance from skin to posterior lumbar epidural space is less than 3 cm in only 0.2% of pregnant women (N = 6,754). Therefore, during mid-line lumbar placement of a needle, loss of resistance before 3 cm rarely identifies the epidural space. The posterior lumbar epidural space is more than 6 cm from the skin in only 11% of parturients. In nonobese parturients, it may be prudent to reinsert epidural needles after passing a depth of 6 cm. Deeper insertion may increase the risk of unilateral block (from entering the lateral epidural space) or dural puncture (18,21). However, in parturients, the risk of dural puncture is greatest when the epidural space is shallow, not deep (22,23).

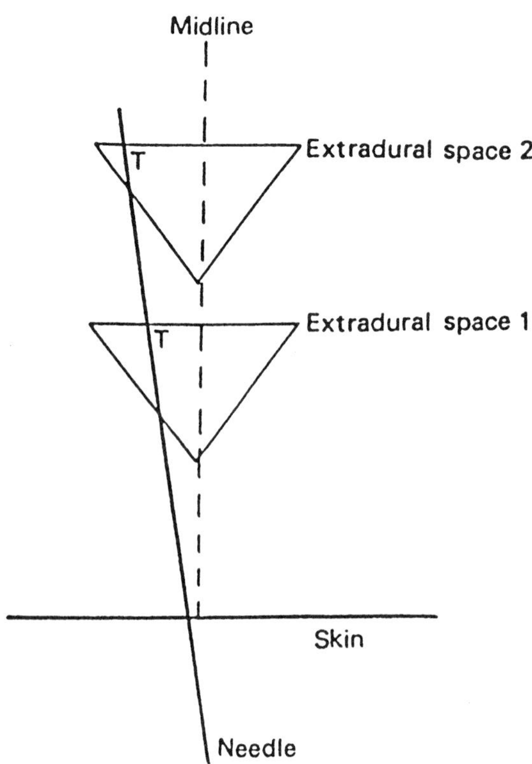

FIG. 2. Lateral displacement errors during lumbar epidural placement increase with larger distances from skin to epidural space. (Reproduced from ref. 21, with permission.)

TABLE 1. *Depth of lumbar posterior epidural space*[a]

Depth (mm)[b]		Patient population	Method
Cranial:	6.0 ± 1.4	Nonobstetric: men and women	MRI
Midpoint:	6.2 ± 1.3		MRI
Caudal:	4.0 ± 1.1		
	5.8	Nonobstetric: women	MRI
	6.3 ± 1.5	Obstetric	MRI
	6.9 ± 4.0	Nonobstetric: men	Needle
	7.0 ± 2.4	Nonobstetric	Needle
	8 ± 0.8	Nonobstetric	MRI

[a]Distance between ligamenta flava and dura mater in posterior midline.
[b]Mean ± SD.
MRI, magnetic resonance imaging.
Data from refs. 9, 10, 25. Bevacqua BK, et al. *Reg Anesth* 1996;21:456; Hoffman VLH, et al. *Reg Anesth* 1997;22:297; Aldrete JA Jr. *J Clin Anesth* 1996;8:84.

In obstetric patients, clinical factors that correlate with the distance from the skin to the posterior lumbar epidural space include:

- Body weight (absolute weight, or weight corrected for height or body surface area),
- Shoe size, and
- Soft tissue edema (15,17,19,20).

Whether this distance varies at different lumbar vertebral interspaces is unclear (15,17,19,20). Ultrasound can be used to measure the distance from skin to posterior epidural space and may be a useful tool in obese parturients (24).

THE PROCEDURE

Prepare the sterile work surface carefully *before* starting the procedure. Neatly lay out all the necessary equipment. This step minimizes the time the patient must spend in an uncomfortable position. Prepare the skin at the back widely. Place a sterile towel beneath the patient.

Approach to the Epidural Space

Mid-line

Raise a skin wheal over the chosen interspace and infiltrate the subcutaneous layers with about 2 mL of local anesthetic. Insert the epidural needle through skin, subcutaneous tissue, supraspinous and interspinous ligaments, and probably ligamentum flavum. Keep the needle in the mid-line and in the sagittal plane, but angle it slightly cephalad (Fig. 4). Penetrating the skin in the rostral portion of the interspace, just below the caudad tip of the cephalad spinous process, will minimize the cephalad angle needed (Fig. 5). Once the tip of the needle enters the ligaments, painful sensation is minimal unless it strays from the mid-line. The tissues (especially the ligamentum flavum) exert significant resistance both to advance of the needle and to injection of fluid. Carefully avoid any sudden advances (see the following section on the LOR technique).

Paramedian

Raise a skin wheal 1.5 cm from the mid-line, opposite the spinous process [whether the center (28), the cephalad (26), or the caudal (27) end matters little]. Infiltrate the subcutaneous tissues, paravertebral muscles, and periosteum of the lamina (the latter is particularly sensi-

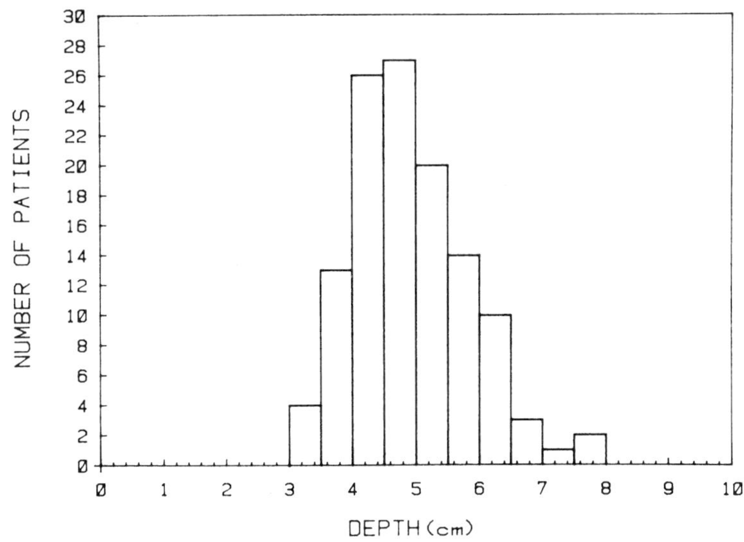

FIG. 3. Histogram showing the distribution frequencies of distances from the skin to the posterior epidural space. (Reproduced from ref. 21, with permission.)

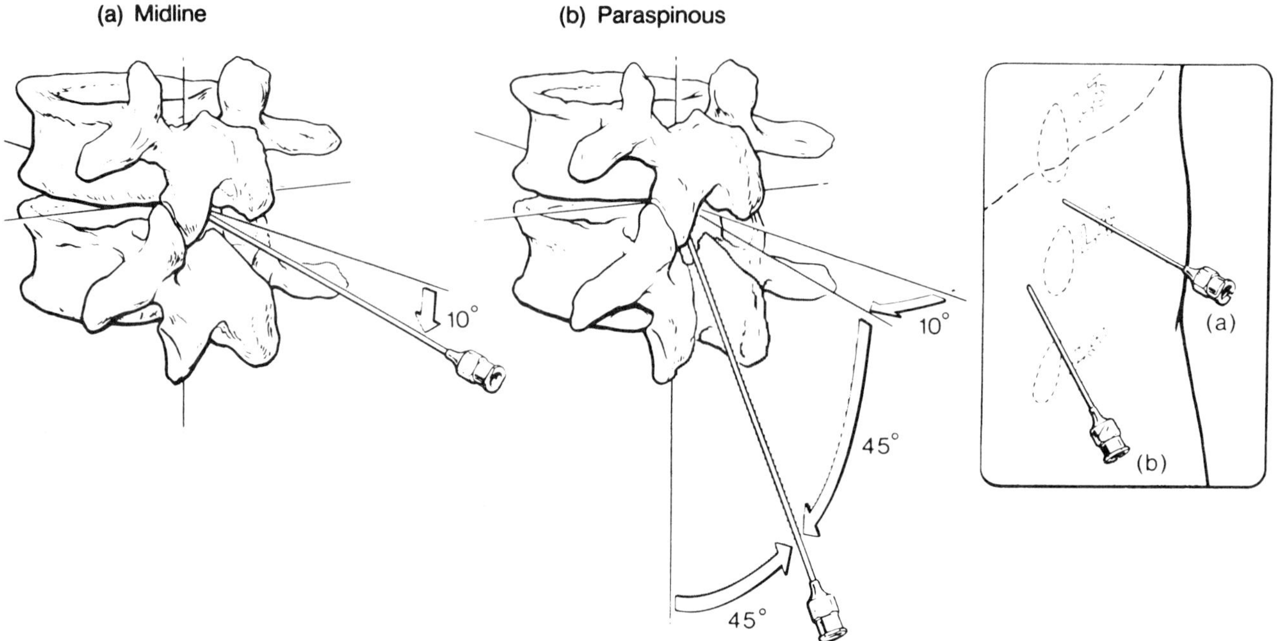

FIG. 4. Sites of needle insertion for lumbar epidural block. **A:** Mid-line. Note insertion closer to the superior spinous process and the slight upward angulation. **B:** Paraspinous (paramedian). Note insertion beside caudad edge of "inferior" spinous process, with 45-degree angulation. (Reproduced from ref. 262, with permission.)

tive) with about 5 mL dilute local anesthetic. Next, insert the epidural needle, initially perpendicular to the skin, until it reaches lamina. Then, withdraw the needle and redirect its tip cephalad until it reaches either upper border of lamina or ligamentum flavum. Alternatively, Bonica (27) recommends inserting the needle at an angle of 15 degrees to the sagittal plane and 135 degrees to the long axis of the patient (Fig. 4). This method requires few passes of the needle, but requires a better understanding of spatial geometry.

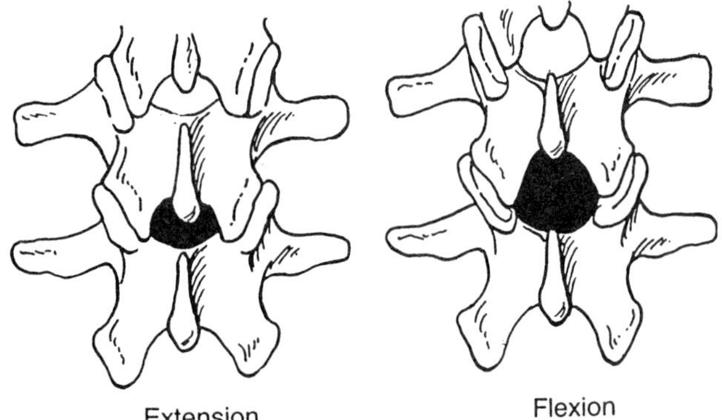

FIG. 5. Extension and flexion of the lumbar spine significantly affect the size and shape of the interlaminar space. Inserting the needle just below the upper spinous process provides the straightest path to the epidural space. (Reproduced from ref. 263, with permission.)

Which Approach?

Both mid-line (median) and paramedian approaches to the posterior epidural compartment can be used. The choice of approach determines the range of possible angles that the epidural needle can take with respect to the skin. With a mid-line approach, needle angles are restricted by the spinous processes to 90 to 110 degrees. Using the paramedian technique allows much steeper needle angles. Bonica (27) recommends 135 degrees. The oblique angle allowed by the paramedian approach may decrease the risk of dural puncture and ease catheter insertion (Fig. 6). Other purported advantages of the paramedian approach include:

- Use of a bony landmark (lamina) to identify the depth of the ligamentum flavum,
- Fewer catheter paresthesias due to improved threading conditions,
- Avoidance of interspinous ligament pathologies such as calcifications or cysts,
- Excellent patient comfort if adequate local anesthetic infiltration is used, and
- Less need for lumbar flexion during needle insertion (28–32).

Small clinical and autopsy studies suggest that the lumbar paramedian approach does encourage cephalad threading of the epidural catheter (33,34).

Three clinical studies have compared these two approaches to the lumbar epidural space. A prospective

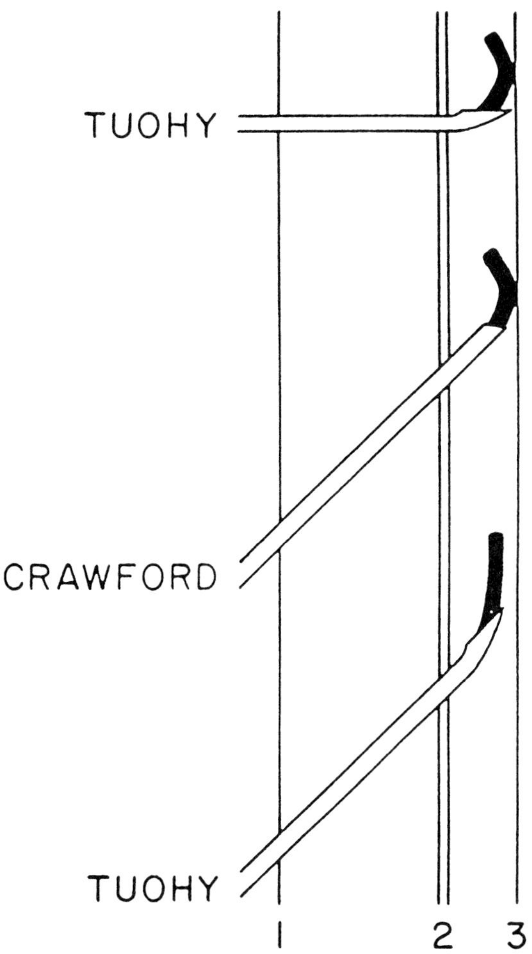

FIG. 6. Epidural needle tip and incident angle affect epidural catheter threading. (Reproduced from ref. 33, with permission.)

randomized comparison that enrolled 165 laboring women reported similar success and complication rates (35). The paramedian group had more pain on needle insertion, but this finding may reflect the study protocol that limited local infiltration in both groups to 2 mL of 1% lidocaine. A retrospective study in pregnant patients (n = 1,010) also reported similar success rates with both approaches (36). The incidence of minor complications (difficulty threading catheter, venous cannulation, paresthesiae with catheter) was higher in the mid-line group. A prospective randomized clinical trial in adult males presenting for urologic surgery (n = 50) found more problems with epidural space identification, catheter threading and injection, and catheter paresthesiae associated with the mid-line approach (37).

Despite the possible advantages of the paramedian approach, the mid-line technique remains more widely used. The primary reason for this preference is probably that teaching the mid-line approach is a simple and trouble-free process (38,39). Moreover, in one clinical trial, when several attempts were necessary, the mid-line approach was more likely to succeed when the paramedian had failed (35). At this point, the data do not permit a clear choice of approach to the lumbar epidural space. Anesthetists should familiarize themselves with the technical aspects of both techniques.

Vertebral Level

Surface landmarks are useful for the correct application of regional anesthesia. For lumbar epidural anesthesia, accurate identification of the individual lumbar vertebrae is helpful for at least two reasons. First, the posterior approach may be blocked by the sacrum if the needle is inserted below the lumbar region. Second, placing the needle caudad to the conus medullaris limits the potential for spinal cord trauma.

The spinal cord terminates at the conus medullaris, and neural elements continue within the dural sac as the cauda equina. The mean level of spinal cord termination is the L_1–L_2 disc. In 95% of patients, the spinal cord terminates above the L_2 vertebrae (40). In a smaller cadaveric dissection series, the mean level of the conus medullaris was one third of a vertebra lower in nonpregnant women than in men (41). The dural sac ends at S_1 or S_2 in 83% of men and nonpregnant women (42). Distally, a thin strand of pia covered with dura, known as the filum terminale, continues to the coccyx. Based on magnetic resonance images of men and nonpregnant women, the mean volume of CSF below T_{11-12} is 43 mL (range 21 to 74 mL) (43). The lumbosacral cauda equina comprises approximately 15% of the lumbosacral subarachnoid space (7.1 to 7.3 mL) (43,44). The cauda equina shows a consistent spatial organization (45–48). There is a progressive rostrocaudal layering of roots from lateral to medial within the cauda equina. The caudal sacral roots occupy a dorsocentral position. This spatial organization is maintained in part by strands of arachnoid mater.

From a practical standpoint, three lumbar interspaces are commonly used for lumbar epidural and spinal anesthesia; L_{4-5}, L_{3-4}, and L_{2-3}. Tuffier's or Jacoby's line, a horizontal line between the two palpated iliac crests, presumably crosses the vertebral column at the L_4 vertebra or the L_4–L_5 interspace (Fig. 7) (49,50). A line drawn between the bony iliac crests intersects with the L_4 vertebra or the L_{4-5} interspace in 79% of supine, nonpregnant patients (51,52). In the lateral decubitus position, a vertical line from upper iliac crest will intersect the vertebral column one half to one segment rostral to a line drawn between the iliac crests (52,53). One factor that probably contributes to this phenomenon is pelvic tilt, which will be accentuated in patients with disparate hip and trunk widths. Additional variability in the location of Tuffier's line is a function of soft tissue overlying the iliac crests and the expected variance in anatomic elements among individuals (54). Alternate methods suggested for accurate identification of lumbar vertebral levels include counting downward from the

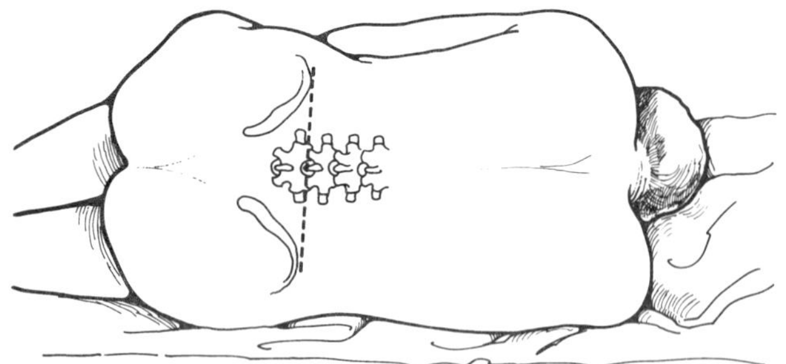

FIG. 7. The line between the two iliac crests is a useful surface landmark for identifying lumbar vertebrae (see text). It is known as Tuffier's or Jacoby's line. (Reproduced from ref. 264, p. 72, with permission.)

most prominent cervical spinous process (C_7) or the intersection with the twelfth rib (T_{12}) (51,55).

Posture

Posture considerations during attempts to identify the lumbar epidural space include body position and vertebral flexion. The two commonly used body positions are sitting and lateral decubitus.

If using the sitting position, have the patient hang her legs over the side of the bed (while sitting as far from the edge as the length of her thighs will allow). Place a pillow on her lap, and encourage her to slouch forward at the waist, not the hips, with her arms folded in front of her on the pillow. An attendant or partner should stand in front of the patient and support her shoulders. Using the partner frees the attendant, but puts the partner in a position to observe the needle insertion. This maneuver does place the partner at risk of fainting, thus producing three patients instead of two.

If the mother is to lie down, she should be in the precise lateral position, with a pillow supporting her head but not beneath her shoulder. Her arms should be in front of her and she should flex her lumbar spine as much as possible. Most women are unable to comply with this request unless they bend their knee up and their head down. Neither move is strictly necessary, except as an aid to lumbar flexion. The partner can sit in front of the patient, where he is unlikely to faint.

Anesthetists vary in their preference for the sitting or lateral position. "The patient position used… is generally related to the personal preference of the anesthetist… (and) is likely to be the position in which he (she) was taught to perform epidurals" (56). A prospective randomized comparison (n = 144) of these two positions during induction of epidural labor analgesia examined the following endpoints: ease of insertion, complications, and maternal comfort (56). The lateral group had a longer time for insertion (10.9 vs 6.6 minutes), greater maternal preference for the alternate position (15% vs 4%), and more frequent need to move to the alternate position (17% vs 1%). A follow-up nonrandomized study (n = 152) found no differences between the sitting and lateral positions (56). The authors concluded "that the anesthetist who is already trained should be permitted the freedom of choice of maternal position and not be encouraged to adopt a less familiar approach." However, anesthetists trained to use the lateral position can more readily adapt to the sitting position than vice versa (56). Training programs should encourage development of clinical skills with both body positions.

A prospective survey of term parturients (n = 50) and their anesthesiologists examined opinions about the sitting and lateral flexed positions (57). Overall, the two positions did not differ in patient comfort or in the ease of L_{3-4} interspace palpation. However, thin patients (body mass index less than 25) preferred the lateral position and obese patients (body mass index greater than 30) preferred the sitting position (Fig. 8).

A prospective randomized study of the sitting and left lateral positions for labor epidural placement (n = 40) found a significantly lower noninvasive cardiac output in the lateral group, presumably due to aortocaval compression from vigorous lumbar flexion (58).

Two studies in parturients compared the distance from the skin to the posterior lumbar epidural space in the sitting and lateral positions (15,17). The results contradict, but one of these studies may be confounded by body weight (15). If the epidural space is nearer the skin in the sitting position, then a catheter fixed to the skin may be pulled out of the epidural space as the patient returns to a reclining position (59,60).

Flexion of the lumbar spine increases the size of the interlaminar space and eases posterior access to the lumbar epidural space (Fig. 5). Lumbar spine flexion also

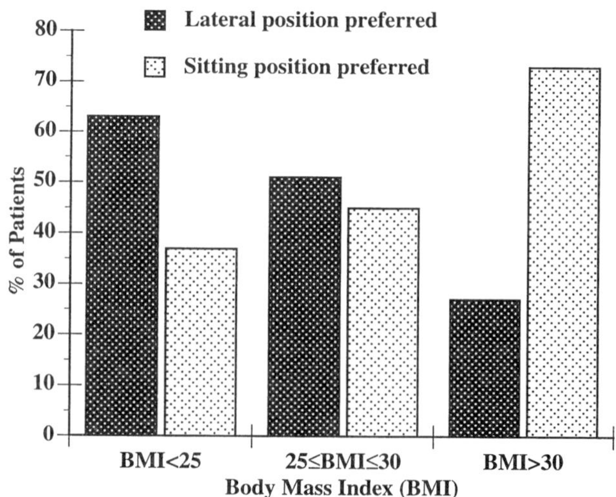

FIG. 8. Patient position preference versus body mass index (Wt/Ht^2). (Redrawn from ref. 57, with permission.)

increases the capacity of the vertebral canal (61,62). In nonpregnant women, lumbar spine flexion changes neither posterior epidural space depth nor the distance from skin to posterior epidural space (10).

In summary, both sitting and lateral positions are satisfactory when attempting to identify the lumbar epidural space. Lumbar flexion improves mid-line access to the posterior epidural compartment, but may cause aortocaval compression in the lateral position.

Epidural Needles

A number of different needle styles have been described and used successfully for lumbar epidural anesthesia. The "Tuohy" needle, named for the anesthesiologist who first popularized its use for a continuous spinal catheter technique, is the predominant needle in current clinical practice (Fig. 9). The true historic origin of the Tuohy needle is controversial (63). Curbelo (64) first reported its use in a continuous epidural catheter technique in 1949. The orifice in the Tuohy needle is designed to minimize dural puncture while maximizing pressure measurements and directionality of catheter threading. Other epidural needle styles include the Hustead, Crawford, Weiss, Cheng, and Crawley needles (65,66).

Commercially available epidural needles are made of stainless steel with the following elements in decreasing percentages: iron, chromium, nickel, manganese, and molybdenum/silicon (67,68). Available Tuohy needles vary in length from 8 to 15 cm. Many epidural needles have alternating 1 cm opaque and polished zones (Fig. 10) to facilitate depth measurement (69,70). Many epidural needles have wings or other hub grip aids to help with control during insertion (65,66).

The diameter or gauge of an epidural needle is a compromise between maximizing needle strength and space for catheter threading versus minimizing local tissue trauma and the risk of postdural puncture headache (PDPH). One prospective randomized study (n = 685) found no difference in the frequency of complications when using 16- or 18-gauge Tuohy needles for induction of labor epidural analgesia (71). These authors recorded pain during needle placement in a subset of their patients (n = 318). Two percent of women reported visual analog scale (VAS) pain scores greater than 70, and 79% reported pain scores less than 30. There were no differences between the 16- and 18-gauge groups (71). Despite the absence of evidence, some experts favor the 18-gauge needle over the 16-gauge needle (72), whereas others prefer a 17-gauge needle that may be less likely to kink on deep vertebrae (73).

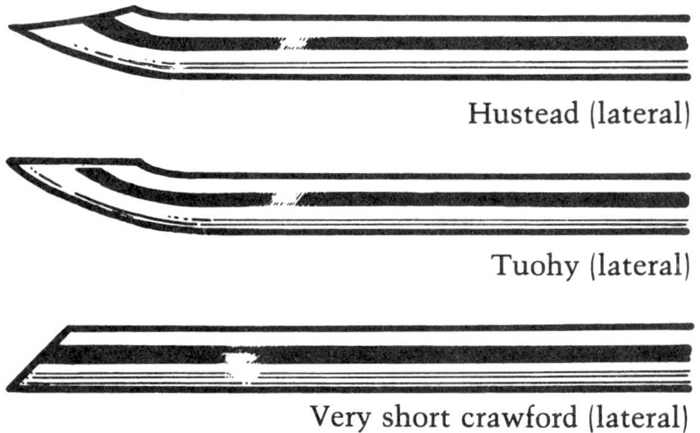

FIG. 9. Selected epidural needle tips. (Reproduced from ref. 264, p. 59, with permission.)

Epidural and spinal needles can be deflected from their intended path of insertion (Fig. 11) (74). The 18-gauge Tuohy needle bends an average of 3 mm toward the orifice for every 5 cm of tissue traversed (74). The magnitude of epidural needle deflection is intermediate between that occurring with pencil point and beveled spinal needles. When redirecting the epidural needle, withdraw it into the subcutaneous tissues each time. This maneuver minimizes lateral forces on the needle and reduces the risk of needle fracture, particularly in obese patients (75–77).

Identifying the Epidural Space

The epidural space should be accurately identified as soon as the tip of the needle passes through the ligamentum flavum. The two most commonly used approaches to identify the epidural space are the hanging-drop and loss of resistance (LOR) techniques. Currently, the hanging-drop technique is less popular than the LOR techniques (78).

Hanging-drop Technique

The hanging-drop technique relies on the negative pressure that develops in most individuals on first entry into the epidural space (79,80). A drop of fluid on the hub of the epidural needle is drawn into the needle upon entering the epidural space (Fig. 12).

Pressure within the epidural space is a key factor in the success of the hanging-drop technique. The pressure in the epidural space is affected by several physiologic variables including arterial pulse, respiration, hypercarbia, and intrathoracic or intraabdominal pressures (81–85). In labor, skeletal muscle activity and increased intraabdominal pressure raise lumbar epidural pressure during painful uterine contractions and maternal expulsive efforts (81,86). Effective analgesia blunts these responses. In nonpregnant patients with lumbar stenosis, upright body positions and lumbar extension are associated with increased lumbar epidural pressure (87). Studies in pregnant and nonpregnant patients show that the pressure in the undisturbed epidural space is positive, not negative (81–84,86,88–90). However, the initial entry pressure may be negative if the ligamenta flava

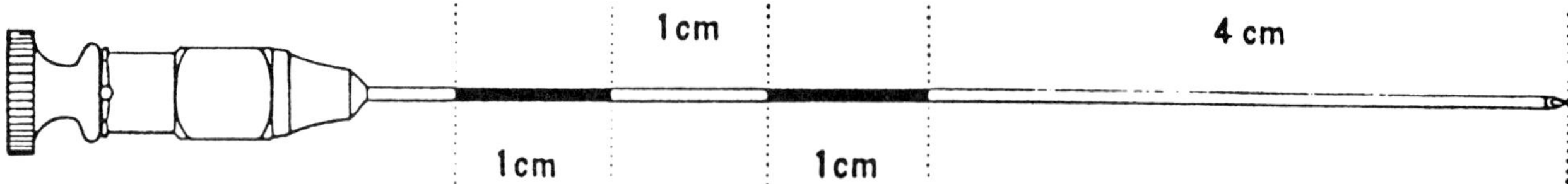

FIG. 10. One-centimeter segments of an epidural needle, with alternating appearance, to aid in depth assessment. (Reproduced from ref. 69, with permission.)

bow forward and snap back along the epidural needle or the tip of the needle indents or "tents" the dura (Fig. 13) (91–93).

Loss of Resistance Technique

There is almost complete resistance to injection through an epidural needle as it passes through the dense interspinous ligament or ligamentum flavum. As the needle tip emerges into the epidural space, the resistance to injection disappears abruptly. The LOR technique can be done using air or saline within the syringe. If saline is used, the epidural needle can be advanced directly by pressure on the shaft or hub or indirectly by pressure on the plunger of the syringe.

Using the mid-line approach, insert the epidural needle, with its stylet in place, until its tip lodges firmly in the interspinous ligament. (When using the paramedian approach, advance the needle until it reaches the ligamentum flavum.) Then, remove the stylet and attach a syringe containing 3 to 5 mL of air or saline.

Loss of Resistance Technique Using Air

This technique is commonly practiced with the patient sitting and using a winged needle. Attach an air-filled syringe to the needle hub. Brace both hands against the patient's back. Hold the wings of the needle and advance it in a series of quantal steps. Pause between each step to apply pressure on the plunger. If the plunger bounces, advance the needle another step before testing again for LOR.

Some anesthesiologists use a hybrid technique in which they hold and advance the needle using one hand and hold the syringe in the other. This is slightly less tedious, as bounce may be elicited repeatedly without having to pause between advances. Alternately, apply continuous pressure to the plunger of the syringe while advancing the needle with the nondominant hand (Fig. 14) (65).

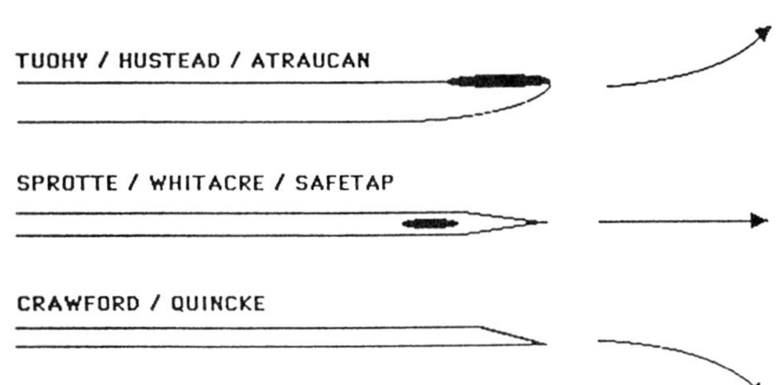

FIG. 11. Deflection of epidural and spinal needles by tissue during placement. Direction of deflection depends on the design of the needle tip. (Reproduced from ref. 74, with permission.)

Loss of Resistance Technique Using Saline

Using a liquid-filled syringe, the epidural needle may be advanced solely by pressure on the plunger of the syringe (94). Advance the syringe slowly and steadily by using the dominant hand to push on the plunger. Apply inertia or breaking force by bracing the nondominant hand against the patient's back and holding the hub of the needle. Once you reach the epidural space, injection of fluid becomes possible and forward movement of barrel of the syringe and needle stop automatically. As soon as LOR occurs, release the pressure on the plunger, so that you inject only a minimal amount of saline. Then detach the syringe; any drip back of saline is transient and readily distinguished from CSF.

A modification of this technique may be necessary in the very occasional patient whose ligaments do not provide absolute resistance to injection of saline. As before, the nondominant hand prevents sudden movement. Now, however, provide forward motion by gripping the barrel of the syringe with the finger tips of the dominant hand. Simultaneously, use the palm of that hand to apply more modest pressure to the plunger. You will feel and see the plunger move forward on entry into the epidural space. This, the true Doughty technique, also prevents the inappropriate injection of saline into ligaments and paravertebral muscles (95,96).

If unsure whether LOR has occurred, use a small air-filled syringe. Pressure on the plunger will elicit bounce if the needle tip is in ligament or muscle. Tilting the needle in the direction opposite its bevel also can help differentiate false from true LOR (Fig. 15). [If the needle is in ligament or soft tissue, resistance to injection will increase. If the needle is in the epidural space, resistance will not change (97).]

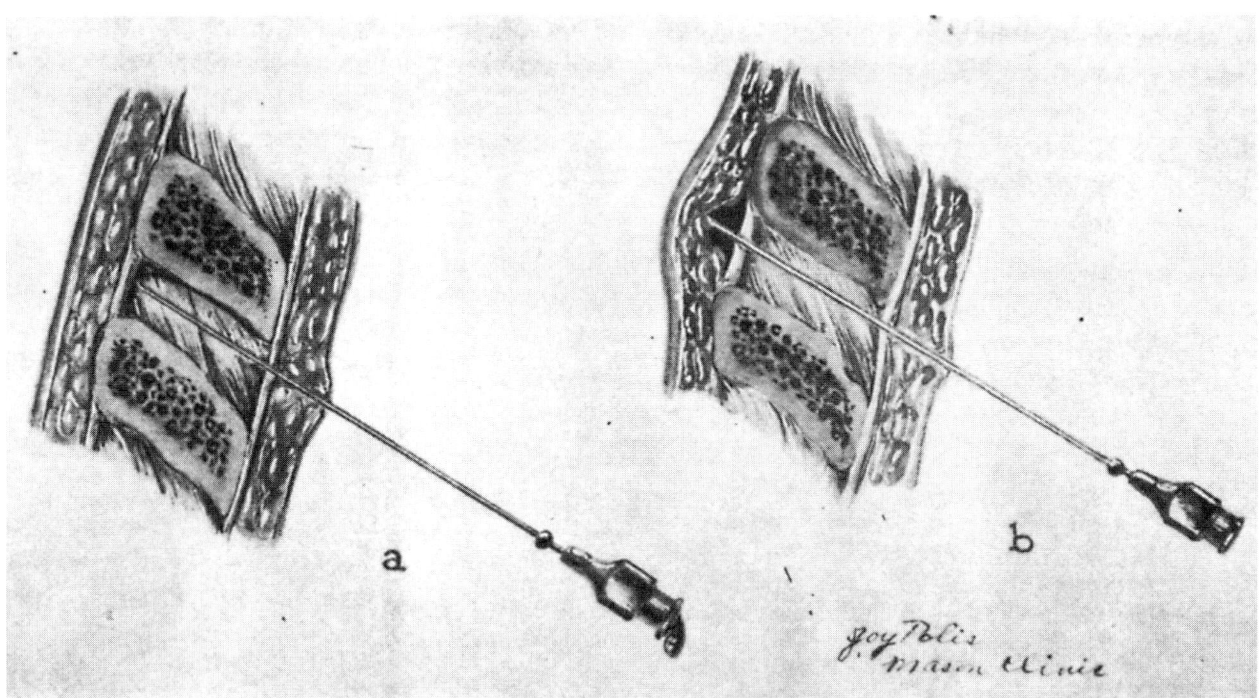

FIG. 12. Hanging-drop technique for identification of the epidural space. (Reproduced from ref. 265, with permission.)

Air or Saline?

The major controversy about the LOR technique surrounds the relative merit of air or saline in the syringe. Both fluids are in common clinical use (78,98). One prospective randomized study (n = 50) identified the epidural space using 4 mL of air or saline in laboring women (99). More women in the air group had unblocked segments after an initial 8 mL of 0.5% bupivacaine (32% vs 8%). Additional local anesthetic provided effective analgesia in all women. Other block characteristics were similar between the two groups. Case reports and laboratory data have suggested an association between epidural air injection and "patchy" epidural blocks (100–102). Other potential complications of using air for the LOR technique include: pneumocephalus, nerve root or spinal cord compression, subcutaneous emphysema, and venous air embolism (103). The volume of saline initially injected into the epidural space also may affect the spread of a subsequent local anesthetic dose (111).

Pneumocephalus typically presents as an immediate headache after dural puncture and intrathecal air injection (104–107). Computed tomography or magnetic resonance imaging can document intracranial air. Treatment of pneumocephalus is primarily supportive and may include supplemental oxygen administration and avoiding nitrous oxide.

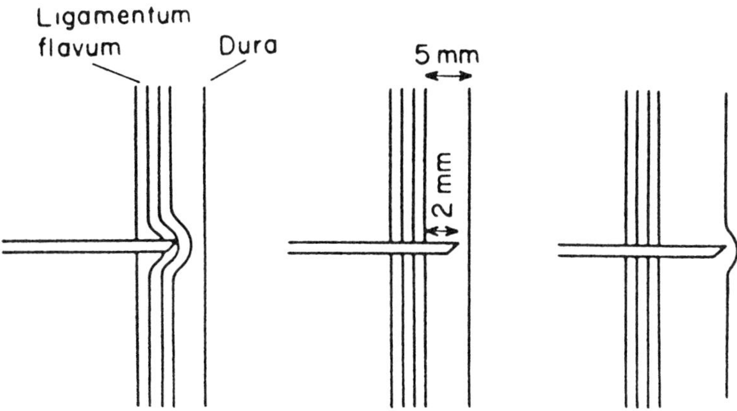

FIG. 13. Contributions of ligamenta flava and dura to "negative" epidural space pressure. (Reproduced from ref. 92, with permission.)

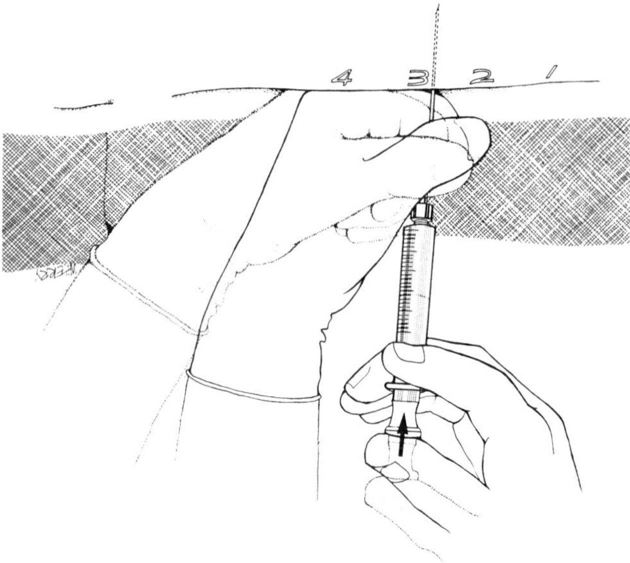

FIG. 14. Loss of resistance: grip the needle with the nondominant hand. Extend the wrist and rock forward on the knuckles to drive the needle forward under rigid control. The thumb of the dominant hand applies constant pressure to the plunger of the syringe. (Reproduced from ref. 65, with permission.)

Case reports of lumbar root compression or paraplegia following the use of air in the LOR syringe have unusual clinical circumstances (i.e., very large air volumes) that limit their implications for routine clinical practice (108,109).

A retrospective study and expert opinion suggest that saline in the LOR syringe is associated with a lower rate of dural puncture than air (78,110). However, a large prospective study in nonpregnant patients found no difference in dural puncture with air or saline (104). Aida et al. (104) alternated weekly between air (n = 1,812) and saline (n = 1,918) when using LOR to identify the epidural space in patients with low back pain or herpes zoster. Neither air nor saline was associated with a greater risk of accidental dural puncture (2.6% vs 2.7%). More patients in the air group (66.7%) complained of PDPH compared with those in the saline group (9.8%). Computed tomography examination showed intrathecal air in most air group patients suffering PDPH. There was no intrathecal air after accidental dural puncture in the saline group patients. Headaches related to intrathecal air were faster in onset and shorter in duration than headaches following accidental dural puncture (Figs. 16 and 17) (104).

When using a mid-line approach with any LOR technique, degenerative cysts within the interspinous ligament may produce a false LOR. These cysts are more common in elderly patients (112).

The Syringe

Glass and plastic syringes are commercially available to use with the LOR technique (113,114). The ideal LOR syringe would have low inherent resistance, low cost, and no instances of the plunger sticking inside the barrel. Glass syringes have less inherent resistance than plastic ones (115). Sticking, however, sometimes occurs with glass syringes (115). A laboratory study found that "dry polishing" a glass syringe led to less inherent resistance than wetting the same syringe with saline (116). A dual-chambered plastic LOR syringe with a proximal air compartment and a distal saline compartment combines aspect of both fluids (117).

A wide variety of devices have been described for use with the hanging-drop and LOR techniques (118–122). Complex equipment also has been developed (123–125). "There appear to be as many variations on identifying the epidural space as there are anesthesiologists!" (126).

In summary, LOR techniques currently are more popular than the hanging-drop technique for identifying the lumbar epidural space. Either air or saline is acceptable to use in the LOR syringe (127). With either medium, limit the injected volume after entering the epidural space.

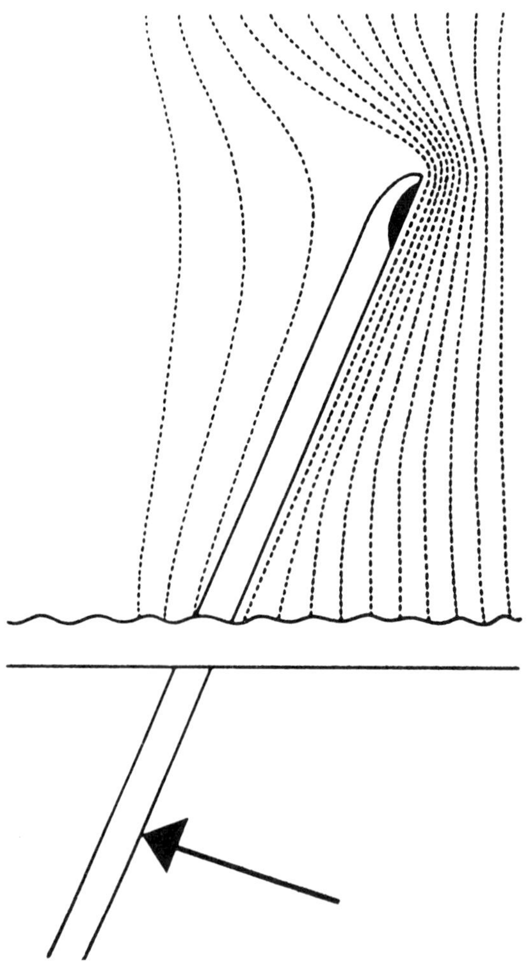

FIG. 15. Tilting the needle during insertion compresses soft tissue, increasing resistance to injection. (Modified from ref. 97.)

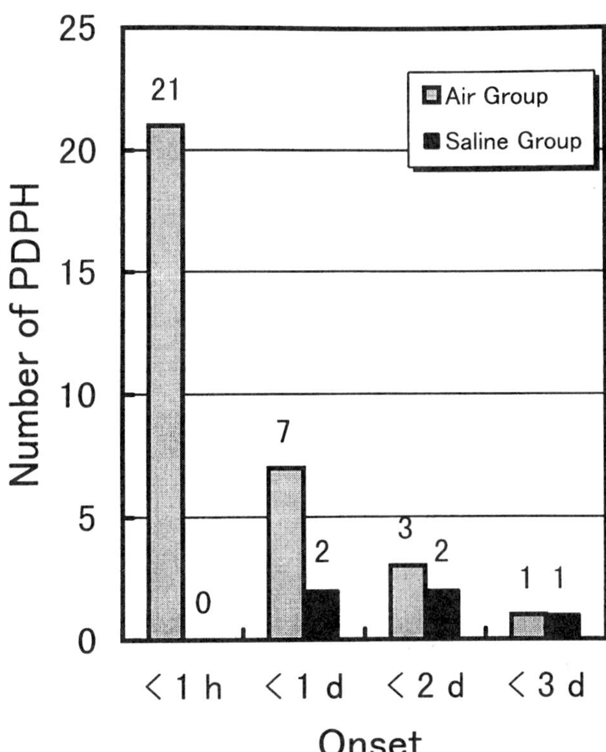

FIG. 16. Onset of postdural puncture headache *(PDPH)* after attempted epidural block using either air or saline for loss of resistance *(LOR)*. Symptoms occurred significantly sooner when air was used for LOR. (Reproduced from ref. 104, with permission.)

Epidural Needle Bevel Orientation

The primary clinical concerns about epidural needle bevel orientation are:

- Dural puncture and PDPH,
- Epidural catheter threading, and
- Needle deflection during placement.

The incidence of PDPH following accidental dural puncture with 16- or 18-gauge Tuohy or Hustead epidural needles is 43% to 80% (128–131). Orienting the bevel of a cutting-tipped spinal needle parallel to the longitudinal axis of the back markedly decreases the incidence of PDPH in nonpregnant patients (132–135). Identifying the epidural space with the needle bevel parallel to the longitudinal axis of the back decreases the risk of moderate-to-severe headache after accidental dural puncture (24% vs 70%) (128).

Once the epidural space is located with a longitudinal oriented needle bevel, should the needle then be rotated 90 degrees to a transverse bevel position (cephalad or caudad) before threading the epidural catheter? Theoretically, rotating the epidural needle will ease catheter threading and help ensure appropriate catheter position. However, there is little evidence that the orientation of the epidural needle bevel significantly affects the final destination of an epidural catheter. For example, catheters commonly coil near the epidural entry site. Forty to one hundred percent of lumbar epidural catheters placed with a cephalad bevel with coil on insertion (136–139). In orthopedic patients, only 64% of catheters were oriented in the same direction as the lumbar epidural needle bevel (140). Needle bevel direction has little or no effect on the spread of local anesthetic injected either through the needle or through an epidural catheter (140–143). It is easier to thread a catheter through a transverse needle bevel than through a laterally directed one (Fig. 18). In one randomized, prospective trial (n = 534), more catheters were passed on first attempt through a cephalad versus laterally directed Tuohy needle (90% vs 77%) (144). Paresthesiae also were more common in the longitudinal bevel group (31% vs 23%). Most catheters were eventually sited in the epidural space, and needle bevel orientation did not alter overall catheter success (144). A similar study found easier catheter insertion, more dermatomal segments blocked, fewer one-sided blocks, and more patients comfortable at 30 minutes with cephalad needle bevel direction (145).

Instead of attempting to pass a catheter through a longitudinally directed needle, some recommend rotating the needle to orient its bevel cephalad within the epidural space (128). This practice has stimulated a lively debate

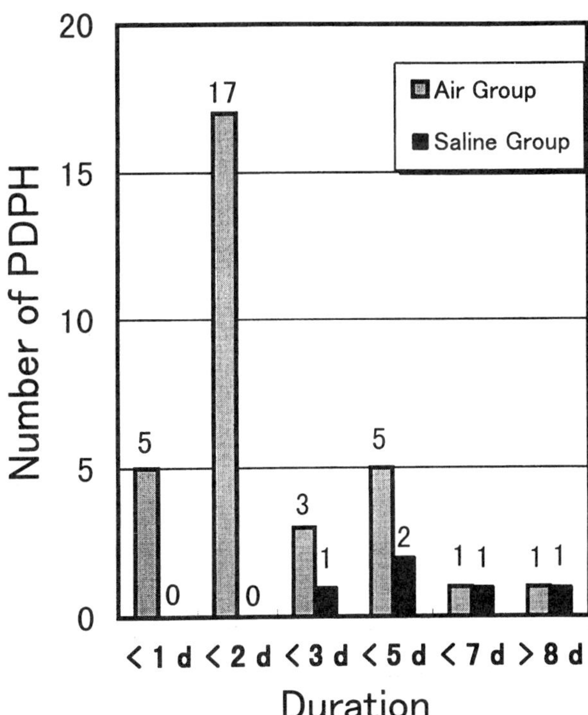

FIG. 17. Duration of postdural puncture headache *(PDPH)* after attempted epidural block using either air or saline for loss of resistance *(LOR)*. PDPH lasted significantly longer when saline was used for LOR. (Reproduced from ref. 104, with permission.)

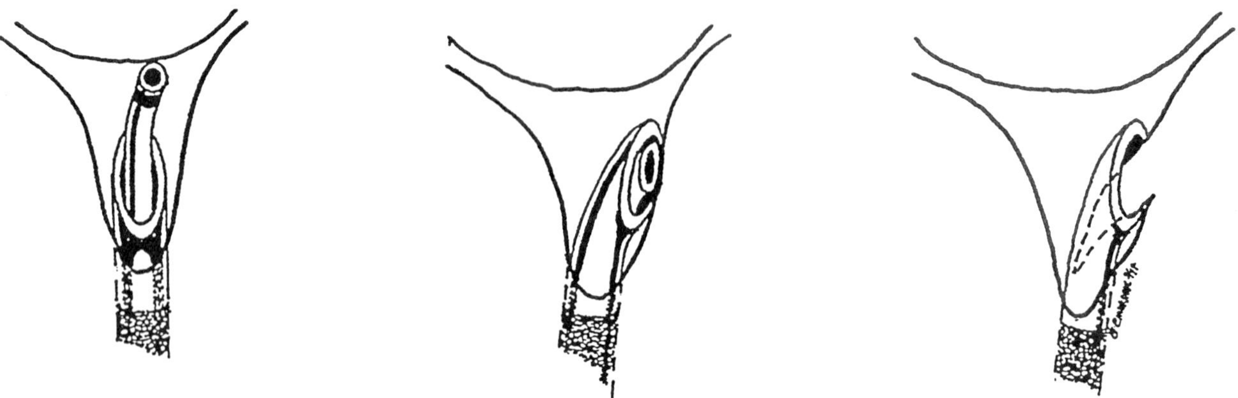

FIG. 18. Longitudinal bevel orientation of a Tuohy needle may favor occlusion of the needle opening by the ligamenta flava. (Reproduced from ref. 144, with permission)

(146–159). The argument against needle rotation rests almost entirely on a perceived increased risk of dural puncture with this maneuver. The clinical and laboratory data supporting this position are limited. Carter et al. (160) studied 30 CSE anesthetics for cesarean section with 180-degree rotation of the Hustead needle after removing the spinal needle. This maneuver resulted in a 20% rate of dural puncture with the epidural needle or catheter. However, the role of spinal needle withdrawal in positioning the dura against the tip of the epidural needle is not known. Hollway and Telford (161) made a series of observations while placing lumbar CSF drains with Tuohy needles. After identifying the epidural space, the following cycle of events was repeated until CSF was seen: advance Tuohy needle 1 cm, aspirate, rotate Tuohy needle 360 degrees, and reaspirate. Using this protocol, 10% of the CSF identifications were made during needle rotation. Meiklejohn (162) studied the force needed to puncture postmortem thoracolumbar dura with and without rotation of a Tuohy needle. Ninety-degree rotation decreased the dural puncture force by 16% to 19% during rotation compared to a nonrotated needle. On the other hand, in laboring women (n = 1,558), 90-degree needle rotation did not increase the risk of dural puncture (128). In a smaller study (n = 160), rotating the needle as much as 270 degrees did not increase the risk of dural puncture (145).

In summary, the risk of PDPH is decreased when the epidural space is identified with the bevel of the epidural needle parallel to the longitudinal axis of the back. Epidural catheter threading is likely to be successful regardless of the epidural needle bevel orientation. Rotating the epidural needle within the epidural space remains controversial among experts, although the risks are mainly theoretical.

Epidural Catheters

After the tip of the epidural needle has been placed into the posterior lumbar epidural compartment, a catheter is threaded to allow intermittent or continuous administration of medications. Currently, most epidural catheters are 18, 19, or 20 gauge and composed of nylon, polyurethane, or Teflon. Some catheters contain removable wire stylets, which may increase the risk of paresthesia, and venous or dural puncture. In the absence of a stylet, epidural catheters are unlikely to pierce intact dura (163,164). A small needle hub insert that minimizes catheter buckling can markedly ease the threading of an epidural catheter (165). On occasion, the catheter will not thread because only the tip of the needle has entered the epidural space. Here, advancing the epidural needle a few millimeters will allow the catheter to clear the bevel (166).

Single Hole versus Multihole

Current epidural catheters have two basic designs: single lumen (open end) and multiorifice (blunt tip). Both catheters have been used safely, although each type of catheter has theoretical advantages and disadvantages. Multiorifice catheters may have ports in several adjacent anatomic compartments (i.e., subarachnoid, subdural, epidural), and multicompartment block has been reported (167,168). However, three prospective randomized studies in obstetric patients found superior clinical performance with multiorifice versus single-lumen epidural catheters (169–171). One study found no differences between catheter types (172). With multiorifice catheters, injection pressure determines the port from which drugs will exit. With low injection pressures, drug exits primarily through the most proximal port. With more vigorous injection, drug exits more uniformly from all ports (173).

Catheter Threading

Several techniques have been proposed to help insert the catheter into the tissues of the lumbar posterior epidural space. In a small study of 32 parturients, injecting 10 mL of air into the epidural space decreased subsequent catheter paresthesiae (49% vs 29%) (174). In a larger study of 200 laboring women, injection of 10 mL of liquid before catheter insertion decreased the incidence of blood vessel puncture (175). Injection of saline or air lacked any effect on epidural catheter complications or block quality in three other studies (176–178). Voluntary hyperventilation just before epidural catheter insertion also lacks a significant impact on catheter complications (179).

Depth of Insertion

Current epidural catheters usually have permanent markings that allow measurement of the length of catheter within the epidural space (180–182). The length of catheter inserted into the epidural space may influence its efficacy and risks. In 1993, most obstetric anesthesiologists inserted only 3 to 5 cm of catheter into the epidural space (183). However, two more recent prospective randomized studies of catheters placed for labor analgesia (one each with a single-lumen or multiorifice catheter) suggest that 5 to 6 cm is the optimal insertion depth (Table 2) (184,185). Catheters inserted only a few centimeters may dislodge, whereas those inserted more deeply are more likely to enter a vein. These depths may need to be modified for individual patients. Deeper insertion may be appropriate for ambulatory or obese patients (59,186–190).

The distance from the skin to the epidural space often increases as the patient moves from the upright, flexed position to a relaxed sitting posture to the lateral position (59). This change can be as much as 4 cm and is greater in obese as compared with thin women. If a catheter is taped to the skin with the patient in the upright, flexed position, it may be pulled out of the epidural space as she lies down (59).

Removal

Usually, epidural catheters are easily removed. Patient position may alter lumbar epidural catheter withdrawal forces (191,192). The force needed to remove a catheter is reportedly less in either the original placement position or in the lateral flexed position. One nonrandomized study reported easier removal in the lateral decubitus versus the sitting position (193). Normally, there is a considerable margin between the force needed to remove an epidural catheter and that needed to break it (191–195). Occasionally, an epidural catheter is very difficult to remove due to "trapping" by vertebrae or ligaments. Suggested maneuvers include:

- Return to the original epidural placement position,
- Lateral decubitus position,
- Spinal flexion,
- Spinal extension, or
- Injection of saline through the catheter during withdrawal (191–193,196–200).

Rarely, epidural catheters knot in situ (201–204). The relationship between knot formation and depth of epidural catheter insertion remains conjectural.

In summary, blunt-tip multiorifice epidural catheters surpass open-end single-lumen catheters in terms of adequate lumbar epidural analgesia without any significant differences in safety. Injection of liquid or air into the epidural space does not consistently improve subsequent epidural catheter insertion. For labor epidural analgesia, threading the catheter 5 to 6 cm into the epidural space is appropriate for most patients. Changing the patient's position will make it easier to remove a "trapped" epidural catheter.

TABLE 2. *Insertion depth and frequency of complications and inadequate analgesia*

	Insertion depth (cm)		
	3	5	7
Number of patients	35	32	33
Intravenous catheters	2.8%	3.0%	17.5%*
Inadequate analgesia	31.4%	6.3%*	33.3%

*$p < 0.05$ vs. other groups.

Laboring women had multiorifice catheters inserted 3, 5, or 7 cm into the epidural space.

All patients initially received 13 mL of 0.25% bupivacaine in divided doses.

Data from ref. 184.

Faulty Equipment

Manufacturing errors have been reported for equipment used in lumbar epidural placement including epidural needles (205–216), loss of resistance syringes (217,218), and epidural catheters (219–226). Also, correctly manufactured equipment may be incorrectly assembled into epidural kits with incompatible contents (227,228). A consistent theme in this literature is the need for a brief inspection of each epidural kit before its use.

THE COMBINED SPINAL–EPIDURAL TECHNIQUE

The CSE technique began as an anesthetic curiosity (229). Then, in the 1980s, several authors described the currently popular needle-through-needle technique (230,231). The popularity of this technique has since grown remarkably. Today, it is used in a wide variety of anesthetic settings. In many centers, this technique is widely used to provide labor analgesia. The following sections describe some technical aspects to consider when performing the CSE technique and some of the real and theoretical risks inherent with this approach. As with any new technique, much remains to be learned about

CSE. As our experience grows, so will our understanding of the risks and benefits of this unique approach to neuraxial analgesia.

Why Combined Spinal–Epidural Technique?

Intrathecal injection can rapidly provide profound clinical effects with minimal amounts of drug. Unfortunately, current techniques are limited to a single injection and, hence, a finite duration of drug action. Multiple drugs can be injected over prolonged periods using an epidural catheter. However, safe and effective epidural blockade requires more time and more drug than intrathecal techniques. The CSE technique provides the rapid onset and greater drug potency of spinal anesthesia with the flexibility of epidural blockade. This combination has proven especially useful when providing labor analgesia.

Advantages of Combined Spinal–Epidural Technique for Labor Analgesia

The greatest single advantage of CSE labor analgesia is the rapid onset of pain relief obtained with intrathecal injection of small amounts of opioids and local anesthetics (see Chapter 16). A CSE technique that uses intrathecal opioids and epidural administration of dilute local anesthetic/opioid mixtures affords effective labor analgesia with a high degree of patient satisfaction. Patients like both the rapid onset of analgesia and the minimal degree of motor blockade that this approach provides (232). Some studies also suggest that CSE labor analgesia is associated with fewer forceps deliveries than traditional epidural analgesia (233).

COMBINED SPINAL–EPIDURAL TECHNIQUES

There are four main varieties of CSE technique, each requiring different equipment and offering different advantages and limitations:

- The single-needle–single-interspace technique (229, 234): A needle is placed in the epidural space and local anesthetic injected. Then, the needle is advanced through the arachnoid and dura and additional local anesthetic is injected intrathecally.
- The double-needle–double-interspace technique (235, 236): The epidural needle and catheter are inserted at one interspace before the spinal injection at another.
- The needle-through-needle–single-interspace technique (230,237): This approach has become the most popular variety of CSE. It requires a longer than usual spinal needle to protrude past the tip of the epidural needle (see following).
- The needle-beside-needle–single interspace technique (238,239): Several devices are available with a spinal needle guide attached to, or incorporated into, the shaft of the epidural needle.

The Needle-Through-Needle Technique

Because its popularity and its associated theoretical or potential problems, this technique will be discussed in some detail.

Equipment

To successfully enter the subarachnoid space from within the epidural space, the spinal needle must extend beyond the tip of the epidural needle (Fig. 18). Too short or too long a protrusion may both lead to failure. Factors that determine the length of protrusion include the lengths of both the spinal and epidural needles and the design of the needle hubs. Although the ideal length of protrusion is unknown, manufacturers have been quick to provide matching spinal and epidural needles for this technique. Most have settled on a maximum protrusion of 10 to 15 mm.

Technique

- Identify the epidural space.
- Insert the spinal needle through the epidural needle. You will often feel a "pop" as the spinal needle penetrates the dura. Remove the stylet from the spinal needle and observe for CSF. The spinal needle may perforate the dura before it is fully extended beyond the tip of the epidural needle. Continuing to advance the spinal needle once it enters the dura may increase the risk of transient paresthesia (240). In addition, if the spinal needle has traversed the dura lateral to the midline, or tangentially, it may pass out of the subarachnoid space if inserted further (Fig. 19) (241). (If using the saline LOR technique to identify the epidural space, clear liquid in the hub of the spinal needle may be CSF or saline. Usually, CSF appears promptly and will fill and drip from the hub of the spinal needle. Saline appears more slowly and in smaller quantities.)
- Fix the position of the spinal needle. The ligamentum flavum helps prevent excessive movement of a spinal needle inserted by itself. With the needle-through-needle technique, the epidural needle traverses the ligamentum flavum, and the spinal needle moves freely. The hub design of some needle-through-needle combinations allows the spinal needle to seat securely within the epidural needle. I pinch the hubs of the spinal and epidural needles together using the thumb and index finger of my nondominant hand.
- Inject appropriate drug (see Chapter 16). Although many experts recommend aspiration of CSF to confirm needle location before, during, or after intrathecal drug injection, I usually skip this step when

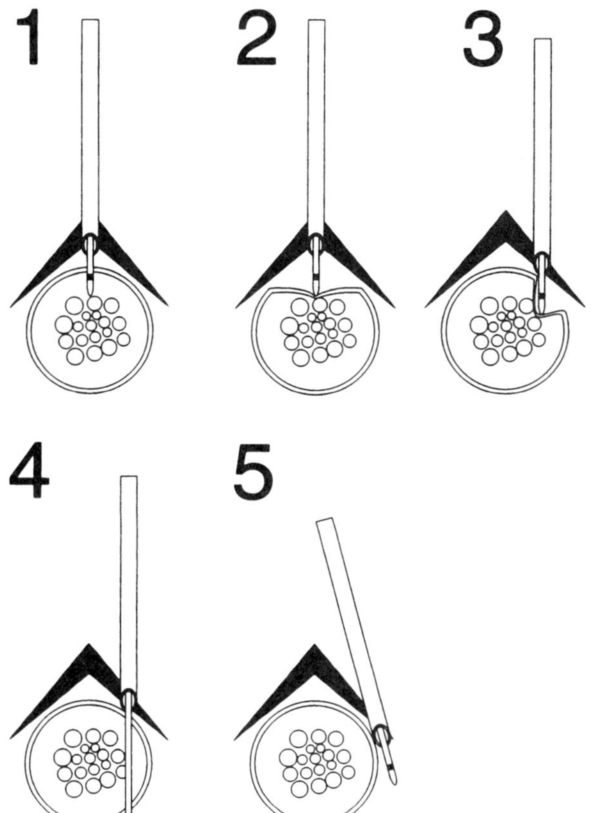

FIG. 19. Diagrammatic representation of different needle positions in vertebral canal. **1:** Ideal situation; mid-line epidural needle guides spinal needle into subarachnoid space. **2:** Spinal needle too short; indents but does not pierce dura. **3:** Spinal needle too short and too lateral; longer needle might have produced successful dural puncture. **4:** Spinal needle too long; has passed through dural sac and out again anteriorly. **5:** Spinal needle too lateral; epidural needle in epidural space but guides spinal needle lateral to dural sac. (Reproduced from ref. 241, with permission.)

using the CSE technique for labor analgesia for two reasons. First, the needle manipulation with aspiration may cause additional dural trauma. Second, the results of aspiration rarely change my management. If initial aspiration is positive, I inject the drug. If initial aspiration is negative, I inject the drug anyway. Because the primary advantage of CSE labor analgesia is its rapid onset, it makes little sense to me to spend additional time trying to perform the technique. If CSF appears spontaneously in my spinal needle, at least part of my injection will enter the subarachnoid space. If the patient does not obtain adequate pain relief, I inject additional drug through the epidural catheter, regardless of my ability to aspirate CSF. Aspirating mid-way through injection strikes me as a good way to dislodge an appropriately placed needle. Aspiration at the end of injection does nothing other than reassure or upset the operator.

- Remove the spinal needle and insert the epidural catheter.

Problems

Failure to Obtain Cerebrospinal Fluid

Patient Position. Initial success is greater if the patient is sitting rather than lying on her side. However, in one study, the ultimate ability to obtain CSF did not depend on the patient's position (Fig. 20). The higher initial success rate in sitting patients presumably relates to the greater lumbar CSF pressure and narrower epidural space in that position. Alternatively, epidural needles placed with the patient in the lateral position may more likely be directed away from the mid-line, thus aiming the spinal needle away from the dura (Fig. 19).

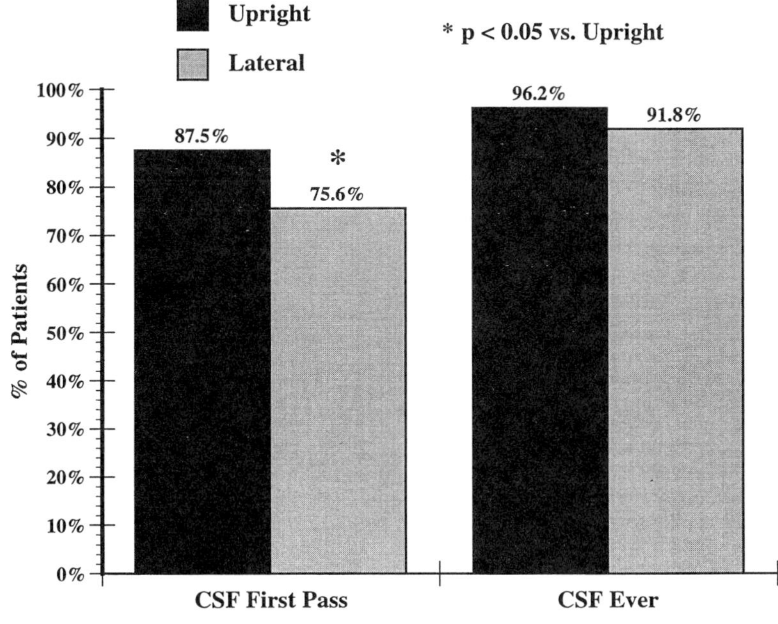

FIG. 20. Patient position versus success of dural puncture during induction of combined spinal-epidural *(CSE)* analgesia. Patients were positioned at the discretion of the anesthetist. After obtaining loss of resistance, a 119- to 120-mm pencil point needle was passed through the epidural needle. The ultimate success of CSE did not differ between the two positions, but cerebrospinal fluid *(CSF)* was more likely to appear during the first attempt if the patient was sitting. (Reproduced from ref. 242, with permission.)

TABLE 3. *Paresthesiae and success of the combined spinal epidural technique with four spinal needles*

Needle	Number of patients	Maximum protrusion (mm)	% Paresthesiae	% Success
27-gauge Whitacre	103	10	17	95
27-gauge Durasafe™	102	12	19	95
25-gauge Durasafe™	102	12	27	95
26-gauge Gertie Marx™	100	15	29	97

Durasafe™ from Becton Dickinson; Gertie Marx™ from International Medical Devices.
Patients were sitting for all procedures.
Data from ref. 240.

Needles. The spinal needle must penetrate the dura. As the dura is not a fixed structure, a needle will first tent, then perforate it (hence, the "pop" as the needle traverses the tensed dura). The likelihood that a properly aimed needle will penetrate the dura depends on both tip configuration and the extent of protrusion. Cutting point needles require less protrusion (but produce more headaches) than pencil point needles. Most pencil point needles designed for use with the CSE technique protrude 10 to 15 mm beyond the tip of the epidural needle. Although needles that extend 15 mm past the tip of the epidural needle theoretically would increase the frequency of dural puncture, such an advantage remains unproven (Table 3) (240).

Technique. If the epidural needle is not in the epidural space, it is extremely unlikely that the spinal needle will find the subarachnoid space.

The epidural needle may be in the epidural space but the spinal needle is not in the subarachnoid space because it is too short, too long, or too lateral (Fig. 19). If too short, the spinal needle tip may indent, but not pierce, the dura mater; if too long, it may transfix the dural sac and pass out again anteriorly; if too lateral, it may pass the dural sac tangentially without piercing it.

If the epidural needle is properly cited, the spinal needle will sometimes "bounce" off the dura (especially if the patient is lying on her side). Rotating the spinal needle 360 degrees or advancing the epidural needle 1 to 2 mm often solves this problem.

Dural Puncture with Epidural Needle

Two studies suggest that using the CSE technique may decrease the risk of accidental dural puncture (Table 4) (242,243). These data come from teaching institutions and may be unique to residents in training. When confronted with an equivocal LOR, the anesthetist using the needle-through-needle technique can use the spinal needle as a probe. If CSF returns, the epidural needle is properly cited and need not be advanced. When faced with a similar situation during induction of epidural analgesia, the operator may be tempted to advance the epidural needle further and unintentionally enter the subarachnoid space.

TABLE 4. *Risk of accidental dural puncture: epidural vs combined spinal epidural*

	Epidural	Combined spinal epidural	Blood patch
Norris et al. [242]	4.2%	1.7%	<1%
Birnbach et al. [243]	1.4%	0.4%	

Data from refs. 242 and 243.

Metallic Particles

Passing spinal needles through Tuohy or Hustead needles creates a small groove on the inside of the tip of the epidural needle (Fig. 21) (244,245). This groove, and concern about the possibility of depositing intrathecal metallic fragments, spurred the development of the needle-beside-needle–single-interspace technique (244). Unused Tuohy needles exposed to magnetic fields always have metal filings at their edges. But, no microscopic

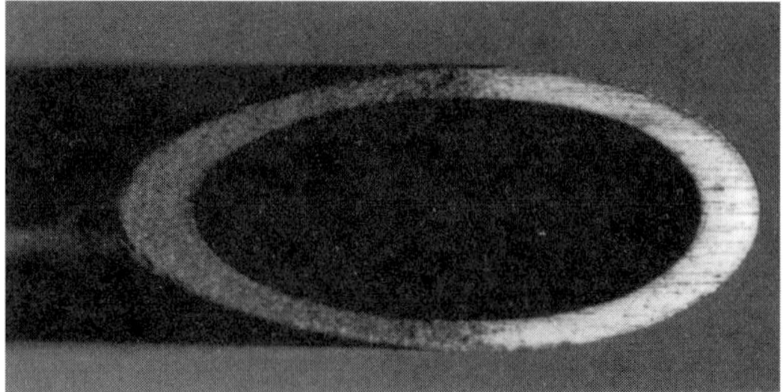
A

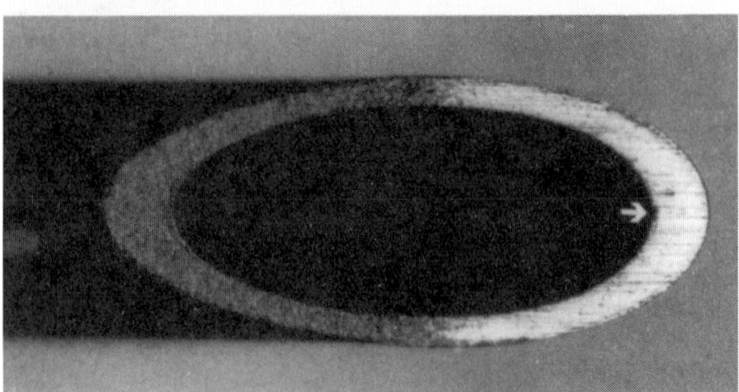
B

FIG. 21. Photomicrographs of the orifice of an 18-gauge Hustead needle before **(A)** and after **(B)** passage of a 24-gauge Sprotte needle. Original magnification ×24. *Arrow* in B denotes notching along the track of the spinal needle. (Reproduced from ref. 266, with permission.)

metallic particles were found in saline used to flush the epidural needles (245). Scanning electron microscope examination with energy dispersive x-ray analysis also found no metal filings in saline injected through epidural needles after passage of a long spinal needle (246). In short, there is no scientific evidence to suggest that the needle-through-needle CSE technique deposits metal fragments intrathecally.

Subarachnoid Catheter

Another concern about the needle-through-needle technique of CSE is that the epidural catheter may pass into the subarachnoid space through the hole made by the spinal needle. Studies in cadavers and laboring women suggest that this risk is negligible. In an epiduroscopic study, Holmström and his colleagues (247) found it impossible, even under direct vision, to pass either a 16- or 18-gauge catheter through the dural puncture made by a 25-gauge Quincke needle. A catheter could be inserted with some difficulty if multiple dural punctures were made. Catheters passed readily through dural punctures made by 17-gauge needles.

In clinical practice, the risk of passing an epidural catheter through a 24-gauge or smaller dural hole is very small. In one series of 506 parturients receiving CSE labor analgesia, only once was CSF first seen in the epidural catheter. This catheter may have passed through the 24-gauge dural hole or through an unrecognized hole made by the epidural needle. When inducing epidural labor analgesia, dural puncture also is occasionally (1 of 375) detected only by seeing CSF in the catheter after insertion (242). Thus, insertion of any epidural needle may damage the dura. A catheter may subsequently pass through the weakened part into the subarachnoid space.

Some epidural needles have a hole in the convex part of the curved Tuohy tip (a "back-eye" needle). In theory, the spinal needle will pass through this hole and pierce the dura in line with the Tuohy needle shaft, whereas the epidural catheter, being too large to pass through the back-eye, travels out of the tip of the Tuohy needle and strikes the dura some distance from the small dural hole. Although an ingenious idea, the evidence indicates that back-eyes anticipate a problem that does not occur. If using one of these needles, do not be misled into thinking that the epidural catheter cannot pass intrathecally, as this is an inherent risk with *any* epidural technique.

Facilitated Spread

Spinal Anesthesia. Early users of the CSE technique noted that small amounts of epidural local anesthetic could significantly increase the level of sensory blockade (248,249). Several factors contribute to this increased spread. Merely injecting normal saline (10 mL) into the epidural space can increase the level of sensory blockade (250–252). Epidural saline causes cephalad displacement of intrathecal contrast medium, presumably by increasing the volume within the epidural space (252). This effect of saline is most pronounced when injected shortly after (5 minutes) the spinal anesthetic (250). If the level of spinal anesthesia has stabilized by the time of injection, epidural saline produces a small (2.0 ± 2.0 segment) rise in sensory level. However, epidural bupivacaine still increases the level of blockade significantly (Fig. 22) (251). Epidural saline no longer increases the level of sensory blockade once the level of spinal anesthesia begins to regress (253). Even after the spinal blockade has regressed, epidural local anesthetics will produce higher sensory blockade in the presence of a dural hole than after epidural injection alone (254,255).

Epidural Drugs. The presence of a 24- or 27-gauge dural hole may allow enhanced intrathecal passage of drugs injected into the epidural space. In animals, dural puncture significantly increases the flux of morphine and lidocaine through meningeal tissue (256). The degree of this effect correlates with the size of the dural hole (Fig. 23) (254). In laboring women, epidural injection of 13 mL of 0.25% bupivacaine blocked 13.6 dermatomes in the absence of a previous dural puncture. This same

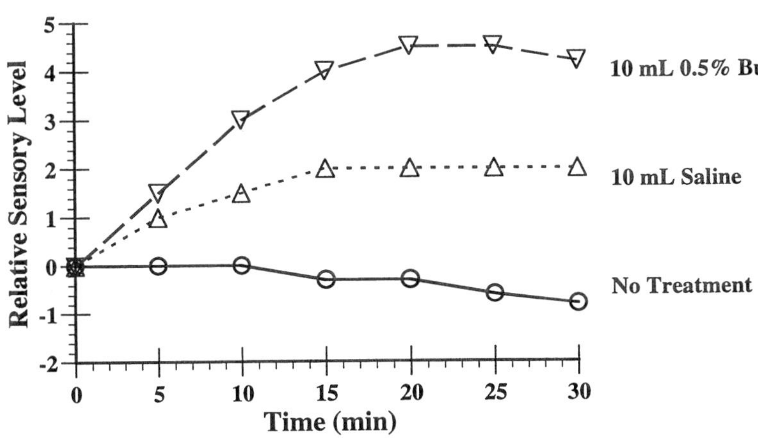

FIG. 22. Nonpregnant patients received 10 mg of 0.5% plain bupivacaine intrathecally. After the maximum level of sensory blockade had been achieved, patients received either 10 mL of epidural bupivacaine 0.5% (▽), 10 mL of epidural saline (△), or nothing (○). (Modified from ref. 251, with permission.)

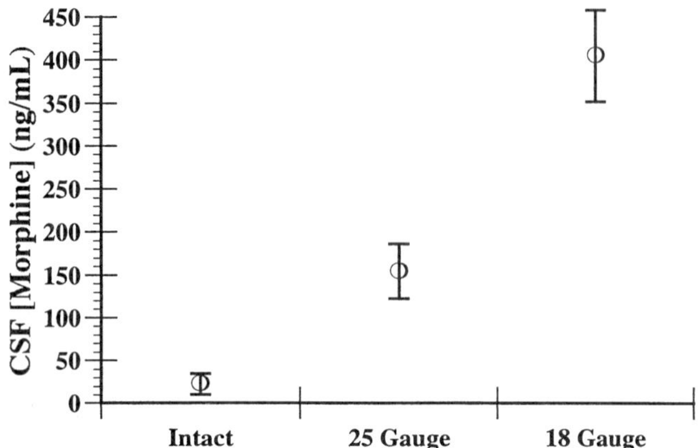

FIG. 23. Cerebrospinal fluid morphine concentration measured at the cisternal magna 6 hours after lumbar epidural injection of 0.2 mg/kg morphine in sheep. Dural puncture was performed one interspace above the insertion site of the epidural catheter, 1 hour before morphine injection. (Data from ref. 254.)

dose of drug blocked 16.6 dermatomes when injected 53 to 235 minutes after dural puncture with a 24- or 27-gauge pencil point needle (Fig. 24) (255). The observed range of sensory blockade was very large. Several patients in each group had fewer than five or more than 20 dermatomes anesthetized. Although the sensory level difference between the groups was statistically significant, it is unlikely to be clinically important given the degree of interpatient variation.

Efficacy

Although the needle-through-needle CSE technique is an effective way to deliver intrathecal drugs, the efficacy of a concurrently placed epidural catheter is unknown. Many hesitate to use this technique in laboring women at high risk for cesarean delivery because, in an acute emergency, such an "untested" catheter may fail to provide adequate operative anesthesia. A recent systematic evaluation of 1,492 multiorifice catheters placed for epidural (n = 545) or CSE (n = 947) labor analgesia provides some information about this issue: 1.2% of epidural catheters failed to produce any analgesia or sensory change; only 0.2% of CSE catheters failed (p <0.05) (257). Catheters placed as part of a CSE technique in laboring women are at least as reliable as those placed as part of epidural labor analgesia.

Headache

The incidence of headache after uncomplicated CSE labor analgesia is low. Fewer than 8% of women report any headache, and fewer than 3% have positional headaches (Fig. 25). The incidence of epidural blood patch is no different than after labor epidural analgesia (0.4%) (242). Approximately 1 in 500 parturients require therapeutic epidural blood patch after uncomplicated needle-through-needle CSE (242,243).

Infection

Both meningitis and epidural abscess have been reported after CSE anesthesia (258–260). These rare complications also are reported after spinal or epidural anesthesia (261). *Viridans streptococci*, a common oropharyngeal bacteria, have emerged as major pathogens of meningitis after spinal anesthesia (261). Routinely wearing a face mask during dural puncture may decrease the risk of this serious complication.

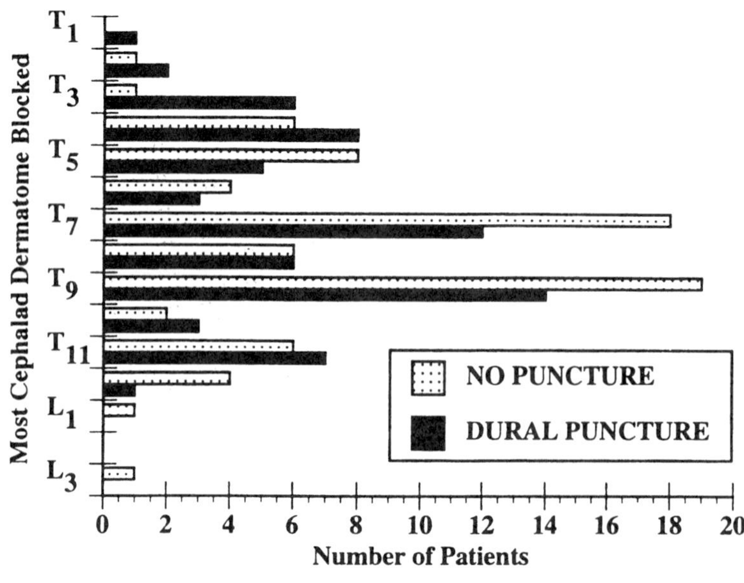

FIG. 24. Most cephalad dermatome blocked on either side in patients receiving 27- or 24-gauge dural puncture and intrathecal sufentanil or no dural puncture before epidural injection of 13 mL of bupivacaine 0.25%. More patients with a dural puncture had sensory blockade to T_4 or higher (17 of 70 vs 8 of 77; $p < 0.05$). (Reproduced from ref. 255, with permission.)

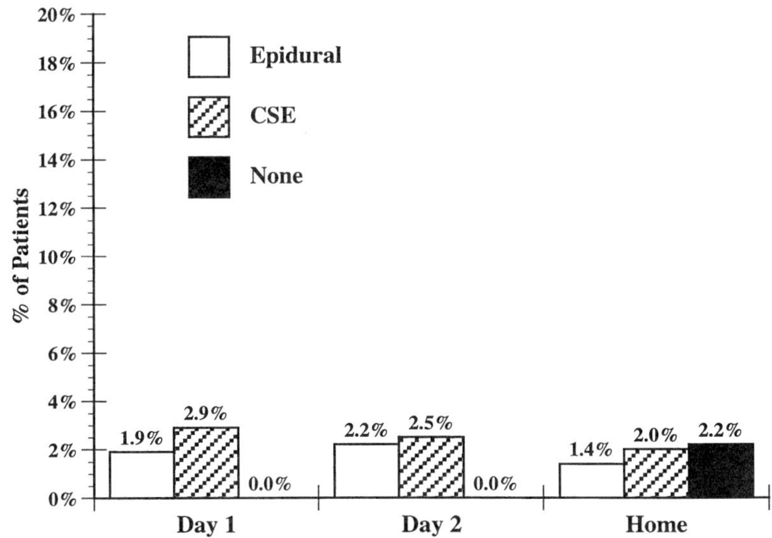

FIG. 25. Incidence of positional headache after delivery in women requesting epidural, combined spinal–epidural *(CSE)*, or no labor analgesia. Patients were visited daily while in the hospital and phoned at home within 2 weeks of delivery. (Data from ref. 242.)

REFERENCES

1. Parkin IG, Harrison GR. The topographical anatomy of the lumbar epidural space. *J Anat* 1985;141:211.
2. Nakagawa H, Mikawa Y, Watanabe R. Elastin in the human posterior longitudinal ligament and spinal dura: a histologic and biochemical study. *Spine* 1994;19:2164.
3. Tencer AF, Allen BL Jr, Ferguson RL. A biomechanical study of thoracolumbar spine fractures with bone in the canal. Part III. Mechanical properties of the dura and its tethering ligaments. *Spine* 1985; 10:741.
4. Patin DJ, Eckstein EC, Harum K, Pallares VS. Anatomic and biomechanical properties of human lumbar dura mater. *Anesth Analg* 1993; 76:535.
5. Reina MA, Dittman M, Garcia AL, van Zundert A. New perspectives in the microscopic structure of human dura mater in the dorsolumbar region. *Reg Anesth* 1997;22:161.
6. Hogan QH. Lumbar epidural anatomy: a new look by cryomicrotome section. *Anesthesiology* 1991;75:767.
7. Hogan QH. Epidural anatomy examined by cryomicrotome section: influence of age, vertebral level and disease. *Reg Anesth* 1996;21:395.
8. Reynolds AF Jr, Roberts PA, Pollay M, Stratemeier PH. Quantitative anatomy of the thoracolumbar epidural space. *Neurosurgery* 1985; 17:905.
9. Westbrook JL, Renowden SA, Carrie LES. Study of the anatomy of the extradural region using magnetic resonance imaging. *Br J Anaesth* 1993;71:495.
10. Capogna G, Celleno D, Simonetti C, Lupoi D. Anatomy of the lumbar epidural region using magnetic resonance imaging: a study of dimensions and a comparison of two postures. *Int J Obstet Anesth* 1997;6:97.
11. Hogan Q. The true epidural space: possible consequences for administered material-based drug delivery systems—reply. *Anesthesiology* 1992;76:866.
12. Zarzur E. Anatomic studies of the human lumbar ligamentum flavum. *Anesth Analg* 1984;63:499.
13. Naffziger HC, Inman V, Saunders JBCM. Lesions of the intervertebral disc and ligamenta flava: clinical and anatomical studies. *Surg Gynecol Obstet* 1938;66:288.
14. Olszewski AD, Yaszemski MJ, White AA III. The anatomy of the human lumbar ligamentum flavum: new observations and their surgical importance. *Spine* 1996;21:2307.
15. Segal S, Beach M, Eappen S. A multivariate model to predict the distance from the skin to the epidural space in an obstetric population. *Reg Anesth* 1996;21:451.
16. Currie JM. Measurement of the depth to the extradural space using ultrasound. *Br J Anaesth* 1984;56:345.
17. Hamza J, Smida M, Benhamou D, Cohen SE. Parturient's posture during epidural puncture affects the distance from skin to epidural space. *J Clin Anesth* 1995;7:1.
18. Harrison GR. The depth of the lumbar epidural space from the skin. *Anaesthesia* 1985;40:685.
19. Meiklejohn BH. Distance from skin to the lumbar epidural space in an obstetric population. *Reg Anesth* 1990;15:134.
20. Palmer SK, Abram SE, Maitra AM, von Colditz JH. Distance from the skin to the lumbar epidural space in an obstetric population. *Anesth Analg* 1983;62:944.
21. Narang VPS, Linter SPK. Failure of extradural blockade in obstetrics: a new hypothesis. *Br J Anaesth* 1988;60:402.
22. Sutton DN, Linter SPK. Depth of extradural space and dural puncture. *Anaesthesia* 1991;46:97.
23. Hamza J, Benhamou D. Dural puncture and depth of the extradural space. *Anaesthesia* 1992;47:169.
24. Wallace DH, Currie JM, Gilstrap LC, Santos R. Indirect sonographic guidance for epidural anesthesia in obese pregnant patients. *Reg Anesth* 1992;17:233.
25. Hirabayashi Y, Shimizu R, Fukuda H, Saitoh K, Igarashi T. Soft tissue anatomy within the vertebral canal in pregnant women. *Br J Anaesth* 1996;77:153.
26. Gaynor PA. The lumbar epidural region: anatomy and approach. In: Reynolds F, ed. *Epidural and spinal blockade in obstetrics.* London: Bailliere Tindall, 1990:3.
27. Bonica J. Continuous peridural block. *Anesthesiology* 1956;17:626.
28. Carrie LES. The approach to the extradural space. *Anaesthesia* 1971; 26:252.
29. Armitage EN. The paramedian approach to lumbar epidural analgesia. *Anaesthesia* 1976;31:1287.
30. Carrie LES. The paramedian approach to the epidural space: technique and choice of needle. *Anaesthesia* 1977;32:670.
31. Chapman GM. The paramedian approach to the epidural space: endorsement. *Anaesthesia* 1977;32:671.
32. Uncles DR, Carrie LES. Pain and the paramedian approach to epidural catherisation. *Anaesthesia* 1993;48:641.
33. Barretto C, Hook R, Seah CH. Use of the Tuohy needle in paramedian approach for peridural block. *Anesth Analg* 1997;56:582.
34. Blomberg RG. Technical advantages of the paramedian approach for lumbar epidural puncture and catheter introduction: a study using epiduroscopy in autopsy subjects. *Anaesthesia* 1988;43:837.
35. Griffin RM, Scott RPF. Forum: a comparison between the midline and paramedian approaches to the extradural space. *Anaesthesia* 1984;39: 584.
36. Jaucot J. Paramedian approach of the peridural space in obstetrics. *Acta Anaesthesiol Belg* 1986;37:187.
37. Blomberg RG, Jaanivald A, Walther S. Advantages of the paramedian approach for lumbar epidural analgesia with catheter technique: a clinical comparison between midline and paramedian approaches. *Anaesthesia* 1989;44:742.
38. Macdonald R. Dr Doughty's technique for the location of the epidural space [Letter]. *Anaesthesia* 1983;38:71.

39. Reynolds F. Avoiding accidental dural puncture [Letter]. *Br J Anaesth* 1988;61:515.
40. Reimann AF, Anson BJ. Vertebral level of termination of the spinal cord with report of a case of sacral cord. *Anat Rec* 1944;88:127.
41. Thompson A. Untitled. *J Anat Physiol* 1894;29:45.
42. Larsen JL, Olsen KO. Radiographic anatomy of the distal dural sac: a myelographic investigation of dimensions and termination. *Acta Radiol* 1991;32:214.
43. Hogan QH, Prost R, Kulier A, Taylor ML, Liu S, Mark L. Magnetic resonance imaging of cerebrospinal fluid volume and the influence of body habitus and abdominal pressure. *Anesthesiology* 119;84: 1341.
44. Hogan Q. Size of human lower thoracic and lumbosacral nerve roots. *Anesthesiology* 1996;85:37.
45. Wall EJ, Cohen MS, Massie JB, Rydevik B, Garfin SR. Cauda equina anatomy I: intrathecal nerve root organization. *Spine* 1990;15:1244.
46. Cohen MS, Wall EJ, Brown RA, Rydevik B, Garfin SR. Cauda equina anatomy II: extrathecal nerve roots and dorsal root ganglia. *Spine* 1990;15:1248.
47. Wall EJ, Cohen MS, Abitbol JJ, Garfin SR. Organization of intrathecal nerve roots at the level of the conus medullaris. *J Bone Joint Surg* 1990;72A:1495.
48. Cohen MS, Wall EJ, Kerbe CW, Abitbol JJ, Garfin SR. The anatomy of the cauda equina on CT scans and MRI. *J Bone Joint Surg* 1991; 73B:381.
49. Kubota Y, Toyoda Y, Kubota H. Jacoby's line rather than Tuffier's line as a guide to lumbar puncture. *Anesth Analg* 1992;74:939.
50. Vandam LD. On the origins of intrathecal anesthesia. *Int Anesthesiol Clin* 1989;27:2.
51. Render CA. The reproductibility of the iliac crest as a marker of lumbar spine level. *Anaesthesia* 1996;51:1070.
52. Ievins FA. Accuracy of placement of extradural needles in the L3-4 interspace: comparison of two methods of identifying L4. *Br J Anaesth* 1991;66:381.
53. Van Gessel EF, Forster A, Gamulin Z. Continuous spinal anesthesia: where do spinal catheters go? *Anesth Analg* 1993;76:1004.
54. Hogan QH. Tuffier's line: the normal distribution of anatomic parameters. *Anesth Analg* 1994;78:194.
55. Thavasothy M. The reproducibility of the iliac crest as a marker of lumbar spinal level [Letter]. *Anaesthesia* 1997;52:797.
56. Stone PA, Kilpatrick AWA, Thorburn J. Posture and epidural catheter insertion: the relationship between skill, experience and maternal posture on the outcome of epidural catheter insertion. *Anaesthesia* 1990;45:920.
57. Vincent RD, Chestnut DH. Which position is more comfortable for the parturient during induction of epidural anesthesia? *Int J Obstet Anesth* 1991;1:9.
58. Andrews PJD, Ackerman WE, Juneja MM. Aortocaval compression in the sitting and lateral decubitus positions during extradural catheter placement in the parturient. *Can J Anaesth* 1993;40:320.
59. Hamilton CL, Riley ET, Cohen SE. Changes in the position of epidural catheters associated with patient movement. *Anesthesiology* 1997;86:778.
60. Webster SG. Migration of epidural catheters. *Anaesthesia* 1986;41: 654.
61. Liyang D, Yinkan X, Wenming Z, Zhihua Z. The effect of flexion-extension motion of the lumbar spine on the capacity of the spinal canal: an experimental study. *Spine* 1989;14:523.
62. Inufusa A, An HS, Lim T-H, Hasegawa T, Haughton VM, Nowicki BH. Anatomic changes of the spinal canal and intervertebral foramen associated with flexion-extension movement. *Spine* 1996;21:2412.
63. Eldor J. Huber needle and Tuohy catheter. *Reg Anesth* 1995;20:252.
64. Curbelo MM. Continuous peridural segmental anesthesia by means of a ureteral catheter. *Anesth Analg* 1949;28:13.
65. Bromage PR. *Epidural analgesia.* Philadelphia: WB Saunders, 1978: 329.
66. Bell GC. Improved epidural needle. *Obstet Gynecol* 1975;46:487.
67. Kumar B, Messahel FM. Evaluation of epidural needles. *Acta Anaesthesiol Scand* 1987;31:96.
68. Herman N, Molin J, Knape KG. No additional metal particle formation using the needle-through-needle combined epidural/spinal technique. *Acta Anaesthesiol Scand* 1996;40:227.
69. Lee JA. Specially marked needle to facilitate extradural block. *Anaesthesia* 1960;15:186.
70. Pither CE. The Lee modification of the Tuohy needle—a useful adjunct to gauging the depth of the epidural space. *Anesth Analg* 1984; 63:1048.
71. McNeill MJ, Thorburn J. Cannulation of the epidural space: a comparison of 18- and 16-gauge needles. *Anaesthesia* 1988;43:154.
72. Moore DC. Sixteen-gauge Tuohy needles should be abandoned. *Anesthesiology* 1980;53:269.
73. Lipov EG, McCarthy RJ, Ivankovich AD. Severe kinking of an epidural needle. *Anesth Analg* 1994;78:607.
74. Kopacz DJ, Allen HW. Comparison of needle deviation during regional anesthetic techniques in a laboratory model. *Anesth Analg* 1995;81:630.
75. Dunn SM, Steinberg RB, O'Sullivan PS, Goolishian WT, Villa EA. A fractured epidural needle: case report and study. *Anesth Analg* 1992; 75:1050.
76. Hershan DB, Rosner HL. An unusual complication of epidural analgesia in a morbidity obese parturient. *Anesth Analg* 1996;82:217.
77. Patt RB, Reddy SK. Walk, don't run: alternative methods of changing needle direction. *Anesth Analg* 1995;80:1067.
78. Stride PC, Cooper GM. Dural taps revisited: a 20-year survey from Birmingham Maternity Hospital. *Anaesthesia* 1993;48:247.
79. Odom CB. Epidural anesthesia. *Am J Surg* 1936;34:547.
80. Bromage PR. The "hanging-drop" sign. *Anaesthesia* 1953;8:237.
81. Messih MNA. Epidural space pressures during pregnancy. *Anaesthesia* 1981;36:775.
82. Shah JL. Forum: influence of cerebrospinal fluid on epidural pressure. *Anaesthesia* 1981;36:627.
83. Thomas PS, Gerson JI, Strong G. Analysis of human epidural pressures. *Reg Anesth* 1992;17:212.
84. Shah JL. Positive lumbar epidural space pressure. *Br J Anaesth* 1994; 73:309.
85. Usubiaga JE, Wikinski JA, Usubiaga LE. Epidural pressure and its relation to spread of anesthetic solutions in epidural space. *Anesth Analg* 1967;46:440.
86. Galbert MW, Marx GF. Extradural pressures in the parturient patient. *Anesthesiology* 1974;40:499.
87. Takahashi K, Miyazaki T, Takino T, Matsui T, Tomita K. Epidural pressure measurements: relationship between epidural pressure and posture in patients with lumbar spinal stenosis. *Spine* 1995;20:650.
88. Bromage PR. Continuous lumbar epidural analgesia for obstetrics. *Can Med Assoc J* 1961;85:1136.
89. Johnston GM, Rodgers RC, Tunstall ME. Alteration of maternal posture and its immediate effect on epidural pressure. *Anaesthesia* 1989; 44:750.
90. Shah JL. Effect of posture on extradural pressure. *Br J Anaesth* 1984; 56:1373.
91. Eaton LM. Observations on the negative pressure in the epidural space. *Proc Staff Meet Mayo Clin* 1938;14:566.
92. Zarzur E. Genesis of the "true" negative pressure in the lumbar epidural space: a new hypothesis. *Anaesthesia* 1984;39:1101.
93. Telford RJ, Hollway TE. Observations on deliberate dural puncture with a Tuohy needle: pressure measurements. *Anaesthesia* 1991;46:725.
94. Sicard JA, Forestier J. Radiographic method for exploration of the extradural space using lipiodol. *Rev Neurol* 1921;28:1264.
95. Macdonald R. Dr. Doughty's technique for the location of the epidural space [Letter]. *Anaesthesia* 1983;38:71.
96. Reynolds F. Avoiding accidental dural puncture [Letter]. *Br J Anaesth* 1988;61:515.
97. Brandstater B. The needle tilt test: an aid to epidural needle insertion. *Anesthesiology* 1989;70:366.
98. Davies MW, Harrison JC, Ryan TDR. Current practice of epidural analgesia during normal labour: a survey of maternity units in the United Kingdom. *Anaesthesia* 1993;48:63.
99. Valentine SJ, Jarvis AP, Shutt LE. Comparative study of the effects of air or saline to identify the extradural space. *Br J Anaesth* 1991; 66:224.
100. Dalens B, Bazin J-E, Haberer J-P. Epidural bubbles as a cause of incomplete analgesia during epidural anesthesia. *Anesth Analg* 1987; 66:679.
101. Boezaart AP, Levendig BJ. Epidural air-filled bubbles and unblocked segments. *Can J Anaesth* 1989;36:603.
102. Stevens R, Mikat-Stevens M, van Clief M, Schubert A, Weinstein Z. Deliberate epidural air injection in dogs: a radiographic study. *Reg Anesth* 1989;14:180.

103. Saberski LR, Kondamuri S, Osinubi OYO. Identification of the epidural space: is loss of resistance to air a safe technique? A review of the complications related to the use of air. *Reg Anesth* 1997;22:3.
104. Aida S, Taga K, Yamakura T, Endoh H, Shimoji K. Headache after attempted epidural block: the role of intrathecal air. *Anesthesiology* 1998;88:76.
105. Kreitzer JM, Reed AP, Dauro AT, Brodman ML, Bronster DJ. Ascending back pain and headache during attempted epidural placement. *J Clin Anesth* 1991;3:414.
106. Ash KM, Cannon JE, Biehl DR. Pneumocephalus following attempted epidural anaesthesia. *Can J Anaesth* 1991;38:772.
107. Gonzalez-Carrasco FJ, Aguilar JL, Llubia C, Nogues S, Vidal-Lopez ZF. Pneumocephalus after accidental dural puncture during epidural anesthesia. *Reg Anesth* 1993;18:193.
108. Kennedy TM, Ullman DA, Harte FA, Saberski LR, Greenhouse BD. Lumbar root compression secondary to epidural air. *Anesth Analg* 1988;67:1184.
109. Nay PG, Milaszkiewicz R, Jothilingam S. Extradural air as a cause of paraplegia following lumbar analgesia. *Anaesthesia* 1993;48:402.
110. Reynolds F. Dural puncture and headache: avoid the first but treat the second. *BMJ* 1993;306:874.
111. Iwama H. Injection volume of slaine with loss of resistance may affect the spread of epidural anesthesia. *Anesthesiology* 1997;86:507.
112. Sharrock NE. Recording of, and an anatomical explanation for, false positive loss of resistance during lumbar extradural analgesia. *Br J Anaesth* 1979;51:253.
113. Williams RAJ. A syringe for extradural analgesia. *Anaesthesia* 1975;30:788.
114. Bricker SRW, Coleman P. Variations in the gliding characteristics of 10-ml plastic syringes used to locate the extradural space by "loss of resistance" techniques. *Br J Anaesth* 1988;61:776.
115. Butler BD, Warters RD, Elk JR, Davies I, Abouleish E. Loss of resistance technique for locating the epidural space: evaluation of glass and plastic syringes. *Can J Anaesth* 1990;37:438.
116. Leiman BC, Katz J, Salzarulo H, Warters RD, Butler BD. A comparison of different methods of lubrication of glass syringes used to identify the epidural space. *Anaesthesia* 1988;43:397.
117. Candido KD, Winnie AP. A dual-chambered syringe that allows identification of the epidural space using the loss of resistance technique with air and with saline. *Reg Anesth* 1992;17:163.
118. Tillman HA, Bhatia KN. Another, yet simpler device for the identification of the epidural space. *Anesthesiology* 1984;60:79.
119. Michel MZ, Lawes EG. Identification of epidural space by drip method. *Reg Anesth* 1991;16:236.
120. Eldor J, Guedj P. Combined hanging drop-loss of resistance technique for identification of the epidural space. *Reg Anesth* 1991;16:299.
121. Glantz L, Gozal Y, Gertel M. A loss-of-resistance technique using both air and saline. *Reg Anesth* 1994;19:294.
122. Barros S. Loss-of-resistance technique using both air and saline. *Reg Anesth* 1995;20:462.
123. Singh A, Elloy MA. An epidural introducer. *Br J Anaesth* 1972;44:1105.
124. Rocco AG, Reisman RM, Lief PA, Ferrante FM. A two-person technique for epidural needle placement and medication infusion. *Reg Anesth* 1989;14:85.
125. Rocco AG, Palombi D. Additional advantages of a two-person technique for epidural needle placement and medication infusion. *Reg Anesth* 1991;16:285.
126. Ostheimer GW. Editorial comment. *Reg Anesth* 1991;16:300.
127. Scott DB. Identification of the epidural space: loss of resistance to air or saline? *Reg Anesth* 1997;22:1.
128. Norris MC, Leighton BL, DeSimone CA. Needle bevel direction and headache after inadvertent dural puncture. *Anesthesiology* 1989;70:729.
129. Hehre FW, Sayig JM. Continuous lumbar peridural anesthesia in obstetrics. *Am J Obstet Gynecol* 1960;80:1173.
130. Kalas DB, Hehre FW. Continuous lumbar peridural anesthesia in obstetrics VIII: further observations on inadvertent lumbar puncture. *Anesth Analg* 1972;51:192.
131. Craft JB, Epstein BS, Coakley CS. Prophylaxis of dural-puncture headache with epidural saline. *Anesth Analg* 1973;52:228.
132. Mihic DN. Postspinal headache and relationship of needle bevel to dural fibers. *Reg Anesth* 1985;10:76.
133. Thorsen G. Neurological complications after spinal anesthesia, and results from 2493 follow-up cases. *Acta Chirurg Scand* 1947;[Suppl 121]:95;1.
134. Lybecker H, Moller JT, May O, Nielsen HK. Incidence and prediction of post-dural puncture headache: a prospective study of 1021 spinal anesthesias. *Anesth Analg* 1990;70:389.
135. Tarkkila PJ, Heine H, Tervo PR. Comparison of Sprotte and Quincke needles with respect to post dural puncture headache and backache. *Reg Anesth* 1992;17:283.
136. Sanchez R, Acuna L, Rocha F. An analysis of the radiological visualization of the catheters placed in the epidural space. *Br J Anaesth* 1967;39:485.
137. Bridenbaugh LD, Moore DC, Bagdi P, Bridenbaugh PO. The position of plastic tubing in continuous-block techniques: an x-ray study of 552 patients. *Anesthesiology* 1968;29:1047.
138. Muneyuki M, Shirai K, Inamoto A. Roentgenographic analysis of the positions of catheters in the epidural space. *Anesthesiology* 1970;33:19.
139. Zaaijman JDT, Slabber CF. The position of epidural catheters in obstetric regional anaesthesia. *S Afr Med J* 1979;55:915.
140. Tiso RL, Thomas PS, Macadaeg K. Epidural catheter direction and local anesthetic dose. *Reg Anesth* 1993;18:308.
141. Baskovski N, Lewinski A. The effect of the direction of the needle bevel in lumbar analgesia. *Anaesthesia* 1982;37:216.
142. Park WY, Poon KC, Massengale MD, MacNamara TE. Direction of the needle bevel and epidural anesthetic spread. *Anesthesiology* 1982;57:327.
143. Munoz HR, Dagnino JA, Allende M, Bugedo GJ, Montes JM, Cherres OG. Direction of catheter insertion and incidence of paresthesias and failure rate in continuous epidural anesthesia: a comparison of cephalad and caudad catheter insertion. *Reg Anesth* 1993;18:331.
144. Richardson MG, Wissler R. Tuohy needle bevel orientation during epidural catheter placement: effect on analgesic success during labor. *Anesthesiology* 1996;85:A908.
145. Huffnagle SL, Norris MC, Arkoosh VA, et al. The effect of epidural needle bevel orientation on spread of sensory blockade in the laboring parturient. *Anesth Analg* 1998;87:326.
146. Toomey PJ. A technique to avoid dural puncture by the epidural catheter. *Anaesthesia* 1992;47:79.
147. Eldor J. Do not rotate the epidural needle. *Anesth Analg* 1994;78:606.
148. Duffy BL. "Don't turn the needle!" *Anaesth Intens Care* 1993;21:328.
149. Norris MC, Leighton BL. "Don't turn the needle!"—a reply. *Anaesth Intens Care* 1993;21:900.
150. Anderson AJ. To turn or not to turn! *Anaesth Intens Care* 1993;21:901.
151. Barratt SM. — and turning. *Anaesth Intens Care* 1993;21:901.
152. Jordan MJ. Rotating needle increases risk. *BMJ* 1993;306:1339.
153. Reynolds F. Epidural analgesia during childbirth: minimizing headache after dural puncture. *BMJ* 1993;307:63.
154. Redick LF. Rotating the epidural needle: a caution. *Anesth Analg* 1993;77:1079.
155. Moore DC. Rotating the epidural needle: a caution—where is the clinical proof? *Anesth Analg* 1994;79:810.
156. Bromage PR. Rotation of the epidural needle: a caution. *Anesth Analg* 1995;81:209.
157. Moore DC. Rotation of the epidural needle: a caution—in response. *Anesth Analg* 1995;81:209.
158. Norris MC. On rotating the epidural needle. *Anesth Analg* 1996;82:429.
159. Bromage PR. On rotating the epidural needle—in response. *Anesth Analg* 1996;82:430.
160. Carter LC, Popat MT, Wallace DH. Epidural needle rotation and inadvertent dural puncture with catheter. *Anaesthesia* 1992;47:447.
161. Hollway TE, Telford RJ. Observations on deliberate dural puncture with Tuohy needle: depth measurements. *Anaesthesia* 1991;46:722.
162. Meiklejohn BH. The effect of rotation of an epidural needle: an in vitro study. *Anaesthesia* 1987;42:1180.
163. Hardy PAJ. Force exerted by epidural catheters. *Anaesthesia* 1986;41:306.
164. Hardy PAJ. Can epidural catheters penetrate dura mater? An anatomical study. *Anaesthesia* 1986;41:1146.
165. Pinchak AC, Podlipski HM, Hagen JF. Mechanical aspects of epidural catheter insertion—prevention of catheter buckling by means of a needle hub insert. *Anesthesiology* 1983;59:549.
166. Hofer RE, Lennon RL, Didier P. "Just a little bit more." *Anesth Analg* 1989;69:691.
167. Beck H, Brassow F, Doehm M, Bause H, Dziadzka A, Schulte am

Esch J. Epidural catheters of the multi-orifice type: dangers and complications. *Acta Anaesthesiol Scand* 1986;30:549.
168. Sals-Blanch X, Martinez-Palli G, Agusti-Lasus M, Nalda-Felipe A. Case report: misplacement of multihole epidural catheters—a report of two cases. *Anaesthesia* 1996;51:386.
169. Michael S, Richmond MN, Birks RJS. A comparison between open-end (single hole) and closed-end (three lateral holes) epidural catheters. *Anaesthesia* 1989;44:578.
170. Collier CB, Gatti SP. Epidural catheters for obstetrics: terminal hole or lateral eyes? *Reg Anesth* 1994;19:378.
171. D'Angelo R, Foss ML, Livesay CH. A comparison of multiport and uniport epidural catheters in laboring patients. *Anesth Analg* 1997; 84:1276.
172. Morrison LMM, Buchan AS. Comparison of complications associated with single-holed and multi-holed extradural catheters. *Br J Anaesth* 1990;64:183.
173. Power I, Thorburn J. Differential flow from multihole epidural catheters. *Anaesthesia* 1988;43:876.
174. Philip BK. Effect of epidural air injection on catheter complications. *Reg Anesth* 1985;10:21.
175. Verniquet AJW. Vessel puncture with epidural catheters: experience in obstetric patients. *Anaesthesia* 1980;35:360.
176. Sarna MC, Smith I, James JM. Paraesthesia with lumbar epidural catheters: a comparison of air and saline in a loss-of-resistance technique. *Anaesthesia* 1990;45:1077.
177. Rolbin SH, Halpern SH, Braude BM, Kapala D, Unger R, Radhakrisnan S. Fluid through the epidural needle does not reduce complications of epidural catheter insertion. *Can J Anaesth* 1990;37:337.
178. Skidmore AL. A retrospective analysis of epidural vein trauma. *Anaesthesia* 1991;45:516.
179. Rolbin SH, Relle A, Hew EM. Hyperventilation does not affect the incidence of paresthesiae and blood vessel cannulation during epidural catheter insertion. *Can Anaesth Soc J* 1985;32:568.
180. Lee JA. A new catheter for continuous extradural analgesia. *Anaesthesia* 1962;17:248.
181. Doughty A. A precise method of cannulating the lumbar epidural space. *Anaesthesia* 1974;29:63.
182. Jawalekar SR, Santos HB. A procedure for measuring the length of the catheter in the epidural space. *Anesthesiology* 1982;57:67.
183. Plumer MH, Rottman R. How anesthesiologists practice obstetric anesthesia—responses of practicing obstetric anesthesiologists at the 1993 meeting of the Society for Obstetric Anesthesia and Perinatology. *Reg Anesth* 1996;21:49.
184. Beilin Y, Bernstein HH, Zucker-Pinchoff B. The optimal distance that a multiorifice epidural catheter should be threaded into the epidural space. *Anesth Analg* 1995;81:301.
185. D'Angelo R, Berkebile BL, Gerancher JC. Prospective examination of epidural catheter insertion. *Anesthesiology* 1996;84:88.
186. Bielin Y. Epidural catheter insertion and satisfactory analgesia. *Anesthesiology* 1996;84:1524.
187. D'Angelo R. Epidural catheter insertion and satisfactory analgesia—in reply. *Anesthesiology* 1996;84:1524.
188. Moore DC. Epidural catheter insertion and satisfactory analgesia—the mobile versus the immobile patient. *Anesthesiology* 1997;86:747.
189. Beilin Y. Epidural catheter insertion and satisfactory analgesia—the mobile versus the immobile patient—in reply. *Anesthesiology* 1997; 86:748.
190. D'Angelo R, Gerancher JC. Epidural catheter insertion and satisfactory analgesia—the mobile versus the immobile patient—in reply. *Anesthesiology* 1997;86:749.
191. Boey SK, Carrie LES. Withdrawal forces during removal of lumbar extradural catheters. *Br J Anaesth* 1994;73:833.
192. Morris GN, Warren BB, Hanson EW, Mazzeo FJ, DiBenedetto DJ. Influence of patient position on withdrawal forces during removal of lumbar extradural catheters. *Br J Anaesth* 1996;77:419.
193. Blackshear RH, Gravenstein N, Radson E. Tension applied to lumbar epidural catheters during removal is much greater with patient sitting versus lying. *Anesthesiology* 1991;75:A833.
194. Blackshear RH, Gravenstein N, Wissler RN, Bjoraker DG. Comparison of tensile strengths of seven types of epidural catheters. *Anesthesiology* 1990;73:A961.
195. Davies R, Vaughn RS, Richards J. Epidural catheters: breaking and extraction forces. *Anaesthesia* 1993;48:900.
196. Gravenstein N, Blackshear RIT, Wissler RN. An approach to spinal or epidural catheters that are difficult to remove. *Anesthesiology* 1991; 75:544.
197. Sia-Kho E, Kudlak TT. How to dislodge a severely trapped epidural catheter. *Anesth Analg* 1992;74:929.
198. Ballance JHW. Difficulty in the removal of an epidural catheter. *Anaesthesia* 1981;36:71.
199. Gadalla F. Removal of a tenacious epidural catheter. *Anaesthesia* 1992;75:1071.
200. Day C. Difficult removal of an epidural catheter. *Anaesthesia* 1993; 48:448.
201. Browne RA, Politi VL. Knotting of an epidural catheter: a case report. *Can Anaesth Soc J* 1979;26:142.
202. Blass NH, Roberts RB, Wiley JK. The case of the errant epidural catheter. *Anesthesiology* 1981;54:419.
203. Moscovici R, Prego G. A trapped epidural catheter. *Anaesthesia* 1993; 45:536.
204. Gozal D, Gozal Y, Beilin B. Removal of knotted epidural catheters: case reports. *Reg Anesth* 1996;21:71
205. Odom NJ, Health ML. A dangerous disposable epidural needle. *Anaesthesia* 1977;32:75.
206. LeDez K, Kneeling P. "Malalignment" of epidural needles. *Anaesthesia* 1984;39:1255.
207. Shribman AJ. A defective Tuohy needle. *Anaesthesia* 1986;41:880.
208. Schlake PT, Peleman RR, Winnie AP. Separation of the hub from the shaft of a disposable epidural needle. *Anesthesiology* 1988;68:611.
209. Vohra A, Pollard BJ. Failure to cannulate the epidural space. *Can J Anaesth* 1989;36:598.
210. Eldor J, Guedj P. Too long plastic obturator of 18-G Portex epidural needle. *Anaesthesia* 1990;45:1098.
211. Cozanitis DA. Faulty Portex epidural needle. *Anaesthesia* 1991;46:516.
212. Lansing SJ, Ward JB. Wet tap due to epidural needle defect. *Anesth Analg* 1992;75:633.
213. Wilson AT, Hawthorne L. Faulty Tuohy needle and dural puncture. *Anaesthesia* 1992;47:1096.
214. Bamber MJ. Unusual defect in a Tuohy needle. *Anaesthesia* 1993;48:743.
215. Norman EA, Ahmad I, Norman DM. Failure of an epidural needle. *Anesth Analg* 1994;79:394.
216. Mackie D, Cranfield J, Boddu K. Unexpected loss of resistance. *Anaesthesia* 1994;49:458.
217. McBeth C. Faulty loss of resistance syringe. *Anaesthesia* 1995;50:186.
218. Stableforth C. Faulty loss of resistance syringe. *Anaesthesia* 1995;50: 668.
219. Deen SM, Marx GF. Fusion between catheter and stylet: an unusual complication of extradural analgesia. *Anesth Analg* 1980;59:516.
220. Simpson PM. Defective epidural cannulae. *Anaesthesia* 1981;36:72.
221. Rutter TW. On passage of catheters through epidural needles. *Anesth Analg* 1990;70:337.
222. Cohen S, Amar D. Defect in the integrity of an epidural catheter. *Reg Anesth* 1990;15:272.
223. Yau G, Ewart MC, Oh TE. Duplicate markings on an epidural catheter. *Anaesthesia* 1991;46:795.
224. Wee LH. Another cause for failed epidural. *Anaesthesia* 1994;49:270.
225. Williams G, Howell P. Equipment failure during epidural catheter placement. *Anaesthesia* 1995;50:831.
226. Stacey BR, Mizikar WE. Defective nylon catheter. *Reg Anesth* 1996;21:377.
227. Patterson KW. Epidural kits: incompatible contents. *Anesth Analg* 1992;74:474.
228. Seitman DT, Shapiro BE. Inability to thread epidural catheter through epidural needle. *Anesth Analg* 1989;69:267.
229. Soresi AL. Episubdural anesthesia. *Anesth Analg* 1937;16:306.
230. Coates MB. Combined subarachnoid and epidural techniques. *Anaesthesia* 1982;37:89.
231. Mumtaz MH, Daz M, Kuz M. Another single space technique for orthopedic surgery. *Anaesthesia* 1982;37:90.
232. Collis RE, Davies DWL, Aveling W. Randomised comparison of combined spinal-epidural and standard epidural analgesia in labour. *Lancet* 1995;345:1413.
233. Nageotte MP, Larson D, Rumney PJ, Sidhu M, Hollenbach K. Epidural analgesia compared with combined spinal-epidural analgesia during labor in nulliparous women. *N Engl J Med* 1997;337:1715.
234. Sprotte G, Schedel R, Pajunk H. Eine "atraumatische." Universalkanöle für einzeitige Regionalanaesthesien. *Reg Anaesth* 1987;10:104.

235. Curelaru I. Long-term subarachnoid anaesthesia with continuous epidural block. *Praktische Anaesthesie* 1979;14:71.
236. Brownridge P. Epidural and subarachnoid analgesia for elective Caesarean section. *Anaesthesia* 1980;36:70.
237. Carrie LES, O'Sullivan G. Subarachnoid bupivacaine 0.5% for Caesarean section. *Eur J Anaesthesiol* 1984;1:275.
238. Torrieri A, Aldrete JA. Regional anesthesia technics. *Acta Anaesthiol Belg* 1988;39:65.
239. Eldor J, Chaimsky G. Combined spinal-epidural needle (CSEN). *Can J Anaesth* 1988;35:537.
240. Herbstman CH, Jaffe JB, Tuman LK, Newman LM. An in vivo evaluation of four spinal needles used for the combined spinal-epidural technique. *Anesth Analg* 1998;86:520.
241. Carrie LES. Combined spinal-epidural anesthesia for cesarean section. *Tech Reg Anesth Pain Manage* 1997;1:118.
242. Norris MC, Grieco WM, Borkowski M, et al. Complications of labor analgesia: Epidural versus combined spinal epidural techniques. *Anesth Analg* 1994;79:529.
243. Birnbach DJ, Stein DJ, Hartman JK, Danzier BI, Thys DM. Complications of combined spinal epidural (CSE) analgesia compared with lumbar epidural analgesia. *Anesthesiology* 1996;85:A860(abst).
244. Eldor J, Brodsky V. Danger of metallic particles in the spinal-epidural spaces using the needle-through-needle approach [Letter]. *Acta Anaesthesiol Scand* 1991;35:461.
245. Herman NL, Molin J, Knape KG. No additional metal particle formation using the needle-through-needle combined spinal/epidural technique. *Acta Anaesth Scand* 1996;40:227.
246. Hargreaves J. Metal particle generation caused by the combined spinal-epidural technique [Letter]. *Br J Anaesth* 1993;70:706.
247. Holmström B, Rawal N, Axelsson K, Nydahl P-A. Risk of catheter migration during combined spinal epidural block: percutaneous epiduroscopy study. *Anesth Analg* 1995;80:747.
248. Carrie LES. Epidural versus combined spinal epidural block for caesarean section. *Acta Anaesthesiol Scand* 1988;32:595.
249. Rawal N, Schollin J, Wesström G. Epidural versus combined spinal epidural block for cesarean section. *Acta Anaesthesiol Scand* 1988; 32:61.
250. Blumgart CH, Ryall D, Dennison B, Thompson-Hill LM. Mechanism of extension of spinal anaesthesia by extradural injection of local anaesthetic. *Br J Anaesth* 1992;69:457.
251. Stienstra R, Dahan A, Alhadi BZR, van Kleep JW, Burm AGL. Mechanism of action of an epidural top-up in combined spinal epidural anesthesia. *Anesth Analg* 1996;83:382.
252. Takiguchi T, Okana T, Egawa H, Okubo Y, Saito K, Kitajima T. The effect of epidural saline injection on anesthetic level during combined spinal and epidural anesthesia assessed clinically and myelographically. *Anesth Analg* 1997;85:1097.
253. Trautman WJ 3rd, Liu SS, Kopacz DJ. Comparison of lidocaine and saline for epidural top-up during combined spinal-epidural anesthesia in volunteers. *Anesth Analg* 1997;84:574.
254. Swenson JD, Wisniewski M, McJames S, Ashburn MA, Pace NL. The effect of prior dural puncture on cisternal cerebrospinal fluid morphine concentrations in sheep after administration of lumbar epidural morphine. *Anesth Analg* 1996;83:523.
255. Leighton BL, Arkoosh VA, Huffnagle S, Huffnagle HJ, Kinsella SM, Norris MC. The dermatomal spread of epidural bupivacaine with and without prior intrathecal sufentanil. *Anesth Analg* 1996;83:526.
256. Bernards CM, Kopacz DJ, Michel MZ. Effect of needle puncture on morphine and lidocaine flux through the spinal meninges of the monkey in vitro. Implications for combined spinal-epidural anesthesia. *Anesthesiology* 1994;80:853.
257. Norris MC. Are combined spinal epidural catheters reliable? Society for Obstetric Anesthesia and Perinatology. *Anesthesiology* [Suppl.] 1998:A11.
258. Harding SA, Collis RE, Morgan BM. Meningitis after combined spinal-extradural anaesthesia in obstetrics. *Br J Anaesth* 1994;73:545.
259. Cascio M, Heath G. Meningitis following a combined spinal-epidural technique in a laboring term parturient. *Can J Anaesth* 1996;43:399.
260. Schroter J, Wa Djamba D, Hoffmann V, Bach A, Motsch J. Epidural abscess after combined spinal epidural block. *Can J Anaesth* 1997; 44:300.
261. Schneeberger PM, Janssen M, Voss A. Alpha-hemolytic streptococci: a major pathogen of iatrogenic meningitis following lumbar puncture. Case reports and a review of the literature. *Infection* 1996;24:29.
262. Cousins MJ, Bromage PR. Epidural neural blockade. In: Cousins MJ, Bridenbaugh PO, eds. *Neural blockade in clinical anesthesia and management of pain,* 2nd ed. Philadelphia: JB Lippincott, 1987:323.
263. Bonica JJ, McDonald JS. *Principles and practice of obstetric analgesia and anesthesia,* 2nd ed. Baltimore: Williams & Wilkins, 1995:404.
264. Mulroy MF. *Regional anesthesia: an illustrated procedural guide.* Boston: Little, Brown, 1989.
265. Moore DC. *Regional block: a handbook for use in the clinical practice of medicine and surgery*, 4th ed. Springfield: CC Thomas, 1965:44.
266. Leighton BL. Complications of the combined spinal–epidural technique. *Tech Reg Anesth Pain Manage* 1997;1:137.

Obstetric Anesthesia, second edition,
edited by Mark C. Norris.
Lippincott Williams & Wilkins, Philadelphia © 1999.

CHAPTER 16

Neuraxial Analgesia for Labor

Part II: Intrathecal Drugs

Valerie A. Arkoosh

The ideal labor analgesic should have the following:

- A localized site of action,
- No effects on motor function or the progress of labor,
- A small dose requirement,
- Low maternal–fetal drug exposure,
- Minimal maternal–fetal side effects, and
- Reversibility.

Analgesics administered into the intrathecal space fulfill many of these criteria. The purpose of this chapter is to review the development of intrathecal labor analgesics, discuss current applications of intrathecal opioids and local anesthetics for labor analgesia, and consider the potential use of nonopioid analgesics.

RATIONALE FOR SPINAL ANALGESIA IN OBSTETRICS

The many advantages of the intrathecal approach include:

- Reliable identification of the subarachnoid space,
- Small drug requirement, which greatly decreases the chance of systemic drug toxicity,
- Rapid, bilateral analgesia, and
- Increased efficacy of nonlocal anesthetic agents, minimizing maternal motor blockade.

A continuous spinal technique allows incremental drug injection to a specific endpoint. Currently, opioids and local anesthetics, alone or in various combinations, are the most commonly used intrathecal analgesics in laboring women.

V. A. Arkoosh: Department of Anesthesiology, Allegheny University Hospital for Women, Philadelphia, Pennyslvania 19131.

Intrathecal opioids are particularly attractive for the obstetric anesthesiologist. In parturients, intrathecal opioids produce dose-dependent analgesia without significant changes in autonomic function, voluntary motor function, or response to innocuous stimuli. In gravid rats and rabbits, intrathecal morphine lacks effect on the onset of labor, maternal or fetal respiratory rate, or fetal viability (1). Naloxone antagonizes subarachnoid opioid analgesia in a dose-dependent fashion.

Small doses of intrathecal isobaric local anesthetics provide adequate but brief labor analgesia with little hypotension or motor blockade (2,3). Intrathecal local anesthetics provide excellent analgesia for the second stage of labor and potentiate the action of intrathecal opioids.

Bilateral analgesia develops rapidly after intrathecal injection of a lipid soluble opioid. In laboring parturients at less than 7-cm cervical dilation, intrathecal sufentanil 10 μg provided better analgesia than epidural bupivacaine 30 mg during the first 30 minutes after injection (Fig. 1) (4). This rapid onset also is apparent in patients in advanced labor. In 38 patients with a mean cervical dilation of 6 cm, sufentanil 10 μg plus bupivacaine 2.5 mg produced satisfactory analgesia in less than 5 minutes (5). Twenty-three of the 38 patients delivered without additional analgesics. In a similar study of 32 parturients at 7-cm dilation, patients were comfortable within 5 minutes of receiving sufentanil 10 μg plus bupivacaine 2.5 mg (6). Effective duration was approximately 130 minutes, and 68% of the patients who delivered vaginally required no additional analgesics.

The quality of opioid analgesia is such that parturients can be comfortable yet ambulate and participate fully in the second stage of labor. Even the addition of small amounts of local anesthetic to the intrathecal opioid pro-

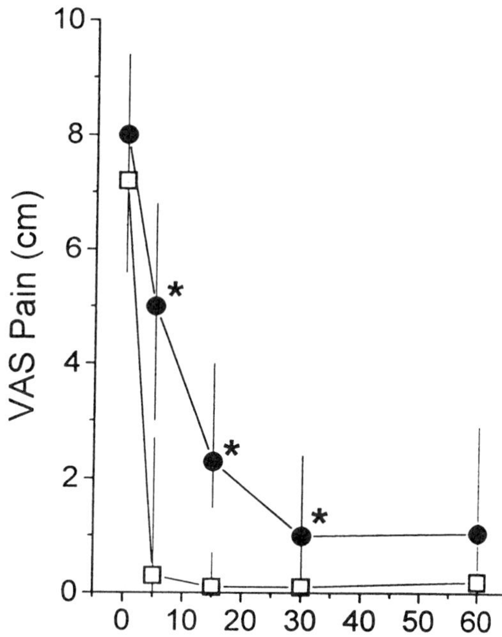

FIG. 1. Maternal pain relief following intrathecal sufentanil 10 μg (□) versus epidural bupivacaine 30 mg (●). (From ref. 4, with permission.)

duces minimal motor impairment. In a series of 300 patients who received intrathecal bupivacaine 2.5 mg plus fentanyl 25 μg as a part of a combined spinal–epidural (CSE) technique, 141 got out of bed to a chair or walked with assistance in the delivery room area (7). Additionally, 43 of 50 patients rated CSE analgesia much better than their previous labor epidural block; none rated it worse. In a subsequent prospective, randomized study, women in the intrathecal (CSE) group reported faster onset of analgesia, and significantly more parturients were satisfied with their analgesia at 20 minutes than those in the epidural bupivacaine group (8). On a postpartum questionnaire, overall satisfaction, feelings of self-control, and report of no leg heaviness during labor were significantly higher in the intrathecal group (8).

Other medications also hold promise for intrathecal labor analgesia. Intrathecal clonidine, an α_2-adrenergic agonist, produces labor analgesia, although accompanied by hypotension, in doses of 100 or 200 μg (9). When combined with sufentanil 2 or 7 μg, clonidine 100 or 200 μg increased the duration of labor analgesia from 2 hours to 2 hours and 40 minutes, and also increased the incidence of hypotension (9). Smaller doses of intrathecal clonidine may be more appropriate. Clonidine 30 μg produced adequate analgesia with a mean duration of 65 ± 27 minutes in 8 of 10 parturients in labor with less than 5-cm cervical dilation (10). Intrathecal clonidine 30 μg and sufentanil 5 μg produced analgesia for 145 ± 43 minutes (10). Analgesia in approximately 50% of these patients was accompanied by a moderate decrease in maternal blood pressure. None required ephedrine or experienced an abnormal fetal heart rate pattern during the episode of hypotension.

Although not yet adequately tested in humans, other medications may eventually be used to enhance intrathecal analgesia produced by opioid or α_2-adrenergic agonists. Intrathecal neostigmine, an acetyl cholinesterase inhibitor, enhances analgesia produced by morphine or clonidine and modulates side effects of coadministered bupivacaine in animals (11,12). Intrathecal magnesium, which does not produce analgesia when injected alone, potentiates morphine-induced analgesia (13).

MECHANISMS OF SPINAL ANALGESIA

Multiple spinal receptor systems are involved in nociceptive processing. These include: opioid, α-adrenergic, serotonergic, cholinergic, γ-aminobutyric, and adenosine receptor agonist systems (14). N-methyl-D-aspartate (NMDA) receptor antagonists inhibit behavior induced by a noxious stimulus. Acetylcholine, calcitonin, neurotensin, serotonin, somatostatin, neuropeptide Y, and ketamine have antinociceptive effects after intrathecal administration in animals (14,15).

Opioids

Identification of opiate receptors in the central nervous system (16) and subsequent localization of these receptors in the substantia gelatinosa of the dorsal horn of the spinal cord (17) stimulated the study of regional analgesia using intraspinal opioids. Several classes of opioid receptors with differing pharmacologic profiles exist. In a chronic spinal dog model, Martin and colleagues (18) originally proposed the μ, k, and σ opioid-receptor classes. Subsequent reports have described ε opioid receptors as well as subclasses of some receptor types (Table 1) (19). Opiate receptors also are located in the brainstem, periventricular gray matter, and thalamus. In humans, epidural opioids produce segmental spinal analgesia (20). Although unproven, intrathecal opioids also presumably act at spinal sites (21). Intrathecal opioids also may produce analgesia by acting at supraspinal sites. Hyperbaric sufentanil, which presumably remains confined to the spinal cord, produces less analgesia than isobaric sufentanil, which may ascend rapidly to the brain (22,23). Rostral spread of intrathecally injected opioid also accounts for many of the nonanalgesic effects of this class of medications.

Stimulation of peripheral nociceptors activates thinly myelinated (A_δ) and unmyelinated (C) afferent nerve fibers. These primary afferents enter the spinal cord in the lateral portion of the dorsal root and bifurcate into both rostral and caudal branches (Fig. 2). They synapse with both second-order neurons in the substantia gelatinosa of the dorsal horn and dendrites of more deeply lying cells. These second-order neurons process and transmit the nociceptive message to supraspinal centers

TABLE 1. *Opioid receptor classification*

Receptor	Analgesia	Naloxone sensitivity	Actions
μ_1	Supraspinal	High	Prolactin release ↓ Acetylcholine turnover Pruritus Induction of catalepsy
μ_2	Spinal and supraspinal	High	Respiratory depression ↓ Dopamine turnover ↓ Gastrointestinal motility
k (may have subtypes)	Spinal, ?supraspinal	Moderate	↓ Antidiuretic hormone release Sedation
d (may have subtypes)	Spinal, ?supraspinal	Low	

Data from ref. 25.

(19). Modulation of the synapse between the primary afferent and the second-order neuron can alter the central passage of painful information. This control can be exercised at several points:

- Inhibition of afferent neurotransmitter release,
- Blockade of the effector mechanism by which the neurotransmitters released from primary afferents act, and
- Alteration of the excitability of the second-order link.

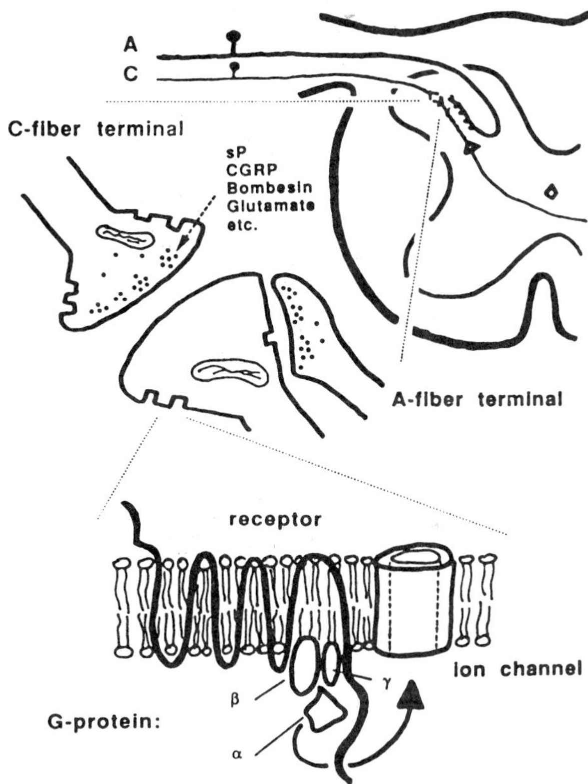

FIG. 2. The synapse of primary afferents in the substantia gelatinosa of the dorsal horn. The C-fiber, but not the A-fiber, terminals have opioid receptors. Opioids also bind postsynaptically on the dendrites of neurons receiving A-fiber and C-fiber excitatory input. Agonist occupation of the presynaptic opioid receptor reduces the release of neurotransmitters from the C-terminal and postsynaptically decreases the excitability of the neuron. At the membrane level, agonist–receptor binding activates the G-protein. The α subunit, which contains the guanine nucleotide binding site, dissociates from the β and γ subunits, increasing potassium permeability. (From ref. 15, with permission.)

Intrathecal opioids appear to act at sites before and after the synapse between the primary afferent and the second-order neuron. A∂ and C fiber stimulation releases substance P, a putative nociceptive neurotransmitter. Presynaptic actions of intrathecal opioids inhibit the release of substance P (24). Intrathecal opioids also hyperpolarize the postsynaptic cell membrane by increasing potassium conductance, thereby decreasing the excitability of the neuron (25). This effect appears mediated by the G-protein that couples the opioid receptor directly to the potassium channel (Fig. 2).

Other mechanisms also may be involved in opioid modulation of nociceptive impulse transmission. Studies have suggested that morphine stimulates the release of adenosine from primary afferent nerves (26,27). Occupation of adenosine receptors produces mild analgesia (28). Additionally, high concentrations of morphine, fentanyl, meperidine, and sufentanil produce a weak local anesthetic effect on isolated nerves (29,30). Recorded A and C fiber action potential amplitude decreases following opioid administration.

α_2-Adrenergic Agonists

α_2-Adrenergic receptors are located on primary afferent terminals at both peripheral and spinal nerve endings, on neurons in the superficial laminae of the spinal cord, and within several brainstem nuclei (9). Most experimental work in humans supports a primarily spinal site of action for these drugs. α_2-Adrenergic agonists, in part, produce analgesia by spinal cholinergic activation (31,32). Descending noradrenergic pathways release norepinephrine, which produces analgesia directly and stimulates acetylcholine release, also causing analgesia. Epidural clonidine increases acetylcholine concentrations in lumbar cerebrospinal fluid (CSF) (33,34). Additionally, in volunteers, epidural clonidine analgesia is increased in an additive fashion by intrathecal neostigmine injection (35).

In summary, intrathecally administered medications suppress the processing of nociceptive stimuli via several mechanisms culminating in depressed neuronal excitability and decreased secretion of nociceptive transmitters (24). Through these mechanisms, intrathecal analgesics alter rostral transmission of nociceptive information and ultimately a patient's perception of pain.

Local Anesthetics

The physiologic effects of local anesthetics are well known to most practitioners. Besides inhibiting pain pathways, local anesthetics also block sympathetic, sensory, and motor nerve conduction. Effects at these sites produce hypotension, urinary retention, and sensory and motor blockade. The intensity and extent of these effects depend upon the amount and concentration of local anesthetic injected. Small intrathecal doses of dilute local anesthetic solutions block mainly the small A_∂ and C fibers, resulting in decreased pain perception but little motor blockade or hypotension.

PHARMACOKINETICS

Once injected into the subarachnoid space, analgesic drugs undergo redistribution via three mechanisms: diffusion, vascular transport, and bulk flow within the CSF (19,36). Initially, drug moves by diffusion into the spinal cord, nerve roots, perineural fat, and across the dura into the epidural space. The drug is absorbed from these areas into the systemic vasculature. Drugs also undergo rostral–caudal movement within the CSF. The predominant mechanism of redistribution for each drug depends upon the lipid solubility, ionization, and molecular weight of the drug.

Lipid Solubility

Lipid solubility is the most important characteristic of a drug. It effects uptake, clearance, and likelihood of rostral spread of both opioids and local anesthetics. Increasing opioid lipid solubility permits rapid uptake into the spinal cord, resulting in a faster analgesic onset. A somewhat lipid-insoluble drug, such as morphine, has an analgesic latency ranging from 15 to 60 minutes. The more lipid soluble opioids, such as fentanyl or sufentanil, begin to produce analgesia within 5 to 10 minutes. High lipid solubility also results in rapid redistribution within the CSF. In dogs, sufentanil is detectable in the cisterna magna 1 minute after a 50-μg epidural injection (37). Cisternal sufentanil concentrations peak 21 minutes after epidural injection and are greater than plasma concentrations at all times (37). Clearance through systemic vascular absorption also is rapid, reducing the duration of a lipid-soluble drug.

With systemic administration of opioids, potency correlates directly with lipid solubility. More lipid soluble drugs (i.e., sufentanil) are more potent than a hydrophilic drug such as morphine. For drugs given intrathecally, however, lipid solubility relates inversely to opioid potency. McQuay et al. (38) showed that, when given intrathecally, two poorly lipid-soluble opioids, morphine and normorphine, are more potent than two highly soluble opioids, meperidine and methadone. They hypothesize that significant nonspecific tissue binding of highly lipid-soluble opioids within the spinal cord limits the amount of drug available for binding at specific opioid receptors.

Clinically, this concept is important when determining equianalgesic intrathecal opioid doses. Clinicians or investigators may use systemic opioid potency ratios to estimate equipotent intrathecal opioid doses. However, the ability of a drug to cross the blood–brain barrier and gain access to opioid receptors influences its systemic potency. Because spinally injected drugs avoid the blood–brain barrier, the intrathecal potency ratio of two drugs may not correlate with the systemic potency ratio. Indeed, high lipid solubility, which implies high systemic potency, results in a less potent intrathecal drug. For instance, sufentanil (octanol:water partition coefficient 1,757) is 12 to 15 times more potent than fentanyl (octanol:water partition coefficient 816) intravenously (39). Intrathecally, however, sufentanil is only five to seven times more potent than fentanyl (40,41,41a).

Ionization and Molecular Weight

In their nonionized form, opioids and local anesthetics cross membranes and interact with specific receptors (19,36). Commonly used opioids and local anesthetics have a pK_a of 7.5 or greater. Therefore, these drugs will exist mainly in the ionized form within the CSF.

Movement of molecules across the dura and into tissues is inversely related to the molecular weight and molecular configuration. Opioids and local anesthetics used for labor analgesia have similar molecular weights but different molecular configurations. Both types of drugs readily cross dural and tissue membranes.

NONANALGESIC PHYSIOLOGIC EFFECTS OF INTRATHECAL OPIOIDS

Besides analgesia, stimulation of intrathecal opioid receptors also can affect bladder, motor, gastrointestinal, and respiratory function and cause pruritus. Most side effects are brief in duration and easily treated (Table 2). Animal studies and clinical reports provide evidence for a receptor-specific suppression of the micturition reflex that involves both bladder contractility and sphincter tone (42,43). High doses of μ-receptor agonists can induce skeletal muscle rigidity due to a receptor-specific interaction in brainstem centers (44). In the presence of spinal spasticity, low doses of intrathecal morphine can reduce motor tone (45). Painless muscular spasm of the lower

TABLE 2. *Side effects of intrathecal opioids and their treatment*

Problem	Treatment	Comment
Pruritus	Nalbuphine 5–10 mg i.v., naloxone 40 μg i.v., propofol 10 mg i.v., diphenhydramine 25 mg i.v.	Pruritus is usually self-limited, but may be severe with morphine
Nausea and vomiting	Metoclopramide 5–10 mg i.v., nalbuphine 5–10 mg i.v., naloxone 40 μg i.v., propofol 10 mg i.v. (111)	Nausea is most frequent after meperidine, usually self-limited
Urinary retention	Catheterization prn	Resolves as analgesia diminishes
Hypotension	Intravenous fluids, ephedrine 5–10 mg i.v.	Significant hypotension is rare, most likely with meperidine or when opioids are used in combination with intrathecal local anesthetics
Respiratory depression	Naloxone 100 μg i.v., may need to repeat	
Postpartum prophylaxis	Naltrexone 25 mg p.o.	Consider after morphine

limbs, lasting 3 to 7 minutes, has been reported following the intrathecal injection of sufentanil 10 μg with epinephrine 200 μg in laboring parturients (46).

The mechanism for nausea and vomiting is most likely related to an action on the chemoemetic trigger zone in the dorsal medulla (47). Nausea is fairly rare with the lipid-soluble opioids [except meperidine (3)], but is seen more frequently and often postpartum with morphine (48–50). If morphine is avoided, side effects are generally mild and easily treated. If using morphine for labor analgesia, consider giving postpartum naltrexone, 25 mg by mouth, to parturients who deliver within 12 hours of intrathecal morphine injection (50).

Respiratory Depression

Potential respiratory effects of spinally administered opioids include a decrease in minute ventilation due to decreased rate and tidal volume, a rightward shift of the CO_2 response curve, and a decreased response to hypoxia (51,52). Respiratory depression is likely due to action at the chemosensitive anterolateral surface of the medulla (52). Respiratory depression can occur with either the lipid-soluble or lipid-insoluble opioids. The time course, however, is very different.

Following intrathecal injection of a lipid-soluble opioid, rapid redistribution of drug within the CSF produces early respiratory effects. Respiratory depression, responsive to stimulation and oxygen, has been reported in a laboring parturient 10 minutes after intrathecal sufentanil 15 μg (53). Respiratory arrest occurred 20 minutes after a second dose (4 hours apart) of sufentanil 12.5 μg (54). This patient responded promptly to naloxone. Respiratory arrest also occurred within 5 minutes of intrathecal sufentanil 10 μg in a parturient who had received intravenous meperidine 2 hours earlier (55). Finally, respiratory arrest, responsive to naloxone, occurred in a parturient 10 to 15 minutes after intrathecal injection of sufentanil 10 μg with bupivacaine 2.5 mg (56). In one series, the risk of respiratory arrest after intrathecal sufentanil 10 μg was estimated to be 1 in 5,000 (55). Sufentanil undergoes very rapid redistribution within the CSF (37). In parturients, presumed cephalad spread of sufentanil or fentanyl has been associated with clinical complaints of dysphagia or facial tingling (57,58). Although respiratory arrest is a rare occurrence, patients should be watched closely for at least 30 minutes after injection of a lipid-soluble opioid.

Delayed respiratory effects are seen following the injection of a lipid-insoluble opioid such as morphine. In this case, rostral spread of drug is slow, and effects may not be seen until 6 to 9 hours after injection (59).

Pruritus

Pruritus is the most common side effect seen in parturients following intrathecal injection of opioids. It is experienced, in varying degrees of severity, in 50% to 90% of patients (48,60). When using a lipid-soluble opioid alone, the pruritus is usually mild and transient. Intrathecal morphine, when used for labor analgesia, has been associated with more severe pruritus, which can persist postpartum (48–50). Although practitioners have reported the successful use of antihistamines to treat intrathecal opioid-induced pruritus, histamine release is not the mechanism of this side effect. Rather, facial pruritus results from a direct opioid receptor effect in the medulla (61,62). Pruritus in other locations is often segmental in distribution and related to the level of opioid injection, implying spinal cord involvement (62). Morphine excites nonnociceptive neurons in the anterior and posterior horns of the spinal cord and may be stimulating pruritus through these pathways (62,63). Therefore, opioid-induced pruritus is best treated with a small dose of an opioid receptor antagonist (Table 2). Of interest, intravenous propofol, 10 to 20 mg, has been reported to relieve pruritus associated with epidural or intrathecal morphine injection in surgical patients (64,65), but not pruritus following intrathecal morphine injection in cesarean delivery patients (66). Propofol may exert its effect by direct suppression of the nonnociceptive spinal neuron systems implicated in the production of pruritus (64).

Do Intrathecal Opioids Cause Hypotension?

Whether or not intrathecal opioids cause maternal hypotension is an area of some controversy. The incidence of a greater than 20% decrease in systolic blood pressure after intrathecal opioid injection in laboring women has been reported to range from 0% (3) to 14% (60). Yet, intrathecal fentanyl does not affect maternal blood pressure, heart rate, or ejection fraction in prehydrated (1.2-L Ringer's lactate), nonlaboring term parturients (67). The degree of hypotension reported in various studies may be a function of the baseline blood pressure used. In a prospective study of 100 nonprehydrated parturients receiving intrathecal sufentanil ± nalbuphine, no patient had a greater than 20% fall in blood pressure if a *prenatal* blood pressure was used as baseline (68). Intrathecal fentanyl caused no change in stoke index, end-diastolic index, or ejection fraction in laboring parturients who had received a 500-mL fluid bolus (69). However, these patients did have a decrease in mean arterial pressure, heart rate, and cardiac index. These authors concluded that the decrease in blood pressure was due to the analgesic effect of intrathecal fentanyl rather than a decrease in preload due to sympathetic blockade.

Two recent studies support the view that any blood pressure fall associated with intrathecal opioid labor analgesia is not sympathetically mediated. The extent of sensory changes in parturients who received intrathecal sufentanil 10 μg does not correlate with changes in systolic blood pressure (70). Also, central temperature and calf-to-toe temperature gradients do not change after intrathecal sufentanil 10 μg. This result indicates that sympathetically induced vasodilatation does not occur after intrathecal opioid injection (71). Finally, intrathecal fentanyl labor analgesia produces a significant decrease in maternal plasma epinephrine concentrations within 5 minutes of injection, coincident with the onset of analgesia (72). In sum, parturients may experience a fall in blood pressure when comparing the postprocedure to the preprocedure pressure and should be monitored appropriately. This decrease is likely due to analgesia, not sympathetic blockade.

Significant hypotension, however, can develop in women who receive combined opioid/local anesthetic injections. D'Angelo and Eisenach (73) reported one such patient who experienced a fall in blood pressure from 135/80 to 68/33 mm Hg during the 12 minutes following intrathecal injection of sufentanil 7.5 μg with bupivacaine 2.5 mg. The patient responded to ephedrine, 60 mg total dose, fluids, and oxygen.

Fetal and Neonatal Effects

Transient fetal heart rate changes following both intrathecal fentanyl and sufentanil have been reported with an incidence of 10% to 15% (7,60). Recently, five episodes of fetal bradycardia associated with uterine hyperactivity have been reported following intrathecal fentanyl 50 μg (74). Resolution of the bradycardia followed terbutaline administration in some of the patients. Although bradycardia has been reported following intrathecal opioids, it also occurs with epidural local anesthetic injection. In a prospective study of 281 parturients receiving either CSE or epidural analgesia (patient choice) and randomly allocated to labor in either the full lateral position or with 30-degree left uterine displacement, there was no difference in the incidence of subsequent fetal bradycardia (3.9% vs 3.8%) (74a). A similar study comparing intrathecal sufentanil 10 μg with epidural bupivacaine found an equivalent incidence of clinically significant fetal heart tracing abnormalities between the two groups within the first hour of administration (75). In a retrospective comparison between patients who received intrathecal opioids and patients who received only systemic opioids or no medication, the incidence of emergency cesarean delivery was 1.3% vs 1.4%, respectively (76). Emergency cesarean section for nonreassuring fetal heart tracings within 90 minutes of intrathecal sufentanil injection only occurred in association with obstetric factors such as a nuchal cord.

As intravenous opioid administration is rarely associated with fetal bradycardia, it is unlikely that fetal bradycardia following intrathecal opioid injection is due to a specific drug effect. Most likely, bradycardia following either intrathecal or epidural drug administration is related to the onset of analgesia. The intensity of uterine contractions depends upon the balance between forces that encourage contraction (i.e., oxytocin) and forces that inhibit contraction (i.e., β-adrenergic agonists, catecholamines). One can postulate that the rapid fall in plasma catecholamines (72) associated with the onset of analgesia might transiently upset this balance in favor of uterine contractile forces, resulting in uterine hyperactivity and potentially decreased blood flow to the fetus. As expected and as is seen clinically, the balance is usually quickly restored either through iatrogenic interventions (i.e., turning off oxytocin, giving terbutaline) or through maternal physiologic mechanisms. It is rare that these episodes of bradycardia last more than 3 to 5 minutes or require operative intervention.

Neonatal welfare appears unaffected and placental transfer minimal following a single dose of intrathecal fentanyl and subsequent epidural bupivacaine fentanyl infusion (77). Maternal–fetal sufentanil transfer is lessened by increased maternal protein binding and enhanced by fetal acidosis (78). The placenta also may accumulate sufentanil (79), thus buffering the fetus when maternal concentration is high or serving as a reservoir when maternal concentration falls.

Obstetric Outcome

Compared with epidural analgesia, intrathecal sufentanil labor analgesia combined with subsequent epidural analgesia lacks effect on the use of cesarean delivery for dystocia (80). In this study of nulliparous women in spontaneous labor, the group that received combined CSE analgesia had significantly higher rates of spontaneous vaginal delivery and lower rates of instrumental vaginal delivery. In addition, those women in the CSE group who required cesarean delivery for dystocia had a greater degree of cervical dilation when the operation was performed. Currently, there are no studies comparing intrathecal opioids alone, or as part of a CSE technique, to systemic or no analgesia.

PATIENT SELECTION

Patients who are candidates for neuraxial labor analgesia are candidates for intrathecal opioid administration. Additionally, intrathecal opioids have proven effective in a subset of patients who, due to coexisting disease, might not tolerate the hemodynamic changes induced by lumbar epidural local anesthetic blockade. This list includes patients with severe pulmonary hypertension (81), severe pulmonary stenosis (82), Wolff-Parkinson-White syndrome (83), and a single ventricle (84). Likewise, a patient with allergy to local anesthetics obtained adequate analgesia with continuous intrathecal meperidine administration (85).

I consider most patients as candidates for intrathecal opioids. In particular, patients in early labor (less than 3 to 4 cm), those whose fetus is high in the pelvis, those who say they do not like "feeling numb," or patients who wish to deliver their baby with minimal analgesic intervention, are offered this technique. Patients who are in the advanced stages of labor and requesting analgesia also benefit from this technique. These patients achieve excellent analgesia quickly, with minimal motor blockade and often deliver without any additional analgesia (5,6). Additionally, this technique is offered to any parturient whose medical condition is such that it would be difficult for her to tolerate a sympathetic blockade.

The CSE technique should be used with caution in parturients at high risk for cesarean delivery, as the technique does not guarantee a working epidural (86). In these patients, either the catheter should be tested soon after insertion or epidural analgesia administered.[1] Intrathecal opioids may prove ineffective in patients known to abuse narcotics. In addition, acute withdrawal could be precipitated by naloxone administration should a serious side effect, such as respiratory depression, occur in these women. Contraindications to this technique include patient refusal, infection at the puncture site, and significant coagulation defects.

CHOICE OF AGENT

Available data support the use of several opioids (morphine, fentanyl, sufentanil, and meperidine) for intrathecal labor analgesia (Table 3). The addition of local anesthetics can enhance intrathecal opioid labor analgesia. This section will review the published data as well as our experience with both opioids and local anesthetics.

Opioids

In 1980, Scott et al. (87) first described the use of intrathecal morphine 1.5 mg in 12 parturients. This dose abolished pain in the first stage of labor in all patients. Second stage pain was relieved in four patients and lessened in three. Scott et al. noted no change in hemodynamic or respiratory parameters and no evidence of motor weakness. All women experienced facial itching. Nine parturients felt nauseated; five vomited. Four subjects required catheterization for urinary retention. All infants did well.

Baraka and colleagues (88) administered either 1 or 2 mg of intrathecal morphine to 20 primiparous patients in active labor. All reported relief within 15 to 60 minutes. Time from intrathecal injection to delivery ranged from 2.0 to 10.5 hours in the 1-mg group and 3.0 to 14.5 hours in the 2-mg group. All parturients, except three in the 2-mg group, were pain-free until delivery. The three women experiencing pain did so after 8 hours. Patients in the 2-mg group required more use of oxytocin. At delivery, all parturients received supplemental analgesia via either local infiltration, pudendal block, or epidural block. Equally high percentages of patients in each group experienced itching, nausea, vomiting, and somnolence. All fetuses exhibited normal neurobehavioral responses when tested during the first 24 hours postpartum.

Mok and Tsai (89) described seven parturients who obtained 75% to 90% labor pain relief lasting 20 to 36 hours after intrathecal morphine 2 mg in 4 mL of 0.9% saline solution. These authors, however, chose not to pursue this technique due to the high incidence of pruritus (73%), vomiting (66%), somnolence (60%), and urinary retention (40%).

Although pleased with the analgesic effects of intrathecal morphine, most investigators are unhappy with the high incidence of side effects. To lessen the side effects, Abboud et al. (90) studied smaller doses of morphine. Intrathecal morphine 0.5 or 1.0 mg in hyperbaric solution produced analgesia beginning 15 to 60 minutes after injection. Maximum pain relief developed by 90 to 120 minutes after injection (90). Analgesia lasted 6 to 8 hours.

[1]Editor's note: A recent report systematically evaluated catheters placed as part of an epidural or CSE technique in laboring women. If CSF was seen in the spinal needle when using the needle-through-needle technique and the epidural catheter was not intravascular, 99% of multiorifice catheters (934 of 945) were in the epidural space and produced bilateral sensory change and analgesia. In this study, 97% (531 of 545) of catheters placed after locating only the epidural space also provided good analgesia. However, only 95% of catheters placed using either technique provided adequate anesthesia for cesarean section. (Norris MC. Are CSE catheters reliable? Abstracts of Scientific Papers. *Society for Obstetric Anesthesia and Perinatology*, 1998.)

TABLE 3. *Suggestions for single injection intrathecal labor analgesia*[a]

Medication	Dose	Duration	When	Comment
Sufentanil	5–10 μg	105–115 min	Early labor Active labor add LA	
Fentanyl	25–35 μg	85–95 min	Early labor Active labor add LA	
Meperidine	10–15 mg	100–110 min	Throughout labor	More nausea and vomiting Good if LA allergy
Bupivacaine	2.5 mg	60 min	Add to sufentanil or fentanyl	More hypotension
Morphine	0.2–0.3 mg	Prolongs opioid ± LA	Early labor	Consider naltrexone postpartum
Epinephrine	100–200 μg	Prolongs opioid + LA	Active labor with opioid and LA	Does not prolong opioid alone

[a]All medications must be preservative-free and diluted with preservative-free saline.
LA, local anesthetic.

Overall, mild-to-moderate pruritus occurred in 80% of patients, nausea or vomiting in 53%, drowsiness or dizziness in 43% and urinary retention in 43%. The two doses produced analgesia of similar duration. The lower, 0.5-mg dose caused less pruritus.

Morphine–phenylpiperidine Combinations

Besides the high incidence of side effects produced by intrathecal morphine, this drug has a long analgesic latency. Many parturients are not comfortable for up to 1 hour after intrathecal administration. To bridge the latency gap, a more lipid-soluble opioid can be given in combination with morphine. In a study of 15 healthy parturients, Leighton et al. (50) gave intrathecal fentanyl 25 μg with morphine 0.25 mg in 2-mL normal saline. All patients had significant pain relief within 5 minutes of drug injection (Fig. 3). Nine patients delivered vaginally with supplemental pudendal block anesthesia mean of approximately 200 minutes after intrathecal injection. Six patients had lumbar epidural analgesia induced 140 ± 51 minutes after opioid injection. Moderate-to-severe postpartum itching and vomiting occurred in seven of eight patients given either no prophylactic opioid antagonists or oral naltrexone 12.5 mg after delivery. Three of five patients given a continuous infusion of naloxone 0.2 mg per hour had mild postpartum itching or nausea. Two patients given oral naltrexone 25 mg had no postpartum side effects.

A subsequent study compared sufentanil 10 μg or fentanyl 25 μg as adjuncts to intrathecal morphine 0.25 mg (91). These parturients underwent simultaneous epidural catheter placement. At patient request, we injected local anesthetic through the epidural catheter. Mean time to epidural local anesthetic injection in the sufentanil group was 162 versus 130 minutes in the fentanyl group (not significant, Fig. 4). Thus, there is little clinical difference between these two drug combinations.

A comparison between epidural analgesia and intrathecal fentanyl and morphine analgesia found the incidence of pruritus and nausea and vomiting to be significantly higher in the intrathecal opioid group. These authors found little to recommend the technique (48).

In summary, intrathecal morphine labor analgesia is accompanied by a high incidence of side effects, which often persist postpartum. Decreasing the dose of morphine shortens the duration of analgesia but does not limit the frequency or severity of side effects. Intrathecal morphine will, however, prolong the duration of the lipid-soluble opioids slightly (49). In my practice, I reserve the use of intrathecal morphine labor analgesia for patients in whom I am planning multiple intrathecal injections (i.e., a patient with Harrington rods). In this case, I give morphine 0.25 to 0.3 mg in the first injection. If the patient delivers within 12 hours of this injection, I prescribe naltrexone 25 mg by mouth after delivery.

Sufentanil

Intrathecal sufentanil alone or in combination with bupivacaine or epinephrine is typically used in doses of 5 to 10 μg (6,49,91–96). The dose of intrathecal sufentanil that provided adequate labor analgesia (pain score = 25)

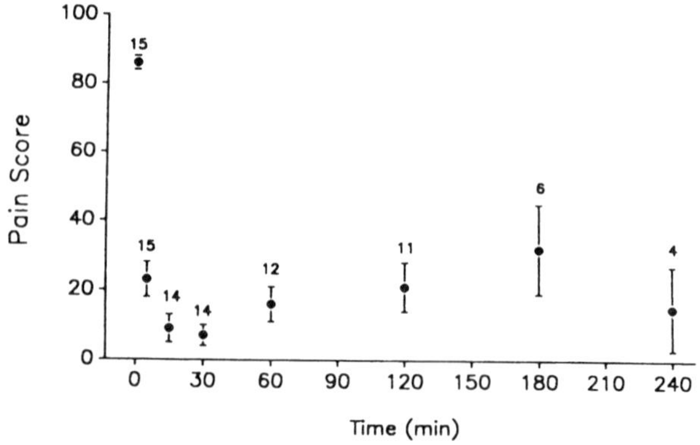

FIG. 3. Mean ± SEM pain scores after intrathecal injection of fentanyl 25 μg and morphine 0.25 mg. The number of patients still laboring with intrathecal opioid analgesia appears above each value. (From ref. 50, with permission.)

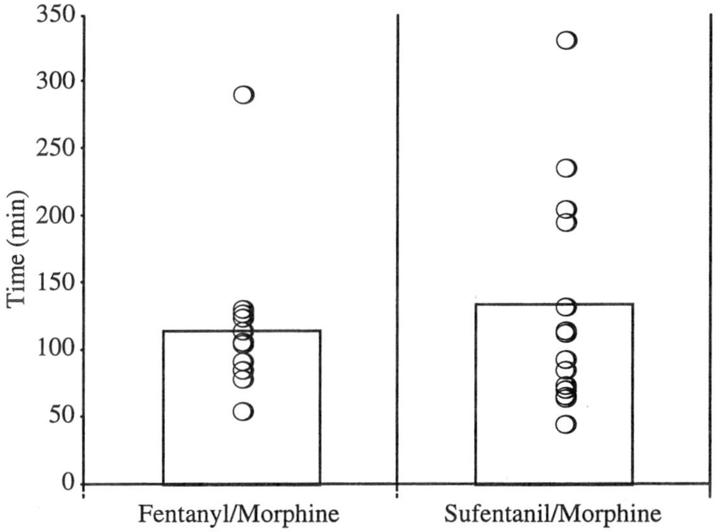

FIG. 4. Mean time (minutes) ± SEM from intrathecal opioid injection to epidural injection of local anesthetic. Each circle represents one patient. Fentanyl/morphine = fentanyl 25 μg + morphine 0.25 mg. Sufentanil/morphine = sufentanil 10 μg + morphine 0.25 mg. (From ref. 91, with permission.)

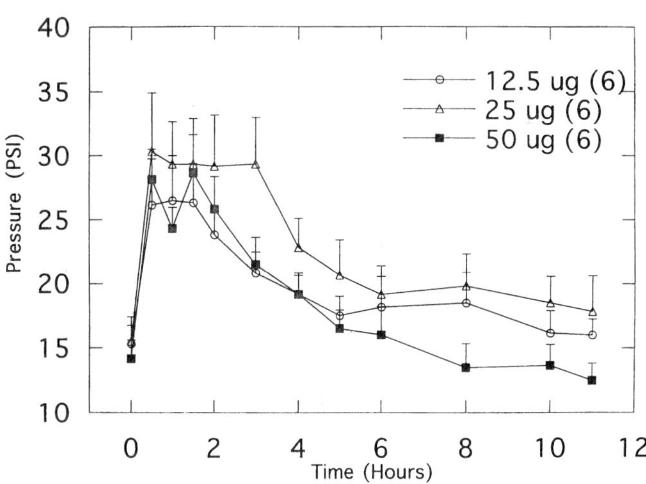

FIG. 5. Algometer pressure (psi) needed to produce a visual analog pain score of 5 vs time (hours) after intrathecal sufentanil (ITS) injection in nonpregnant female volunteers. Numbers in parentheses are the number of subjects included in the figure. Values are mean ± SEM. Multivariate analysis of variance indicated statistically significant changes for all groups for 6 hours. There was no statistically significant dose-dependent effect of ITS on pressure algometry. (From ref. 97, with permission.)

in 50% (ED_{50}) and 95% (ED_{95}) of healthy parturients at 6-cm cervical dilation was 2.6 μg (1.8 to 3.2 μg, 95% confidence interval) and 8.9 μg (7.5 to 11.5 μg, 95% confidence interval), respectively (40). In a similar study, the dose of intrathecal sufentanil that produced acceptable pain relief in 50% of nulliparous patients (ED_{50}) in spontaneous labor at less than 5-cm cervical dilation was 1.8 μg (0.54 to 2.96 μg, 95% confidence limits) (41a). Although doses as high as 15 μg of intrathecal sufentanil have been reported in clinical use, the dose–response curve in female volunteers flattens after 12.5 μg (Fig. 5) (97). Higher doses fail to produce proportionate increases in the duration or intensity of analgesia.

Fentanyl

Intrathecal fentanyl alone or in combination with local anesthetic is typically used in doses ranging from 25 to 50 μg (50,74). A dose of 25 μg produced maximum analgesia in nulliparous patients in active labor. Doses of 35 or 45 μg did not produce any more profound or prolonged analgesia (41).

Meperidine

Meperidine, 10 to 20 mg, provides adequate labor analgesia (3). Because meperidine has local anesthetic effects, it is more effective as a sole agent in later stages of labor (3). Unfortunately, this analgesia is accompanied by a relatively high incidence of vomiting. Because of this bothersome side effect, I rarely use meperidine in my practice. It remains, however, an excellent choice for a parturient with documented local anesthetic allergy (85).

Local Anesthetics

Bupivacaine

Intrathecal bupivacaine 2.5 to 5 mg produces labor analgesia with little motor blockade for approximately 1 hour (2,3). A continuous intrathecal infusion of bupivacaine 0.125% has been used with some success (98). Four of 20 women experienced persistent perineal pain, which was relieved by injection of hyperbaric bupivacaine. Unfortunately, this intervention resulted in profound motor blockade. Given the utility of the bupivacaine opioid combinations, there is little reason to use this drug as the sole analgesic.

VOLUME OF DILUENT

Sufentanil 10 μg has been studied in diluent volumes ranging from 1 to 10 mL (70,99). Despite the volume difference, there are no clinically measurable differences in the resulting hemodynamic, respiratory, pain, nausea, pruritus, motor blockade, or sensory change outcomes. In my practice, I dilute the injectate to 2 mL.[2]

PROLONGING DURATION

The combination of sufentanil 10 μg plus bupivacaine 2.5 mg has a mean duration of 148 ± 27 minutes compared with 114 ± 26 minutes and 70 ± 34 minutes for

[2]Editor's note: I usually inject undiluted sufentanil 0.2 mL.

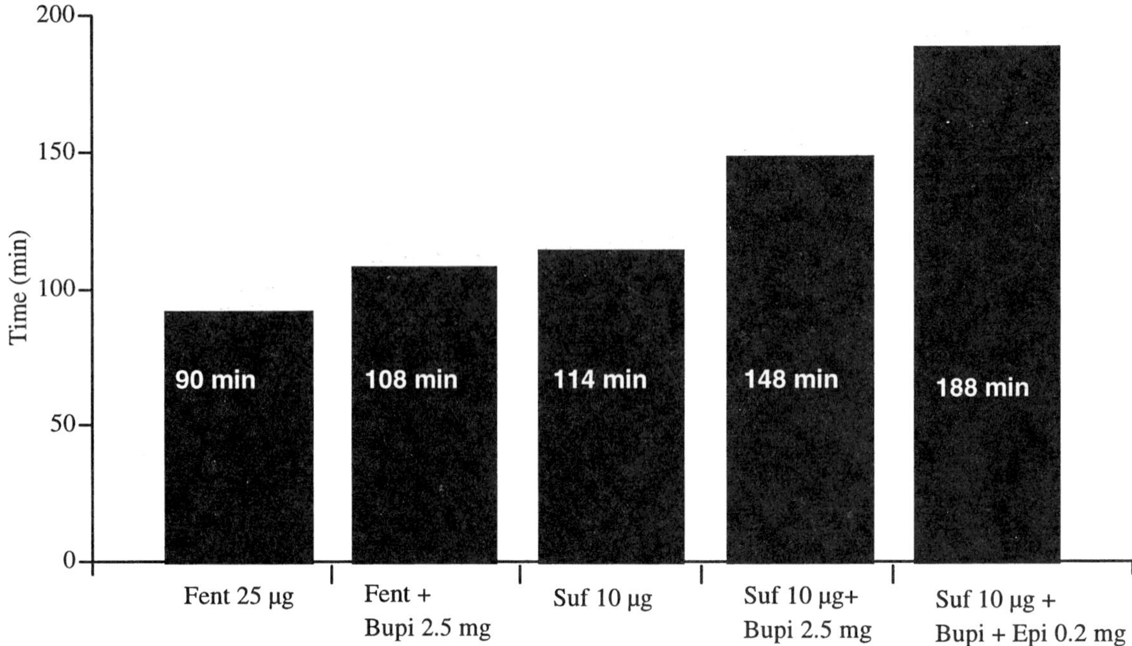

FIG. 6. Duration of various combinations of drugs used for intrathecal labor analgesia versus time. (Compiled from refs. 41,93,94,112.)

sufentanil and bupivacaine alone (93). Patients who receive a single, small dose of bupivacaine do not have significant motor weakness. Adding epinephrine 200 µg has little to no effect on the duration of sufentanil 10 µg (49,92). However, the triple combination of bupivacaine 2.5 mg, sufentanil 10 µg, and epinephrine 200 µg produces analgesia lasting 188 ± 25 minutes in nulliparous patients at less than or equal to 5-cm cervical dilation (Fig. 6) (94).

CONTINUOUS SPINAL ANALGESIA

The development of 28-gauge catheters that can pass through a 22-gauge needle produced a resurgence of interest in continuous spinal analgesia for labor. A continuous technique overcomes many of the limitations of single injections. It allows repeated opioid injection during labor and offers the option of using local anesthetics for vaginal or cesarean delivery. Other potential advantages of continuous spinal analgesia include:

- Dependable catheter placement,
- The ability to provide analgesia and anesthesia rapidly,
- Minimal drug requirement, and
- Symmetric, bilateral sensory blockade.

The unfortunate reports of cauda equina syndrome that followed the widespread introduction of small-gauge spinal catheters (100) led the Food and Drug Administration to mandate their removal from the market (101).

Spinal catheters may predispose to maldistribution of local anesthetic, exposing nerve roots to toxic concentrations of drug. Local anesthetic injected through larger-gauge spinal needles disperses widely throughout the CSF. In contrast, drug injected through small-bore spinal catheters pools near the site of injection or flows with gravity. Should a spinal catheter be directed caudally, high concentrations of drug may arise in the region of the cauda equina (102). Hyperbaric drug appears more likely than isobaric local anesthetics to pool in dependent regions of the spinal cord and damage nerve roots. This risk may not be limited to continuous spinal anesthesia. Hyperbaric 5% lidocaine, in particular, is neurotoxic in some laboratory preparations (103–105). Uncomplicated, single injection spinal anesthesia with hyperbaric 5% lidocaine can produce transient signs of neurological toxicity (106).

Currently, the safety and efficacy of continuous spinal labor analgesia with a 28-gauge catheter are under study by the Food and Drug Administration. If accidental dural puncture occurs, I will frequently insert the epidural catheter into the intrathecal space, rather than make a repeat attempt to locate the epidural space. In this setting, either intermittent injection or continuous infusion of opioids provides good labor analgesia. Table 4 shows a recommended dosing regimen. Intrathecal sufentanil usually provides good pain relief until late in the active or second stage of labor. At this point, I administer isobaric (0.25%) bupivacaine in 1-mL doses. Limit the total dose of bupivacaine injected to 5 to 7.5 mg. If blockade

TABLE 4. *Suggestions for managing a spinal catheter with sufentanil*

Preparation
1. Administer an intravenous fluid bolus of 250–500 mL
2. Dilute sufentanil with preservative-free saline to:
   5 μg/mL for bolus
   1 μg/mL for infusion

Induction
1. Insert intrathecal catheter 3–4 cm (further insertion may risk direct nerve trauma)
2. Inject sufentanil 5 μg (with 20-gauge catheter, flush with 1-mL saline)
3. Position patient with left uterine displacement and monitor blood pressure every 2–3 minutes for 15 min
4. Treat inadequate analgesia with bupivacaine (0.25%) 2.5 mg, may repeat ×1
5. If no analgesia, consider malpositioned catheter and remove
6. Begin sufentanil infusion at 5 μg/h
7. For breakthrough pain, administer bupivacaine 2.5 mg, may repeat ×1 and
   Consider increasing sufentanil infusion to 6–7 μg/h (higher than this risks maternal sedation)
   For repeated episodes of breakthrough pain, add bupivacaine to infusion to run at 1–2 mg/h

Cesarean section
1. Prehydrate as needed
2. Administer bupivacaine (0.5%) in 5-mg doses to achieve T_4 level
3. May give preservative-free morphine as per usual practice

Do not use lidocaine of any concentration or baricity through an intrathecal catheter. Use hyperbaric bupivacaine only if necessary (this will be rare). Titrate in 3.75-mg doses.

does not spread as expected, suspect a malpositioned catheter. Try to reposition the patient or catheter to encourage wider spread of drug. If these maneuvers fail, remove the spinal catheter and switch to an alternative anesthetic technique.

CLINICAL ISSUES

Intrathecal Labor Analgesia and the Epidural Test Dose

Injection of an intrathecal opioid ± local anesthetic results in sensory changes in many parturients. These sensory changes may interfere with the ability to subsequently detect intrathecal location of an epidural catheter. Corba et al. (107) administered an epidural test dose of either bupivacaine 7.5 mg or lidocaine 60 mg with epinephrine 15 μg, 20 minutes after intrathecal injection of either sufentanil 10 μg or sufentanil 10 μg with bupivacaine 2.5 mg (107). The extent of sensory blockade increased in most patients after the test dose. No patient experienced a change in heart rate or blood pressure, and 98% had no change in motor blockade. All catheters functioned as if located in the epidural space. These authors concluded that sensory changes alone are unreliable to rule out intrathecal location of an epidural catheter. Clinicians must also check for hemodynamic and motor function changes when testing an epidural catheter 20 minutes after intrathecal labor analgesia.

Baricity of Injectate and Maternal Position

In the absence of dextrose, all commonly used intrathecal opioid and local anesthetic solutions are hypobaric relative to CSF (Table 5) (108). Thus, maternal posture can influence spread of sensory block. When parturients were randomly allocated to the sitting or lateral position during intrathecal injection of fentanyl 25 μg with bupivacaine 2.5 mg, those in the sitting position had significantly higher maximal cephalad extent of sensory block: T_3 versus T_6 (109). When asymmetry was observed in the lateral group, the greater spread occurred on the side that was nondependent during injection. Despite differences in sensory analgesia, time to request for additional analgesia did not differ between the groups.

In an attempt to decrease intrathecal opioid side effects, most of which are due to cephalad spread of drug, investigators have provided labor analgesia with hyperbaric sufentanil (22,23). Although pruritus is lessened, so is the duration and quality of analgesia (Figs. 7 and 8).

TABLE 5. *Densities of dextrose-free intrathecal medications*

Anesthetic solution	Density at 37°C (g/mL)
Bupivacaine 0.25%	0.99912 ± 0.00002
Bupivacaine 0.5%	0.99937 ± 0.00001
Fentanyl 50 μg/mL	0.99333 ± 0.00002
Sufentanil 50 μg/mL	0.99332 ± 0.00001
Morphine 1 mg/mL (Astramorph, Astra)	0.99983 ± 0.00002
Sodium chloride 0.9%	0.99951 ± 0.00001

Density of cerebrospinal fluid (CSF) at 37°C in term parturients: 1.00030 ± 0.00018. Drugs with densities <1.00018 are hypobaric relative to CSF in parturients.
From ref. 107.

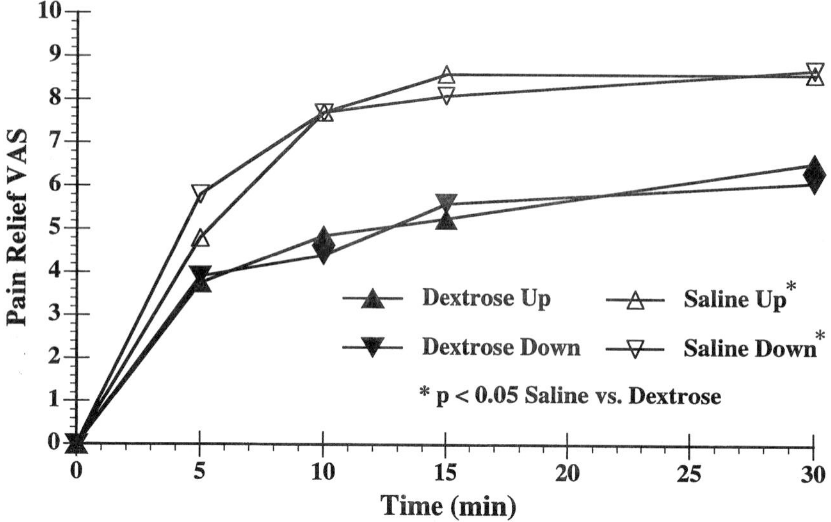

FIG. 7. Pain relief visual analog scores *(VAS)* after intrathecal injection of 10-µg sufentanil mixed with either dextrose or saline via a 24-gauge Sprotte needle with the aperture facing either cephalad (up) or caudad (down). Patients in the dextrose groups had significantly less pain relief than did those in the saline groups. (From ref. 22, with permission.)

Ambulation

Many parturients can safely ambulate after receiving intrathecal opioids alone or in combination with small doses of bupivacaine and epinephrine (7,8,94,96,110). Following intrathecal fentanyl 25 µg with bupivacaine 2.5 mg, all women who experienced a fall in blood pressure did so within the first 30 minutes after injection (110). Then, patients were able to walk without any change in blood pressure. Test each patient for motor weakness before she ambulates. Ability to do a partial deep knee bend or step up on a small step stool without assistance are good predictors of ability to ambulate. Parturients should walk with an accompanying person and should be wearing nonslip footwear. Whether or not ambulation improves obstetric outcome is unclear, but it may improve maternal feelings of well-being and self-
•6• control during labor.

SUMMARY

Spinal labor analgesia is a rapidly expanding area of interest to the obstetric anesthesiologist. Spinal administration of opioids in particular fulfills many of the desiderata of labor analgesia. The list includes bilateral analgesia of rapid onset, low risk of systemic drug toxicity, minimal effect upon maternal expulsive efforts, no appreciable effect upon the neonate, and reversibility. Options for administration range from a single injection to a continuous spinal technique.

Areas for further study include the effect of intrathecal opioids and low-dose local anesthetics on the progress of labor, further refinement of drug doses and combinations to maximize the duration of a single dose of analgesia, and investigation of potential analgesic agents that work via nonopioid receptor mechanisms. Additionally, a continuous spinal technique using an

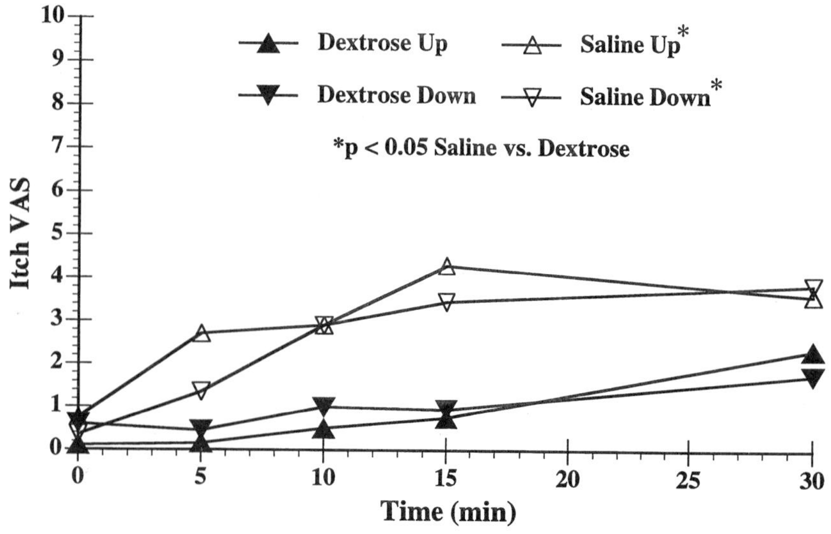

FIG. 8. Pruritus visual analog scores *(VAS)* after intrathecal injection of 10-µg sufentanil mixed with either dextrose or saline via a 24-gauge Sprotte needle with the aperture facing either cephalad (up) or caudad (down). Patients in the saline groups had significantly more itching than did those in the dextrose groups. (From ref. 22, with permission.)

infusion of opioid analgesics for the duration of labor continues to be appealing.

REFERENCES

1. Yaksh TL, Wilson PR, Kaiko RF, Inturrisi CE. Analgesia produced by a spinal action of morphine and effects upon parturition in the rat. *Anesthesiology* 1979;51:386.
2. Benedetti C, Tiengo M. Continuous subarachnoid analgesia in labour. *Lancet* 1990;335:225.
3. Honet JE, Arkoosh VA, Norris MC, Huffnagle HJ, Silverman NS, Leighton BL. Comparison among intrathecal fentanyl, meperidine, and sufentanil for labor analgesia. *Anesth Analg* 1992;75:734.
4. D'Angelo R, Anderson MT, Philip J, Eisenach JC. Intrathecal sufentanil compared to epidural bupivacaine for labor analgesia. *Anesthesiology* 1994;80:1209.
5. Abouleish A, Abouleish E, Camann W. Combined spinal-epidural analgesia in advanced labour. *Can J Anaesth* 1994;41:575.
6. Viscomi CM, Rathmell JP, Mason SB, Livermore M, Schaprio H. Analgesic efficacy and side effects of subarachnoid sufentanil-bupivacaine administered to women in advanced labor. *Reg Anesth* 1996; 21:424.
7. Collis RE, Baxandall ML, Srikantharajah ID, Edge G, Kadim MY, Morgan BM. Combined spinal epidural (CSE) analgesia: technique, management, and outcome of 300 mothers. *Int J Obstet Anesth* 1994; 3:75.
8. Collis RE, Davies DWL, Aveling W. Randomized comparison of combined spinal-epidural and standard epidural analgesia in labour. *Lancet* 1995;345:1413.
9. Eisenach JC, De Kock M, Klimscha W. α2-Adrenergic agonists for regional anesthesia. *Anesthesiology* 1996;85:655.
10. Gautier PE, De Kock M, Fanard L, Van Steenberge A, Hody J. Intrathecal clonidine combined with sufentanil for labor analgesia. *Anesthesiology* 1998;88:651.
11. Abram SE, Winnie RP. Intrathecal acetyl cholinesterase inhibitors produce analgesia that is synergistic with morphine and clonidine in rats. *Anesth Analg* 1995;81:501.
12. Carp H, Jayaram S, Morrow D. Intrathecal cholinergic agonists lessen bupivacaine spinal-block-induced hypotension in rats. *Anesth Analg* 1994;79:112.
13. McCarthy RJ, Kroin JS, Ivankovich AD. Synergistic analgesia and attenuation of morphine tolerance by intrathecal co-infusion of magnesium sulfate and morphine. *Anesthesiology* 1997;87:A813.
14. Solomon RE, Gebhart GF. Synergistic antinociceptive interactions among drugs administered to the spinal cord. *Anesth Analg* 1994; 78:1164.
15. Sosnowski M, Yaksh TL. Spinal administration of receptor-selective drugs as analgesics: new horizons. *J Pain Symptom Manage* 1990; 5:204.
16. Pert CB, Snyder SH. Opiate receptor: demonstration in nervous tissue. *Science* 1973;179:1011.
17. Atweh SF, Kuhar MJ. Autoradiographic localization of opiate receptors in rat brain. I. Spinal cord and lower medulla. *Brain Res* 1977; 124:53.
18. Martin WR, Eades CG, Thompson JA, Huppler RE, Gilbert PE. The effects of morphine- and nalorphine-like drugs in the non-dependent and morphine-dependent chronic spinal dog. *J Pharmacol Exp Ther* 1976;197:517.
19. Sabbe MB, Yaksh TL. Pharmacology of spinal opioids. *J Pain Symptom Manage* 1990;5:191.
20. Coda BA, Brown MC, Schaffer R, et al. Pharmacology of epidural fentanyl, alfentanil, and sufentanil in volunteers. *Anesthesiology* 1994;81:1149.
21. Camann WR, Denny RA, Holby ED, Datta S. A comparison of intrathecal, epidural, and intravenous sufentanil for labor analgesia. *Anesthesiology* 1992;77:884.
22. Ferouz F, Norris MC, Arkoosh VA, Leighton BL, Boxer LM, Corba RJ. Baricity, needle direction, and intrathecal sufentanil labor analgesia. *Anesthesiology* 1997;86:592.
23. Gage JC, D'Angelo R, Miller R, Eisenach JC. Does dextrose affect analgesia or the side effects of intrathecal sufentanil. *Anesth Analg* 1997;85:826.
24. Yaksh TL, Noueihed R. The physiology and pharmacology of spinal opiates. *Ann Rev Pharmacol Toxicol* 1985;25:433.
25. Minami M, Satoh M. Molecular biology of the opioid receptors: structures, functions and distributions. *Neurosci Res* 1995;23:121.
26. Sweeney MI, White TD, Sawynok J. Involvement of adenosine in the spinal antinociceptive effects of morphine and noradrenaline. *J Pharmacol Exp Ther* 1987;243:657.
27. Sawynok J, Sweeney MI, White TD. Adenosine release may mediate spinal analgesia by morphine. *TIPS* 1989;10:186.
28. Sosnowski M, Stevens CW, Yaksh TL. Assessment of the role of A1/A2 adenosine receptors mediating the purine antinociception, motor and autonomic function in the rat spinal cord. *J Pharmacol Exp Ther* 1989;250:915.
29. Power I, Brown DT, Wildsmith JAW. The effect of fentanyl, meperidine and diamorphine on nerve conduction in vitro. *Reg Anesth* 1991; 16:204.
30. Gissen AJ, Gugino LD, Datta S, Miller J, Covino BG. Effects of fentanyl and sufentanil on peripheral mammalian nerves. *Anesth Analg* 1987;66:1272.
31. Gordh T Jr, Jansson I, Hartvig P, Gillberg PG, Post C. Interactions between noradrenergic and cholinergic mechanisms involved in spinal nociceptive processing. *Acta Anaesthesiol Scand* 1989;33:39.
32. Detweiler DJ, Eisenach JC, Tong C, Jackson C. A cholinergic interaction in alpha2 adrenoceptor-mediated antinociception in sheep. *J Pharmacol Exp Ther* 1993;265:536.
33. Eisenach J, Detweiler D, Hood D. Hemodynamic and analgesic actions of epidurally administered clonidine. *Anesthesiology* 1993; 78:277.
34. Eisenach JC, Hood DD, Tuttle R, Shafer S, Smith T, Tong C. Computer-controlled epidural infusion to targeted cerebrospinal fluid concentrations in humans: clonidine. *Anesthesiology* 1995;83:33.
35. Hood DD, Mallak KA, Eisenach JC, Tong C. Interaction between intrathecal neostigmine and epidural clonidine in human volunteers. *Anesthesiology* 1996;85:315.
36. Greene N. Uptake and elimination of local anesthetics during spinal anesthesia. *Anesth Analg* 1983;62:1013.
37. Stevens RA, Petty RH, Hill HF, et al. Redistribution of sufentanil to cerebrospinal fluid and systemic circulation after epidural administration in dogs. *Anesth Analg* 1993;76:323.
38. McQuay HJ, Sullivan AF, Smallman K, Dickenson AH. Intrathecal opioids: potency and lipophilicity. *Pain* 1989;36:111.
39. Scott JC, Cooke JE, Stanski DR. Electroencephalographic quantitation of opioid effect: comparative pharmacodynamics of fentanyl and sufentanil. *Anesthesiology* 1991;74:34.
40. Herman NL, Calicott R, Van Decar TK, Conlin G, Tilton J. Determination of the dose-response relationship for intrathecal sufentanil in laboring patients. *Anesth Analg* 1997;84:1256.
41. Palmer CM, Cork RC, Hays R, Van Maren G, Alves D. The dose-response relation of intrathecal fentanyl for labor analgesia. *Anesthesiology* 1998;88:355.

41a. Arkoosh VA, Cooper M, Norris MC, et al. Intrathecal dose response in nulliparous patients. *Anesthesiology* 1998;89:364.

42. Durant PAC, Yaksh TL. Drug effects of urinary bladder tone during spinal morphine-induced inhibition of the micturition reflex in unanesthetized rats. *Anesthesiology* 1988;68:325.
43. Rawal N, Mollefors K, Axelsson K, Lingårdh G, Widman B. An experimental study of urodynamic effects of epidural morphine and of naloxone reversal. *Anesth Analg* 1983;62:641.
44. Havemann U, Lechoslaw T, Kuschinsky K. Role of opioid receptors in the substantia nigra in morphine-induced muscular rigidity. *Life Sci* 1982;31:2319.
45. Erickson DL, Blacklock JB, Michaelson M, Sperling KB, Lo JN. Control of spasticity by implantable continuous flow morphine pump. *Neurosurgery* 1985;16:215.
46. Newman LM, Patel RV, Krolick T, Ivankovich AD. Muscular spasm in the lower limbs of laboring patients after intrathecal administration of epinephrine and sufentanil. *Anesthesiology* 1994;80:468.
47. Costello DJ, Borison HL. Naloxone antagonizes narcotic self-blockade of emesis in the cat. *J Pharmacol Exp Ther* 1977;203:222.
48. Caldwell LE, Rosen MA, Shnider SM. Subarachnoid morphine and fentanyl for labor analgesia. *Reg Anesth* 1994;19:2.
49. Grieco WM, Norris MC, Leighton BL, et al. Intrathecal sufentanil labor analgesia: the effects of adding morphine or epinephrine. *Anesth Analg* 1993;77:1149.

50. Leighton BL, DeSimone CA, Norris MC, Ben-David B. Intrathecal narcotics for labor revisited: the combination of fentanyl and morphine intrathecally provides rapid onset of profound, prolonged analgesia. *Anesth Analg* 1989;69:122.
51. Atchison SR, Durant PA, Yaksh TL. Cardiorespiratory effects and kinetics of intrathecally injected d-ala-d-leu-enkephalin and morphine in unanesthetized dogs. *Anesthesiology* 1986;65:609.
52. Etches RC, Sandler AN, Daley MD. Respiratory depression and spinal opioids. *Can J Anaesth* 1989;36:165.
53. Hays RL, Palmer CM. Respiratory depression after intrathecal sufentanil during labor. *Anesthesiology* 1994;81:511.
54. Baker MN, Sarna MC. Respiratory arrest after second dose of intrathecal sufentanil. *Anesthesiology* 1995;83:231.
55. Ferouz F, Norris MC, Leighton BL. Risk of respiratory arrest after intrathecal sufentanil. *Anesth Analg* 1997;85:1088.
56. Greenhalgh CA. Respiratory arrest in a parturient following intrathecal injection of sufentanil and bupivacaine. *Anaesthesia* 1996;51:173.
57. Hamilton CL, Cohen SE. High sensory block after intrathecal sufentanil for labor analgesia. *Anesthesiology* 1995;83:1118.
58. Currier DS, Levin KR, Campbell C. Dysphagia with intrathecal fentanyl. *Anesthesiology* 1997;87:1570.
59. Abouleish E. Apnoea associated with the intrathecal administration of morphine in obstetrics. A case report. *Br J Anaesth* 1988;60:592.
60. Cohen SE, Cherry CM, Holbrook H Jr, El-Sayed YY, Gibson RN, Jaffe RA. Intrathecal sufentanil for labor analgesia-sensory changes, side effects, and fetal heart rate changes. *Anesth Analg* 1993;77:1155.
61. Thomas DA, Williams GM, Iwata K, Kenshalo DR Jr, Dubner R. A site of action of morphine in producing facial scratching in monkeys. *Anesthesiology* 1993;79:548.
62. Ballantyne JC, Loach AB, Carr DB. Itching after epidural and spinal opiates. *Pain* 1988;33:149.
63. Belcher G, Ryall RW. Differential excitatory and inhibitory effects of opiates on nonnociceptive and nociceptive neurones in the spinal cord of the cat. *Brain Res* 1978;145:303.
64. Saiah M, Borgeat A, Wilder-Smith OHG, Rifat K, Suter PM. Epidural morphine induced pruritus: propofol versus naloxone. *Anesth Analg* 1994;78:1110.
65. Borgeat A, Wilder-Smith OHG, Saiah M, Rifat K. Subhypnotic doses of propofol relieve pruritus induced by epidural and intrathecal morphine. *Anesthesiology* 1992;76:510.
66. Beilin Y, Bernstein HH, Zucker-Pinchoff B, Zahn J, Zenzen WJ. Subhypnotic doses of propofol do not relieve pruritus induced by intrathecal morphine after cesarean section. *Anesth Analg* 1998;86:310.
67. Grant GJ, Susser L, Cascio M, Moses M, Zakowski MI. Hemodynamic effects of intrathecal fentanyl in nonlaboring term parturients. *J Clin Anesth* 1996;8:99.
68. Newman LM, Wlodarski JC, Tanck EN, Ivankovich D. Neither intrathecal sufentanil nor intrathecal sufentanil plus nalbuphine cause hypotension in laboring parturients. *Anesthesiology* 1994;81:A1153.
69. Mandell GL, Jamnback L, Ramanathan S. Hemodynamic effects of subarachnoid fentanyl in laboring parturients. *Reg Anesth* 1996; 21:103.
70. Riley ET, Ratner EF, Cohen SE. Intrathecal sufentanil for labor analgesia: do sensory changes predict better analgesia and greater hypotension? *Anesth Analg* 1997;84:346.
71. Riley ET, Walker D, Hamilton CL, Cohen SE. Intrathecal sufentanil for labor does not cause a sympathectomy. *Anesthesiology* 1997;87: 874.
72. Cascio M, Pygon B, Bernett C, Ramanathan S. Labour analgesia with intrathecal fentanyl decreases maternal stress. *Can J Anaesth* 1997;44: 605.
73. D'Angelo R, Eisenach JC. Severe maternal hypotension and fetal bradycardia after a combined spinal epidural anesthetic. *Anesthesiology* 1997;87:166.
74. Clarke VT, Smiley RM, Finster M. Uterine hyperactivity after intrathecal injection of fentanyl for analgesia during labor: a cause of fetal bradycardia? *Anesthesiology* 1994;81:1083.
74a. Eberle RL, Norris MC, Eberle AM, et al. The effect of maternal position on fetal heart rate during epidural or intrathecal labor analgesia. *Am J Obstet Gynecol* 1998;179:150.
75. Nielsen PE, Erickson JR, Abouleish EI, Perriatt S, Sheppard C. Fetal heart rate changes after intrathecal sufentanil or epidural bupivacaine for labor analgesia: incidence and clinical significance. *Anesth Analg* 1996;83:742.
76. Albright GA, Forster RM. Does combined spinal-epidural analgesia with subarachnoid sufentanil increase the incidence of emergency cesarean delivery. *Reg Anesth* 1997;22:400.
77. Fernando R, Bonello E, Gill P, Urquhart J, Reynolds F, Morgan B. Neonatal welfare and placental transfer of fentanyl and bupivacaine during ambulatory combined spinal epidural analgesia for labour. *Anaesthesia* 1997;52:517.
78. Johnson RF, Johnson HV, Arney TL, Paschall RL, Herman N, Downing JW. Sufentanil transfer across the human term placenta: the effect of fetal pH. *Society of Obstetric Anesthesia and Perinatology 1995 Annual Meeting,* 1995:58.
79. Zakowski M, Grant GJ, Turndorf H. Uptake and transfer of sufentanil in human placenta during in vitro perfusion. *Society of Obstetric Anesthesia and Perinatology 1994 Annual Meeting,* 1994:82.
80. Nageotte MP, Larson D, Rumney PJ, Sidhu M, Hollenbach K. Epidural analgesia compared with combined spinal-epidural analgesia during labor in nulliparous women. *N Engl J Med* 1997;337:1715.
81. Abboud TK, Noueihed R, Daniel J. Intrathecal morphine for relief of labor pain in a parturient with severe pulmonary hypertension. *Anesthesiology* 1983;59:477.
82. Ransom DM, Leicht CH. Continuous spinal analgesia with sufentanil for labor and delivery in a parturient with severe pulmonary stenosis. *Anesth Analg* 1995;80:418.
83. Brizgys RV, Shnider SM. Hyperbaric intrathecal morphine analgesia during labor in a patient with Wolff-Parkinson-White syndrome. *Obstet Gynecol* 1984;64:44S.
84. Copel JA, Harrison D, Whittemore R, Hobbins JC. Intrathecal morphine analgesia for vaginal delivery in a women with a single ventricle. *J Reprod Med* 1986;31:274.
85. Johnson MD, Hurley RJ, Gilbertson LI, Datta S. Continuous microcatheter spinal anesthesia with subarachnoid meperidine for labor and delivery. *Anesth Analg* 1990;70:658.
86. Patel SD, Arkoosh VA, Storey AM, et al. Does the combined spinal epidural technique guarantee a working epidural? *Anesthesiology* 1995;83:A962.
87. Scott PV, Bowen FE, Cartwright P, et al. Intrathecal morphine as sole analgesic during labor. *Br Med J* 1980;281:351.
88. Baraka A, Noueihid R, Hajj S. Intrathecal injection of morphine for obstetric analgesia. *Anesthesiology* 1991;54:136.
89. Mok MS, Tsai SK. More experience with intrathecal morphine for obstetric analgesia [Letter]. *Anesthesiology* 1981;55:481.
90. Abboud TK, Shnider SM, Dailey PA. Intrathecal administration of hyperbaric morphine for the relief of pain in labour. *Br J Anaesth* 1984;56:1351.
91. Arkoosh VA, Sharkey SJ, Norris MC, Isaacson W, Honet JE, Leighton BL. Subarachnoid labor analgesia: fentanyl and morphine versus sufentanil and morphine. *Reg Anesth* 1994;19:243.
92. Camann WR, Minzter BH, Denney RA, Datta S. Intrathecal sufentanil for labor analgesia. *Anesthesiology* 1993;78:870.
93. Campbell DC, Camann WR, Datta S. The addition of bupivacaine to intrathecal sufentanil for labor analgesia. *Anesth Analg* 1995;81:305.
94. Campbell DC, Banner R, Crone LA, Gore-Hickman W, Yip RW. Addition of epinephrine to intrathecal bupivacaine and sufentanil for ambulatory labor analgesia. *Anesthesiology* 1997;86:525.
95. Kartawiadi SL, Vercauteren MP, Van Steenberge AL, Adriaensen HA. Spinal analgesia during labor with low-dose bupivacaine, sufentanil, and epinephrine. *Reg Anesth* 1996;21:191.
96. Gautier PE, Debry F, Fanard L, Van Steenberge A, Hody J. Ambulatory combined spinal-epidural analgesia for labor: influence of epinephrine on bupivacaine-sufentanil combination. *Reg Anesth* 1997;22:143.
97. Lu JK, Schafer PG, Gardner TL, et al. The dose-response pharmacology of intrathecal sufentanil in female volunteers. *Anesth Analg* 1997;85:372.
98. McHale S, Mitchell V, Howsam S, Carli F. Continuous subarachnoid infusion of 0.125% bupivacaine for analgesia during labor. *Br J Anaesth* 1992;69:634.
99. Isaacson W, Arkoosh VA, Kinsella SM, et al. Intrathecal sufentanil labor analgesia: the effect of diluent volume. *Anesthesiology* 1994;81:A1154.
100. Rigler ML, Drasner K, Krejcie TC, et al. Cauda equina syndrome after continuous spinal anesthesia. *Anesth Analg* 1991;72:275.
101. Food and Drug Administration. Cauda equina syndrome associated with the use of small-bore catheters in continuous spinal anesthesia. *FDA Safety Alert,* May 29, 1992.
102. Rigler ML, Drasner K. Distribution of catheter-injected local anesthetic in a model of the subarachnoid space. *Anesthesiology* 1991;75:684.

103. Lambert LA, Lambert DH, Strichartz GR. Irreversible conduction block in isolated nerve by high concentrations of local anesthetics. *Anesthesiology* 1994;80:1082.
104. Sakura S, Chan V, Ciriales R, Drasner K. Intrathecal infusion of lidocaine in the rat results in dose-dependent, but not concentration-dependent, sacral root injury. *Anesthesiology* 1993;79:A851.
105. Strichartz GR, Manning T, Datta S. Irreversible conduction block in mammalian nerves by direct application of 2% and 5% lidocaine. *Reg Anesth* 1994;19[2S]:21.
106. Schneider M, Ettlin T, Kaufmann M, et al. Transident neurologic toxicity after hyperbaric subarachnoid anesthesia with 5% lidocaine. *Anesth Analg* 1993;76:1154.
107. Corba RJ, Arkoosh VA, Leighton BL, Huffnagle HJ, Huffnagle S. What is the effect of intrathecal labor analgesia on the reliability of a subsequent epidural local anesthetic test dose? *Society for Obstetric Anesthesia and Perinatology 1997 Annual Meeting,* 1997:91.
108. Richardson MG, Wissler RN. Density of dextrose-free local anesthetics, opioids, and combinations measured at 37°C. *Anesth Analg* 1997; 84:95.
109. Richardson MG, Thakur R, Abramowicz JS, Wissler RN. Maternal posture influences the extent of sensory block produced by intrathecal dextrose-free bupivacaine with fentanyl for labor analgesia. *Anesth Analg* 1996;83:1229.
110. Shennan A, Cooke V, Lloyd-Jones F, Morgan B, de Swiet M. Blood pressure changes during labour and whilst ambulating with combined spinal epidural analgesia. *Br J Obstet Gynecol* 1995;102:192.
111. Borgeat A, Wilder-Smith OHG, Saiah M, Rifat K. Subhypnotic doses of propofol possess direct antiemetic properties. *Anesth Analg* 1992; 74:539.
112. Palmer CM, Van Maren G, Nogami WM, Marquez RC, Alves D. Bipivacaine augments intrathecal fentanyl for labor analgesia. *Reg Anesth* 1996;21:S6.

Obstetric Anesthesia, second edition,
edited by Mark C. Norris.
Lippincott Williams & Wilkins, Philadelphia © 1999.

CHAPTER 17

Neuraxial Analgesia for Labor

Part III: Epidural Drugs

Edward T. Riley

The perfect labor analgesic would relieve pain but:

- Would not impair maternal motor function,
- Would have no adverse fetal effects,
- Would not alter the course of labor,
- Would be effective throughout labor, and
- Could be readily used to provide anesthesia for cesarean delivery.

Although intrathecal opioids can provide good analgesia with no motor block (1), they have their limitations:

- Finite duration, usually 1 to 2 hours (2,3).
- Repeated dural puncture or intrathecal catheter is needed for repeat doses.
- Opioids alone are often inadequate for the second stage of labor (4).

Continuous epidural analgesia remains the technique of choice for relieving labor pain. A lumbar epidural catheter can be used to provide analgesia throughout labor and, should the need arise, anesthesia for surgical delivery.

Currently, epidural analgesia can be tailored to closely approximate the properties of the ideal labor analgesic. Continuous infusion techniques, neuroselective local anesthetics, and dilute solutions of local anesthetics combined with opioids and other adjuvants can provide excellent maternal analgesia without significantly impairing maternal motor function or fetal and neonatal physiology. This chapter will briefly discuss the anatomy of labor pain and some local anesthetic pharmacology pertaining to labor epidural analgesia. Then follows a review of commonly used local anesthetics, opioids and other adjuvants, and a discussion of a clinical approach for providing lumbar epidural analgesia for labor pain relief.

E. T. Riley: Department of Anesthesia, Stanford University School of Medicine, Stanford, California 94305-5640.

ANATOMY OF LABOR PAIN

During labor and delivery, noxious stimuli are transmitted from the uterus, vagina, and perineum to the central nervous system along discrete neural pathways. Understanding the location of these pathways provides a rational basis for analgesic interventions. Uterine contractions and cervical dilation are the primary source of pain during the first stage of labor. The afferent nerves from the uterus and cervix include somatic and visceral sensory fibers that travel with uterine sympathetic nerves. These fibers pass through the paracervical tissue, along the uterine artery, and then through the inferior, middle, and superior hypogastric plexi to the sympathetic chain. Then, impulses enter the spinal cord with the T_{10} to L_1 or L_2 spinal nerves. Pain during the second stage of labor is due to descent of the fetal presenting part into the pelvis, stretching tissues innervated by the pudendal nerve. These somatic nerves enter the spinal cord at the second, third, and fourth sacral roots.

In theory, blockade of the T_{10} to L_2 dermatomes should relieve pain during the first stage of labor. Second stage pain can be managed by extending the block to S_4. In practice, labor pain is not always so easily managed. During the first stage of labor, the fetal presenting part can compress and stretch the lumbosacral plexus, causing pain below the L_2 dermatome. In the second stage of labor, areas outside of the distribution of the pudendal nerve can be stimulated and blockade of somatic nerve roots beyond $S_{2\text{-}4}$ may be needed.

The lumbar region of the spine is the best place for an epidural catheter for labor pain. Here, nerve roots from T_{10} to L_2 are consistently blocked with small volumes of local anesthetics. Lumbar injection sometimes fails to block the sacral nerve roots effectively without using relatively large volumes of local anesthetic (which may worsen motor block). Sacral block is more easily accomplished with a caudal catheter. However, caudal catheters are inadequate for blocking the pain from the first stage of labor. A two-catheter system (lumbar and caudal) has been proposed. However, the extra work and risk associated with placing two catheters probably outweighs the benefits. This technique has never seen wide use.

PHARMACOLOGY OF CONDUCTION BLOCKADE

Epidurally administered local anesthetics produce analgesia by inhibiting nerve conduction in the afferent fibers transmitting painful stimuli to the spinal cord. Most available evidence suggests that this effect occurs at the level of the nerve root.

Pharmacologically, epidural local anesthetics bind to voltage-gated sodium channels. In the normal state, resting nerve cells are polarized, with a slightly negative transmembrane potential. When an action potential is propagated along a nerve, sodium channels open and allow nerve cell depolarization. Once a threshold transmembrane potential is reached, the action potential is propagated along the nerve. Local anesthetics slow depolarization and block propagation of the action potential (Fig. 1).

Local anesthetics act inside the axon. To gain access to its site of action, the local anesthetic molecule must first diffuse into the axon and then enter the sodium channel. Experimentally, external application of quaternary analogs of local anesthetics does not produce conduction blockade because these permanently charged molecules cannot diffuse across cell membranes. Direct intracellular injection of quaternary analogs does block nerve conduction (5,6).

Thus, local anesthetics must initially assume a lipophilic (uncharged) form to cross the axonal membrane and then become hydrophilic (charged) to bind to the sodium channel. Clinically useful local anesthetics are weak bases consisting of a lipophilic benzene ring and a tertiary amine. The tertiary amine can exist in either a charged, hydrophilic, or an uncharged, lipophilic, form (Fig. 2).

In solution, local anesthetic molecules exist in both charged and uncharged states. The balance between these two forms of drug is determined by the relationship between the pK_a of the local anesthetic and the pH of the solution. The pK_a of a given compound is the pH at which there are equal amounts of charged and uncharged drug. The pK_a of clinically useful local anesthetics, which are weak bases, is above 7.0 (Table 1). Commercially available local anesthetic solutions are buffered to a low (acidic) pH. In these solutions, the vast majority of local anesthetic molecules are charged (the ratio of charged to uncharged molecules is 10^3 to 10^4:1). One approach to speeding the onset of local anesthetic blockade is to raise the pH (i.e., with $NaHCO_3$) of the injected solution. As the pH of the solution approaches the pK_a of the drug, more local anesthetic is in its uncharged, diffusible form.

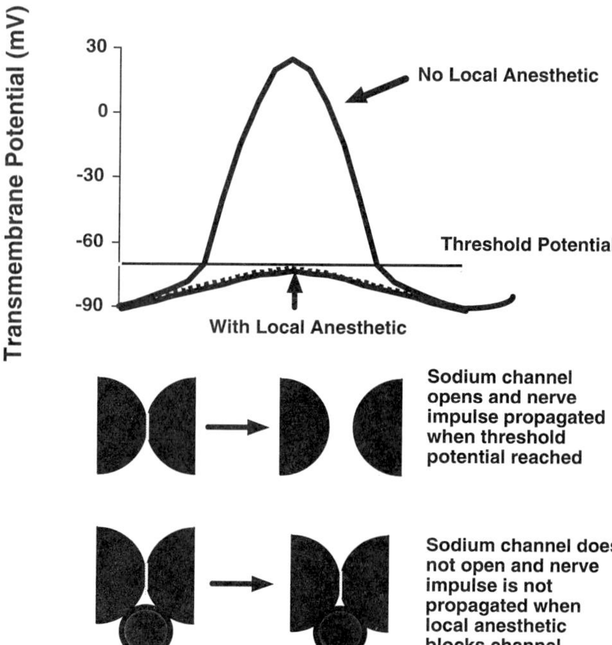

FIG. 1. Sodium channels are stimulated to open when the threshold potential of the cell is exceeded. The action potential is then propagated along the nerve. Local anesthetics prevent the threshold potential from being exceeded and block propagation of the action potential.

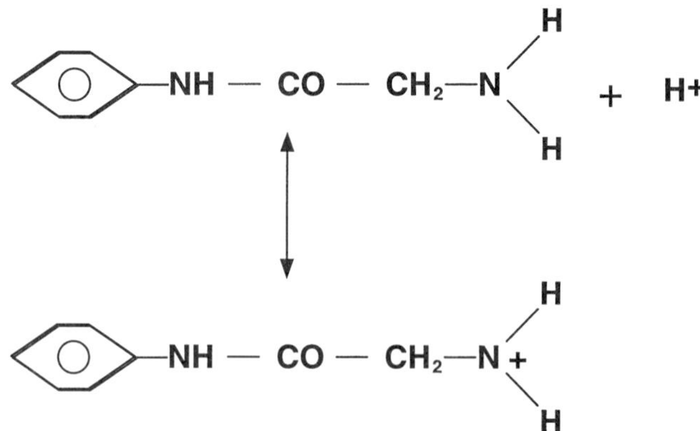

FIG. 2. A generic amide local anesthetic in equilibrium between the charged quaternary amine form and the uncharged tertiary amine form. To diffuse into the nerve, the molecule must be in the uncharged tertiary amine configuration and is active in the receptor as a quaternary amine.

TABLE 1. *Pharmacology of the local anesthetics commonly used for epidural analgesia in obstetrics*

Drug	Class	Onset	Duration	pK_a	Partition coefficient (lipid solubility)	Protein binding (%)	Motor sparing
Bupivacaine	Amide	Slow	Long	8.1	27	95	Yes
Ropivacaine	Amide	Slow	Long	8.1	6	94	Yes
Lidocaine	Amide	Fast	Medium	7.8	3	65	No
2-Chloroprocaine	Ester	Fast	Short	8.7	1	—	No

Another important feature of local anesthetics is their differential effects on nerve conduction. Clinically, pain transmission is more susceptible to local anesthetic blockade than light touch sensation, which in turn is more susceptible than motor function. The mechanism of this phenomena is poorly understood. Axon size may have some role. Smaller nerve fibers are more susceptible to local anesthetic blockage than larger fibers (7). Thus, the small-diameter A_δ (1 to 4 μm) and C fibers (0.4 to 1.2 μm) that conduct pain sensation are more easily blocked than large A_α fibers (6 to 22 μm) that transmit motor impulses and proprioceptive information. However, in some studies, larger fibers are more susceptible to local anesthetic blockade (8,9). In mice, ventral root axons (motor neurons) are more readily blocked than dorsal root axons (sensory neurons) (10). Other mechanisms (anatomic site of blockade, location of the fibers within the nerve bundle, frequency-dependent blockade, etc.) may ultimately explain why lower concentrations of local anesthetics seem to preferentially block pain transmission over motor transmission.

Local anesthetics also differ among themselves in the relative amounts of sensory and motor blockade they produce. The ideal local anesthetic for labor analgesia would block pain transmission but leave motor function untouched. Of the commonly used drugs, bupivacaine and ropivacaine seem to produce less motor block than equianalgesic concentrations of lidocaine or 2-chloroprocaine. However, systematic comparisons of motor block produced by the dilute solutions of local anesthetics commonly used for labor analgesia are just beginning (11,12). Until this important work is completed, we must rely on clinical experience and observation when choosing local anesthetics for labor analgesia.

Lipid solubility and protein binding are important factors in determining a local anesthetic's potency, onset, and duration. Increased lipid solubility allows the drug to diffuse rapidly into the axon and then to its site of action. Increased protein binding leads to a stronger bond between drug and receptor. However, the relationship among potency, onset, duration, lipid solubility, and protein binding is not simple. Potency, onset, and duration also are affected by other physiochemical properties (pK_a, metabolism, etc.). Additionally, there are detrimental effects of increased lipid solubility and protein binding. If lipid solubility is too high, the drug may quickly diffuse away from its site of action. Nonspecific binding to epidural fat may limit the amount of drug that reaches the site of action. Too much protein binding also may hinder diffusion to the site of action. Although it is possible to make some predictions about a drug based on its lipid solubility and protein binding, clinical testing will likely reveal surprises.

LOCAL ANESTHETICS

Theoretically, the best local anesthetic for labor analgesia will:

- Have a fast onset,
- Have a long duration,
- Be rapidly titratable,
- Preferentially block pain compared to motor function, and
- Have low toxicity.

In practice, no local anesthetic fulfills all these requirements. In practice, one must prioritize among these categories when choosing a drug for labor epidural analgesia. Most often, minimizing motor blockade takes precedence over onset. Unlike epidural anesthesia for cesarean section, toxicity is less important during labor because most anesthesiologists use very low doses of drug in this setting. Following is a summary of the clinically important features of commonly used local anesthetics (Table 1). This information is based on studies of local anesthetics alone for labor analgesia. The use of adjuvants will be discussed later.

Bupivacaine

Bupivacaine is the most commonly used local anesthetic for labor analgesia (13). There are several reasons for this popularity.

- Bupivacaine produces relatively less motor blockade compared to most other local anesthetics.
- It is widely available.
- It has a relatively long duration.

Used alone, bupivacaine will provide adequate labor analgesia at concentrations of 0.125% to 0.25% (14,15). In a systematic study of labor pain relief, Columb and Lyons (11) found that 20 mL of 0.065% plain bupivacaine provided adequate labor analgesia (pain score less than 10 on a scale of 0 to 100) in 50% of patients (EC_{50}).

Twenty milliliters of 0.129% bupivacaine will provide adequate analgesia in 95% of laboring women (EC_{95}) (Table 2).

Bolus injection of 12.5- to 50-mg bupivacaine (10 to 20 mL of 0.125% to 0.25% solution) or infusions of around 25 mg/hour (20 mL/hour of 0.125% bupivacaine) carry a very low risk of maternal systemic toxicity. Although epidural bupivacaine readily crosses the placenta, no adverse effects were noted in neonates whose mothers received epidural infusion of 0.125% bupivacaine at 10 mL/hour for up to 15 hours (16).

Fetal heart rate changes have been associated with bupivacaine labor analgesia (17–19). Because these changes do not occur with larger doses of bupivacaine used for elective cesarean section, it is unlikely that they are due to a direct drug effect on the fetal heart (20). Instead, they are usually associated with uterine hypertonus and probably represent the effects of a sudden decrease in plasma catecholamine concentration associated with the onset of analgesia (17). Catecholamines have a tocolytic effect, and the decrease in their concentration may lead to temporary uterine hypertonus, decreased placental perfusion, and fetal asphyxia (21,22). These fetal heart rate changes are transient and lack effect on the outcome of the labor or the neonate.

Lidocaine

Lidocaine has proven safe and effective for labor analgesia (19). Clinically, lidocaine produces more intense motor block and less analgesia than bupivacaine (Table 1). The EC_{50} of epidural lidocaine in labor is 0.37% and the EC_{95} is 0.52% (Table 2) (11). These data suggest a potency ratio of lidocaine to bupivacaine of 4:1 (0.52%/0.129%). A study comparing 0.75% lidocaine to 0.125% bupivacaine for labor analgesia (a ratio of 6:1) found better analgesia with bupivacaine (23). Similarly, epidural infusion of 0.75% lidocaine during the second stage of labor produced no better analgesia than epidural infusion of saline (24). In contrast, epidural infusion of 0.125% bupivacaine produced good or excellent second-stage analgesia in 82% of patients studied (25). However, lidocaine has a faster onset than bupivacaine and can be useful in certain situations (e.g., emergency forceps delivery).

TABLE 2. *Relative potency of epidural local anesthetics in laboring women*

Drug	EC_{50}[a]	EC_{95}[b]
Bupivacaine	0.065%	0.129%
Lidocaine	0.37%	0.52%
2-Chloroprocaine	0.43%	0.83%
Ropivacaine	0.111%	0.143%

[a]Concentration of local anesthetic that provided adequate labor analgesia (pain score <10 on a scale of 0 to 100) in 50% of patients.

[b]Concentration of local anesthetic that provided adequate labor analgesia (pain score <10 on a scale of 0 to 100) in 95% of patients.

Data from refs. 11, 12, 41.

2-Chloroprocaine

2-Chloroprocaine is currently the only ester local anesthetic used for epidural anesthesia. It has little toxicity and a rapid onset. In obstetric anesthesia, it often is used to provide epidural anesthesia for emergency operative delivery. Several problems limit its usefulness for labor analgesia:

- It is a short-acting drug and, unless used as a continuous infusion, requires frequent reinjections.
- Doses that provide adequate labor analgesia are accompanied by significant motor block.
- It impairs the action of epidural bupivacaine and opioids (26). Although epidural 2-chloroprocaine rapidly provides labor analgesia, it markedly shortens the duration of subsequently injected epidural bupivacaine (Fig. 3) (27).
- Epidural 2-chloroprocaine also inhibits the effect of subsequent epidural fentanyl. After cesarean delivery, epidural fentanyl provides a shorter and lesser degree of analgesia after 2-chloroprocaine than after lidocaine (28). However, 2-chloroprocaine has less of an inhibitory effect on the efficacy of fentanyl when they are given together for labor analgesia. Epidural fentanyl (60 μg) decreases the EC_{50} of 2-chloroprocaine 0.43% to 0.26% (40%) (12). This dose of fentanyl decreases the EC_{50} of epidural bupivacaine by 55% (Fig. 4) (29).

The in vivo half-life of 2-chloroprocaine in maternal plasma is 3 minutes (30). In most cases, this rapid destruction by plasma esterases limits the risk of systemic

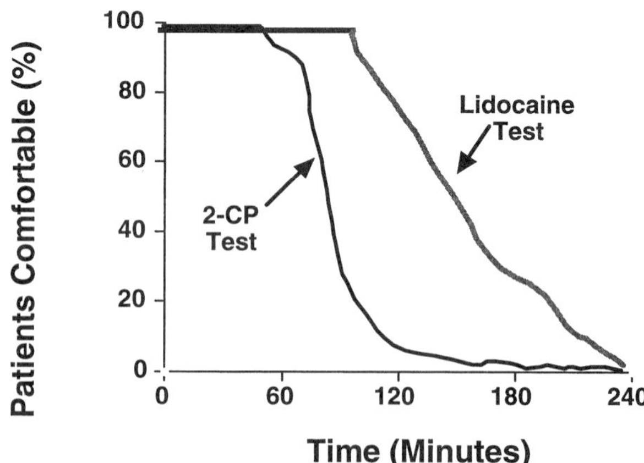

FIG. 3. The effect of a "test dose" of either 2% lidocaine or 2-chloroprocaine (2-CP) on the duration of epidural analgesia provided by 10 mL of 0.25% bupivacaine, fentanyl 50 μg, and epinephrine 3.33 μg/mL given to laboring women. (Data from ref. 27.)

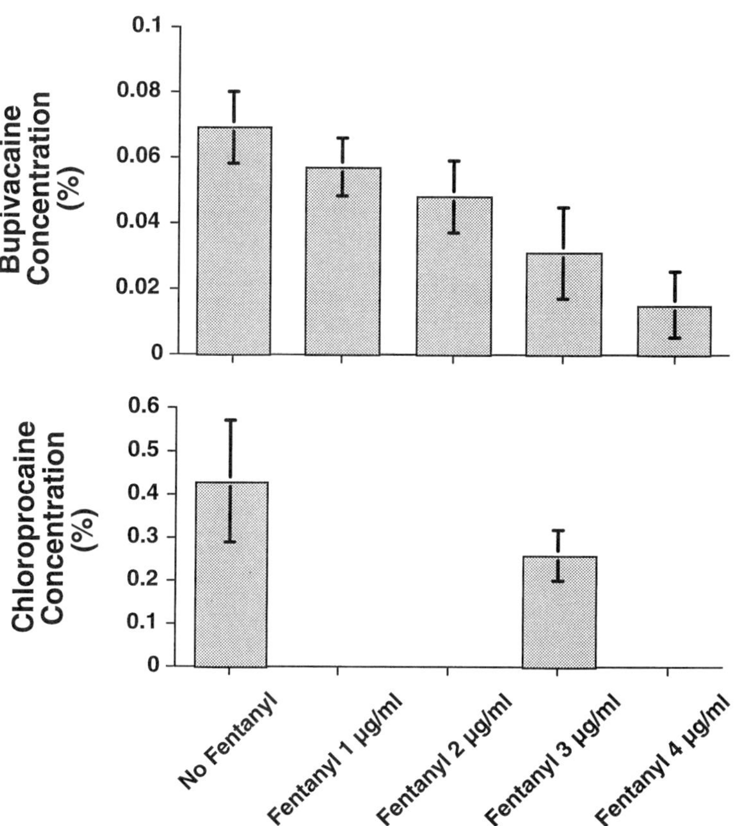

FIG. 4. The effect of epidural opioids on the minimum local anesthetic concentration for labor analgesia (bars are the 50% effective concentration and the error bars are the 95% confidence intervals). (Data from refs. 12 and 29.)

toxicity. However, in patients with atypical pseudocholinesterase, 2-chloroprocaine can cause prolonged block (31). In these women, toxicity after systemic absorption also may occur.

2-Chloroprocaine has a history of causing nerve injury and back pain. These problems are probably related to the preservatives, not the drug itself. Neurological damage was reported after accidental intrathecal injection of 2-chloroprocaine containing sodium bisulfite (32,33). In 1987, sodium bisulfite was replaced with disodium ethylenediaminetetraacetic acid (EDTA). This additive caused back pain, probably from muscle spasm related to hypocalcemia (EDTA chelates calcium) (34,35). Currently, 2-chloroprocaine is marketed without preservatives and shelf life is prolonged by using dark bottles to protect the drug from light. Although these changes hopefully will decrease the morbidity associated with 2-chloroprocaine, they will not make the drug more useful for labor analgesia.

Ropivacaine

Ropivacaine is a new amide local anesthetic that is structurally similar to bupivacaine. Lipid solubility, pK_a, and protein binding also resemble that of bupivacaine. Purportedly, ropivacaine is less cardiotoxic (36,37) and causes less motor blockade than bupivacaine (38). The lack of cardiotoxicity has little impact on ropivacaine's use for labor analgesia. The small bolus injections and dilute infusion mixtures that currently are used in laboring women make cardiac toxicity from unrecognized intravenous bupivacaine very unlikely. However, less motor blockade may be advantageous. No prospective trial has shown changes in the incidence of forceps and vacuum delivery, but a meta-analysis of several studies found fewer instrumental deliveries with ropivacaine versus bupivacaine (39).

If ropivacaine does cause less motor block and fewer instrumental deliveries, it may become the local anesthetic of choice for labor epidural analgesia. However, the currently available data suffer from two limitations. First, most studies to date have assumed that bupivacaine and ropivacaine are equipotent. Other data suggest that bupivacaine is more potent. Comparisons in nonpregnant patients find that 0.75% bupivacaine is as effective as 1.0% ropivacaine (40). In laboring women, the EC_{50} of bupivacaine is half that of ropivacaine (0.061% vs 0.111%) (Table 2) (41). Thus, bupivacaine would be expected to produce more motor block (and more analgesia) than the same dose of ropivacaine.

The second issue that needs further study is the interaction of ropivacaine and epidural opioids. Lipid-soluble opioids significantly potentiate the effects of epidural bupivacaine (29). Because of this interaction, labor analgesia can be provided with very low concentrations of epidural bupivacaine. Many of these dilute opioid/local anesthetic mixtures produce little or no clinically detectable motor block. Similar studies need to be done with ropivacaine before we can determine its role in labor epidural analgesia.

Meperidine

Meperidine is most commonly used as an intramuscular or intravenous analgesic. However, it also has local anesthetic-like properties (42) and is an effective spinal anesthetic for labor analgesia, tubal ligation, cesarean section, and urologic procedures (43–46). In labor, epidural meperidine 100 mg is as effective as 0.25% bupivacaine (47). Epidural meperidine produced more sedation, itching, and nausea but less motor and sensory blockade. No studies have compared epidural meperidine with bupivacaine/opioid combinations.

ADJUVANTS

Opioids

Epidural opioids alone (with the exception of meperidine) do not provide adequate labor analgesia. However, epidural opioids allow the concentration of local anesthetic to be decreased without altering the quality of pain relief. Epidural local anesthetic/opioid mixtures can provide good labor analgesia with minimal maternal motor blockade. The lipid-soluble opioids (fentanyl, sufentanil, and alfentanil) are most effective. Morphine's slow onset limits its use during labor. Although multiple studies show that a lower concentration of local anesthetic plus an opioid provide labor analgesia that is comparable to a higher concentration of local anesthetic alone, very few studies have systematically quantitated the local anesthetic sparing effect of epidural opioids. Fentanyl markedly decreases the EC_{50} of both epidural bupivacaine and 2-chloroprocaine in laboring women (Fig. 4) (12,29). Epidural sufentanil also has a dose-dependent local anesthetic sparing effect when used with bupivacaine (48).

Multiple studies have shown that commonly used doses of epidural opioids during labor have few detrimental maternal or fetal side effects (49). Several important questions have yet to be answered clearly:

- What is the optimal dose of epidural opioid?
- What is the upper limit of opioid that can be used safely during labor?
- Is one opioid better than the others?

Few studies have systematically evaluated differing doses of epidural opioids and local anesthetic. Epidural sufentanil 30 μg and a lidocaine/epinephrine "test dose" provide adequate analgesia in early, but not later, labor (48). Epidural fentanyl 1 to 4 μg/mL progressively decreases the EC_{50} of bupivacaine in laboring women (29). The authors recommended 3 μg/mL because the incidence of itching increased significantly at 4 μg/mL. Thus, the optimal dose of epidural sufentanil or fentanyl represents a tradeoff between analgesia and side effects (nausea, pruritus, neonatal depression) (Table 3).

There are few differences among fentanyl, alfentanil, and sufentanil as adjuvants to epidural local anesthetics. Because of sufentanil's larger volume of distribution, it will have less effect on the fetus than equipotent doses of the other two (50).

Sodium Bicarbonate

To block conduction, local anesthetic must first diffuse across the nerve cell membrane in its uncharged form. The closer the pH of a local anesthetic solution to that drug's pK_a, the greater the proportion of uncharged drug (Fig. 2). Because commercially available local anesthetic solutions are buffered to a low pH, adding sodium bicarbonate should raise the pH of these solutions and may speed the onset of analgesia. Unfortunately, raising the pH of a local anesthetic solution also may increase the intensity of (motor) blockade. So, I rarely use bicarbonate for labor analgesia. Adding bicarbonate to epidural lidocaine will speed the onset of anesthesia for operative delivery.

When adding bicarbonate to local anesthetics, it is important not to add so much that the drug precipitates. It is safe to add bicarbonate to lidocaine or 2-chloroprocaine in a ratio of 1:10. However, bupivacaine will precipitate if you exceed a ratio of about 1:100.

Epinephrine

Epinephrine enhances analgesia and shortens onset when added to local anesthetic solutions (51,52). Epinephrine is a mixed α_1- and β-adrenergic agonist. Its ability to potentiate epidural local anesthetics is probably related to its α_1-agonist actions. Local α_2-agonist–mediated vasoconstriction may limit systemic absorption and keep more local anesthetic at its site of action. Stimulation of spinal cord α_2 receptors also can produce analgesia and contribute to epinephrine's effects. Epidural epinephrine increases motor block associated with local anesthetics (53). Local vasoconstriction and enhanced

TABLE 3. *Recommended doses of epidural opioids for labor analgesia*

Drug	Bolus injection[a]	Continuous infusion[b]
Fentanyl	50–100 μg	2–4 μg/mL
Sufentanil	10–15 μg	0.3–0.4 μg/mL

[a]Mix with 10–20 mL of 0.125% bupivacaine.
[b]Mix with 0.0625%–0.083% bupivacaine and infuse at 10–20 mL/h.

local anesthetic blockade probably explain this effect. The β-agonist action of epinephrine can inhibit uterine contractions and significantly slow labor. Dounas et al. (54) found that 10 mL of 0.25% bupivacaine mixed with 5 μg/mL of epinephrine significantly slowed labor compared with plain bupivacaine and bupivacaine mixed with epinephrine 1.66 μg/mL. Other potential adverse effects such as maternal tachycardia or decreased uterine blood flow are not clinically significant (55). In sum, epinephrine has little to offer as an adjuvant for labor epidural analgesia.

Clonidine

Clonidine is now available for epidural use in the United States. Epidural clonidine has been used in Europe for several years, and there are a few published reports of its use for labor analgesia. Epidural clonidine potentiates local anesthetics (improved pain scores, longer duration) without increasing motor block (56,57). Maternal and neonatal hemodynamic side effects are minimal and not clinically significant. Experience with this drug will determine its role in labor epidural analgesia.

TEST DOSES

Unrecognized intrathecal or intravascular injection of large doses of local anesthetic could have devastating consequences. To minimize these risks, many experts recommend injecting a "test dose," usually containing lidocaine and 15 μg epinephrine before giving the therapeutic dose of epidural local anesthetic (58). However, when inducing labor epidural analgesia, a separate "test dose" usually is unnecessary and may be detrimental. The local anesthetic content of most "test doses" (45 to 60 mg of lidocaine or 7.5 to 12.5 mg of bupivacaine) approaches or exceeds the amount used to induce labor epidural analgesia (Table 4). The extra local anesthetic (and epinephrine) included in the "test dose" increases the risk of a motor block. Giving the initial bolus in small increments will safeguard against unrecognized intrathecal injection.

Intravascular catheters often are detected by injecting epinephrine 15 μg. Tachycardia or subjective symptoms following this "test dose" are highly suggestive of intravascular injection. However, the major risk of unrecognized intravenous injection or infusion of dilute local anesthetic/opioid mixtures for labor epidural analgesia is inadequate pain relief, not systemic local anesthetic toxicity. Thus, the potential risks of epinephrine (increased motor block and decreased uterine activity) may outweigh its benefits in this setting. If the initial bolus of local anesthetic and opioid does not provide adequate analgesia, suspect an intravascular catheter. Look closely for changes in pinprick or temperature sensation. If present, try more local anesthetic. If absent, the catheter could be intravascular or simply not in the epidural space. In either case, replace it. By looking for signs and symptoms of epidural blockade, rather than simply injecting a "test dose" to rule out intrathecal or intravascular catheter location, one can safely provide labor epidural analgesia without unneeded local anesthetic or epinephrine (59).

TABLE 4. *Suggested techniques for labor analgesia*

Clinical Situation	Local Anesthetic	Adjuvants
Very early labor with mild pain (cervical dilation = 2 cm)	Bolus: None Infusion: 0.0625% bupivacaine 12–15 mL/h	Bolus: sufentanil 10–15 μg Infusion: sufentanil 0.33 μg/mL
Active labor, predicted time to second stage >1 h	Bolus: 0.125% bupivacaine 10–15 mL Infusion: 0.0625% bupivacaine 12–15 mL/h	Bolus: sufentanil 10–15 μg Infusion: sufentanil 0.33 μg/mL
Active phase of labor, predicted time to second stage <1 h	Bolus: 0.25% bupivacaine 10–15 mL Infusion: may hold or 0.0625% bupivacaine 12–15 mL/h	Bolus: sufentanil 10–15 μg Infusion: if used, sufentanil 0.33 μg/mL
Patient previously comfortable, still ≥ 1 h until pushing	Bolus: 0.25% bupivacaine 7–10 mL Infusion: increase rate by 20%	Bolus: ± sufentanil 5–10 μg
Patient requiring frequent top ups[a]	Bolus: 0.25% bupivacaine 7–10 mL Infusion: 0.125% bupivacaine 10–12 mL/h	Bolus: none if extra boluses of sufentanil already given Infusion: sufentanil 0.33 μg/mL ± epinephrine 1:200,000 and bicarbonate 0.5% by volume.
Patient entering second stage[a]	Severe pain with delivery expected within 45 min: 1% lidocaine 10–12 mL Moderate pain: 0.25% bupivacaine 10–12 mL	If lidocaine: bicarbonate (10% by volume)
Forceps delivery	1% or 2% Lidocaine	Bicarbonate (10% by volume)

[a]Assuming the catheter is correctly placed and provides for a good distribution of the local anesthetic (i.e., block not one sided, block will not move down to sacral roots, etc.). Unless you have evidence of good distribution of the local anesthetic, replace the catheter.

WALKING EPIDURAL

Ambulation may speed labor, and patients like the idea of being able to walk after receiving labor pain relief. These points explain much of the current fascination with "walking epidurals." Ambulation may be compatible with any epidural technique that minimizes motor block.

There are several questions that should be answered before allowing parturients to walk after induction of labor epidural analgesia:

- How much motor block is acceptable? We have tried to measure leg strength in an attempt to predict ability to ambulate. Only a trial of walking seems sufficiently sensitive and specific.
- Does impaired sensation, especially proprioception, make walking unsafe? People with dorsal column lesions can ambulate adequately. Despite detectable posterior column sensor impairment, patients can ambulate safely with epidural analgesia (60).
- Is hypotension a concern? Epidural local anesthetics decrease lower extremity sympathetic tone. In clinical practice, postural hypotension is rarely a problem. In one study, laboring women received intrathecal fentanyl 25 μg and bupivacaine 2.5 mg followed by intermittent epidural injections of 10 to 15 mL of 0.1% bupivacaine with 2 μg/mL fentanyl. Mean heart rate increased from 85 to 90 beats/min with ambulation, but blood pressure did not change significantly. Blood pressure fell below 100 mm Hg in only 1 of 35 women who ambulated (61).
- How badly do laboring women want to walk? In my experience, by the time most labor patients receive epidural analgesia, they are ready to stay in bed. Not once have I had a patient ask to walk outside her labor room. However, patients appreciate being able to walk to the bathroom or sit in a chair. Even if the patient does not ambulate, minimizing maternal motor blockade may improve satisfaction. These women need less assistance to change position in the bed and appear to push better in the second stage of labor.

If a patient does want to ambulate after induction of labor epidural analgesia, strive to minimize motor block. Use the lowest effective concentration of local anesthetic (preferably either bupivacaine or ropivacaine). Avoid epinephrine. Check blood pressure for orthostatic changes. Assess motor function (patients should be able to do a "modified deep knee bend"). Have an attendant walk with the patient.

CONTINUOUS INFUSIONS

Continuous epidural infusion techniques overcome many of the limitations of intermittent injection labor epidural analgesia. Compared with intermittent bolus techniques, continuous techniques require fewer interventions and provide greater patient satisfaction (62–65). Thus, continuous infusions benefit both anesthesiologist and patient.

Continuous infusions have a few potential limitations. Over the course of labor, continuous epidural infusions deliver more drug than intermittent bolus injections. However, the amount of drug remains well within safe limits for both mother and fetus (66). Continuous infusion of relatively concentrated local anesthetic solutions also may produce excessive maternal motor blockade. Using dilute local anesthetic/opioid mixtures minimizes this risk. Dilute local anesthetic/opioid mixtures are as effective as more concentrated solutions. For instance, laboring women who received an infusion of fentanyl and 0.0625% bupivacaine required no more top-ups than women who received an infusion of fentanyl and 0.125% bupivacaine (67). When using continuous epidural infusions for labor analgesia, evaluate the extent of sensory and motor block every 2 to 3 hours and change infusion rate or concentration if necessary.

PATIENT-CONTROLLED EPIDURAL ANALGESIA

Patient-controlled epidural analgesia (PCEA) is a relatively new technique that allows the patient to self-medicate and titrate to a desired level of pain relief. The usual practice is to induce epidural analgesia in the usual manner and then begin a "background" infusion of a dilute local anesthetic/opioid mixture (usually 6 to 8 mL/hour). Patients then self-medicate with additional drug as needed (usually 3- to 6-mL boluses every 15 to 30 minutes).

PCEA has been compared with continuous infusion techniques. With PCEA, patients use less drug, have similar levels of analgesia and satisfaction, and no differences in labor outcome or need for physician intervention (62,63,68). Compared to intermittent bolus techniques, pain control and satisfaction often are better with PCEA, but there are no differences in the amount of drug used (62,63,69,70). One study found an increased risk of instrumental vaginal deliveries with PCEA compared with intermittent boluses of local anesthetic (69).

In my opinion, any advantages of PCEA are rather insignificant compared to the cost of investing in new pumps. Additionally, I prefer the presence of a trained professional during bolus injections. There is a trend toward more episodes of hypotension with PCEA (62). Clinical experience will determine how prevalent this method will become in anesthetic practice.

SUGGESTED TECHNIQUES

The technique of labor epidural analgesia should be tailored to each patient. No single drug combination works in all clinical situations. Some important variables to consider include:

- Stage of labor,
- Acceptable degree of motor block,
- Patient expectations,
- Drug cost and availability, and
- Availability of qualified anesthetic personnel.

The following recommendations are based on my clinical practice. The obstetric suite at Stanford University Hospital is a hybrid academic/private practice. We have approximately 4,500 deliveries per year and about 30 obstetricians and obstetric residents. Only a couple of obstetricians object to early epidural anesthesia, and all prefer minimal motor block. Our cesarean section rate averages 15%. We provide continuous coverage with at least one anesthesia resident and one anesthesiologist. Our goal is to provide good analgesia with little motor block and minimal need for additional intervention (Table 4).

Most patients receive epidural analgesia in early labor (≤ 3-cm cervical dilation). At this point, pain is readily relieved by segmental block from T_{10} to L_2. Here, we induce analgesia with 12 to 15 mL of 0.125% bupivacaine with 10 μg of sufentanil. More dilute concentrations of bupivacaine often are inadequate. After the initial bolus, I begin a continuous infusion of 0.0625% bupivacaine with sufentanil 0.33 μg/mL at 12 to 15 mL/hour. I treat inadequate analgesia with 5 to 10 mL of 0.125% to 0.25% bupivacaine depending on the amount of pain and stage of labor.

I vary from this routine based on the clinical situation. I will initiate the block with 0.25% bupivacaine if the patient is close to the second stage of labor. Conversely, I will initiate the block with just opioid if the patient is in very early labor. If I need to rapidly provide analgesia for spontaneous or forceps delivery, I often give lidocaine with bicarbonate.

For the patient who does not get comfortable with these doses, I use bicarbonate and epinephrine to increase the analgesic potency of the local anesthetic/opioid mixture. I have a low threshold for replacing the epidural catheter. I believe that some patients have higher drug requirements, not because of differences in pain tolerance or drug sensitivity, but because of malpositioned catheters. In my experience, a patient who is requiring frequent top-ups and concentrated local anesthetics will respond to my usual drug mixtures after replacing the catheter.

REFERENCES

1. Cohen SE, Cherry CM, Holbrook RH, El-Sayed YY, Gibson RN, Jaffe RA. Intrathecal sufentanil for labor analgesia—sensory changes, side effects, and fetal heart rate changes. *Anesth Analg* 1993;77:1155.
2. Riley ET, Ratner EF, Cohen SE. Intrathecal sufentanil for labor analgesia: do sensory changes predict better analgesia and greater hypotension? *Anesth Analg* 1997;84:346.
3. Camann WR, Minzter BH, Denney RA, Datta S. Intrathecal sufentanil for labor analgesia. Effects of added epinephrine. *Anesthesiology* 1993;78:870.
4. Honet J, Arkoosh V, Norris M, et al. Comparison among intrathecal fentanyl, meperidine, and sufentanil for labor analgesia. *Anesth Analg* 1992;75:734.
5. Narahashi T, Frazier DT. Site of action and active form of local anesthetics. *Neurosci Res* 1971;4:65.
6. Strichartz GR, Ritchie JM. The action of local anesthetics on ion channels of excitable tissues. In: Strichartz GR, ed. *Local anesthetics. Handbook of experimental pharmacology, vol 81.* Berlin: Springer-Verlag, 1987:21.
7. Gasser HS, Erlanger J. The role of fiber size in the establishment of a nerve block by pressure or cocaine. *Am J Physiol* 1929;88:581.
8. Rosenberg PH, Heinonen E. Differential sensitivity of A and C nerve fibers to long-acting amide local anesthetics. *Br J Anaesth* 1983;55:163.
9. Wildsmith JAW, Gissen AJ, Takman B, Covino BG. Differential blockade: ester v. amides and the influence of pKa. *Br J Anaesth* 1987; 59:379.
10. Dietz FB, Jaffee RA. Bupivacaine preferentially blocks ventral root axons in rats. *Anesthesiology* 1997;86:172.
11. Columb MO, Lyons G. Determination of the minimum local analgesic concentrations of epidural bupivacaine and lidocaine in labor. *Anesth Analg* 1995;81:833.
12. Polley LS, Columb MO, Lyons G, Nair SA. The effect of epidural fentanyl on the minimum local analgesic concentration of epidural chloroprocaine in labor. *Anesth Analg* 1996;83:987.
13. Burger G. Audience Responses SOAP 97. *Society for Obstetric Anesthesia and Perinatology Newsletter.* Fall 1997.
14. Belfrage P, Berlin A, Raabe N, et al. Lumbar epidural analgesia with bupivacaine in labor. *Am J Obstet Gynecol* 1975;123:839.
15. Crawford JS. Lumbar epidural block in labour: a clinical analysis. *Br J Anaesth* 1972;44:66.
16. Bader AM, Fragneto R, Terui K, Arthur GR, Loferski B, Datta S. Maternal and neonatal fentanyl and bupivacaine concentrations after epidural infusion during labor. *Anesth Analg* 1995;81:829.
17. Steiger RM, Nageotte MP. Effect of uterine contractility and maternal hypotension on prolonged decelerations after bupivacaine epidural anesthesia. *Am J Obstet Gynecol* 1990;163:808.
18. Eddleston JM, Maresh M, Horsman EL, et al. Comparison of the maternal and fetal effects associated with intermittent or continuous infusion of extradural analgesia. *Br J Anaesth* 1992;69:154.
19. Abboud TK, Khoo SS, Miller F, et al. Maternal, fetal, and neonatal responses after epidural anesthesia with bupivacaine, 2-chloroprocaine, or lidocaine. *Anesth Analg* 1982;61:638.
20. Loftus JR, Holbrook RH, Cohen SE. Fetal heart rate after epidural lidocaine and bupivacaine for elective cesarean section. *Anesthesiology* 1991;75:406.
21. Clarke VT, Smiley RM, Finster M. Uterine hyperactivity after intrathecal injection of fentanyl for analgesia during labor: a cause of fetal bradycardia. *Anesthesiology* 1994;81:1083
22. Nielsen PE, Erickson JR, Abouleish EI, Perriatt S, Sheppard C. Fetal heart rate changes after intrathecal sufentanil or epidural bupivacaine for labor analgesia: incidence and clinical significance. *Anesth Analg* 1996;83:742.
23. Milaszkiewicz R, Payne N, Loughnan B, et al. Continuous extradural infusion of lignocaine 0.75% vs. bupivacaine 0.125% in primiparae: quality of analgesia and influence on labour. *Anaesthesia* 1992;47:1042.
24. Chestnut DH, Bates JN, Choi WW. Continuous infusion epidural analgesia with lidocaine: efficacy and influence during the second stage of labor. *Obstet Gynecol* 1987;69:323.
25. Chestnut DH, Vandewalker GE, Owen CL, Bates JN, Choi WW. The influence of continuous epidural bupivacaine analgesia on the second stage of labor and method of delivery in nulliparous women. *Anesthesiology* 1987;66:774.
26. Corke BC, Carlson CG, Dettbarn WD. The influence of 2-chloroprocaine on the subsequent analgesic potency of bupivacaine. *Anesthesiology* 1984;60:25.
27. Grice SC, Eisenach JC, Dewan DM. Labor analgesia with epidural bupivacaine plus fentanyl: enhancement with epinephrine and inhibition with 2-chloroprocaine. *Anesthesiology* 1990;72:623.
28. Camann WR, Hartigan PM, Gilbertson LI, et al. Chloroprocaine antag-

onism of epidural fentanyl: a receptor-specific phenomenon? *Anesthesiology* 1990;73:860.
29. Lyons G, Columb M, Hawthorne L, Dresner M. Extradural pain relief in labour: bupivacaine sparing by extradural fentanyl is dose dependent. *Br J Anaesth* 1997;78:493.
30. Kuhnert BR, Kuhnert PM, Philipson EH, et al. The half-life of 2-chloroprocaine. *Anesth Analg* 1986;65:273.
31. Kuhnert BR, Philipson EH, Pimental R, Kuhnert PM. A prolonged chloroprocaine epidural block in a postpartum patient with abnormal pseudocholinesterase. *Anesthesiology* 1982;56:477.
32. Ravindran RS, Bond VK, Tasch MD, Gupta CD, Luerssen TG. Prolonged neural blockade following regional analgesia with 2-chloroprocaine. *Anesth Analg* 1980;59:447.
33. Reisner LS, Hochman BN, Plumer MH. Persistent neurologic deficit and adhesive arachnoiditis following intrathecal 2-chloroprocaine injection. *Anesth Analg* 1980;59:452.
34. Stevens RA, Urmey WF, Urquhart BL, Kao TC. Back pain after epidural anesthesia with chloroprocaine. *Anesthesiology* 1993;78:492.
35. Hynson JM, Sessler DI, Glosten B. Back pain in volunteers after epidural anesthesia with chloroprocaine. *Anesth Analg* 1991;72:253.
36. Santos AC, Arthur GR, Wlody D, De Armas P, Morishima HO, Finster M. Comparative systemic toxicity of ropivacaine and bupivacaine in nonpregnant and pregnant ewes. *Anesthesiology* 1995;82:734.
37. Feldman HS, Dvoskin S, Halldin MH, Ask AL, Doucette AM. Comparative local anesthetic efficacy and pharmacokinetics of epidurally administered ropivacaine and bupivacaine in the sheep. *Reg Anesth* 1997;22:451.
38. Zaric D, Nydahl PA, Philipson L, Samuelsson L, Heierson A, Axelsson K. The effect of continuous lumbar epidural infusion of ropivacaine (0.1%, 0.2%, and 0.3%) and 0.25% bupivacaine on sensory and motor block in volunteers: a double-blind study. *Reg Anesth* 1996;21:14.
39. Cederholm I. Preliminary risk-benefit analysis of ropivacaine in labour and following surgery. *Drug Saf* 1997;16:391.
40. Wood MB, Rubin AP. A comparison of epidural 1% ropivacaine and 0.75% bupivacaine for lower abdominal gynecologic surgery. *Anesth Analg* 1993;76:1274.
41. Polley LS, Columb MS, Naughton NN, et al. Relative analgesic potencies of ropivacaine and bupivacaine for epidural analgesia in labor. *Anesth Analg* 1998;86:S384.
42. Sandu L, Mungie C, Ionescu C, et al. Clinical and experimental data on conduction anesthesia and analgesia with pethidine. *Chirurgie* 1983; 32:75.
43. Honet J, Arkoosh V, Norris M, et al. Comparison among intrathecal fentanyl, meperidine, and sufentanil for labor analgesia. *Anesth Analg* 1992;75:734.
44. Patel D, Janardhan Y, Merai B, et al. Intrathecal meperidine in endoscopic urologic procedures: a comparative study with local anesthetic. *Reg Anesth* 1989;14:49.
45. Famewo C, Naguib M. Spinal anaesthesia with meperidine as the sole agent. *Can Anaesth Soc J* 1985;32:533.
46. Acalovschi I, Ene V, Lorinczi E, Nicolaus F. Saddle block with pethidine for perineal operations. *Br J Anaesth* 1986;58:1012.
47. Baraka A, Maktabi M, Noueihid R. Epidural meperidine-bupivacaine for obstetric analgesia. *Anesth Analg* 1982;61:652.
48. Steinberg RB, Dunn SM, Dixon DE, Rehm KL, Pastides H, Hu X. Comparison of sufentanil, bupivacaine, and their combination for epidural analgesia in obstetrics. *Reg Anesth* 1992;17:131.
49. Vettermann J, Thomas H, Lischke V, Asskali F. Repeated addition of fentanyl to bupivacaine peridural analgesia in labor. Clinical action and fentanyl plasma level. *Anaesthesist* 1996;45:428.
50. Loftus JR, Hill H, Cohen SE. Placental transfer and neonatal effects of epidural sufentanil and fentanyl administered with bupivacaine during labor. *Anesthesiology* 1995;83:300.
51. Eisenach JC, Grice SC, Dewan DM. Epinephrine enhances analgesia produced by epidural bupivacaine during labor. *Anesth Analg* 1987;66:447.
52. Abboud TK, Sheik-ol-Eslam A, Yanagi T, et al. Safety and efficacy of epinephrine added to bupivacaine for lumbar epidural analgesia in obstetrics. *Anesth Analg* 1985;64:585.
53. Yarnell RW, Ewing DA, Tierney E, et al. Sacralization of epidural block with repeated doses of 0.25% bupivacaine during labor. *Reg Anesth* 1990;15:275.
54. Dounas M, O'Kelly B, Jamali S, Mercier FJ, Benhamou D. Maternal and fetal effects of adrenaline with bupivacaine (0.25%) for epidural analgesia during labour. *Eur J Anaesthesiol* 1996;13:594.
55. Albright GA, Jouppila R, Hollm SS, et al. Epinephrine does not alter human intervillous blood flow during epidural anesthesia. *Anesthesiology* 1981;54:131.
56. Cigarini I, Kaba A, Bonnet F, et al. Epidural clonidine combined with bupivacaine for analgesia in labor. Effects on mother and neonate. *Reg Anesth* 1995;20:113.
57. O'Meara ME, Gin T. Comparison of 0.125% bupivacaine with 0.125% bupivacaine and clonidine as extradural analgesia in the first stage of labour. *Br J Anaesth* 1993;71:651.
58. Mulroy MF, Norris MC, Liu SS. Safety steps for epidural injection of local anesthetics: review of the literature and recommendations. *Anesth Analg* 1997;85:1346.
59. Norris MC, Fogel ST, Dalman H, et al. Labor epidural analgesia without an intravascular "test dose." *Anesthesiology* 1998;88:1495.
60. Buggy D, Hughes N, Gardiner J. Posterior column sensory impairment during ambulatory extradural analgesia in labour. *Br J Anaesth* 1994; 73:540.
61. Shennan A, Cooke V, Lloyd-Jones F, Morgan B, de Swiet M. Blood pressure changes during labour and whilst ambulating with combined spinal epidural analgesia. *Br J Obstet Gynaecol* 1995;102:192.
62. Tan S, Reid J, Thorburn J. Extradural analgesia in labour: complications of three techniques of administration. *Br J Anaesth* 1994;73:619.
63. Purdie J, Reid J, Thorburn J, Asbury AJ. Continuous extradural analgesia: comparison of midwife top-ups, continuous infusions and patient controlled administration. *Br J Anaesth* 1992;68:580.
64. Smedstad KG, Morison DH. A comparative study of continuous and intermittent epidural analgesia for labour and delivery. *Can J Anaesth* 1988;35:234.
65. Hicks JA, Jenkins JG, Newton MC, Findley IL. Continuous epidural infusion of 0.075% bupivacaine for pain relief in labour. A comparison with intermittent top-ups of 0.5% bupivacaine. *Anaesthesia* 1988;43:289.
66. Jones G, Paul DL, Elton RA, McClure JH. Comparison of bupivacaine and bupivacaine with fentanyl in continuous extradural analgesia during labour. *Br J Anaesth* 1989;63:254.
67. Stoddart AP, Nicholson KEA, Popham PA. Low dose bupivacaine/fentanyl epidural infusions in labour and mode of deliverly. *Anaesthesia* 1994;49:1087.
68. Ferrante FM, Rosinia FA, Gordon C, Datta S. The role of continous background infusions in patient-controlled epidural analgesia for labor and delivery. *Anesth Analg* 1994:79:80.
69. Paech MJ, Pavy TJG, Sims C, Westmore MD, Storey JM, White C. Clinical experience with patient-controlled and staff-administered intermittent bolus epidural analgesia in labor. *Anaesth Intens Care* 1995;23:459.
70. Gambling DR, Huber CJ, Berkowitz J, et al. Patient-controlled epidural analgesia in labour: varying bolus dose and lockout interval. *Can J Anaesth* 1993;40:211.

Obstetric Anesthesia, second edition,
edited by Mark C. Norris.
Lippincott Williams & Wilkins, Philadelphia © 1999.

CHAPTER 18

Neuraxial Analgesia for Labor

Part IV: Effects on Progress and Outcome of Labor

Robert L. Eberle and Mark C. Norris

Obstetricians and anesthesiologists have long been debating the impact of epidural analgesia on the progress and outcome of labor. Sparking this dispute is the clear association between epidural labor analgesia and:

- Duration of the first stage of labor,
- Frequency of oxytocin use,
- Duration of the second stage of labor,
- Malpresentation,
- Instrumental delivery, and
- Cesarean delivery for dystocia.

Although many claim that epidural labor analgesia causes these problems, it is equally plausible that a preexisting condition, which creates prolonged, abnormal labor (with the attendant increased risk of cesarean delivery), also generates the request for effective pain relief (i.e., epidural analgesia).

This chapter discusses many aspects of this dispute. We review the studies reporting a relationship between epidural analgesia and the length of the first stage of labor, oxytocin use, the length of the second stage of labor, the use of forceps for delivery, the incidence of fetal malpresentation, and the frequency of cesarean delivery. We examine the many confounding variables that may affect both the course of labor and the request for epidural analgesia. In the end, maternal and fetal factors, plus variations in obstetric management, have a much greater impact on the progress and outcome of labor than does epidural analgesia. We hope to provide insight into the difficulties surrounding attempts to study this topic and to prepare you to critically interpret future studies on this important topic.

R. L. Eberle: Department of Anesthesiology, Albany Medical Center, Albany, New York 12208-3412.

M. C. Norris: Department of Anesthesiology, Washington University School of Medicine, St. Louis, Missouri 63110-1083.

METHODOLOGY

Nonrandomized Studies

This dispute persists partly because of the limitations inherent in the methodologies used to study it. Nonrandomized, retrospective comparisons usually report longer, more complicated labors in women who chose epidural analgesia versus those who do not (1–7). Because these authors sometimes assume that women who request epidural analgesia are similar to those who do not, they conclude that epidural analgesia impedes the progress of labor. However, women who request epidural analgesia often have signs of abnormal labor before any anesthetic intervention. Statistical models (multivariate or regression analysis) used to correct this problem often fail to include all known and unknown preexisting conditions (confounding variables). The following paragraphs review some of the confounding variables that can influence the outcome of nonrandomized studies.

Selection Bias

Selection bias can occur when patients are not randomly assigned to a treatment group. A confounding variable causes a patient to choose one treatment (i.e., epidural analgesia) over another (i.e., systemic opioids). These confounding variables can include inherent maternal and fetal characteristics as well as differences in anesthetic availability, and technique or obstetric management. Nonrandomized studies that attempt to control these variables with statistical tests are limited by our imperfect knowledge of the determinants of the progress and outcome of labor. Authors often fail to measure variables that can have profound effects on the progress of labor and the request for epidural analgesia.

Maternal Characteristics

Many readily measured maternal characteristics are associated with abnormal labor. Some of these variables include:

- Advanced age (8–12),
- Shorter height (9–11),
- Weight and body mass index (7,10–12),
- Ethnicity (13), and even
- Shoe size (14,15).

Parity is a recognized risk factor, and nulliparae are significantly more likely to have prolonged labor and cesarean delivery due to dystocia (1,12,16–21).

Other important maternal characteristics that correlate with abnormal labor are less readily measured and rarely considered in nonrandomized studies. For example, small pelvic outlet, determined by radiographic pelvimetry, predicts both occiput posterior presentation and the use of epidural labor analgesia (22). Presumably, posterior presentation produces more maternal pain than the more common occiput anterior and transverse positions. These women, then, are more likely to request epidural analgesia, producing a correlation between epidural block and occiput posterior presentation.

Maternal anxiety is another potential cause of prolonged labor (23–25). Anxiety can result from poor coping skills, concerns for safety, or pain (23). Anxiety in early labor correlates with elevated maternal catecholamine concentrations (23,24). These two variables correlate inversely with uterine activity and directly with the duration of labor (23,25). The severity of pain during the latent phase of labor predicts the duration of labor and the frequency of instrumental delivery (Figs. 1 and 2) (25). So pain or anxiety can be risk factors for complicated labor and are the major indications for requesting epidural labor analgesia.

Fetal Characteristics

Fetal size potentially affects the progress of labor (1,3,7,9,26,27). Larger infants require operative delivery more often. Infant age (9,10,28) and sex (11) also affect the progress of labor, possibly because of their effect on size.

Obstetric Characteristics

Some variables are difficult to label as maternal or fetal characteristics, but result from the interaction between fetal and maternal characteristics.

Cervical dilation on admission to the hospital correlates with the use of epidural analgesia. In most nonrandomized studies, women who eventually request epidural labor analgesia are admitted at lesser cervical dilation than those who request systemic or no analgesia (1,3,5–7, 9,10,26,27,29). Higher station of the fetal presenting part on admission correlates with both the later request for epidural analgesia (18,26) and the risk of cesarean delivery (9). Inducing epidural analgesia with the presenting part at high station predicts malpresentation at delivery when compared to placement at low station (27), but nonrandomized studies cannot determine if early epidural analgesia causes malpresentation or if preexisting malpresentation produced more pain at high station.

Dysfunctional or slow labor causes instrumental or cesarean delivery independent of the method of labor analgesia (18). In one study, inadequate uterine contractions were the most common cause of cesarean delivery (30).

The fetal–pelvic index, which compares fetal head and abdominal circumferences with respective maternal inlet and mid-pelvic circumferences, is a means of identifying the presence or absence of fetal–pelvic disproportion. A fetal–pelvic index greater than 1 is a more sensitive predictor of eventual dystocia cesarean section than pelvic outlet or infant size alone (31). Fetal–pelvic index correlates with the risk of operative delivery (both cesarean and forceps) in multiple patient populations (Table 1) (32–36). Intuition might predict that a tighter fitting fetus would produce more tissue destruction during labor and more pain. As yet, no studies have evaluated the ability of fetal–pelvic index to predict a request for epidural analgesia.

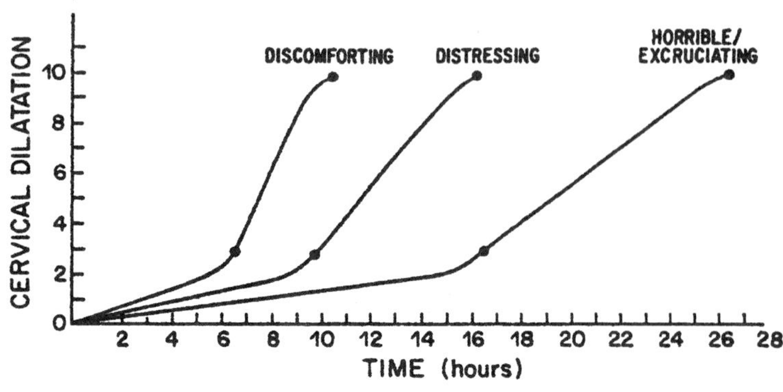

FIG. 1. Relationship between pain in latent labor and the rate of cervical dilation. (From ref. 25, with permission.)

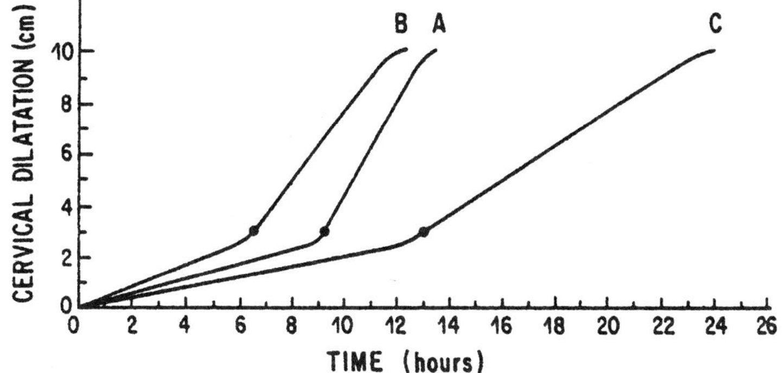

FIG. 2. Relationship between cognitive activity and rate of cervical change. *A,* coping related; *B,* equally coping related and distress related; *C,* distress related. (From ref. 25, with permission.)

Anesthetic Management

The specific technique of epidural labor analgesia may affect the progress of labor. Epidural local anesthetics cause motor blockade in a dose-dependent fashion (37–40). Motor block from concentrated local anesthetics may prolong the second stage of labor (37) and increase the need for forceps delivery (37–39). More concentrated local anesthetics may increase the risk of malpresentation (40). There are no data that suggest that more concentrated local anesthetics increase the risk of dystocia or cesarean section.

Epidural labor analgesia also can have indirect effects on the progress and outcome of labor. Intravenous fluids associated with induction of epidural analgesia can transiently decrease uterine activity (Fig. 3) (41,42). Epinephrine is commonly added to epidural local anesthetic solutions. Some studies report that epidural epinephrine, presumably because of its β-agonist activity, decreases the frequency of uterine contractions (43–45). Although these effects are transient and might not alter eventual outcome, they may affect the duration of labor (43).

Maternal position can alter uterine activity. Allowing the patient to lie supine results in more frequent, less intense, uterine contractions and increases basal uterine tone. Positioning a laboring woman on her side produces less frequent, but more effective, uterine contractions (46). Changes in uterine activity related to maternal position may be a result of altered hemodynamics from aortocaval compression (47).

Maternal position also may affect the course of labor independent of uterine activity. In one study, allowing the mother to walk with epidural analgesia resulted in fewer forceps deliveries and episiotomies (48). Maternal position can change pelvic inlet and outlet diameters (49–51). Both gravity and changes in pelvic geometry may produce the theoretical benefits of maternal upright position and ambulation.

Obstetric Management

Obstetric management too can alter the course of labor. "Active management of labor," which includes the

TABLE 1. *Fetal pelvic index >1 predicts the risk of cesarean delivery for dystocia*

Population	Number of patients	Sensitivity	Specificity	Positive predictive value	Negative predictive value	Accuracy
Mixed (32)	75[a]	85%	92%			89%
		87%	100%	100%	92%	
Macrosomia (estimated fetal weight >4,000 g) (33)	34	94%	94%	94%	94%	94%
Labor induction (34)	49	86%	100%	100%	95%	96%
	Nulliparae	85%	100%			93%
	Multiparae	100%	100%			100%
Abnormal labor requiring augmentation (35)	46	71%	95%	94%	75%	83%
	Protracted	88%	100%			94%
	Arrested	71%	80%			75%
Trial of labor after cesarean section (31)	65	72%	100%	100%	90%	
Nulliparae (37)	137	75%	97%			85%

Sensitivity, true positives/true positives + false negatives; specificity, true negatives/true negatives + false positives; positive predictive value, true positives/true positives + false positives; negative predictive value, true negatives/true negatives + false negatives; accuracy, correct results/all tests.

[a]Results reported differently in refs. 32, 37.

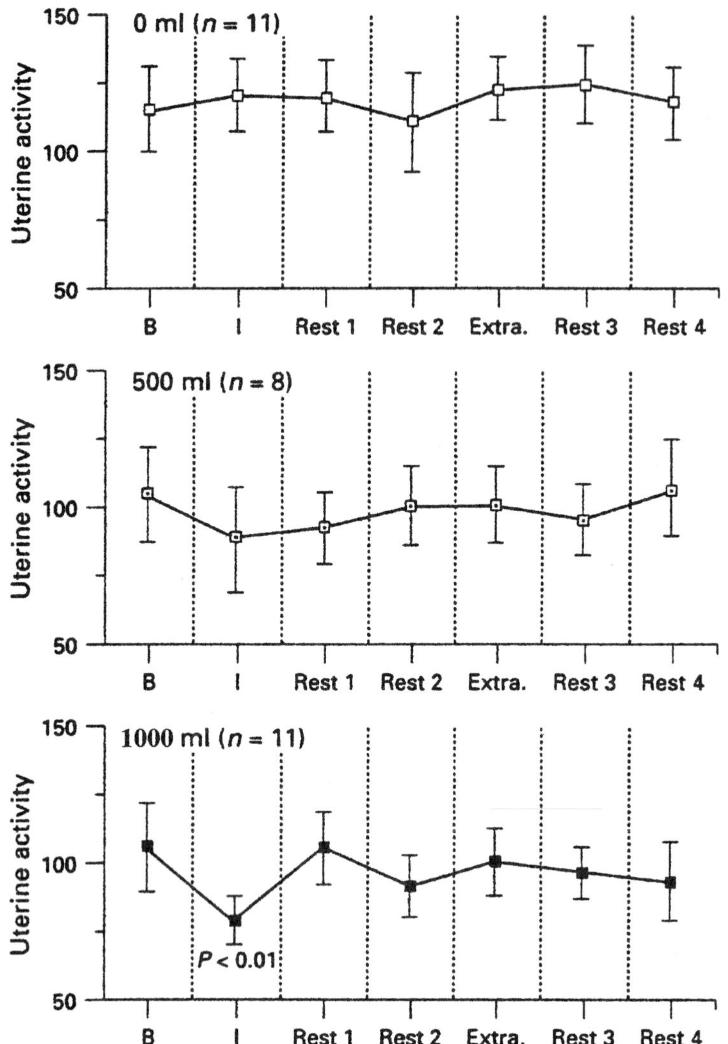

FIG. 3. Uterine activity (mean ± SD) after varying amounts of intravenous fluids. *B,* baseline; *I,* infusion; *Extra,* epidural injection. (From ref. 43, with permission.)

aggressive use of oxytocin and artificial rupture of membranes (AROM), is associated with a reduced frequency of cesarean delivery in some institutions (30,52–54). After the introduction of the active management of labor (catastrophe analysis), Akoury et al. (53) report a reduction in cesarean deliveries for nulliparae from 13% to 4.3% and a reduction in forceps deliveries from 29% to 7%, whereas the use of epidural labor analgesia remained constant (26% and 24%, respectively). In a randomized study, active management of labor reduced cesarean deliveries from 14.1% to 10.5% with no change in operative deliveries (cesarean plus instrumental deliveries) (54). The use of epidural analgesia was equal for both groups (72% and 70%). In another study, active management of labor shortened the duration of labor but did not decrease the frequency of cesarean delivery (55).

Other obstetric interventions can influence the progress of labor. For instance, Casey et al. (56) randomly assigned patients to receive a prostaglandin suppository followed in 4 hours by AROM, or immediate AROM and oxytocin stimulation (56). Patients who received prostaglandins had a shorter first stage of labor and less oxytocin requirement (56).

The use of cesarean section varies widely among obstetricians. In one hospital, where epidural analgesia was not readily available, the cesarean delivery rate ranged from 19.1% to 42.3% (21). Obstetrician, behind parity, was the second most important risk factor for cesarean delivery (21). Physician convenience can influence obstetric decisions. In another study, most cesarean deliveries for dystocia were performed in the early evening, after office hours (57). Guillemette and Fraser (58) compared obstetric outcomes between three obstetricians with low rates of cesarean section for dystocia with two others having higher rates. The two groups did not differ in their use of epidural analgesia or oxytocin. Obstetricians with lower rate of cesarean section intervened earlier in the second stage with forceps or vacuum.

Practice setting can alter the cesarean delivery rate (9,59,60). A retrospective study of 65,647 patients across four hospitals compared private and clinic patients (59). Private patients consistently had more cesarean deliveries (59). This risk persisted after adjusting for obstetric risk and birth weight (59). Another retrospective study reported marked differences in the use of cesarean section between private and clinic patients despite similar use of epidural labor analgesia (60). Cesarean delivery rates also differ by region (11).

Physician bias affects the use of epidural labor analgesia. Some obstetricians encourage labor epidural analgesia whereas others do not. Patients managed by obstetricians are more likely to receive epidural labor analgesia than those managed by family practice physicians and midwives (61). This difference may reflect the higher-risk population presumably seen by obstetricians compared to other health care providers, or a philosophical difference concerning labor pain or epidural analgesia among health care providers or patients. Another form of physician bias can exist if the presence of epidural analgesia affects obstetrician management. Here the question arises: Is an obstetrician more likely to perform an operative delivery simply because an epidural catheter is in place? Also, do patients at high risk for cesarean delivery alter anesthetic practice? Here a different question arises: Do anesthesiologists recommend epidural labor analgesia if they believe a cesarean section will be required?

Socioeconomic Factors

Socioeconomic factors correlate with both cesarean delivery (11,62) and epidural analgesia (61). These effects are likely indirect and due to differences in patient education and desires, or patient or fetal characteristics. Physician economic gain is another possible indirect socioeconomic effect. In one study, epidural analgesia was used more often for patients with private insurance (61). In another study, cesarean delivery was less frequent for patients with an income less than $11,000 per year (62).

Retrospective Analysis with Historical Controls

Another observational approach to this problem is "catastrophe" analysis. These studies examine the impact of sudden increase (or decrease) in the availability of epidural analgesia on the progress and outcome of labor and use historic, not contemporary, controls. Here, the risk of cesarean delivery does not correlate with the frequency of epidural labor analgesia (16,19,63–65). However, within each time period, patients receiving epidural analgesia are often at greater risk of cesarean delivery than those who do not (65). The risk of cesarean delivery associated with epidural labor analgesia often decreases with increases in the use of this technique (65). Presumably, when the availability of anesthetic care is limited, only patients with severe pain and prolonged labors receive epidural labor analgesia. When the use of epidural labor analgesia increases, lower-risk patients also receive this intervention (Tables 2 and 3).

As reassuring as these studies may be to the obstetric anesthesiologist, they too have their limitations. Concurrent, unrecognized changes in patient risk factors, nursing care, or obstetric management also may influence the risk of cesarean delivery. It may be difficult to retrospectively determine the true indication for a given cesarean delivery. Finally, the true effect of epidural analgesia on the progress and outcome of labor may become lost in the variation normally seen in any patient population.

Prospective Studies

The prospective randomized clinical trial is the most widely accepted method to determine the causative nature of an observed correlation. Here, however, even this approach has its limitations. Small studies lack statistical power to convincingly prove no difference (66–68). It is unethical to deny pain relief, so epidural analgesia is often compared to systemic narcotics (with the assumption that narcotics have no effects on the progress of labor). Other studies suffer from a high incidence of noncompliance and cross-over (patients randomized to one treatment group either decline any treatment or demand the alternative therapy) (68,69). Even if these problems could be eliminated, it is impossible to blind the obstetrician to the type of analgesia a patient receives. Thus, conscious or unconscious bias on the part

TABLE 2. *Impact of 24-h availability of epidural labor analgesia on maternal outcome*

Descriptor	Before[a] (n = 373)	After[a] (n = 421)	*p* Value
Operative deliveries	118 (31.6%)	147 (34.9%)	0.328
Operative vaginal deliveries	77 (20.6%)	105 (24.9%)	0.151
Operative vaginal deliveries for fetal concerns	25 (6.7%)	31 (7.4%)	0.717
Cesarean sections	41 (11.8%)	42 (10.0%)	0.641
Cesarean sections for fetal concerns	11 (2.9%)	18 (4.3%)	0.320
Cesarean sections for arrested labor	29 (7.8%)	22 (5.2%)	0.143
Third- or fourth-degree and cervical lacerations	47 (12.6%)	47 (11.2%)	0.532
Shoulder dystocia	18 (4.8%)	26 (6.2%)	0.407
Chorioamnionitis	14 (3.8%)	35 (8.3%)	0.008

[a]Before, 13.1% use epidural labor analgesia; after, 58.7% epidural labor analgesia.
Data from ref. 66.

TABLE 3. *Maternal outcome among patients receiving epidural labor analgesia*

Descriptor	Group 1E[a] (n = 49)	Group 2E[a] (n = 247)	*p* Value
Operative deliveries	30 (61.2%)	113 (45.7%)	0.048
Operative vaginal deliveries	12 (24.5%)	78 (31.6%)	0.324
Operative vaginal deliveries for fetal concerns	2 (4.1%)	18 (7.3%)	0.546
Cesarean sections	18 (36.7%)	35 (14.2%)	0.0002
Cesarean sections for fetal concerns	4 (8.2%)	13 (5.3%)	0.497
Cesarean sections for arrested labor	13 (26.5%)	20 (8.1%)	0.0002
Third- or fourth-degree and cervical lacerations	7 (14.3%)	26 (10.5%)	0.445
Shoulder dystocia	3 (6.1%)	19 (7.7%)	1.00
Chorioamnionitis	6 (12.2%)	33 (13.4%)	0.833

[a]Group 1E, patients receiving epidural labor analgesia *before* institution of a 24-h labor epidural service (13.1% use epidural labor analgesia); group 2E, patients receiving epidural labor analgesia *after* institution of a 24-h labor epidural service (58.7% use epidural labor analgesia). Group 2E includes more low-risk women; thus, the "effect" of epidural labor analgesia on outcome appears less.

Data from ref. 66.

of the patient or her medical care providers could influence obstetric outcome.

Summary

Retrospective analysis and nonrandomized observational studies have limited ability to show causality because of the failure to account for confounding variables. Studies using historical controls consistently find no impact of epidural analgesia on the incidence of cesarean delivery, but may miss small or unrecorded effects. The currently available randomized prospective trials are often too small or have a high cross-over rate. Still, considerable data concerning epidural analgesia and the progress and outcome of labor are currently available. The following sections will review these studies in an attempt to discern if epidural analgesia does cause prolonged labor, the need for oxytocin, malpresentation, and operative delivery. In reading the following sections, remember: "generally accepted criteria to define causality include strength of the association, consistency, biologic plausibility, specificity, dose-response gradient and temporality" (70).

EPIDURAL ANALGESIA AND THE FIRST STAGE OF LABOR

Several nonrandomized retrospective studies report a strong relationship between epidural analgesia and the duration of the first stage of labor (1,3–7). Some of these authors suggest that epidural analgesia causes prolonged labor (1,4,5,7).

A typical nonrandomized study retrospectively examined the impact of several factors on the risk of prolonged labor in 147 nulliparae who received epidural analgesia and a nonrandom matched control group of 147 women who did not (7). The authors reported a 5.9-fold increase in the risk of prolonged labor associated with epidural analgesia. The risk of prolonged labor increased by a factor of 42.5 if epidural analgesia was induced before 2 cm of cervical dilation. Maternal body mass index, cervical dilation on admission, oxytocin use, and birth weight also predicted prolonged labor. Multivariate conditional logistic regression analysis determined that epidural analgesia, induction of epidural analgesia before 2-cm cervical dilation, cervical dilation less than 2 cm on admission, and birth weight greater than 4,000 g were independent risk factors for prolonged labor. The authors concluded that early epidural placement and less advanced cervical dilation on admission were the most important predictors of prolonged labor. They suggest that epidural analgesia should be delayed until the cervix is more dilated to reduce the incidence of prolonged labor. (They did not make the equally plausible, but more obviously irrational, recommendation that hospital admission be delayed to prevent prolonged labor.) Remember, severe pain in early labor (i.e., less than 2-cm cervical dilation) is an independent predictor of prolonged labor (25) and, thus, women requesting epidural analgesia early in labor are already at increased risk of cesarean delivery. Delaying effective analgesia will only result in more pain, not a shorter labor.

In most of these nonrandomized, retrospective reports, women who requested epidural analgesia already had signs of abnormal labor before they received any anesthetic intervention. Patients who received epidural analgesia had less cervical dilation on admission and slower rates of cervical dilation before epidural placement (1,2,5,18). Other preexisting factors may influence both the request for epidural analgesia and the duration of the first stage of labor. Women who request epidural labor analgesia are carrying bigger fetuses than those who do not (3,7).

The correlation between epidural analgesia and prolonged first stage of labor is inconsistent. Some studies show no correlation (18,71) and others a shortening of the first stage associated with epidural analgesia (1,72,73). Thus, although some studies find a strong association between epidural analgesia and prolonged labor, the presence of so many confounding variables limits the plausibility of any cause-and-effect relationship.

Nonrandomized, prospective studies also report that epidural analgesia correlates with a prolonged first stage of labor (2,29,40). However, "this (correlation) may be due to the fact that patients who accepted the proposed epidural analgesia were most likely those destined to go through a protracted painful labor (2).

Any effect of epidural analgesia on labor must have a plausible biologic mechanism. In the case of prolonged first stage of labor, this mechanism would most likely involve the effects of epidural block on uterine contractility. However, neither in vitro nor clinical studies consistently show any effect of local anesthetics (47,74,75) or epidural analgesia on uterine activity.

Newton et al. (29) conducted a nonrandomized trial that attempted to address this issue. They used standardized oxytocin therapy to maintain cervical dilation rates. Patients receiving epidural analgesia were matched with control patients of the same parity. Myometrial activity was compared during the hour before induction of epidural analgesia (or the hour before control patients reached that same cervical dilation—the "reference point"), 1 hour after the reference point, and from the reference point to complete dilation. Myometrial activity was determined from rates of cervical dilation, uterine activity, oxytocin use, and operative delivery. Patients who received epidural labor analgesia had slower rates of cervical dilation *before* the reference point. After stratifying patients into those with initial cervical dilation rates of less than or greater than 1 cm/hour, rates of cervical dilation after the reference point were compared. Epidural analgesia did not affect uterine activity, but was associated with slower rates of cervical dilation. This effect was greatest in women who had an initial rate of dilation of less than 1 cm/hour. Patients in the epidural group had more operative deliveries.

This study confirms the association between epidural analgesia and prolongation of the first stage of labor. However, the authors made certain assumptions that may have predetermined their conclusion that epidural analgesia hindered cervical dilation. Two questions need to be answered to illustrate their assumptions. Were their patient groups comparable? If not, does their analysis support the contention that epidural analgesia was the cause of any subsequent differences? The answer to the first question is obviously "no." The patient groups were different from the start. Women who requested epidural analgesia already had slower rates of cervical dilation. That women having slow labor before the induction of epidural analgesia continue to have slow labor after the induction epidural analgesia is not surprising (18).

Even if epidural analgesia does not impair uterine activity, it may decrease the efficiency of uterine contractions. Nielson et al. (75) evaluated the effect of epidural analgesia on the pressure gradient between the upper and lower uterine segments (fundal dominance) (Fig. 4). They found a significant *increase* in fundal dominance after induction of epidural analgesia with 0.25% bupivacaine (Fig. 5) (75).

Not only have no studies shown that epidural analgesia inhibits uterine contractility, some have reported that

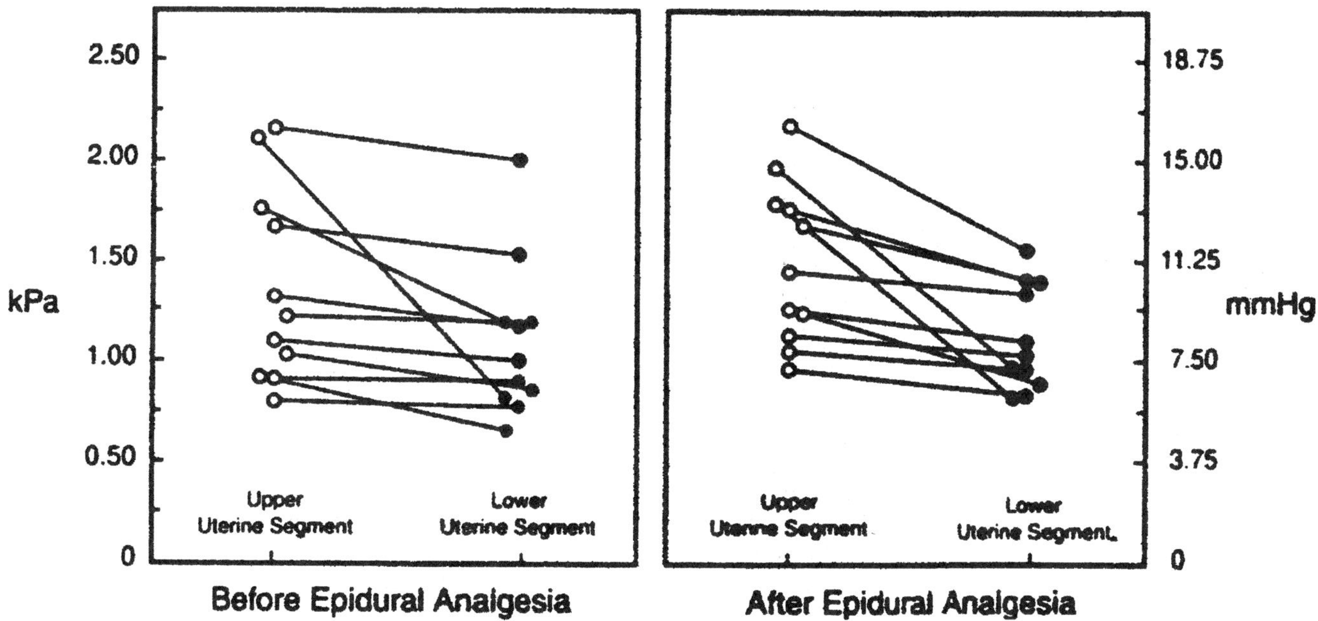

FIG. 4. Fundal dominance before and after epidural analgesia. Mean upper uterine segment pressure exceeds lower segment pressures both before and after induction of epidural labor analgesia (p <0.01). (From ref. 75, with permission.)

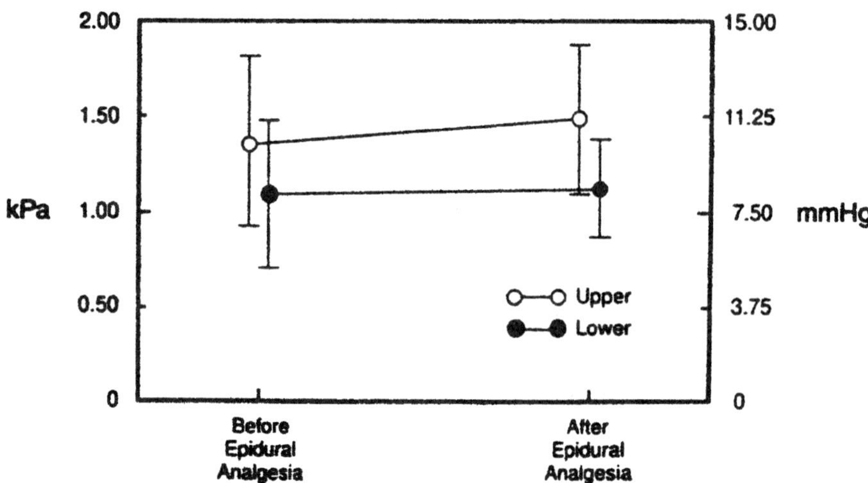

FIG. 5. The effect of epidural analgesia on fundal dominance. A significant increase in fundal dominance occurred after induction of epidural analgesia (p <0.001). (From ref. 75, with permission.)

epidural analgesia improves the efficiency of uterine contractions. In one study, the rate of cervical dilation increased after induction epidural analgesia in 6 of 9 primiparae and 5 of 9 multiparae (76). The authors suggest that pain relief could cause these improvements. Because this study lacked a control group, an alternative explanation, that the rate of cervical dilation and uterine efficiency improve as labor progresses, also is plausible. Still, this study suggests that epidural analgesia *per se* does not have any adverse effects on uterine activity.

If epidural analgesia alters the progress of labor, the effect should be consistent. A nonrandomized, prospective study compared 100 patients who received epidural analgesia to 100 patients who did not (77). Here, primiparae often had abnormal labor patterns before induction of epidural analgesia. Afterwards, the progress of labor "normalized" and there were no differences between the epidural and nonepidural groups.

Prospective randomized studies often report longer labors in women receiving epidural compared with systemic analgesia (66,69,78). These studies are either too small to allow firm conclusions (66,67) or compare labor duration only in protocol compliant women (69,78). (This issue is important. Eliminating women who progress too rapidly to receive their allocated epidural analgesia will prolong the apparent duration of labor in that group. Eliminating women assigned to the systemic medication group who demand epidural analgesia will shorten the average duration of labor in that group. Eliminating women who have little pain and may be at low risk for complicated labor will miss any effects that epidural labor analgesia has on uncomplicated labor.) One study with few cross-over patients did report a longer first stage of labor associated with epidural analgesia (260 vs 199 minutes) (78).

The effects of epidural analgesia on the first stage of labor are unclear. Although there is a strong association between epidural analgesia and the duration of labor, this finding is inconsistent and lacks a plausible biologic basis. Although nonrandomized studies often implicate epidural analgesia as a cause of prolonged labor, it is equally plausible that some women who request epidural analgesia are already having painful, dysfunctional labors.

OXYTOCIN USE AND EPIDURAL ANALGESIA

In retrospective studies, oxytocin use during the first stage of labor is strongly associated with epidural analgesia (1,3,5,60). This effect is especially strong when epidural analgesia is induced with the fetus at high station (27). Because oxytocin use is often associated with more painful labor, epidural analgesia may be induced before planned oxytocin augmentation in anticipation of increased pain (6,65). This factor adds to the many difficulties that surround the interpretation of data from nonrandomized studies (see previous). In a nonrandomized prospective study, despite equal use of oxytocin before induction, patients who received epidural analgesia more often required oxytocin augmentation with greater drug doses than matched controls (29). Although this study shows a strong association between epidural analgesia and oxytocin augmentation, it was not randomized. It is possible (but unknowable) that patients in the epidural group would have required additional oxytocin even without anesthetic intervention. One prospective, randomized comparison of epidural and systemic labor analgesia also reported more use of oxytocin augmentation after induction of analgesia in patients in the epidural group (33% vs 15%) (78).

EPIDURAL ANALGESIA AND MALPRESENTATION

Malpresentation of the fetal head is a potential cause of dystocia and may prolong the second stage of labor and increase the need for forceps or cesarean delivery. Epidural labor analgesia has been implicated as a cause of malpresentation (3,5). Epidural local anesthetics can

TABLE 4. *Method of delivery in women receiving differing concentrations of epidural local anesthetic*

	Control (n = 40)	High-dose infusion (n = 40)	Low-dose infusion (n = 38)
Spontaneous vaginal delivery	30	15[a]	19[a]
Neville-Barnes forceps	6	5	13[b]
Kiellands forceps	0	11[c]	2
Ventouse extraction	2	5	1
Cesarean section	2	4	3

High-dose infusion, 0.125% bupivacaine + 1 µg/mL fentanyl at 10 mL/h; low-dose infusion; 0.0625% bupivacaine + 1 µg/mL fentanyl at 10 mL/h.
[a]$p < 0.05$ vs control; [b]$p < 0.05$ vs high-dose infusion; [c]$p < 0.01$ vs low-dose infusion.
Data from ref. 41.

produce motor blockade and muscle weakness. The resultant relaxation of pelvic floor muscles may contribute to malrotation of the fetal head as labor progresses. Nonrandomized studies often report a higher incidence of malpresentation among patients receiving epidural compared with systemic analgesia (3,5). However, differences in maternal pelvic capacity can influence both the request for epidural analgesia and the incidence of malpresentation (22). Women with small pelvises are more likely to have persistent malpresentations. Pain related to malrotation then increases their use of epidural analgesia.

Still, anesthetic management can have an impact on the frequency of malpresentation. Stoddart et al. (40) induced epidural labor analgesia with 0.5% bupivacaine and then randomly assigned women to receive an epidural infusion of either 0.125% bupivacaine or 0.0625% bupivacaine plus fentanyl. Patients in the 0.0625% bupivacaine group received less bupivacaine and required fewer rotational forceps, suggesting a lower incidence of malpresentation. The use of Kiellands rotational forceps was the same in the 0.0625% bupivacaine group as in a matched, no analgesia control group, but more patients still required Neville-Barnes outlet forceps in the epidural group (Table 4). Thus, epidural analgesia using dilute local anesthetic/opioid mixtures may not increase the risk of malpresentation and rotational forceps. However, more concentrated local anesthetic solutions may. Alternatively, preexisting malpresentation may produce more pain and the eventual request for effective labor analgesia. Then, epidural analgesia with minimal motor block allows spontaneous correction of malpresentation, but does not reduce the requirement for operative delivery (reflecting the more complicated labors in women who request epidural labor analgesia).

EPIDURAL ANALGESIA AND THE SECOND STAGE OF LABOR

The second stage of labor starts at full cervical dilation and ends with delivery. As with the issues discussed previously, considerable controversy surrounds the role of epidural analgesia and the progress and outcome of the second stage of labor. In nonrandomized studies, epidural analgesia is usually associated with a longer second stage (1,4–6,18,40,73). Many studies report this correlation regardless of the duration of the first stage of labor or the use of oxytocin (18,73). Some authors report that this prolongation persists even if no additional epidural medications are given during the second stage of labor (allowing the epidural to "wear off") (6). Many authors argue that this correlation reflects a direct effect of epidural analgesia (1,2,5,29). Epidural labor analgesia may impair internal rotation of the fetal head by abolishing the maternal pushing reflex and relaxing the pelvic floor (1). One nonrandomized study did not find an increase in the duration of the second stage of labor associated with epidural analgesia, but the strength of such a negative result is limited because few patients were studied (i.e., the study had inadequate power to detect any true difference) (77).

One nonrandomized study using a historical control group has examined the impact of a sudden *decrease* in the use of epidural analgesia on the duration of the second stage of labor. In a hospital in Tennessee, the use of epidural labor analgesia in primiparae fell from 80% to 33% after changes in insurance coverage (19). The mean duration of the second stage of labor was reduced from 84 to 46 minutes. For multiparae, the epidural rate changed from 63% to 40%, and the second stage of labor was shortened from 40 to 17 minutes. Lyon et al. (65) report a 10-minute increase in the duration of the second stage of labor after the introduction of an elective epidural service in a military hospital (the epidural rate increased from 13.1% to 58.7%).

Evidence that epidural analgesia can prolong the second stage of labor also is apparent in prospective randomized studies that compare different epidural analgesia management techniques. In one such study, nulliparae with functioning epidural catheters randomly received a continuous infusion of either 0.125% bupivacaine or saline after 8-cm cervical dilation (37). Patients in the saline group had more pain, less motor block, a shorter second stage of labor, and fewer forceps deliveries (Table 5). There were no differences in the use of rotational forceps or the number of cesarean deliveries

TABLE 5. *Effect of epidural analgesia (0.125% bupivacaine) on the second stage of labor*

	Bupivacaine (n = 46)	Saline (n = 46)	*p* Value
Duration of active phase of first stage (min)[a]	354 ± 236	331 ± 182	NS
Duration of known bupivacaine infusion (min)[a]	173 ± 126	221 ± 138	NS
Bupivacaine dosage before start of study solution (mg)[a]	82 ± 42	94 ± 40	NS
Bupivacaine dosage after start of study solution (mg)[a]	49 ± 28	0	
Total bupivacaine dosage (mg)[a]	132 ± 60	94 ± 40	<0.005
Duration of second stage (min)[a,b]	124 ± 70	94 ± 54	<0.05
Motor block at start of study solution			
None	23 (50%)	26 (57%)	NS
Partial	19 (41%)	16 (35%)	
Almost complete	4 (9%)	4 (9%)	
Complete	0 (0%)	0 (0%)	
Motor block before delivery			
None	24 (52%)	41 (89%)	<0.0005
Partial	18 (39%)	4 (9%)	
Almost complete	4 (9%)	1 (2%)	
Complete	0 (0%)	0 (0%)	
Position of vertex immediately before delivery			NS
Occiput anterior	39 (85%)	40 (87%)	
Occiput posterior	6 (13%)	5 (11%)	
Occiput transverse	1 (2%)	1 (2%)	

Patients in the bupivacaine group received epidural infusion of 0.125% bupivacaine until delivery. Women in the saline group received epidural saline infusion after 8-cm cervical dilation.

NS = not significant.

[a]Mean ± SD.

[b]Excluding six women in each group who underwent cesarean delivery.

Data from ref. 38.

TABLE 6. *Effect of epidural analgesia (0.125% bupivacaine) on the method of vaginal delivery*

	Bupivacaine (n = 40)	Saline (n = 40)	*p* Value
Spontaneous	19 (48%)	29 (73%)	<0.05
Low forceps	12 (30%)	7 (18%)	
Mid vacuum followed by low forceps	6 (15%)	0 (0%)	
Mid forceps	3 (8%)	4 (10%)	

Patients in the bupivacaine group received epidural infusion of 0.125% bupivacaine until delivery. Women in the saline group received epidural saline infusion after 8-cm cervical dilation.

Data from ref. 38.

TABLE 7. *Effect of epidural analgesia (0.0625% bupivacaine with 2 μg/mL fentanyl) on the second stage of labor*

	Bupivacaine-fentanyl (n = 29)	Saline (n = 34)
Duration of active phase of first stage (min)[a]	316 ± 188	317 ± 199
Duration of known bupivacaine-fentanyl infusion (min)[a]	227 ± 159	215 ± 164
Bupivacaine dosage before start of study solution (mg)[a]	47 ± 30	44 ± 29
Bupivacaine dosage after start of study solution (mg)[a]	16 ± 13	0
Fentanyl dosage before start of study solution (μg)[a]	169 ± 80	161 ± 84
Fentanyl dosage after start of study solution (μg)[a]	50 ± 41	0
Duration of second stage (min)[b]	53 (5–283)	63 (16–181)
Position of vertex immediately before delivery		
Occiput anterior	27 (93%)	31 (91%)
Occiput posterior	1 (3%)	3 (9%)
Occiput transverse	1 (3%)	0 (0%)

Nulliparous women had epidural labor analgesia with a continuous infusion of 0.0625% bupivacaine + fentanyl 2 μg/mL. At complete cervical dilation, patients received a blinded infusion of either 0.0625% bupivacaine + fentanyl 2 μg/mL (bupivacaine-fentanyl) or saline.

[a]Mean ± SD.

[b]Median (range) (excluding one woman in the bupivacaine-fentanyl group who underwent cesarean section after full cervical dilation).

Data from ref. 80.

TABLE 8. *Effect of epidural analgesia (0.0625% bupivacaine with 2 μg/mL fentanyl) on the method of vaginal delivery*

	Bupivacaine-fentanyl (n = 28)	Saline (n = 34)
Spontaneous	22 (79%)	29 (85%)
Outlet forceps	0 (0%)	0 (0%)
Low forceps	2 (7%)	4 (12%)
Mid forceps	2 (7%)	1 (3%)
Mid vacuum followed by low forceps	2 (7%)	0 (0%)

Nulliparous women had epidural labor analgesia with a continuous infusion of 0.0625% bupivacaine + fentanyl 2 μg/mL. At complete cervical dilation, patients received a blinded infusion of either 0.0625% bupivacaine + fentanyl 2 μg/mL (bupivacaine-fentanyl) or saline.
Data from ref. 80.

(Table 6). A similar study substituted saline for 0.0625% bupivacaine with 2 μg/mL fentanyl at full cervical dilation (79). With this dilute local anesthetic/opioid mixture, the vast majority of patients (97%) had no detectable motor block. Continuing the bupivacaine/fentanyl infusion provided better pain relief without any increase in the duration of labor or the use of forceps for delivery compared with saline (Tables 7 and 8). Six patients, five in the bupivacaine/fentanyl group and one in the saline group, had a prolonged second stage of labor (greater than 180 minutes).

One prospective, randomized study compared epidural and intravenous analgesia during the second stage of labor (78). Although there were no differences in the duration of the second stage of labor, more women in the epidural group had an instrumental delivery. Obstetric intervention is an important variable to consider when evaluating studies of the impact of epidural analgesia on the second stage of labor.

Most observational studies find a correlation between epidural analgesia and the duration of the second stage of labor. Although epidural analgesia seems to prolong the second stage of labor, the role of obstetric intervention and anesthetic technique must be considered. Prospective randomized studies suggest that epidural infusion of dilute local anesthetic/opioid mixtures have little effect on the duration of the second stage of labor.

EPIDURAL ANALGESIA AND INSTRUMENTAL DELIVERY

Forceps or vacuum extraction can facilitate vaginal delivery. Instrumental delivery is classified as outlet, low forceps, or mid forceps, based on the station of the fetal skull (80). Vacuum extraction often is used in place of forceps delivery. In addition, instrumental rotation may be used for failure of spontaneous internal rotation of the fetal head and is considered basic for rotations of less than 45 degrees and complex if greater than 45 degrees (80). Prerequisites for placement of forceps include complete dilation and a fetal head engaged in the pelvis (80). Pudendal block, epidural block, spinal block, or occasionally general anesthesia may be necessary (80). Indications for instrumental delivery vary. Fetal indications include a nonreassuring fetal status, failure to deliver after a prolonged second stage of labor with an indication to shorten the second stage, and failure to deliver after an appropriately managed second stage (80). Maternal indications include avoiding voluntary expulsive effort (cardiac or cerebrovascular disease) or inability to push effectively due to neuromuscular disease, exhaustion, lack of cooperation, or excessive anesthesia (80). Operative delivery (instrumental or cesarean delivery) may be considered in nulliparae for a second stage longer than 2 hours, or 3 hours with a regional anesthetic (80). For multiparae, operative delivery may be considered after 1 hour, or 2 hours with a regional anesthetic (80). A longer second stage is permissible provided appropriate fetal monitoring is used and the fetal status is reassuring (81).

Determining the effects of epidural analgesia on the frequency of instrumental delivery can be complex. Effective epidural analgesia makes it easier to perform an instrumental delivery (1). Differences in obstetric and anesthetic management may influence the use of instrumental delivery.

Nonrandomized, retrospective studies most often report a strong correlation between epidural analgesia and instrumental delivery (1,4,5,73,82,83). This association is seen with primiparous and multiparous patients. In some settings, this correlation probably reflects the philosophy that "a simple forceps delivery as early as possible in the second stage of labor is outstandingly the most advantageous for both mother and infant" (73). Although a prolonged second stage is cited as the most common reason to deliver with forceps, it is apparent from the previous quotation that many forceps deliveries for "prolonged second stage" may, in reality, be elective. In many of these studies, intervention for prolonged second stage occurred at 2 hours, not the currently recommended 3 hours (82,83). Retrospective studies often fail to clearly identify the indications for forceps delivery, and the type of forceps delivery and anesthetic technique used. As a result, they are of little use in determining the cause(s) of the association between epidural analgesia and instrumental delivery.

Prospective, nonrandomized studies using "matched" control patients also show an increase in instrumental delivery associated with epidural analgesia (2,10,17,29). These studies often fail to identify an allowable length of the second stage (2,10,17,29), the fetal presentation (2,29), or the type of instrumental delivery (2,29). A typical example prospectively analyzed 925 nulliparae (10). Multiple logistic regression analysis concluded that epidural analgesia increased the relative risk of operative delivery (mid forceps and cesarean delivery). As with all nonrandomized studies, regression analysis cannot control for unmeasured or unknown variables (see previous). These authors failed to define clearly the allowable length of the second stage of labor or fetal presentation. They also combined forceps and cesarean delivery, limiting our ability to interpret their results.

Hawkins et al. (28) retrospectively reviewed 14,804 deliveries before and after the introduction of an epidural service. Epidural analgesia was strongly associated with instrumental delivery both when the epidural rate was 3% and after it rose to 27%. Interestingly, the association between epidural analgesia and instrumental delivery was greater for multiparae than nulliparae. Hawkins et al. (28) also report data from a prospective case controlled study. Patients having an instrumental delivery were matched with patients who did not. Stage two of labor typically was allowed to last 2 to 3 hours, and patients frequently pushed for more than 2 hours. Instrumental delivery was not separated by type and included vacuum extraction, low outlet, or mid pelvic forceps. Several variables were associated with instrumental delivery, including gravity, parity, gestational age, duration of stage two, malposition (occiput posterior or transverse), infant weight, prior cesarean delivery, and epidural analgesia. The authors used multivariate analysis in an attempt to control for confounding factors. Again, epidural analgesia was associated with instrumental delivery, especially in multiparae. Four other variables also were independently associated with instrumental delivery: gestational age, duration of stage two, presentation, and prior cesarean delivery. Hawkins et al. (28) concluded that epidural analgesia is associated with instrumental delivery, but they could not determine causation.

The application of forceps is a clinical decision. Variables that influence this decision include expedited delivery for "fetal distress," teaching, physician convenience, physician preference, and ease of application due to the superior analgesia that epidural block provides. Some of these variables may be inaccurately measured or skewed because of reporting bias.

Obstetric and anesthetic management can have significant effects on the duration of the second stage and the frequency of instrumental delivery rates. Some authors believe that simply allowing the second stage to last longer lessens the need for rotational forceps delivery (18). Randomized studies also show the impact of obstetric or anesthetic management on the incidence of instrumental deliveries. Delayed pushing allows more spontaneous vaginal deliveries and fewer forceps deliveries without any fetal compromise (84). Starting oxytocin at the beginning of the second stage shortens its duration and reduces nonrotational forceps deliveries (85). Lower concentrations of epidural local anesthetics, presumably by reducing motor block, improving the urge or ability to push, or reducing pelvic floor relaxation allowing improved rotation of the fetal head, result in more spontaneous vaginal deliveries and fewer forceps deliveries (38–40).

The association between epidural analgesia and instrumental delivery is common in observational studies. Although the relationship is strong, too many variables exist for nonrandomized studies to determine if epidural analgesia causes instrumental deliveries, if it merely influences the decision to use forceps, or if there is some other unknown factor that causes both epidural analgesia and instrumental delivery.

EPIDURAL ANALGESIA AND CESAREAN DELIVERY

Nonrandomized Studies

Epidural analgesia correlates with cesarean delivery in nonrandomized studies (2–6,9,10,26). Nonrandomized studies are prone to selection bias, so regression analysis often is used to control for measured confounding variables (3,26). Thorp et al. (3) retrospectively analyzed 711 nulliparae who delivered following actively managed labors. The cesarean delivery rate for dystocia was 10.3% for patients who received epidural analgesia and 3.8% for those that did not (3). Patients who received epidural analgesia also had lesser cervical dilation on admission, more oxytocin use, higher birth weights, and longer labors (3). After using regression analysis to compensate for age, race, gestational age, cervical dilation on admission, oxytocin use, duration of oxytocin use, maximum infusion rate of oxytocin, duration of labor, presence of meconium, and birth weight, the correlation between epidural analgesia and cesarean delivery due to dystocia remained (3). Among the important confounding variables not considered in their analysis were fetal–pelvic index, and maternal pain and anxiety (see previous).

Thorp et al. (5) published a follow-up study that attempted to identify factors that increase the risk of cesarean delivery in nulliparae receiving epidural analgesia. Five hundred term, nulliparae with spontaneous labor and cervical dilation less than 5 cm were included. All labors were actively managed (5). Patients with similar cervical dilation on admission were further subdivided by the rate of cervical dilation and cervical dilation at epidural placement (for a total of six subgroups) (5). Comparisons were made between subgroups with similar patient characteristics. Overall, the cesarean delivery rate was 15.6% for patients who received epidural analgesia and 2.4% for those who did not. After comparing different subgroups, the correlation between epidural analgesia and cesarean delivery for dystocia was greatest when initial cervical dilation was slow and the epidural was placed before 3 cm of cervical dilation (5).

Thorp et al. offer several theories to explain the impact of epidural labor analgesia on the cesarean delivery rate. These possibilities include decreased uterine activity, prolongation of the first stage of labor, relaxation of the pelvic diaphragm predisposing to minor malpresentation, decreased maternal urge to push, decreased ability to push, and prolonged second stage with an increased incidence of instrumental delivery (with cesarean delivery being chosen over instrumental delivery due to medical legal concerns). As seen previously, there is little evidence to support any effect of epidural analgesia on uterine activity or the first stage of labor. Although epidural analgesia may prolong the second stage of labor, the decision to perform an operative delivery is highly subjective and can be influenced by the very presence of an epidural block.

As with the other issues discussed in this chapter, unmeasured or unknown confounding factors may produce the association between epidural analgesia and cesarean section seen in these nonrandomized studies. For example, women with positive fetal–pelvic indexes may have more severe labor pain and be more likely to request epidural labor analgesia and to eventually require a cesarean delivery (31).

Lieberman et al. (26) also attempted to evaluate the association between epidural analgesia during the first stage of labor and cesarean delivery in a retrospective study of 1,733 low-risk nulliparae in spontaneous labor. Patients who received epidural analgesia had larger infants, were admitted earlier in labor, and were dilating more slowly than those who required no or systemic labor analgesia. These authors attempted to "simulate randomization" by dividing patients into quintiles based on how likely they were to receive epidural labor analgesia (Tables 9 and 10). Measured maternal, pregnancy, and labor characteristics were similar within each quintile. They then compared patients who did and did not receive epidural analgesia within each quintile. Cesarean delivery was highest in the quintile with the most frequent use of epidural analgesia and lowest in the quintile with the least frequent use. Within each quintile, epidural analgesia was associated with cesarean delivery (Fig. 6). This association existed regardless of the timing of analgesia, but was greatest when the block was placed at low dilation and high station.

The authors recognize that within their nonrandomized study, patients who requested epidural analgesia may have been inherently different from those who did not. Still, they conclude that epidural analgesia increases the risk of cesarean delivery. They argue that any factor causing slow abnormal labor, severe pain, the request for epidural analgesia, and eventual cesarean delivery could only occur in a few patients. Almost two-thirds of their patients received epidural analgesia, yet not all of those women had dysfunctional labor. (This argument misses the point. In any patient population, a fixed number of women will have dysfunctional labor and may require cesarean section for dystocia. Because severe pain is a symptom of dystocia, these women will be more likely to request epidural analgesia. However, not all women who request epidural analgesia have severe pain, nor is all severe labor pain due to dystocia. Thus, women who request labor epidural analgesia are more likely to have dystocia than those who do not, but not all women who request epidural analgesia suffer from dystocia.) Many of the variables that predict the request for epidural labor analgesia also are independent risk factors for cesarean section (i.e., maternal age, weight, rate of cervical dilation). Thus, these data may merely indicate that women at high risk for cesarean section are likely to undergo cesarean section. As with other nonrandomized studies, unmeasured (i.e., pelvic capacity, fetal–pelvic index) or unknown variables may confound their results.

TABLE 9. *Variables examined to predict the likelihood of use of epidural labor analgesia among 1,733 low-risk nulliparae*

Maternal demographic/physical characteristics
Maternal age
Maternal race: white,[a] black, Hispanic, other
Insurance: private, public, other
Maternal prepregnant weight[a]
Maternal height[a]
Pregnancy and labor characteristics
Infant birth weight[a]
Gestational duration[a]
Male infant
Dilation at admission (cm)[a]
Initial rate of cervical dilation (cm/h)[a]
Station of the fetal head at admission[a]
Treated with active management of labor[a]
Ruptured membranes at admission
Maternal chronic hypertension
Maternal pregnancy-induced hypertension

[a]Selected by stepwise regression for model to predict likelihood of receiving epidural labor analgesia.
Data from ref. 26.

The correlation between epidural analgesia and cesarean delivery is not universal (6,18,83). One very large retrospective study (7,317 patients) failed to find any association between these two variables (83).

Prospective nonrandomized studies are inconsistent as well. One study concluded that epidural analgesia increases the risk for cesarean delivery with either active or traditional management of labor (9). A similar study

TABLE 10. *Characteristics of women according to use of epidural analgesia*

Characteristic	Epidural (n = 991)	No epidural (n = 742)
Demographic and physical characteristics		
Mean maternal age (yr)	29.4	29.2
White maternal race[a]	73%	67%
Private insurance	88%	85%
Mean prepregnant weight (lb)[a]	133.9	131.4
Mean maternal height (in.)[a]	64.5	65.0
Pregnancy/labor characteristics		
Mean birth weight (g)[a]	3463	3378
Mean gestational age (wk)[a]	40.2	39.9
Male infant	51%	52%
Mean dilation at first exam (cm)[a]	2.8	3.9
Mean initial rate of dilation (cm/h)[a]	0.5	1.2
Fetal station at admission -2 or -3[a]	27%	13%
Treated with active management of labor[a]	27%	34%
Cesarean delivery[a]	17%	4%

[a] p <0.05.
Data from ref. 26.

also found a correlation between epidural analgesia and operative delivery (cesarean delivery, mid forceps, and rotational forceps) (10). These authors did not conclude that epidural analgesia causes operative delivery because several important confounding variables were not measured (the progress of labor before epidural placement, timing of epidural placement, etc.) (10). Another prospective study examined factors that contribute to the use of epidural analgesia (6). Here, too, there was a correlation between epidural analgesia and cesarean delivery, but significance was lost when considering the type of labor (spontaneous, augmented, or induced) (6).

Several studies have used historical control groups to study the impact of a sudden change in the use of labor epidural analgesia on the frequency of cesarean delivery. With the introduction of 24-hour obstetric anesthesia coverage, the use of labor epidural analgesia increases. If a cause-and-effect relationship exists, the frequency of dystocia should rise with the increased use of labor epidural analgesia. In these studies, the rates of cesarean or operative delivery remain stable (Table 11) (16,19,65,86).

Decreasing the use of labor epidural analgesia also does not reduce the frequency of cesarean delivery (19). Johnson and Rosenfeld (19) report a constant cesarean

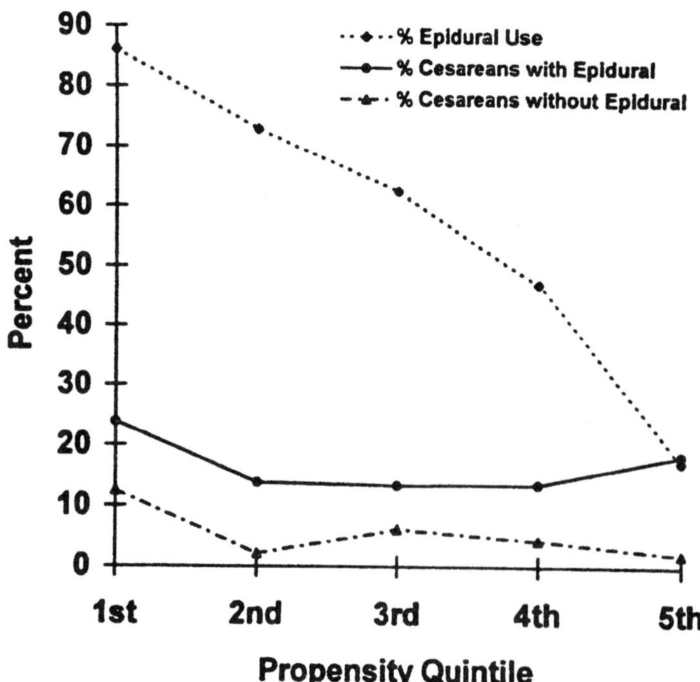

FIG. 6. Percentage of cesarean deliveries according to the use of epidural analgesia and propensity quintile. See text and Tables 9 and 10. (From ref. 26, with permission.)

TABLE 11. *Cesarean delivery rates before and after a sudden change in the use of epidural labor analgesia in four institutions*[a]

First author (reference)	n: before vs after	Parity	Epidural Rate (%): before vs after	Cesarean Delivery Rates (%): Total: before vs after	Dystocia: before vs after	Dystocia: after epidural vs after no epidural
Johnson (19)	116 vs 103	Mixed	71 vs 21[d]	17.2 vs 18.4[b]	—	—
Lyon (66)	373 vs 421	Nulliparae	13 vs 59[d]	11.8 vs 10.0	7.8 vs 5.2	8.1 vs 1.1[d]
Gribble (16)[c]	526 vs 425	Nulliparae	0 vs 61[d]	16.7 vs 16.0	14.4 vs 14.4	18.8 vs 7.9
Gribble (16)[c]	772 vs 659	Multiparae	0 vs 38[d]	3.8 vs 3.2	2.6 vs 1.5	2.8 vs 0.7
Gribble (16)	1,298 vs 1,084	Mixed	0 vs 47[d]	9.0 vs 8.2	7.4 vs 6.5	11.2 vs 2.8
Fogel (87)	3,195 vs 3,733	Mixed	1 vs 29[d]	9.1 vs 9.7	3.0 vs 3.1	8.0 vs 1.0[d]

[a]Dystocia cesarean delivery rates in the parturients who did and did not choose epidural analgesia when available.
[b]Calculated from raw data: 20/116 vs 19/103.
[c]Rows 3 and 4 are subsets of row 5.
[d]$p < 0.01$.
After ref. 87.

delivery rate as the use of epidural analgesia decreased from 71% to 27%. These studies suggest that factors other than epidural analgesia are much more important in determining risk of cesarean delivery. However, historical controls also are imperfect. Concurrent changes in obstetric and anesthetic practice may counteract the effect of epidural analgesia on dystocia.

Although the rate of cesarean delivery for dystocia does not change with changes in the availability of epidural analgesia, patients who receive epidural blocks are more likely to undergo cesarean delivery for dystocia. The rate of cesarean delivery for dystocia is four- to eightfold higher in the patients receiving epidural analgesia compared with those who do not (Table 11) (16,65,86). As noted previously, there is a finite incidence of dystocia within any patient population. When obstetric anesthesia services are readily available, women with dystocia will select epidural labor analgesia (65). As epidural analgesia utilization increases, more low-risk women receive epidural labor analgesia and the risk of dystocia associated with epidural analgesia decreases (Table 3) (65).

Finally, Hemminki and Jensen (20) reviewed the Finnish birth registry from 1991 to 1993. Within hospitals, there was an association between epidural labor analgesia and cesarean delivery (20). However, there was no correlation between cesarean deliveries and epidural use between institutions. The authors concluded that unaccounted confounding factors exist that cause cesarean deliveries.

Randomized Trials

To date, only a few randomized prospective trials have examined the impact of epidural analgesia on the risk of cesarean delivery for dystocia. As with nonrandomized studies, their results are inconsistent. Limitations of these trials include small sample sizes and a high incidence of protocol noncompliance.

Philipsen et al. (67) randomly assigned 111 patients to receive either epidural analgesia or intramuscular meperidine. Epidural catheters were not dosed after 8-cm cervical dilation. For both groups, second-stage analgesia was supplemented with nitrous oxide and pudendal blocks. There were no differences in the duration of the first or second stage of labor, the number of spontaneous vaginal deliveries, instrumental deliveries, or cesarean deliveries. Unfortunately, the small number of patients enrolled in this study limits the power of their negative result. (The statistically insignificant 1.6 times greater risk of cesarean section in the epidural group may have become significant had they studied more patients.)

Thorp et al. (66) randomly assigned 93 nulliparae in spontaneous labor to epidural or intravenous meperidine analgesia. Epidural infusions consisted of 0.125% bupivacaine after an initial bolus of 0.25% bupivacaine. The use of epidural analgesia increased the rate of cesarean delivery for dystocia from 2.2% to 16.7%. They terminated their study after 93 patients, contending that it was unethical to continue to subject women to the "risks" of epidural analgesia. Aside from the questionable validity of this choice (87), this study also may have suffered from a failure of randomization. The duration from admission to randomization and from admission to first analgesia was consistently greater for the epidural group (204 vs 170 minutes, and 316 vs 258 minutes, respectively). Thus, women who were randomly assigned to the epidural group may have already been at greater risk for dystocia than women assigned to the meperidine group.

A recent randomized study found no difference between those patients who received epidural analgesia or intravenous butorphanol (68). This study had a narrow patient population consisting of nulliparae in spontaneous labor with a cervical dilation of at least 4 cm and effacement of 80%. Epidural labor analgesia was induced with 0.25% bupivacaine plus fentanyl followed by an

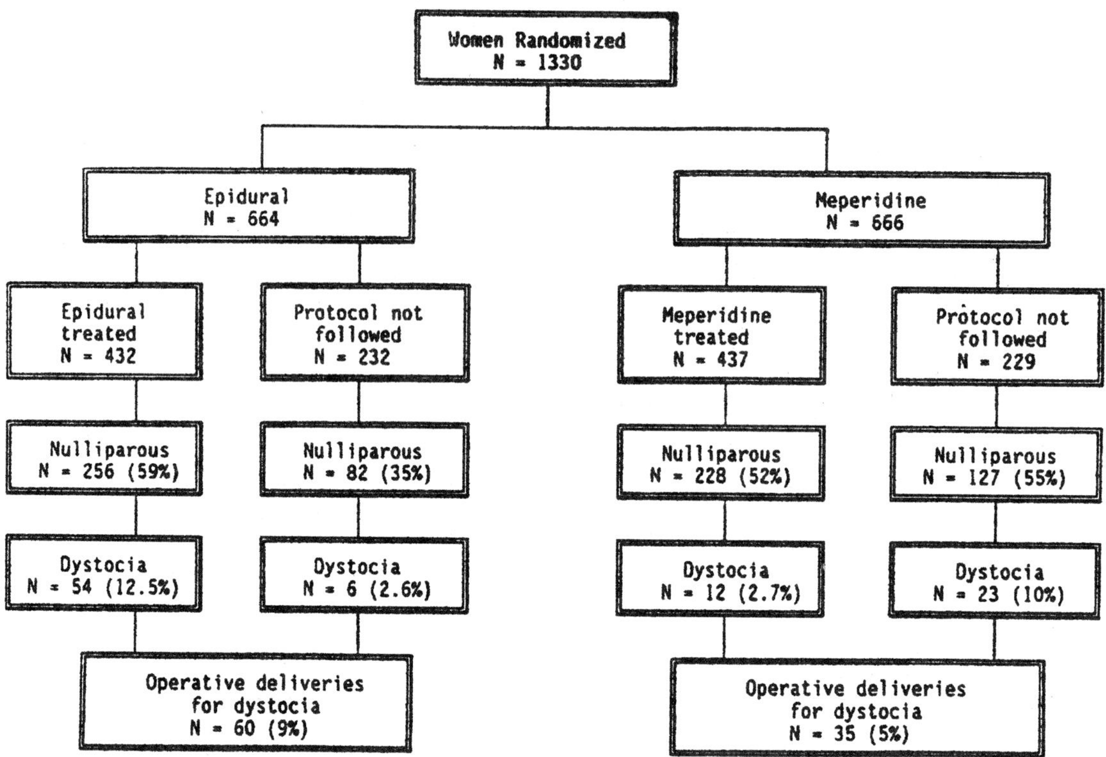

FIG. 7. Incidence of operative delivery (forceps and cesarean section) in women randomly assigned to receive either epidural block or intravenous meperidine for labor analgesia. Protocol compliant women in the epidural group ("epidural treated") were more likely to develop dystocia than protocol compliant women in the meperidine group ("meperidine treated"). The relative risk of dystocia was less, but still significant among all women assigned to the epidural group, regardless of their actual treatment (intention-to-treat analysis). (From ref. 69, with permission.)

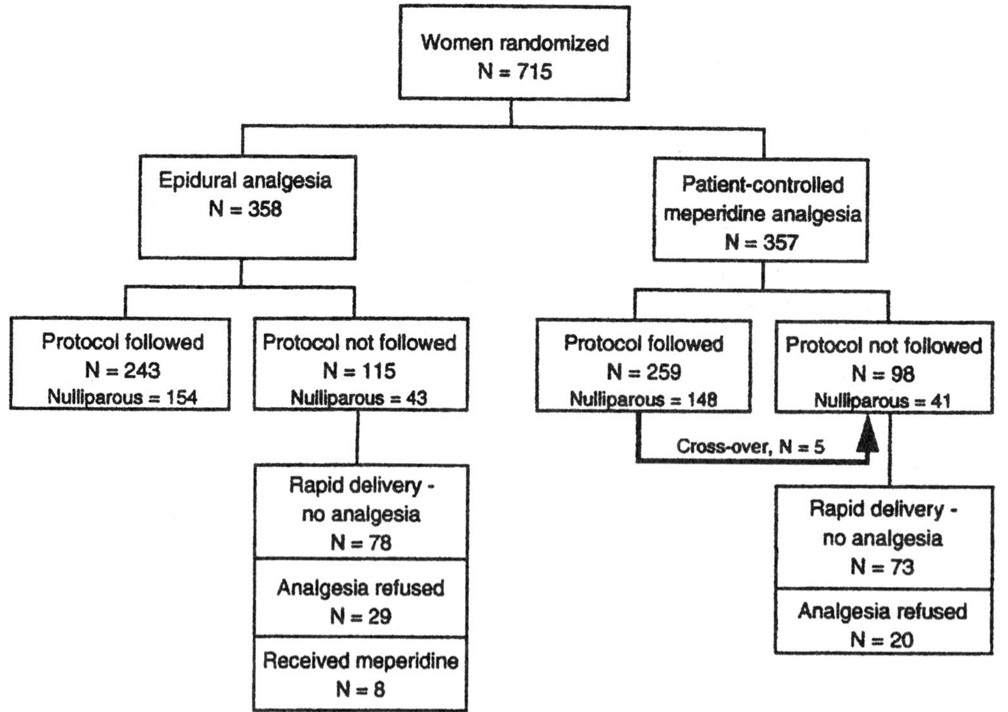

FIG. 8. Distribution of women randomly allocated to receive either epidural or patient-controlled intravenous meperidine analgesia during labor. "Protocol followed" includes women who received only their selected analgesia until delivery. "Protocol not followed" includes women who delivered before receiving analgesia, refused their allocated method of analgesia, or demanded epidural analgesia because of inadequate pain relief with intravenous meperidine. (From ref. 78, with permission.)

infusion of 0.125% bupivacaine plus fentanyl. In this study, many women crossed over from systemic to epidural analgesia due to inadequate pain relief (12 of 51). In spite of this relatively large selective reduction in the systemic analgesia group, no differences were found in dystocia-related cesarean deliveries. This study was stopped early, after 100 patients. The authors determined that 2,500 patients would be needed to establish a statistically significant difference in cesarean delivery rates (8% and 6%, respectively).

Another prospective study randomly assigned 1,330 patients to receive either epidural or intravenous meperidine labor analgesia (Fig. 7) (69). Epidural labor analgesia was induced with 0.25% bupivacaine followed with an infusion of 0.125% bupivacaine plus fentanyl. Protocol compliant patients (i.e., women randomized to the epidural group who received epidural block and those randomized to the meperidine group who received only meperidine) were more likely to require cesarean delivery for dystocia if they were in the epidural group. However, many patients did not receive their allocated treatment (232 of 664 in the epidural group and 229 of 666 in the meperidine group). This high rate of noncompliance could have skewed their results. Women in the epidural group most often were noncompliant because they delivered rapidly or declined epidural analgesia (i.e., they were at low risk of abnormal labor). Women in the meperidine group most often were noncompliant because they received inadequate pain relief from their assigned treatment and demanded epidural analgesia (i.e., they were at high risk of abnormal labor) (Fig. 7). When these data were examined using "intent-to-treat analysis," the risk associated with epidural analgesia was much lower. Epidural analgesia increased the incidence of operative delivery (both forceps and cesarean delivery) from 5% to 9%. These authors did not report the results of their intent-to-treat analysis of the impact of epidural labor analgesia on the risk of *cesarean* delivery.

In an attempt to overcome the limitations of the previous study, Sharma et al. (78) randomly assigned 715 women to epidural analgesia or patient-controlled intravenous meperidine analgesia (Fig. 8). Epidural analgesia was maintained with 0.125% bupivacaine with fentanyl infusion after an initial bolus of 0.25% bupivacaine. Epidural analgesia was continued through stage two (the infusion was halved or turned off after 1 hour or dosed for inadequate pain relief). Approximately equal numbers of patients in each group received their assigned treatment. Based on intention-to-treat analysis, there were no differences in spontaneous vaginal deliveries, instrumental deliveries (low and outlet), or cesarean deliveries (dystocia and nonreassuring fetal heart rate tracings) between the groups. Epidural labor analgesia did not increase the risk of cesarean delivery when either all patients or only treatment-compliant patients were analyzed (Tables 12 and 13).

Only two prospective randomized studies have evaluated the timing of epidural analgesia on the course of labor for nulliparae (88,89). Women in either spontaneous or oxytocin-stimulated labor requesting analgesia between 3- and 5-cm cervical dilation were randomly assigned to receive either epidural labor analgesia with 0.25% bupivacaine or intravenous nalbuphine. After 5-cm cervical dilation, all women received epidural analgesia that was maintained with an infusion of 0.125% bupivacaine. "Early" epidural analgesia did not prolong labor, increase the need for oxytocin, or increase the risk of operative delivery (88,89). Although the differences in cervical dilation between the two study groups was small, these results do suggest that inducing epidural labor analgesia before 5-cm cervical dilation does not increase the risk of dystocia.

TABLE 12. *Epidural vs intravenous meperidine for labor analgesia; effect on method of delivery (intent-to-treat analysis)*

Method of delivery	Epidural analgesia (n = 358)	Patient-controlled intravenous meperidine analgesia (n = 357)	*p* Value
Spontaneous	319 (89)	326 (91)	NS
Instrumental vaginal			
Total	26 (7)	15 (4)	NS
Low forceps[a]	22 (6)	12 (3)	NS
Outlet forceps[b]	4 (1)	3 (1)	NS
Cesarean delivery			
Total	13 (4)	16 (5)	NS
Dystocia	9 (3)	10 (3)	NS
Nonreassuring FHR tracing	4 (1)	6 (2)	NS
Total operative delivery	39 (11)	31 (9)	NS

Data are n (%).
FHR, fetal heart rate.
[a]Low forceps, +2 cm to +4 cm below the ischial spines.
[b]Outlet forceps, fetal head at the perineum.
Data from ref. 78.

TABLE 13. *Epidural vs intravenous meperidine for labor analgesia: effect on method of delivery (protocol compliant women)*

Method of delivery	Epidural analgesia (n = 243)	Patient-controlled intravenous meperidine analgesia (n = 259)	*p* Value
Spontaneous	209 (86)	236 (91)	NS
Instrumental vaginal			
Total	22 (9)	9 (3)	0.01
Low forceps[a]	18 (7)	8 (3)	<0.05
Outlet forceps[b]	4 (2)	1	NS
Cesarean delivery			
Total	12 (5)	14 (6)	NS
Dystocia	8 (3)	10 (4)	NS
Nonreassuring FHR tracing	4 (2)	4 (2)	NS
Total operative delivery	34 (14)	23 (9)	NS

Data are n (%).
FHR = fetal heart rate.
[a]Low forceps, +2 cm to +4 cm below the ischial spines.
[b]Outlet forceps, fetal head at the perineum.
Data from ref. 78.

CONCLUSION

There is a consistent association between epidural analgesia and abnormal labor. Women who receive epidural analgesia may have longer labors, require more oxytocin, have persistent malrotation of the fetal head, and need instrumental or cesarean delivery. Many investigators claim that epidural labor analgesia causes these abnormalities. However, women do not request epidural analgesia randomly. Many women request epidural block only after failing to obtain adequate relief from other methods of analgesia. Severe pain is a symptom of abnormal labor. Careful review of the data shows that pain associated with abnormal labor leads many women at high risk for dystocia to request epidural analgesia.

Epidural analgesia can prolong the second stage of labor and may increase the frequency of malpresentation and instrumental delivery. A few studies suggest that using dilute local anesthetic/opioid mixtures can minimize the impact of epidural analgesia on the second stage of labor.

REFERENCES

1. Willdeck-Lund G, Lindmark G, Nilsson BA. Effect of segmental epidural block on the course of labour and the condition of the infant during the neonatal period. *Acta Obstet Gynecol Scand* 1979;23:301.
2. Diro M, Beydoun SN. Segmental epidural analgesia in labor: a matched control study. *J Natl Med Assoc* 1985;78:569.
3. Thorp JA, Parisi VM, Boylan PC, Johnston DA. The effect of continuous epidural analgesia on cesarean section for dystocia in nulliparous women. *Am J Obstet Gynecol* 1989;161:670.
4. Pello LC, Rosevear SK, Dawes GS, Moulden M, Redman CW. Computerized fetal heart rate analysis in labor. *Obstet Gynecol* 1991;78:602.
5. Thorp JA, Eckert LO, Ang MS, Johnston DA, Peaceman AM, Parisi VM. Epidural analgesia and cesarean section for dystocia: risk factors in nulliparas. *Am J Perinatol* 1991;8:402.
6. Cammu H, Verlaenen H, Amy JJ, DeKoster K, Derde M-P, Buekens P. Epidural analgesia in active management of labor. *Acta Obstet Gynecol Scand* 1994;73:235.
7. Malone FD, Geary M, Chelmow D, Sronge J, Boylan P, D'Alton ME. Prolonged labor in nulliparas: lessons from the active management of labor. *Obstet Gynecol* 1996;88:211.
8. Mor-Yosef S, Samueloff A, Modan B, Navot D, Schenker JG. Ranking the risk factors for cesarean: logistic regression analysis of a nationwide study. *Obstet Gynecol* 1990;75:944.
9. Peaceman AM, Lopez-Zeno JA, Minogue JP, Socol ML. Factors that influence route of delivery—active versus traditional labor management. *Am J Obstet Gynecol* 1993;169:940.
10. Turcot L, Marcoux S, Fraser WD. Multivariate analysis of risk factors for operative delivery in nulliparous women. *Am J Obstet Gynecol* 1997;176:395.
11. Harlow BL, Frigoletto FD, Cramer DW, et al. Epidemiologic predictors of cesarean section in nulliparous patients at low risk. *Am J Obstet Gynecol* 1996;172:156.
12. Brost BC, Goldenberg RL, Mercer BM, et al. The preterm prediction study: association of cesarean delivery with increases in maternal weight and body mass index. *Am J Obstet Gynecol* 1997;177:333.
13. Johnson NP, Lewis J, Ansell DA. Does ethnicity influence obstetric intervention? *N Z Med J* 1995;108:511.
14. Frame S, Moore J, Peters A, Hall D. Maternal height and shoe size as predictors of pelvic disproportion: an assessment. *Br J Obstet Gynaecol* 1995;92:1239.
15. Kennedy JL, Greenwald E. Correlation of shoe size and obstetric outcome: an anthropometric study. *Am J Obstet Gynecol* 1981;140:466.
16. Gribble RK, Meier PR. Effect of epidural analgesia on the primary cesarean rate. *Obstet Gynecol* 1991;78:231.
17. Hoult IJ, MacLennan AH, Carrie LES. Lumbar epidural analgesia in labour: relation to fetal malposition and instrumental delivery. *Br Med J* 1977;1:14.
18. Studd JWW, Crawford JS, Duignan NM, Rowbotham CJF. The effect of lumbar epidural analgesia on the rate of cervical dilatation and the outcome of labour of spontaneous onset. *Br J Obstet Gynaecol* 1980; 87:1013.
19. Johnson S, Rosenfeld J. The effect of epidural anesthesia on the length of labor. *J Fam Pract* 1995;40:244.
20. Hemminki E, Gissler M. Epidural analgesia as a risk factor for operative delivery. *Int J Gynaecol Obstet* 1996;53:125.
21. Goyert GL, Bottoms SF, Marjorie TC, Nehra PC. The physician factor in cesarean birth rates. *N Engl J Med* 1989;320:706.
22. Floberg J, Belfrage P, Ohlsen H. Influence of the pelvic outlet capacity on fetal head presentation at delivery. *Acta Obstet Gynecol Scand* 1987;66:127.
23. Lederman RP, Lederman E, Work B Jr, McCann DS. Anxiety and epinephrine in multiparous women in labor: relationship to duration of labor and fetal heart rate pattern. *Am J Obstet Gynecol* 1985;153:870.

24. Lederman RP, Lederman E, Work BA, McCann DS. The relationship of maternal anxiety, plasma catecholamines, and plasma cortisol to progress in labor. *Am J Obstet Gynecol* 1978;132:495.
25. Wuitchik M, Bakal D, Lipshitz J. The clinical significance of pain and cognitive activity in latent labor. *Obstet Gynecol* 1989;73:35.
26. Lieberman E, Lang JM, Cohen A, D'Agostino R, Datta S, Frigoletto FD. Association of epidural analgesia with cesarean delivery in nulliparas. *Obstet Gynecol* 1996;88:993.
27. Robinson CA, Macones GA, Roth NW, Morgan MA. Does station of the fetal head at epidural placement affect the position of the fetal vertex at delivery? *Am J Obstet Gynecol* 1996;175:991.
28. Hawkins JL, Hess KR, Kubicek MA, Joyce TH III, Morrow DH. A reevaluation of the association between instrument delivery and epidural analgesia. *Reg Anesth* 1995;20:50.
29. Newton ER, Shroeder BC, Knape KG, Bennet BL. Epidural analgesia and uterine function. *Obstet Gynecol* 1995;85:749.
30. O'Driscoll K, Foley M, MacDonald D. Active management of labor as an alternative to cesarean sections for dystocia. *Obstet Gynecol* 1984;63:485.
31. Morgan MA, Thurnau GR, Fishburne JI Jr. The fetal-pelvic index as an indicator of fetal-pelvic disproportion: a preliminary report. *Am J Obstet Gynecol* 1986;155:608.
32. Morgan MA, Thurnau GR. Efficacy of the fetal-pelvic index for delivery of neonates weighing 4000 grams or greater: a preliminary report. *Am J Obstet Gynecol* 1988;158:1133.
33. Morgan MA, Thurnau GR. Efficacy of the fetal-pelvic index in patients requiring labor induction. *Am J Obstet Gynecol* 1988;159:621.
34. Thurnau GR, Morgan MA. Efficacy of the fetal-pelvic index as a predictor of fetal-pelvic disproportion in women with abnormal labor patterns that require labor augmentation. *Am J Obstet Gynecol* 1988;159:1168.
35. Thurnau GR, Scates DH, Morgan MA. The fetal-pelvic index: a method of identifying fetal-pelvic disproportion in women attempting vaginal birth after previous cesarean delivery. *Am J Obstet Gynecol* 1991;165:353.
36. Morgan MA, Thurnau GR. Efficacy of the fetal-pelvic index in nulliparous women at high risk for fetal-pelvic disproportion. *Am J Obstet Gynecol* 1992;166:810.
37. Chestnut DH, Vandewalker GE, Owen CL, Bates JN, Choi WW. The influence of continuous epidural bupivacaine analgesia on the second stage of labor and method of delivery in nulliparous women. *Anesthesiology* 1987;66:774.
38. Thorburn J, Moir DD. Extradural analgesia: the influence of volume and concentration of bupivacaine on the mode of delivery, analgesic efficacy and motor block. *Br J Anaesth* 1981;53:933.
39. Vertommen JD, Vandermeulen E, Van Aken H, et al. The effects of the addition of sufentanil to 0.125% bupivacaine on the quality of analgesia during labor and on the incidence of instrumental deliveries. *Anesthesiology* 1991;74:809.
40. Stoddart AP, Nicholson KEA, Popham PA. Low dose bupivacaine/fentanyl epidural infusions in labour and mode of delivery. *Anaesthesia* 1994;49:1087.
41. Zamora JE, Rosaeg OP, Lindsay MP, Crossan M. Haemodynamic consequences and uterine contractions following 0.5 or 1.0 litre crystalloid infusion before obstetric epidural analgesia. *Can J Anaesth* 1996;43:347.
42. Cheek TD, Samuels R, Miller F, Tobin M, Gutsche BB. Normal saline i.v. fluid load decreases uterine activity in active labour. *Br J Anaesth* 1996;77:632.
43. Gunther RE, Bauman J. Obstetrical caudal anesthesia: a randomized study comparing 1% mepivacaine with 1% mepivacaine plus epinephrine. *Anesthesiology* 1972;37:288.
44. Craft JB, Epstein BS, Coakley CS. Effect of lidocaine with epinephrine versus lidocaine (plain) on induced labor. *Anesth Analg* 1972;51:243.
45. Matadial L, Cibils LA. The effect of epidural anesthesia on uterine activity and blood pressure. *Am J Obstet Gynecol* 1976;125:846.
46. Caldetro-Barcia R, Noriega-Guerra L, Cibils LA, et al. Effect of position changes on the intensity and frequency of uterine contractions during labor. *Am J Obstet Gynecol* 1960;80:284.
47. Schellenberg JC. Uterine activity during lumbar epidural analgesia with bupivacaine. *Am J Obstet Gynecol* 1977;127:26.
48. Asselineau D. Does ambulation under epidural analgesia during labor modify the conditions of fetal extraction? (in French). *Contracept Fertil Sex* 1996;24:505.
49. Lilford RJ, Glanville JN, Gupta JK, Shrestha R, Johnson N. The action of squatting in the early postnatal period marginally increases pelvic dimensions. *Br J Obstet Gynaecol* 1989;96:964.
50. Russel JGB. Moulding of the pelvic outlet. *J Obstet Gynaecol Br Emp* 1969;76:817.
51. Borrel V, Fernstrom I. The movements to the sacro-iliac joints and their importance to changes in the pelvic dimensions during parturition. *Acta Obstet Gynecol Scand* 1957;36:42.
52. Turner MJ, Brassil M, Gordon H. Active management of labor associated with a decrease in the cesarean section rate in nulliparas. *Obstet Gynecol* 1988;71:150.
53. Akoury HA, Brodie G, Caddick R, McLaughin VD, Pugh PA. Active management of labor and operative delivery in nulliparous women. *Am J Obstet Gynecol* 1988;158:255.
54. Lopez-Zeno JA, Peaceman AM, Adashek JA, Socol ML. A controlled trial of a program for the active management of labor. *N Engl J Med* 1992;326:450.
55. Frigoletto FD, Leiberman E, Lang JM, et al. A clinical trial of active management of labor. *N Engl J Med* 1995;333:745.
56. Casey C, Kehoe J, Mylotte MJ. Vaginal prostaglandins for the ripe cervix. *Int J Gynaecol Obstet* 1994;44:21.
57. Fraser W, Usher RH, McLean FH, et al. Temporal variation in rates of cesarean section for dystocia: does convenience play a role? *Am J Obstet Gynecol* 1987;156:300.
58. Guillemette J, Fraser WD. Differences between obstetricians in cesarean section rates and the management of labour. *Br J Obstet Gynaecol* 1993;99:105.
59. Haynes de Regt R, Mindoff HL, Feldman J, Schwarz RH. Relation of private or clinic care to the cesarean birth rate. *N Engl J Med* 1986; 315:619.
60. Neuhoff D, Burke MS, Porreco RP. Cesarean birth for failed progress in labor. *Obstet Gynecol* 1989;73:915.
61. Hueston WJ, McClaflin RR, Mansfield CJ, Rudy M. Factors associated with the use of intrapartum epidural analgesia. *Obstet Gynecol* 1994; 84:579.
62. Gould JB, Davey B, Stafford RS. Socioeconomic differences in rates of cesarean section. *N Engl J Med* 1989;321:233.
63. Bailey PW, Chir B, Howard FA. Epidural analgesia and forceps delivery: laying a bogey. *Anaesthesia* 1983;38:282.
64. Ong B, Cohen MM, Cummings M, Palahniuk RJ. Obstetrical anaesthesia at Winnipeg Women's Hospital 1975-1983: anaesthetic techniques and complications. *Can J Anaesth* 1987;34:294.
65. Lyon DS, Knuckles G, Whitaker E, Salgado S. The effect of instituting an elective labor epidural program on the operative delivery rate. *Obstet Gynecol* 1997;90:135.
66. Thorp JA, Hu DH, Albin RM, et al. The effect of intrapartum epidural analgesia on nulliparous labor: A randomized, controlled, prospective trial. *Am J Obstet Gynecol* 1993;160:851.
67. Philipsen T, Jensen N-H. Epidural block or parenteral pethidine as analgesic in labour: a randomized study concerning progress in labour and instrumental deliveries. *Eur J Obstet Gynecol Reprod Biol* 1989; 30:27.
68. Bofill JA, Vincent RD, Ross EL, Martin PF, Werhan CF, Morrison RW. Nulliparous active labor, epidural analgesia, and cesarean delivery for dystocia. *Am J Obstet Gynecol* 1997;177:177.
69. Ramin SM, Gambling DR, Lucas MJ, Sharma SK, Sidawi JE, Leveno KJ. Randomized trial of epidural versus intravenous analgesia during labor. *Obstet Gynecol* 1995;86:783.
70. The environment and disease: associations or causation? *Proceedings of the Annual Meeting of the Royal Society of Medicine.* London: Bradford-Hill, 1965:295.
71. Phillips JC, Hochberg CJ, Petrakis JK, VanWinkle JD. Epidural analgesia and its effects on the "normal" progress of labor. *Am J Obstet Gynecol* 1977;129:316.
72. Crawford JS. Lumbar epidural block in labour: a clinical analysis. *Br J Anaesth* 1972;44:66.
73. Crawford JS. The second thousand epidural blocks in an obstetric hospital practice. *Br J Anaesth* 1972;44:1277.
74. Zuspan FP, Cibils LA, Pose SV. Myometrial and cardiovascular responses to alterations in plasma epinephrine and norepinephrine. *Am J Obstet Gynecol* 1962;84:841.
75. Nielsen PE, Abouleish E, Meyer BA, Parisi VM. Effect of epidural analgesia on fundal dominance during spontaneous active-phase nulliparous labor. *Anesthesiology* 1996;84:540.

76. Henry JS, Kingston MB, Maughan GB. The effect of epidural anesthesia on oxytocin-induced labor. *Am J Obstet Gynecol* 1967;97:359.
77. Jouppila R, Jouppila P, Karinen JM, Hollem A. Segmental epidural analgesia in labour: related to the progress of labour, fetal malposition and instrumental delivery. *Acta Obstet Gynecol Scand* 1979;58:135.
78. Sharma K, Sidawi JE, Ramin M, Lucas MJ, Leveno KJ, Cunningham FG. A randomized trial of epidural versus patient-controlled meperidine analgesia during labor. *Anesthesiology* 1997;87:487.
79. Chestnut DH, Laszewski LJ, Pollack KL, Bates JN, Manago NK, Choi WW. Continuous epidural infusion of 0.0625% bupivacaine-0.0002% fentanyl during the second stage of labor. *Anesthesiology* 1990;72:613.
80. ACOG. Technical Bulletin No. 196. August 1994.
81. Cohen WR. Influence of the duration of second stage of labor on perinatal outcome and puerperal morbidity. *Obstet Gynecol* 1977;49:226.
82. Kaminski HM, Stafl A, Aiman J. The effect of epidural analgesia on the frequency of instrumental obstetric delivery. *Obstet Gynecol* 1987;69:770.
83. Ploeckinger B, Ulm MR, Chalubinski K, Gruber W. Epidural anaesthesia in labour: influence on surgical delivery rates, intrapartum fever and blood loss. *Gynecol Obstet Invest* 1995;39:24.
84. Maresh M, Choong K-H, Deard RW. Delayed pushing with lumbar epidural analgesia in labour. *Br J Obstet Gynaecol* 1983;90:623.
85. Saunders NJ, Spiby H, Gilbert L, et al. Oxytocin infusion during second sage of labour in primiparous women using epidural analgesia: a randomized double blind placebo controlled trial. *Br Med J* 1989;299:1423.
86. Fogel ST, Shyken JM, Leighton BL, Mormol JS, Smeltzer JS. Epidural labor analgesia and the incidence of cesarean section. *Anesth Analg* 1998;87:119.
87. Grossman RA. The peril of hasty analysis. *Am J Obstet Gynecol* 1994;171:1387.
88. Chestnut DH, Vincent RD Jr, McGrath JM, Choi WW, Bates JN. Does early administration of epidural analgesia affect obstetric outcome in nulliparous women who are receiving intravenous oxytocin. *Anesthesiology* 1994;80:1193.
89. Chestnut DH, McGrath JM, Vincent RD Jr, et al. Does early administration of epidural analgesia affect obstetric outcome in nulliparous women who are in spontaneous labor? *Anesthesiology* 1994;80:1201.

Obstetric Anesthesia, second edition,
edited by Mark C. Norris.
Lippincott Williams & Wilkins, Philadelphia © 1999.

CHAPTER 19

Indications for Cesarean Delivery

Jaye M. Shyken

In the United States (U.S.), cesarean section is the most commonly performed surgical procedure in women of child-bearing age. The contribution of cesarean delivery to maternal morbidity, without a clearly attributable improvement in neonatal outcome, sparked a national public health initiative to bring about the safe reduction in their number. With this commitment came resistance, debate, and the necessity to scrutinize operative obstetric practices.

HISTORICAL PERSPECTIVE

The name of the procedure, "cesarean section," is widely held to have derived from the surgical birth of Julius Caesar, although historians dispute the veracity of this event. The term more likely evolved from the Latin verb "caedare," to cut, and the term "caesones," which referred to infants born by postmortem cesarean section. Initial cesarean deliveries were performed to rescue an infant from a dead or dying mother. One of the first documented reports of a successful cesarean section, resulting in the survival of both mother and infant, was reported some 82 years after the event in 1500. James Miranda Stuart Barry, some time between 1815 and 1821, performed the first successful cesarean section in the British Empire (1).

Before 1846, physicians performed cesarean sections without benefit of anesthesia. William T.G. Morton's introduction of diethyl ether transformed the practice of surgical delivery, allowing obstetricians the luxury to operate with care, cleanse the surgical layers, and spare women surgical agony and shock. Cesarean section then replaced destructive fetal procedures, which until then were necessary to accomplish vaginal delivery in women with arrested labor. Recognition of the germ theory in the second half of the nineteenth century, with the introduction of aseptic techniques and antiseptic agents, improved infectious morbidity and mortality. Surgical techniques, such as using sutures on the incised uterus and the low cervical transverse cesarean section, also served to lower maternal morbidity. The most important event to advance the safety of cesarean section was the discovery of penicillin in 1928. Penicillin was purified for use as a drug in 1940 and became generally available thereafter (1). The increasing safety and ease of surgery allowed the later trend toward liberal use of cesarean delivery.

TRENDS IN THE UNITED STATES CESAREAN DELIVERY RATE

The rate of cesarean delivery in the U.S. is among the highest for industrialized nations, ranking third among 21 countries studied. Only Brazil and Puerto Rico surpassed the cesarean section rate in the U.S. in 1987 (Fig. 1). Although the rate of cesarean section increased in other countries during the 1970s and 1980s, the rate of increase was not as dramatic in Canada, England and Wales, Sweden, and The Netherlands as in the U.S. (2).

In 1970, 5.5% of babies in the U.S. were born by cesarean section. The use of cesarean section rose dramatically in subsequent decades (Fig. 2). The peak in cesarean delivery rate occurred in 1988 at 24.7%. Since that time, the rate has slowly and steadily declined (3). The 1995 birth statistics from the National Center for Health Statistics indicate a national cesarean section rate of 20.8% for all births, a 9% drop since 1989 (4). Despite the persistent reduction in the rate of cesarean birth over a 6-year period, the use of cesarean section remains over threefold greater than in 1970 and over fourfold higher than in 1965.

Within the U.S., cesarean delivery rates vary greatly by region (Fig. 3) (5,6), by institution (5–7), and by patient demographics. Rates of cesarean delivery are highest in hospitals with fewer than 100 beds compared to larger

J. M. Shyken: Department of Obstetrics and Gynecology, Washington University School of Medicine, St. Louis, Missouri 63110.

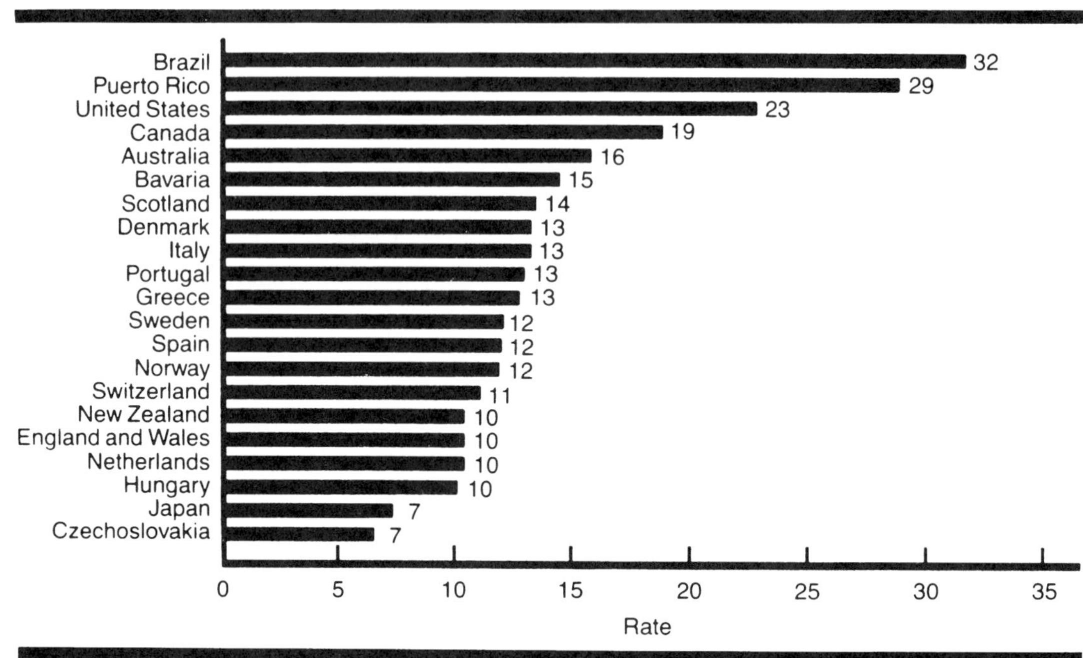

FIG. 1. Cesarean section rates per 100 hospital deliveries in selected countries for 1985 or most recent year for which data are available. Data are incomplete for Australia, Bavaria, Portugal, Spain, and Switzerland. (Reprinted from ref. 2.)

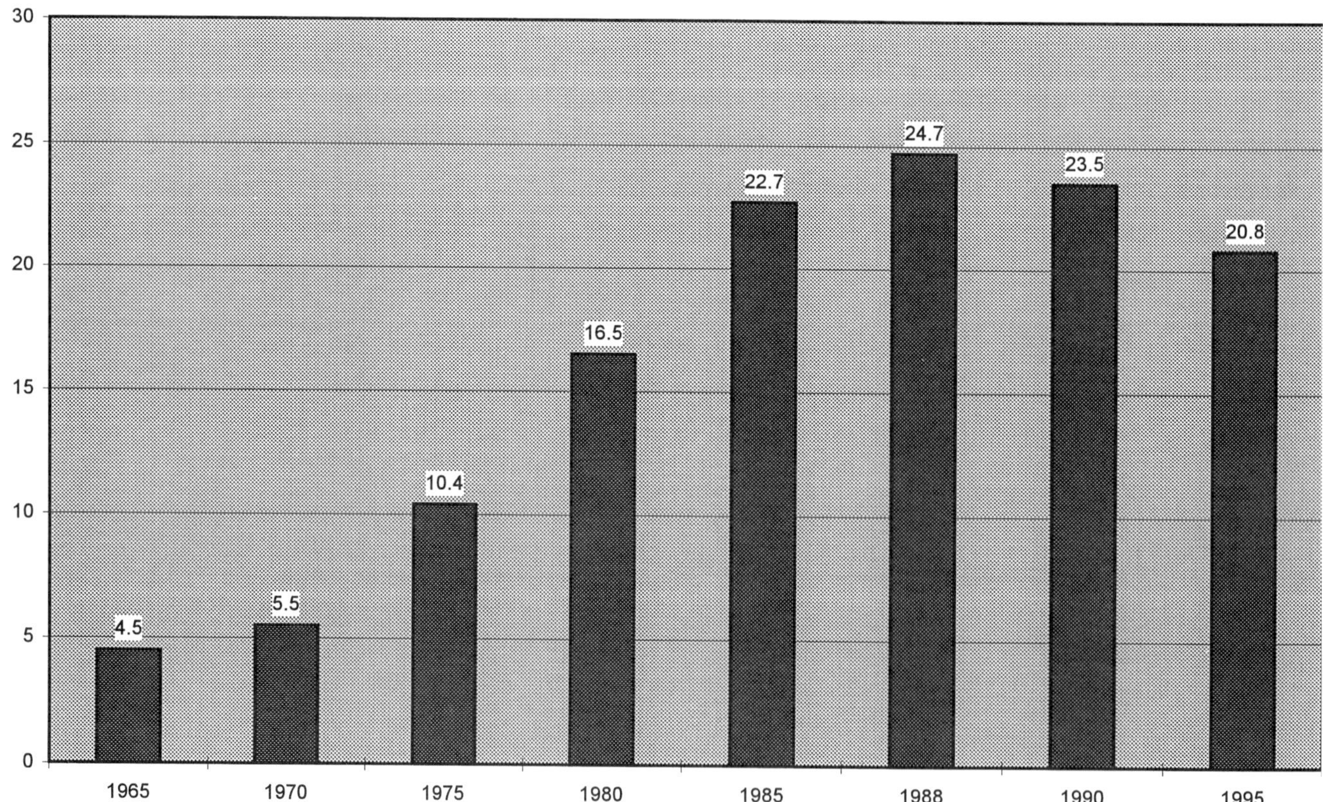

FIG. 2. United States cesarean deliveries per 100 births for selected years from 1965 through 1995. (Data from ref. 3 and the National Center for Health Statistics.)

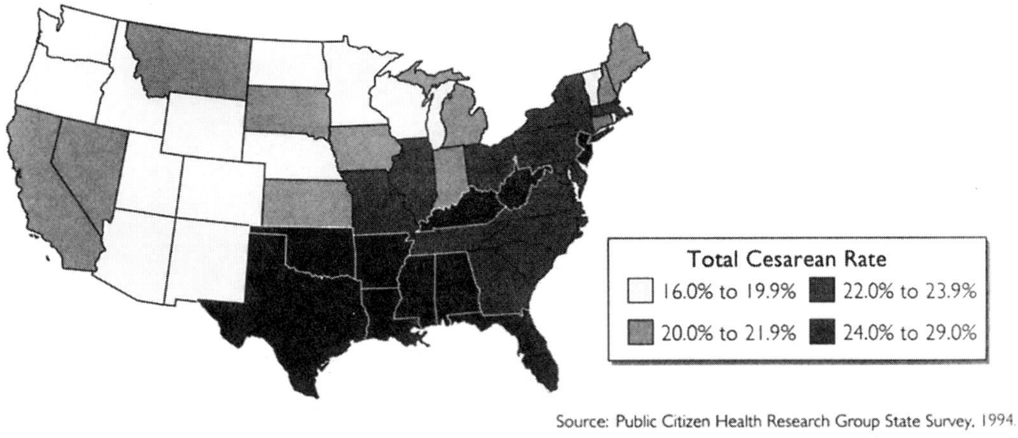

Total Cesarean Rate
16.0% to 19.9%
22.0% to 23.9%
20.0% to 21.9%
24.0% to 29.0%

Source: Public Citizen Health Research Group State Survey, 1994

FIG. 3. Regional variation in cesarean delivery rate. (Reprinted from ref. 100, with permission.)

facilities, and in proprietary, for-profit institutions compared to nonprofit, state, or governmental entities (3). Women of higher socioeconomic status are more likely to have a cesarean delivery than women of lower socioeconomic status (8). Even after controlling for birth weight and obstetric risk factors, patients of private physicians are at greater risk of cesarean delivery than patients of resident or teaching attending physicians (9).

Figure 4 shows the relative contribution of primary cesarean delivery to the overall cesarean delivery rate. The rate of primary cesarean deliveries also peaked in 1988 and then slowly declined (3). From 1980 to 1985,

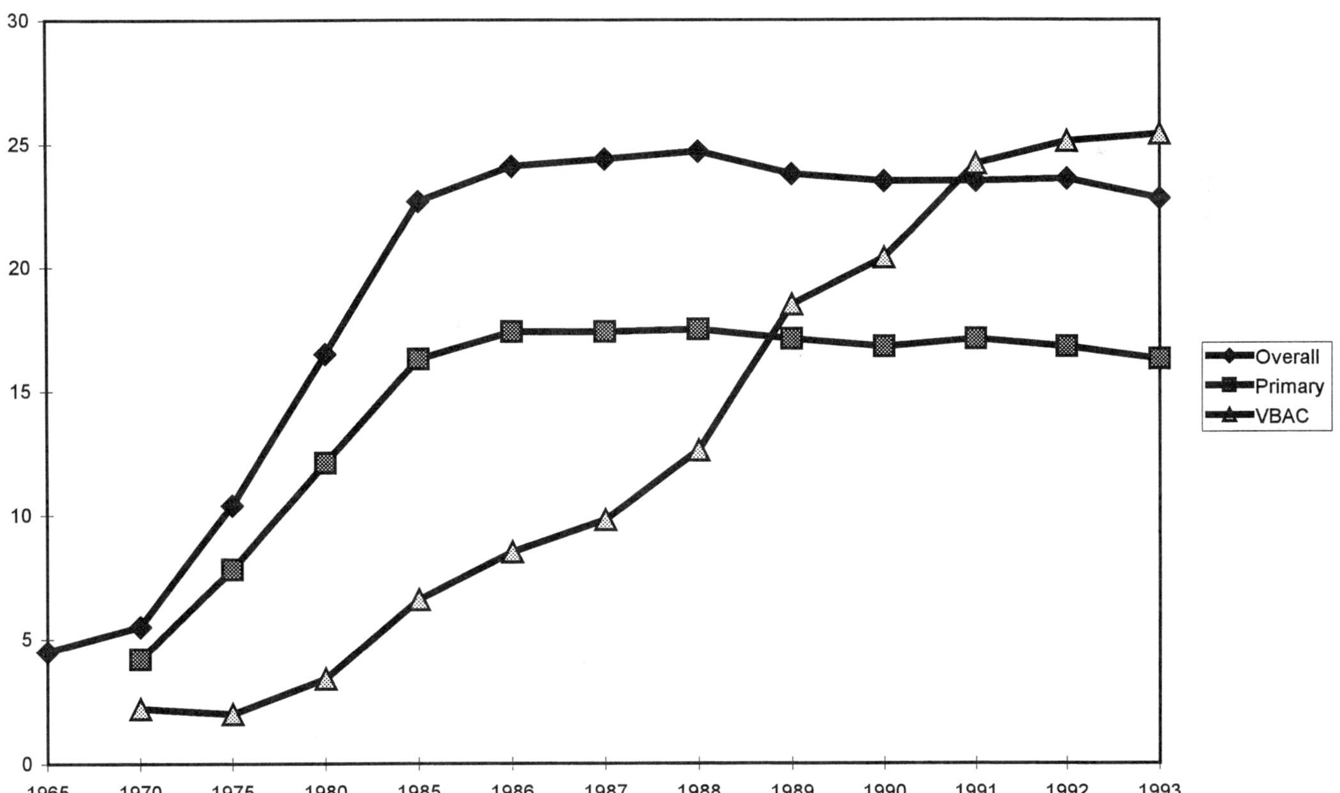

FIG. 4. Trend in the United States cesarean delivery rate and vaginal birth after cesarean section (VABC) rate. Overall cesarean section rate is the number of cesarean deliveries per 100 births, the primary rate is the rate of first cesarean sections per 100 births, and the VBAC rate is the number of vaginal births per 100 women with a previous cesarean section. (Reprinted from ref. 3.)

dystocia and previous cesarean section accounted for the largest contribution to the increased overall rate (10). In 1991, indications for cesarean deliveries were:

- Previous cesarean (35%),
- Dystocia (30.4%),
- Breech presentation (11.7%),
- Fetal distress (9.2%), and
- Other unspecified indications (13.7%) (11).

Elective, repeat cesarean sections are declining as a growing number of women undergo a trial of labor following vaginal delivery. The vaginal birth after cesarean section (VBAC) rate is the percentage of women who had a previous cesarean section but deliver vaginally in a subsequent pregnancy. The current VBAC rate in the U.S. is 25.4%, a precipitous increase over the rate of 3.4% in 1980 (Fig. 4) (3). The plateau of the overall cesarean section rate is largely attributable to the growing rate of trial of labor following cesarean section, making the relative contribution of primary cesarean sections of growing importance.

The perinatal mortality rate is the number of fetal deaths (after 22 weeks' gestation) plus neonatal deaths (in the first 28 days of life) per 1,000 total births (12). Between 1950 and 1980, the U.S. perinatal mortality rate declined dramatically from 39.0 per thousand to 17.5 per thousand coincident with a large increase in the cesarean section rate (13). The subsequent fall in perinatal mortality to 13.3 per thousand in 1990 (14) was modest compared to the accompanying dramatic rise in cesarean sections. In Dublin, Ireland, a similar fall in the perinatal mortality was not associated with an increase in cesarean deliveries, which remained below 5% (15). Although the Dublin and U.S. experiences are not entirely comparable, it is clear that an increase in cesarean section rate of the magnitude seen in this country should be questioned. The perinatal mortality rate continues to fall despite a modest reduction in the rate of cesarean delivery (14).

FACTORS CONTRIBUTING TO THE USE OF CESAREAN DELIVERY

Repeat Cesarean Sections

By 1980, 97% of women in the U.S. with a previous cesarean delivery underwent repeat cesarean section, in sharp contrast to European and Scandinavian countries that never subscribed to the dictum "once a cesarean, always a cesarean." Notzon and colleagues (10) identified repeat cesarean section as one of the major factors in the increase in the cesarean section rate from 1980 to 1985 and to a lesser extent between 1985 and 1990. In response to the climbing national cesarean section rate, in 1980, the National Institute of Child Health and Human Development Conference on Childbirth, after reviewing available data, concluded that VBAC was an appropriate and safe alternative to repeat cesarean section (16). Despite the growing enthusiasm for a trial of labor following cesarean section over the second half of the decade, in 1990, 80.5% of women with a previous cesarean section were delivered by a repeat cesarean section (10). The potential impact of achieving the Healthy People 2000 goal of a VBAC rate of 35 or greater per 100 eligible women is substantial.

Malpractice Concerns

Obstetricians cite malpractice fears as a principal source of unnecessary cesarean sections. In the current hostile medical–legal climate, lawsuits frequently are prompted by the birth of a baby with an abnormal outcome. Mothers of infants who had permanent perinatal injuries or deaths and had closed malpractice claims in Florida were interviewed. When asked to identify what was wrong with the care they received, 53% percent of respondents alleged failure to recognize fetal distress, 57% alleged failure to manage fetal distress appropriately, and 33% alleged failure to perform a cesarean section (17). The majority of lawsuits, therefore, appear to be a result of failure to perform, or a delay in the performance of, a cesarean section. A positive association exists between the rate of cesarean delivery and perceived and actual malpractice claims risk. After controlling for clinical risk of cesarean delivery, physicians with higher malpractice premiums and physicians who practice in hospitals experiencing a greater number of malpractice claims had a higher likelihood of performing cesarean sections. In addition, physician's *perceptions* about the probability of being sued were positively associated with the cesarean delivery rate (7). It does not appear that major strides in the reduction in cesarean deliveries will occur until these concerns are addressed.

Births to Older Women

Older maternal age appears to be an independent risk factor for cesarean section among parous and nulliparous women (18–21). Dystocia, fetal distress, preeclampsia, and abruptio placentae occur more frequently in women 35 or older, and account for the majority of cesarean deliveries in these patients. Women over 35 are twice as likely to have a cesarean delivery as those between 20 and 29 (19). A comparison of these two groups did not find significant differences in labor management. However, increased maximum oxytocin requirements, increased incidence of dystocia with birth weight 3,600 g or more, and a trend toward larger birth weights with advancing maternal age suggest that maternal and fetal factors contribute to the increased risk of cesarean section. Although pregnancy complications increase with advancing maternal age, an intrinsic uterine factor also may be important. Perhaps there is an unidentified age-related decrement in myometrial response due to decreased oxytocin receptor concentration or inherent myometrial contractility. The concept of a "premium" pregnancy among older nulliparous or previously infertile older women may constitute a social drive toward cesarean delivery.

Birth rates for women in their thirties continue to increase. The birth rate for women aged 40 to 44 years rose 20% between 1990 and 1995, and increased by 74% from 1981 to 1995 (4). Parrish and co-workers (21) examined the effects of maternal age and parity on the primary cesarean section rate. They estimated that delayed childbearing accounted for 18% of the increase in the primary cesarean rate from 1970 to 1987 through 1990. These changing demographic characteristics of the obstetric population should be considered when evaluating the overall trend in the cesarean birth rate.

Dystocia

Many of the cesarean sections performed for dystocia do not represent true cephalopelvic disproportion. Diagnoses included under the heading of dystocia include failed induction of labor, hypotonic uterine dysfunction, prolonged latent phase, and fetal cephalic malposition. It is appropriate to perform cesarean sections for labor arrest disorders, which include arrest of dilation or arrest of descent in the active phase of labor. These disorders are diagnosed in the active phase of labor, at ≥ 4 cm of cervical dilation. The diagnosis of labor arrest disorders requires the absence of change in dilation or descent of the presenting fetal part for 2 hours in the presence of adequate uterine contractions. It is inappropriate to perform abdominal delivery for labor protraction disorders or for hypotonic uterine contractions, which are more appropriately treated with a dilute oxytocin infusion (22). Coincident obstetric complications and slow progress in labor may lead to improper surgical interventions.

Epidural Analgesia and Dystocia

Epidural analgesia in labor and cesarean delivery for dystocia are strongly associated (23,24). It is not clear that the epidural block itself causes the increase in cesarean deliveries or is merely a marker for the presence of abnormal labor (see Chapter 18). Retrospective studies examining this association are plagued with selection bias. Women who requested epidural analgesia in one retrospective study by Thorp and colleagues (25) differed from women who did not request epidural by having less cervical dilation on admission, a higher risk of oxytocin administration, longer duration of oxytocin use, and higher birth weights. Even after correction for these and other risk factors, the relationship between epidural analgesia and a higher rate of cesarean delivery held (25). This correlation does not constitute causation.

Wuitchik and colleagues (26) demonstrated that women who reported excruciating, horrible pain in the latent phase of labor had the greatest likelihood of cesarean delivery (26.3%) compared to women who reported distressing pain (7.1%) or merely discomfort (0%). The intensity of pain positively correlated with the durations of both the latent and active phases of labor (26). Thus, dysfunctional labor may be more painful and more likely to result in a plea for pain relief.

The prospective, randomized studies to date suggest an association between cesarean section and epidural labor analgesia, but are hampered by small sample size (27), lack of blinding of care providers to the presence or absence of epidural analgesia (27,28), and a high rate of crossover from intravenous to epidural analgesia (28). A recent prospective controlled trial comparing epidural to patient-controlled meperidine analgesia, in which adequate relief was attained in both groups, found no difference in the cesarean section rates (29).

Several authors studied the impact of instituting an on-demand labor epidural service on the cesarean delivery rate. When the use of epidural analgesia increased from 13.1% to 58.7% in a military population, neither the overall cesarean delivery rate (11.8% vs 10.0%) nor the dystocia cesarean delivery rate (7.8% vs 5.2%) changed (30). Studies by Gribble and Meier (31) and Fogel and co-workers (32) confirm these findings. The rate of cesarean delivery for dystocia did not change in our institution after the establishment of an elective epidural service (3.0% vs 3.1%). However, women who received labor epidural analgesia, when available, were more likely to have cesarean deliveries for dystocia than women who did not (8.0% vs 1.0%) (32). Again, women with painful, dysfunctional labor may choose epidural analgesia. The widespread use of epidural analgesia, therefore, does not appear to contribute to the increase in cesarean delivery.

Forceps Delivery

From 1980 to 1987, while the cesarean section rate increased by 48%, the rate of forceps procedures declined by 43% and the rate of vacuum delivery increased modestly from 0.6% to 3.3% (33). Clearly, residency training programs offer fewer opportunities for gaining facility with operative vaginal delivery. The safety of low and outlet forceps procedures is well established (34,35). Mid forceps deliveries are performed at fewer programs (36), in the face of controversy about associated maternal and neonatal morbidity (34,37). The most recent American College of Obstetricians and Gynecologists (ACOG) Educational Bulletin addressing operative vaginal delivery continues to recognize the importance of these technical skills and supports training in, and performance of, forceps and vacuum-assisted deliveries (38). Physicians inclined to liberal use of forceps in training tend to become less aggressive in private practice. The combination of fewer training opportunities and lack of maintenance of learned skills results in fewer operative vaginal deliveries. It is important, then, to maintain these skills as the alternative is an increased rate of maternal morbidity through cesarean section.

In 1991, over 30% of cesarean sections were performed for dystocia (11). This diagnosis actually accounts for a greater fraction of the total number of operations performed when one considers that dystocia may have been an indication for the first cesarean section among women having a repeat procedure. Given the growth in the rate of primary cesarean sections, in which dystocia plays a prominent role, an effort to reduce the number of cesarean sections for dystocia will have a powerful impact.

Breech

The rate of cesarean delivery for breech increased in almost every country between 1980 and 1985 (2). Advances in neonatal and obstetric care, which improved neonatal survival, moved the limit of fetal viability from less than 32 weeks in 1970, to 23 to 24 weeks' gestational age. The rate of malpresentations in pregnancies between 24 and 32 weeks is high, and contributes to the cesarean delivery rate.

The utility of cesarean delivery for breech-presenting fetuses has not been established (39). Although needed, the sufficiently large, prospective randomized controlled trials to address this issue appear infeasible (40). At a time when 80% to 90% of breech-presenting fetuses are delivered abdominally, it is unlikely that physicians will gain enough expertise and comfort with breech delivery to change this trend. Moreover, breech presentation accounts for only 3% to 4% of singleton deliveries. A targeted effort to increase the number of vaginal breech deliveries would be of dubious benefit.

Fetal Distress

The term *fetal distress* is poorly defined and its diagnosis is subjective. The term implies fetal decompensation leading to asphyxia. The intent of electronic fetal monitoring (EFM) is to identify an asphyxial condition early, before the onset of central nervous system damage or fetal death. The use of electronic fetal heart rate monitoring increased dramatically during the time that cesarean section use increased and a concomitant decline in stillbirths and perinatal mortality occurred. Whether EFM accounts for the reduction in perinatal mortality is controversial (41,42). However, EFM frequently is blamed for an increase in cesarean sections. Some suggest that the inability to detect improvement in neonatal outcome in randomized trials comparing EFM to intermittent fetal auscultation is due to insufficient sample sizes to detect a rare outcome, and our lack of standardization and understanding of the technology (43,44). A meta-analysis of the randomized trials comparing electronic fetal heart rate monitoring to intermittent fetal heart rate auscultation found a significantly increased cesarean section rate [odds ratio (OR) 1.53, 95% confidence interval (CI) 1.17 to 2.01] and a higher cesarean delivery rate for fetal distress (OR 2.55, 95% CI 1.81 to 3.53) associated with EFM. The authors also showed a significant reduction in perinatal deaths due to fetal hypoxia in the EFM group of 0.7 per 1,000, compared to the auscultated group of 1.8 per 1,000 (OR 0.41, 95% CI 0.17 to 0.98) (45).

The U.S. rate of cesarean section for fetal distress is roughly 2% of deliveries or about 9% of cesarean deliveries (11). The contribution of this diagnosis to the cesarean delivery rate is relatively minor. It is unlikely that the practice of EFM will change dramatically given fears of malpractice liability, or that a change in this practice will have a significant impact on the rate of cesarean birth.

Other

Since 1980, the rate of twin births increased 42% and the number of higher-order multifetal gestations rose by 272%. This growth is thought to be due to increasing maternal age at delivery and the use of fertility-enhancing medications (46). Although multiple births are more likely to be delivered abdominally, their impact on the overall cesarean delivery rate is small. "Other" indications for cesarean delivery, which include such diagnoses as multiple birth, placenta previa, malpresentation, abruptio placenta, and fetal malformations, account for only 3.5% of total births (47).

Physician Factors

The rate of cesarean delivery is determined in part by physician factors. Demott and Sandmire (48,49) suggested that the individual physician's style of labor management was the main determinant of the likelihood of cesarean section for private patients in their institutions. The authors found no differences in obstetric, fetal, or socioeconomic risks for cesarean delivery and postulated that the difference in cesarean section rates between physicians was due to individual's susceptibility to medical–legal liability pressure (49). When nonprogressive labor was considered, physicians who had low cesarean section rates were more inclined to use oxytocin liberally, allow a longer second stage labor, and allow a longer duration of ruptured membranes before surgery (48). A temporal pattern for cesarean section for stage I dystocia has been reported, suggesting the influence of physician convenience not only on the decision to perform, but the timing of cesarean delivery. The peak time epoch to perform cesarean sections coincides with times outside of office hours and before traditional sleeping time (50). Of course, staffing patterns and operating room availability vary throughout the day and night and also may influence the timing of operative intervention for dystocia.

MATERNAL AND FETAL INDICATIONS FOR CESAREAN DELIVERY

The major indications for cesarean delivery in the U.S. are previous cesarean section, breech, dystocia, and fetal distress. The common indications for cesarean section generally fall into maternal, fetal, or maternal and fetal reasons (Table 1). Many indications for cesarean delivery are controversial within the obstetric community, making decisions whether or not to deliver by cesarean somewhat subjective. The case of breech presentation, whether term or preterm, is but one example.

The rate of congenital anomalies in the U.S. is stable, but our ability to reach an antepartum diagnosis through ultrasound and maternal serum screening is increasing. Fetuses with lethal anomalies generally are not delivered by cesarean section, but fetuses with sublethal and uncertain prognoses pose management dilemmas. Unfortunately, there are no prospective, randomized trials to provide direction. The benefit of elective cesarean delivery for vertex-presenting fetuses with the diagnosis of isolated neural tube defect is not proven. Three retrospective studies show no benefit (51–53), but one retrospective study suggests a better prognosis at age 2 after elective cesarean delivery before labor (54). Although not proven to prevent permanent neurological damage, ACOG states that cesarean section should be considered for these babies (55). Vaginal delivery appears appropriate for infants with isolated hydrocephalus with macrocephaly (56), anterior abdominal wall defects (57,58), sacrococcygeal teratomas less than 5 cm (59), and fetal ovarian cysts (60). Fetuses who cannot be monitored appropriately during labor, such as those with complete heart block, and those with associated nonreassuring signs are better served by abdominal delivery.

Desire for elective, permanent surgical sterilization is not an indication for either repeat or primary cesarean delivery. The morbidity associated with cesarean delivery and intrapartum bilateral tubal ligation is greater than that of vaginal delivery followed by postpartum tubal ligation through a minilaparotomy incision.

TABLE 1. *Commonly reported indications for cesarean section*

Fetal Indications
- Fetal distress
- Transverse lie
- Breech, frank and complete*
- Breech, incomplete
- Breech, preterm*
- Active herpes simplex virus
- Selected fetal congenital anomalies*
- Triplets*
- High order multifetal gestation
- Monoamniotic twins

Maternal and Fetal Indications
- Cephalopelvic disproportion
- Failure to progress
- Placenta previa
- Abruptio placenta with excessive blood loss or fetal distress
- Severe preeclampsia or eclampsia remote from delivery
- Fetal macrosomia > 5,000 grams without maternal Diabetes mellitus
- Fetal macrosomia > 4,500 grams with maternal Diabetes mellitus
- Previous classical cesarean delivery

Maternal Indications
- Failed induction of labor
- Obstructive lesions
- Invasive cervical cancer
- Abdominal cervical cerclage
- Prior rectovaginal fistula repair* or colporrhaphy
- Conjoined twins
- Unrepaired maternal cerebrovascular anomalies*

*Controversial.

COMPLICATIONS

Cesarean delivery is associated with greater mortality than vaginal delivery. The leading causes of direct obstetric maternal mortality are pulmonary embolism, hemorrhage, and infection. Other causes such as amniotic fluid embolism, anesthetic complications, and preeclampsia are less frequent (61). The major sources of maternal mortality are clearly associated with cesarean delivery, although the risk of maternal mortality is quite low, 0.13 to 0.53 per 1,000 cesarean births (62). The relative risk of death associated with cesarean section is 6.7 and includes indirect maternal deaths, women with medical disorders, and life-threatening complications. When only direct maternal mortality is considered in previously healthy women, the relative risk of death attributable to cesarean section versus vaginal delivery is 4.7. Emergency and intrapartum cesarean delivery carries an approximately 1.5-fold increased risk of mortality compared to elective cesarean delivery (63).

A 10-year review of cesarean section morbidity showed an overall intraoperative complication rate of 14.8% among 2,647 cases. The most common intraoperative complications were bleeding from uterine corpus lacerations (10.1%), blood loss greater than 1 L (7.3%), fetal lacerations (1.3%), bladder laceration (0.8%), lacerations of other organs or vessels (0.3%), and other complications (1.9%). Intraoperative complications were significantly more common in women having repeat cesarean deliveries compared to primary cases (23.4% vs 7.4%, $p < 0.001$). The overall postoperative complication rate was 35.7%, of which major complications occurred in 4.5% and minor complications occurred in 31.2%. Major complications included postpartum hemorrhage greater than 1,500 mL, repeat laparotomy, pelvic infection, thrombosis, pneumonia, sepsis, coagulopathy, and other complications. The most common minor postoperative complication was fever in 24.6%. Other minor complications included postpartum hemorrhage of 1,000 to 1,500 mL, hematoma, urinary tract infection, thrombophlebitis, wound infection, ileus, endometritis, and bladder paralysis (64).

Infectious and hemorrhagic morbidity is an important source of lengthened postoperative hospitalization and increased cost of care. The postoperative wound infection rate is about 4.5% to 8% (65–67), and the endomyometritis rate is about 1.0% to 7% (64,67). Blood transfusions are necessary in 1.4% to 3.4% of cases (68,69). As expected, emergency cesarean delivery is associated with greater intraoperative and postoperative risk than elective procedures.

In addition to intraoperative and postoperative complications, effects of cesarean section on future pregnancies are possible. Women with a previous cesarean delivery appear to have an increased risk of ectopic pregnancy, abruptio placenta, and placenta previa (70). Women who have a previous cesarean birth and parity of 3 or greater are at increased risk (OR 1.7, 95% CI 0.7 to 4.2) of placenta previa (71). The risk of rupture of a low transverse incision in a future labor is approximately 0.3% (68).

RATIONALE FOR LOWERING THE NATIONAL CESAREAN DELIVERY RATE

Although the cesarean section rate in the U.S. is no longer rising, it remains excessive (72). Curtailing unnecessary cesarean sections prevents avoidable maternal morbidity and mortality, shortens hospital stays, prevents long-term complications, and saves billions of dollars in health care costs. The potential cost savings from a reduction in the cesarean section rate can be gleaned from the 1991 CDC National Hospital Discharge Survey data. In 1991, the average cost for a cesarean delivery was $7,826 compared with $4,720 for a vaginal birth. These supplementary costs represent additional physician fees and additional hospital charges due to longer hospital stays and increased maternal morbidity. Had the national cesarean delivery rate been 15% rather than the recorded 23.5%, the number of cesarean births avoided would have been 349,000, saving more than one billion dollars (11). The goal of reducing the number of unnecessary cesarean sections from the perspective of morbidity and cost is a worthy one.

What is the ideal cesarean section rate? The ideal rate has yet to be determined, and a national goal may be neither feasible nor even desirable. Nonetheless, achieving the U.S. Department of Health objective of a national cesarean section rate of no more than 15% of all deliveries in the year 2000 (73) will require a reduction of about 160,000 cesarean deliveries each year.

METHODS TO LOWER THE CESAREAN DELIVERY RATE

Hospital programs to reduce the number of unnecessary cesarean deliveries are gaining popularity (Table 2). Socol and colleagues (74), at a primarily private university hospital, acheived a decline in the cesarean delivery rate from 27.3% to 16.9% over 5 years. Both primary and repeat cesarean operations decreased, while the perinatal mortality rate was halfed (74). They encouraged VBAC, provided individuals with feedback about their cesarean delivery rate, and began an active management of labor program.

TABLE 2. *Methods to reduce the cesarean section rate*

1. Encourage a trial of labor following one or more low transverse cesarean deliveries.
2. Educate patients and the community about the value of VBAC.
3. Institute practice guidelines to minimize individual physicaian differences in the rate of cesarean delivery for dystocia.
4. Provide reliable, accurate data to physicians regarding their cesarean delivery rate.
5. Provide reliable, accurate data to nurses regarding their cesarean delivery rate.
6. Consider a peer review process for VBAC, induction, and cesarean delivery for dystocia.
7. Make the diagnosis of fetal distress with care.
8. Make the safe reduction of the cesarean delivery rate a departmental and organizational priority.

Others achieved similar successes through quality assurance, peer review, and specific labor management guidelines (75). Recently, Porreco and Thorp (76) reviewed the literature regarding the causes of the rise in unnecessary cesarean deliveries in the U.S. and offer some suggestions to address the cesarean "epidemic." Fruitful measures will address elective repeat cesarean section and primary cesarean deliveries for dystocia and breech.

Vaginal Birth after Cesarean Section

A trial of labor after cesarean delivery is a safe alternative to elective repeat cesarean section and can be expected to be successful in 60% to 80% of cases (68,77,78). Flamm and co-workers (78) found a shorter length of hospital stay, fewer postpartum transfusions, and less postpartum febrile morbidity among women attempting a trial of labor. This reduction in maternal morbidity was not associated with a change in perinatal mortality (78). That a trial of labor is not risk-free is demonstrated by McMahon and co-workers (68). In their comparison of trial of labor with elective repeat cesarean section, the rate of maternal complications was not different between groups. However, those who had a failed trial of labor were at greater risk of intraoperative injury and twice as likely to have major complications (68). The risk of uterine rupture is less than 1% (68,77). VBAC is clearly supported after a single, low transverse cesarean section.

The enthusiasm for VBAC in the U.S is growing (Fig. 4). Certain conditions previously thought controversial do not necessarily constitute contraindications to trials of labor. A judicious trial of cesarean scar is warranted in the presence of two or more previous low transverse incisions (79), suspected fetal macrosomia (80), and an unknown scar unless the history indicates a high likelihood of classic uterine incision (81). In some conditions, a trial of labor has been demonstrated safe in small trials, but there are insufficient data to warrant the routine recommendation of VBAC. These conditions include a previous low vertical cesarean scar, twin gestation, and breech presentation. There also are insufficient data to routinely recommend external cephalic version or prostaglandin E_2 gel for cervical ripening in a scarred uterus. On the other hand, ACOG supports the use of oxytocin for the induction and augmentation of labor and the use of epidural analgesia for VBAC, as the safety is established (82).

Patient demand is still a major factor in the determination of route of delivery after previous cesarean section. Kline and Arias (83) found that of 121 women who had an elective repeat cesarean section, 31.6% were scheduled on the basis of patient demand, in the absence of obstetric indication for repeat cesarean delivery. Most patient fears about VBAC are not supported by evidence. Much of the decision for a repeat, scheduled cesarean delivery is driven by memories of a prolonged and painful labor and a desire for convenient scheduling (84). It is necessary for physicians and hospitals to coordinate education along the continuum of care. Education about VBAC begins at the time of the initial cesarean section. During the following pregnancy, after documentation of a previous low transverse cesarean scar by review of the operative note, VBAC literature should be provided. VBAC classes or education should be encouraged in order to address risks and benefits as well as individual concerns. Finally, these measures should be followed by physician advocation for a trial of labor.

Active Management of Labor and Other Dystocia Strategies

The diagnosis of dystocia accounts for a large percentage of primary cesarean deliveries and contributes to the repeat cesarean delivery problem. A program of "active management of labor" is designed to prevent dystocia in nulliparous women (see Chapter 11) (85). Although several centers report a reduction in their cesarean delivery rate after initiation of an active management program (74,86,93), two prospective randomized trials give conflicting results (87,88). A meta-analysis of the highest quality randomized and nonrandomized trials indicate a 34% reduction in cesarean delivery associated with active management without an increase in neonatal morbidity (89). This program differs from the traditional approach and requires investments in patient and provider education and nursing support. Cost savings are realized, however, through the reduction in unnecessary surgical deliveries.

Physician factors may have an important role in the decision to perform cesarean delivery. When physicians have large discrepancies in their cesarean section rates, without demonstrable differences in fetal outcome, a program that selects a "best practice model" for emulation can be important. Practice guidelines are the core of some institutional efforts to decrease cesarean delivery and improve patient care (74), whereas others rely on second opinions and peer review (75). Provision of accurate, reliable data to physicians regarding their personal cesarean delivery rate in relationship to their peers allows the process of quality improvement to begin.

Alternative institutional strategies to reduce cesarean deliveries for dystocia are under investigation. One hospital noted a reduction in the rate of total and repeat primary cesarean section from 24.9% to 21.7% and from 17.6% to 15.3%, respectively, after the introduction of mandatory in-hospital coverage by attending physicians. The authors postulate that fewer time-related cesarean sections for dystocia and fetal distress were performed because external pressures related to social, family, and professional commitments were removed (90). Other efforts include one-on-one labor support (91) midwifery, alternative pain management strategies, and increased ambulation in labor. The impact of nursing care on the decision to perform cesarean delivery should not be underestimated. Nurses spend a greater amount of time with laboring women and a difficult labor may be stressful for mother and nurse alike. Little mention is made of the fact that decisions about cesarean delivery are made after considerable nursing input.

External Cephalic Version

Over 80% of breech-presenting infants are delivered by cesarean section. External cephalic version (ECV) should result in a success rate of about 58% allowing labor in a cephalic presentation (92). A randomized controlled trial demonstrated a reduction in cesarean deliveries in women undergoing ECV (93). The success of a version attempt appears to be augmented with the use of a tocolytic agent, such as ritodrine, in nulliparous women (94), but the utility in parous women is debatable (92). Serious complications of ECV are unusual, occurring in fewer than 1% of cases. Reported adverse effects include abruptio placenta, preterm labor, and transient fetal heart rate changes. Although infrequent, the possibility of complications prompted the ACOG to recommend ECV be performed in conjunction with pre- and postprocedure fetal assessment and in a venue in which cesarean delivery can be performed readily (92). A recent small, randomized, trial of epidural analgesia for ECV suggests that this modality safely improves version success (95). Routine external cephalic version will not bring about a substantial reduction in the national cesarean delivery rate but can be of benefit to individual women. Gifford and co-workers (96) presented an analysis predicting that a program of ECV can reduce the cesarean rate for breech from 89% to 32% (even without performing breech deliveries) at a cost savings of $1,500 per case.

Diagnose Fetal Distress Carefully

Fetal distress and "other" indications account for a minority of the total cesarean delivery rate. However, all avoidable and unnecessary cesarean deliveries should be addressed. The diagnosis of fetal distress should be made with care. Techniques such as intrapartum fetal scalp stimulation (97), vibroacoustic stimulation (98), and assessment of fetal acid–base status via scalp blood sampling can provide reassurance to continue labor. Amnioinfusion is used to reduce the frequency and intensity of variable decelerations and decrease the number of cesarean deliveries (99).

SUMMARY

The ideal cesarean delivery rate has yet to be determined. The Healthy People 2000 benchmark of a total cesarean section rate of 15% and a 12% primary cesarean section rate is achievable, but clearly not by the millennium. The key to the safe reduction in the national cesarean section rate will be through implementation of institutional efforts to reduce repeat procedures and address the diagnosis of dystocia. The approach will involve patient and provider education, and multidisciplinary quality improvement. However, as long as fears of malpractice claims abound, "defensive" cesarean deliveries will continue to be performed.

REFERENCES

1. Sewell JE. *Cesarean section: a brief history.* Washington, DC: The American College of Obstetricians and Gynecologists, 1993.
2. Notson FC. International differences in the use of obstetric interventions. *JAMA* 1990;263:3286.
3. Anonymous. Rates of cesarean delivery—United States, 1993. *MMWR* 1995;44:303.
4. Ventura SJ, Martin JA, Curtin SC, Mathews TJ. Report of final natality statistics, 1995. Monthly Vital Statistics Report 1997;45:11 [Suppl], PHS 97-1120.
5. Hueston WJ. Site-to-site variation in the factors affecting cesarean section rates. *Arch Fam Med* 1995;4:346.
6. Rock SM. Variability and consistency of rates of primary and repeat cesarean sections among hospitals in two states. *Public Health Rep* 1993;108:514.
7. Localio AR, Lawthers AG, Bengtson JM, et al. Relationship between malpractice claims and cesarean delivery. *JAMA* 1993;269:366.
8. Gould JB, Davey B, Stafford RS. Socioeconomic differences in rates of cesarean section. *N Engl J Med* 1989;321:233.
9. Haynes De Regt R, Minkoff HL, Feldman J, Schwarz RH. Relation of private or clinic care to the cesarean birth rate. *N Engl J Med* 1986; 315:619.
10. Notzon FC, Cnattingius S, Bergsjo P, et al. Cesarean section delivery in the 1980s: international comparison by indication. *Am J Obstet Gynecol* 1994;170:495.
11. Anonymous. Rates of cesarean delivery-United States, 1991. *MMWR* 1993;42:285.
12. ACOG Committee on Obstetric Practice. Perinatal and infant mortality statistics. ACOG Committee Opinion No. 167. Washington, DC: American College of Obstetricians and Gynecologists, 1995.
13. Bottoms SF, Rosen MG, Sokol RJ. The increase in the cesarean birth rate. *N Engl J Med* 1980;302:559.
14. Perinatal mortality. Vital Statistics of the United States 1992, Vol. II, Mortality, Part A, PHS 96-1101.
15. O'Driscoll K, Foley M. Correlation of decrease in perinatal mortality and increase in cesarean section rates. *Obstet Gynecol* 1983;61:1.
16. U.S. Department of Health and Human Services; Public Health Service; National Institutes of Health. Repeat cesarean birth. In: Cesarean childbirth. Washington, DC: U.S. Government Printing Office; 1981; NIH Publication 82-2067.
17. Hickson GB, Clayton EW, Githens PB, Sloan FA. Factors that prompted families to file medical malpractice claims following perinatal injuries. *JAMA* 1992;267:1359.
18. Harlow BL, Frigoletto FD, Cramer DW, et al. Epidemiologic predictors of cesarean section in nulliparous patients at low risk. RADIUS study group. Routine Antenatal Diagnostic Imaging with Ultrasound Study. *Am J Obstet Gynecol* 1995;172:156.
19. Adashek JA, Peaceman AM, Lopez-Zeno JA, Minogue JP, Socol ML. Factors contributing to the increased cesarean birth rate in older parturient women. *Am J Obstet Gynecol* 1993;169:936.
20. Martel M, Wacholder S, Lippman A, Brohan J, Hamilton E. Maternal age and primary cesarean section rates: a multivariate analysis. *Am J Obstet Gynecol* 1987;156:305.
21. Parrish KM, Holt VL, Easterling TR, Connell FA, LoGerfo JP. Effect of changes in maternal age, parity, and birth weight distribution on primary cesarean delivery rates. *JAMA* 1994;271:443.
22. ACOG. Dystocia and the augmentation of labor. ACOG Technical Bulletin No. 218. Washington, DC: American College of Obstetricians and Gynecologists, 1995.
23. Lieberman E, Lang JM, Cohen A, D'Agostino R, Datta S, Frigoletto FD. Association of epidural analgesia with cesarean delivery in nulliparas. *Obstet Gynecol* 1996;88:993.
24. Morton SC, Williams MS, Keller EB Kahn K. Effect of epidural analgesia for labor on the cesarean delivery rate. *Obstet Gynecol* 1994;83: 1045.
25. Thorp JA, Parisi VM, Boylan PC, Johnston DA. The effect of continuous epidural analgesia on cesarean section for dystocia in nulliparous women. *Am J Obstet Gynecol* 1989;161:670.
26. Wuitchik M, Bakal D, Lipshitz J. The clinical significance of pain and cognitive activity in latent labor. *Obstet Gynecol* 1989;73:35.
27. Thorp JA, Hu DH, Albin RM, et al. The effect of intrapartum epidural analgesia on nulliparous labor: a randomized, controlled, prospective trial. *Am J Obstet Gynecol* 1993;169:851.
28. Ramin SM, Gambling DR, Lucas MJ, Sharma SK, Sidawi JE, Leveno KJ. Randomized trial of epidural versus intravenous analgesia during labor. *Obstet Gynecol* 1995;86:783.
29. Sharma SK, Sidawi JE, Ramin SM, Lucas MJ, Leveno KJ, Cunningham G. Cesarean delivery: a randomized trial of epidural versus patient-controlled meperidine analgesia during labor. *Anesthesiology* 1997;87:487.
30. Lyon DS, Knuckles G, Whitaker E, Salgado S. The effect of instituting an elective labor epidural program on the operative delivery rate. *Obstet Gynecol* 1997;90:135.
31. Gribble RK, Meier PR. Effect of epidural analgesia on the primary cesarean rate. *Obstet Gynecol* 1991;78:231.
32. Fogel ST, Shyken JM, Leighton BL, Mormol JS, Smeltzer JS. Epidural labor analgesia and the incidence of cesarean delivery for dystocia. *Anesth Analg* 1998;87:119.
33. Zahniser SC, Kendrick JS, Franks AL, Saftlas AF. Trends in obstetric operative procedures, 1980 to 1987. *Am J Public Health* 1992;82: 1340.
34. Robertson PA, Laros RK, Zhao R-L. Neonatal and maternal outcome in low-pelvic and midpelvic operative deliveries. *Am J Obstet Gynecol* 1990;162:1436.
35. Gray DL, Nelson M. Cord blood acid-base status in neonates delivered by silastic vacuum cup extraction: comparison with forceps and spontaneous deliveries. *Obstet Gynecol* 1988;71:76.
36. Ramin SM, Little BB, Gilstrap LC. Survey of forceps delivery in North America. *Obstet Gynecol* 1993;81:307.
37. Bashore RA, Philips WH Jr, Brinkman CR III. A comparison of the morbidity of midforceps and cesarean delivery. *Am J Obstet Gynecol* 1990;162:1428.
38. ACOG. Operative vaginal delivery. ACOG Technical Bulletin No. 196. Washington, DC: American College of Obstetricians and Gynecologists, 1994.
39. Cheng M, Hannah M. Breech delivery at term: a critical review of the literature. *Obstet Gynecol* 1993;82:605.
40. Eller DP, VanDorsten JP. Route of delivery for the breech presentation: a conundrum. *Am J Obstet Gynecol* 1995;173:393.
41. Vintzileos AM, Antsaklis A, Varvarigos I, Papas C, Sofatzis I, Montgomery JT. A randomized trial of intrapartum electronic fetal heart

rate monitoring versus intermittent auscultation. *Obstet Gynecol* 1993;81:899.
42. Luthy DA, Shy KK, Van Belle G, et al. A randomized trial of electronic fetal monitoring in preterm labor. *Obstet Gynecol* 1987;69:687.
43. Parer JT, Livingston EG. What is fetal distress? *Am J Obstet Gynecol* 1990;162:1421.
44. Cibils LA. On intrapartum fetal monitoring. *Am J Obstet Gynecol* 1996;174:1382.
45. Vintzileos AM, Nochimson DJ, Guzman ER, Knuppel RA, Lake M, Schifrin BS. Intrapartum electronic fetal heart rate monitoring versus intermittent auscultation: a meta-analysis. *Obstet Gynecol* 1995;85:149.
46. Guyer B, Martin JA, MacDorman MF, Anderson RN, Strobino DM. Annual summary of vital statistics—1996. *Pediatrics* 1997;100:905.
47. Paul RH, Miller DA. Cesarean birth: how to reduce the rate. *Am J Obstet Gynecol* 1995;172:1903.
48. DeMott RK, Sandmire HF. The Green Bay cesarean section study. II. The physician factor as a determinant of cesarean birth rates for failed labor. *Am J Obstet Gynecol* 1992;166:1799.
49. DeMott RK, Sandmire HF. The Green Bay cesarean section study. I. The physician factor as a determinant of cesarean birth rates. *Am J Obstet Gynecol* 1990;162:1593.
50. Fraser W, Usher RH, McLean FH, et al. Temporal variation in rates of cesarean section for dystocia: does "convenience" play a role? *Am J Obstet Gynecol* 1987;156:3.
51. Bensen JT, Dillard RG, Burton BK. Open spina bifida: does cesarean section improve prognosis? *Obstet Gynecol* 1988;71:532.
52. Sakala EP, Andree I. Optimal route of delivery for meningomyelocele. *Obstet Gynecol Surv* 1990;45:209.
53. Hill AE, Beattie F. Does cesarean section delivery improve neurological outcome in open spina bifida. *Eur J Pediatr Surg* 1994;4:32.
54. Luthy DA, Wardinsky T, Shurtleff DB, et al. Cesarean section before the onset of labor and subsequent motor function in infants with meningomyelocele diagnosed antenatally. *N Engl J Med* 1991;324:662.
55. ACOG. Maternal serum screening. ACOG Educational Bulletin No. 228. Washington, DC: American College of Obstetricians and Gynecologists, 1996.
56. Kuller JA, Katz VL, Wells SR, Wright LN, McMahon J. Cesarean delivery for fetal malformations. *Obstet Gynecol Surv* 1996;51:371.
57. Moretti M, Khoury A, Rodriquez J, Lobe T, Shaver D, Sibai B. The effect of mode of delivery on the perinatal outcome in fetuses with abdominal wall defects. *Am J Obstet Gynecol* 1990;163:833.
58. Kirk EP, Wah RM. Obstetric management of the fetus with omphalocele or gastroschisis: a review and report of one hundred twelve cases. *Am J Obstet Gynecol* 1983;146:512.
59. Gross SJ, Benzie RJ, Sermer M, Skidmore MB, Wilson SR. Sacrococcygeal teratoma: prenatal diagnosis and management. *Am J Obstet Gynecol* 1987;56:393.
60. Sakala EP, Leon ZA, Rouse GA. Management of antenatally diagnosed fetal ovarian cysts. *Obstet Gynecol Surv* 1991;46:407.
61. Jacob S, Bloebaum L, Shah G, Varner MW. Maternal mortality in Utah. *Obstet Gynecol* 1988;91:187.
62. Schuitemaker N, van Roosmalen J, Dekker G, van Dongen P, van Geijn H, Gravenhorst JB. Maternal mortality after cesarean section in the Netherlands. *Acta Obstet Gynecol Scand* 1996;75:332.
63. Lilford RJ, Van Coeverden De Groot HA, Moore PJ, Bingham P. The relative risks of caesarian section (intrapartum and elective) and vaginal delivery: a detailed analysis to exclude the effects of medical disorders and other acute pre-existing physiological disturbances. *Br J Obstet Gynecol* 1990;97:883.
64. Van Ham MAPC, van Dongen PWJ, Mulder J. Maternal consequences of caesarean section: a retrospective study of intraoperative and postoperative maternal complications of caesarean section during a 10-year period. *Eur J Obstet Gynecol Reprod Biol* 1998;74:1.
65. Nice C, Feeney A, Godwin P, et al. A prospective audit of wound infection rates after caesarean section in five West Yorkshire hospitals. Journal of Hospital Infection 1996;33:55-61.
66. Martens MG, Kolrud BL, Faro S, Maccato M, Hammill H. Development of wound infection or separation after cesarean delivery: a prospective evaluation of 2,431 cases. *J Reprod Med* 1995;40:171.
67. Henderson E, Love EJ. Incidence of hospital-acquired infections associated with caesarean section. *J Hosp Infect* 1995;29:245.
68. McMahon MJ, Luther ER, Bowes WA, Olshan AF. Comparison of a trial of labor with an elective second cesarean section. *N Engl J Med* 1996;335:689.
69. Hillan EM. Postoperative morbidity following cesarean delivery. *J Adv Nurs* 1995;22:1035.
70. Hemminki E, Merilainen J. Long-term effects of cesarean sections: ectopic pregnancies and placental problems. *Am J Obstet Gynecol* 1996;174:1569.
71. McMahon MJ, Li R, Schenck AP, Olshan AF, Royce RA. Previous cesarean birth: a risk factor for placenta previa? *J Reprod Med* 1997;42:409.
72. Flamm BL, Quilligan EJ. *Cesarean section:* guidelines for appropriate utilization. New York: Springer-Verlag, 1995.
73. U.S. Department of Health Services. Healthy People 2000. Washington, DC: USDHS, 1991; PHS 91-50212.
74. Socol ML, Garcia PM, Peaceman AM, Dooley SL. Reducing cesarean births at a primarily private university hospital. *Am J Obstet Gynecol* 1993;168:1748.
75. Myers SM, Gleicher N. A successful program to lower cesarean-section rates. *N Engl J Med* 1988;319:1511.
76. Porreco RP, Thorp JA. The cesarean birth epidemic: trends, causes, and solutions. *Am J Obstet Gynecol* 1996;175:369.
77. Cowan RK, Kinch RA, Ellis B, Anderson R. Trial of labor following cesarean delivery. *Obstet Gynecol* 1994;83:933.
78. Flamm BL, Goings JR, Liu Y, Wolde-Tsadik G. Elective repeat cesarean delivery versus trial of labor: a prospective multicenter study. *Obstet Gynecol* 1994;83:927.
79. Asakura H, Meyers SA. More than one previous cesarean delivery: a 5-year experience with 435 patients. *Obstet Gynecol* 1995;85:924.
80. Flamm BL, Goings JR. Vaginal birth after cesarean section: is suspected fetal macrosomia a contraindication? *Obstet Gynecol* 1989;74:694.
81. Pruett KM, Kirshon B, Cotton DB. Unknown uterine scar and trial of labor. *Am J Obstet Gynecol* 1988;159:807.
82. ACOG. Vaginal delivery after previous cesarean birth. ACOG Practice Patterns No. 1. Washington, DC: American College of Obstetricians and Gynecologists, 1995.
83. Kline J, Arias F. Analysis of factors determining the selection of repeated cesarean section or trial of labor in patients with histories of prior cesarean delivery. *J Reprod Med* 1993;38:289.
84. Abitbol M, Castillo I, Taylor UB, Rochelson BL, Shmoys S, Monheit AG. Vaginal birth after cesarean section: the patient's point of view. *Am Fam Physician* 1993;47:129.
85. Peaceman AM, Socol ML. Active management of labor. *Am J Obstet Gynecol* 1996;175:363.
86. Akoury HA, Brodie G, Caddick R, McLaughin VD, Pugh PA. Active management of labor and operative delivery in nulliparous women. *Am J Obstet Gynecol* 1988;158:255.
87. Frigoletto FD, Lieberman E, Lang JM, et al. A clinical trial of active management of labor. *N Engl J Med* 1995;333:745.
88. Lopez-Zeno JA, Peaceman AM, Adashek JA, Socol ML. A controlled trial of a program for the active management of labor. *N Engl J Med* 1992;326:450.
89. Glantz JC, McNanley TJ. Active management of labor: a meta-analysis of cesarean delivery rates for dystocia in nulliparas. *Obstet Gynecol Surv* 1997;52:497.
90. Klasko SK, Cummings RV, Balducci J, DeFulvio JD, Reed JF. The impact of mandated in-hospital coverage on primary cesarean delivery rates in a large nonuniversity teaching hospital. *Am J Obstet Gynecol* 1995;172:637.
91. Zhang J, Bernasko JW, Leybovich E, Fahs M, Hatch MC. Continuous labor support from labor attendant for primiparous women: a meta-analysis. *Obstet Gynecol* 1996;88:739.
92. ACOG. External cephalic version. ACOG Practice Patterns No. 4. Washington, DC: American College of Obstetricians and Gynecologists, 1997.
93. Mahomed K, Seeras R, Coulson R. External cephalic version at term. A randomized controlled trial using tocolysis. *Br J Obstet Gynaecol* 1991;98:8.
94. Marquette GP, Boucher M, Theriault D, Rinfret D. Does the use of a tocolytic agent affect the success rate of external cephalic version? *Am J Obstet Gynecol* 1996;175:859.

95. Schorr SJ, Speights SE, Ross EL, et al. A randomized trial of epidural anesthesia to improve external cephalic version success. *Am J Obstet Gynecol* 1997;177:1133.
96. Gifford DS, Keeler E, Kahn KL. Reductions in cost and cesarean rate by routine use of external cephalic version: a decision analysis. *Obstet Gynecol* 1995;85:930.
97. Clark SL, Gimovsky ML, Miller FC. The scalp stimulation test: a clinical alternative to fetal scalp blood sampling. *Am J Obstet Gynecol* 1984;148:274.
98. Polzin GB, Blakemore KJ, Petrie RH, Amon E. Fetal vibro-acoustic stimulation: magnitude and duration of fetal heart rate accelerations as a marker of fetal health. *Obstet Gynecol* 1988;72:621.
99. Miyazaki FS, Nevarez F. Saline amnioinfusion for relief of repetitive variable decelerations: a prospective randomized study. *Am J Obstet Gynecol* 1985;153:301.
100. Medical Leadership Council. *Coming to term:* innovations in safety reducing cesarean rates. Washington, DC: The Advisory Board Company, 1996.

Obstetric Anesthesia, second edition,
edited by Mark C. Norris.
Lippincott Williams & Wilkins, Philadelphia © 1999.

CHAPTER 20

General Anesthesia for Cesarean Delivery

Andrew M. Malinow

In United States, 15% to 22% of cesarean deliveries are accomplished under general anesthesia (1). The frequency of general anesthesia for cesarean delivery varies greatly between individual hospitals. Several of the factors that influence the use of general anesthesia are:

- Patterns of labor analgesia (a higher use of epidural analgesia for labor increases the use of epidural anesthesia for cesarean delivery),
- Patient populations (high-risk obstetric centers with more stressed and distressed fetuses needing immediate delivery may use general anesthesia more commonly), and
- Obstetrician and anesthesiologist practice patterns (the diagnosis of fetal distress and, therefore, the need for emergency delivery vary from institution to institution).

INDICATIONS

Although the use of general anesthesia for elective cesarean delivery is no longer routine, the technique must be available at any time to facilitate obstetric intervention. In modern practice, general anesthesia for cesarean delivery is reserved for limited situations (Table 1). Coexisting maternal diseases, which contraindicate regional anesthesia and rapid deterioration of fetal well-being, are the most common of these indications. In addition, not every regional anesthetic proves adequate for the entire surgical procedure. Oversedation, resulting in loss of maternal airway reflexes, may lead to disaster. In the face of inadequate regional anesthesia, I prefer intraoperative induction of general anesthesia with tracheal intubation.

There has been recent interest in identifying the factors that influence a patient's choice of general anesthesia over regional anesthesia for cesarean delivery (2–4). In one study, women who opted for general anesthesia were slightly older, of higher parity, of lower socioeconomic class, or had a previous pregnancy loss (2). Patients choosing general anesthesia for cesarean delivery also scored differently from those choosing regional anesthesia when given psychometric tests for anxiety and depression (2).

The anesthesiologist, by providing patients with clear, concise information, has a role to play in the selection process. A brief discussion with the anesthesiologist will mollify initial fears about regional anesthesia in one-fifth of parturients who initially refuse regional anesthesia for cesarean delivery (3). Another survey suggested that 43% of women given general anesthesia for cesarean delivery were not given a choice of their anesthesia, although it must be noted that almost one-half these of patients presented for emergent cesarean deliveries (4).

ADVANTAGES

General anesthesia produces rapid, reproducible conditions for cesarean delivery. General anesthesia has a long record of fetal and relative maternal safety. Success of general anesthesia is independent of a patient's anxiety

TABLE 1. *Indications for general anesthesia for cesarean delivery*

Acute severe fetal distress
Epidural catheter not in situ
Relative and absolute contraindications to regional anesthesia
Maternal hemodynamic instability
Severe maternal hemorrhage
Coexisting maternal cardiac disease (e.g., severe right-to-left shunt, fixed primary pulmonary hypertension, severe aortic stenosis)
Maternal coagulopathy
Maternal infection
Superficial to the lumbosacral spine
Sepsis
Patient refusal of regional anesthesia
Regional anesthesia inadequate for surgery

A. M. Malinow: Department of Anesthesiology, University of Maryland, Baltimore, Maryland 21201.

about remaining "awake." Stoicism is not a factor in the patient under general anesthesia.

DISADVANTAGES

Disadvantages of general anesthesia center on airway management (Table 2). Anatomic and physiologic changes of pregnancy increase the risk of failed intubation. Parturients are at high risk for aspiration of gastric contents. The often hectic and tumultuous conditions surrounding emergent cesarean delivery may compromise preoperative evaluation of the parturient with a potentially difficult airway.

Today, an anesthesiologist routinely uses a multitude of drugs during a general anesthetic. The obstetric suite is an ideal site for drug substitution or other misuse. Anesthetic medications often are prepared, labeled, and left unattended on an operating room anesthesia cart. Later, they may be used immediately to induce general anesthesia.

Owing to the frequent use of regional anesthesia in the labor and delivery suite, anesthesia machines are used less often than in the general surgical suite. These anesthesia machines may receive less frequent routine maintenance. The possibility of undetected machine malfunction increases. All anesthetic machines in the labor and delivery suite should be checked out daily and after every use in anticipation of emergency induction of general anesthesia.

Finally, the physiologic consequences of the induction of general anesthesia and tracheal intubation may prove deleterious to the mother with coexisting medical conditions (e.g., cardiac or neurologic).

PREPARATION FOR GENERAL ANESTHESIA

Airway Assessment

Preoperative evaluation begins with a thorough evaluation of the airway. The following factors contribute to difficult tracheal intubation in the parturient:

TABLE 2. *Disadvantages of general anesthesia for cesarean delivery*

Maternal airway management
Failed intubation
Trauma
Increased number of anesthetic drugs needed/drug substitution
Anesthesia machine failure
Physiologic consequences of general anesthesia
Stress response and coexisting disease (i.e., increased intracranial pressure at induction, tracheal intubation, emergence, tracheal extubation)
Pharmacologic response to general anesthesia
Anesthetic agents have desired effects (i.e., intraoperative anesthesia) and undesired effects (i.e., hyperkalemic response to succinylcholine in patients with paraplegia)

- The often emergent nature of cesarean delivery limits the time for preanesthetic evaluation and preparation.
- Medical personnel who can help with a difficult airway are relatively scarce.
- Anatomic airway changes in the gravida, perhaps exacerbated by obesity or preeclampsia/eclampsia, increase the technical difficulty of tracheal intubation.
- Inexperienced anesthesiology personnel are often assigned to the labor and delivery suite.

Importance of Airway Assessment

Maternal Mortality

By 1988 to 1990, anesthetic-related maternal mortality had decreased to 1.7 per 1,000,000 live births from 4.3 per 1,000,000 live births a decade earlier (5). The use of regional anesthesia for cesarean delivery has greatly increased (5). The absolute number of deaths due to regional anesthesia has decreased by 80%, down to 1.9 per 1,000,000 regional anesthetics (5).

The absolute number of deaths involving general anesthesia (due most frequently to airway problems) was stable over that decade (5). However, fewer general anesthetics for cesarean delivery were administered. The risk of maternal mortality is now 32 per 1,000,000 general anesthetics, a 17-fold increase in relative risk compared to patients receiving regional anesthesia for cesarean delivery (5). The incidence of failed intubation in the obstetric population is 1 of 250, approximately ten times more frequent than in the general surgical patient population (6). Disturbingly, this number has not decreased over the last 10 years (6).

Identifying the Patient "At Risk"

The Confidential Enquiry Into Perioperative Death (1987) found that preanesthetic assessment did not occur in 10% of the mortality reviewed. Regular review of patients admitted to the labor and delivery suite can anticipate 87% of urgent or emergent cesarean deliveries (7,8). The anesthesiologist must identify the parturient with a potentially difficult airway soon after her admission to the labor and delivery suite. Look for the presence of the many different indicators of difficult airway (i.e., ability to open the mouth, mandibular length, and loose dentition). Attempt to visualize the normal oropharyngeal anatomy (soft palate, uvula, and tonsillar fossae).

Factors Associated with Difficult Airway

Anatomic Abnormalities

Samsoon and Young (9) retrospectively reviewed a group of seven parturients who previously experienced failed intubation. At the first posthospital discharge visit, they confirmed their immediate antepartum conclusion that external examination of the head and neck would not hint at difficult tracheal incubation. However, visual inspection of the oropharynx in six of these seven women revealed partial or total obliteration of anatomic detail (the seventh women had normal structure but was already diagnosed with tracheal stenosis). On laryngoscopy, the glottic aperture and posterior arytenoid cartilage were not visualized in five of these six women (9). In another retrospective review of failed tracheal intubation at cesarean delivery, over 60% of the patients had an abnormal examination of the airway recorded in the preoperative evaluation; the most common anatomic findings recorded were a receding jaw, limited mouth opening, and prominent teeth (6).

In a prospective study of 277 obstetric patients presenting for cesarean delivery under general anesthesia, 264 had Mallampati scores of 1 or 2 (all structures visible including the tonsillar fauces or with only partial obliteration of the epiglottis, respectively) (10). Of those 264 patients, only four were later judged as a difficult tracheal intubation. Two of the 13 patients assigned a Mallampati score of 3 or 4 were later judged as a difficult tracheal intubation (10).

Rocke et al. (11) evaluated over 1,500 patients presenting for general anesthesia for cesarean delivery. Their report examined the commonly stated anatomic risk factors for difficult tracheal intubation. They calculated the relative risk of difficulty at tracheal intubation versus a Mallampati class 1 airway (Table 3) (11).

These studies suggest that the relative absence of normal anatomic detail (soft palate, uvula, and tonsillar fauces) on visual inspection of the oropharynx correlates with possible difficult incubation in obstetric patients. Airway evaluation must be a routine part of the preanesthetic evaluation of the parturient (see Chapter 32).

Obesity

In one review, obesity complicated 80% of anesthetic-related maternal deaths (12). Forty-seven percent of cases involved general anesthesia for cesarean delivery (12). One-half of the deaths were directly due to failure to establish an adequate airway (12). Obesity (body mass index greater than 23) doubles the incidence of partially obliterated oropharyngeal anatomy (13). The cesarean delivery rate (and, therefore, the incidence of anesthetic intervention) increases from 18% to 30% (13). In the morbidly obese parturient (greater than 300 lb), the cesarean delivery rate exceeds 50% (14). One-half these operations are done during labor. In one series, 24% of cesarean deliveries were accomplished under general anesthesia. One-third of the tracheal intubations were difficult, with a failed tracheal intubation rate of 6% (1 of 17 patients) (14).

TABLE 3. *Relative risk of factors associated with difficulty at tracheal intubation as compared with an uncomplicated Mallampati class 1 evaluation*

Anatomic feature	Relative risk
Mallampati 4	11.30
Receding mandible	9.71
Protruding maxillary incisors	8.00
Mallampati 3	7.58
Short neck	5.01
Mallampati 2	3.23
Mallampati 1	1.00

From ref. 11, with permission.

Pregnancy-induced Hypertension

Pregnancy-induced hypertension also may predispose to difficult intubation. Women with pregnancy-induced hypertension (a population at high risk of cesarean delivery) are twice as likely as normotensive parturients to have poorly visible oropharyngeal structures (15).

Avoiding Trouble with the Difficult Airway

Early Induction of Epidural Analgesia

Early induction of labor analgesia usually precludes the need for general anesthesia should cesarean delivery later become necessary. However, not every epidural anesthetic proves adequate for cesarean delivery. Intraoperative induction of general anesthesia may be required should unanticipated intraoperative events delay closure of the abdomen and create distress in the awake (and aware) parturient. For example, massive hemorrhage (with possible hemodynamic instability), unplanned uterine repair, or hysterectomy occurs in 1.3% to 1.6% of repeat cesarean deliveries in women given a trial of labor (16). In addition, an epidural catheter placed during labor sometimes fails to provide adequate anesthesia for emergent cesarean delivery. Morgan at al. (7) had to convert 14% of already established epidural anesthetics to general anesthesia before emergent cesarean delivery. When the decision-to-delivery time was less than 10 minutes, 50% of these women received general anesthesia (7). Routine use of rapidly acting local anesthetics (i.e., 3% 2-chloroprocaine) may further decrease the need for general anesthesia among women already receiving epidural labor analgesia. At the University of Maryland, we use alkalinized 3% 2-chloroprocaine or 2% lidocaine with epinephrine to extend and intensify epidural anesthesia for emergent cesarean delivery. Fewer than 3% of epidural anesthetics for cesarean delivery are converted to general anesthesia at some time during surgery. Most often, we use general anesthesia only for emergent cesarean delivery of a severely distressed fetus (i.e., when the decision-to-incision time is less than 5 minutes).

Developing a Plan

Identifying the parturient with a potentially difficult airway helps ensure adequate time to plan and to communicate with the obstetrician before the need for general anesthesia. Appropriate planning may include awake intubation, fiberoptic bronchoscopy-assisted intubation, surgical control of the airway, or retrograde intubation. Such intervention requires time to collect personnel and equipment.

Experienced Personnel

Finally, the experience of the anesthesiologist plays an important role in the incidence of anesthetic-related maternal mortality (17). Expertise, especially relating to the prediction and management of the difficult airway, is acquired during training and is not innate to the unsupervised junior trainee. In a recent review of obstetric patients who had experienced failed tracheal intubation, most incidents occurred at night or on weekends when the patients were cared for by less experienced anesthesiologists. In this review of failed tracheal intubation, almost all of the anesthesiologists observed cricoarytenoid cartilage but not glottic aperture at laryngoscopy (6). These facts suggest that more experience in dealing with the difficult airway (e.g., use of gum elastic bougies, light wands, etc.) on the part of the anesthesiologist might have converted a failed tracheal intubation into a successful one.

Acid-aspiration Prophylaxis

Pharmacologic methods of acid-aspiration prophylaxis are part of the planning for every general anesthetic for cesarean delivery. Drug trials in humans provide conflicting data on which regimen is best. No one agent (or combination of agents) will ensure a nonfatal aspiration. Even the accepted criteria of critical intragastric volume (less than 0.4 mL/kg) and acidity (pH greater than 2.5) (18) have not been rigorously developed. Acidity of the aspirate may be more crucial than volume (19). This fact is important, especially in pharmacologic preparation of the nonfasted parturient presenting for urgent or emergent cesarean delivery. Risk factors vary among patients and institutions. Obstetric practices about the ingestion of food and liquids differ greatly, particularly in the latent phase of labor. In addition, labor analgesia practices using parenteral and epidural opioids, known inhibitors of gastric motility, also vary. Applying study data to the clinical situation requires careful interpretation. The urgency of the clinical situation often precludes certain agents. Clinicians use antacids, H_2-receptor antagonists, and metoclopramide in varying combinations in a search for the optimally prepared "full stomach."

Urgent or Emergent Cesarean Delivery

Adequate preparation of gastric contents in the laboring patient differs from that of the fasted parturient presenting for elective delivery. Women may eat just before admission. Labor significantly slows or eliminates physiologic gastric emptying, resulting in a true "full stomach." No acid-aspiration prophylaxis regimen reliably reduces the volume and raises the pH of gastric contents in the laboring patient. Mechanically emptying the stomach before induction of anesthesia for cesarean delivery is no better than a single dose of sodium citrate at decreasing the number of patients at risk for aspiration pneumonitis (20). This cruel punishment, awake passage of a gastric tube, has, I hope, been abandoned in the modern practice of obstetric anesthesia.

Antacid

Administration of 0.3 M of sodium citrate quickly and reliably increases the pH of intragastric contents (Figs. 1 and 2B) (21–23). There is mild controversy over the dose (15 or 30 mL) of sodium citrate. In some studies, the larger dose produces a greater rise in pH (5.7 ± 0.8 vs 4.6 ± 1.1) (23). In addition, 30 mL maintains pH above 2.5 for a longer time (24) without significantly increasing intragastric volume (23) compared to the smaller dose (Table 4). Sodium bicarbonate has been used as a single-dose antacid in parturients with questionable efficacy (25).

Ranitidine

The coadministration of single-dose ranitidine (50 mg) intravenously and 0.3 M sodium citrate orally maintains intragastric alkalinization longer than antacid alone; however, this effect becomes significant only 2 hours after treatment (20,26). Ranitidine does not reduce intragastric

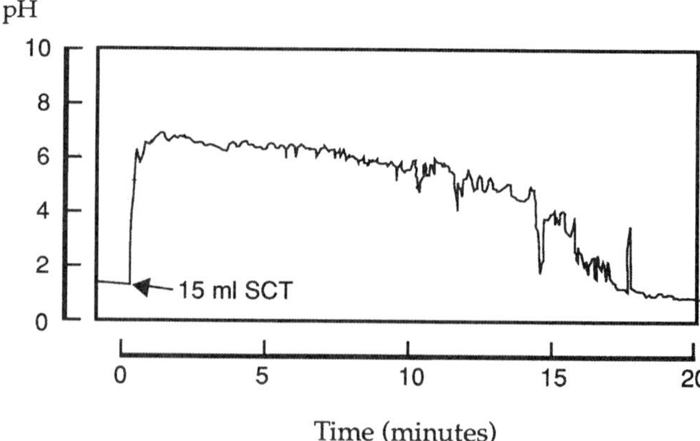

FIG. 1. Intragastric pH change after the administration of 15 mL of 0.3 M sodium citrate (SCT) to a woman in labor. (From ref. 22, with permission.)

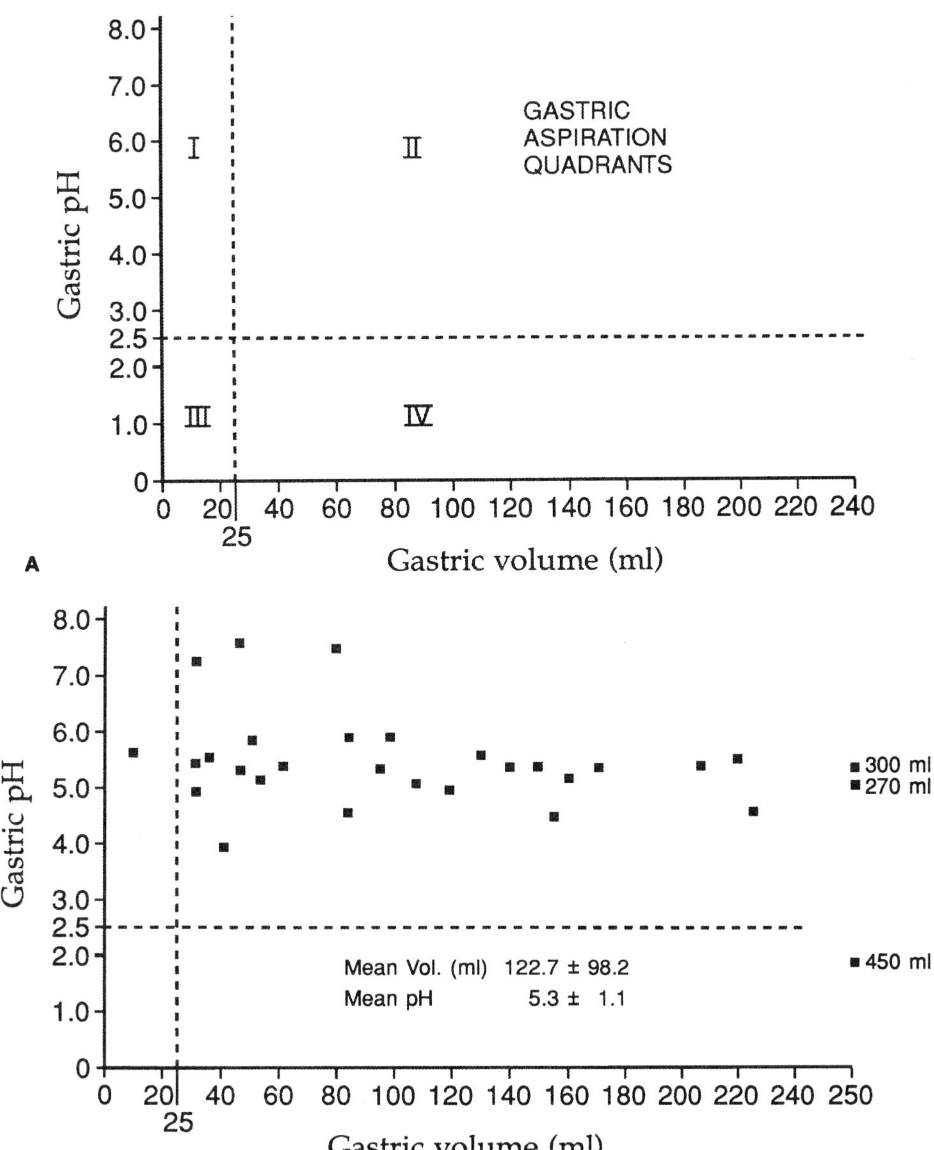

FIG. 2. A: Division of gastric pH and volume coordinates into four quadrants indicating risk level. Patients in quadrant IV (pH less than 2.5 and volume greater than 25 mL) should be at greatest risk for the development of acid pneumonitis after aspiration of gastric contents. **B:** Gastric volume and pH in laboring parturients receiving only 0.3 M sodium citrate before emergency cesarean delivery. Fifteen received 15 mL of Na citrate and 15 received 30 mL. **C:** Gastric volume and pH at cesarean delivery in laboring parturients receiving ranitidine 50 mg i.m. every 6 hours during labor. **D:** Gastric volume and pH at cesarean delivery in laboring parturients receiving ranitidine 50 mg i.m. every 6 hours during labor and one dose of 0.3 M Na citrate 15 mL immediately before the induction of anesthesia. (From ref. 23, with permission.)

volume (20,26); therefore, the coadministration of single-dose intravenous ranitidine and oral antacid is of little practical use in the parturient presenting for emergent or urgent cesarean delivery under general anesthesia. Regularly scheduled parenteral ranitidine doses do not adequately prepare the gastric contents of the laboring parturient presenting for emergent or urgent cesarean delivery under general anesthesia (Fig. 2C) (20,26). At the very least, give an oral antacid before inducing general anesthesia for urgent or emergent cesarean delivery (Table 5). Famotidine (20 mg p.o.) appears to be an acceptable substitute for ranitidine (150 mg p.o.) (27).

Effervescent Cimetidine/Sodium Citrate

Effervescent cimetidine/sodium citrate (400 mg/0.9 M, respectively, in 15 mL of water) effectively alkalinizes intragastric contents (28). This combination will maintain

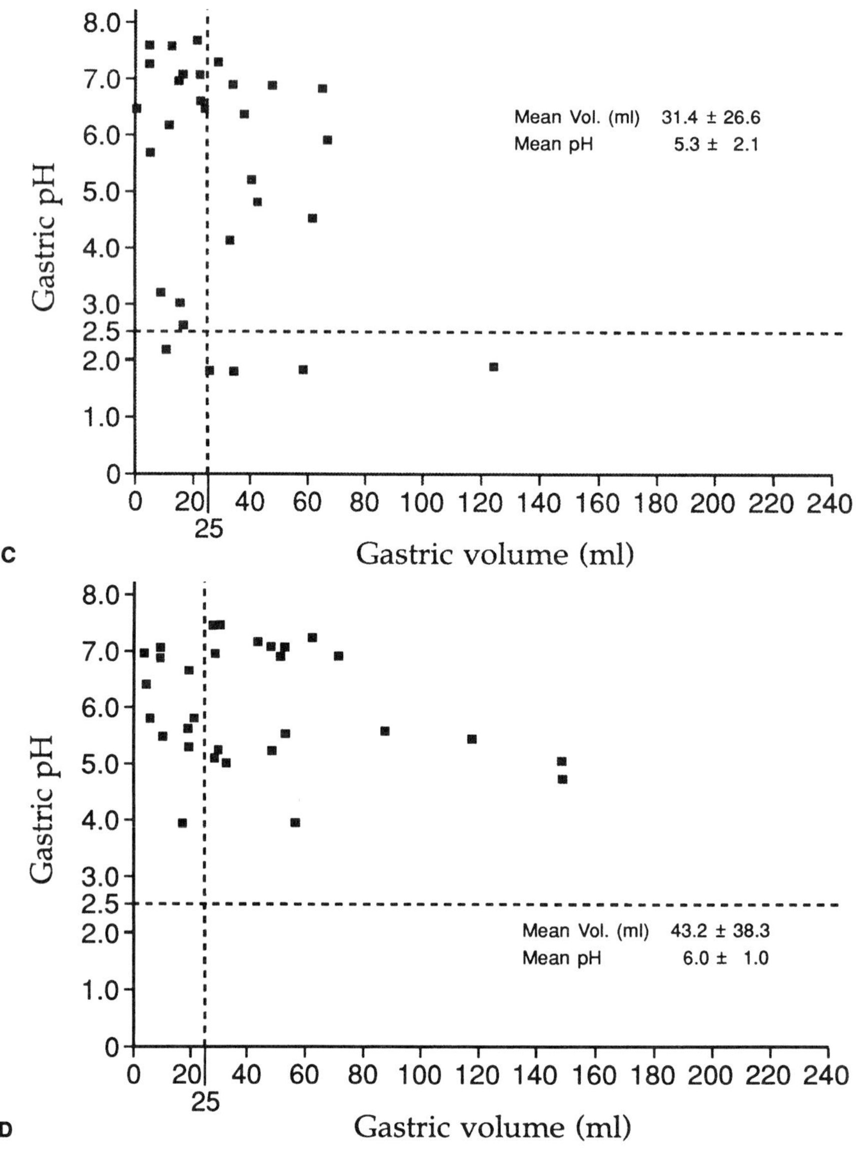

FIG. 2. (Continued).

TABLE 4. *Alkalinization of gastric contents by 0.3 M sodium citrate, as measured by noninvasive radiotelemetry*

	Median basal pH (range)	Median maximum pH (range)	Mean time to peak pH (range)[a]	Mean time pH >3.0 (range)[a]
15-mL sodium citrate (in labor)	2 (1.4–2.5)	6.8 (5.4–7.9)	1.0 (0.6–2.81)	84[b] (11.8–195.8)[c]
15-mL sodium citrate (term but not in labor)	1.4 (1.3–2.8)	6.8 (5.9–7.5)		26.6 (17.8–104.3)[c]
30-mL sodium citrate (term but not in labor)	2 (1.6–2.5)	6.8 (5.8–8.3)		42.1 (6.6–97.5)[c]

[a]Values given in minutes.
[b]Prolonged duration patients in labor; probably due to effects of labor decreasing gastrointestinal motility.
[c]Note wide range of duration.
Data from refs. 22, 24.

TABLE 5. *Suggested acid-aspiration prophylaxis*

Scheduled elective cesarean delivery (assuming a fasted patient for scheduled 7:30 a.m. surgery)	
Ranitidine	150 mg p.o. at 10 p.m., 50 mg i.v. at 6 a.m. (for scheduled 7:30 a.m. surgery)
Ranitidine	300 mg p.o. 3 h before scheduled surgery
Urgent cesarean delivery (patient may or may not be in labor; at least 5 min available before induction of anesthesia)	
Metoclopramide	10 mg slow i.v.
0.3 M sodium citrate	30 mL p.o. before moving to operating room table
Ranitidine	Consider 50 mg i.v. if 30–60 min will elapse until induction of anesthesia
Emergent cesarean delivery (<5 min until induction of anesthesia)	
0.3 M sodium citrate	30 mL p.o. before moving to operating room table

intragastric pH significantly higher than antacid alone at 1 hour after treatment and beyond. In addition, fewer patients have gastric aspirates with pH less than 2.5 at 20 minutes (1.6%) and at 60 minutes (1.6%) compared to antacid treatment alone (14% and 10% at 20 and 60 minutes, respectively). These results are similar to those seen after the coadministration of intravenous ranitidine and oral sodium citrate (Fig. 2D). Additional studies may confirm that this promising oral combination drug is superior to oral antacid alone.

Omeprazole

Omeprazole, which blocks the proton pump in the parietal cell, effectively reduces both intragastric volume and acidity after a double-dose oral regimen (40 mg at night and early morning) in women fasted before elective cesarean delivery (29). Double-dose omeprazole yields intragastric volumes and acidity that are similar to those provided by double-dose oral ranitidine (150 mg). However, the incidence of treatment failures was nil compared to 6% in parturients receiving ranitidine. Omeprazole seems a promising oral alternative to oral and parenteral combinations. Single-dose omeprazole provides inadequate preparation of gastric contents.

Metoclopramide

Metoclopramide often is given before the induction of general anesthesia for urgent cesarean delivery. It will increase lower esophageal sphincter tone within 2 to 5 minutes of parenteral administration (30). Compared to placebo, intravenous metoclopramide (10 mg) decreases mean residual intragastric volume (59.5 ± 61 mL vs 19.0 ± 13 mL). In addition, fewer patients have volumes greater than 25 mL (75% vs 36%) (31).

Narcotic administration inhibits the effects of metoclopramide (32). A dose of metoclopramide at induction or during general anesthesia in hope of emptying the stomach before extubation is therefore of questionable value. In addition, the use of metoclopramide is not without risk (33–35). Therefore, I give metoclopramide only to parturients who present for urgent or emergent cesarean delivery soon after eating (Table 5).

Elective Cesarean Delivery

The patient scheduled for cesarean delivery should routinely fast for at least 8 hours before induction of general anesthesia. Feeding women clear liquids just before a 4-hour fast doubles the volume of gastric aspirate compared with patients conventionally fasted (65 ± 21 mL vs 33 ± 22 mL, respectively) (36). Antacid ingestion adequately alkalinized gastric aspirates in all patients (36). In the conventionally fasted patient presenting for elective cesarean delivery, two doses of ranitidine (150 mg p.o. then 50 mg i.m.) or cimetidine (400 mg PO then 200 mg IM) over 6 to 8 hours will decrease intragastric volume (to 9 ± 7.2 mL) and increase pH (to 6.2 ± 0.8) (23,37). In these studies, no patient had a gastric aspirate volume greater than 25 mL or pH less than 2.5. Further alkalinization of the stomach (at the expense of increased intragastric volume) increases the risk in an already acceptably "prepared" patient. The use of a double-dose (orally, then intramuscularly) H_2-receptor antagonist regimen therefore avoids the need for routine use of oral antacid (or intravenous metoclopramide). Single-dose oral ranitidine (150 mg) yields similar mean intragastric volume and pH as a double-dose oral regimen in women presenting for cesarean delivery (26,38). However, the incidence of "treatment failures" (or those patients exceeding acceptable intragastric volume or acidity criteria) is increased with a single- or double-dose oral ranitidine regimen (3%) compared with a double-dose (orally, then intramuscularly) ranitidine regimen (0%). Parenteral metoclopramide eliminated treatment failures in patients given double-dose oral ranitidine (38).

If a double-dose H_2-receptor antagonist regimen has not been followed on the fasted patients, then there are two remaining options. First, ingesting an increased dose of H_2-receptor antagonist (ranitidine 300 mg or famotidine 40 mg) will effectively decrease the number of patients at risk for aspiration (compared with placebo) at 3 hours after treatment (27). An alternative regimen would include oral antacid ingestion followed by parenteral administration of metoclopramide before induction of anesthesia (Table 5).

Cost-effectiveness

The cost-effectiveness of acid-aspiration prophylaxis often is questioned. There are few answers. An abstract presented at the 1985 Annual Meeting of the Society of Obstetric Anesthesia and Perinatology modeled the cost-effectiveness of three acid-aspiration prophylaxis regimens

(0.3 M sodium citrate, double-dose parenteral cimetidine, and the combination of these two drugs) (39). For elective cesarean deliveries, the combination of antacid and H_2-receptor antagonist reduced mortality to almost nil, with an incremental cost of $130,000 per life saved compared with antacid alone. In the laboring parturient, antacid was both more effective and less costly than cimetidine. Antacid therapy reduced mortality by almost 90% when compared to no intervention, at a cost of $57,000 per life saved. Combination therapy further reduced mortality at the great incremental cost of $40,000,000 per life saved. Results from this model support the routine use of H_2-receptor antagonist therapy before elective cesarean delivery. Results from this model cast added doubt (about cost efficacy) to my skepticism about the routine use of H_2-receptor antagonist therapy during labor.

Positioning

Uterine Displacement

Always provide uterine displacement to avoid supine hypotension. Methods of uterine displacement are not as important as their routine and vigilant practice.

Operating Position

Venous air emboli occur commonly during cesarean delivery (44% to 62%) (40–42) and are unrelated to the type of anesthesia (41). Venous air emboli at cesarean delivery only rarely are hemodynamically significant, although their occurrence has been associated with cardiorespiratory collapse (43). Positioning the table in a 5-degree reverse Trendelenburg's position decreases the incidence of venous air emboli to less than 8% (41). I routinely place the patient in a slight head-up position at the start of surgery and avoid Trendelenburg's position during cesarean delivery.

Optimal Airway Management

No matter how emergent the need for delivery, take time before the induction of general anesthesia to ensure optimal alignment of the shoulders, neck, and head ("sniffing" position). This step will maximize the chances of successful intubation and help emergency airway management, should it become necessary. Blankets are ubiquitous in the delivery suite. Even the extremely obese parturient can be optimally positioned using folded and stacked blankets to support the upper back and maternal occiput (see Chapter 25, Fig. 6).

Monitoring and Equipment

The parturient undergoing cesarean section requires the same types of intraoperative monitoring as any patient having emergency intraabdominal surgery.

Airway/Breathing

End-tidal gas analysis is essential in the management of the patient under general anesthesia. Measuring end-tidal nitrogen (or oxygen) can document adequate denitrogenation before rapid sequence induction of anesthesia. Capnography helps confirm proper position of the tracheal tube. Intraoperative capnometry aids in monitoring maternal ventilation. In the gravid ewe, intermittent positive-pressure hyperventilation decreases uteroplacental perfusion (although this animal model may not reproduce the effects of hyperventilation during the short interval between tracheal intubation and delivery of the human fetus). The resultant hypocapnia may hinder placental exchange of oxygen and carbon dioxide owing to a change in oxyhemoglobin affinity (44). In the term parturient, decreased alveolar dead space and increased alveolar ventilation (45) combine to lower the end-tidal/arterial carbon dioxide gradient toward zero (Fig. 3) (46,47). A tidal volume of 10 mL/kg at 10 breaths per minute using a semiclosed circle system will provide the least change in fetal acid–base balance, will not increase the incidence of low Apgar scores, and will provide maternal normocapnia (48). Monitoring maternal exhaled carbon dioxide with capnometry will document normocapnia.

Circulation

Establish sufficient intravenous access to allow rapid replacement of large fluid volumes. A free-flowing, securely fastened, large-bore (at least 18-gauge) peripheral intravenous catheter should be in situ before induction of general anesthesia for anticipated routine cesarean delivery. Certain high-risk conditions as well as changing intra-

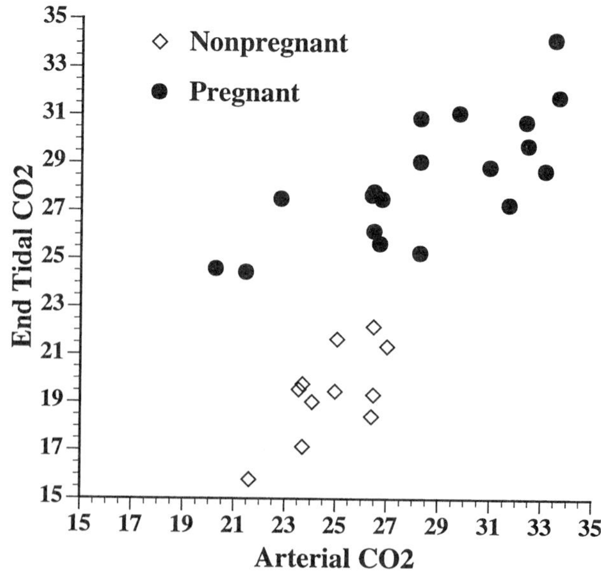

FIG. 3. End-tidal to arterial CO_2 gradient during general anesthesia in nonpregnant and pregnant women. (Data from ref. 46.)

operative surgical conditions may demand additional intravenous access to allow rapid transfusion (*vide infra*). Have equipment available to allow rapid infusion of warmed, intravenous fluids in the hemorrhaging parturient.

Today, with increasing frequency, the anesthesiologist is encountering the parturient with peripheral intravenous access made difficult (or impossible) from a long history of drug abuse. Keep an adequate supply of disposable central venous access kits immediately available. Sonography can help locate the internal jugular vein. Such equipment is available in almost every labor and delivery suite. Sometimes, however, the anesthesiologist is faced with the need to provide general anesthesia immediately in a parturient without obvious venous access. In such dire emergencies, I have found that cannulation of the femoral vein is relatively easy with a catheter of proper length. Difficulty in securing the catheter and infectious complications are drawbacks to this approach. Later, alternate routes of venous access can be obtained at a (hopefully) less harried pace.

The ability to transduce intraarterial and central venous pressures, as well as to measure cardiac output, is vital in the management of certain obstetric or coexisting medical disease.

Temperature

I use forced hot air circulation blankets in my routine anesthetic practice at cesarean delivery. I find these devices useful in maintaining intraoperative maternal body temperature. Besides obvious intraoperative benefit, normothermia enhances maternal "bonding" in the postanesthesia care unit.

Fetus

In the parturient presenting for cesarean delivery, I monitor fetal heart rate electronically until surgical preparation of the abdomen or even induction of anesthesia (if an internal scalp electrode is already in place). Any change in fetal heart rate can be evaluated by the perinatal team and may alert them to significant changes in fetal condition. Signs of rapid intrauterine deterioration can increase the urgency of delivery. Conversely, the diagnosis of acute fetal distress can be reevaluated upon arrival in the operating room, sometimes eliminating the need for immediate surgery.

Preoxygenation and Denitrogenation

Pregnancy-related alterations in respiratory physiology greatly influence the preparation of the parturient for induction of general anesthesia. Filling the lungs with oxygen prolongs the interval from onset of apnea to hypoxemia and is a critical part of a rapid sequence induction for any emergent surgical patient.

The gravida has multiple reasons for a decreased apnea to hypoxemia time (49). At term, oxygen consumption increases 20% to 30% (50). In labor, oxygen consumption may rise by 80% (51). Especially in the supine position, airway closure occurs during tidal breathing (52), increasing shunt fraction and producing hypoxemia.

Functional residual capacity is smaller in parturients (53–55), whereas minute ventilation rises (56). These physiologic alterations speed nitrogen washout and oxygenation while breathing 100% oxygen.

Two methods of preoxygenation and denitrogenation are commonly used in the operating room: four vital capacity breath hyperventilation and 3-minute tidal volume breathing. Both produce a similar rise in arterial pO_2 and a similar fall in oxygen saturation desaturation during apnea (an average duration of 50 seconds). However, unless a tight mask fit is ensured, hyperventilation predisposes to room air (and, therefore, nitrogen) entrainment. Alveolar oxygen concentration then becomes unpredictable (57).

Using a circle system (common in the United States) and oxygen flows of 5 to 6 L/min, Norris and Dewan (58) showed that four vital capacity breath hyperventilation and 3-minute tidal volume breathing produced similar levels of arterial oxygenation during rapid sequence induction of general anesthesia. In a follow-up study, Norris et al. (59) showed that parturients needed a mean 55 seconds of tidal breathing to reach 5% end-tidal nitrogen, compared to 111 seconds for nonpregnant women. Four vital capacity breath hyperventilation does not wash out nitrogen as effectively as 3-minute tidal volume breathing (5% end-tidal nitrogen as compared to 1%, respectively) (Fig. 4). The extra margin of safety (10 to 15 additional seconds of apnea) provided before hypoxemia, however, is clinically insignificant (59).

From these studies, it becomes evident that the additional 2.5-minute wait for tidal volume breathing preoxygenation may give added, although slight, benefit in the nonemergent situation. In the emergent situation, four vital capacity breath hyperventilation of high-flow oxygen will safely suffice if proper attention is given to mask fit and patient instruction.

Pretreatment/Defasiculation

Fasiculation

The need for a defasiculating (or pretreatment) dose of nondepolarizing neuromuscular relaxant before the intubating dose of succinylcholine is questionable. Between 68% and 100% of nonpregnant surgical patients experience vigorous fasiculation in response to succinylcholine (60–63). However, pregnancy, as early as in the first trimester, decreases the incidence and severity of fasiculation (60). At term, the incidence of fasiculation decreases to 9% (64). Pretreatment with d-tubocurarine (0.05 mg/kg) does not further reduce this incidence (64).

Myalgia

The incidence of postoperative myalgia is 20% in first-trimester women compared with 30% to 40% in nonpregnant patients (60,65). At term, 7.5% to 13% of

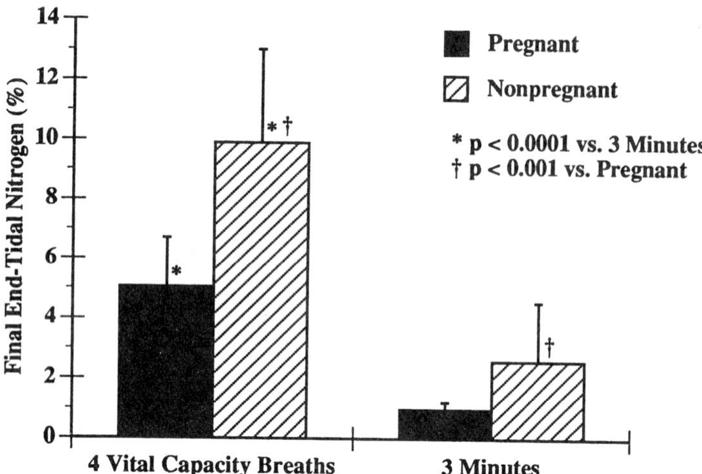

FIG. 4. Final end-tidal nitrogen concentration (%) following 3 minutes of tidal breathing or four deep breaths of 100% oxygen in ten healthy parturients and nine healthy nonpregnant women. (Redrawn from ref. 59, with permission.)

women report postoperative myalgia (64–66). Pretreatment with d-tubocurarine does not decrease the incidence of postoperative myalgia (64–66). Hormonal effects on skeletal muscle may explain this low risk of myalgia during gestation (65,66).

Action of Succinylcholine

In term parturients, pretreatment with d-tubocurarine does not alter the onset of succinylcholine neuromuscular blockade (time to 100% twitch depression) (64). However, paralysis lasts 120 to 150 seconds longer, increasing from 7 to 9 minutes in nonpretreated patients (64). This prolongation of neuromuscular paralysis is of questionable clinical significance. The time to recovery is short enough to have the patient begin spontaneous (or assisted) ventilation before the end of surgery, but it is still far longer than a patient will tolerate apnea during a difficult intubation. Interestingly, decreasing the dose of succinylcholine by 30% in nonpretreated parturients decreases the recovery time toward the duration found in pretreated parturients, but does not prolong the onset time (64). I see no benefit to pretreatment, as it does not decrease the incidence of fasciculation or postoperative myalgia, and I omit it when inducing general anesthesia for cesarean delivery.

INTRAVENOUS INDUCTION AGENTS

Many induction agents used for cesarean delivery were studied in an era when maintenance techniques of general anesthesia (i.e., predelivery maternal inspired oxygen concentrations of 30% to 100%, with or without the use of a volatile agent) were very different from today. Comparison of two or more studies of neonatal outcome after maternal induction with one of these agents requires caution.

Thiopental/Thiamylal

In the United States, thiopental (or its analog, thiamylal) is the most frequently used drug for induction of general anesthesia for cesarean delivery (Table 6). In the parturient, the mean dose of thiopental needed to induce general anesthesia (3.5 mg/kg pregnant body weight) is 35% less than the mean induction dose needed in nonpregnant patients (67–69). Thiopental appears in fetal blood within 45 seconds of maternal administration. Fetal drug concentrations peak 1.5 to 3.0 minutes after induction (69–72).

Rapid maternal redistribution and nonuniform intervillous blood flow lead to a wide variability in measured umbilical venous (UV) and maternal venous (MV) blood thiopental concentration ratios (UV/MV) (73). At delivery, neither UV nor MV thiopental concentrations correlate with induction-to-delivery times (70). However, UV and MV thiopental concentrations closely correlate with each other, and the UV/MV ratio is usually below 1 (70). Uptake by the fetal liver and dilution with systemic venous blood further decrease fetal arterial thiopental concentration (69).

Varying a single bolus of thiobarbiturate from 4 to 7 mg/kg does not affect Apgar scores (70,72). A maternal induction dose of 8 mg/kg will increase the number of Apgar scores less than 7 (40%) compared with lower doses of thiobarbiturate (10%) (72). Barbiturate can still be measured in the maternal blood up to 9 hours after delivery and is measurable (though in minute concentrations) in the colostrum (74).

In my practice, thiopental/thiamylal 4 mg/kg is the standard induction dose for general anesthesia for cesarean delivery. I sometimes increase the dose by 25% to 50% (or supplement it with adjuvant agents) when inducing general anesthesia for parturients who may be compromised by the hypertensive response to induction or intubation.

Methohexital

Methohexital is 2.5 to 3 times as potent as thiopental (69). An induction dose of methohexital greater than 1 mg/kg has been associated with an increased number of

TABLE 6. *General anesthesia for cesarean delivery: induction agents*

Drug	Dose	Maternal effects	Neonatal effects
Thiopental/thiamylal	4 mg/kg		Increased low Apgar scores with dose >7 mg/kg
Methohexital	1 mg/kg		Increased incidence of low Apgar scores,[a] prolonged time to sustained respiration[a]
Ketamine	1–1.5 mg/kg	Possibly augmented hypertensive response to intubation, decreased recall, increased dreaming	>2 mg/kg increased neonatal depression
Etiomidate	0.3 mg/kg	Pain on injection, myoclonus	Slightly increased umbilical venous base deficit,[a] possible neonatal adrenal suppression
Midazolam	0.2–0.3 mg/kg	0 (%) recall, slight hypotensive effect[a]	± Increased incidence of low 1-min Apgar scores,[a] transient postdelivery hypotonus
Propofol	2.0–2.8 mg/kg	Cutaneous rash, pain on injection, slight decrease in heart rate[a]	± Transient neurobehavioral changes

[a]Vs thiopental/thiamylal, 3–4 mg/kg.

low Apgar scores and a delayed time to sustained respiration (Table 6) (75).

Ketamine

Many anesthesiologists use intravenous ketamine (1 mg/kg) to induce general anesthesia in the following clinical situations:

- Significant maternal hemorrhage,
- Parturients with asthma (potential salutary effects of peripheral catecholamine release on bronchospasm), and
- Cesarean delivery for fetal distress.

Some routinely use ketamine for induction (Table 6). This drug appears to lower the incidence of intraoperative maternal awareness (*vide infra*) (76).

Ketamine produces dose-dependent maternal hypertension in humans (77) and animals (78). Although perhaps best avoided in parturients who may not tolerate hypertension at induction (i.e., preeclampsia or coexisting neurosurgical disease), in elective cesarean delivery, ketamine 1 mg/kg does not increase maternal blood pressure at induction/intubation any higher than thiopental 4 mg/kg (78).

Ketamine concentrations in umbilical blood peak 1 to 2 minutes after maternal intravenous administration (69,79). Apgar scores are similar in neonates delivered abdominally after induction of anesthesia with ketamine 1 mg/kg or thiopental 3 mg/kg (76). Induction of general anesthesia with ketamine 2 mg/kg is associated with neonatal depression (69). Some experts advocate ketamine as the anesthetic induction drug of choice for cesarean delivery of the distressed fetus. In the gravid ewe, ketamine maintains uteroplacental blood flow without deleterious effects on fetal cardiovascular or blood acid–base measurements (80). In sheep with induced fetal asphyxia, neither cerebral and myocardial blood flow nor acid–base measurements deteriorate after ketamine (81). In a similar model, induction of anesthesia with ketamine better preserved fetal blood pressure and cerebral blood flow than did thiopental (81).

Compared to thiopental, induction of general anesthesia with ketamine may decrease postoperative morphine requirements (24.3 vs 35 mg) (82). This effect probably relates to ketamine's ability to stimulate N-methyl-D-aspartate receptors and block their activation in response to noxious input (82).

Etomidate

Etomidate has found limited popularity as an induction drug for general anesthesia at cesarean delivery. Etomidate, which rapidly induces anesthesia, is quickly hydrolyzed to an inactive substance, limiting its duration (83). In addition, etomidate produces little cardiorespiratory change.

Etomidate can be used as an induction agent at cesarean delivery (Table 6) (83–85). However, it frequently produces pain on injection and myoclonus (84). The incidence of myoclonus may be lower during rapid sequence induction due to succinylcholine paralysis (83).

Etomidate readily crosses the placenta (84). Compared with thiopental 3.5 mg/kg, etomidate 0.3 mg/kg produces a questionably significant decrease in neonatal time to sustained respiration (85). There is a slight increase in umbilical vein base deficit versus thiopental (–6.5 vs –4.7, respectively) (83). This greater degree of neonatal acidosis also is of questionable clinical significance. The concentration of etomidate in maternal blood is nil at 2 hours postinduction. Only a very small amount of etiomidate is found in colostrum (74).

Early neonatal adrenal suppression also has been reported after maternal etomidate (86). Because of reports of bothersome maternal side effects, possible neonatal effects, and its expense as compared to thiopental and ketamine, I use etomidate as an induction agent at cesarean delivery only in the occasional parturient with significant cardiac disease.

Midazolam

Studies of midazolam, a water-soluble benzodiazepine with a short elimination half-life, as an induction agent for cesarean delivery have yielded mixed results (Table 6) (70,87–89).

Midazolam 0.2 to 0.3 mg/kg is an effective induction agent for cesarean delivery (87,89). A slight (8 mm Hg) increase in maternal diastolic blood pressure during induction (87) is the only hemodynamic difference seen when comparing midazolam 0.2 to 0.3 mg/kg to thiopental 3.5 to 4.0 mg/kg for induction of general anesthesia for cesarean delivery (89). Neither induction time (time to loss of maternal lid reflex after injection of midazolam) nor the duration of postanesthetic recovery differed from thiopental.

Midazolam crosses the placenta less rapidly than thiopental (70). The UV/MV ratio for midazolam is 0.66 (70). One study reported lower 1-minute Apgar scores in neonates delivered abdominally after midazolam compared to those delivered after thiopental induction. Twenty percent (5 of 26) of neonates delivered after induction of general anesthesia with midazolam had low Apgar scores (and three of the five needed tracheal intubation and intermittent positive-pressure ventilation) versus 4% after thiopental (89). This difference in 1-minute Apgar scores was not seen in another comprehensive study of midazolam, although predelivery anesthetic maintenance was different (88). Funic blood acid–base analysis was similar in neonates delivered after induction of general anesthesia with either drug (89). Time to sustained neonatal respiration was similarly independent of the drug used for maternal induction (89). There was a significant interaction between body temperature, general body tone, and arm recoil in neonates delivered abdominally to mothers who had received midazolam induction (89). This alteration in neurobehavioral scores disappeared within 4 hours of delivery (88,89). The average elimination half-life in neonates is shorter for midazolam than for thiopental (6.3 vs 14.7 hours) (70).

Midazolam is therefore safe for induction of general anesthesia for cesarean delivery. However, maternal hemodynamic changes are very similar to those seen with thiopental. The high incidence of low 1-minute Apgar scores (although funic blood acid–base values are similar with thiopental) and the transient neonatal hypotonus are troublesome. Therefore, I see no place for midazolam induction of general anesthesia in my routine practice of obstetric anesthesia.

Propofol

Intravenous propofol rapidly induces general anesthesia and provides quick recovery owing to its rapid metabolism to inactive substances. Propofol 2.0 to 2.8 mg/kg has been compared to thiopental 4.0 to 5.0 mg/kg for induction of general anesthesia for cesarean delivery (Table 6) (90–98).

Blood pressure tends to fall more after induction with thiopental compared with propofol (91,92). This hypotension corrects with tracheal intubation. Following intubation, maternal systolic arterial blood pressure rises higher and returns to baseline more slowly after thiopental than propofol (Fig. 5A) (91,95,99). After induction of general anesthesia with propofol, maternal blood pressure remains 10 to 12 mm Hg below baseline during the remainder of the predelivery period (Fig. 5A) (91,93,95). Maternal heart rate after induction of general anesthesia with propofol is similar (92) or lower (93) than after thiopental (Fig. 5B). The decrease in maternal heart rate seen after induction of general anesthesia with propofol is evident only after 3 to 4 minutes (93,95). Response to surgical manipulation or hemorrhage may account for the variability in reported heart rate.

Up to 37% of parturients complain of pain on injection of propofol (93) and 7% exhibit a cutaneous rash (92). Propofol does not significantly shorten postanesthetic recovery time in parturients compared with thiopental (93).

Propofol readily crosses the placenta. The UV/MV ratio for propofol is approximately 0.75 (90,91,93,96). Propofol is rapidly cleared from the neonatal circulation (90). The number of neonates with low 1-minute Apgar scores (less than 7) after induction of general anesthesia with propofol is similar to that reported after thiopental (5% to 11%) (90–95,98). Funic blood acid–base analysis is similar in neonates after induction of general anesthesia with propofol or thiopental (91–93,98). Some investigators have reported mildly depressed 1-hour neurobehavioral scores in neonates delivered after induction of general anesthesia with propofol. However, others find no neurobehavioral changes (90). In any case, the neurobehavioral changes are transient (not seen after 2 to 4 hours of life) (94,99).

In my practice, induction of general anesthesia with propofol offers no advantages over thiopental. Unpredictability in maternal hemodynamics is troubling. Currently, the price of propofol does not justify its routine use for an in-patient procedure such as cesarean delivery.

Propofol infusions have been used to maintain general anesthesia with or without nitrous oxide (89,98,99). This technique seems to have no significant advantage and is of increased cost as compared traditional methods.

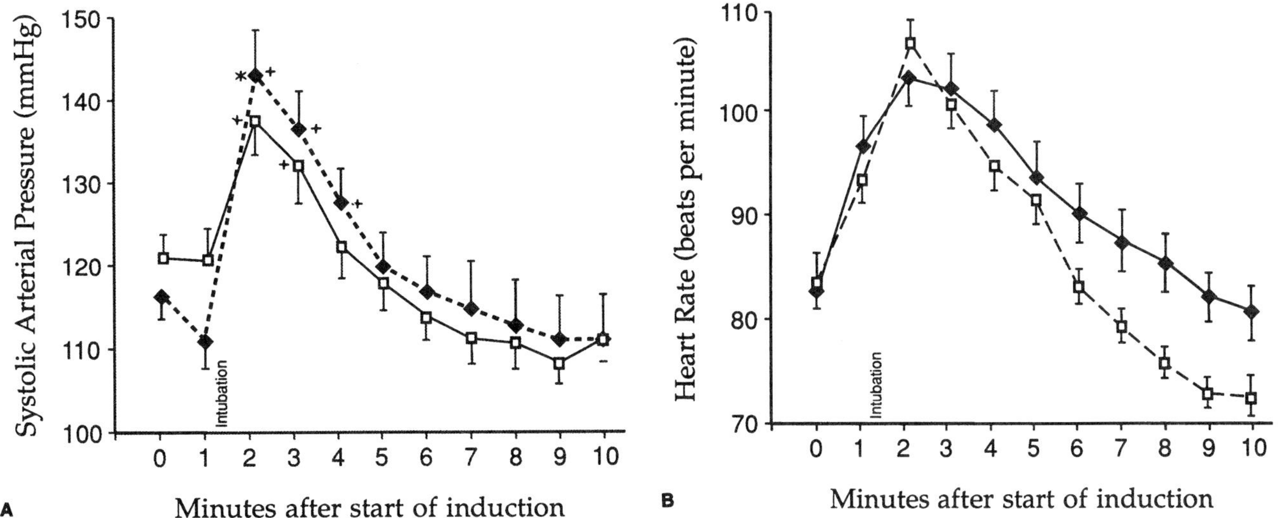

FIG. 5. A: Systolic arterial blood pressure (mean ± SEM) after induction of general anesthesia with propofol 2 mg/kg (n = 20, open boxes) or thiopental 4 mg/kg (n = 20, solid diamonds) for elective cesarean delivery. *p <0.05 versus propofol; +p <0.01 versus baseline. **B:** Maternal heart rate (mean ± SEM) after induction of general anesthesia with propofol 2 mg/kg (n = 20, open boxes) or thiopental 4 mg/kg (n = 20, solid diamonds) for elective cesarean delivery. There are no statistically significant differences between the two groups. (From ref. 95, with permission.)

NEUROMUSCULAR RELAXANTS

All currently used neuromuscular blocking drugs cross the placenta, but their highly ionized, hydrophilic state greatly limits placental transfer. The neonate is clinically affected only under unusual conditions.

Succinylcholine

Succinylcholine 1.0 to 1.5 mg/kg, is the most commonly used drug to facilitate tracheal intubation in a rapid sequence induction of general anesthesia for cesarean delivery. The estimated UV/MV ratio of succinylcholine is 0.04 (100). Although detectable neonatal concentrations of succinylcholine are possible after routine clinical maternal administration, neonatal paralysis has been reported only in an infant homozygous for atypical serum cholinesterase (101).

Nondepolarizing Neuromuscular Relaxants

Common obstetric practice attempts to limit induction-to-delivery times. This practice usually obviates the need for additional predelivery muscle paralysis after the intubating dose of succinylcholine. On occasion, additional muscle paralysis can be provided by using a succinylcholine infusion or the administration of a small dose of nondepolarizing neuromuscular relaxant. Only trace concentrations of d-tubocurarine have been found in the neonate after routine maternal dose (102). The UV/MV ratio of vecuronium is approximately 0.14 (103,104); the UV/MV ratio of atracurium is 0.08 (105). The UV/MV ratio of pancuronium is 0.22 but rises with increasing induction-to-delivery intervals (106). The small doses of nondepolarizing muscle relaxants needed during maintenance of anesthesia for cesarean delivery produce no detectable neonatal effects.

Under certain conditions (i.e., malignant hyperthermia, cholinesterase deficiency, neurological disease with upper motor neuron paresis), succinylcholine is contraindicated. Awake tracheal intubation without sedation can be difficult, unpleasant for both patient and anesthesiologist, and potentially deleterious in certain coexisting disease states. Superior laryngeal nerve blocks are relatively contraindicated because they leave the patient with an unprotected airway. Injection of high-dose vecuronium has been used to facilitate tracheal intubation at cesarean delivery. Vecuronium 0.2 mg/kg given in a rapid sequence before thiopental will provide intubating conditions in 156 seconds. Although not studied directly in comparison to thiopental, there is some evidence that induction of general anesthesia with ketamine hastens the onset of vecuronium-induced neuromuscular block (107). Use of a priming technique to lower the total dose of vecuronium by 45% does not hasten the onset of paralysis. Intubating conditions were judged good or excellent in all parturients given the high-dose vecuronium. Only two patients recalled paresis before loss of consciousness. Paralysis lasted almost 2 hours (103).

Rocuronium 0.6 mg/kg has been used to facilitate tracheal intubation at cesarean delivery (108,109). Onset of 50% neuromuscular block occurs at approximately 45 seconds. At this time, intubating conditions were considered poor in most cases (108). Latencies until 90% and 100% block are approximately 80 and 105 seconds, respectively (108,109). Good to excellent intubating conditions were produced in nearly all patients studied (108,109). Unlike vecuronium, induction of general anesthesia with ketamine does not alter the latency of rocuronium-induced neuromuscular paralysis (108).

I increase the dose of rocuronium to 1.2 mg/kg to shorten the time to 100% neuromuscular block. Either dose of rocuronium (0.6 or 1.2 mg/kg) will produce neuromuscular paralysis for longer period than succinylcholine, a fact to remember if there is any doubt as to the ability to intubate the trachea.

A skilled assistant must maintain cricoid pressure until successful tracheal intubation is confirmed. As always, the possibility of failed intubation and difficult or impossible mask ventilation under cricoid pressure remains a specter in the mind of the anesthesiologist.

After delivery, any of the muscle relaxants already mentioned (e.g., intermediate-acting nondepolarizing agents, succinylcholine infusion) can be used to maintain paralysis. A peripheral nerve stimulator helps manage neuromuscular paralysis and reversal. Although the basic precepts of maintaining and reversing neuromuscular blockade are similar to surgical patients, the parturient may present some differences. For instance, pregnant patients may need less mivacurium to maintain paralysis than nonpregnant patients (110). Yet, reversal is not enhanced with the use of anticholinesterase (110). Again, such phenomena are managed optimally with a peripheral nerve stimulator.

MAINTENANCE OF ANESTHESIA

Volatile Agent

The specific choice of a volatile agent to maintain anesthesia before delivery has little or no effect on mother or fetus. The placental transfer of halothane and enflurane is similar (measured UV/MA ratios of approximately 0.70) (111). The UA/UV ratios for halothane and enflurane are both less than 0.5 (112). Administration of isoflurane, enflurane, halothane, sevoflurane, and desflurane as the volatile agent for general anesthesia for elective cesarean delivery does not alter behavioral or biochemical markers of neonatal outcome (112–117). Administering two-thirds of the minimum alveolar concentration (MAC) of the volatile agent limits the maternal stress response better than lesser concentrations of anesthetic (116).

There is little information about the effects of general anesthetic agents on fetal environment during acute fetal distress. In the acidotic fetus, cerebral vasodilation and a decrease in cerebral metabolic oxygen consumption in the face of a fall in cardiac output help maintain cerebral blood flow. Maternal administration of low-dose halothane supports cerebral blood flow, cerebral oxygen supply, and lowered cerebral metabolic oxygen consumption during the first 15 minutes of asphyxia (118). In animal models subjected to longer periods of fetal asphyxia, halogenated agents sometimes produce decreases in fetal cerebral blood flow (119,120). Conflicting results may be due to slight differences in protocol to produce and maintain fetal acidosis. In the clinical situation, maternal administration of 2/3 MAC isoflurane or halothane in 50% nitrous oxide/oxygen does not alter neonatal outcome as measured by Apgar score or funic blood acid–base analysis (121). Administration of 2% halothane in oxygen lowered 1-minute Apgar score, umbilical vein pO_2, pH, and increased umbilical vein base deficit (122).

Oxygen Concentration

General anesthesia for cesarean delivery usually includes 50% nitrous oxide in oxygen plus 2/3 MAC volatile agent before delivery of the fetus. Increasing maternal p_aO_2 above 280 to 300 mm Hg (corresponding to an F_IO_2 of 0.5 to 0.6) fails to increase umbilical vein blood oxygen tension during general anesthesia for cesarean delivery (123–126). In these studies, however, the inspired maternal concentration of volatile agent was not varied to maintain the same total MAC of anesthetic given (deletion of nitrous oxide from the anesthetic was not accompanied by an increase in the inspired volatile anesthetic concentration). Therefore, an increase in stress-related catecholamines from "lighter" anesthesia could have decreased uteroplacental blood flow.

Other studies have also addressed the effect of both inspired maternal oxygen concentration and total MAC of the anesthetic on fetal outcome. In 35 parturients (mixed obstetric diagnoses, some patients in labor but none with fetal distress) having cesarean delivery under general anesthesia with 2/3 MAC isoflurane, a decrease of maternal F_IO_2 from 0.5 to 0.33 does not significantly change funic blood acid–base values (127).

In another study, 200 patients presenting for elective or emergent cesarean delivery under general anesthesia were randomly assigned to receive either 100% inspired maternal oxygen or 50% inspired maternal oxygen in nitrous oxide (128). Isoflurane, 1.5 MAC, was given for 5 minutes and then decreased to 1 MAC and continued until delivery in parturients who were not receiving nitrous oxide. Induction-to-delivery times were 10 to 12 minutes, even for emergent deliveries! There were no differences in umbilical vein or artery carbon dioxide tension, pH, or base deficit between the women who breathed 100% or 50% oxygen (128). There were no differences between groups in umbilical artery blood oxygen tension (128). However, umbilical vein oxygen tension was increased (to 28 to 35 mm Hg) in the group receiving 100% inspired maternal oxygen being delivered emergently (42% for fetal distress) (128). There were no differences in need for ventilation or intubation, or in Apgar scores in neonates with the lower umbilical vein oxygen tension (128).

TABLE 7. *Suggested technique general anesthesia*

- Premedication
  - Elective delivery
    - Two doses of H_2-receptor antagonist (e.g., ranitidine, 150 mg p.o. at bedtime; ranitidine, 50 mg i.v. in morning)
  - Nonelective delivery or if laboring patient
    - 30 mL of 0.3M sodium citrate (or its equivalent) p.o.; metoclopramide, 10 mg slow i.v. push, optimally 30 min before delivery
- Positioning
  - Uterine displacement
  - Arrange shoulders and neck in "sniffing" position
- Monitors and special equipment
  - Continuous electrocardiography
  - Noninvasive oscillometric blood pressure monitor
  - Pulse oximetry
  - Temperature monitor
  - Penpheral nerve stimulator
  - Oxygen analyzer
  - Mass spectrometer or capnograph
  - Orogastric tube
  - Bladder catheter
  - Forced warm air warming blanket
- *Induction* (in delivery room, after surgeon ready to make incision)
  - Preoxygenation (high-flow 100% oxygen, tight-fitting face mask)
    - Elective delivery
      - 3 min tidal volume breathing
    - Emergency delivery
      - Four vital capacity breath hyperventilation
  - Rapid sequence intravenous induction with cricoid pressure
    - Thiopental 4 mg/kg pregnant body weight (PBW) i.v.
    - Succinylcholine 1.5 mg/kg PBW i.v., to facilitate intubation
  - Tracheal intubation and inflation of cuff, check breath sounds, and check far capnographic evidence of expired carbon dioxide
  - Begin surgery
- Maintenance
  - Before delivery
    - High-flow nitrous oxide/oxygen 50:50 with up to 0.67 MAC volatile agent
    - Succinylcholine, 0.1% infusion, as necessary to maintain muscle relaxation
  - After delivery
    - Decrease gas flows
    - Nitrous oxide/oxygen 70:30
    - Intravenous opioid (i.e., morphine sulfate, 0.2 mg/kg, as tolerated according to maternal hemodynamic status)
    - Intravenous amnestic agent (i.e., diazepam 2.5–5 mg or midazolam 1–2 mg)
    - Succinylcholine infusion (or intermediate duration nondepolarizing neuromuscular blocker) as needed
- Emergence and recovery
  - Extubation
    - Fully reactive and awake
    - 5-sec headlift
  - Supplemental oxygen
  - Monitoring
    - Pulse oximetry
    - Continuous electrocardiography
    - Continual blood pressure
  - Titrate intravenous analgesic to patient comfort, begin intravenous patient-controlled analgesia (PCA) infusion (i.e., morphine sulfate, 2-mg bolus; 10-min lockout; 1-h maximum of 10 mg), PCA protocol orders
  - Discharge from recovery room by usual criteria
  - Patient discharge instructions
  - Follow-up note the next day and thereafter as indicated

Substitution of enflurane or halothane for isoflurane in 100% oxygen in a similar protocol (but now comparing neonatal outcome to a group of parturients receiving 2/3 MAC halothane in 50% nitrous oxide in oxygen) showed no difference in funic blood carbon dioxide tension, pH, Apgar score, or need for resuscitation (129). Umbilical vein oxygen tension was not significantly or consistently higher in any one comparison group, although when all (three) patient groups receiving 100% inspired maternal oxygen were combined, there was a statistically significant increase in umbilical vein oxygen tension from 33.4 to 39.7 mm Hg. The clinical significance of this increase remains obscure. It is therefore of questionable neonatal benefit to increase inspired maternal oxygen concentrations above 50% to 60%. In addition, the use of 100% inspired maternal oxygen may increase the incidence of maternal awareness (*vide infra*).

See Table 7 for a suggested method of general anesthesia for cesarean delivery.

BLOOD LOSS

Mild controversy exists about the effects of general anesthesia on blood loss at cesarean delivery. Volatile anesthetics relax uterine muscle and may produce relative uterine inertia and hemorrhage. In women who have delivered vaginally, oxytocin stimulation produces adequate uterine contraction despite the use of low-dose volatile anesthetic (halothane or enflurane) (130). Clinically, the use of supplemental low-dose volatile anesthetic to help ensure amnesia, especially when administered for only the short time before delivery and then discontinued, does not increase intraoperative blood loss (131–134).

Gilstrap et al. (135) reviewed 239 cesarean deliveries in which the type of anesthesia (regional or general) was not controlled. General anesthesia included a halogenated agent (up to 1.0% halothane for longer than 10 minutes) in most patients. There were no differences in pre- and postdelivery hematocrit in either group of women (Table 8). But, 35% of women receiving the halogenated agent had a drop in hematocrit greater than 8 vol %, and one-half of these women received a transfusion versus only 1% of women receiving regional anesthesia.

A more recent review of blood loss in cesarean delivery under regional or general anesthesia divided patients into those whose postoperative hematocrit was more or less than 5% lower than preoperative hematocrit (136). Again, although average blood loss was similar in each group, there were more patients whose hematocrit dropped more than 5% in the general anesthesia group (136). However, no patient required transfusion (136).

Transfusion therapy has evolved as physicians (and the public) focus on the transmission of blood-borne pathogens. Camann and Datta (137) reported a series of 9,596 cesarean deliveries of which 336 were complicated by a need for red cell transfusion. During the 4-year study period (1984 to

TABLE 8. *Effects of general anesthesia for cesarean delivery on blood loss*

	Regional anesthesia (n = 150)	General anesthesia with halogenated agent (n = 114)[a]	Statistical significance (*p* value)
Hematocrit			
Predelivery	37.1	37.3	NS
Postdelivery	33.4	30.8	NS
Percentage of patients with hematocrit decrease ≥8 vol %	10%	35%	<0.05
Percentage of patients receiving red blood cells	1%	18%[b]	<0.05

[a]Fifty-nine percent of patients exposed to halogenated agent for >11 min. Eighty-five percent of patients received halothane 0.5%–1%.
[b]Sixty-seven percent of the patients received halogenated agent for >15 min.
NS, not significant.
Data from ref. 135.

1987), the need for transfusion was halved to an incidence of 3.2% per year. The need for massive transfusion (8% of transfusions were more than 5 U of packed red cells) was usually complicated by a coexisting obstetric conditions associated with hemorrhage, including abnormality of placentation, coagulopathy after abruption or with preeclampsia, and emergency surgery (137). Of high-risk parturients needing transfusion at cesarean delivery, almost 70% received general anesthesia (137). Of low-risk parturients (including elective cesarean delivery, breech, and nonobstetric reasons for cesarean delivery) needing transfusion at cesarean delivery, only 31% received general anesthesia (137). Type of anesthesia did not alter blood requirements in this low-risk population, although the incidence of transfusion in these patients was low (0.53%) (137). Because the use of general anesthesia for cesarean section is dwindling, only high-risk patients receive this technique. It will be increasingly difficult to discern whether it is the general anesthetic or indications for emergent cesarean delivery that increases the risk of blood loss requiring transfusion.

AWARENESS

Drug dose for general anesthesia during cesarean delivery is chosen to limit potential neonatal effects. In addition, the short induction-to-incision time often leaves the anesthesiologist with a "lightly" anesthetized mother. Maternal awareness and, more importantly, recall are possible. Awareness, dreaming, and recall have been described in the parturient under general anesthesia. The anesthesiologist must differentiate between these entities. Carefully distinguish between dreaming and recall when dealing with complaints in the postpartum period. The incidence of these potentially unpleasant effects varies greatly among reports. The following factors seem to influence the reported incidence of unpleasant effects:

- Choice of induction agent,
- Technique for anesthetic maintenance before delivery of the fetus,
- Time from anesthetic induction to delivery,
- The possible emergency nature of delivery, and
- The method of detection of intraoperative awareness.

Thiopental and Ketamine

The use of 0.67 MAC volatile agent to supplement 50% nitrous oxide/oxygen or 100% oxygen for general anesthesia before delivery of the fetus is associated with an incidence of maternal awareness, as detected by purposeful movements of an isolated limb, as high as 60% after an induction with thiopental 4 mg/kg (138,139). The addition of ketamine 0.5 mg/kg, thiopental 2 mg/kg for induction reduces the incidence of awareness by half. Ketamine 1 to 1.5 mg/kg induction reduces the incidence of awareness to 0% to 20% (140). Electroencephalographic (EEG) spectral analysis also has shown a smaller decrease (i.e., lighter anesthesia) in power after thiopental 4 mg/kg induction versus ketamine 1 mg/kg (140).

The reported incidence of dreaming varies between 0% and 25% (141,142). The incidence of dreaming seems to depend on the emergent nature of the delivery and perhaps the emotional state of the mother before induction of general anesthesia.

Maternal recall is potentially damaging to both the mother (psychologically) and the anesthesiologist (medical–legally as well as psychologically). The incidence of recall is reported to be 0% to 18% (138,139,141–143,145). The incidence of recall is seemingly unaffected by the choice of ketamine or thiopental as the induction agent but again may be increased after the induction of general anesthesia for emergency cesarean delivery.

Propofol

Anesthetic induction with propofol 2.3 to 2.5 mg/kg followed by maintenance with low-dose halothane in 50% nitrous oxide/oxygen is associated with a 40% incidence of intraoperative awareness (90). This rate may have been affected by discontinuation of all anesthetic agents between uterine incision and delivery. Recall was reported by 0% to 20% of women after induction of general anesthesia with propofol 2.1 to 2.3 mg/kg followed by 50%

nitrous oxide/oxygen and low-dose isoflurane and 0% to 5% after induction with thiopental 4 to 5 mg/kg (90–93).

Midazolam

Recall is uncommon after induction of general anesthesia with midazolam 0.2 mg/kg, followed by maintenance of anesthesia with low-dose halothane and 50% nitrous oxide/oxygen (146).

Practical Considerations

Isolated limb techniques, lower esophageal contractility, and EEG spectral analysis (140,147) monitors reveal awareness or "light" anesthesia but are poor predictors of maternal recall (142). If "light" anesthesia is detected, there may not be any pharmacologic intervention that can "erase" the event. Although explicit recall of stimuli under general anesthesia for cesarean delivery is rare, there is evidence that auditory processing of perioperative stimuli and explicit learning can occur (147). The prudent anesthetist would consider all parturients at least "aware" of the auditory environment in the operating room. Limit casual conversation in the operating room. Quiet verbal reassurance of the parturient by the anesthesiologist is perhaps justified until delivery of the baby, and the opportunity to "deepen" the anesthetic.

NEONATAL EFFECTS OF GENERAL ANESTHESIA

Many variables, including the method of neonatal evaluation, surgical technique and timing, and preexisting fetal condition, confound the study of neonatal effects of general anesthesia. Most studies include only neonates born at elective cesarean deliveries.

Neonatal Evaluation

In many prospective studies (with relatively small numbers of patients), general anesthesia produces a similar incidence of depressed neonates (reflected by low 1- and 5-minute Apgar scores) as regional anesthesia (148–151). Amiel-Tyson/Barrier/Shnider Neurological and Adaptive Capacity Scores (NACS) have been performed on neonates born of mothers under general anesthesia. Analysis reveals lower scores on test items for adaptive capacity, passive tone, active tone, primary reflexes, and total scores at 15 minutes and 2 hours of life but not beyond, compared to neonates born under regional anesthesia (151). Using Scanlon Early Neonatal Neurobehavioral Score (ENNS), neonates born to mothers under general anesthesia scored lower on habituation and orientation items at 3 hours but were similar at 24 hours of life and beyond compared to neonates born under regional anesthesia (149).

Hormonal Evaluation

Neonatal hormones have been measured in attempts to quantify the influence of anesthetic technique in the neonatal stress response. Funic epinephrine concentrations are higher after epidural versus general anesthesia (152). Maternally administered ephedrine might be responsible for this difference. There is no correlation between fetal epinephrine concentration and umbilical blood pH. There are no differences in neonatal β-endorphin concentrations in babies born after epidural anesthesia compared with general anesthesia (153).

Pre-existing Fetal Condition

Two large series of patients undergoing cesarean delivery have yielded seemingly conflicting data. A recent analysis of almost 41,000 patients undergoing elective cesarean delivery found a higher frequency of fetal umbilical arterial blood pH less than 7.10 associated with regional anesthesia (154). The relative risk of low pH was 4.7- and 2.4-fold higher during spinal and epidural anesthesia versus general anesthesia. Apgar scores between 5 and 7 were increasingly likely in patients receiving regional compared with general anesthesia. These data are in contrast with another study of neonatal outcome in 3,940 elective and nonelective cesarean deliveries (Table 9). Compared to infants born under regional anesthesia, neonates born under general anesthesia had a higher inci-

TABLE 9. *Neonatal outcome after cesarean section by anesthetic technique*

Indications for cesarean section	Anesthetic technique	Infants with 1-min Apgar scores 0 to 4 (%)	Infants with 5-min Apgar scores 0 to 4 (%)	Neonates requiring oxygen by mask (%)	Neonates requiring intubation and ventilation (%)	Neonatal deaths (%)
Elective	Regional	2.0	0.2	10.1	1.7	0.5
	General	6.5[a]	0.4	16.3[b]	0.8	1.2
Fetal distress	Regional	18.5	2.8	19.7	19.0	3.3
	General	43.5[b]	8.3	18.0	42.5[c]	6.5
Cephalopelvic disproportion	Regional	9.1	0.5	14.5	10.4	0.7
	General	23.0[c]	3.4	24.0[c]	19.0[c]	1.4

[a] $p \leq 0.05$ vs regional anesthesia.
[b] $p \leq 0.01$ vs regional anesthesia.
[c] $p \leq 0.001$ vs regional anesthesia.
Data from ref. 155.

dence of low (less than 4) 1-minute Apgar scores after elective cesarean deliveries, cesarean deliveries with a diagnosis of cephalopelvic disproportion, and cesarean deliveries with a diagnosis of fetal distress (155). Neonates born under general anesthesia have a higher incidence of low (less than 4) 5-minute Apgar scores after cesarean deliveries with a diagnosis of fetal distress. Neonates born under general anesthesia after nonelective cesarean delivery also were more likely to need oxygen and intubation. However, anesthetic technique did not correlate with neonatal mortality (155). Although the results of these two large studies seemingly conflict, they may suggest that immediate neonatal outcome for a nonstressed (i.e., elective abdominal delivery) fetus is unrelated to anesthetic choice.

Timing of Delivery

There is a difference of opinion about the optimal time for delivery of the fetus after induction of general anesthesia. Traditional teaching has stressed minimizing induction-to-delivery (I–D) intervals. However, no correlation between clinical or biochemical indexes of neonatal outcome and I–D interval has been reported (156,157).

Datta et al. (156) have suggested that long uterine incision-to-delivery (U–D) intervals also influence neonatal outcome. Possible reasons for deterioration in neonatal status with increasing U–D interval include the following:

- An acute decrease in uteroplacental perfusion due to uterine artery spasm or venocaval compression during uterine manipulation,
- Inhalation of amniotic fluid by the fetus during prolonged delivery, and
- Fetal head compression during difficult delivery.

The data, however, are confusing. An I-D interval longer than 8 minutes with a U-D interval longer than 3 minutes is associated with a significant decrease in funic blood pH (156,157). The values for the mean umbilical artery pH (7.22 ± 0.01) and mean umbilical vein pH (7.30 ± 0.01), however, are not considered acidotic. In one study, maternal vein-to-umbilical vein pH gradient increased significantly in the long I–D, long U–D interval patients. This finding suggests decreased uteroplacental oxygen delivery and resultant fetal acidosis perhaps from maternal hyperventilation during this time (156). A U–D interval longer than 3 minutes also correlates with a greater incidence of low 1-minute Apgar scores (141,156,157). There are no differences, however, in funic blood oxygen tensions with prolonged I–D and U–D intervals (156).

Another study has challenged the importance of U–D intervals (158). Multivariate regression analysis of a group of 204 parturients delivered abdominally relates low 1- and 5-minute Apgar scores to the presence of fetal distress and preeclampsia (158). The presence of meconium-stained amniotic fluid also correlated with low 1-minute Apgar scores. This finding may be due to neonatal cardiorespiratory response to tracheal suction (158). These investigators found no relationship of I–D interval or U–D interval to Apgar scores or umbilical vein blood pH (158).

Controversy still exists over the proper timing of delivery of the neonates under general anesthesia. In our institution, we routinely induce general anesthesia after surgical preparation and draping of the patient is complete. Sacrifice of surgical technique for speed of delivery has occasionally led to unexpected maternal and even fetal trauma. Our obstetricians attempt to minimize both I–D and U–D intervals after induction of general anesthesia, but not at the sacrifice of surgical technique. Pediatricians are present at all cesarean deliveries to provide prompt attention to the neonate. Time of induction of general anesthesia, skin incision, uterine incision, and delivery as well as Apgar scores and results of funic blood acid–base analysis are recorded in the anesthesia record.

SUMMARY

The scientific basis of the practice of general anesthesia for cesarean delivery is based on human and animal data, but routine practice is more often dictated by tradition, cost, or the choice of the individual anesthesiologist. Choice of induction agent probably is based on cost and tradition. Thiopental and ketamine are inexpensive and have a long record of safety. Development of newer drugs to induce general anesthesia has had little practical application in obstetric anesthesia. There is no alternative at present to the use of succinylcholine to facilitate rapid sequence induction and tracheal intubation. The volatile agents in routine use today are interchangeable. Within the guidelines of routine anesthetic care, fetal outcome may depend mostly on preexisting fetal status at the time of cesarean delivery, that is, a healthy term fetus can withstand anesthesia and delivery better than a distressed, preterm fetus.

Techniques of general anesthesia have long proven safe for the mother; however, prevention of anesthetic-related maternal morbidity and mortality today centers on management of the difficult or impossible airway. Many investigators are attempting to prevent maternal hypoxemia and the sequelae of acid aspiration. There will always be a need for general anesthesia in the delivery suite, and there will always be "difficult" airways, which may lead to failed intubation. However, one must continue to focus on increasing the margin of safety at the time of induction of general anesthesia. The methods of prediction, identification, and management of the difficult airway must improve. Better methods of acid-aspiration prophylaxis also may have considerable impact in reducing maternal morbidity and mortality. Continuing education of anesthesia personnel (as well as our obstetric and nursing colleagues) in the safe practice of obstetric anesthesia is mandatory.

REFERENCES

1. Hawkins JL, Gibbs C, Orleans M, Martin-Salvaj G, Beaty B. Obstetric Anesthesia Workforce Survey, 1981 vs 1992. *Anesthesiology* 1997;87:135.
2. Holdcroft A, Parshall AM, Knowlesh G, Waite KE, Morgan BM. Factors associated with mothers selecting general anesthesia for lower segment cesarean section. *J Psychosomat Obstet Gynecol* 1995;16:167.
3. Gajraj NM, Sharma SK, Souter AJ, Pole Y, Sidawi JE. A survery of obstetric patients who refuse regional anaesthesia. *Anaesthesia* 1995; 50:740.
4. Kee WDN, Hung VYS, Roach VJ, Law TK. A survery of factors influencing patients choices of anaesthesia for caesarean section. *Aust N Z J Obstet Gynaecol* 1997;37:300.
5. Hawkins JL, Koonin LM, Palmer SK, Gibbs CP. Anesthesia-related deaths during obstetric delivery in the United States 1979–1990. *Anesthesiology* 1997;86:277.
6. Hawthorne L, Wilson R, Lyons G, Dressner M. Failed intubation revisited: 17 year experience in a teaching maternity unit. *Br J Anaesth* 1996;76:680.
7. Morgan BM, Magni V, Goroszeniuk T. Anaesthesia for emergency caesarean section. *Br J Obstet Gynecol* 1990;97:420.
8. Morgan M. Anaesthetic contribution to maternal mortality. *Br J Anaesth* 1987;59:842.
9. Samsoon GLT, Young RB. Difficult tracheal intubation: a retrospective study. *Anaesthesia* 1987;42:487.
10. Yeo SW, Chang JL, Thomas E. Difficult intubation: a prospective study. *Singapore Med J* 1992;33:362.
11. Rocke DA, Murray WB, Rout CC, Gouwns E. Relative risk analysis of factors associated with difficult intubation in obstetric anesthesia. *Anesthesiology* 1992;77:67.
12. Endler GC, Mariona FG, Sokal RJ, Stevenson LB. Anesthetic-related maternal mortality in Michigan, 1972–1984. *AM J Obstet Gynecol* 1988;159:187.
13. Dupont X, Hamza J, Jullien P, Narchi P. Risk factors associated with difficult airways in normotensive parturients. *Anesthesiology* 1990;73:A999(abst).
14. Hood DD, Dewan DM, Ashten K. Anesthesia in the morbidly obese parturient. *Anesthesiology* 1993;79:1210.
15. Dupont X, Hamza J, Jullien P, Narchi P. Is pregnant reduced hypertension a risk factor for difficult intubation? *Anesthesiology* 1990;73:A985(abst).
16. Chazotte C, Cohen WR. Catastrophic complications of previous cesarean section. *Am J Obstet Gynecol* 1990;738:163.
17. Morgan M. Anaesthetic contribution to maternal mortality. *Br J Anaesth* 1987;59:842.
18. Roberts B, Shirley A. Reducing the risk of acid aspiration at cesarean section. *Anesth Analg* 1974;53:859.
19. James CF, Modell JH, Gibbs CP, Kuck EJ, Ruiz C. Pulmonary aspiration-effects of volume and pH in the rat. *Anesth Analg* 1984;63:665.
20. Brock-Utne JG, Rout C, Moodley J, Mayat N. Influence of perioperative gastric aspiration on the volume and pH of gastric contents on obstetric patients undergoing cesarean section. *Br J Anaesth* 1989; 62:397.
21. Gibbs CP, Spohr L, Schmidt D. The effectiveness of sodium citrate as an antacid. *Anesthesiology* 1982;57:44.
22. O'Sullivan GM, Bullingham RE. Non-invasive assessment by radiotelemetry of antacid effect during labor. *Anesth Analg* 1985; 64:95.
23. Colman ED, Frank M, Loughran BA, Cohen DG, Cattermole R. Use of IM ranitidine for the prophylaxis of aspiration pneumonitis in obstetrics. *Br J Anaesth* 1988;61:720.
24. O'Sullivan GM, Bullingham RES. Does twice the volume of antacid have twice the effect in pregnant women at term? *Anesth Analg* 1984; 63:752.
25. Matthews ML, Moore J. Sodium bicarbonate as a single dose antacid in obstetric anaesthesia. *Anaesthesia* 1989;44:590.
26. Thompson M, Loughran PG, McAuley DM, Wilson CM, Moore J. Combined treatment with ranitidine and saline antacids prior to obstetric anaesthesia. *Anaesthesia* 1984;39:1086.
27. Lin C-J, Huang C-L, Hsu H-W, Chen TL. Prophylaxis against and aspiration in regional anesthesia for elective cesarean section: a comparison between oral single dose ranitidine, famotidine and omeperazole assessed with fiberoptic gastric aspiration. *Acta Anaesthesiol Sin* 1996;34:179.
28. Ormezano X, Francois TP, Viaud J-Y, et al. Aspiration pneumonitis prophylaxis in obstetric anaesthesia: a comparison of effervescent cimetidine-sodium citrate mixtures and sodium citrate. *Br J Anaesth* 1990;64:503.
29. Ewart MC, Yau G, Gin T, Kotur CF, Oh TE. A comparison of the effects of omeprazole and ranitidine on gastric secretion in women undergoing elective cesarean section. *Anaesthesia* 1990;45:527.
30. Cohen S, Morris DW, Schoen HG, Dimarino AJ. The effects of oral and intravenous metoclopramide on human lower esophageal pressure. *Gastroenterology* 1976;70:484.
31. Bylsma-Howell M, Riggs KW, McMorland GH, et al. Placental transfer of metoclopramide: assessment of maternal and neonatal effects. *Can Anaesth Soc J* 1983;30:487.
32. Nimmo WS, Wilson J, Prescott F. Narcotic analgesia and delayed gastric emptying during labour. *Lancet* 1975;1:890.
33. Manchikanti L. Metoclopramide's role in anesthetic practice. *Anesthesiol Rev* 1984;17:8.
34. Caldwell C, Rains G, McKiterick K. An unusual reaction to preoperative metoclopramide. *Anesthesiology* 1987;67:854.
35. Bevacqua A. Supraventricular tachycardia associated with postpartum metoclopramide administration. *Anesthesiology* 1988;68:124.
36. Lewis M, Crawford JS. Can one risk fasting the obstetric patient for less than 4 hours? *Br J Anaesth* 1987;59:312.
37. Frank M, Evans M, Flynn P, Aun C. Comparison of the prophylactic use of magnesium trisilicate mixture B.P.C., sodium citrate mixture or cimetidine in obstetrics. *Br J Anaesth* 1984;56:355.
38. O'Sullivan GM, Sear W, Bullingham RE, Carrie LES. The effect of magnesium trisilicate mixture, metoclopramide and ranitidine on gastric pH, volume and serum gastrin. *Anaesthesia* 1985;40:246.
39. Koren MJ, Freiberg HV, Ostheimer GW. Prophylaxis against acid aspiration during general anesthesia in obstetric patients: a cost-effectiveness analysis. Proceedings of the Annual Meeting of the Society of Obstetric Anesthesia and Perinatology. 1985:96.
40. Malinow AM, Naulty JS, Hunt CO, Datta S, Ostheimer GW. Venous air emboli at cesarean delivery. *Anesthesiology* 1987;66:816.
41. Fong J, Gadalla F, Druzin M. Venous air emboli occurring during cesarean section: the effect of patient position. *Can J Anaesth* 1991;38:191.
42. Vartikar JV, Johnson MD, Datta S. Precordial Doppler monitoring and pulse oximetry during cesarean delivery with detection of venous air embolism. *Reg Anesth* 1989;14:145.
43. Robinson DA, Albin M. Venous air embolism and cesarean sections [Letter]. *Anesthesiology* 1987;66:93.
44. Levinson G, Shnider SM, de Lorimier M, et al. Effects of maternal hyperventilation on uterine blood flow and fetal oxygenation and acid-base status. *Anesthesiology* 1974;40:340.
45. Shankar KB, Mosely H, Vemula V, Kumar Y. Physiologic dead space during general anaesthesia for cesarean section. *Can J Anaesth* 1987;34:373.
46. Shankar KB, Mosely H, Kumar Y, Vemula V. Arterial to end-tidal carbon dioxide tension difference during caesarean section anaesthesia. *Anaesthesia* 1986;41:698.
47. Rampton AJ, Mallaiah S, Garrett P. Increased ventilation requirements during obstetric general anaesthesia. *Br J Anaesth* 1988;61:730.
48. Burger GA, Datta S, Chantigian C, et al. Optimal ventilation in general anesthesia for cesarean delivery. *Anesthesiology* 1983;59: A420(abst).
49. Archer GW, Marx GF. Arterial oxygen tension during apnea in parturient women. *Br J Anaesth* 1974;46:358.
50. Pernoll MC, Metcalfe J, Schlenker TL, Welch JE, Matsumoto JA. Oxygen consumption at rest and during exercise in pregnancy. *Respir Physiol* 1975;25:285.
51. Hagerdal M, Morgan CW, Sumner AK, Gutsche BB. Minute ventilation and oxygen consumption during labor with epidural analgesia. *Anesthesiology* 1983;59:425.
52. Awe RJ, Nicotra MB, Newsom TD, Viles R. Arterial oxygenation and alveolar-arterial gradients in term pregnancy. *Obstet Gynecol* 1979;53:182.
53. Baldwin GR, Moorthi DS, Welton A, Macdonald KF. New lung functions and pregnancy. *Am J Obstet Gynecol* 1977;127:235.

54. Cugell DW, Frank NR, Grensler ER, Badger TL. Pulmonary function in pregnancy. I. Serial observations in normal women. *Am Rev Tuberc* 1953;67:568.
55. Gee JBL, Packer BS, Millen JE, Robin ED. Pulmonary mechanics during pregnancy. *J Clin Invest* 1967;46:945.
56. Byrne F, Odeno-Dominah A, Kipling R. The effect of pregnancy on pulmonary nitrogen washout: a study of preoxygenation. *Anaesthesia* 1987;42:148.
57. Russell GN, Smith CL, Snowden SL, Bryson THL. Preoxygenation and the parturient patient. *Anaesthesia* 1987;42:346.
58. Norris MC, Dewan DM. Preoxygenation for cesarean section: a comparison of two techniques. *Anesthesiology* 1985;67:827.
59. Norris MC, Kirkland R, Torjman MC, Goldberg ME. Denitrogenation in pregnancy. *Can J Anaesth* 1989;36:523.
60. Datta S, Crocker J, Alper MH. Muscle pain following administration of suxamethonium to pregnant and nonpregnant patients undergoing tubal ligation. *Br J Anaesth* 1977;49:625.
61. Cullen DJ. The effect of pretreatment with nondepolarizing muscle relaxants on the neuromuscular blocking action of succinylcholine. *Anesthesiology* 1971;35:572.
62. Blitt CD, Carlson GL, Rolling GD, Hameroff R, Otto CW. A comparative evaluation of the pretreatment with nondepolarizing neuromuscular blockers prior to the administration of succinylcholine. *Anesthesiology* 1981;55:687.
63. Manchikanti L. Diazepam does not prevent succinylcholine-induced fasiculations and myalgia—a comparative evaluation of the effect of diazepam and d-tubocurarine pretreatments. *Acta Anesthesiol Scand* 1984;28:523.
64. Cook WF, Schultetus RR, Caton D. A comparison of d-tubocurarine pretreatment and no pretreatment in obstetric patients. *Anesth Analg* 1987;66:756.
65. Thind GS, Bryson THL. Single-dose suxamethonium and muscle pain in pregnancy. *Br J Anaesth* 1983;55:745.
66. Crawford JS. Suxamethonium muscle pains and pregnancy. *Br J Anaesth* 1971;43:677.
67. Christensen JH, Andreasen F, Jansen JA. Pharmacokinetics of thiopentone in cesarean section. *Acta Anaesth Scand* 1981;25:174.
68. Christensen JH, Andreasen F, Jansen JA. Pharmacokinetics of thiopentone in a group of young women and a group of young men. *Br J Anaesth* 1980;52:913.
69. Chantigian RC, Ostheimer GW. Effects of maternally administered drugs in the fetus and newborn. In: Friedman E, ed. *Advances in perinatal medicine,* vol. 5. New York: Plenum, 1986:181.
70. Bach V, Carl P, Ravlo O, et al. A randomized comparison between midazolam and thiopental for elective cesarean section anesthesia. III. Placental transfer and elimination in neonates. *Anesth Analg* 1989;68:238.
71. McKechnie FB, Converse G. Placental transmission of thiopental. *Am J Obstet Gynecol* 1955;71:369.
72. Kosah Y, Takahashi T, Mark LC. Intravenous thiobarbituate anesthesia for cesarean section. *Anesthesiology* 1969;31:489.
73. Datta S, Alper MA. Anesthesia for cesarean section. *Anesthesiology* 1980;53:142.
74. Esener Z, Sarihara B, Given H, Ustun E. Thiopental and etiomidate concentrations in maternal and umbilical plasma and in colostrum. *Br J Anaesth* 1992;69:586.
75. Holdcroft A, Robinson MT, Gordon H, Whitman JG. Comparison of effect of two induction doses of methohexitone on infants delivered by elective caesarean section. *Br Med J* 1974;2:472.
76. Pelk B, Sinclair DM. Induction agents for caesarean section—a comparison of thiopentone and ketamine. *Anaesthesia* 1973,28:37.
77. Meer FM, Downing W, Coleman AJ. An intravenous method of anaesthesia for caesarean section. Part II. Ketamine. *Br J Anaesth* 1973;45:191.
78. Pickering BG, Palahnink RJ, Cote J, Wade JG, Pash MG. Cerebral vascular response to ketamine and thiopentone during foetal acidosis. *Can Anaesth Soc J* 1982;29:463.
79. Haram X, Sagen A, Solheim E. Transplacental passage of ketamine after intravenous administration. *Acta Anesth Scand* 1977;21:41.
80. Levinson G, Shnider SM, Gildea E, deLorimier M. Maternal and foetal cardiovascular and acid-base changes during ketamine anaesthesia in pregnant ewes. *Br J Anaesth* 1973;45:1111.
81. Swartz J, Cumming M, Biehl D. The effect of ketamine anaesthesia in the acidotic foetal lamb. *Can J Anaesth* 1987;34:233.
82. Ngan-Kee WD, Khaw KS, Ma ML, Mainland PA, Gin T. Postoperative analgesic requirements after cesarean section: a comparison of anesthetic induction with ketamine or thiopental. *Anesth Analg* 1997;85:1294.
83. Downing JW, Bailey RJR, Brock-Utne JG, Boulton JG. Etomidate for induction of anesthesia at cesarean section: comparison with thiopentone. *Br J Anaesth* 1979,51:135.
84. Suresh MS, Solanaki R Andrews JJ, et al. Comparison of etomidate with thiopental for induction of anesthesia at cesarean section. *Anesthesiology* 1986;65:A400(abst).
85. Houlton PJ, Downing JW, Buley RJ, Brock-Utne JO. Anaesthetic induction for caesarean section with etomidate compared with thiopentone. *S Afr Med J* 1978;54:773.
86. Reddy BK, Pizer B, Bull PT. Neonatal serum cortisol suppression by etomidate. *Eur J Anesth* 1988;5:171.
87. Crawford ME, Carl P, Bach V, Ravlo O, Mikkelsen BO, Werner M. A randomized comparison between midazolam and thiopental for elective cesarean section. I. Mothers. *Anesth Analg* 1989;68:229.
88. Ravlo O, Carl P, Crawford ME, Bach V, Mikkelsen BO, Nielsen HK. A randomized comparison between midazolam and thiopental for elective cesarean section anesthesia. II. Neonates. *Anesth Analg* 1989;68:234.
89. Bland BAR, Lawes KG, Duncan PW, Warnell I, Downing JW. Comparison of midazolam and thiopental for rapid sequence induction for elective cesarean section. *Anesth Analg* 1987;66:1165.
90. Dailland P, Cockshott ID, Lirzin JD, et al. Intravenous propofol during cesarean section. Placental transfer, concentrations in breast milk, and neonatal effects. A preliminary study. *Anesthesiology* 1989;71:827.
91. Moore J, Bill KM, Flynn RJ, McKeating KT, Howard PJ. A comparison between propofol and thiopentone as induction agents in obstetric anaesthesia. *Anaesthesia* 1989;44:753.
92. Capogna G, Celleno D, Sebastiani M, et al. Propofol and thiopentone or caesarean section revisited. Maternal effects and neonatal outcome. *Int J Obstet Anaesth* 1991;1:19.
93. Valtonen M, Kanto J, Rosenberg P. Comparison of propofol and thiopentone for induction of anaesthesia for elective caesarean section. *Anaesthesia* 1989;44:758.
94. Celleno D, Capogna G, Tomassetti M, Constantino P, Di Feo G, Nisini R. Neurobehavioral effects of propofol on the neonate following elective cesarean section. *Br J Anaesth* 1989;62:649.
95. Gin T, Gregory MA, Oh TE. The haemodynamic effects of propofol and thiopentone for the induction of caesarean section. *Anaesth Intens Care* 1990;18:175.
96. Gin T, Gregory MA, Chan K, Oh TE. Maternal and fetal levels of propofol at caesarean section. *Anaesth Intens Care* 1990;18:180.
97. Gin T, Gregory MA, Chan K, Buckley T, Oh TE. Pharmacokinetics of propofol in women undergoing elective caesarean section. *Br J Anaesth* 1990;64:148.
98. Gregory MA, Gin T, Yaw G, Leung RKW, Chan K, Oh TE. Propofol infusion for caesarean section. *Anaesthesia* 1990;37:514.
99. Abboud TK, Zhu J, Richardson M, Peres da Silva E, Donovan M. Intravenous propofol vs thiamylal-isoflurane for cesarean section: comparative maternal and neonatal effects. *Acta Anaesth Scand* 1995:39:205.
100. Drabkhova J, Crul JF, van der Kleijn E. Placental transfer of 14C-labelled succinylcholine in near term macaca mulatta monkeys. *Br J Anaesth* 1973;45:1087.
101. Baraka A, Hatoun S, Bassili M, et al. Response of the newborn to succinylcholine injection in homozygotic atypical mothers. *Anesthesiology* 1975;43:115.
102. Cohen EN, Paulson WJ, Wall J, et al. Thiopental, curare and nitrous oxide anesthesia for cesarean section with studies on placental transmission. *Surg Obstet Gynecol* 1953;97:456.
103. Hawkins J, Johnson TD, Kubicek MA, Skjonsby BS, Morrow DH, Joyce TH. Vecuronium for rapid-sequence intubation for cesarean section. *Anesth Analg* 1990;71:185.
104. Demtriou M, Depoix JP, Diakite B, Fromartin M, Duvaldstein P. ORG N 45 in women undergoing cesarean section. *Br J Anaesth* 1982;54:643.
105. Flynn RI, Frank M, Hughes R. The use of atracurium in caesarean section. *Br J Anaesth* 1984;56:599.
106. Duvaldestin P, Demtriou M, Henzel D, et al. The placental transfer of pancuronium and its pharmacokinetics during caesarian section. *Acta Anaesthesiol Scand* 1978;22:327.
107. Baraka A, Tabbosh Z, Bijjani A. Onset of vecuronium neuromuscular blocks is more rapid in patients undergoing cesarean section. *Can J Anaesth* 1992;34:135.

108. Baraka AS, Sayyid SS, Assouf BA. Thiopental-rocuronium for regional sequence intubation in parturients undergoing cesarean section. *Anesth Analg* 1997;84:104.
109. Abouleish E, Abboud T, Lechevalier T, Zhu J, Chalian A, Alford K. Rocuronium (ORG 9426) for cesarean section. *Br J Anaesth* 1994;73:336.
110. Jan GSK, Tong WN, Chan AMH, Hui TWC, Lo JWR. Recovery from mivacurium block with or without anticholinesterase following continuous infusion in obstetric patients. *Anaesth Intens Care* 1996;24:585.
111. Dwyer R, Tee JPH, Moore J. Uptake of halothane and isoflurane by mother and baby during cesarean section. *Br J Anaesth* 1995;74:379.
112. Abboud TK, Kim SH, Henriksen EH, et al. Comparative maternal and neonatal effects of halothane and enflurane for cesarean section. *Acta Anesthesiol Scand* 1985;29:663.
113. Abboud TK, Zhu J, Richardson M, et al. Desflurane: a new volatile anesthetic for cesarean section: maternal and neonatal effects. *Acta Anaesthesiol Scand* 1995;39:723.
114. Wallace DH, Armstrong A, Damas A, et al. The effect of desflurane or low dose enflurane on uterine tone at cesarean delivery: placental transfer and recovery. *Anesthesiology* 1993;79:310.
115. Gambling DR, Sharma SK, White PF, Bereson TV, Bala AS, Gouldson R. Use of sevoflurane during elective cesarean birth: a comparison with isoflurane and spinal anesthesia. *Anesth Analg* 1995;81:90.
116. Abboud TK, D'Onofrio L, Reyes A, et al. Isoflurane or halothane for cesarean section. Comparative maternal and neonatal effects. *Acta Anesthesiol Scand* 1989;33:578.
117. Tunstall ME, Sheikh A. Comparison of 1.5% enflurane with 1.25% Isoflurane in oxygen for cesarean section: avoidance of awareness without nitrous oxide. *Br J Anaesth* 1989;62:138.
118. Cheek DBC, Hughes SC, Dailey PA, et al. Effect of halothane on regional cerebral blood flow and cerebral metabolic oxygen consumption in the fetal lamb in utero. *Anesthesiology* 1987;67:361.
119. Palahniuk RJ, Doig GA, Johnson GN, Pash MP. Maternal halothane anesthesia reduces cerebral blood flow in the acidotic sheep fetus. *Anesth Analg* 1980;59:35.
120. Yarnell R, Biehl DR, Tweed WA, Gregory GA, Siter D. The effect of halothane anaesthesia on the asphyxiated foetal lamb in utero. *Can Anaesth Soc J* 1983;30:474.
121. Mokriski BLK, Malinow AM. Neonatal acid-base status following general anesthesia with halothane or isoflurane for emergent abdominal delivery. *J Clin Anesth* 1992;4:97.
122. Pedersen JE, Fernandes A, Christensen M. Halothane 2% for cesarean section. *Eur J Anesthesiol* 1992;9:319.
123. Marx GF, Mateo CV. Effects of different oxygen concentrations during general anaesthesia during caesarean section. *Can Anaesth Soc J* 1971;18:587.
124. Baraka A. Correlation between maternal and foetal PO_2 and PCO_2 during caesarean section. *Br J Anaesth* 1970;42:434.
125. Rorke NJ, Davey DA, DuToit HJ. Foetal oxygenation during caesarean section. *Anaesthesia* 1968;23:585.
126. Perreault C, Blaise GA, Meloche R. Maternal inspired oxygen concentration and fetal oxygenation during caesarean section. *Can J Anaesth* 1992;39:155.
127. Lawes EG, Newman B, Campbell MJ, et al: Maternal inspired oxygen concentration and neonatal status for caesarean section under general anesthesia: a comparison of effects of 33% or 50% oxygen in nitrous oxide. *Br J Anaesth* 1988;61:250.
128. Piggott SE, Bogod DG, Rosen M, Rees GAD. Isoflurane with either 100% oxygen or 50% nitrous oxide in oxygen for caesarean section. *Br J Anaesth* 1990;65:325.
129. Bogod DG, Rosen M, Rees GAD. Maximum FIO_2 during caesarean section. *Br J Anaesth* 1988;61:255.
130. Marx GF, Young IK, Lin CC, et al. Postpartum uterine pressure under halothane or enflurane anesthesia. *Obstet Gynecol* 1978;57:695.
131. Moir DD. Anaesthesia for caesarean section. *Br J Anaesth* 1970;42:136.
132. Coleman AJ, Downing JW. Enflurane anesthesia for cesarean section. *Anesthesiology* 1975;42:354.
133. Abboud TK, Kim SH, Henriksen EH, et al. Comparative maternal and neonatal effects of halothane and enflurane for cesarean section. *Acta Anesth Scand* 1985;29:663.
134. Warren TM, Datta S, Ostheimer GW, et al. Comparison of the maternal and neonatal effects of halothane, enflurane and isoflurane for cesarean delivery. *Anesth Analg* 1983;62:516.
135. Gilstrap LC, Hauth JC, Hankins DV, Patterson AR. Effect of the type of anesthesia on blood loss at cesarean section. *Obstet Gynecol* 1987;69:328.
136. Andrews WW, Ramin SM, Maberry MC, Shearer V, Black S, Wallace DH. Effect of type of anesthesia on blood loss at elective repeat cesarean section. *Am J Perinatol* 1992;9:197.
137. Camann WR, Datta S. Red cell use during cesarean delivery. *Transfusion* 1991;31:12.
138. Stilettos RR, Hill CR, Dharamaj CM, Banner TE, Berman J. Wakefulness during cesarean section after anesthetic induction with ketamine, thiopental, or ketamine and thiopental combined. *Anesth Analg* 1986;65:723.
139. Baraka A, Louis F, Nouchid R, Diab M, Dabbous A, Sibai A. Awareness following different techniques of general anesthesia for cesarean section. *Br J Anaesth* 1989;62:645.
140. Gaitini L, Vaida S, Collins G, Somri M, Sabo E. Awareness detection during caesrean section under general anaesthesia using EEG spectrum analysis. *Can J Anaesth* 1995;42:377.
141. Baraka A, Fack L, Dalleh R. Maternal awareness and neonatal outcome after ketamine anaesthesia for caesarean section. *Can J Anaesth* 1990;37:641.
142. Bogod DG, Orton K, Yaw HM, Oh TE. Detecting awareness during general anaesthetic caesarean section: A comparison of two methods. *Anaesthesia* 1990;45:279.
143. Warren TM, Datta S, Ostheimer GW, Naulty S, Weiss JB, Morrison JA. Comparison of the maternal and neonatal effects of halothane, enflurane and isoflurane for cesarean delivery. *Anesth Analg* 1983;62:516.
144. Moir DD. Anaesthesia for cesarean section. An evaluation of a method using low flow concentrations of halothane end 50% oxygen. *Br J Anaesth* 1970;42:136.
145. Morgan BM, Aulakh JM, Barker JP, Goroszeniuk T, Trojanowski A. Anaesthesia for cesarean section. A medical audit of junior anaesthetic staff practice. *Br J Anaesth* 1983;55:885.
146. Bland BAR, Lawes KG, Duncan PW, Warnell L, Downing JW. Comparison of midazolam and thiopental for rapid sequence anesthetic induction for elective cesarean section. *Anesth Analg* 1987;66:1165.
147. Lubke GH, Kerssens C, Gershon RY, Sebal DS. Bispectral index (BIS) in relation to direct and indirect memory function during cesarean sections. *Anesth Analg* 1998;86:S216.
148. Zagorzycki MT, Brinkman CR. The effect of general and epidural anesthesia upon neonatal Apgar scores in repeat cesarean section. *Surg Gynecol Obstet* 1982;155:641.
149. Kangos-Saarela T, Koivisto M, Joupilla R, Joupilla P, Hollmen A. Comparison of the effect of general and epidural anesthesia for cesarean section on the neurobehavioral responses of newborn infants. *Acta Anaesth Scand* 1989;33:313.
150. Downing JW, Houlton PC, Barclay A. Extradural analgesia for cesarean section: a comparison with general anaesthesia. *Br J Anaesth* 1979;51:367.
151. Abboud TK, Naggappala S, Murakawa K, et al. Comparison of the effect of general and regional anesthesia for general anesthesia for cesarean section. *Br J Anaesth* scores. *Anesth Analg* 1985;64:996.
152. Akturk G, Kiral N, Bailak A, Jolak M, Ozen I, Ereiges N. The choice of anaesthetic technique for caesarean section does not affect plasma beta-endorphin level in the neonate. *Eur J Anesthesiol* 1995;12:525.
153. Adams HA, Biscoping J, Baumans P, Birgmann A, Herpelmann B. Maternal and fetal stress responses during cesarean section. *Reg Anaesth* 1989;12:87.
154. Mueller MD, Bruhuiler H, Schupfer GK, Luscher KP. Higher rate of fetal academia after regional anesthesia for elective cesarean delivery. *Obstet Gynecol* 1997:90:131.
155. Ong BY, Cohen MM, Palahniuk RL. Anesthesia for cesarean section: effects on neonates. *Anesth Analg* 1989;68:270.
156. Datta S, Ostheimer GW, Weiss JB, Brown WU, Alper MH. Neonatal effect of prolonged anesthetic induction. *Obstet Gynecol* 1981;58:331.
157. Crawford JS, James FM III, Crawley M. A further study of general anesthesia cesarean section. *Br J Anaesth* 1976;48:661.
158. Andersen HE, Auster GH, Marx GF, Merkatz IR. Neonatal status in relation to incision intervals, obstetric factors and anesthesia at cesarean delivery. *Am J Perinatol* 1987;4:279.

Obstetric Anesthesia, second edition,
edited by Mark C. Norris.
Lippincott Williams & Wilkins, Philadelphia © 1999.

CHAPTER 21

Epidural Anesthesia for Cesarean Delivery

Robert R. Gaiser

Because of the growing popularity of epidural analgesia for labor, the use of epidural anesthesia for cesarean section has increased in recent decades. Although it is now common to use an epidural catheter placed during labor to provide cesarean section anesthesia, this practice is a relatively recent development. Only in 1973 was it shown that labor epidural analgesia could be extended for cesarean section (1). Anesthesiologists were worried that epidural anesthesia would be inadequate for major intra-abdominal surgery in an awake, unmedicated parturient. Using an epidural block for cesarean section is a stringent test of the technique because deficiencies in analgesia cannot be covered by the free use of depressant drugs (1). In this first review, the authors reported excellent anesthesia by using 14 to 16 mL of local anesthetic, usually 2% lidocaine with 1:200,000 epinephrine, in 182 cases: 170 patients felt no discomfort, and only 12 required supplemental sedation. The biggest problem was the surgeon's ability to tolerate an awake patient who at times coughed or vomited. Since then, epidural block has become a well-accepted, established way to provide anesthesia for cesarean section. Despite its considerable popularity, epidural anesthesia has its limitations. Some key issues include:

- Maternal hypotension,
- Neonatal acidosis,
- Postdural puncture headache,
- Quality of anesthesia, and
- Failure rate (2).

However, with a thorough understanding of these issues and meticulous technique, we can use epidural block to provide excellent, safe maternal anesthesia for both elective and emergency cesarean section.

R.R. Gaiser: Department of Anesthesiology and Pharmacology, University of Pennsylvania, Philadelphia, Pennsylvania 19104.

ADVANTAGES OF EPIDURAL ANESTHESIA FOR CESAREAN SECTION

Flexibility is one of the most important advantages of epidural anesthesia. With an epidural catheter, the block can be adjusted, prolonged, and even reinitiated, as the clinical situation demands. We can control the level and density of sensory block by altering the selection, volume, and concentration of injected drug(s). Thus a parturient can receive labor analgesia with a dilute local anesthetic/opioid mixture. Later, incremental injection of more concentrated local anesthetics can rapidly provide surgical anesthesia for cesarean delivery.

Another important advantage of epidural anesthesia is the ability to prolong the block. This factor is important when the duration and extent of surgery are uncertain. Such cases may include repeated cesarean section or potential cesarean hysterectomy. Chestnut et al. (3) reviewed 3 years' experience with elective and emergency cesarean hysterectomies. Of the 46 patients identified, 12 received epidural anesthesia. Despite an average operative time of more than 2 hours and an estimated blood loss ranging from 1,300 to 2,600 mL, no parturient with a functioning epidural catheter required intraoperative conversion to general anesthesia. Repeated epidural injections of local anesthetic maintained maternal comfort throughout the operation. In addition to intraoperative anesthesia, an epidural catheter also can be used for postoperative analgesia (see Chapter 38).

The gradual onset of epidural blockade may help limit the frequency and severity of maternal hypotension (4). This approach may prove especially useful in certain clinical settings. Epidural anesthesia has proven safe for the woman with severe preeclampsia (5–7). Similarly, parturients with certain cardiac lesions (i.e., severe aortic stenosis) have a limited ability to respond to sudden hemodynamic changes. Slowly inducing epidural anesthesia while maintaining maternal blood pressure with fluids and vasopressors is a very effective way to manage these potentially unstable patients (see Chapter 27) (8–10).

CONTRAINDICATIONS

Patient refusal and infection at the site of needle insertion are absolute contraindications to epidural anesthesia. Other clinical situations may represent relative contraindications to epidural block (Table 1).

Neurological Disease

Some avoid epidural anesthesia when it might be blamed for a postoperative exacerbation of an existing neurological problem. The limited existing information that addresses this question is reassuring. Women with multiple sclerosis have the same risk of postpartum relapse with general or epidural anesthesia (11). The use of more concentrated local anesthetic solutions correlates with the risk of relapse. However, this association probably reflects the greater stresses of a labor and (cesarean) delivery that produce the need for more concentrated drug, not a neurotoxic effect of local anesthetics.

Hypovolemia

Do not induce epidural anesthesia in a patient who is hypovolemic from acute blood loss. The combination of sympathectomy and hypovolemia can produce profound hypotension. However, epidural anesthesia is a safe choice if intravascular volume can be restored and maintained.

Coagulopathy

Think twice before inducing epidural anesthesia in a patient with a coagulopathy or thrombocytopenia (i.e., women with preeclampsia, sepsis, intrauterine fetal demise, amniotic fluid embolism, and dilutional coagulopathy after massive hemorrhage and crystalloid infusion). Unchecked bleeding within the epidural space can cause permanent neurological injury. Severe back pain, bladder dysfunction, and progressive sensory and motor deficit may be symptoms of an epidural hematoma. Between 1966 and 1995, 51 cases of hematoma associated with epidural anesthesia were published (12). Fourteen of the 51 occurred in patients with a preexisting coagulopathy; all were general surgical patients. None of the obstetric patients were coagulopathic. Neurological outcome was directly related to the time between the onset of clinical symptoms and surgical decompression. Complete or good recovery occurred only when surgical decompression took place within 8 hours. If inducing epidural anesthesia in the patient at risk for an epidural hematoma, use a short-acting local anesthetic to allow early detection of symptoms.

TABLE 1. *Epidural anesthesia for cesarean section*

Indications
Flexibility
Delayed onset of blockade
Ability to extend blockade
Contraindications
Absolute
Patient refusal
Coagulopathy
Infection at site
Relative
Hypovolemia
Sepsis
Preexisting neurologic disease
Spinal abnormalities

Preeclampsia-induced thrombocytopenia is the most common coagulation abnormality in parturients. Although considerable debate surrounds the lower limit of platelet count that will allow safe induction of epidural anesthesia (13), otherwise healthy women with platelet counts well below 100,000/mm^3 have received epidural block without complication (14). There is a growing consensus that a woman with preeclampsia, but without clinical signs of abnormal bleeding, is an appropriate candidate for epidural block even if her platelet count is low.

Low-dose aspirin therapy during pregnancy may help prevent preeclampsia and fetal growth retardation (15,16). The enzyme cyclooxygenase converts arachidonic acid into the first prostaglandin G_2. All subsequent prostaglandins are derived from this initial compound. Aspirin permanently blocks cyclooxygenase activity in platelets. A single dose of aspirin will inhibit this enzyme for the 8- to 11-day life span of the platelet. The resulting platelet dysfunction may increase the risk of bleeding complications in parturients receiving regional anesthesia. Historically, bleeding time has been used to assess platelet function. However, a critical reevaluation of this test showed that it fails to predict the risk of bleeding (17). Thromboelastography, another test of the coagulation system, cannot distinguish parturients taking low-dose aspirin from normal controls (18). Fortunately, a collaborative study of more than 9,000 parturients reported no anesthetic-related bleeding complications associated with a daily dose of aspirin (60 mg) (19).

Back Pain

Neither intervertebral disc herniation nor back pain precludes epidural anesthesia. Epidural anesthesia does not increase severity of preexisting back pain or the incidence of new postoperative backache (see Chapter 39) (20,21).

Infection

The epidural catheter may serve as a site of abscess formation in the patient with sepsis. In parturients, chorioamnionitis is the most common cause of maternal bacteremia and sepsis (see Chapter 29). One retrospective review of 10,047 deliveries over a 1-year period found 319 cases of chorioamnionitis. Eight of these patients had positive blood cultures, and three of them received epidural anesthesia (22). There were no cases of epidural abscess. However, there is a report of maternal death after epidural anesthesia for cesarean section in a parturient with unsuspected sepsis (23). Death was thought to result from induction of epidural anesthesia in a profoundly hypovolemic patient in septic shock.

COMPARISON OF EPIDURAL AND SPINAL BLOCKADE

Although there are obvious similarities between epidural and spinal blockade, there are clinically important differences.

Mechanism of Blockade

Spinal blockade is achieved by injection of local anesthetic in the cerebrospinal fluid (CSF). Drug dose and baricity are the key determinants of the extent and duration of spinal anesthesia. With epidural anesthesia, baricity is not a factor, as there is no CSF in the epidural space. The extent of block appears to be related to the volume of the drug injected, whereas the density is related to the total mass of drug (24).

Liu et al. (25) injected 300 mg of 3% (10 mL) and a 1% (30 mL) 2-chloroprocaine in a randomized, double-blind, crossover study in 12 healthy volunteers. The 1% solution produced more extensive sensory effects. It blocked two more dermatomes to pinprick, touch, and cold than did the 3% concentration. However, the intensity of sensory and motor block at the hip and knee was unaffected by the concentration of 2-chloroprocaine.

Efficiency

Epidural anesthesia for cesarean section may require more time and resources than spinal block. Riley et al. (26) examined the costs of these two techniques for elective cesarean section. Forty-seven parturients had an epidural catheter inserted and dosed in the operating room, whereas 47 received spinal anesthesia. Patients in the epidural group spent more time in the operating room (101 vs 83 minutes). This difference was mostly due to time spent before surgical incision (46 vs 11 minutes). The indirect costs associated with the longer time spent in the operating room were responsible for greater patient charges in the epidural group (Fig. 1). The conclusion that spinal anesthesia is more cost efficient than epidural block for elective cesarean section is premised on a protocol of inserting and injecting epidural catheters in the expensive operating room. Inducing anesthesia in the patient's room is considerably less costly and could alter the conclusions of this study.

Although safe induction of the dense sensory and motor block required for cesarean section does take longer with epidural than with spinal anesthesia, the two techniques have multiple similarities. Both require preanesthetic evaluation, patient consent, intravenous access, proper positioning, insertion of the needle, and injection of the local anesthetic. At this point, the techniques diverge because of the slower onset of epidural anesthesia. However, with careful selection of local anesthetic and adjuvant agents, the difference in onset can be as short as 10 minutes.

Complications

Riley et al. (26) also examined the complications associated with spinal and epidural anesthesia in a teaching institution. Women in the epidural group were more likely to require intraoperative anxiolytics and analgesics. Six patients in the epidural group and none in the spinal group had other complications. These were:

- One dural puncture,
- One intrathecal catheter,
- One intravascular needle and catheter, and
- Three inadequate blocks.

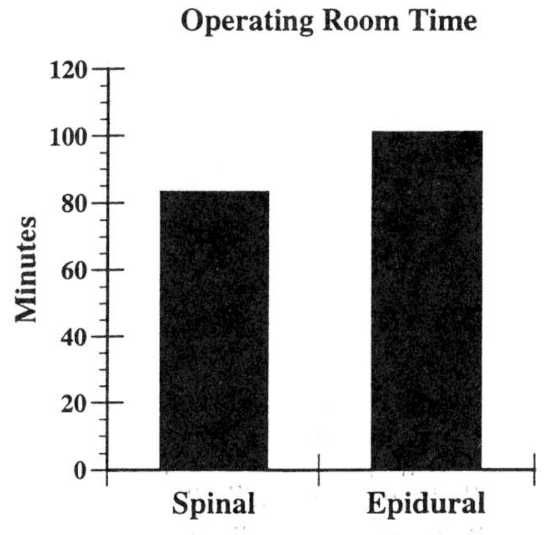

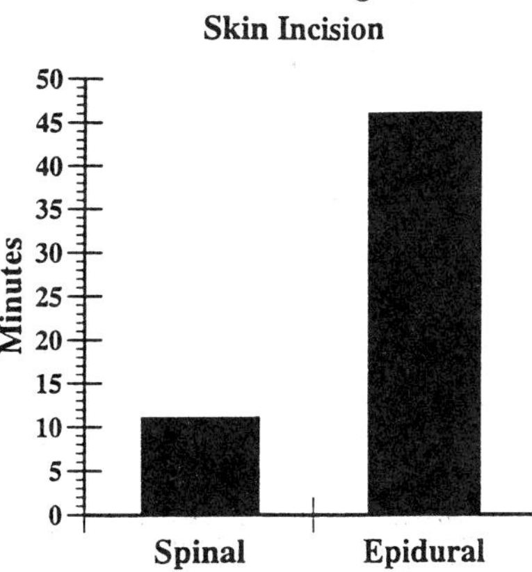

FIG. 1. Epidural anesthesia for elective cesarean section requires more intraoperative time than does spinal anesthesia. The primary reason for this increase is the longer period from entering the operating room to surgical incision. There are ways to decrease this time period, such as placement of the epidural catheter in a preoperative holding area or the labor room. (Adapted from ref. 26, with permission.)

It would be interesting to know if a similar complication rate exists when epidural anesthesia is initiated by fully trained anesthesiologists.

Duration

Despite its many advantages, single injection spinal anesthesia has one major limitation: its finite duration. Because epidural anesthesia can be induced and maintained by using an indwelling catheter, it remains the best choice when flexibility and prolonged duration are required.

PHYSIOLOGY OF EPIDURAL BLOCKADE

Mechanism of Action

Local anesthetics produce reversible neural blockade by preventing the passage of sodium ions through the nerve membrane (27). When injected into the epidural space, most drug diffuses into the circulation where is it redistributed to other tissues for metabolism and eventual excretion (28). Some is retained in fatty tissue within the epidural space, whereas the rest reaches target nerve fibers within the spinal nerves and nerve roots (29). Two mechanisms account for neural blockade during epidural anesthesia. One is direct blockade at the spinal nerve root. Another is local anesthetic diffusion through the dura, arachnoid, and pia mater to reach the spinal cord itself. The concentrations of local anesthetic in the CSF during epidural anesthesia are similar to those found during spinal anesthesia (24). With time, epidural blockade comes to resemble spinal blockade.

Cardiovascular

The major circulatory effect of extensive epidural local anesthetic–induced sensory block is related to the accompanying sympathetic blockade. A mid-thoracic level of sympathetic blockade causes vasodilation in both lower extremities and the splanchnic circulation. The resultant reduction in venous return to the heart decreases cardiac output, which then reduces blood pressure. Decreased arteriolar tone plays a lesser role. Although the decline in cardiac output is largely attributed to a reduction in venous return, a sympathetic blockade to T_4 also impairs left ventricular contractility by inhibiting conduction in afferent cardiac sympathetic nerves. Echocardiography reveals altered left ventricular contractility after high thoracic epidural anesthesia, even in patients without myocardial disease (Fig. 2) (30). If the block extends to T_1 (completely blocking cardiac sympathetic nerve fibers), heart rate may slow.

Pulmonary

Uncomplicated epidural blockade rarely causes respiratory complications. It has no effect on inspiratory function. Expiratory pressures and flow rates are decreased in relation to the degree of impairment of abdominal muscle function. (Peak expiratory pressure correlates with the ability to cough effectively by generating high intrapulmonary pressures against a closed glottis.) Mid-thoracic blockade by using 2% lidocaine with epinephrine decreases peak expiratory pressure by 45%. In contrast, 0.5% bupivacaine, which produces less motor blockade than does lidocaine, decreases expiratory pressure by only 10% (Fig. 3) (31). Epidural blockade itself has little effect on forced expiratory flow rate, but once cesarean section begins, expiratory flow rates decrease considerably (32).

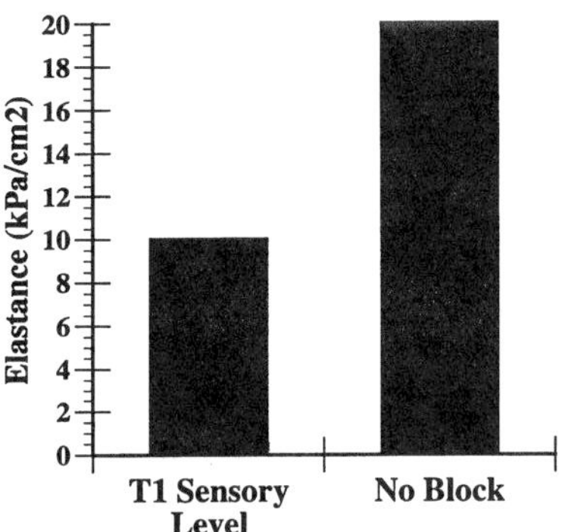

FIG. 2. Elastance is the slope of the end-systolic pressure length relation of the left ventricle, as measured during transesophageal echocardiography. Elastance may be used as a measure of ventricular contractility, and it is relatively insensitive to ventricular loading conditions. In this study, left ventricular contractility, as measured as the maximal elastance of the left ventricle, was grossly reduced during high thoracic sensory levels with epidural anesthesia. (Adapted from ref. 30, with permission.)

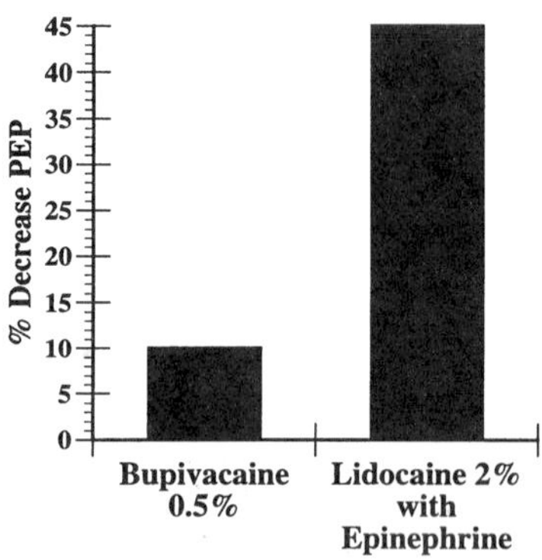

FIG. 3. One of the simplest pulmonary-function tests to obtain is peak expiratory pressure (PEP), which is measured with a variable-orifice flowmeter. Because the peak pressure occurs early in a forced expiration, flow limitation does not occur in the airways and thus is highly dependent on abdominal musculature. PEP is decreased by 45% with 2% lidocaine with epinephrine administered epidurally compared with a 10% reduction for 0.5% bupivacaine. Peak airway pressure is important for effective coughing. (Adapted from ref. 31, with permission.)

Subjective dyspnea may develop if the level of sensory blockade exceeds T_2. About 5% of women having epidural anesthesia for cesarean section reported this symptom (33). Its etiology is probably the lack of proprioceptive input from the chest wall and intercostal musculature. Reassurance is the most appropriate treatment.

Endocrine

Epidural anesthesia blunts the endocrine stress response to cesarean section. Increases in plasma concentrations of cortisol, catecholamines, and blood glucose are less with epidural compared with general anesthesia (Fig. 4) (34).

Hematologic

In orthopedic patients, epidural anesthesia decreases the risk of venous thrombosis and postoperative pulmonary embolism (35). The mechanism of this effect is not fully understood. Perhaps sympathetic nervous system blockade decreases venous stasis by increasing lower extremity blood flow. Epidural block also may directly affect the coagulation system (36). In one study, 95 patients undergoing elective lower extremity vascular reconstruction were randomized to either general anesthesia or epidural anesthesia with 0.75% bupivacaine. There was a lower incidence of postoperative arterial thrombosis in the epidural group. The plasma concentration of type 1 plasminogen activator inhibitor (PAI) also was lower in the epidural group. Type 1 PAI is a rapid and specific inhibitor of both tissue- and urokinase-type plasminogen activators and may represent the primary regulator of plasminogen activation.

Epidural anesthesia also decreases intraoperative blood loss compared with general anesthesia (37). Epidural anesthesia–related hypotension only partially explains this effect, as blood loss does not always correlate with intraoperative blood pressure.

Obstetric

Fetal oxygenation depends on both uterine and umbilical blood flow. Multiple approaches have been used to examine the effects of epidural anesthesia on these variables. Radioactive isotopes can be used to measure uterine blood flow. Skoeldebrand et al. (38,39) showed that epidural anesthesia with bupivacaine did not change uterine blood flow, but bupivacaine with epinephrine 1:400,000 significantly decreased uterine blood flow by 34%. Pulsed Doppler ultrasound measures blood-flow velocity. Studies using this technique have shown that uterine blood flow does not change or increases under epidural anesthesia, provided epinephrine is not added and hypotension is avoided (40). Intervillous and umbilical blood flows are unchanged (41–43).

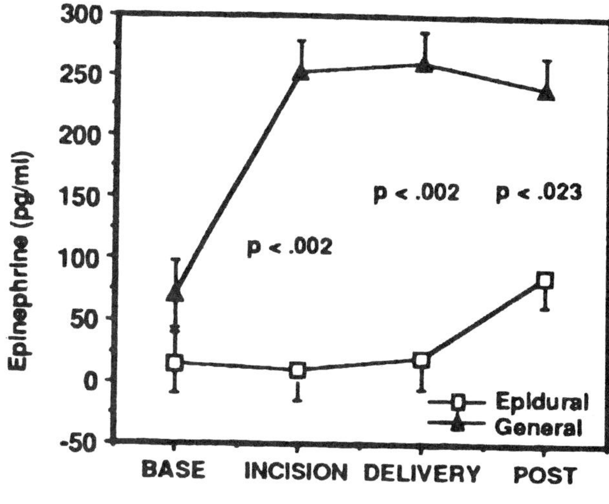

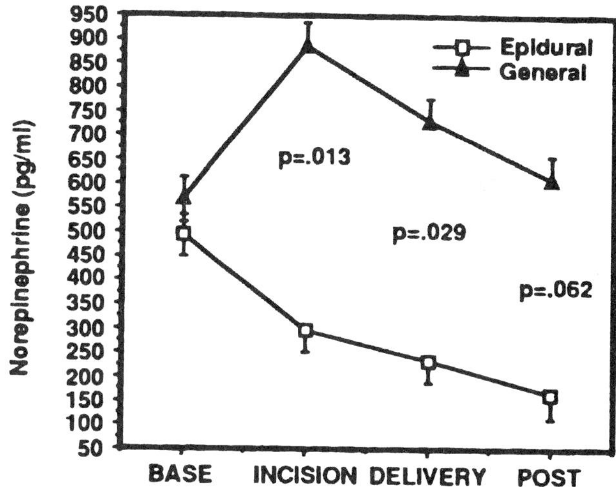

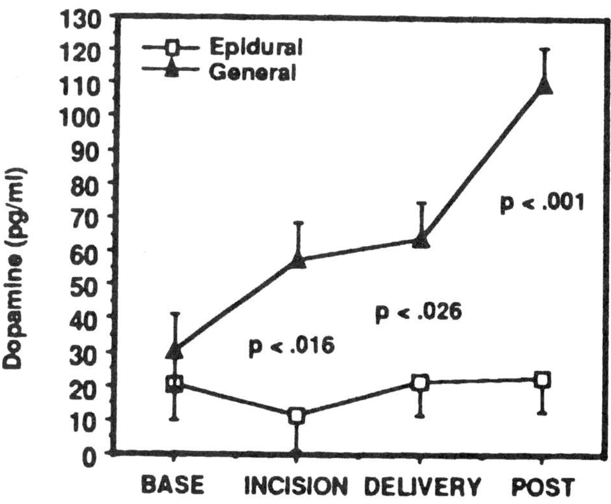

FIG. 4. Surgical incision is accompanied by a stress response that includes an increase in the plasma concentrations of epinephrine and norepinephrine. This stress response is not seen with epidural anesthesia compared with general anesthesia. (Reprinted from ref. 34, with permission.)

LOCAL ANESTHETIC

Amides

Although many local anesthetics are available for epidural anesthesia, not all are suitable for use in obstetrics. Mepivacaine and prilocaine, like lidocaine, rapidly induce profound anesthesia of moderate duration. Mepivacaine produces less vasodilation than does lidocaine. This effect delays its absorption from the epidural space and prolongs its duration. However, metabolism of mepivacaine is markedly prolonged in the fetus, and significant neonatal neurobehavioral effects have been reported, so it is rarely used in parturients (44). Large doses of prilocaine (>600 mg) can cause methemoglobinemia, ruling out its use for cesarean section (45). Etidocaine rapidly produces long-lasting sensory and motor blockade, but profound motor block can long outlast sensory analgesia. As result, it is rarely used for cesarean section (46).

Lidocaine

Lidocaine was the first amide local anesthetic to be introduced into clinical practice. Its potency, rapid onset, and moderate duration make it one of the most commonly used drugs for epidural anesthesia. Both 1.5% and 2% concentrations are used for cesarean section. Intrathecal lidocaine may be neurotoxic (47).

Cauda equina syndrome has been reported after the use of 2% lidocaine with misplaced catheters (48,49). Lidocaine was injected through an intended epidural catheter that proved to be subdural or intrathecal. These cases emphasize the importance of intrathecal test doses and the need for careful management of recognized spinal catheters.

Bupivacaine

Epidural bupivacaine provides anesthesia of slow onset and long duration. It is both potent and toxic. Epidural bupivacaine produces relatively greater-intensity sensory than motor blockade. A 0.5% concentration is used for cesarean section. Although a 0.75% concentration is available, the Food and Drug Administration (FDA) rescinded its approval for use in obstetrics because of a high incidence of cardiac complications.

Bupivacaine is more cardiotoxic than lidocaine. Both bupivacaine and lidocaine depress intracardiac conduction by blocking sodium channels. However, bupivacaine binds to the open sodium channel for much longer than lidocaine, making bupivacaine 16 times more potent than lidocaine in reducing cardiac contractility and conductivity (50). Initial studies suggested that pregnancy enhanced the cardiac toxicity of bupivacaine (51,52). However, carefully controlled, blinded follow-up studies found no difference in the susceptibility of nonpregnant and pregnant sheep to the cardiotoxic effects of bupivacaine (53). The high maternal mortality associated with unrecognized intravenous injection of bupivacaine probably relates to the difficulties involved in resuscitating a parturient, not to greater intrinsic toxicity of bupivacaine in this population.

Ropivacaine

Ropivacaine is a new amide local anesthetic structurally similar to mepivacaine and bupivacaine (Fig. 5). It is the first local anesthetic prepared as the pure *s*-enantiomer. Previous amide local anesthetics have been prepared as racemic mixtures. (Although both enantiomers

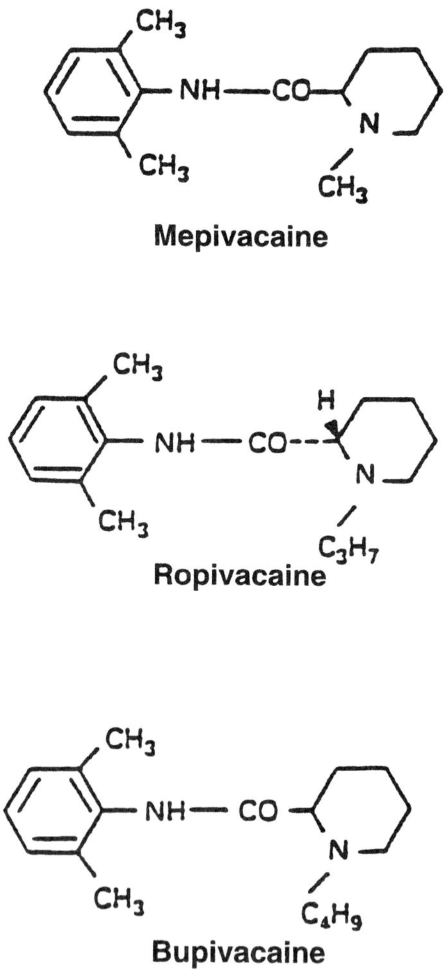

FIG. 5. Ropivacaine is an amide local anesthetic in the same family as mepivacaine and bupivacaine. One basic structural difference is seen on the piperidine nitrogen of the respective molecules, as bupivacaine has a butyl group, mepivacaine, a methyl group, and ropivacaine, a propyl group. A second important distinction relates to the fact that this group of drugs are chiral, with an asymmetric carbon atom in the amine ring, resulting in two mirror-image forms of the compounds. Both mepivacaine and bupivacaine are racemic mixtures, containing equal amounts of the *r* and *s* enantiomers, whereas ropivacaine is produced solely as the *s* form.

of bupivacaine have similar local anesthetic actions, the *d*-enantiomer is considerably more cardiotoxic (54). The *s*-enantiomer preparation of ropivacaine is markedly less cardiotoxic than racemic bupivacaine (55–58). Ropivacaine is available in 0.2%, 0.5%, 0.75%, and 1.0% concentrations. The FDA approved only the 0.5% concentration for cesarean section. In parturients, both ropivacaine, 0.5%, and bupivacaine, 0.5%, produce similar sensory anesthesia. The duration of motor block is significantly shorter after ropivacaine. Neonatal outcome and umbilical cord blood–gas tensions are similar (59). Ropivacaine lacks effect on uteroplacental or fetal circulations, as assessed by Doppler ultrasound (60).

Esters

The only clinically useful ester local anesthetic for cesarean section under epidural anesthesia is 3% 2-chloroprocaine. This drug is short-acting, not very potent, and unlikely to cause systemic toxicity. When used for elective cesarean section, 2-chloroprocaine has no detectable adverse maternal or neonatal effects (61). The in vitro maternal and fetal plasma half-lives of 2-chloroprocaine are 11 and 15 seconds, respectively. The in vivo half-life in maternal plasma is 3 minutes (62). Because fetal acidosis does not increase the placental transfer of 2-chloroprocaine, it may be a good choice for the mother with a possibly asphyxiated fetus (63).

In the 1980s, prolonged neurological deficits were reported after unrecognized subarachnoid injection of large volumes of 2-chloroprocaine (64). Gissen et al. (65) found that 2-chloroprocaine, at low pH, when combined with sodium bisulfite, produced irreversible conduction blockade in isolated nerve fibers. 2-Chloroprocaine alone or sodium bisulfite, 0.2%, at physiologic pH produced no signs of irreversible toxicity. They suggested that sulphur dioxide liberated from the bisulfite at a low pH diffused into the nerve membrane and formed sulfurous acid, which caused the damage. The same workers also reported that the rapid administration of large volumes of fluid into the subarachnoid space, in the presence of systemic hypotension, decreased spinal cord perfusion and produced signs of cord ischemia (65).

The manufacturer replaced the sodium metabisulfite preservative with the calcium chelator, EDTA. Unfortunately, binding of calcium by EDTA produced hypocalcemic tetany in the paraspinous muscles and reports of severe spasmodic back pain after large doses of this preparation of 2-chloroprocaine (66). A new preservative-free preparation is now available.

2-Chloroprocaine impairs the analgesic efficacy of subsequently administered epidural opioids. This effect is seen with both morphine and fentanyl (67–69). Camann et al. (68) showed that 2-chloroprocaine prevented the analgesic effects of fentanyl, even after the local anesthetic induced epidural block had been allowed to recede. Although the mechanism of this effect is unclear, Coda et al. (70) showed, in guinea-pig hippocampal slices, that 2-chloroprocaine binds to, but does not activate, mu and kappa receptors.

2-Chloroprocaine also impairs the action of bupivacaine if the two agents are used together or sequentially. Cohen and Thurlow (71) reported that a mixture of 2-chloroprocaine and bupivacaine produced shorter-acting epidural analgesia than did bupivacaine alone. In the isolated rat sciatic nerve, a metabolite of 2-chloroprocaine persists after recovery from neural blockade and interferes with the subsequent action of bupivacaine (72).

ADJUVANT AGENTS

Many anesthesiologists add a variety of compounds to the local anesthetic used for cesarean section epidural anesthesia. These drugs aim to speed the onset, enhance the quality, and prolong the duration of epidural local anesthetic blockade.

Epinephrine

Local anesthetics exhibit a biphasic effect on vascular smooth muscle. In low concentrations, they promote vasoconstriction. In the typically used higher concentrations, vasodilation occurs. The resulting increased blood flow speeds vascular uptake and removal of drug from the epidural space (73). The vasoconstrictor epinephrine decreases the rate of vascular absorption of some local anesthetics. Epinephrine, when added to achieve a concentration of 1:200,000 (5 μg/mL), reduced the mean peak plasma concentrations of epidural lidocaine by 23% and epidural bupivacaine by 28% but did not alter the time to peak concentrations (74). This effect allows more anesthetic to reach sites of action within the nerve membrane and improves the density and duration of anesthesia.

Brose and Cohen (75) attempted to determine the optimal concentration of epinephrine for use with epidural lidocaine during cesarean section. Forty parturients were randomly assigned to receive 20 mL of 2% lidocaine alone or with epinephrine in concentrations of 1:400,000, 1:300,000, or 1:200,000. Patients in the plain lidocaine group had the most intraoperative pain and the highest plasma lidocaine concentrations. The three concentrations of epinephrine were equally effective in improving the quality of epidural blockade. Whereas plain 2% lidocaine is inadequate for epidural anesthesia for cesarean section, bupivacaine and ropivacaine produce satisfactory anesthesia without the addition of epinephrine.

Some controversy surrounds use of epinephrine-containing local anesthetics in obstetrics (76). In the rat sciatic nerve, a single dose of epinephrine produces prolonged vasoconstriction and reduces neural blood flow by 40% (77). Ischemic neural damage may follow. It is reassuring, however, that epidural epinephrine has been used extensively in humans for nearly 90 years without reported neurological sequelae. In fact, intrathecal epinephrine, 0.4 to 1.0 mg, produced no neurological complications, and 1.0 mg provided complete labor analgesia for 120 minutes (78). Systemic absorption of epidurally injected epinephrine induces hemodynamic changes related to the drug's β-agonist action. Vasodilation decreases systemic vascular resistance and blood pressure. Heart rate increases in response to the decrease in blood pressure as well as to epinephrine's direct chronotropic action. Although β-agonist effects predominate, we also can see α-agonist actions. Epidural injection of epinephrine-containing local anesthetics in patients with underlying uteroplacental insufficiency increases placental vascular resistance (79). In women with severe preeclampsia, epidural epinephrine may contribute to maternal hypertension (80). Whenever I use lidocaine for my epidural local anesthetic, I add epinephrine at a concentration of 1:400,000 (2.5 μg/mL). I do not add epinephrine to 2-chloroprocaine, bupivacaine, or ropivacaine.

Commercially available epinephrine-containing local anesthetic solutions are buffered to a pH of 3.5 to prevent oxidation of the epinephrine. Solutions without epinephrine are buffered to a higher pH (5.0) and have a shorter latency. The onset of lidocaine with epinephrine can be hastened either by adding epinephrine to the plain drug shortly before use or by increasing the pH of the commercial preparation with sodium bicarbonate (see the following). Clinical studies suggest that these two approaches are equally effective (81) (Fig. 6).

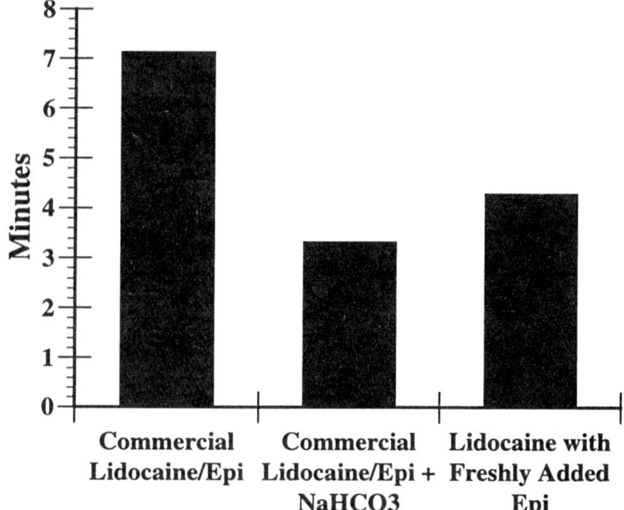

FIG. 6. Two ways exist to hasten the onset of sensory block of lidocaine. One was is to add sodium bicarbonate to the commercial lidocaine/epinephrine mixture. The other way is to add the epinephrine yourself. Either way results in comparable onset of blockade, which is much faster than the commercial mixture without sodium bicarbonate. (Adapted from ref. 81, with permission.)

Other a2 Agonists

In addition to its vasoconstrictor action, epinephrine enhances epidural local anesthetics by a direct action on α_2-adrenergic receptors in the dorsal horn of the spinal cord (82). Other α_2 agonists also produce analgesia after epidural injection. The most extensively studied of these drugs is clonidine. Most studies of this drug focused on postoperative analgesia. A single epidural bolus of clonidine, 800 μg, provides approximately 6 hours of pain relief. For longer periods of analgesia, a continuous infusion is required (83). The choice of local anesthetic also influences the efficacy of epidurally injected α_2 agonists. After cesarean section with epidural bupivacaine, clonidine produced effective analgesia with either a 400- or 800-μg bolus followed by a 40 μg/hour infusion. In contrast, providing surgical anesthesia with epidural 2-chloroprocaine diminishes analgesia from 800 μg and abolishes it from 400 μg of epidural clonidine (84). Epidural clonidine does not alter residual bupivacaine sensory blockade but does prolong the duration of motor blockade. Epidural clonidine decreases maternal heart rate and blood pressure. With larger doses, maternal sedation, which can be associated with snoring, obstructive apnea, and episodes of arterial oxygen desaturation, occurs (85).

Opioids

The use of epidural opioids in combination with local anesthetics has gained increasing popularity. A single dose of epidural morphine can provide prolonged postoperative analgesia. Continuous infusion of lipid-soluble opioids (i.e., fentanyl) may produce analgesia by either a direct spinal action or by systemic absorption and blood-borne delivery to the brain.

Fentanyl and Sufentanil

Epidural fentanyl and sufentanil both improve intraoperative analgesia and provide some postoperative analgesia. Both fentanyl and sufentanil are more lipid soluble than morphine and have a more rapid onset. One double-blind study of 60 healthy women reported that fentanyl, 100 μg, did not change the onset or duration of sensory or motor blockade produced by 0.5% bupivacaine. However, fentanyl significantly improved the quality of intraoperative analgesia, as assessed by both the parturients and the anesthesiologist, without any adverse maternal or neonatal effects (86). Others showed that the sensory onset of epidural bupivacaine can be shortened by 3 to 4 minutes with the addition of 1 μg/kg fentanyl without any effect on neonatal neurobehavioral scores (87,88). Similar studies using sufentanil have been published. In one, 45 parturients were randomized to receive sufentanil, 80, 50, or 0 μg, with epidural lidocaine. Superior analgesia was obtained with both doses of sufentanil. The infants born to those mothers who received 80 μg sufentanil showed a mild neurobehavioral depression, whereas 50 μg had no significant neonatal side effects (89). Studies in animals suggested that visceral nociceptors are more sensitive than somatic ones to the synergistic interaction of local anesthetics and opioids (90). Maternal side effects of epidural fentanyl and sufentanil include drowsiness, nausea, and pruritus.

Morphine

Unlike fentanyl and sufentanil, morphine is not lipid soluble and has a longer latency. When injected during the induction of epidural blockade for cesarean section, morphine, 3 mg, fentanyl, 75 μg, or sufentanil, 50 μg, improved intraoperative analgesia. However, morphine provided the longest pain-free interval after delivery (91) (Fig. 7). Morphine is primarily used for analgesia after cesarean section. Palmer et al. (92) showed that the duration of analgesia with epidural morphine plateaus after 3.75 mg. Larger doses of morphine did not prolong analgesia but did increase the incidence and severity of side effects including respiratory depression, urinary retention, nausea, and pruritus.

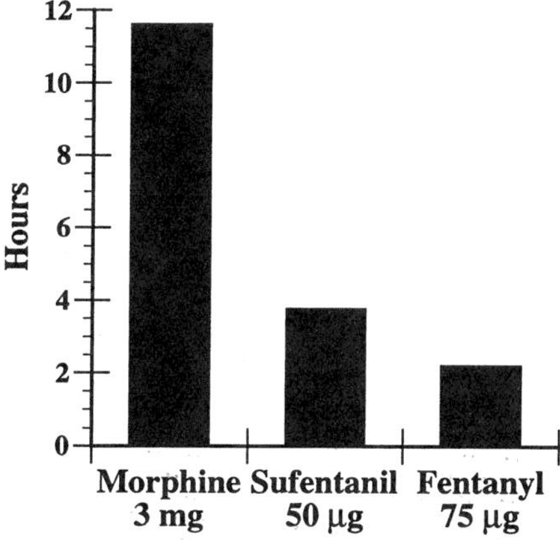

FIG. 7. Either morphine, 3 mg, sufentanil, 50 μg, or fentanyl, 75 μg, was added to the local anesthetic at the beginning of epidural anesthesia for elective cesarean section. All improved intraoperative analgesia. However, morphine provided the longest pain-free interval after delivery but also resulted in a higher number of patients with pruritus and vomiting. (Adapted from ref. 91, with permission.)

Other Opioids

Whereas morphine, fentanyl, and sufentanil are the most commonly used drugs, other opioids have been studied. Large doses (30 μg/kg) of epidural alfentanil produced neonatal hypotonia (93). A continuous epidural infusion of alfentanil at 0.2 mg/hour can provide analgesia after cesarean section (94), but more cost-effective therapies are available. Epidural meperidine, 100 mg, has a rapid onset and provides analgesia of 6 hours (95,96). Although it has a slower onset than meperidine, morphine remains the longest lasting epidural opioid.

For elective cesarean section, I always add 1 μg/kg fentanyl to my epidural local anesthetic. Fentanyl improves and may hasten the onset of block without adversely affecting mother or neonate. For urgent cesarean section, fentanyl is usually not immediately obtainable, and I do not include it in my initial injection. When it does become available, I include it in a subsequent dose.

Sodium Bicarbonate

2-Chloroprocaine and lidocaine are readily alkalinized to near physiologic pH without precipitation by adding sodium bicarbonate. Bupivacaine precipitates with the addition of small amounts of sodium bicarbonate (97). Increasing the pH of the local anesthetic speeds the onset of bupivacaine, lidocaine, and 2-chloroprocaine neural blockade (Table 2) (98). Initially, the mechanism of this effect was thought to be related to the change in pH. Sodium bicarbonate brings the pH of the solution closer to the pK_a of the local anesthetic, increasing the relative concentration of uncharged molecules and shortening the latency (99). The actual mechanism may be different. Sodium bicarbonate alters the sodium channel, making it more susceptible to local anesthetic blockade. Carbonic anhydrase converts sodium bicarbonate to carbon dioxide. Carbon dioxide diffuses across the nerve membrane and decreases the intracellular pH, which in turn increases the charged fraction of intracellular local anesthetic. This ionized drug cannot leave the cell, and a concentration gradient is established for nonionized drug, which draws more local anesthetic into the neuron. This ion trapping produces profound block more rapidly compared with local anesthetic without sodium bicarbonate (Fig. 8) (100).

TABLE 2. *Amount of sodium bicarbonate for alkalinization of local-anesthetic solutions*

Local anesthetic (pK_a)	HCO_3 required (mEq/20 mL)
Chloroprocaine (8.7)	1.92
Lidocaine (7.9)	1.92
Bupivacaine (8.1)	0.05
Ropivacaine (8.1)	0.05

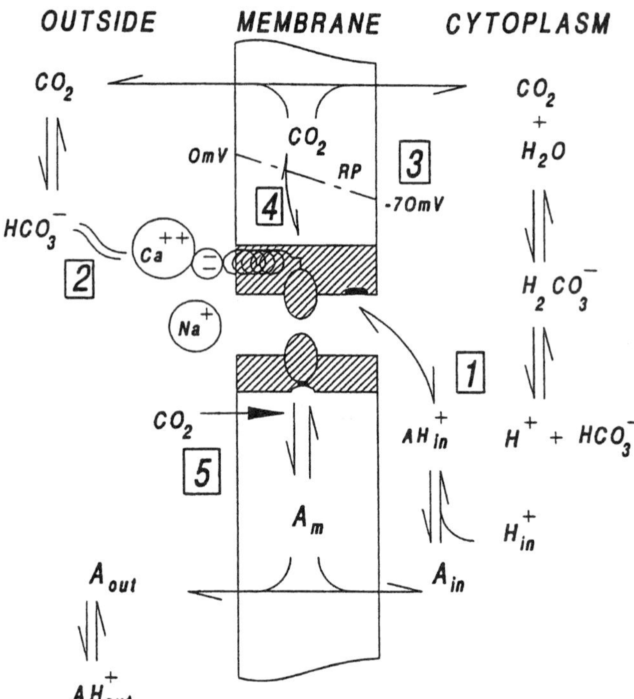

FIG. 8. Sodium bicarbonate increases the speed of onset of local anesthetics not by increasing the pH of the solution closer to the pK_a, as had been previously thought, but by increasing the acidity of the nerve cytoplasm, leading to trapping of the cationic form of local anesthetic. The carbon dioxide formed also modifies the sodium channel, influencing binding. Bicarbonate leads to sodium channel inactivation, a channel conformation known to bind local anesthetic more tightly. (Reprinted from ref. 99, with permission.)

SOME TECHNICAL CONSIDERATIONS

Anatomy

The spinal canal lies within the vertebral column between the foramen magnum and the sacral hiatus, bound anteriorly by the vertebral bodies, laterally by the pedicles, and posteriorly by the laminae. The spinal cord extends within the canal from the brainstem to its termination at the $L_{1\text{-}2}$ vertebral level. The remaining lower lumbar and sacral nerve roots continue within the spinal canal as the cauda equina. Three membranes cover the spinal cord, creating three spaces. The three membranes are the pia mater, arachnoid mater, and the dura mater. The three spaces are subarachnoid, subdural, and epidural. The epidural space is bound by the posterior longitudinal ligament anteriorly and the ligamentum flavum posteriorly; it extends from the base of the skull to the sacral hiatus (see Chapter 14).

The Appropriate Sensory Level

The recommended level of sensory blockade for cesarean section varies from T_8 to T_2 (101–104). Although some of this dissimilarity is explained by operative technique (exteriorizing the uterus for repair requires a higher level of block), the range is still great. Pain sensations from pelvic organs enter the spinal cord at T_{10} to L_1, but more extensive blockade is required for cesarean section because some pelvic nerves accompany sympathetic fibers through the various intra-abdominal plexi and the greater splanchnic nerve to reach the spinal cord as high as T_4 (105). Visceral pain also arises from other intra-abdominal structures, such as the peritoneum, which are innervated by sensory afferents that enter the spinal cord as far cephalad as T_4.

Most available data suggest that the higher the level of sensory block, the more comfortable the patient. Under spinal anesthesia, patients are more likely to be comfortable when the level of sensory block exceeds T_5 (106). In another study of 220 women undergoing cesarean section under regional anesthesia, the only patients experiencing pain were those who had anesthesia (loss of ability to perceive touch) below T_5 (107). No patient with anesthesia above T_5 experienced pain. This level was approximately two dermatomes lower than the level of analgesia (loss of sharpness to pin-prick).

The lower extent of sensory blockade also is important for patient comfort. Another cause of visceral pain during cesarean section is incomplete block of the large nerve roots of L_5 to S_2. Blocking of these roots is required to prevent pain from traction on the uterosacral ligaments or bladder.

Perioperative Management

Step 1: Preoperative Evaluation

As with all anesthetics, evaluate parturients who are to receive epidural anesthesia preoperatively. Assess their physical status and appropriateness for epidural anesthesia. Explain the procedure and possible complications and obtain informed consent. Inspect the patient's spine for evidence of infection, previous surgery, or scoliosis (which may make the procedure technically more difficult).

Step 2: Aspiration Prophylaxis

All parturients are at high risk of regurgitation and aspiration of stomach contents. Whereas choosing regional over general anesthesia will decrease this risk, it does not eliminate it. Blocks fail. Excessive sensory blockade or profound maternal hypotension can impair airway reflexes and consciousness. Thus patients having a regional anesthetic for their cesarean section require some form of acid aspiration prophylaxis. I always give 30 mL sodium citrate before induction of epidural anesthesia for cesarean section. Others also administer an H_2 blocker to decrease stomach acidity and metoclopramide to improve gastric emptying (a delayed effect), increase gastroesophageal junction pressure (an immediate effect), and decrease intraoperative nausea and vomiting (108,109)

Step 3: Equipment and Setting

Have appropriate resuscitation equipment available. Essentials are a means of positive-pressure ventilation, an oxygen source, and suction. Monitoring consists of blood pressure, heart rate, and pulse oximetry. The electrocardiogram (ECG) is usually applied after completion of the epidural catheter placement. Have a vasopressor, usually ephedrine, prepared and readily available.

Step 4: Insert Epidural Catheter

Patient Position

Positioning depends on patient comfort and the anesthesiologist's preference. Thin patients often prefer the lateral position (110). In obese women, identifying the midline and other landmarks may be easier in the sitting position.

Choose an Interspace

Usually a line joining the iliac crests passes through the $L_{4\text{-}5}$ interspace. However, in the term parturient, the lumbar lordosis of the spine increases. As a result, the line joining the iliac crests may be more cephalad, crossing the $L_{3\text{-}4}$ interspace. I usually choose the $L_{2\text{-}3}$ or $L_{3\text{-}4}$ interspace.

Local Infiltration

Inject local anesthetic intradermally to raise a skin wheal. Then by using a thin 1.5-inch needle, infiltrate the subcutaneous tissues and probe for bony landmarks.

Insert the Epidural Needle

The epidural needle has a blunt tip to reduce the chance of puncturing the dura. The side-facing orifice at the tip allows the passage of a catheter. Insert the needle until it is firmly seated in the interspinous ligament.

Locate the Epidural Space

Remove the stylet and attach an air- or liquid-filled syringe with a freely mobile plunger. Brace the dorsum of the nondominant hand on the parturient's back. Grasp the needle shaft or hub with your thumb and index or middle finger. The nondominant hand controls the advancement of the epidural needle in 2-mm increments, while the thumb of the dominant hand continuously or intermittently depresses the plunger of the syringe. While the tip of the needle lies in ligament, the plunger of the syringe cannot be easily depressed. When the needle tip enters the compliant epidural space, there is a loss of resistance, and the plunger is easily depressed.

Practitioners often have strong preferences about the choice of an air- or saline-filled syringe. The sensation felt on the syringe plunger is different for the two. Air is compressible. Saline is not. Although some question the safety of air for the loss-of-resistance technique (111), the rarity of complications and the absence of irreversible damage suggests that either air or saline is appropriate, provided the user's success rate is acceptable.

A possible alternative to loss of resistance is the hanging-drop technique. A drop of sterile fluid is placed in the open needle hub. When the needle enters the epidural space, the fluid is drawn into the needle by negative pressure. This negative pressure results from tenting of the dura primarily and transmission of negative intrathoracic pressure secondarily. I do not use this technique in parturients because compression by the enlarged uterus increases the pressure within the epidural space (112).

Pass the Catheter

Pass a catheter through the needle into the epidural space and then remove the needle over the catheter. The ideal depth of insertion depends on the type of catheter, 5 cm for a multiport catheter (113) and 6 cm for an single-holed one (114). Have the patient sit straight before securing the catheter with tape. When the patient unflexes her back after epidural insertion, the folds of her back move around the catheter. If secured when the spine is flexed, the catheter moves out of the epidural space as much as 2 cm when the parturient unflexes her back. This movement is greatest in obese women (115).

Step 9: The Test Dose

Unrecognized intrathecal or intravenous injection of local anesthetics can prove fatal. To detect unrecognized intrathecal or intravascular injection anesthetists often inject some form of test dose before the bulk of the epidural local anesthetic. Before injecting any drug into the epidural catheter, look for spontaneous blood return; then gently aspirate. If using a multiport catheter, these steps alone will detect the vast majority (>95%) of intravenous catheters (116).

I routinely test catheters with 3 mL of lidocaine, 1.5%, with epinephrine 1:200,000. If injected intravenously, the patient's heart rate increases (117). If it is given intrathecally, the patient rapidly develops a sensory level. If it is administered epidurally, the patient experiences no discernible symptoms.

No matter which test dose is used, a negative test dose does not guarantee correct placement. Epidural local anesthetics should be injected incrementally, with contin-

---

Editor's note: I agree that 30 mL of 0.3 *M* sodium citrate alone is adequate acid aspiration prophylaxis before cesarean section.

uous patient monitoring for symptoms of intrathecal or intravascular injection.

Step 10: Patient Position

Have the parturient lie supine with left uterine displacement. In the supine position, the gravid uterus obstructs the aorta and vena cava, impeding uterine artery blood flow, decreasing venous return and cardiac output. Decreased uterine perfusion can produce fetal acidosis (118).

Step 11: Monitor the Fetus

Monitor the fetus during epidural placement. Document fetal heart tones after induction of anesthesia but before preparation of the surgical site for incision.

Step 12: Prehydration

Marx et al. (119) first described the use of fluid preloading to prevent hypotension during induction of regional anesthesia. Both crystalloid and colloid have been used, with neither having an advantage.

The intravenous solution should not contain dextrose. Rapid dextrose infusion produces maternal hyperglycemia, hyperinsulinemia, and an increase in blood lactate. Neonatal hyperglycemia and then hypoglycemia follow shortly after delivery (120).

Rout et al. (121) questioned the role of volume in the prevention of hypotension for elective cesarean section. Prehydration with 20 mL/kg of crystalloid decreased the incidence of hypotension by 16%; from 71% to 55%. With aggressive treatment with ephedrine and additional intravenous fluids, there were no differences in neonatal umbilical blood gas values or Apgar scores between infants born of mothers who developed hypotension and those born of mothers who remained normotensive (121).

For urgent cesarean section, I do not delay the surgery for fluid preload. For elective cesarean section, I still give 1,500 to 2,000 mL of crystalloid before injecting local anesthetic.

Step 13: Choose a Local Anesthetic

For elective cesarean section, bupivacaine, ropivacaine, or lidocaine with epinephrine are appropriate choices depending on the desired speed of onset. Give one of these drugs in 5-mL aliquots until a T_4 sensory level is achieved. Bupivacaine and ropivacaine require 30 minutes to achieve a T_4 sensory level. Larger volumes of local anesthetic increase the spread of blockade. Usually 20 to 30 mL of drug will produce an adequate level of sensory block for cesarean section (122).

For urgent cesarean section, I use either lidocaine 1.5% with epinephrine, 1:400,000, and sodium bicarbonate or 3% 2-chloroprocaine. Inject the drug in divided doses over 2 to 3 minutes, while constantly questioning the patient about symptoms of intravascular or intrathecal injection. Always aspirate before each incremental injection. Check the level of sensory block 2 minutes after injecting 20 mL of drug. If the sensory level is not T_4, give additional 5-mL aliquots.

In laboring women receiving a continuous epidural infusion of local anesthetic and opioid, lidocaine 2% or 1.5% with epinephrine produces surgical anesthesia in approximately 4 minutes. 2-Chloroprocaine has a faster onset, approximately 2 to 3 minutes (123,124).

Step 14: Supplemental Oxygen

Giving supplemental oxygen to the mother before delivery will increase umbilical p_aO_2. Umbilical venous and arterial p_aO_2 progressively increase as maternal inspired oxygen concentration is increased from 21% to 100%. Fears that a high maternal p_aO_2 may cause uterine vasoconstriction or affect the fetus are unfounded (125). For elective cesarean section, nasal prongs are better tolerated by the patient. For urgent cesarean section, I use a nonrebreathing mask.

Step 15: Intraoperative Problems

Pain

Intraoperative discomfort frequently complicates epidural anesthesia for cesarean section. The reported percentage of patients experiencing intraoperative pain varies from 10% to 50% (126).

Causes of Intraoperative Pain.

- Breakthrough pain: pain that is perceived despite the presence of bilateral sensory blockade. Epidural local anesthetics do not completely block afferent nerve conduction. High-intensity stimuli may overcome otherwise adequate sensory blockade. Available local anesthetics vary in their ability to produce dense sensory block. Lidocaine requires the addition of epinephrine; 0.5% bupivacaine and ropivacaine are often inadequate as sole agents.
- Pain conducted through unblocked nerves. A T_4 upper sensory level as well as excellent sacral anesthesia is important. However, in some individuals, peritoneal stimulation may require a sensory block up to T_1 (30).

  The presence of blood or amniotic fluid in the subdiaphragmatic region leads to shoulder pain in up to 6% of patients. Because the sensory innervation of the diaphragm is via the phrenic nerve, it cannot be blocked safely. Some recommend placing the operating table in 5 to 10 degrees head-up tilt (reverse Trendelenberg position) to reduce the cephalad spread of blood and amniotic fluid (127).

- Inadequate or uneven sensory blockade. Inadequate block may be due to a misplaced catheter or to an inadequate dose of local anesthetic. Asato and Goto (128) examined unilateral blocks by epidurography. In these cases, the catheter was located either in the anterior epidural space or had exited the epidural space through a foramen. In one case of transforaminal passage, the tip of the catheter was in the paravertebral region. It seems that the common denominator in unilateral epidural block is catheter-tip misplacement. With anterior epidural catheter placement, medial spread of local anesthetic is inhibited by trabeculations between the ventral aspect of the dura and the posterior longitudinal ligament. In the event of unilateral anesthesia, the catheter should be removed and replaced.

  Unblocked segments are much less common than either unilateral block or a block that does not rise high enough. Unrecognized sensory block regression during surgery is another cause of intraoperative pain.

Prevention and Treatment of Intraoperative Pain. Dense sensory blockade extending from the sacral dermatomes to at least T_4 is an important first step to limiting intraoperative pain. Treatment of intraoperative pain depends on the duration and the intensity of pain. Nitrous oxide in oxygen in a ratio of 50%:50% provides effective analgesia of rapid onset and offset (129). Intravenous ketamine, 0.2 to 0.4 mg/kg, and fentanyl, 1 µg/kg, also are effective (130,131). In low doses, neither has any detectable effects in the infant. Epidural fentanyl, 100 µg, improves intraoperative analgesia without affecting maternal respirations or neurobehavior in healthy term infants (132).

First, distinguish between pain and anxiety and determine whether pharmacologic treatment is needed. I usually begin with small amounts of intravenous fentanyl and then add supplemental nitrous oxide if needed. However, if the epidural block is insufficient to provide adequate anesthesia, these maneuvers should not be used to delay the inevitable use of general or spinal anesthesia.

Shivering

Approximately 30% of women shiver during cesarean section under epidural anesthesia (133). Current work suggests that shivering arises as part of the normal thermoregulatory response to cooling. Warming the intravenous fluids infused, epidural fentanyl, and intravenous meperidine or clonidine all reduce the incidence of shivering (134–136).

Nausea and Vomiting

Nausea and vomiting frequently occur during cesarean section under epidural anesthesia. Nausea and vomiting from cerebral hypoperfusion are often the first symptoms of hypotension. Other causes of intraoperative nausea and vomiting include peritoneal manipulation and opioid medications. Preventing hypotension reduces the likelihood of nausea and vomiting. Pretreatment with metoclopramide and droperidol are valuable in the prophylaxis of intraoperative emesis (137,138). Ondansetron, a potent selective serotonergic receptor antagonist, also limits nausea and vomiting (139).

CONDITION OF THE NEWBORN

Epidural anesthesia for cesarean section requires the use of large doses of local anesthetic, which readily cross the placenta and could have significant effects in the newborn. Most studies found that 1-minute Apgar scores are higher in infants born of mothers who received epidural anesthesia compared with those born of mothers who receive general anesthesia (140,141). This difference most likely represents placental transfer of medications required for general anesthesia. Usually by 5 minutes, the difference in Apgar scores disappears. Some authors reported no differences in 1-minute Apgar scores between regional and general anesthesia. All 52 infants in one study scored more than 7 at both 1 and 5 minutes (142).

Obstetricians commonly sample umbilical cord blood at delivery for evaluation of acid–base status. Various workers reported differing results when attempting to correlate Apgar scores with acid–base values (143,144). Most studies showed no significant differences between epidural and general anesthesia for elective cesarean delivery (145,146).

Although maternal drugs may not depress Apgar scores, they can produce subtle changes in newborn behavior. In 1961, Brazelton (147) noted that maternal medication affected newborn behavior after normal delivery. He then devised a method of detecting these changes during the first week of life. This test became known as the Brazelton Neonatal Behavioral Assessment Scale (NBAS). The examination has 49 parameters and is thorough, exhaustive, and time consuming (approximately 45 minutes). Like all neurobehavioral tests, it must be performed by an appropriately trained observer.

Another commonly used test to detect the effects of obstetric medications is the Early Neonatal Neurobehavioral Scale (ENNS, described by Scanlon) (44). The ENNS uses noxious or aversive stimuli and does not provide for any given baby a single number that can immediately identify a depressed or vigorous neonate. The Neurologic and Adaptive Capacity Score (NACS) was developed by Amiel-Tison et al. (148). NACS screens for central nervous system depression caused by drugs and differentiates such effects from those seen after perinatal asphyxia. The NACS assesses 20 criteria in five basic areas: active tone, adaptive capacity, general assessment, passive tone, and primary reflexes. A total NACS of 35 to 40 indicates a neurologically normal neonate. It is currently the most popular test for assessing neonatal neurobehavioral status.

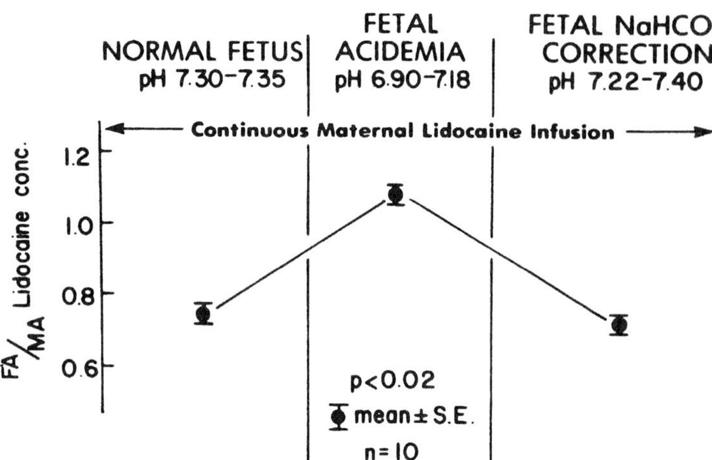

FIG. 9. With acidosis, serum concentrations of lidocaine in the fetus are higher compared with a nonacidotic state with continuous maternal lidocaine infusion. (Reprinted from Biel D, Shnider SM, Levinson G, Callender K. *Anesthesiology* 1978;48:409, with permission.)

Several studies compared neurobehavioral scores in babies delivered by elective cesarean section under epidural or general anesthesia. Most reported better scores for infants delivered under epidural anesthesia, although these differences usually disappear by 24 hours (149). Comparing individual local anesthetics, there are no differences in scores among babies whose mothers received epidural lidocaine, bupivacaine, 2-chloroprocaine, or ropivacaine (150,151).

Urgent cesarean section for fetal asphyxia is a different situation. With fetal asphyxia, fetal acidosis develops as blood is redistributed to vital organs such as the heart and brain, and other areas maintain metabolism by the anaerobic pathway (152). Local anesthetic concentrations may be higher in the acidotic fetus compared with nonacidotic fetus. The uncharged form of local anesthetic readily crosses the placenta, becoming positively charged in the acidotic fetus. As the local anesthetic is now in the charged form, it is unable to recross the placenta and return to the maternal circulation. The ionic form of the local anesthetic has become trapped within the placenta and fetus (Fig. 9) (153). In acidotic fetal lambs, lidocaine and bupivacaine reversed some of the cardiovascular responses to asphyxia (154). In preterm acidotic lambs, lidocaine is associated with progressive deterioration and further decreases in pH, mean arterial pressure, and blood flow to the brain, heart, and adrenals (155). Should lidocaine be avoided in these situations? This question has been studied both retrospectively and prospectively. In the retrospective analysis, there was no difference in newborn outcome if lidocaine was used as the local anesthetic for urgent cesarean section (156). Prospectively, lidocaine concentrations in the distressed fetus were not higher than in the nondistressed fetus (124). Although there is the concern of ion trapping, the rapid delivery of the fetus before significant absorption from the epidural space limits placental transfer. Lidocaine is not contraindicated for urgent cesarean delivery.

CONCLUSION

The popularity of epidural anesthesia for cesarean section has increased with the steadily increasing use of epidural analgesia in labor. A functioning epidural catheter offers the ability to vary the extent, density, and duration of epidural blockade. These advantages often outweigh the slow onset of epidural local anesthetics. With the appropriate choice of local anesthetic and additives, this onset can be shortened. Dense sensory blockade extending from the sacral dermatomes to at least T_4 will help ensure maternal comfort during surgery. Expecting and appropriately managing the physiologic consequences of extensive sensory and sympathetic blockade help ensure safe use of this technique, allowing an awake, comfortable mother and nondepressed infant.

REFERENCES

1. Milne M, Lawson JIM. Epidural analgesia for caesarean section: a review of 182 cases. *Br J Anaesth* 1978;45:1206.
2. Lyons G. Epidural is an outmoded form of regional anaesthesia for elective caesarean section. *Int J Obstet Anesth* 1995;4:34.
3. Chestnut D, Dewan D, Redick L. Anesthetic management for obstetric hysterectomy: a multi-institutional study. *Anesthesiology* 1989;70:607.
4. Lussos SA, Datta S. Anesthesia for caesarean delivery. Part 1: general considerations and spinal anesthesia. *Int J Obstet Anesth* 1992;1:79.
5. Gaiser RR, Antonik L. Successful epidural anesthesia in a patient with an arachnoid cyst, preeclampsia, and triplets. *Reg Anesth* 1996;21:592.
6. O'Kelly SW, Handel JM. Caesarean section for the preeclamptic. *Br J Hosp Med* 1993;49:202.
7. Willdeck-Lund G. General anaesthesia versus epidural block for caesarean section in patients with preeclampsia. *Acta Obstet Gynecol Scand Suppl* 1984;118:117.
8. Carp H, Jayaram A, Vadhera R, et al. Epidural anesthesia for cesarean delivery and vaginal birth after maternal Fontan repair: report of two cases. *Anesth Analg* 1994;78:1190.
9. Brian JE Jr, Seifen AB, Clark RB, et al. Aortic stenosis, cesarean delivery, and epidural anesthesia. *J Clin Anesth* 1993;5:154.
10. Colclough GW. Epidural anesthesia for cesarean delivery in a parturient with aortic stenosis. *Reg Anesth* 1990;15:273.
11. Bader AM, Hunt CO, Datta S, et al. Anesthesia for the obstetric patient with multiple sclerosis. *J Clin Anesth* 1988;1:21.
12. Wulf H. Epidural anaesthesia and spinal hematoma. *Can J Anaesth* 1996;43:1260.
13. Schindler M, Gatt S, Isert P, et al. Thrombocytopenia and platelet

functional defects in preeclampsia: implications for regional anaesthesia. *Anaesth Intens Care* 1990;18:169.

14. Rasmus K, Rottman R, Kotello D, Wright W. Unrecognized thrombocytopenia and regional anesthesia in parturients: a retrospective review. *Obstet Gynecol* 1989;73:943.
15. Wallenburg HCS. Low dose aspirin therapy in obstetrics. *Curr Opin Obstet Gynecol* 1995;7:135.
16. Uzan S, Beaeufils M, Breart G, et al. Prevention of fetal growth retardation with low dose aspirin: findings of the EPREDA trial. *Lancet* 1991;337:1427.
17. Rodgers R, Levin J. A critical reappraisal of bleeding time. *Semin Thromb Hemost* 1990;16:1.
18. Ortikowski CE, Payne AJ, Moodley J, Rocke DA. Thromboelastography after aspirin ingestion in pregnant and nonpregnant subjects. *Br J Anaesth* 1992;69:159.
19. CLASP Collaborative Group. CLASP: a randomized trial of low dose aspirin for the prevention and treatment of preeclampsia among 9364 pregnant women. *Lancet* 1994;353:619.
20. Breen TW, Ransil BJ, Groves PA, Oriol NE. Factors associated with back pain after childbirth. *Anesthesiology* 1994;81:29.
21. Macarthur AJ, Macarthur C, Weeks SK. Is epidural anesthesia in labor associated with chronic low back pain? A prospective cohort study. *Anesth Analg* 1997;85:1066.
22. Bader AM, Gilbertson L, Kirz L, Datta S. Regional anesthesia in women with chorioamnionitis. *Reg Anesth* 1992;17:84.
23. Morgan PJ. Maternal death following epidural anaesthesia for caesarean section delivery in a patient with unsuspected sepsis. *Can J Anaesth* 1995;42:330.
24. Bromage PR. Mechanism of action of extradural local anaesthetics. *Br J Anaesth* 1975;47:199.
25. Liu SS, Ware PD, Ragendran S. Effects of concentration and volume of 2-chloroprocaine on epidural anesthesia in volunteers. *Anesthesiology* 1997;86:1288.
26. Riley ET, Cohen SE, Marcario A, et al. Spinal versus epidural anesthesia for cesarean section: a comparison of time efficiency, costs, charges, and complications. *Anesth Analg* 1995;80:709.
27. Butterworth JR, Strichartz GR. Molecular mechanisms of local anesthesia: a review. *Anesthesiology* 1990;72:711.
28. Braid DP, Scott DB. The systemic absorption of local analgesia drugs. *Br J Anaesth* 165;37:394.
29. Bromage PR. Spread of analgesia solutions in the epidural space and their site of actions: a statistical study. *Br J Anaesth* 1962;34:161.
30. Goertz AW, Seeling W, Heinrich H, Lindner KA, Shirmer U. Influence of high thoracic epidural anesthesia on left ventricular contractility as assessed using end-systolic pressure-length relationship. *Acta Anaesth Scand* 1993;37:38.
31. Yun E, Topulos GP, Body SC, et al. Pulmonary function changes during epidural anesthesia for cesarean delivery. *Anesth Analg* 1996;82:750.
32. Gamil M. Serial peak expiratory flow rates in mothers during caesarean section under extradural anaesthesia. *Br J Anaesth* 1989;62:415.
33. Capogna G, Celleno D. Improving epidural anesthesia during cesarean section: causes of maternal discomfort or pain during surgery. *Int J Obstet Anesth* 1994;3:149.
34. Ramanathan J, Coleman P, Sibaii B. Anesthetic modification of hemodynamic and neuroendocrine stress responses to cesarean delivery in women with severe preeclampsia. *Anesth Analg* 1991;73:772.
35. Haas SB. Effects of epidural anesthesia on the incidence of venous thromboembolism following joint replacement. *Orthopedics* 1994;17(suppl):18.
36. Rosenfeld BA, Beattie C, Christopherson R, et al. The effects of different anesthetic regimens on fibrinolysis and the development of postoperative arterial thrombosis: Perioperative Ischemia Randomized Anesthesia Trial Study Group. *Anesthesiology* 1993;79:435.
37. Ploeckinger B, Ulm MR, Chalubinski K, Gruber W. Epidural anaesthesia in labour: influence of surgical delivery rates, intrapartum fever, and blood loss. *Gynecol Obstet Invest* 1995;39:24.
38. Skjoeldebrand A, Eklund J, Johansson H, et al. Uteroplacental blood flow measured by placental scintigraphy during epidural anaesthesia for caesarean section. *Acta Anaesthesiol Scand* 1990;34:79.
39. Skjoeldebrand A, Eklund J, Lunell NO, et al. The effect on uteroplacental blood flow of epidural anaesthesia containing adrenaline for caesarean section. *Acta Anaesthesiol Scand* 1990;34:85.
40. Giles WB, Lah F, Trudinger BJ. The effect of epidural anaesthesia for caesarean section on maternal uterine and fetal umbilical artery blood flow velocity waveforms. *Br J Obstet Gynaecol* 1987;94:55.
41. Halpern S, Glanc P, Myhr T, et al. Uterine and umbilical blood flow velocity during epidural anaesthesia for cesarean section. *Can J Anaesth* 1994;41:1057.
42. Hollmen AI, Jouppila R, Albright GA, et al. Intervillous blood flow during caesarean section with prophylactic ephedrine and epidural anaesthesia. *Acta Anaesthesiol Scand* 1984;8:396.
43. Marquette GP, Mechas I, Charest J, Rey E. Epidural anaesthesia for elective caesarean section does not influence fetal umbilical artery blood flow indices. *Can J Anaesth* 1994;41:1053.
44. Scanlon JW, Brown WU, Weiss JB, Alper MH. Neurobehavioral responses of newborn infants after maternal epidural anesthesia. *Anesthesiology* 1974;40:121.
45. Arens JF, Carrera AE. Methemoglobin levels following peridural anesthesia with prilocaine for vaginal deliveries. *Anesth Analg* 1970;49:219.
46. Bromage PR, Datta S, Dunford LA. Etidocaine: an evaluation in epidural analgesia for obstetrics. *Can Anaesth Soc J* 1974;21:535.
47. Drasner K. Lidocaine spinal anesthesia: a vanishing therapeutic index? *Anesthesiology* 1997;87:469.
48. Drasner K, Rigler ML, Sessler DI, Stoller AL. Cauda equina syndrome following intended epidural anesthesia. *Anesthesiology* 1992;76:582.
49. Cheng ACK. Intended epidural anesthesia as a possible cause of cauda equina syndrome. *Anesth Analg* 1994;78:157.
50. Moller R, Covino BG. Cardiac electrophysiologic properties of bupivacaine and lidocaine compared with those of ropivacaine, a new amide local anesthetic. *Anesthesiology* 1990;72:322.
51. Santos AC, Pedersen H, Harmon TW, et al. Does pregnancy alter the systemic toxicity of local anesthetics? *Anesthesiology* 1989;70:991.
52. Morishima HO, Pederson H, Finster M, et al. Bupivacaine toxicity in pregnant and nonpregnant ewes. *Anesthesiology* 1985;63:134.
53. Santos AC, Arthur GR, Wlody D, et al. Comparative systemic toxicity of ropivacaine and bupivacaine in nonpregnant and pregnant ewes. *Anesthesiology* 1995;82:734.
54. Reynolds F. Does the left hand know what the right hand is doing? An appraisal of single enantiomer local anesthetics. *Int J Obstet Anesth* 1997;6:257.
55. Reiz S, Haeggmark S, Johansson G, Nath S. Cardiotoxicity of ropivacaine: a new amide local anaesthetic agent. *Acta Anaesthesiol Scand* 1989;33:93.
56. Feldman HS, Arthur GR, Covino BG. Comparative systemic toxicity of convulsant and supraconvulsant doses of intravenous ropivacaine, bupivacaine, and lidocaine in the conscious dog. *Anesth Analg* 1989;69:794.
57. Santos AC, Arthur GR, Pedersen H, et al. Systemic toxicity of ropivacaine during ovine pregnancy. *Anesthesiology* 1991;75:137.
58. Scott DB, Lee A, Fagan D, et al. Acute toxicity of ropivacaine compared with that of bupivacaine. *Anesth Analg* 1989;69:563.
59. Datta S, Camann W, Bader A, Vanderburgh L. Clinical effects and maternal and fetal plasma concentrations of epidural ropivacaine versus bupivacaine for cesarean section. *Anesthesiology* 1995;82:1346.
60. Alahuhta S, Rasmen J, Jouppila P, et al. The effects of epidural ropivacaine and bupivacaine for cesarean section on uteroplacental and fetal circulation. *Anesthesiology* 1995;83:23.
61. Datta S, Corke BC, Alper MH, et al. Epidural anesthesia for cesarean section: a comparison of bupivacaine, chloroprocaine, and etidocaine. *Anesthesiology* 1980;52:48.
62. Kuhnert BR, Kuhnert PM, Philipson EH, et al. The half-life of 2-chloroprocaine. *Anesth Analg* 1986;65:273.
63. Philipson EH, Kuhnert BR, Syracuse CD. Fetal acidosis, 2-chloroprocaine, and epidural anesthesia for cesarean section. *Am J Obstet Gynecol* 1985;151:322.
64. Ravindran RS, Bond VK, Tasch MD, et al. Prolonged neural blockade following regional anesthesia with 2-chloroprocaine. *Anesth Analg* 1980;59:447.
65. Gissen AJ, Datta S, Lambert D. The chloroprocaine controversy. II. Is chloroprocaine neurotoxic? *Reg Anesth* 1984;9:135.
66. Allen RW, Fee JP, Moore J. A preliminary assessment of epidural chloroprocaine for day procedures. *Anaesthesia* 1993;48:773.
67. Eisenach JC, Schlaret TJ, Dobson CE, Hood DH. Effect of prior anesthetic solution on epidural morphine analgesia. *Anesth Analg* 1991;73:119.

68. Camann WR, Hartigan PM, Gilbertson LI, Johnson MD, Datta S. Chloroprocaine antagonism of epidural opioid analgesia: a receptor specific phenomenon? *Anesthesiology* 1990;73:860.
69. Grice SC. Eisenach JC, Dewan DM. Labor analgesia with epidural bupivacaine plus fentanyl: enhancement with epinephrine and inhibition with 2-chloroprocaine. *Anesthesiology* 1990;72:623.
70. Coda B, Bausch S, Haas M, Chaukin C. The hypothesis that antagonism of fentanyl analgesia by 2-chloroprocaine is mediated by direct action on opioid receptor. *Reg Anesth* 1997;22:43.
71. Cohen SE, Thurlow A. Comparison of a chloroprocaine-bupivacaine mixture with chloroprocaine and bupivacaine used individually for obstetric epidural analgesia. *Anesthesiology* 1979;51:288.
72. Corke BC, Carlson CG, Dettbarn WD. The influence of 2-chloroprocaine on the subsequent analgesic potency of bupivacaine. *Anesthesiology* 1984;60:25.
73. Blair MR. Cardiovascular pharmacology of local anesthetics. *Br J Anaesth* 1975;47S:247.
74. Burm AGL, Van Kleck JW, Gladines M, Olthof G, Spierdijk J. Epidural anesthesia with lidocaine and bupivacaine: effects of epinephrine on the plasma concentration profiles. *Anesth Analg* 1986; 65:1281.
75. Brose WG, Cohen SE. Epidural lidocaine for cesarean section: effect of varying epinephrine concentration. *Anesthesiology* 1988;69:436.
76. Moore JK. There is no place for adrenaline in the epidural or subarachnoid space. *Int J Obstet Anesth* 1994;3:54.
77. Partridge BL. The effects of local anesthetics and epinephrine on rat sciatic nerve blood flow. *Anesthesiology* 1989;71:757.
78. Priddle HD, Andros GJ. Primary spinal anesthetic effects of epinephrine. *J Curr Anesth Analg* 1950;29:156.
79. Marx GF, Elstein ID, Schuss M, Anaegbunam A, Fleischer A. Effects of epidural block with lignocaine and lignocaine-adrenaline on umbilical artery velocity wave ratios. *Br J Obstet Gynaecol* 1990;97:517.
80. Hadzic A, Vloka J, Patel N, Birnbach D. Hypertensive crisis after a successful placement of an epidural anesthetic in a hypertensive parturient. *Reg Anesth* 1995;20:156.
81. DiFazio CA, Carron H, Grosslight KR, et al. Comparison of pH-adjusted lidocaine solutions for epidural anesthesia. *Anesth Analg* 1986;65:760.
82. Eisenach J, Detweiler D, Hood D. Hemodynamics and analgesic actions of epidurally administered clonidine. *Anesthesiology* 1993;78:277.
83. Mendez R, Eisenach JC, Kashta K. Epidural clonidine analgesia after cesarean section. *Anesthesiology* 1990;73:848.
84. Huntoon M, Eisenach JC, Boese P. Epidural clonidine after cesarean section: appropriate dose and effect of prior local anesthetic. *Anesthesiology* 1992;76:187.
85. Narchi P, Benhamou D, Hamza J, Bouaziz H. Ventilatory effects of epidural clonidine during the first 3 hours after cesarean section. *Acta Anaesthesiol Scand* 1992;36:791.
86. Paech MJ, Westmore MD, Speirs HM. A double-blind comparison of epidural bupivacaine and bupivacaine-fentanyl for caesarean section. *Anaesth Intens Care* 1990;18:22.
87. Noble DW, Morrison LM, Brockway MS. Adrenaline, fentanyl, or adrenaline and fentanyl as adjuncts to bupivacaine for extradural anaesthesia in elective caesarean section. *Br J Anaesth* 1991;66:645.
88. Preston PG, Rosen MA, Hughes SC, et al. Epidural anesthesia with fentanyl for cesarean section: maternal effects and neonatal outcome. *Anesthesiology* 1988;68:938.
89. Capogna G, Celleno D, Tomassetti M. Maternal analgesia and neonatal effects of epidural sufentanil for cesarean section. *Reg Anesth* 1989;14:282.
90. Maves TJ, Gebhart GF. Antinociceptive synergy between intrathecal morphine and lidocaine during visceral and somatic nociception in the rat. *Anesthesiology* 1992;76:91.
91. Celleno D, Capogna G, Sebastian M. Epidural analgesia during and after cesarean delivery: comparison of five opioids. *Reg Anesth* 1991; 16:79.
92. Palmer C, Petty J, Nogami W, et al. What is the optimal dose of epidural morphine for post-cesarean analgesia? A dose-response study. *Anesthesiology* 1996;85:A909.
93. Heytas L, Cammu H, Cammu F. Extradural analgesia during labour using alfentanil. *Br J Anaesth* 1987;59:331.
94. Chrubas KJ, Wuest H, Schulte-Moentin J, et al. Relative analgesia potency of epidural fentanyl, alfentanil, and morphine in the treatment of postoperative pain. *Anesthesiology* 1988;68:929.
95. Ngan Kee WD, Lam KK, Chen PP, Gin T. Epidural meperidine after cesarean section: a dose-response study. *Anesthesiology* 1996;85:289.
96. Glynn CJ, Mather LE, Cousins MJ, et al. Peridural meperidine in humans: analgesic response, pharmacokinetics, and transmission into CSF. *Anesthesiology* 1981;55:520.
97. Peterfreund RA, Datta S, Ostheimer GW. pH Adjustment of local anesthetic solutions with sodium bicarbonate: laboratory evaluation of alkalinization and precipitation. *Reg Anesth* 1989;14:265.
98. Ackerman WE III, Ware TR, Junega M. The air-liquid interface and the pH and pCO_2 of alkalinized local anesthetic solutions. *Can J Anaesth* 1992;39:387.
99. Wong K, Strichartz GR, Raymond SA. On the mechanisms of potentiation of local anesthetics by bicarbonate buffer: drug structure-activity studies on isolated peripheral nerve. *Anesth Analg* 1993;76:131.
100. Ackerman WE, Denson DD, Junega MM, et al. Alkalinization of chloroprocaine for epidural anesthesia: effects of pCO_2 at constant pH. *Reg Anesth* 1990;15:89.
101. Wylie WD, Churchill-Davidson HC. *A practice of anaesthesia,* 3rd ed. Chicago: Year Book Medical Publishers, 1972.
102. Dripps RD, Eckenhoff JE, Van Damm LD. *Introduction to anesthesia: the principles of safe practice,* 3rd ed. Philadelphia: WB Saunders, 1961.
103. Craft JB, Roizen MF, Dao SD, et al. A comparison of T4 and T7 dermatomal levels of analgesia for caesarean section using the lumbar epidural technique. *Can Anaesth Soc J* 1982;29:264.
104. Ness TJ, Gebhart G. Visceral pain: a review of experimental studies. *Pain* 1990;41:167.
105. Bonica JJ. Autonomic innervation of the viscera in relation to nerve block. *Anesthesiology* 1968;29:793.
106. Chantigian RC, Datta S, Burger GA, Naulty JS, Lambert DH, Ostheimer GW. Anesthesia for cesarean delivery utilizing spinal anesthesia: tetracaine vs. tetracaine and procaine. *Reg Anesth* 1984;9:195.
107. Russell IF. Levels of anaesthesia and intraoperative pain at caesarean section under regional block. *Int J Obstet Anesth* 1995;4:71.
108. Hodgkinson R, Glassenberg R, Joyce TH III, et al. Comparison of cimetidine (Tagamet) with antacid for safety and effectiveness in reducing gastric acidity before elective cesarean section. *Anesthesiology* 1983;59:86.
109. Lussos SA, Bader AM, Thornhill ML, Datta S. The antiemetic efficacy and safety of prophylactic metoclopramide for elective cesarean delivery during spinal anesthesia. *Reg Anesth* 1992;17:126.
110. Vincent RD, Chestnut DH. Which position is more comfortable for the parturient during identification of the epidural space. *Int J Obstet Anesth* 1991;1:9.
111. Saberski LR, Kondamuri S, Osinubi OYO. Identification of the epidural space: is loss of resistance to air a safe technique? A review of the complications related to the use of air. *Reg Anesth* 1997;22:3.
112. Messih H. Epidural space pressures during pregnancy. *Anaesthesia* 1981;36:775.
113. Beilin Y, Bernstein HH, Zucker-Pinchoff B. The optimal distance that a multiorifice epidural catheter should be threaded into the epidural space. *Anesth Analg* 1995;81:301.
114. D'Angelo R, Berkebile B, Gerancher J. Prospective examination of epidural catheter insertion. *Anesthesiology* 1996;84:88.
115. Hamilton CL, Riley ET, Cohen SE. Changes in the position of epidural catheters associated with patient movement. *Anesthesiology* 1997;86:778.
116. Norris MC, Fogel ST, Dalman H, et al. Labor analgesia without an intravascular "test dose." *Anesthesiology* 1998;88:1495.
117. Moore DC, Batra MS. The components of an effective test dose prior to epidural block. *Anesthesiology* 1981;55:693.
118. Baheti DK. Epidural analgesia with left lateral tilt for caesarean section. *Anaesthesia* 1975;30:396.
119. Marx GF, Cosmi EV, Wollman SB. Biochemical status and clinical condition of mother and infant at cesarean section. *Anesth Analg* 1969;48:986.
120. Philipson EH, Kalhan SC, Riha MM, Pimentel R. Effects of maternal glucose infusion on fetal acid-base status in human pregnancy. *Am J Obstet Gynecol* 1987;157:866.
121. Rout CC, Rocke DA, Levin J. A reevaluation of the role of crystalloid preload in the prevention of hypotension associated with spinal anesthesia for elective cesarean section. *Anesthesiology* 1993;79:262.
122. Thorburn J, Moir DD. Epidural analgesia for elective caesarean section: technique and its assessment. *Anaesthesia* 1980;35:3.

123. Price ML, Reynolds F, Morgan BM. Extending epidural blockade for emergency caesarean section: evaluation of 2% lignocaine with adrenaline. *Int J Obstet Anesth* 1991;1:13.
124. Gaiser RR, Cheek TG, Adams HK, Gutsche BB. Epidural lidocaine for the cesarean delivery of the distressed fetus. *Int J Obstet Anesth* 1998;7:27.
125. Ramanathan S, Gandhi S, Arismendy J, et al. Oxygen transfer from mother to fetus during cesarean section under epidural anesthesia. *Anesth Analg* 1982;61:576.
126. Crawford JS, Davies P, Lewis M. Some aspects of epidural block provided for elective caesarean section. *Anaesthesia* 1976;41:1039.
127. Capogna G, Celleno M. Improving epidural anesthesia during cesarean section: causes of maternal discomfort or pain during surgery. *Int J Obstet Anesth* 1994;3:149.
128. Asato F, Goto F. Radiographic findings of unilateral epidural block. *Anesth Analg* 1996;83:519.
129. Piggott SE, Bogod DG, Rosen M, et al. Isoflurane with either 100% oxygen or 50% nitrous oxide in oxygen for caesarean section. *Br J Anaesth* 1990;65:325.
130. Downing JW, Mahomedy MC, Teal DE, Allen PJ. Anaesthesia for caesarean section with ketamine. *Anaesthesia* 1976;31:883.
131. Rayburn WF, Smith CV, Parriott JE, Woods RE. Randomized comparison of meperidine and fentanyl during labor. *Obstet Gynecol* 1989; 74:604.
132. Gaffus MP, Bansal P, Lawton C, et al. Surgical analgesia for cesarean delivery with epidural bupivacaine and fentanyl. *Anesthesiology* 1986; 65:331.
133. Sessler DI, Ponte J. Shivering during epidural anesthesia. *Anesthesiology* 1990;72:816.
134. Johnson MD, Sevarino FB, Lema MJ. Cessation of shivering and hypothermia associated with epidural sufentanil. *Anesth Analg* 1989; 68:70.
135. Workhoven MN. Intravenous fluid temperature, shivering, and the parturient. *Anesth Analg* 1986;65:496.
136. Capogna G, Celleno D. IV clonidine for post-extradural shivering in parturients: a preliminary study. *Br J Anaesth* 1993;71:294.
137. Chestnut DH, Vandewalker GE, Owne CL, et al. Administration of metoclopramide for prevention of nausea and vomiting during epidural anesthesia for elective cesarean section. *Anesthesiology* 1987; 66:563.
138. Pan PH, Moore CH. Intraoperative antiemetic efficacy of prophylactic ondansetron versus droperidol for cesarean section patients under epidural anesthesia. *Anesth Analg* 1996;83:982.
139. McKenzie R, Kovac A, O Connor T, et al. Comparison of ondansetron versus placebo to prevent postoperative nausea and vomiting in women undergoing ambulatory gynecologic surgery. *Anesthesiology* 1993; 78:21.
140. Marx GF, Luykz WM, Cohen S. Fetal-neonatal status following caesarean section for fetal distress. *Br J Anaesth* 1984;56:1009.
141. Evans CM, Murphy JF, Gray OP, Rosen M. Epidural versus general anaesthesia for elective caesarean section: effect on Apgar score and acid-base status of the newborn. *Anaesthesia* 1989;44:778.
142. Abboud TK, Nagappala S, Murakawa K, et al. Comparison of the effects of general and regional anesthesia for cesarean section on neonatal neurologic and adaptive capacity scores. *Anesth Analg* 1985; 64:996.
143. Crawford JS, Davies P, Pearson JE. Significance of the individual components of the Apgar score. *Br J Anaesth* 1973;45:148.
144. Marx GF, Mahajan S, Miclat MN. Correlation of biochemical data with Apgar scores at birth and at one minute. *Br J Anaesth* 1977; 49:831.
145. Palahniuk RJ, Scatliff J, Biehl D, et al. Maternal and neonatal effects of methoxyflurane, nitrous oxide and lumbar epidural anaesthesia for caesarean section. *Can Anaesth Soc J* 1977;24:586.
146. James FM, Crawford JS, Hopkinson R, Davies P, Naiem H. A comparison of general anesthesia and lumbar epidural analgesia for elective cesarean section. *Anesth Analg* 1977;56:228.
147. Brazelton TB. Psychophysiologic reactions in the neonate. II. Effect of maternal medication on the neonate and his behavior. *J Pediatr* 1961;58:513.
148. Amiel-Tison C, Barrier G, Shnider SM, et al. A new neurologic and adaptive capacity scoring system for evaluating obstetric medications in full-term newborns. *Anesthesiology* 1982;56:340.
149. Hodgkinson R, Bhatt M, Kim SS, Grewal G, Marx GF. Neonatal neurobehavioral tests following cesarean section under general and spinal anesthesia. *Am J Obstet Gynecol* 1978;132:670.
150. Abboud TK, Kyung CK, Noueihed R, et al. Epidural bupivacaine, chloroprocaine or lidocaine for cesarean section-maternal and neonatal effects. *Anesth Analg* 1983;62:914.
151. Stienstra R, Jonker TA, Bourdrez P, et al. Ropivacaine 0.25% versus bupivacaine 0.25% for continuous epidural analgesia in labor: a double-blind comparison. *Anesth Analg* 1995;80:285.
152. Jones MD, Sheldon RE, Petter LL, et al. Fetal cerebral oxygen consumption at different levels of oxygenation. *J Appl Physiol* 1977; 43:1080.
153. Morishima HO, Santos AC, Pedersen H, et al. Effect of lidocaine on the asphyxial responses in the mature fetal lamb. *Anesthesiology* 1987;66:502.
154. Santos AC, Yun EM, Bobby PD, Noble G, Arthur GR, Finster M. The effects of bupivacaine, L-nitro-arginine-methyl ester and phenylephrine on cardiovascular adaptations to asphyxia in the preterm fetal lamb. *Anesth Analg* 1997;85:1299.
155. Morishima HO, Pedersen H, Santos AC, et al. Adverse effects of maternally administered lidocaine on the asphyxiated preterm fetal lamb. *Anesthesiology* 1989;71:110.
156. Gaiser RR, Cheek TG, Gutsche BB. Epidural lidocaine vs 2-chloroprocaine for fetal distress requiring urgent cesarean section. *Int J Obstet Anesth* 1994;3:208.

Obstetric Anesthesia, second edition,
edited by Mark C. Norris.
Lippincott Williams & Wilkins, Philadelphia © 1999.

CHAPTER 22

Spinal Anesthesia for Cesarean Delivery

Mark C. Norris

"Cesarean section in an awake patient is undoubtedly a major test of regional anesthesia. The operation may be lengthy, profound blockade of many nerves is required, strong visceral stimulation is present, sudden cardiovascular changes are compounded by posture, and fetal well-being may be influenced by several physiologic variables and drugs" (1). Spinal anesthesia is perhaps the most elegant approach to this challenge. With one small needle, and an almost homeopathic amount of drug, the anesthesiologist can readily provide profound anesthesia and excellent operating conditions for major intra-abdominal surgery.

Spinal anesthesia has seen intermittent use in obstetrics since 1900 (2). In the past, a high incidence of hypotension and the risk of headache were serious limitations (3). By the early 1980s, experts often recommended epidural rather than spinal blockade for cesarean section. Currently, spinal anesthesia is regaining popularity (4). Although hypotension is still common, routine use of left uterine displacement and ephedrine have limited its severity and neonatal impact. The advent of pencil-point spinal needles has greatly reduced the risk of postdural puncture headache (see Chapter 39) (5). In some centers, spinal anesthesia also has proven more cost effective than epidural block (6). As a result, many anesthesiologists prefer spinal anesthesia for cesarean delivery (Fig. 1).

This chapter reviews the use of spinal blockade for cesarean delivery. It examines the maternal and fetal hemodynamic effects of spinal anesthesia. It discusses ways to minimize the incidence and impact of maternal hypotension. There follows a discussion of some technical issues including drug selection and dosage. Last, the chapter briefly considers combined spinal epidural anesthesia for cesarean section and the use of spinal anesthesia in patients having a preexisting, but inadequate, epidural block.

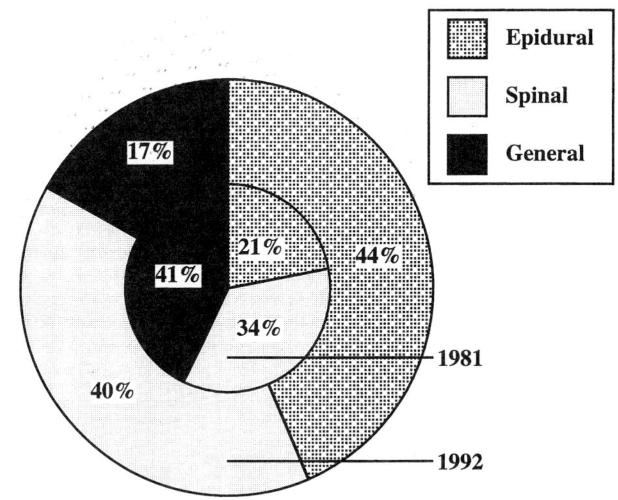

FIG. 1. Anesthesia for cesarean section, 1981 vs 1992. (Data from ref. 4, with permission.)

ADVANTAGES/DISADVANTAGES

Advantages

Spinal anesthesia has several advantages over epidural blockade for cesarean section. The technique is safe, simple, and quick. In contrast, epidural anesthesia is a technically complex, potentially dangerous, and time-consuming procedure. Epidural anesthesia places the patient at risk of dural puncture with a large-gauge needle. It involves the injection of potentially lethal doses of local anesthetic. The safe induction of epidural anesthesia requires time. Drugs are injected in small boluses at 2- to 3-minute intervals. Onset of surgical anesthesia can take more than 30 minutes (7). In contrast, spinal anesthesia produces extensive, profound blockade with a single injection of only 5% to 10% of the amount of drug required for epidural blockade. Maternal systemic absorption produces blood drug concentrations of about

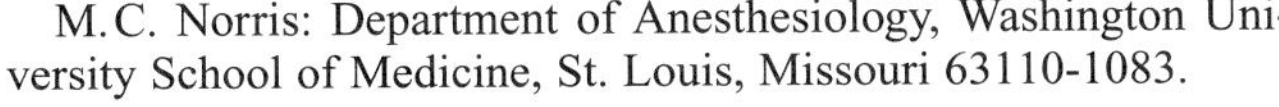
M.C. Norris: Department of Anesthesiology, Washington University School of Medicine, St. Louis, Missouri 63110-1083.

5% of those developing with epidural blockade. The fetus is exposed to only minute amounts of drug (8). Once you have located the subarachnoid space and injected an appropriate amount of local anesthetic, you are virtually assured of good, dense, bilateral sensory blockade. [In one series, the failure rate of spinal anesthesia for cesarean section was only 2.8% (9). At Barnes–Jewish Hospital, in 1997, all of the 170 spinal anesthetics performed for cesarean section produced adequate block for skin incision and delivery.] Surgery can begin within 5 to 10 minutes of drug injection (6,10). Spinal anesthesia's inherent efficiency can save both time and money (Fig. 2) (6).

Spinal anesthesia usually produces better operating conditions than does epidural block. One study compared 150 women having cesarean section by using 10 to 17.5 mg hyperbaric bupivacaine with 70 women receiving 0.5% bupivacaine or 2% lidocaine with 1:200,000 epinephrine. Of patients in the spinal group, 87% versus 67% in the epidural group were pain free (11).

Patients prefer spinal anesthesia. In one survey, patients undergoing elective cesarean section under spinal anesthesia reported less discomfort than those receiving epidural block. Eighty percent of women having had both epidural and spinal anesthesia preferred the spinal anesthetic (12).

Disadvantages

Although spinal anesthesia is a safe, reliable anesthetic technique, it does have risks and limitations. Sensory blockade occasionally ascends into the cervical region. These high levels of block can impair maternal respiration. Fortunately, diaphragmatic function usually remains intact, and only minor changes in respiratory function develop (13). Only rarely do sensory and motor block extend high enough to warrant endotracheal intubation.

Spinal headache is inseparable from this anesthetic technique. The recent introduction of small-gauge, pencil-point spinal needles has markedly decreased this risk (5).

Maternal hypotension frequently follows subarachnoid injection of local anesthetics. Profound, prolonged hypotension can harm both mother and infant. Fortunately, both the severity and the consequences of maternal hypotension can be limited. Prehydration, careful attention to left uterine displacement, and the judicious use of ephedrine can minimize this problem.

Finally, a single subarachnoid injection provides only a finite period of anesthesia. Sometimes surgery outlasts the anesthetic. With careful selection of drug and dosage, we can reliably provide up to 2 hours of good operating conditions. Combined spinal epidural anesthesia is an alternative for possibly prolonged procedures.

Neonatal Outcome

For the infant, the quality of the maternal anesthetic usually matters more than the specific technique. There are, however, some reported differences in early neonatal status among anesthetics. Most studies reported that babies born under general anesthesia have lower 1-minute Apgar scores and are more likely to require assisted ventilation at birth than are those delivered with regional anesthesia (14–17). Studies of umbilical acid–base values report either no differences between anesthetic techniques or a higher incidence of acidemia in infants born with regional versus general anesthesia (14,16–19). Infants born with maternal general anesthesia also often score lower on neurobehavioral examination (18,20). Some of these differences persist for the first 2 days of life (20). In one study, infants born of mothers receiving spinal anesthesia had better neurobehavioral scores than did those whose mothers received epidural block (18). A recent study comparing spinal anesthesia with isoflurane-

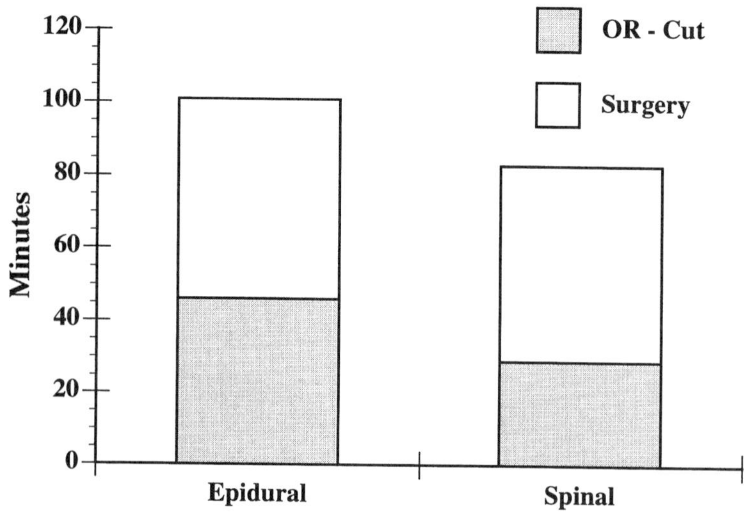

FIG. 2. Operating room times associated with spinal and epidural anesthesia for cesarean delivery. Ninety-four patients had either spinal (n = 47) or epidural (n = 47) anesthesia for cesarean delivery. All blocks were done in the operating room. Hyperbaric 0.75% bupivacaine was used for spinal anesthesia; 2% lidocaine with epinephrine (n = 43) or 0.5% bupivacaine (n = 1) was used for epidural block. Three patients in the epidural group eventually received a spinal anesthetic because of a failed epidural (n = 2) or accidental dural puncture (n = 1). *OR cut time,* time from entering OR until surgical incision; *surgery time,* time for surgical incision until leaving OR; OR cut time was significantly shorter in patients receiving spinal anesthesia. (Reprinted from ref. 6, with permission.)

or sevoflurane-supplemented general anesthesia reported no difference in neurobehavioral scores among the groups. Infants in all groups scored higher at 24 hours than at 2 hours after birth (16).

Fetal catecholamine secretion plays an important role in the adaptation to extrauterine life. Infants born by cesarean section have lower plasma catecholamine concentrations than do infants delivered vaginally. However, infants whose mothers receive regional anesthesia for cesarean section have higher plasma catecholamine concentrations than do infants whose mothers receive general anesthesia (21).

Maternal hypotension may have an impact on neonatal outcome (see the following). Significant maternal hypotension may risk both umbilical acidosis and depressed neurobehavioral scores. Infants whose mothers experienced 4 to 8 minutes of hypotension during the induction of epidural anesthesia for cesarean section had abnormal neurobehavioral tests for 2 days (22). Still, with good maternal hydration and careful blood pressure (BP) monitoring, brief episodes of maternal hypotension do not adversely affect neurobehavioral scores (23).

INDICATIONS/CONTRAINDICATIONS

There are few absolute contraindications to spinal anesthesia. Some of these include:

- Maternal refusal,
- Uncorrected hypovolemia,
- Coagulopathy, and
- Infection at the site of needle puncture.

Many also hesitate to induce spinal anesthesia in a variety of other situations (Table 1).

The most significant of these "relative contraindications" to spinal anesthesia is its use in the presence of a nonreassuring fetal heart rate (FHR) tracing. Although some argue for the rapid induction of general anesthesia in this setting, spinal anesthesia is often a safe alternative and may have significant advantages. General anesthesia offers speed, but induction and intubation impair uterine blood flow (24). In gravid ewes, uterine vascular resistance increases and fetal condition deteriorates during barbiturate–nitrous oxide anesthesia (25). In contrast, in laboring women, spinal anesthesia for cesarean section decreases plasma norepinephrine concentrations (26). This effect may improve uterine artery blood flow and fetal oxygen supply. Induction of general anesthesia also compromises maternal airway reflexes. If the patient proves difficult to intubate, both maternal and fetal hypoxemia may follow.

Maternal hypotension brought on by spinal blockade can worsen fetal condition. In laboring women, however, this complication is unlikely. One group of investigators reported a 50% incidence of hypotension during induction of spinal blockade in nonlaboring women. In contrast, none of their laboring patients (n = 14) experienced a significant decrease in blood pressure (26).

Marx et al. (14) examined neonatal outcome in 126 parturients undergoing emergency cesarean section with regional or general anesthesia. All women were carrying acutely distressed fetuses (persistent, severe, late FHR decelerations, scalp pH less than 7.20 or decreasing steadily) (Table 2). In all cases, surgery began within 20 minutes of the last scalp pH. The women selected either general or regional anesthesia. Those choosing general anesthesia received either ketamine or thiopental followed by 40% nitrous oxide in oxygen. Fifty-five parturients picked regional anesthesia. In the 22 with indwelling epidural catheters, sensory block was extended with 3% 2-chloroprocaine. Thirty-three women received a tetracaine spinal anesthetic. All spinal injections were done by the most senior person available, using a 22-gauge needle. All women in the regional group received at least 800 mL of crystalloid during induction of anesthesia and oxygen, 6 L/min, until delivery. In the regional group, blood pressure did not decrease below 100 mm Hg. Infants in both groups had similar umbilical blood gas values. Infants in the regional group had better 1-minute Apgar scores (Table 3). The authors suggested that the beneficial effects of regional anesthesia on maternal catecholamine secretion and uterine blood flow explained their results.

TABLE 1. *Contraindications to spinal anesthesia for cesarean section*

Absolute contraindications
Maternal refusal
Uncorrected hypovolemia
Clinically apparent coagulopathy
Infection at the site of needle insertion
Relative contraindications
Potential hypovolemia (Placenta previa/accreta)
Laboratory coagulopathy
Systemic infection
Neurological disease
Back pain
Nonreassuring fetal heart-rate tracing
Severe preeclampsia

TABLE 2. *Indications for delivery in 168 parturients for emergency cesarean section*

Etiology	General anesthesia (n = 71) (%)	Regional anesthesia (n = 55) (%)
Late decelerations	26	29
Variable decelerations	9	12
Persistent bradycardia	34	31
Persistent tachycardia	7	8
Acidosis	14	8
Thick meconium, first stage of labor	10	12

From ref. 14, with permission.

TABLE 3. *Outcome: induction to delivery intervals, fetal and neonatal data in 126 cases of cesarean section for fetal distress with either general or regional anesthesia*

Parameter	General anesthesia (n = 71)	Regional anesthesia (n = 55)
Scalp pH	7.204 ± 0.053	7.198 ± 0.043
Induction to skin incision	67.0 ± 12.0 s	5.3 ± 0.5 min
Skin incision to delivery	7.0 ± 2.8 min	7.8 ± 2.9 min
Uterine incision to delivery	68.3 ± 42.7 s	74.0 ± 40.3 s
UVpH	7.286 ± 0.050	7.282 ± 0.054
UApH	7.221 ± 0.057	7.220 ± 0.053
Apgar score >7 (%)		
1 min	51	78*
5 min	85	98

UV, umbilical vein; UA, umbilical artery.
*p <0.05 vs general anesthesia.
From ref. 14, with permission.

PHYSIOLOGIC EFFECTS OF SPINAL ANESTHESIA

Spinal anesthesia for cesarean section induces extensive sensory, motor, and sympathetic neural blockade. This action has significant effects on maternal central nervous system, cardiovascular, and respiratory physiology.

Central Nervous System

Although intrathecal injection of local anesthetic blocks both efferent and afferent nerve conduction, the site and degree of this effect remain unclear. Spinal anesthesia produces efferent blockade of both motor and sympathetic impulses. Motor weakness is common with even small doses of intrathecal local anesthetics. Sometimes, however, even dense abdominal surgical anesthesia may not completely block motor function in the lower extremities (27).

Spinal anesthesia produces significant blockade of efferent sympathetic impulses. Small, thinly myelinated, preganglionic sympathetic nerve fibers are more susceptible to local anesthetic blockade than are larger, more heavily myelinated sensory fibers. So, in the cephalad regions of blockade, low concentrations of local anesthetic may block sympathetic but not sensory impulses. The exact extent of this "zone of differential blockade" is uncertain. In humans, estimation of efferent sympathetic nervous system activity is difficult (28). Differing methods yield different results. Blockade of the ability to perceive cold extends two to three segments above the level of sensory blockade (29,30). Thermographic measurements of changes in skin temperature suggest that it extends even higher, six or more segments above the level of sensory block (31).

Other methods suggest that spinal anesthesia produces incomplete sympathetic blockade. Sweat glands are regulated by the sympathetic nervous system. Their activity can be assessed by measuring changes in skin conductance (32). These studies suggest that sympathetic nerve activity persists below the level of sensory block (33). The hemodynamic and catecholamine responses to a cold pressor test (plunging a hand in a bucket of ice-cold water for 2 minutes) also can serve as an index of sympathetic nervous system function. Upper thoracic sensory block does not change the heart-rate response to the cold pressor test and blunts, but does not eliminate, the blood pressure and cardiac index changes (28,34). Plasma epinephrine and norepinephrine concentrations increase in some, but not all patients (28,34). Incomplete blockade of the sympathetic nervous system also could explain the occurrence of tourniquet and visceral pain despite the presence of adequate levels of sensory block (35,36).

Most important, spinal anesthesia produces afferent sensory blockade. As with the sympathetic nervous system, somatosensory activity may persist despite the presence of surgical anesthesia. Intrathecal bupivacaine prolongs the latency and decreases the amplitude of, but does not eliminate, somatosensory evoked potentials elicited below the level of block (37). Direct spinal cord stimulation can be perceived in the presence of profound peripheral anesthesia (38). Unlike epidural anesthesia, spinal block inhibits central temporal summation of repeated noxious stimuli (39). These results suggest that the primary site of spinal anesthesia–induced conduction blockade lies within the dorsal root ganglia and spinal rootlets, not in the spinal cord itself (38,40).

Cardiovascular System

Spinal anesthesia profoundly alters maternal hemodynamics. Hypotension, the most clinically significant hemodynamic effect of spinal anesthesia, can occur rapidly. If untreated, hypotension can be severe and harm both mother and infant (Fig. 3) (41).

Incidence and Severity

The incidence of maternal hypotension varies with definition, frequency of measurement, method of measurement (manual vs automatic cuff), and prophylactic therapy (if any). Significant hypotension complicates 50% to 60% of spinal anesthetics in nonlaboring parturients (42). Hypotension develops less often in laboring women (26,43). In supine parturients, not receiving intravenous

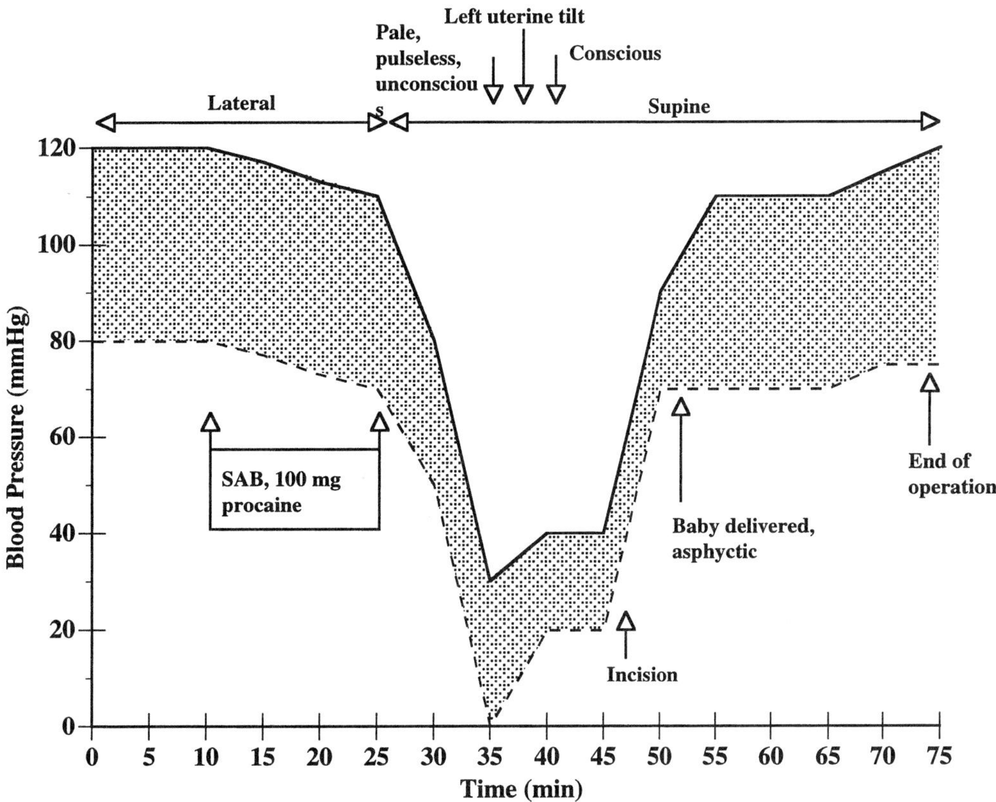

FIG. 3. Hemodynamic effect of subarachnoid block in supine patient. Marked hypotension caused loss of consciousness. Patient regained consciousness with left uterine tilt. Blood pressure did not recover fully until delivery. Note infant born markedly depressed. (Redrawn from ref. 41, with permission.)

fluids, maternal blood pressure decreases by an average of 44% after subarachnoid injection of local anesthetics (Fig. 4) (44).

Etiology

Maternal hypotension develops in proportion to the extent of sympathetic blockade, which increases venous capacitance, decreases arteriolar tone, and decreases cardiac output (Fig. 5) (45). Mesenteric venodilation from sympathetic blockade of the splanchnic circulation is the most important cause of this increased venous capacitance, which in turn decreases central venous pressure (CVP) and left ventricular end diastolic volume (Fig. 6) (46). After CVP decreases, cardiac output, stroke volume, and therefore, blood pressure decrease (Fig. 7) (47–49). All these effects are more pronounced if the mother lies supine without left uterine displacement (Figs. 3 and 7).

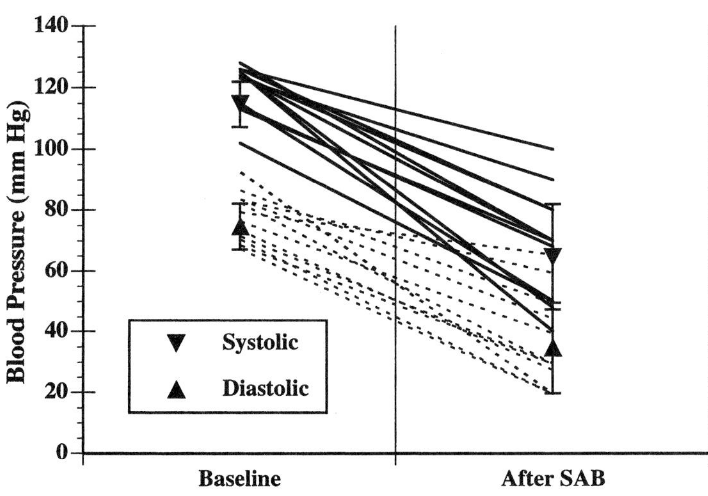

FIG. 4. Change in blood pressure in 12 healthy term parturients after subarachnoid injection of 0.2% procaine. All women lay supine, and none received intravenous fluids. Systolic pressure decreased by 44 ± 14%, whereas diastolic pressure decreased by 54 ± 18%. (Data from ref. 44, with permission.)

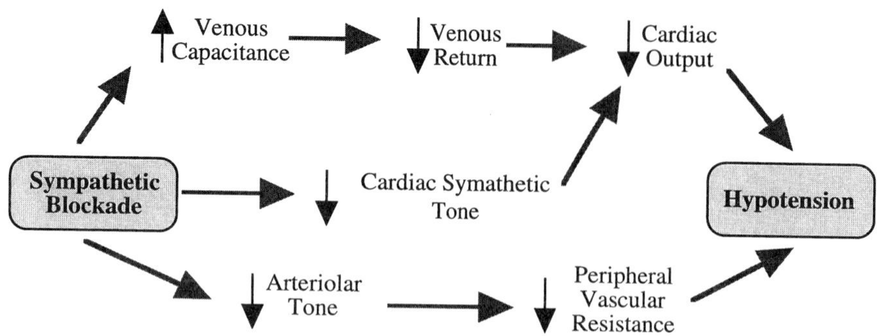

FIG. 5. Mechanism of hypotension during spinal anesthesia.

Both decreased venous return and blockade of sympathetic fibers to the heart (T_1 to T_4) contribute to the decline in cardiac output. Although the exact contribution of cardiac sympathectomy to hypotension during spinal anesthesia is unclear, significant hypotension is more common in patients with sensory blockade above T_5 and hence significant blockade of cardiac sympathetic nerves (50). Clinically, some degree of cardioaccelerator fiber blockade develops whenever the level of sensory block extends above T_6 to T_8. In this setting, compensatory tachycardia does not accompany decreases in blood pressure (30,48). More commonly, heart rate decreases as blood pressure decreases (51,52).

Fetal Effects of Spinal Anesthesia

Uterine/Placental Blood Flow

Spinal anesthesia also may alter uterine and placental blood flow. Although these parameters cannot be directly measured in humans, they can be indirectly evaluated by using radioactive tracers or ultrasound.

Investigators in Sweden examined intravillous blood flow (IVBF) during spinal anesthesia by using xenon 133. Their patients received 1.5 to 2.0 L of crystalloid before spinal anesthesia, and investigators treated "incipient" hypotension with an ephedrine infusion. In only one of nine patients did blood pressure decrease more than 30 mm Hg. IVBF did not change significantly in seven of their parturients. In one woman with preeclampsia, IVBF increased by 193%. In another, with diabetes, it decreased 72%. The investigators found no correlation between the change in IVBF and the change in maternal blood pressure. They suggested that, in their well-hydrated parturients, the increased maternal blood volume compensated for small changes in blood pressure (53).

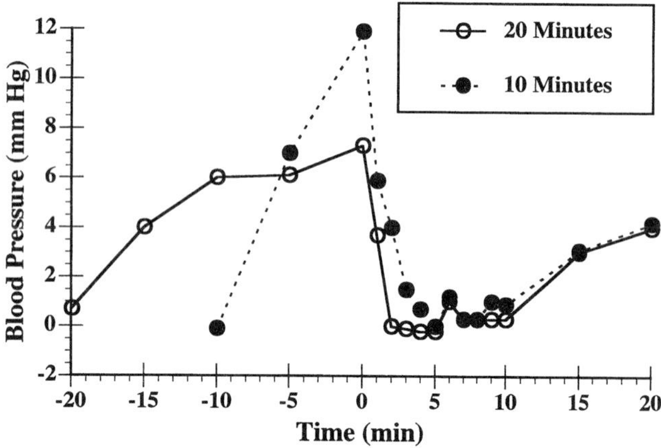

FIG. 6. Change in central venous pressure during 20 mL/kg crystalloid preload over 10 or 20 minutes and spinal anesthesia for elective cesarean delivery. (Redrawn from ref. 78, with permission.)

The same group has examined the effects of spinal anesthesia on uterine artery pulsatility index (increases in pulsatility index reflect vasoconstriction). These patients received 1.0 L lactated Ringer's solution before block. Despite a high incidence of maternal hypotension (62%), there were no consistent changes in pulsatility index. In some patients, there were transient increases in pulsatility index after block. These changes did not correlate with any hemodynamic event and had no impact on Apgar scores or umbilical artery pH (54).

Fetal Blood Flow

The maternal hemodynamic response to subarachnoid anesthesia could indirectly affect fetal blood flow. By using ultrasound and pulsed Doppler measurements, Lindblad et al. (55) measured vessel diameter and blood-flow velocity in the descending fetal aorta and umbilical artery and vein. They made these measurements before and then 15 and 30 minutes after induction of spinal anesthesia in 15 term parturients. All women received 2.0 L of crystalloid before blockade. In addition, an ephedrine infusion maintained blood pressure. Maternal spinal anesthesia produced no changes in fetal aortic or umbilical blood flows. The rising slope, a measure of myocardial contractility, also did not change. At 30 minutes, a moderate decrease in umbilical pulsatility index developed. The pulsatility index reflects peripheral, and here, possibly placental resistance. These results suggest that slight placental vasodilation develops after maternal spinal anesthesia. Because this change occurred late (30 minutes after induction), these authors postulated that it reflected an effect of the ephedrine. Another study looking at umbilical artery flow velocity wave forms reported no significant changes 15 minutes after spinal blockade (56).

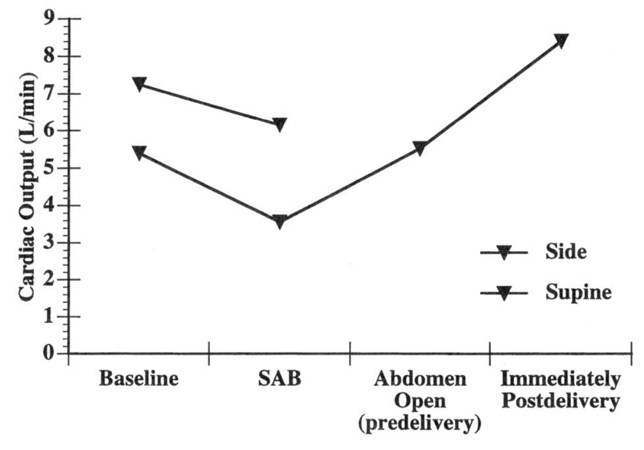

A

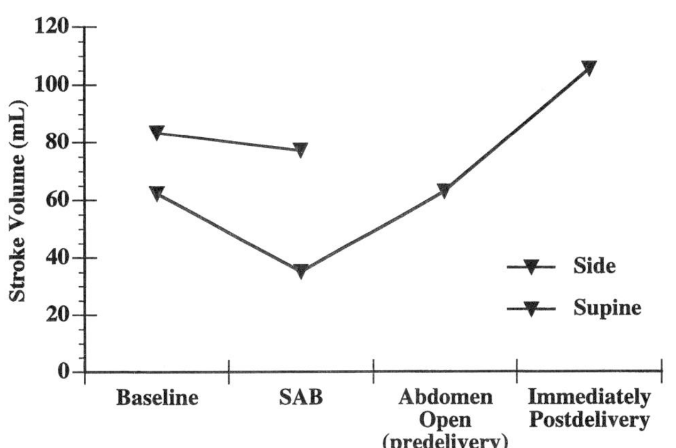

B

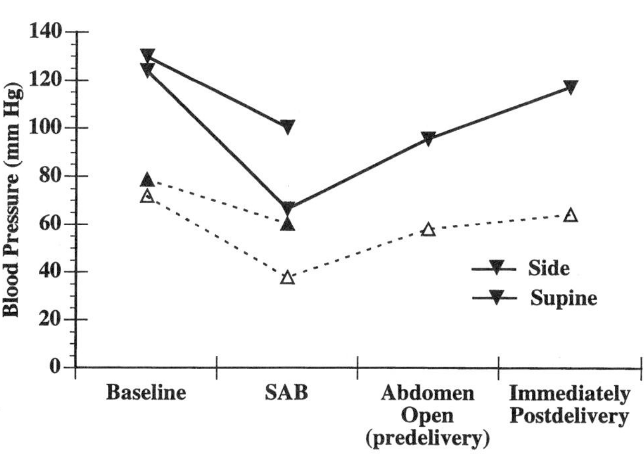

C

FIG. 7. Hemodynamic effects of spinal anesthesia in the term parturient. **A:** Cardiac output after spinal blockade in 12 patients undergoing cesarean section. Relieving aortocaval compression, by turning the patient to her side, or with delivery, significantly ameliorates the effects of spinal anesthesia. Note that cardiac output is significantly lower in the supine position even before induction of spinal anesthesia. **B:** Stroke volume after spinal blockade in 12 women at cesarean section. Relieving aortocaval compression, by turning the patient to her side, or with delivery, significantly eases the effects of spinal anesthesia. Note that stroke volume is significantly lower in the supine position even before induction of spinal anesthesia. **C:** Blood pressure (solid line, systolic; dashed line, diastolic) decreases precipitously after spinal blockade when term parturients remain supine. Relieving aortocaval compression by turning the patient to her side or by delivering the infant significantly alters the hemodynamic response to spinal anesthesia. (Redrawn from ref. 48, with permission.)

Fetal/Neonatal Effects of Maternal Hypotension

The effect of maternal hypotension on the fetus/neonate varies with its severity and duration. Maternal position, volume status, and drug therapy also may alter the consequences of hypotension.

Severe, prolonged hypotension can harm the fetus. In a small series, Ebner (3) reported fetal bradycardia only when maternal systolic pressure decreased below 50 mm Hg for more than 12 minutes. A follow-up study further investigated the relation between maternal hypotension and fetal bradycardia. Twenty-nine women were positioned supine after receiving a spinal anesthetic for elective cesarean section. The investigators monitored maternal blood pressure and fetal electrocardiogram for 15 minutes after induction of blockade. No fetal bradycardia occurred in the 13 women whose systolic blood pressure remained above 70 mm Hg. Among those whose systolic blood pressure decreased below 70 mm Hg, the severity and the duration of maternal hypotension correlated with the incidence of fetal bradycardia (Table 4) (57). Thus severe, prolonged maternal hypotension can cause significant fetal bradycardia.

The fetal effects of transient maternal hypotension are less clear. Marx et al. (58) reported that maternal hypotension (systolic blood pressure less than 96 mm Hg, duration undefined) was associated with a prolonged time to sustained respiration. Infants of nonhypotensive mothers developed sustained respirations in 20.0 seconds. Babies born of hypotensive mothers did not breathe consistently until 48.8 seconds after delivery. Babies in the hypotensive group also had statistically insignificantly lower umbilical artery pH values.

TABLE 4. *Relation between the severity and duration of maternal hypotension after induction of spinal anesthesia and the incidence of fetal bradycardia*

Minimal maternal systolic BP after spinal anesthesia (mm Hg)	No. of patients	Incidence of fetal bradycardia (%)
>100	9	0
90–99	1	0
80–89	0	0
70–79	3	0
60–69	5	20
50–59	8	38
<50	3	67
Duration of maternal systolic BP <80 mm Hg (min)		
0–1.9	8	0
2–3.9	8	0
4–5.9	3	33
>6	9	44

From ref. 57, with permission.

This study is difficult to evaluate. Women who became hypotensive were a mixed group who received several different "prophylactic" measures or no prophylaxis at all. The authors did not report the duration of hypotension. All women in this study received dextrose-containing fluids. [Maternal dextrose infusion decreases umbilical artery pH (59) and worsens the fetal response to hypotension (60).] Patients received only a single bolus of ephedrine. It is unclear that "time to sustained respiration" is a meaningful measure of neonatal condition.

Datta and Brown (61) reported a study of 15 healthy term parturients. All received 1 L of dextrose-containing crystalloid before induction of anesthesia. All were placed supine with left uterine displacement and received oxygen by face mask. These investigators defined hypotension as a systolic blood pressure less than 100 mm Hg or a decrease of more than 30 mm Hg from baseline. If hypotension developed, they treated it promptly with ephedrine until the systolic blood pressure was at least 100 mm Hg. Hypotension occurred in eight of the 15 women. In all cases, hypotension lasted less than 3 minutes. This transient hypotension was associated with a slightly lower umbilical artery pH (7.26 vs 7.30) (61). A follow-up study using a similar protocol produced comparable results. "Babies born to mothers with hypotension were significantly more acidotic than controls although acid–base levels were still within normal limits." Neurobehavioral studies were normal in both groups (62). Again, however, the use of dextrose-containing fluids may have influenced these results.

Other investigators found no correlation between transient maternal hypotension and neonatal acidosis. In one study, parturients received 1 L of crystalloid before induction. Those who experienced hypotension (systolic blood pressure less than 100 mm Hg) received 10-mg increments of ephedrine. These authors found no difference between infants of hypotensive and normotensive mothers in uterine artery or uterine vein pH values (63). Other studies reported similar results (54,64–66). In one such study, women were prehydrated with 1.5 to 2.0 L of non–dextrose-containing crystalloid. Neither mild (blood pressure less than 100 mm Hg) nor moderate (blood pressure less than 90 mm Hg) hypotension increased the frequency or severity of neonatal acidosis (Fig. 8) (65).

Thus although severe maternal hypotension may have significant fetal implications, transient decreases in maternal blood pressure are well tolerated. Infants of diabetic mothers may be more sensitive to the maternal hemodynamic effects of spinal anesthesia (61,67).

Factors Influencing the Severity of Maternal Hypotension

The magnitude of the maternal hemodynamic response to spinal anesthesia depends on both patient and anesthetic factors. Labor and left uterine displacement probably have the most significant effects on the incidence of hypotension. Anesthesiologists used a variety of strategies to lower the incidence and impact of maternal hypo-

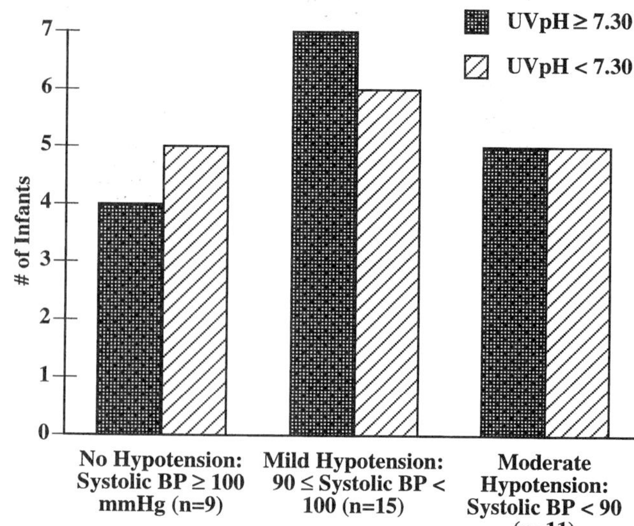

FIG. 8. Number of infants with umbilical vein pH (UVpH) greater and less than 7.30 after no, mild, or moderate maternal hypotension. (Redrawn from ref. 65, with permission.)

tension (42). Some investigators tried giving large amounts of fluid. Others tried to minimize the size of the maternal circulation with leg-compression devices. Vasopressors also are widely used.

Risk

The severity of maternal hypotension varies widely. Little is known about the variables that influence an individual patient's risk of significant hypotension, but some differences have been observed between women who do or do not develop hypotension with regional block. Parturients with initial systolic blood pressures more than 140 mm Hg or those with increased systemic vascular resistance are more likely to develop hypotension (20% decrease in systolic blood pressure) (68). [This observation is interesting because other studies suggested no increase, or even a decrease, in the risk of hypotension among women with preeclampsia (44,69).] Women who are more sensitive to the supine position (as shown by heart-rate increases or leg flexion) also are more likely to develop severe hypotension (blood pressure less than 70% of baseline) (70). Thus intrinsic differences in cardiovascular responsiveness among patients may play a role in determining an individual's risk of significant hypotension during spinal anesthesia.

Labor

Clark et al. (43) noted that laboring patients were less inclined to develop hypotension than were nonlaboring women (43). Other groups of investigators confirmed this observation (26,71). There are several possible explanations for this phenomenon. Laboring women usually receive intravenous fluids while hospitalized. Thus these patients may simply be better hydrated than are those seen for elective cesarean delivery (71).

The protective effect of labor is most marked in conjunction with left uterine displacement (Fig. 9) (43). Descent of the fetal head into the pelvis lessens aortocaval compression. This development may improve the subsequent efficacy of left uterine displacement. In addition, left uterine displacement allows the blood (300 mL) squeezed from the uterus with each contraction to reach the maternal central circulation and help support blood pressure.

Patient Positioning

Uterine Displacement. The hemodynamic effects of spinal anesthesia in the parturient are greatly aggravated by aortocaval compression. Maintaining adequate left uterine displacement is probably the single most important step in minimizing the maternal and fetal impact of spinal anesthesia–induced hypotension. Although no one has prospectively evaluated the effect of left uterine displacement on the frequency and severity of maternal hypotension, this point seems well established. Early reports emphasized the role of aortocaval compression in producing profound hypotension after induction of spinal anesthesia for cesarean section (Fig. 9) (41,72). Left uterine displacement has long been recommended as an initial treatment of maternal hypotension (43,47,72). Subsequent studies consistently reported better neonatal outcome (higher umbilical artery pH and Apgar scores) when the uterus is displaced after induction of anesthesia (73,74).

Head-Down Tilt. Trendelenberg positioning is a traditional treatment for spinal anesthesia–induced hypotension. However, studies in both pregnant and nonpregnant patients showed that 10 to 15 degrees of head-down tilt has little or no effect on the blood pressure response to spinal anesthesia (75,76).

Volume

Crystalloid. Many investigators studied maternal prehydration and the genesis of hypotension. Wollman and Marx (47) evaluated the maternal safety and efficacy of a rapidly infused fluid bolus in 19 laboring and nonlaboring term parturients. All had CVP catheters inserted before the induction of spinal anesthesia. Fourteen of the women received an infusion of 1 L of 5% dextrose in Ringer's lactate (D_5RL) (plus an intramuscular injection of 0.4 mg atropine) before induction of anesthesia. Hydration caused a slight increase in CVP but eliminated hypotension after induction of spinal anesthesia. After delivery, CVP was the same whether or not the women received the fluid bolus (47). These authors concluded that prehydration effectively prevented hypotension during spinal anesthesia for cesarean section. Unfortunately, most subsequent studies suggested that prehydration has only limited ability to prevent maternal hypotension.

In a study of 247 parturients, the combination of left uterine displacement plus fluid prehydration decreased the frequency of hypotension from 92% to 53% (43). In another study, more than half the women receiving 1.5 to 2.0 L of crystalloid before induction of spinal anesthesia, and up to 3.3 L by delivery, experienced transient hypotension (65). Rapid redistribution of crystalloid out of the intravascular space may limit the efficacy of prehydration (Fig. 10) (77). However, Rout et al. (78) found that infusion of 20 mL/kg crystalloid over 10 minutes instead of 20 minutes both failed to decrease the frequency and severity of spinal anesthesia–induced hypotension and markedly increased CVP in some patients (Fig. 6) (78). In another study, 16 (59%) of 27 parturients developed severe hypotension (systolic blood pressure less than 70% of baseline) despite infusion of 2 L crystalloid within 5 minutes of induction of spinal anesthesia (70). Thus despite its ubiquitous use, most studies reported a significant incidence of maternal hypotension after crystalloid prehydration.

Recently several groups of investigators systematically reevaluated the efficacy of prehydration in preventing maternal hypotension during spinal anesthesia for

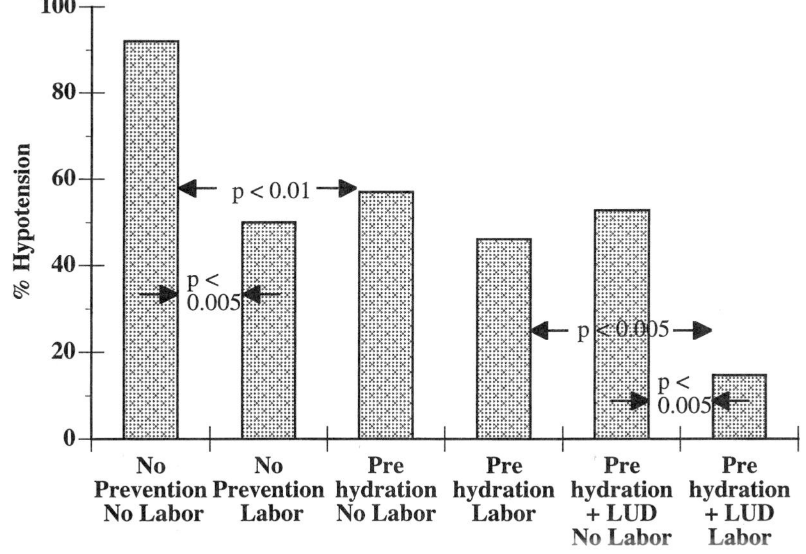

FIG. 9. Incidence of hypotension in laboring and nonlaboring women receiving spinal anesthesia for cesarean section. Women had either no preventive measures, prehydration with 1 L D_5RL, or prehydration plus left uterine displacement (LUD). (Redrawn from ref. 43, with permission.)

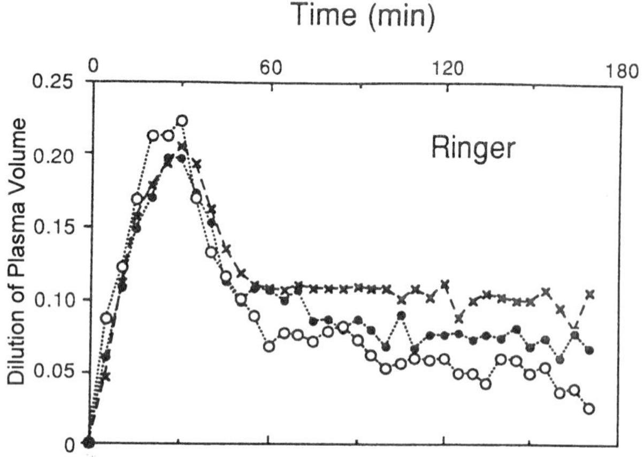

FIG. 10. The blood hemoglobin (solid circle), blood water (open circle), and serum albumin (cross) concentrations as makers of plasma volume dilution during and after intravenous infusion of 25 mL/kg Ringer solution over 30 minutes in eight male volunteers. (Reprinted from ref. 77, with permission.)

cesarean section (Table 5). Rout et al. (79) studied 144 women seen for elective repeated cesarean section. Patients received either no prehydration or 20 mL/kg crystalloid within 20 minutes of induction. Prehydration decreased the incidence of hypotension from 71% to 44%. Park et al. (80) compared 10, 20, and 30 mL/kg prehydration. Although increasing the volume of infused fluid tended to decrease the frequency of hypotension (Table 5), this difference did not achieve statistical significance. These results led some to abandon routine prehydration before spinal anesthesia (81).

Volume loading not only increases maternal CVP but also increases release of atrial natriuretic peptide (ANP; Fig. 11) (82). Vasodilation and diuresis mediated by ANP may help explain the limited ability of prehydration to maintain maternal blood pressure during spinal anesthesia for cesarean section.

Whereas prehydration does not prevent maternal hypotension, it may blunt the fetal repercussions of the maternal hemodynamic response to spinal anesthesia. In one study, increasing the volume of prehydration did not alter incidence or severity of hypotension but did decrease the incidence of umbilical acidemia (uterine vein pH less than 7.20; Table 6) (83). These investigators allocated 64 term parturients to one of two groups. One group received 500 to 999 mL of crystalloid (D_5RL) before the induction of spinal anesthesia. The other group received 1,000 to 1,500 mL. Maternal hypotension, defined as a systolic pressure less than 80% of baseline, occurred with equal frequency in both groups. In the less-hydrated group, the lower the maternal pressure, the lower the uterine vein pH and the greater the umbilical vein base deficit. In contrast, maternal hypotension did not correlate with umbilical acid–base status in the better-hydrated group. In the less-hydrated group, 20% of the neonates were acidotic. Only 8% of the babies in the better-hydrated group were acidotic (Table 6). Severe hypotension (systolic blood pressure less than 70 mm Hg) also developed with equal frequency in both groups, but its gravity and duration were less in the better-hydrated group. In addition, less neonatal acidemia followed severe hypotension in the better-hydrated group (Table 7). These authors concluded that although prehydration may not prevent postspinal hypotension, it does limit the fetal biochemical consequences (83). The use of dextrose-containing fluids complicates the interpretation of these data (see earlier), but they do suggest caution before we conclude that routine prehydration has no benefit. No one has yet examined the effects of varying volumes of dextrose-free prehydration on acid–base status only in infants whose mothers develop hypotension.

Colloid. As with crystalloids, colloid infusion appears to decrease but not to eliminate maternal hypotension during spinal anesthesia for cesarean section. One study comparing equal volumes of 5% albumin and D_5RL reported no hypotension in the albumin group (n = 24) versus a 25% incidence of hypotension in the crystalloid group (systolic blood pressure less than 100 mm Hg) (84). Another study compared prehydration with 500 mL of 6% hetastarch plus 1,000 mL lactated Ringer's to prehydration with 2,000 mL lactated Ringer's (85). Again, the frequency and severity of hypotension were less in the colloid group (45% vs 85%).

Leg Compression

Several groups investigated leg compression as a way to reduce the incidence of maternal hypotension during spinal anesthesia (86–90). Most commonly, these investigators suggested that leg compression can prevent venous pooling in the lower extremities and thereby limit the incidence of hypotension. However, control of venous capacitance lies not in the leg veins, but mostly in the mesenteric venous system (46,91). Instead, leg compression may limit

TABLE 5. *Prehydration and maternal hypotension*

	Volume of prehydration					
Study	None	10 mL/kg	1.0 L	20 mL/kg	30 mL/kg	1.5–2.0 L
Clark et al. (43)[a]	25/27 (92%)		28/53 (53%)			
Rout et al. (79)	44/62 (71%)			43/78 (55%)		
Norris MC (65)						24/35 (69%)
Park et al. (80)		12/18 (67%)		10/18 (56%)	9/19 (47%)	

[a]Prehydration with D_5RL, "None" group positioned supine.

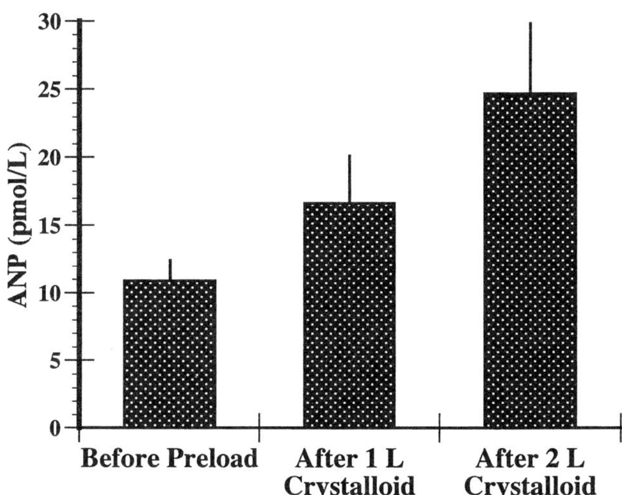

FIG. 11. Atrial natriuretic peptide *(ANP)* response to crystalloid infusion before and during spinal anesthesia for cesarean section. Parturients received 1000 mL crystalloid before and an additional 1000 mL after induction of anesthesia. Values expressed as mean ± SEM. (Reprinted from ref. 82, with permission.)

hypotension by increasing peripheral resistance through compression of postcapillary vessels (91). Consistent with this theory is the finding that leg compression is effective only when relatively high pressures (more than 40 mm Hg) are applied by using either inflatable splints (87) or Esmarch bandages (89,90), not thromboembolic stockings, which produce a maximal pressure of 18 mm Hg (88).

Vasopressors

Ephedrine is the vasopressor of choice in obstetrics. It has been used both to treat and to prevent maternal

TABLE 6. *Effects of volume of crystalloid prehydration on maternal blood pressure and neonatal acid–base status*

Volume of prehydration	500–999 mL (n = 40)	1,000–1,500 mL (n = 24)
Maximal decrease		
Systolic BP (mm Hg)	25 ± 16	28 ± 11
Diastolic BP (mm Hg)	11 ± 10	16 ± 13
Σ (mm Hg)	79 ± 54	70 ± 38
Maximal decrease systolic BP (% of cases)		
>20 mm Hg	69	74
>30 mm Hg	18	29
% requiring vasopressor	62	71
Dose of vasopressor (mg)	12 ± 12	12 ± 10
UVpH	7.32 ± 0.06	7.32 ± 0.03
UApH	7.24 ± 0.05	7.25 ± 0.04
% with umbilical acidemia	20	8[a]

Values expressed as mean ± SD.
S, summed decrease in BP.
[a]$p < 0.05$ vs 500–999 mL.
Modified from ref. 83, with permission.

TABLE 7. *Maternal blood pressure and neonatal acid–base status in cases of severe hypotension (systolic BP <70 mm Hg) after spinal anesthesia: increased fluid prehydration limits the duration and impact of severe maternal hypotension*

Volume of prehydration	500–999 mL (n = 7)	1,000–1,500 mL (n = 7)
Maximum decrease in systolic BP (mm Hg)	49 ± 10	43 ± 5
Σ (mm Hg)	164 ± 53	91 ± 22[a]
Dose of vasopressor (mg)	21 ± 7	13 ± 3[a]
UV		
pH	7.28 ± 0.07	7.31 ± 0.04
Base deficit (mEq/L)	10.5 ± 2.6	6.4 ± 1.5[a]
UA		
pH	7.19 ± 0.08	7.25 ± 0.04
Base deficit (mEq/L)	11.5 ± 2.6	8.0 ± 2.6[a]

Values expressed as mean ± SD.
S, summed decrease BP.
[a]$p < 0.05$ vs 500–999 mL.
Modified from ref. 83, with permission.

hypotension. Several studies have tried to find the optimal timing and route of ephedrine administration.

Prophylactic intramuscular ephedrine does not reliably prevent maternal hypotension. Moya and Smith (92) reviewed their clinical experience with prophylactic ephedrine. Their patients received an intramuscular injection of ephedrine, 50 mg, about 10 minutes before induction of spinal anesthesia. Nonetheless, 46% had a greater than 20% decrease in blood pressure (92). Other investigators confirmed that prophylactic intramuscular injection of ephedrine fails to prevent hypotension reliably during spinal or epidural anesthesia and occasionally induces maternal hypertension (Fig. 12) (64,71,84).

Other investigators reported better success with prophylactic intravenous ephedrine. Datta et al. (93) recommended giving 10 to 30 mg of intravenous ephedrine "as soon as any fall from base line pressure" occurs. This technique "virtually eliminates hypotension." These authors compared this prophylactic ephedrine therapy with giving therapeutic ephedrine only after blood pressure decreased by more than 30 mm Hg or to less than 100 mm Hg. Women in the prophylactic group experienced less nausea and vomiting. Neonates in the prophylactic group had significantly better Apgar scores and acid–base parameters than those in the therapeutic group (93). Unfortunately, methodologic problems make it difficult to interpret these results and apply them to current practice. The groups were studied in sequence, not as a part of a randomized, blinded protocol. Other concurrent changes in clinical practice may have occurred to induce the observed differences. The prophylactic group included patients whose blood pressure decreased slightly, but who would not have become significantly hypotensive. The therapeutic group, in contrast, consisted only of women who actually developed hypotension. In addition, the infants in this study seemed especially sensitive to maternal hypotension. In the thera-

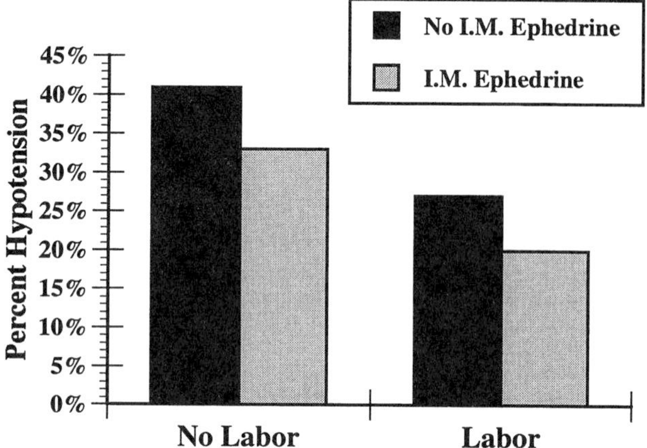

FIG. 12. Prophylactic intramuscular (i.m.) ephedrine does not significantly decrease the incidence of hypotension in laboring and nonlaboring women receiving epidural anesthesia for cesarean section. (Data from ref. 71, with permission.)

peutic group, 83% of the neonates had 1-minute Apgar scores below seven. Part of this may problem may lie in the author's use of dextrose-containing fluid for prehydration. [Maternal dextrose infusion reduces umbilical artery pH (59) and worsens the fetal response to hypotension (60).] Other studies reported no effect of transient maternal hypotension on 1-minute Apgar scores (64–66). Although prophylactic ephedrine seems to limit maternal side effects, the need to use it to ensure a good neonatal outcome remains unclear.

Ephedrine infusions may be more effective than intermittent bolus injections. Kang et al. (66) mixed 50 mg ephedrine with 500 mL of crystalloid. They infused this solution at 50 mL/min for the first 2 minutes after induction of spinal blockade. Then they adjusted the infusion rate to maintain maternal blood pressure above 100 mm Hg. When blood pressure stabilized, they stopped the infusion. A control group of women received 20-mg boluses of ephedrine if their blood pressure decreased below 80% of baseline. Maternal hypotension, nausea, and vomiting occurred less often in the infusion group. Neonates in both groups had good Apgar scores and acid–base values (66). In another study, a fixed-rate ephedrine infusion (0.4 mg/kg/h) limited but did not prevent maternal hypotension (52).

Ephedrine, although effective and seemingly safe, does cross the placenta. It causes fetal tachycardia. It increases fetal catecholamine concentrations and transiently increases neonatal electroencephalogram (EEG) delta wave activity (94).

Summary

- Spinal anesthesia has profound effects on the maternal cardiovascular system.
- Expect significant hypotension.
- Limit the severity and consequences of hypotension by assuring adequate left uterine displacement, infusing dextrose-free intravenous fluids, and using intravenous ephedrine to treat significant decreases in maternal BP.

Respiratory Function

Motor block accompanying the high level of sensory blockade produced by spinal anesthesia for cesarean section significantly alters maternal pulmonary function. Levels of sensory blockade above T_6 produce little change in forced vital capacity but significantly decrease expiratory flow rate (forced expiratory volume in 1 s and peak expiratory flow rate) (95,96). Expiratory flow rates decrease even further with surgery and delivery of the infant (95,96). Epidural anesthesia for cesarean section has similar effects on maternal respiratory function (97,98). The magnitude of these changes is comparable to the effects of surgery itself. Pulmonary function remains depressed into the postoperative period (Fig. 13). Fortunately, spinal anesthesia alone does not impair maternal oxygenation or ventilation (96); however, the interaction between anesthesia, surgery, and maternal respiratory disease may significantly impair the ability of some women to cough and mobilize their airway secretions (97).

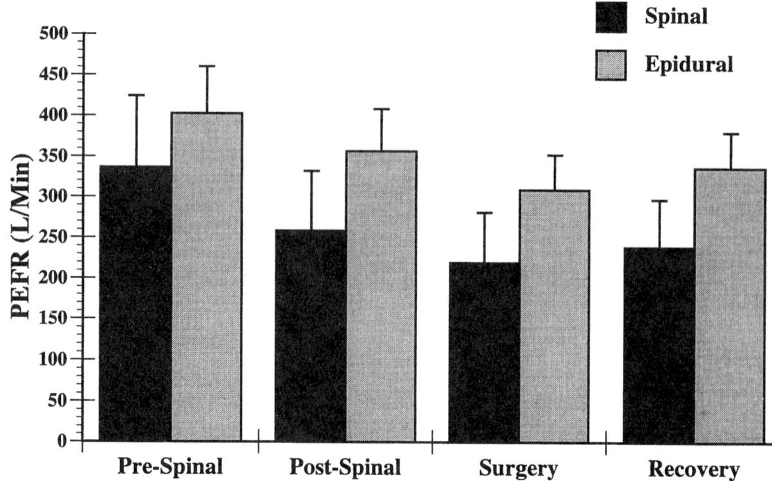

FIG. 13. Changes in peak expiratory flow rate after spinal or epidural anesthesia for cesarean section. All patients had sensory block to at least T_6. (Data from refs. 95 and 97, with permission.)

Conclusions

Spinal anesthesia can present significant threats to maternal and fetal well-being. Extensive sensory blockade, headache, and hypotension are common risks. The chapters on intraoperative and postoperative complications discuss high block and postdural puncture headache. Hydration, left uterine displacement, and ephedrine can limit the incidence and repercussions of hypotension. By understanding the potential hemodynamic consequences of subarachnoid blockade in parturients and by careful attention to preventive and therapeutic measures, the obstetric anesthesiologist can safely use this reliable technique.

SOME TECHNICAL ISSUES

This section discusses, in detail, how to provide spinal anesthesia for cesarean section. It focuses primarily on four issues: the choice of crystalloid solution for prehydration; the level of sensory blockade required; and the selection and dose of drug. Questions addressed in this section include:

- Which drug?
- How much drug?
- What adjuvant drugs might improve the quality of sensory blockade?

Finally, we briefly consider what position the patient should assume during induction of blockade.

Patient Preparation

Venous Access

Patients seen for cesarean section should have a well-functioning, large-bore (at least 18-gauge) intravenous catheter in place. Remember, cesarean section is a major intra-abdominal operation with the potential for significant and rapid blood loss. Women undergoing even routine, elective cesarean delivery lose on average 1,000 mL of blood.

Aspiration Prophylaxis

These women should receive some type of acid aspiration prophylaxis. I give them 30 mL of sodium citrate by mouth on the way to the operating suite.

Prehydration

Attitudes toward prehydration have changed significantly in the past few years (see earlier). I no longer infuse large volumes of crystalloid within a few minutes of induction. Instead, I infuse fluids under gravity during transport to the operating room and while preparing to induce anesthesia. The choice of crystalloid to be infused can have significant impact on neonatal outcome.

Acute maternal infusion of as little as 10 g glucose causes significant maternal and consequently fetal hyperglycemia. The fetus secretes insulin in response to this hyperglycemia. After delivery, with insulin, but not glucose, still present, fetal hypoglycemia can occur (Fig. 14) (59,99). Some authors expressed concern that maternal hypoglycemia might develop if the fasted parturient receives no glucose (60). However, maternal fasting glucose concentrations usually range from 60 to 100 mg/dL (mean ± SD, 80.5 ± 13.1 mg/dL) (100). I rarely give glucose to healthy parturients during cesarean section.

Even without sugar, the choice of crystalloid solution can still affect neonatal outcome. Sodium chloride, although free of glucose, contains a large amount of unbuffered chloride ion. Acute infusion of large volumes of 0.9% NaCl induces a maternal hyperchloremic metabolic acidosis and increases the risk of neonatal acidosis (100). Other available crystalloid solutions contain lactate and acetate as buffers (lactated Ringer's, Plasmalyte®). Theoretically these compounds could upset maternal and fetal carbohydrate metabolism, increasing the risk of neonatal hypoglycemia, but a clinical comparison of Plasmalyte and 0.9% sodium chloride as fluid therapy before and during cesarean section found no differences in maternal or neonatal glucose concentrations (100).

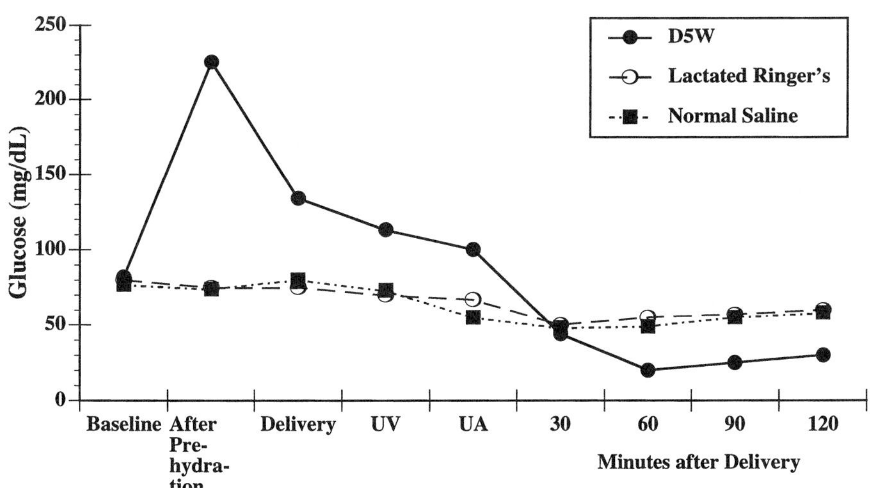

FIG. 14. Changes in blood glucose concentration in mother and infant after intravenous fluid administration. (Redrawn from ref. 99, with permission.)

How High a Level?

A level of sensory blockade above T_{10} will block the somatic sensations of cesarean section. Eliminating visceral pain from peritoneal stimulation and uterine manipulation requires more extensive anesthesia. Whereas patients will often tolerate the procedure with a T_6 to T_8 level of sensory blockade, they will more likely need supplemental systemic analgesics than will those patients who have a higher level of block (101). The level of anesthesia (loss of ability to perceive touch) may be more important than the level of analgesia (loss of sharpness to pinprick). In parturients, analgesia extends up to nine segments higher than does anesthesia (11,102). Only when the level of anesthesia is above T_5 will women be reliably pain free during cesarean section (11).

I strive for a level of sensory blockade between T_4 and T_1. I prefer having the block spread a little too high to not high enough. Occasionally, the level of sensory blockade creeps up into the cervical dermatomes. I then place an extra pillow under the woman's head in an attempt to limit further cephalad spread. I also assess motor function by checking hand-grip strength and respiratory function by asking her to speak and breathe deeply. If the block extends so high that the patient cannot phonate or maintain her O_2 saturation above 95%, I apply cricoid pressure and secure the airway to protect against possible aspiration. Fortunately, this complication occurs only rarely (fewer than 1 per 100 spinal anesthetics).

Drugs

Which Drug?

Bupivacaine, lidocaine, and tetracaine are currently the most commonly used intrathecal local anesthetics. Of these choices, I believe that bupivacaine is most appropriate for spinal anesthesia for cesarean section.

Tetracaine often fails to provide good maternal sensory blockade. Twenty-five percent to 80% of parturients will require supplemental intravenous analgesia (103,104). In addition, tetracaine's motor blockade persists long after the sensory block has regressed (103,104). Substituting 10% procaine for dextrose when using tetracaine for spinal anesthesia will improve the quality of sensory blockade. However, tetracaine plus procaine produces a higher level of sensory blockade than does tetracaine alone, and the problem of persistent motor block remains (104).

Hyperbaric lidocaine also is widely used for spinal anesthesia for cesarean section. However, this drug also has significant limitations. One published study of hyperbaric lidocaine (65 to 75 mg) for spinal anesthesia for cesarean section noted rapid but unpredictable sensory anesthesia (105). Four of 15 women who received 65 mg lidocaine in the lateral position complained of dysphagia and had sensory block to the C_2 dermatome. Another group reported good success with lidocaine, 80 mg, for operations lasting 32 to 70 minutes (mean, 49 minutes). Patients often had significant pain on arrival in the recovery room (106). Lidocaine's duration (less than 60 minutes) limits its usefulness for many cesarean sections. Recent reports of transient neurological symptoms after lidocaine spinal anesthesia in nonpregnant patients have led many anesthesiologists (myself included) to abandon its use (107,108).

Currently hyperbaric bupivacaine is probably the most widely used local anesthetic for spinal anesthesia for cesarean section (109). This popularity exists because bupivacaine overcomes many of the limitations of tetracaine and lidocaine. Bupivacaine produces better sensory block with less motor blockade than does tetracaine (103). In parturients, 10 mg hyperbaric tetracaine and 12.5 mg hyperbaric bupivacaine produced similar levels of sensory blockade, yet women receiving bupivacaine had significantly better intraoperative analgesia and faster regression of sensory and motor block (Table 8) (103).

Hyperbaric bupivacaine also provides better surgical anesthesia than tetracaine in some groups of nonpregnant patients. Early experience with the drug found that the

TABLE 8. *Onset, duration, and quality of blockade at cesarean section*

	Tetracaine (n = 20)	Bupivacaine (n = 20)
Onset	8.95 ± 4.74	6.65 ± 2.83[a]
Duration of blockade		
Sensory	180 ± 80	117 ± 38[a]
Motor	372 ± 140	201 ± 64[a]
Category of intraoperative analgesia		
A (painless)	11	20[a]
B (discomfort, no analgesia)	4	0
C (discomfort/pain, analgesia required)	3	0
D (general anesthesia after surgery begun)	1	0
E (general anesthesia before surgery)	1	0

Parturients received either 10 mg hyperbaric tetracaine or 12.5 mg hyperbaric bupivacaine. All values expressed as mean (min) ± SD.

[a] $p < 0.01$.

From ref. 103, with permission.

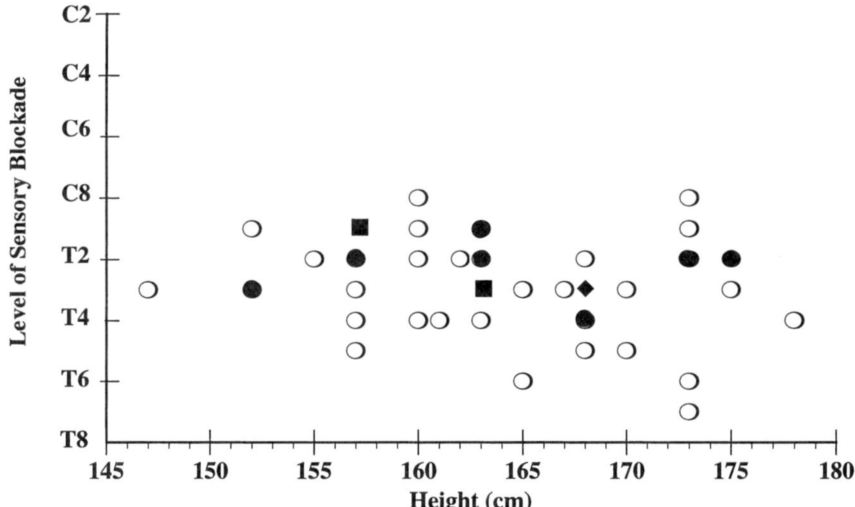

FIG. 15. Sensory blockade after subarachnoid injection of 12 mg hyperbaric bupivacaine in 50 term parturients. Sensory blockade develops independent of patient height. *Open circle,* one patient; *solid circle,* two patients; *square,* three patients; *diamond,* four patients. (Redrawn from ref. 114, with permission.)

patients undergoing vaginal hysterectomy with tetracaine anesthesia had more intraoperative pain than those receiving bupivacaine (110). Another study compared equal doses of tetracaine and bupivacaine in 40 patients undergoing knee surgery with a tourniquet. Tetracaine produced both longer-lasting sensory and motor blockade, but 60% of the patients in the tetracaine group complained of tourniquet pain compared with only 25% in the bupivacaine group (35). High-frequency impulses carried by unmyelinated, slowly conducting C fibers cause tourniquet (and visceral) pain. These fibers may recover more rapidly from tetracaine than from bupivacaine blockade (111).

In my practice, hyperbaric 0.75% bupivacaine, in doses of 12 to 15 mg, provides good sensory blockade to at least the T_6 dermatome. Sensory change begins within 4 to 6 minutes and peaks between 15 and 20 minutes (10). The drug provides good maternal comfort for 60 to 120 minutes of intra-abdominal surgery.

How Much Drug?

For many anesthesiologists, "common sense" and "clinical experience" implied that a given dose of local anesthetic would produce a higher level of sensory blockade in a shorter patient compared with a taller patient (112). This line of thought reasons that a bolus of hyperbaric local anesthetic flows a certain distance from the site of subarachnoid injection. If two patients receive the same dose of local anesthetic, and in both, the drug travels the same distance along the spinal canal, then the shorter patient (or the patient with the shorter vertebral column) should develop a higher dermatomal level of sensory blockade. By following this reasoning, some experts recommended varying the dose of local anesthetic with the height of the patient (104,113). However, in parturients, there is no correlation between the height or vertebral column length and the spread of sensory blockade (Figs. 15 and 16) (102,114, 115). [An important limitation of these studies is the some-

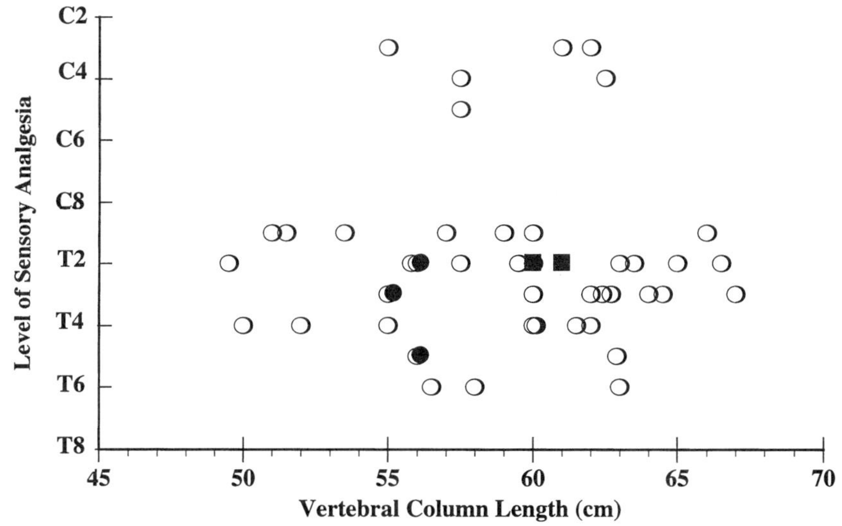

FIG. 16. Maximum level of sensory analgesia to pinprick, measured 15 minutes after subarachnoid injection of 15 mg hyperbaric bupivacaine in 52 term parturients. Sensory blockade develops independent of vertebral column length. *Open circle,* one patient; *solid circle,* two patients; *square,* three patients. (Redrawn from ref. 102, with permission.)

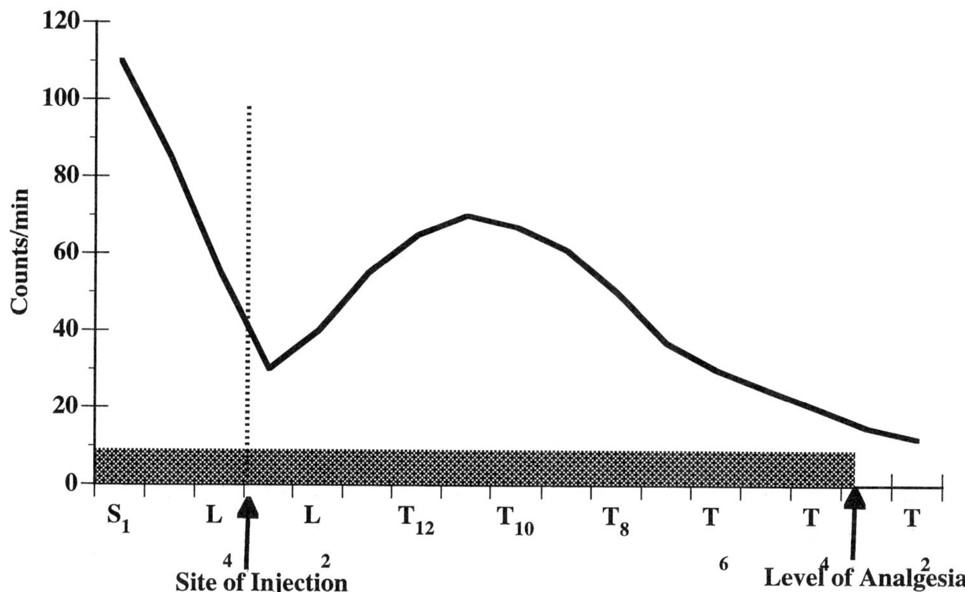

FIG. 17. Spread of iodine 131, mixed with hyperbaric tetracaine, 30 minutes after injection into the subarachnoid space at $L_{3\text{-}4}$ with the patient supine. The hyperbaric solution flows with gravity to the dependent regions of the spinal column. (Redrawn from ref. 117, with permission.)

what narrow range of parturients' heights and vertebral column lengths. Some patients shorter than 147 cm (4 feet 10 inches) or taller than 174 cm (5 feet 8 inches) might develop too high or too low a level of block. I have given 15 mg hyperbaric bupivacaine to women as short as 145 cm without complications.]

Examining the physical properties of the injected local anesthetic solution and the anatomic shape of the spinal column explains the lack of correlation between height and the spread of spinal anesthesia. By using glass tubes and methyl violet dye, Barker (116) showed that hyperbaric local anesthetics pool in dependent regions of the spinal column. Kitahara et al. (117) measured the spread of radioactivity after injecting local anesthetic plus iodine. Radioactivity was greatest in the dependent regions of the spinal column and correlated with the spread of sensory blockade (Fig. 17) (117). When the patient lies supine, the thoracolumbar spine slopes 8 to 12 degrees in the cephalad direction. Hyperbaric solutions pool in the lowest part of the thoracic curvature (T_5 to T_6; Fig. 18). They produce sensory blockade into the upper thoracic dermatomes regardless of the distance between the site of injection and the base of the thoracic curve (118).

Although the level of sensory blockade produced by the hyperbaric drug is independent of patient height, the same may not be true for isobaric drugs. Pitkänen reported a weak, but statistically significant, correlation between height and the spread of 0.5% bupivacaine in nonpregnant patients (119). More recently, Schnider et al. (120) treated the extent and duration of sensory blockade as pharmacodynamic data and derived a population model to examine the effect of patient height on the spread of sensory blockade. Ninety-six nonpregnant patients received 15 or 22.5 mg 0.5% bupivacaine. As with all studies of spinal anesthesia, there was large interindividual variation in the

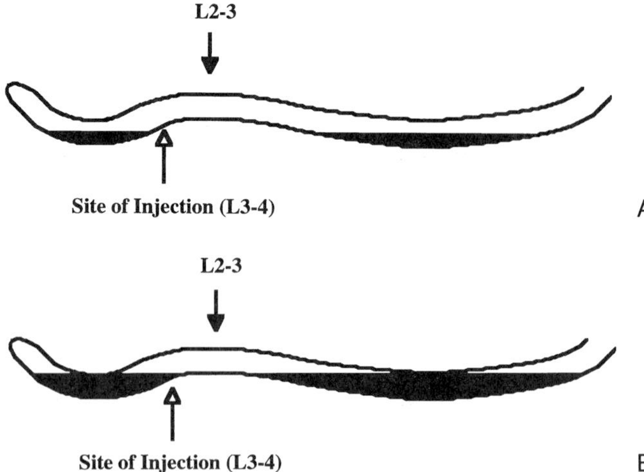

FIG. 18. **A:** Hyperbaric local anesthetics in moderate doses (7.5 to 12 mg 0.75% bupivacaine in 8.25% dextrose or 9 to 15 mg 0.5% tetracaine in 5% dextrose) pool in the lowest region of the thoracic spine. In term parturients, these doses of drug produce mid- to upper-thoracic levels of sensory blockade (median, T_3) regardless of the height of the patient or the dose of drug injected. **B:** When larger doses of drug are injected (15 mg 0.75% bupivacaine in 8.25% dextrose or 18 mg 0.5% tetracaine in 5% dextrose), the capacity of this upper thoracic pool is exceeded, and higher levels (median, T_1) of sensory blockade occur.

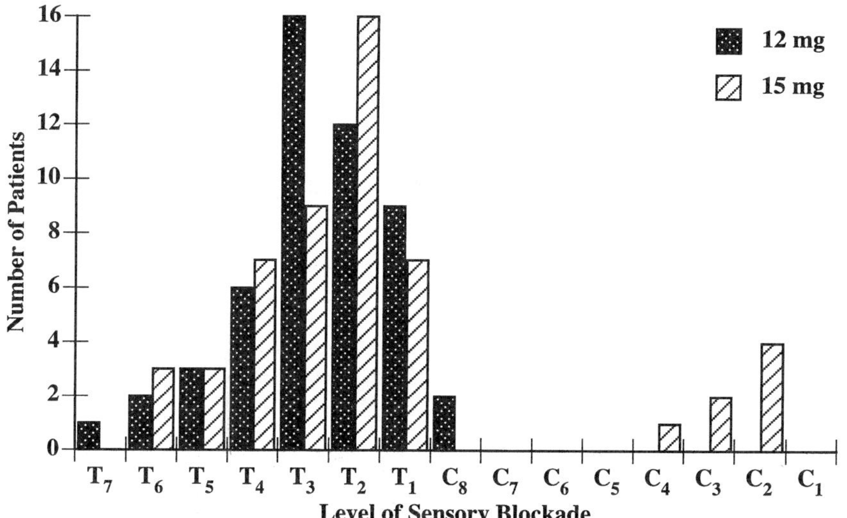

FIG. 19. Maximal level of sensory analgesia to pinprick, measured 15 minutes after subarachnoid injection of 12 or 15 mg hyperbaric bupivacaine in term parturients. The mode shifts from T_3 to T_2 with the larger dose of drug. (Data from refs. 102 and 114, with permission.)

extent and duration of blockade. They found significant correlations between patient height and the onset, extent, and duration of block. Their model suggests that a 10-cm increase in height would be associated with a 1.1-dermatome decrease in the level sensory block.

Within the commonly used range of hyperbaric drug doses (7.5 to 12 mg hyperbaric bupivacaine or 7 to 15 mg hyperbaric tetracaine), similar levels of sensory blockade develop despite varying doses of drug injected (Fig. 18A) (27,121). Baricity, not the amount of drug injected, primarily determines the spread of subarachnoid local anesthetics. Larger doses of drug produce more dense but not more extensive sensory blockade (27,121). When the dose of local anesthetic increases further (15 mg bupivacaine or 18 mg tetracaine), it exceeds the capacity of the upper thoracic curvature, and more extensive dermatomal spread follows (Figs. 18B, 19; Table 9) (27, 121).

Although very large doses of local anesthetic can increase the spread of blockade, the volume in which the drug is diluted appears to have no effect. Injection of 10 mL of 0.125% bupivacaine with 1:800,000 epinephrine (12.5 mg of bupivacaine) produces the same level of sensory block (T_2) as 2.5 mL of 0.5% bupivacaine (51). In term parturients, Russell (122,123) injected 15 mg bupivacaine mixed to progressively greater dilutions. All solutions of drug behaved as if hypobaric. During drug injection, most women developed unilateral sensory blockade on the nondependent side. When they were placed supine, the distribution of block equalized. The volume of injected drug did not alter the level of sensory block attained (median, T_2).

TABLE 9. *Spread of sensory blockade and the quality of analgesia in 88 term parturients*

Dose of tetracaine	9 mg	12 mg	15 mg	18 mg
Number of patients	20	27	25	16
Maximal level of analgesia	T_4	T_4	T_3	C_7[a]
Quality of analgesia (% good)	67	81	96	100

Analgesia was rated good if patients required <100 μg fentanyl and 50 mg meperidine after delivery.
[a]$p < 0.05$.
From ref. 121, with permission.

Improving the Quality of Block

Many investigators, dissatisfied with the degree of patient comfort they obtained with their usual technique, tried a variety of ways to improve the quality of anesthesia during cesarean section. Tetracaine and dextrose alone often prove inadequate for cesarean section. Mixing the tetracaine with an equal volume of 10% procaine instead of dextrose increases the level of sensory blockade and improves the quality of analgesia (104). Procaine may produce better sensory blockade than tetracaine, but the tetracaine–procaine group received more local anesthetic than the tetracaine–dextrose group. Simply injecting more tetracaine, rather than adding a second local anesthetic, has the same effect. Pan et al. (121) injected 9, 12, 15, or 18 mg of hyperbaric tetracaine into a series of parturients. They noted steadily better patient comfort with increasing dose of tetracaine (Table 9).

Other investigators tried to improve patient comfort when using hyperbaric bupivacaine. Increasing the dose of drug injected is probably the simplest way to achieve this end. Pederson et al. (27) compared women who received an average of 8.4 mg of hyperbaric bupivacaine with those who received 10.9 mg. Both groups developed similar levels of sensory blockade, but women in the higher-dose group were much less likely to experience

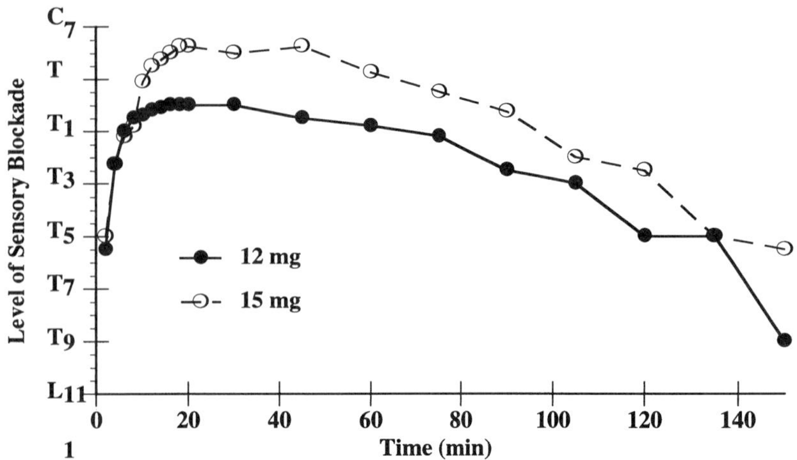

FIG. 20. Onset and duration of sensory blockade in term parturients after subarachnoid injection of either 12 or 15 mg 0.75% bupivacaine with 8.25% bupivacaine. The higher dose of drug blocks significantly more spinal segments for a significantly longer time. Sensory block regressed to T_{10} in 140.6 ± 16.5 minutes (mean ± SD) after 12 mg and in 162.1 ± 33.8 minutes after 15 mg. (Redrawn from ref. 10, with permission.)

moderate to severe pain during surgery (32% vs 71%). De Simone et al. (10) increased the dose of bupivacaine even more. They gave parturients either 12 or 15 mg hyperbaric drug. The 15-mg group had a slightly higher level of sensory blockade (Fig. 20), and all patients had good to excellent intraoperative analgesia (Table 10) (10).

Others have attempted to improve intraoperative analgesia by adding fentanyl, morphine, or epinephrine to hyperbaric bupivacaine. Most studies reported that adding any of these drugs to intrathecal bupivacaine will improve the quality of intraoperative analgesia.

Fentanyl, in doses of at least 6.25 μg, improves intraoperative and postoperative analgesia produced by at least 7.5 mg hyperbaric bupivacaine or 80 mg hyperbaric lidocaine (106,124). Intrathecal fentanyl does not significantly improve the quality of intraoperative analgesia in women receiving 15 mg hyperbaric bupivacaine (125). Higher doses of fentanyl (more than 15 μg) increase the incidence of itching and produce significant maternal sedation and respiratory depression (124,125).

Abouleish et al. (113) conducted a series of studies examining the addition of epinephrine and morphine to intrathecal bupivacaine (Fig. 21). Adding 200 μg epinephrine to an average of 9.3 mg hyperbaric bupivacaine improved the quality of intraoperative analgesia but also increased the intensity of motor block and slightly prolonged the regression of sensory block. One study suggested that epinephrine may slow the onset of sensory blockade as well (126). Intrathecal morphine, 200 μg, both improved quality of intraoperative blockade and provided prolonged postoperative analgesia when added to hyperbaric bupivacaine (127). The combination of epinephrine and morphine is more effective than either drug alone (128). Not surprisingly, however, intrathecal morphine increases the incidence of nausea, vomiting, and itching (128).

Whereas these studies show that patients can be comfortable with lower doses of intrathecal bupivacaine, I prefer the simplicity of using a large dose of a single drug. Hyperbaric bupivacaine, 15 mg, produces excellent operative conditions without the need for additional intrathecal or intravenous supplements (Fig. 22) (125).

TABLE 10. *Quality of intraoperative analgesia: 12 vs 15 mg hyperbaric bupivacaine*

Group	Excellent	Good	Fair	Poor
12 mg	8	5	3	0
15 mg	5	7	0	0

Excellent, no supplemental analgesia; good, <5 mg morphine i.v.; fair, 5–10 mg morphine i.v. ± midazolam; poor, ≥10 mg morphine i.v. or general anesthesia.

From ref. 10, with permission.

Conclusion

Any of the three local anesthetics mentioned can, if given in high enough doses, provide good maternal comfort during cesarean section. Because it provides better sensory blockade at commonly used doses and produces shorter duration of motor block, I prefer hyperbaric bupivacaine for most cesarean sections. I routinely use 15 mg of 0.75% bupivacaine with 8.25% dextrose (Table 11). Those who wish to use smaller doses of local anesthetic should consider adding opioid or epinephrine to improve the quality of sensory blockade.

Maternal Position

Neither the sitting nor the lateral decubitus position offers any clear advantage during induction of spinal anesthesia. Although onset of sensory block is slightly

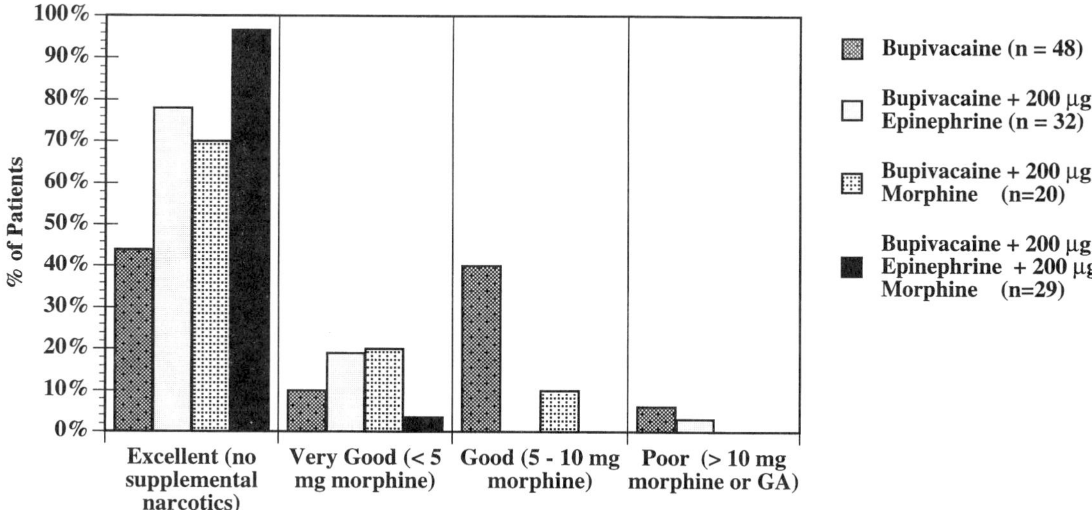

FIG. 21. Quality of intraoperative analgesia in term parturients receiving 0.75% hyperbaric bupivacaine, average dose 9.3 mg, with or without epinephrine or morphine. Adding either drug significantly improves patient comfort. Onset and extent of sensory blockade were similar in all groups. Epinephrine slightly prolonged the duration of sensory blockade. (Data from refs. 113 and 127, with permission.)

faster in the lateral position, the final level is unaffected (129,130). When inducing blockade in the lateral decubitus position, the side on which the patient lies does matter. If the patient assumes the left lateral position for induction and then lies supine with left tilt for uterine displacement, blockade on the right side may not extend high enough for surgery. In contrast, inducing anesthesia with the patient in the right lateral position and then placing her supine with left tilt for uterine displacement helps to assure good bilateral blockade (131).

A similar phenomenon occurs when using isobaric bupivacaine. Here, however, the greater extent of blockade develops on the nondependent side (0.5% bupivacaine is slightly hypobaric) (132,133). Should this problem arise, rolling the patient from side to side evens the spread of analgesia (134).

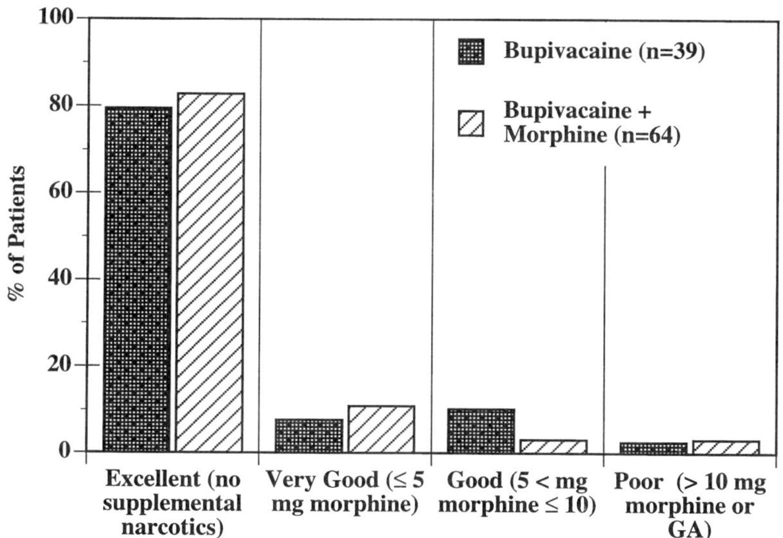

FIG. 22. Quality of intraoperative analgesia in term parturients receiving 15 mg hyperbaric 0.75% bupivacaine with or without 0.15 mg morphine for spinal anesthesia for cesarean section. Adding intrathecal morphine does not improve the quality of analgesia. Most patients in both groups had excellent sensory blockade. (From Norris MC, unpublished data, with permission.)

TABLE 11. *Spinal anesthesia for cesarean section: suggested technique*

Preparation	Large-bore peripheral i.v.
Premedication	30-mL sodium citrate within 15 min of induction.
Prehydration	1.0 L balanced saline solution (i.e., Plasmalyte) within 15–30 min of induction. Infuse under gravity. Do not delay induction for fluid infusion
Positioning	Sitting or right lateral decubitus
Induction	Identify the subarachnoid space
	Small-gauge pencil-point needle (≤ 24 gauge)
	L_{2-3} interspace or lower
	Midline or paramedian approach (paramedian approach often easier when patient is in the lateral decubitus position)
	Inject local anesthetic
	15 mg 0.75% bupivacaine with 8.25% dextrose
	Add morphine if desired for postoperative analgesia
Maintenance	Position patient supine with 10–15 degrees of left uterine tilt
	Administer ≤ 50% O_2 by face mask
	Monitor maternal blood pressure every 1–2 min for 20 min, then every 3–5 min
	Continue fluids until maternal blood pressure stabilizes
Hypotension	Well hydrated
	5–10 mg ephedrine when BP <90 mm Hg or mother symptomatic
	Poorly hydrated
	10 mg ephedrine when BP begins to decrease

BP, blood pressure.

COMBINED SPINAL–EPIDURAL ANESTHESIA

One limitation of spinal anesthesia is its finite duration. Hyperbaric bupivacaine, 15 mg, readily provides 90 to 120 minutes of good operating conditions. Occasionally, however, cesarean section lasts longer. If this situation can be predicted in advance, a combined spinal–epidural anesthetic offers the rapid onset of spinal anesthesia and the flexibility of epidural catheterization. I also use this technique in patients with poor anatomic landmarks in whom I anticipate technical difficulty when attempting to locate the subarachnoid space with a small-gauge spinal needle. In these women (especially the morbidly obese parturient), I find it easier first to find the epidural space with an 18-gauge needle and then to use the needle through needle technique to enter the subarachnoid space (see Chapter 15). Some anesthesiologists use the combined spinal–epidural technique even for routine cesarean sections (69,135,136). There are a few technical issues to consider before using a combined spinal–epidural anesthetic for cesarean section.

Patient Position

With the needle-through-needle technique, the success rate for dural puncture is slightly higher if the patient is sitting, not lying on her side (137). However, if the patient sits, hyperbaric drug will pool caudally while the epidural catheter is being inserted and secured, and then the level of sensory block may not be high enough for surgery. This problem is most significant when smaller (10 mg) doses of hyperbaric drug are used (138). I try to limit this risk by injecting a larger dose of bupivacaine and minimizing the time spent inserting and fixing the epidural catheter. If the level of sensory block is rising too slowly, I place the operating table in 5- to 10-degree head-down tilt as needed. If the level is still inadequate, I dose the epidural catheter (see later).

If the patient lies on her side for the needle-through-needle technique, the level of spinal anesthesia may ascend too high during insertion and fixation of the epidural catheter (135). (In most parturients, the hips are wider than the shoulders. When lying on a horizontal surface, the vertebral column slopes toward the patient's head.) Carrie (135) recommends the "Oxford position" to minimize this risk (Fig. 23) (135).

Epidural Anesthesia in the Presence of Spinal Blockade

There are two things to consider when preparing to inject epidural local anesthetics in the presence of spinal anesthesia. First is the difficulty in detecting a subarachnoid catheter, and the other is the impact of dural puncture and spinal anesthesia on the spread of epidurally injected drugs.

In this setting, subarachnoid injection of additional local anesthetic may produce dangerously high sensory blockade. One way to detect subarachnoid catheter placement is to wait until the spinal sensory level has regressed several segments before injecting a small (i.e., 5 to 10 mg bupivacaine) subarachnoid test dose. Although this approach has its merits, waiting until the spinal begins to recede may increase the risk that the patient will feel pain

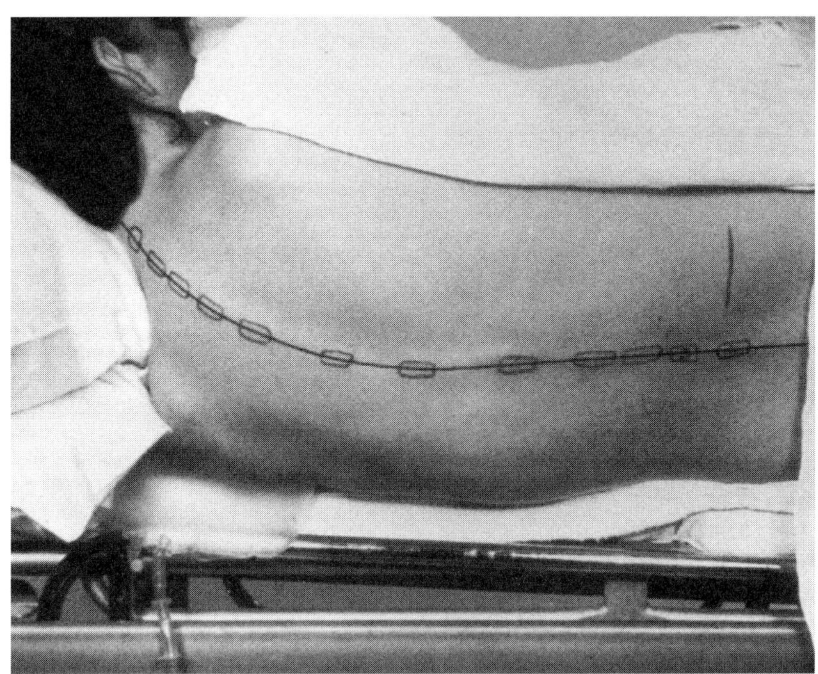

FIG. 23. The "Oxford position." Placing an inflated bag under the shoulder and three pillows under the head produces an uphill slope of the cervical and thoracic spine. Even if final patient positioning is delayed, hyperbaric drug will not ascend to the cervical nerve roots. (Photograph reproduced from ref. 135, with permission.)

before effective epidural anesthesia can be established. Instead, cautiously dose the epidural catheter about 1 hour after the induction of spinal anesthesia. Initially inject a small dose of epidural local anesthetic bupivacaine (1 to 2 mL 0.5%) and watch carefully for any sign of rising blockade (i.e., numbness or weakness of the upper extremities, or, if the patient is heavily sedated, look for a decrease in blood pressure or heart rate, or a change in respiratory pattern). Wait 5 minutes between successive injections of drug. Using small doses and waiting 5 minutes between injections minimizes the risks of unrecognized intrathecal or intravenous injection.

I base the concentration and volume of drug injected on the anticipated remaining duration of surgery. If the operation will be finished in 15 to 30 minutes, and the patient still has at least a T_4 level of sensory blockade, I give 10 mL 0.25% bupivacaine mostly to provide some analgesia in the immediate postoperative period. If I expect extensive or prolonged surgery (i.e., a cesarean hysterectomy), I will "replace" the regressing spinal anesthetic with epidural injection of 15 to 20 mL 0.5% bupivacaine.

When dosing an epidural catheter in the presence of spinal anesthesia, small amounts of epidural local anesthetic can significantly raise the level of sensory blockade (139,140). Several factors contribute to this increased spread. Pressure within the epidural space caused by fluid injection is transmitted to the subarachnoid space and can displace intrathecal local anesthetic and raise the level of sensory blockade. Epidural injection of both saline and local anesthetic can extend the preexisting spinal block by this mechanism (141,142). The dural hole left by the spinal needle allows increased subarachnoid passage of epidurally injected drug (143,144). Clinically, however, extensive sensory block is likely to be a problem only after unrecognized intrathecal injection of local anesthetic.

In sum, even though combined spinal epidural anesthesia can be very useful in selected parturients seen for cesarean section, the technique must be used carefully with a full understanding of its potential risks.

SPINAL ANESTHESIA AFTER FAILED EPIDURAL BLOCK

Occasionally, epidural injection of local anesthetic fails to produce adequate surgical anesthesia. In this setting, the clinician may opt for spinal anesthesia instead of repeating the epidural block or proceeding to general anesthesia. Several recent case reports raised questions about the safety of this choice (145–147). Most often, a patient with unilateral or patchy labor epidural blockade received a spinal anesthetic for cesarean section. Shortly after intrathecal injection of 9 to 15 mg hyperbaric bupivacaine, the patient developed respiratory distress or apnea requiring emergency intubation and ventilation. These reports raise some interesting questions:

- Does performing a spinal anesthetic after a previous epidural increase the risk of dangerously high block?
- What are the mechanisms of this excessive spinal block?
- Is spinal anesthesia contraindicated after a failed epidural?
- Can changes in spinal anesthetic technique reduce the risk of high block?

Most of the authors of these case reports assume that the risk of high spinal anesthesia is greater after failed epidural anesthesia, but few data support this conclusion. Furst and Reisner (146) conducted a retrospective chart review and found an 11% incidence (three of 27) of sensory block above C_8 when spinal anesthesia was induced after a failed epidural compared with 0.2% (one of 643) when spinal block was used as the initial anesthetic. Although these numbers suggest an increased risk of high block when spinal anesthesia follows an attempted epidural, remember the many limitations of retrospective studies. It is also interesting to note that sensory change can often be detected above C_8 after intrathecal injection of hyperbaric bupivacaine, 15 mg, but respiratory compromise and intubation are extremely rare (102). Other clinicians reported no complications in small case series (n = 12 or 30) of spinal anesthesia after failed epidural (148,149).

Several explanations for the apparent increased spread of spinal anesthesia after failed epidural have been offered. Fluid within the epidural space may compress the thecal sac, forcing intrathecally injected drugs to higher levels. The fresh dural hole may allow rapid diffusion of previously injected epidural local anesthetic (149,150). However, in young patients, injected volume readily escapes the epidural space through the intervertebral foramina (151). Thus I doubt that much local anesthetic remains within the space either to change intrathecal pressure or to diffuse across a new dural hole. Alternatively, after epidural injection, local anesthetic diffuses into the subarachnoid space in amounts too small to block nerve conduction. After subsequent intrathecal injection, the epidurally injected drug combines with the spinal drug to extend the upper level of sensory blockade (146).

The publication of these reports of high sensory block after failed epidural block led some anesthesiologists to declare that spinal anesthesia is contraindicated in this situation (147,152). Others, however, believed that spinal anesthesia can still be a safe choice (91,148).

Several approaches may limit the risk of high sensory block after failed epidural anesthesia. While the first impulse may be to use a small dose of intrathecal local anesthetic, this approach risks inadequate intensity and duration of anesthesia (148). Stoneham and Souter (149) recommended performing the block with the patient lying on her side (in the Oxford position: Fig. 23) and then immediately turning her to the opposite side after drug injection. The patient remains in the lateral position for 20 minutes while the table is tilted up and down to keep the level of sensory blockade at T_4. Although this approach has its merits, it is time consuming, and using head-up tilt (reverse Trendelenberg) to control the level of sensory block risks venous pooling and hypotension (40).

Vickers and Wilkey (148) reported 30 patients who received spinal anesthesia for cesarean section after labor epidural analgesia. Spinal anesthesia was induced in either the sitting or lateral position with hyperbaric bupivacaine (usually at least 12.5 mg). No patient had excessive sensory block. Two of four patients who received less than 12.5 mg bupivacaine require supplemental analgesia (including general anesthesia).

Despite this controversy, I usually attempt to use spinal anesthesia for cesarean section after a failed labor epidural. Unless I am concerned about technical difficulty (i.e., a patient with poorly palpable spinous processes), I induce anesthesia in the right lateral position to minimize the risk of postural hypotension in a patient with some preexisting sympathetic blockade. I base my dose of local anesthetic on the extent of the existing epidural block, and I usually use 10 to 15 mg hyperbaric bupivacaine. After drug injection, I carefully position the patient supine with left uterine displacement and place an extra pillow under her head. I monitor the patient's respiration and upper extremity motor function carefully. Despite these precautions, an occasional parturient will develop an excessively high level of sensory blockade. If so, I apply cricoid pressure and rapidly induce general anesthesia with a small dose of thiopental and use succinylcholine to facilitate intubation.

This situation serves most of all as a reminder to monitor patients receiving labor epidural analgesia carefully and immediately replace any catheter that does not function as expected.

CONCLUSION

This chapter reviewed spinal anesthesia for cesarean section. I hope the reader now understands both how to use this technique safely (Table 11) and the reasons behind its use. With proper attention to maternal hemodynamics and to drug selection and dosage, spinal blockade provides profound, reliable, and safe anesthesia for both mother and fetus.

REFERENCES

1. Brownridge P. Central neural blockade and caesarean section. Part 1: review and case series. *Anaesth Intens Care* 1979;7:33.
2. Greene NM, Brull SJ. *Physiology of spinal anesthesia.* Baltimore: Williams & Wilkins, 1993:309.
3. Ebner H. An evaluation of spinal anesthesia in obstetrics. *Anesth Analg* 1959;38:378.
4. Hawkins JL, Gibbs CP, Orleans M, Martin-Salvaj G, Beaty B. Obstetric anesthesia workforce survey: 1981 versus 1992 [Abstract]. *Anesthesiology* 1997;87:135.
5. Lambert DH, Hurley RJ, Hertwig L, Datta S. Role of needle gauge and tip configuration in the production of lumber puncture headache. *Reg Anesth* 1997;22:66.
6. Riley ET, Cohen SE, Macario A, Desai JB, Ratner EF. Spinal versus epidural anesthesia for cesarean section: a comparison of time efficiency, costs, charges and complications. *Anesth Analg* 1995;80:709.
7. Datta S, Camann W, Bader A, VanderBurgh L. Clinical effects and maternal and fetal plasma concentrations of epidural ropivacaine versus bupivacaine for cesarean section. *Anesthesiology* 1995;82:1346.
8. Kuhnert BR, Zuspan KJ, Kuhnert PM, Syracuse CD, Brown DE. Bupivacaine disposition in mother, fetus and neonate after spinal anesthesia for cesarean section. *Anesth Analg* 1987;66:407.

9. Juhani TP, Hannele H. Complications during spinal anesthesia for cesarean delivery: a clinical report of one year's experience. *Reg Anesth* 1993;18:128.
10. De Simone CA, Leighton BL, Norris MC. Spinal anesthesia for cesarean delivery: a comparison of two doses. *Reg Anesth* 1995;20:90.
11. Russell IF. Levels of anaesthesia and intraoperative pain at caesarean section under regional block. *Int J Obstet Anesth* 1995;4:71.
12. Keohane M. Patient comfort: spinal versus epidural anesthesia for cesarean section. *Anesth Analg* 1996;82:219.
13. Norris MC, Torjman M, Leighton BL, DeSimone CA. Respiratory and motor function during bupivacaine spinal anesthesia for cesarean section. *Anesth Analg* 1990;70:S283.
14. Marx GF, Luykx WM, Cohen S. Fetal-neonatal status following caesarean section for fetal distress. *Br J Anaesth* 1984;56:1009.
15. James FM III, Crawford JS, Hopkinson R, Davies P, Naiem H. A comparison of general anesthesia and lumbar epidural analgesia for elective cesarean section. *Anesth Analg* 1977;56:228.
16. Gambling DR, Sharma SK, White PF, Van Beveren T, Bala AS, Gouldson R. Use of sevoflurane during elective cesarean birth: a comparison with isoflurane and spinal anesthesia. *Anesth Analg* 1995;81:90.
17. Roberts SW, Leveno KJ, Sidawi JE, Lucas MJ, Kelly MA. Fetal acidemia associated with regional anesthesia for elective cesarean delivery. *Obstet Gynecol* 1995;85:79.
18. Abboud TK, Nagappala S, Murakawa K, et al. Comparison of the effects of general and regional anesthesia for cesarean section on neonatal neurologic and adaptive capacity scores. *Anesth Analg* 1985; 64:996.
19. Shyken JM, Smeltzer JS, Baxi LV, Blakemore KJ, Ambrose SE, Petrie RH. A comparison of the effect of epidural, general, and no anesthesia on funic acid-base values by stage of labor and type of delivery. *Am J Obstet Gynecol* 1990;163:802.
20. Hodgkinson R, Bhatt M, Kim SS, Grewal G, Marx GF. Neonatal neurobehavioral tests following cesarean section under general and spinal anesthesia. *Am J Obstet Gynecol* 1978;132:670.
21. Irestedt L, Lagercrantz H, Hjemdahl P, Hgnevik K, Belfrage P. Fetal and maternal plasma catecholamine levels at elective cesarean section under general or epidural anesthesia versus vaginal delivery. *Am J Obstet Gynecol* 1982;142:1004.
22. Hollmén AI, Jouppila R, Koivisto M, et al. Neurologic activity of infants following anesthesia for cesarean section. *Anesthesiology* 1978; 48:350.
23. Corke BC, Datta S, Ostheimer GW, Weiss JB, Alper MH. Spinal anaesthesia for caesarean section: the influence of hypotension on neonatal outcome. *Anaesthesia* 1982;37:658.
24. Jouppila P, Kuikka J, Jouppila R, Hollmén A. Effect of induction of general anesthesia for cesarean section on intervillous blood flow. *Acta Obstet Gynecol Scand* 1979;58:249.
25. Palahniuk RJ, Cumming M. Foetal deterioration following thiopentone-nitrous oxide anaesthesia in the pregnant ewe. *Can Anaesth Soc J* 1977;24:367.
26. Abboud TK, Artal R, Henriksen EH, Earl S, Kammula RK. Effects of spinal anesthesia on maternal circulating catecholamines. *Am J Obstet Gynecol* 1983;142:252.
27. Pedersen H, Santos AC, Steinberg ES, Schapiro HM, Harmon TW, Finster M. Incidence of visceral pain during cesarean section: the effect of varying doses of spinal bupivacaine. *Anesth Analg* 1989; 69:46.
28. Stevens RA, Frey K, Liu SS, et al. Sympathetic block during spinal anesthesia in volunteers using lidocaine, tetracaine, and bupivacaine. *Reg Anesth* 1997;22:325.
29. Greene NM. Area of differential block in spinal anesthesia with hyperbaric tetracaine. *Anesthesiology* 1958;19:45.
30. Brull SJ, Greene NM. Time-courses of zones of differential sensory blockade during spinal anesthesia with hyperbaric tetracaine or bupivacaine. *Anesth Analg* 1989;69:342.
31. Chamberlain DP, Chamberlain BDL. Changes in the skin temperature of the trunk and their relationship to sympathetic block during spinal anesthesia. *Anesthesiology* 1986;65:139.
32. Janitzki A, Götte A. Function and behavior of the sympathetic system in regional anesthesia. *Reg Anesth* 1990;13:91.
33. Janitzki A, Götte A. Skin resistance measurements indicating the activity of the sympathetic nervous system in spinal anesthesia. *Reg Anesth* 1986;9:49.
34. Stevens RA, Beardsley D, White JL, Kao T-C, Gantt R, Holman S. Does spinal anesthesia result in a more complete sympathetic block than that from epidural anesthesia? *Anesthesiology* 1995;82:8778.
35. Concepcion MA, Lambert DH, Welch KA, Covino BG. Tourniquet pain during spinal anesthesia: a comparison of plain solutions of tetracaine and bupivacaine. *Anesth Analg* 1988;67:828.
36. Alahuhta S, Kangas-Saarela T, Hollmén AI, Edström HH. Visceral pain during caesarean section under spinal and epidural anaesthesia with bupivacaine. *Acta Anaesthesiol Scand* 1990;34:95.
37. Lund C, Selmar P, Hansen OB, Kehlet H. Effect of intrathecal bupivacaine on somatosensory evoked potentials following dermatomal stimulation. *Anesth Analg* 1987;66:809.
38. Boswell MW, Lacono RP, Guthkelch AN. Sites of action of subarachnoid lidocaine and tetracaine: observations with evoked potential monitoring during spinal cord stimulator implantation. *Reg Anesth* 1992;17:37.
39. Curatolo M, Petersen-Felix S, Arendt-Nielsen L, Zbinden AM. Spinal anaesthesia inhibits central temporal summation. *Br J Anaesth* 1997; 78:88.
40. Greene NM, Brull SJ. *Physiology of spinal anesthesia.* Baltimore: Williams & Wilkins, 1993:1.
41. Holmes F. The supine hypotensive syndrome: its importance to the anesthetist. *Anaesthesia* 1960;15:298.
42. Rout CC, Rocke DA. Prevention of hypotension following spinal anesthesia for cesarean section. *Int Anesth Clin* 1994;32:117.
43. Clark RB, Thompson DS, Thompson CH. Prevention of spinal hypotension associated with cesarean section. *Anesthesiology* 1976;45:670.
44. Assali NS, Prystowsky H. Studies on autonomic blockade. I. Comparison between the effects of tetraethylammonium chloride (TEAC) and high selective spinal anesthesia on blood pressure of normal and toxemic pregnancy. *J Clin Invest* 1950;1950:1354.
45. Greene NM, Brull SJ. *Physiology of spinal anesthesia.* Baltimore: Williams & Wilkins, 1993:85.
46. Hogan QH, Stekiel TA, Stadnicka A, Bosnjak ZJ, Kampine JP. Region of epidural blockade determines sympathetic and mesenteric capacitance effects in rabbits. *Anesthesiology* 1995;83:604.
47. Wollman SB, Marx GF. Acute hydration for prevention of hypotension of spinal anesthesia in parturients. *Anesthesiology* 1968;29:374.
48. Ueland K, Gills RE, Hansen JM. Maternal cardiovascular dynamics. I. Cesarean section under subarachnoid block anesthesia. *Am J Obstet Gynecol* 1968;100:42.
49. Robson SC, Boys RJ, Rodeck C, Morgan B. Maternal and fetal hemodynamic effects of spinal and extradural anaesthesia for elective caesarean section. *Br J Anaesth* 1992;68:54.
50. Shiroyama K, Nakagawa I, Izumi H, Kurokawa H, Kuroda M. Cause of hypotension during spinal anesthesia: the relation between the level of anesthesia and the hypotension. *Masui* 1994;43:697.
51. Van Zundert AA, De Wolf AM, Vaes L, Soetens M. High-volume spinal anesthesia with bupivacaine 0.125% for cesarean section. *Anesthesiology* 1988;69:998.
52. Olsen KS, Feilberg VL, Hansen CL, Rudkjbing O, Pedersen T, Kyst A. Prevention of hypotension during spinal anesthesia for caesarean section. *Int J Obstet Anesth* 1994;3:20.
53. Jouppila P, Jouppila R, Barinoff T, Koivula A. Placental blood flow during caesarean section performed under subarachnoid blockade. *Br J Anaesth* 1984;56:1379.
54. Karinen J, Räsänen J, Alahuhta S, Jouppila R, Jouppila P. Effect of crystalloid and colloid preloading on uteroplacental and maternal haemodynamic state during spinal anaesthesia for caesarean section. *Br J Anaesth* 1995;75:531.
55. Lindblad A, Bernow J, Marsal K. Fetal blood flow during intrathecal anaesthesia for elective caesarean section. *Br J Anaesth* 1988;61:376.
56. Fairlie FM, Kirkwood I, Lang GD, Sheldon CD. Umbilical artery flow velocity waveforms during spinal anesthesia. *Eur J Obstet Gynecol Reprod Biol* 1990;38:3.
57. Ebner H, Barcohana J, Bartoshuk AK. Influence of postspinal hypotension on the fetal electrocardiogram. *Am J Obstet Gynecol* 1960; 80:569.
58. Marx GF, Cosmi EV, Wollman SB. Biochemical status and clinical condition of mother and infant at cesarean section. *Anesth Analg* 1969;48:986.
59. Kenepp NB, Shelley WC, Gabbe SG, Kumar S, Stanley CA, Gutsche BB. Fetal and neonatal hazards of maternal hydration with 5% dextrose before cesarean section. *Lancet* 1982;1:1150.
60. Peng ATC, Shamsi HH, Blancato LS, Shulman SM, Chervenak FA, Castro JL. Euglycemic hydration with dextrose 1% in lactated ringer's

solution during epidural anesthesia for cesarean section. *Reg Anesth* 1987;12:184.

61. Datta S, Brown WU Jr. Acid-base status in diabetic mothers and their infants following general or spinal anesthesia for cesarean section. *Anesthesiology* 1977;47:272.
62. Darchy B, Forceville X, Bavoux E, Soriot F, Domart Y. Clinical and bacteriologic survey of epidural analgesia in patients in the intensive care unit. *Anesthesiology* 1996;85:988.
63. Clark RB, Brunner JA III. Dopamine for the treatment of spinal hypotension during cesarean section. *Anesthesiology* 1980;53:514.
64. Gutsche BB. Prophylactic ephedrine preceding spinal anesthesia for cesarean section. *Anesthesiology* 1976;45:462.
65. Norris MC. Hypotension during spinal anesthesia for cesarean section: does it affect neonatal outcome? *Reg Anesth* 1987;12:191.
66. Kang YG, Abouleish E, Caritis S. Prophylactic intravenous ephedrine infusion during spinal anesthesia for cesarean section. *Anesth Analg* 1982;61:839.
67. Datta S, Kitzmuller JL, Naulty JS, Ostheimer GW, Weiss JB. Acid-base status of diabetic mothers and their infants following spinal anesthesia for cesarean section. *Anesth Analg* 1982;61:662.
68. Ouzounian JG, Masaki DI, Abboud TK, Greenspoon JS. Systemic vascular resistance index determined by thoracic electrical bioimpedance predicts the risk for maternal hypotension during regional anesthesia for cesarean delivery. *Am J Obstet Gynecol* 1996;174:1019.
69. Wallace DH, Leveno KJ, Cunningham FG, Giesecke AH, Shearer VE, Sidawi JE. Randomized comparison of general and regional anesthesia for cesarean delivery in pregnancies complicated by severe preeclampsia. *Obstet Gynecol* 1995;86:193.
70. Kinsella SM, Norris MC. Advance prediction of hypotension at cesarean delivery under spinal anesthesia. *Int J Obstet Anesth* 1996;5:3.
71. Brizgys RV, Dailey PA, Shnider SM, Kotelko DM, Levinson G. The incidence and neonatal effects of maternal hypotension during epidural anesthesia for cesarean section. *Anesthesiology* 1987;67:782.
72. Scott DB. Inferior vena caval occlusion in late pregnancy and its importance in anaesthesia. *Br J Anaesth* 1968;40:120.
73. Crawford JS, Burton M, Davies P. Time and lateral tilt at caesarean section. *Br J Anaesth* 1972;44:477.
74. Ansari I, Wallace G, Clemetson CAB, Mallikarjuneswara VR, Clemetson CDM. Tilt cesarean section. *J Obstet Gynaecol Br Commonw* 1970;77:713.
75. Miyabe M, Sato S. The effect of head-down tilt position on arterial blood pressure after spinal anesthesia for cesarean delivery. *Reg Anesth* 1997;22:239.
76. Miyabe M, Namiki A. Effect of head-down tilt on arterial blood pressure after spinal anesthesia. *Anesth Analg* 1993;76:549.
77. Svensén C, Hahn RG. Volume kinetics of Ringer solution, Dextran 70, and hypertonic saline in male volunteers. *Anesthesiology* 1997;87:204.
78. Rout CC, Akoojee SS, Rocke DA, Gouws E. Rapid administration of crystalloid preload does not decrease the incidence of hypotension after spinal anaesthesia for elective caesarean section. *Br J Anaesth* 1992;68:394.
79. Rout CC, Rocke DA, Levin J, Gouws E, Reddy D. A reevaluation of the role of crystalloid preload in the prevention of hypotension associated with spinal anesthesia for elective cesarean section. *Anesthesiology* 1993;79:262.
80. Park GE, Hauch MA, Curlin F, Datta S, Bader AM. The effects of varying volumes of crystalloid administration before cesarean delivery on maternal hemodynamics and colloid osmotic pressure. *Anesth Analg* 1996;83:299.
81. Jackson R, Reid JA, Thorburn J. Volume preloading is not essential to prevent spinal-induced hypotension at caesarean section. *Br J Anaesth* 1995;75:262.
82. Pouta AM, Karinen J, Vuolteenaho OJ, Laatikainen TJ. Effect of intravenous fluid preload on vasoactive peptide secretion during cesarean section under spinal anesthesia. *Anaesthesia* 1996;51:128.
83. Caritis SN, Abouleish E, Edelstone DI, Mueller-Heubach E. Fetal acid-base state following spinal of epidural anesthesia for cesarean section. *Obstet Gynecol* 1980;56:610.
84. Mathru M, Rao TLK, Kartha RK, Shanmugham M, Jacobs HK. Intravenous albumin administration for prevention of spinal hypotension during cesarean section. *Anesth Analg* 1980;59:655.
85. Riley ET, Cohen SE, Rubenstein AJ, Flanagan B. Prevention of hypotension after spinal anesthesia for cesarean section: six percent hetastarch versus lactated Ringer's solution. *Anesth Analg* 1995;81:838.
86. James FM III, Greiss FC Jr. The use of inflatable boot to prevent hypotension during spinal anesthesia for cesarean section. *Anesth Analg* 1973;52:246.
87. Goudie TA, Winter AW, Ferguson DJM. Lower limb compression using inflatable splints to prevent hypotension during spinal anaesthesia for caesarean section. *Acta Anaesthesiol Scand* 1988;32:541.
88. Sood PK, Cooper PJF, Michel MZ, Wee MYK, Pickering RM. Thromboembolic deterrent stockings fail to prevent hypotension associated with spinal anaesthesia for elective caesarean section. *Int J Obstet Anesth* 1996;5:172.
89. Bhagwangee S, Rocke DA, Rout CC, Koovarhee RV, Brinjball R. Prevention of hypotension following spinal anaesthesia for elective caesarean section by wrapping of the legs. *Br J Anaesth* 1990;65:819.
90. Rout CC, Rocke DA, Gouws E. Leg elevation and wrapping in the prevention of hypotension following spinal anaesthesia for elective cesarean section. *Anaesthesia* 1993;48:304.
91. Hogan QH. Venous capacitance changes in the lower extremities during spinal anesthesia. *Reg Anesth* 1996;21:376.
92. Moya F, Smith B. Spinal anesthesia for cesarean section. *JAMA* 1962; 179:115.
93. Datta S, Alper MH, Ostheimer GW, Weiss JB. Method of ephedrine administration and nausea and hypotension during spinal anesthesia for cesarean section. *Anesthesiology* 1982;56:68.
94. Kangas-Saarela T, Hollmén AI, Tolonen U, et al. Does ephedrine influence newborn neurobehavioral responses and spectral EEG when used to prevent maternal hypotension during cesarean section? *Acta Anaesthesiol Scand* 1990;34:8.
95. Conn DA, Moffat AC, McCallum GDR, Thorburn J. Changes in pulmonary function tests during spinal anaesthesia for cesarean section. *Int J Obstet Anesth* 1993;2:12.
96. Kelly MC, Fitzpatrick KTJ, Hill DA. Respiratory effects of spinal anaesthesia for caesarean section. *Anaesthesia* 1996;51:1120.
97. Gamil M. Serial peak expiratory flow rates in mothers during caesarean section under extradural anaesthesia. *Br J Anaesth* 1989;62:415.
98. Yun E, Topulos GP, Body SC, Datta S, Bader A. Pulmonary function changes during epidural anesthesia for cesarean delivery. *Anesth Analg* 1996;82:750.
99. Philipson EH, Kalhan SC, Riha MM, Pimental R. Effects of maternal glucose infusion on fetal acid-base status in human pregnancy. *Am J Obstet Gynecol* 1987;157:866.
100. Norris MC, Leighton BL, De Simone CA, Goodman DA, Gorman RM. Influence of the choice of crystalloid solution on neonatal acid-base status at cesarean section. *Anesthesiology* 1987;67:A458.
101. Craft JB Jr, Roizen MF, Dao SD, Edwards M, Gilman R. A comparison of T4 and T7 dermatomal levels of analgesia for caesarean section using the lumbar epidural technique. *Can Anaesth Soc J* 1982; 29:264.
102. Norris MC. Patient variables and the subarachnoid spread of hyperbaric bupivacaine in the term parturient. *Anesthesiology* 1990;72:478.
103. Michie AR, Freeman RM, Dutton DA, Howie HB. Subarachnoid anaesthesia for elective caesarean section: a comparison of two hyperbaric solutions. *Anaesthesia* 1988;43:96.
104. Chantigian RC, Datta S, Burger GA, Naulty JS, Lambert DH, Ostheimer GW. Anesthesia for cesarean delivery utilizing spinal anesthesia: tetracaine versus tetracaine and procaine. *Reg Anesth* 1984;9:195.
105. Bembridge M, MacDonald R, Lyons G. Spinal anaesthesia with hyperbaric lignocaine for elective caesarean section. *Anaesthesia* 1986;41:906.
106. Palmer CM, Voulgaropoulos D, Alves D. Subarachnoid fentanyl augments lidocaine spinal anesthesia for cesarean delivery. *Reg Anesth* 1995;20:389.
107. de Jong RH. Last round for a "heavyweight"? *Anesth Analg* 1994;78:3.
108. Drasner K. Lidocaine spinal anesthesia: a vanishing therapeutic index? *Anesthesiology* 1997;87:469.
109. Plumer MH, Rottman R. How anesthesiologists practice obstetric anesthesia: responses of practicing obstetric anesthesiologists at the 1993 meeting of the Society for Obstetric Anesthesia and Perinatology. *Reg Anesth* 1996;21:49.
110. Moore DC. Spinal anesthesia: bupivacaine compared with tetracaine. *Anesth Analg* 1980;59:743.
111. Stewart A, Lambert DH, Concepcion MA, et al. Decreased incidence of tourniquet pain during spinal anesthesia with bupivacaine: a possible explanation. *Anesth Analg* 1988;67:833.

112. Greene NM. Distribution of local anesthetic solutions within the subarachnoid space. *Anesth Analg* 1985;64:715.
113. Abouleish EI. Epinephrine improves the quality of spinal hyperbaric bupivacaine for cesarean section. *Anesth Analg* 1987;66:395.
114. Norris MC. Height, weight and the spread of spinal anesthesia for cesarean section. *Anesth Analg* 1988;67:555.
115. Hartwell BL, Aglio LS, Hauch MA, Datta S. Vertebral column length and spread of hyperbaric subarachnoid bupivacaine in the term parturient. *Reg Anesth* 1991;16:17.
116. Barker AE. A report of clinical experiences with spinal analgesia in 100 cases and some reflections on the procedure. *Br Med J* 1907;1:655.
117. Kitahara T, Kuri S, Yoshida J. The spread of drugs used for spinal anesthesia. *Anesthesiology* 1956;17:205.
118. Smith TC. The lumbar spine and subarachnoid block. *Anesthesiology* 1968;29:60.
119. Pitkänen MT. Body mass and spread of spinal anesthesia with bupivacaine. *Anesth Analg* 1987;66:127.
120. Schnider TW, Minto CF, Bruckert H, Mandema JW. Population pharmacokinetic modeling and covariate detection for central neural blockade. *Anesthesiology* 1996;85:502.
121. Pan PM, Lin Z-F, Lim J, Tung M-C, Wie T-T. The optimal dose of hyperbaric tetracaine for spinal anesthesia for cesarean section. *Anaesth Sinica* 1989;27:349.
122. Russell IF. Spinal anesthesia for cesarean delivery with dilute solutions of plain bupivacaine: the relationship between infused volume and spread. *Reg Anesth* 1991;16:130.
123. Vucevic M, Russell IF. Spinal anaesthesia for caesarean section: 0.125% plain bupivacaine 12 mL compared with 0.5% plain bupivacaine 3 mL. *Br J Anaesth* 1992;68:590.
124. Hunt CO, Naulty JS, Bader AM, et al. Perioperative analgesia with subarachnoid fentanyl-bupivacaine for cesarean delivery. *Anesthesiology* 1989;71:535.
125. Belzarena SD. Clinical effects of intrathecally administered fentanyl in patients undergoing cesarean section. *Anesth Analg* 1992;74:653.
126. Moore CH, Wilhite A, Pan PH, Blass NH. The addition of epinephrine to subarachnoid administered hyperbaric bupivacaine with fentanyl for cesarean delivery: the effect on onset time. *Reg Anesth* 1992; 17:202.
127. Abouleish E, Rawal N, Fallon K, Hernandez D. Combined intrathecal morphine and bupivacaine for cesarean section. *Anesth Analg* 1988; 67:370.
128. Abouleish E, Rawal N, Tobon-Randall B, Rivera-Weiss M, Meyer B, Wu A, Rashad MN. A clinical and laboratory study to compare the addition of 0.2 mg of morphine, 0.2 mg of epinephrine, or their combination to hyperbaric bupivacaine for spinal anesthesia in cesarean section. *Anesth Analg* 1993;77:457.
129. Inglis A, Daniel M, McGrady E. Maternal position during induction of spinal anaesthesia for caesarean delivery. *Anaesthesia* 1995; 50:363.
130. Ferouz F, Norris M, Arkoosh V, Huffnagle S, Leighton B, Huffnagle HJ. The effect of Sprotte needle aperture orientation and patient position on hyperbaric bupivacaine anesthesia [Abstract]. New York State Society of Anesthesiologists, PostGraduate Assembly 1996;P-9108.
131. Sprague DH. Effects of position and uterine displacement on spinal anesthesia for cesarean section. *Anesthesiology* 1976;44:164.
132. Richardson MG, Wissler RN. Densities of dextrose-free intrathecal local anesthetics, opioids, and combinations measured at 37°C. *Anesth Analg* 1997;84:95.
133. Russell IF. Effect of posture during the induction of subarachnoid analgesia for caesarean section: right vs. left lateral. *Br J Anaesth* 1987;59:342.
134. Russell IF. Spinal anaesthesia for caesarean section: the use of 0.5% bupivacaine. *Br J Anaesth* 1983;55:309.
135. Carrie LES. Combined spinal-epidural anesthesia for cesarean section. *Tech Reg Anesth Pain Manage* 1997;1:118.
136. Davies SJ, Paech MJ, Welch H, Evans SF, Pavy TJG. Maternal experience during epidural of combined spinal-epidural anesthesia for cesarean section: a prospective randomized trial. *Anesth Analg* 1997; 85:607.
137. Norris MC, Grieco WM, Borkowski M, et al. Complications of labor analgesia: epidural versus combined spinal epidural techniques. *Anesth Analg* 1994;79:529.
138. Patel M, Samsoon G, Swami A, Morgan B. Posture and the spread of hyperbaric bupivacaine in parturients using the combined spinal epidural technique. *Can J Anaesth* 1993;40:943.
139. Carrie LES. Epidural versus combined spinal epidural block for caesarean section. *Acta Anaesthesiol Scand* 1988;32:595.
140. Rawal N, Schollin J, Wesström G. Epidural versus combined spinal epidural block for cesarean section. *Acta Anaesthesiol Scand* 1988; 32:61.
141. Stienstra R, Dahan A, Alhadi BZR, van Kleep JW, Burm AGL. Mechanism of action of an epidural top-up in combined spinal epidural anesthesia. *Anesth Analg* 1996;83:382.
142. Blumgart CH, Ryall D, Dennison B, Thompson-Hill LM. Mechanism of extension of spinal anaesthesia by extradural injection of local anaesthetic. *Br J Anaesth* 1992;69:457.
143. Swenson JD, Wisniewski M, McJames S, Ashburn MA, Pace NL. The effect of prior dural puncture on cisternal cerebrospinal fluid morphine concentrations in sheep after administration of lumbar epidural morphine. *Anesth Analg* 1996;83:523.
144. Leighton BL, Arkoosh VA, Huffnagle S, Huffnagle HJ, Kinsella SM, Norris MC. The dermatomal spread of epidural bupivacaine with and without prior intrathecal sufentanil. *Anesth Analg* 1996;83:526.
145. Gupta A, Enlund G, Bengtsson M, Sjberg F. Spinal anaesthesia for caesarean section following epidural analgesia in labour: a relative contraindication. *Int J Obstet Anesth* 1994;3:153.
146. Furst SR, Reisner LS. Risk of high spinal anesthesia following failed epidural block for cesarean delivery. *J Clin Anesth* 1995;7:71.
147. Mets B, Broccoli E, Brown AR. Is spinal anesthesia after failed epidural anesthesia contraindicated for cesarean section. *Anesth Analg* 1993;77:629.
148. Vickers R, Wilkey A. Spinal anaesthesia for caesarean section. *Br J Anaesth* 1996;77:301.
149. Stoneham M, Souter A. Spinal anesthesia for caesarean section in women with incomplete extradural analgesia. *Br J Anaesth* 1996; 77:301.
150. Mets B. Spinal anesthesia after failed epidural anesthesia. *Anesth Analg* 1996;82:214.
151. Bromage PR. *Epidural analgesia.* Philadelphia: WB Saunders, 1978: 638.
152. Gupta A. Spinal anesthesia after failed epidural anesthesia. *Anesth Analg* 1996;82:214.

Obstetric Anesthesia, second edition,
edited by Mark C. Norris.
Lippincott Williams & Wilkins, Philadelphia © 1999.

CHAPTER 23

Anesthesia and Cardiac Disease

David Anthony Rocke and C. C. Rout

Maternal cardiac disease complicates 1% to 2% of pregnancies and is a significant cause of maternal mortality (1). The Report on Confidential Enquiries Into Maternal Deaths in the United Kingdom 1991–1993 (2) recorded 41 deaths (including four late deaths) due to cardiac disease, approximately twice the number recorded in each of the previous two triennia. This increase was due mostly to more acquired heart disease (27 cases) including nine cases of ruptured thoracic aortic aneurysm. Migration from developing countries is maintaining the number of cases of rheumatic heart disease. In developed countries, the prevalence of ischemic heart disease in women in the reproductive age group appears to be increasing. Both factors may increase the importance of heart disease as a cause of maternal mortality. Areas of substandard care highlighted by the U.K. report included delay in referral to senior and specialist help, inadequate cooperation between specialists involved in patient care, and a perceived reluctance to perform chest radiographs in pregnancy.

GENERAL CONSIDERATIONS

Because of the increased risks associated with labor and delivery and operative delivery in these patients, it is essential that the obstetric anesthesiologist be involved as early as possible in their care. A plan of analgesic and anesthetic management should be made in consultation with all specialist care providers, clearly documented, and kept under repeated review during the antenatal course.

The cardiac work demanded by pregnancy (Chapter 1) and the hemodynamic instability of labor and delivery increase the maternal risk from anesthetic intervention. The obstetric anesthesiologist faces two principal concerns:

- Can epidural analgesia be safely used for labor and delivery?
- What is the safest method of providing anesthesia for cesarean section? (A debate that usually devolves to a choice between epidural and general anesthesia.)

Regional Anesthesia

Women with most cardiac lesions withstand the hemodynamic effects of a carefully conducted epidural block better than the hemodynamic effects of a labor and delivery without the benefit of effective analgesia.

Patients with valvular stenosis or right-to-left intracardiac shunts may not tolerate the high sympathetic block associated with epidural anesthesia for cesarean delivery. Even women with regurgitant valvular lesions that normally improve with epidural analgesia may not withstand a poorly conducted block (3). Whatever the circumstances, induce epidural blockade by using incremental doses of drug. Monitor the hemodynamic response to block closely. Epidural or spinal opiates can provide excellent analgesia for the first stage of labor and avoid the deleterious effects of sympathetic blockade; however, neuraxial opioids alone rarely provide adequate analgesia for the second stage of labor. They also do not ensure sufficient pain relief for operative delivery. Saddle block (single injection spinal or via intrathecal catheter) or a caudal/epidural can be effective for second-stage analgesia.

Systemic Analgesia for Labor

The most common contraindication to epidural anesthesia in the parturient with cardiac disease is anticoagulant therapy (see Chapter 24). Maternal anticoagulation precludes major conduction analgesia. In these cases, if the patient cannot withstand the hemodynamic effects of labor and delivery without epidural analgesia, it is best to proceed to elective cesarean section under general anesthesia. If the patient is going to labor, the standard regi-

D. A. Rocke and C. C. Rout: Department of Anesthesiology, University of Natal, Durban, South Africa.

men of intermittent intramuscular meperidine provides neither adequate analgesia nor cardiovascular stability. In this circumstance, we recommend a continuous intravenous infusion of alfentanil. Start the drug in early labor with a loading dose of 30 μg/kg over 10 minutes. Then begin an infusion of 1 μg/kg/min. This technique can provide excellent analgesia for the first stage of labor. Additional bolus doses may be required for the second stage. The neonate should receive intravenous naloxone, if necessary on delivery, and be observed closely in a neonatal unit for the first 12 hours of life.

General Anesthesia

An important consideration when planning a general anesthetic is maternal cardiovascular stability. The rapid-sequence induction recommended in obstetric anesthesia induces a profound adrenergic response; however, this reaction can be modified without compromising maternal safety. We find that giving alfentanil, 30 μg/kg, and then etomidate, 0.3 mg/kg, and succinylcholine, 1 mg/kg, usually obtunds the pressor response to intubation. After delivery, most infants have respiratory depression with this dose of alfentanil. They respond promptly to intravenous naloxone. The infant should be observed closely in the neonatal unit and further naloxone given if necessary. Use the inhalational agent most appropriate to the patient's cardiac lesion for maintenance of anesthesia. Avoid nitrous oxide because it increases pulmonary vascular resistance. After delivery, supplemental opiates safely deepen maternal anesthesia. Vecuronium remains an appropriate nondepolarizing muscle relaxant.

Monitoring

Take maximal advantage of noninvasive methods of cardiovascular monitoring. In addition, we recommend central venous pressure monitoring in all but the most trivial cases. In the more severe lesions, we use systemic and pulmonary artery catheters. Continue monitoring into the postdelivery period, if necessary in a critical care unit. The greatest risk of circulatory overload arises during the first 48 hours after delivery as the contracted uterus displaces blood into the systemic circulation. If using epidural anesthesia, continue injecting local anesthetics so that the receding sympathetic block does not compound the increase in blood volume.

Vasoactive Drugs

Exercise caution in the use of vasopressors and oxytoxic agents. Consider using a pure constrictor, such as phenylephrine, in patients with stenotic valvular lesions. Patients with regurgitant valvular lesions or poor left ventricular function should respond better to an agent with inotropic activity, such as ephedrine. If an oxytocic agent is necessary, then an infusion of synthetic oxytocin is best. Avoid bolus doses because significant, albeit transient, systemic hypotension can occur. Ergot alkaloids cause a sustained increase in systemic vascular resistance.

β-Blockers are increasingly used in pregnancy, particularly in the management of mitral stenosis. These drugs may cause intrauterine growth retardation and loss of beat-to-beat variability in the fetus, and bradycardia and hypoglycemia in the neonate (4). However, their use can prevent pulmonary edema in patients with mitral stenosis and decreases the need for closed mitral valvotomy during pregnancy (5). β-Blockers do not contraindicate incremental epidural anesthesia; however, be careful with the high block required for cesarean delivery. Significant bradycardia is possible, and the heart's ability to respond to decreased afterload is impaired.

Antibiotic Prophylaxis

Antibiotic prophylaxis against bacterial endocarditis is necessary for both vaginal and operative deliveries in all patients with valvular or congenital lesions or previous cardiac surgery. The appropriate agents should provide gram-positive and gram-negative coverage.

Other Considerations

Patients with cardiac disease are more vulnerable to the effects of obstetric complications should they occur. Pay particular attention to avoiding aortocaval compression. Give an effective antacid before general anesthesia.

VALVULAR HEART DISEASE

Mitral Stenosis

Of the isolated valvular lesions seen in pregnancy, mitral stenosis is the most common. It also is the dominant lesion in most cases of mixed mitral valve disease. Hemodynamically, it should be regarded as a fixed obstruction to left ventricular filling. Although the maternal mortality during pregnancy is 1%, this risk may increase to 14% to 17% in patients who develop atrial fibrillation (6).

Life-threatening pulmonary edema can develop with remarkable speed in women with previously asymptomatic mitral stenosis. This situation is most likely in immigrants from the developing world who may be unaware that they have heart disease (7). Balloon dilatation has proven successful after failed medical therapy if the valve is pliable with no or minimal regurgitation (8–16). In two published cases (16), patients were able to discontinue medication and deliver vaginally after balloon valvuloplasty. An advantage of balloon valvuloplasty is that the risks to the fetus can be minimized by shielding of the abdomen and pelvis. The use of transesophageal echocardiography shortens fluoroscopic time (9,14).

Evaluation

On examination, determine the New York Heart Association (NYHA) functional classification (Chapter 2) and exclude remediable exacerbating features such as anemia, infection, and tachycardia. Review the patient's medications. Look for features of severe disease (i.e., an opening snap within 80 msec of the second heart sound and features of pulmonary hypertension). The electrocardiogram (EKG) may show atrial fibrillation or, if sinus rhythm, a broad notched P wave in lead II (P mitrale). Evidence of right ventricular hypertrophy on EKG suggests pulmonary hypertension. Radiographic findings in the chest include a straight left-heart border, left atrial enlargement, and Kerley's B lines. Upper-lobe blood diversion is a common finding in pregnancy and is not a helpful sign. Echocardiography will exclude other valvular lesions and allow assessment of left ventricular function (invariably good in isolated mitral stenosis, but decreased in a few patients with mixed valvular lesions). Direct measurement or Doppler flow studies across the valve can provide objective assessment of mitral valve area.

Anesthesia and Analgesia

Avoid maternal tachycardia. The pressure gradient across the valve is inversely proportional to the square of the diastolic filling time (17). A small increase in heart rate (decreased diastolic filling time) will therefore cause a marked increase in left atrial pressure. β-Blockers can control heart rate. Consider starting this therapy in patients with good left ventricular function who are not taking long-term β-blockers.

Use epidural block for labor analgesia unless it is specifically contraindicated. The venous dilation caused by epidural local anesthetics helps attenuate the changes in venous volume associated with the contracting uterus. Do not give extra fluid before induction. Instead, infuse fluid as indicated by central volume status. Use at least a central venous catheter to assess volume status. Strongly consider pulmonary arterial catheterization in NYHA functional classes III and IV.

If epidural analgesia is contraindicated, NYHA functional classes I and II manage well with intermittent parenteral analgesia, provided maternal heart rate is kept under control. Meperidine is not the ideal agent because it may cause a tachycardia. For NYHA grades III and IV, intermittent analgesia is insufficient. In these cases, we recommend alfentanil by infusion.

For cesarean section, NYHA class I and II patients tolerate the higher epidural block required for operative delivery. Monitor cardiac preload and adjust as necessary. Even NYHA grades III and IV may fare better with epidural anesthesia. Although these patients do not tolerate any sudden reduction in cardiac afterload, they are often on the brink of pulmonary edema, with very high pulmonary arterial and venous pressures. Any sudden increase in afterload or heart rate (such as after intubation) may precipitate pulmonary edema and necessitate postoperative intensive respiratory care with mechanical ventilation. The venodilation produced by slow incremental epidural anesthesia is of benefit. In this setting, pulmonary artery pressure must be monitored. Maintain adequate left ventricular preload during the onset of sympathetic blockade. Carefully avoid fluid overload.

If using a general anesthetic, obtund the adrenergic response to intubation with β-blockers, alfentanil, or both. Etomidate is the most suitable intravenous induction agent. Rocuronium may be a more suitable (combining cardiovascular stability with rapid onset) agent than suxamethonium. Maintain anesthesia with halothane or enflurane in air and oxygen. Avoid isoflurane, as it reduces systemic vascular resistance. Nitrous oxide can increase pulmonary artery pressure. After delivery, give a long-acting opiate.

These patients are at the greatest risk of pulmonary edema immediately postpartum. Blood volume expands as the uterus contracts and the vasodilator effects of regional blockade wear off. Because of the high incidence of pulmonary edema in the early postpartum period, we always give furosemide, 20 to 40 mg, intravenously with delivery of the placenta. Then we closely monitor the patient's volume status for the next 24 to 48 hours.

Mitral Regurgitation

Mitral regurgitation usually improves during pregnancy owing to the decreased systemic vascular resistance and increased blood volume. The key to anesthetic management is to encourage forward flow of blood. Reducing systemic vascular resistance, maintaining left ventricular filling pressure, and avoiding bradycardia help to achieve this goal. Epidural anesthesia with fluid preloading provides these conditions. It is the preferred anesthetic technique for both labor with vaginal delivery and cesarean section. Atrial fibrillation, requiring anticoagulant therapy, is comparatively common. If general anesthesia is required, try to avoid the pressor response to intubation and any myocardial depression. A vasodilator infusion may be a useful adjunct to anesthesia. In severe cases, an inotrope may be necessary. The usual monitoring considerations apply.

Mitral Valve Prolapse

The vast majority of patients with this common congenital lesion are asymptomatic and have trivial regurgitation. Decreases in left ventricular volume increase the degree of prolapse. Avoid volume depletion and tachycardia. Patients with significant or symptomatic regurgitation should be managed as for mitral regurgitation.

Mixed Mitral Valve Disease

Manage these patients according to the dominant lesion, as assessed by echocardiography. The combination of both significant stenosis and regurgitation may impair left ventricular function, in which case the patient will not tolerate β-blockade. Here, keep the heart rate between 80 and 100 beats/min by using digoxin. The benefits of epidural labor analgesia and the use of invasive monitoring were recently outlined by Sharma et al. (18).

Aortic Stenosis

Evaluation

This lesion is uncommon in pregnancy. Most patients develop symptoms beyond child-bearing age. Patients with aortic stenosis poorly tolerate any decrease in afterload or diastolic filling time; however, they also do not endure bradycardia well. Ability to compensate for any decrease in systemic vascular resistance by an increase in stroke volume is limited by the severity of the stenosis. Tachycardia may lead to ischemia and cardiac failure. Unlike mitral stenosis, absence of symptoms does not necessarily suggest mild disease. However, women who are asymptomatic before pregnancy, have a normal EKG, good left ventricular function, and who can achieve at least 7 MET on the treadmill without angina, a decrease in blood pressure, or ST-segment depression will have no trouble (19). All patients with aortic valve disease must have echocardiographic evaluation before delivery to assess the pressure gradient across the valve, valve area, and ventricular performance. This should include direct measurement of valve area. Pressure gradients (as assessed by Doppler) can be misleading, as they depend on flow. Doppler output velocity should increase during pregnancy if the left ventricle is coping. Therefore the severity of mild to moderate disease is usually overestimated by gradients during pregnancy. On the other hand, a low gradient does not necessarily imply mild disease and may reflect severely impaired left ventricular function. A decrease in Doppler velocity or the development of tachycardia, dyspnea, or angina is a danger signal. If these occur, hospital admission, bed rest, and β-blocker therapy are needed to provide diastolic time for coronary flow and left ventricular filling.

If possible the pregnancy should be kept going until the fetus is viable and delivered before dealing with the mother's valve. If required earlier, balloon valvulotomy may buy time but at the risk of creating substantial regurgitation (15,20). The valve area and systolic ejection time also should be considered (valve area less than 1 cm^2 implies severe disease; values less than 0.6 cm^2 are critical).

Anesthesia and Analgesia

In mild cases, epidural conduction blockade can be used for both vaginal and abdominal delivery. A continuous-infusion technique minimizes the hemodynamic changes associated with local anesthetic blockade. For severe cases, we recommend avoiding local anesthetic–induced sympathectomy. Neuraxial opioids or intravenous analgesia can be used for labor and delivery. General anesthesia is still probably the safest method for cesarean section in severe cases. Easterling et al. (21) reported the successful use of epidural conduction blockade in four patients with varied degrees of aortic stenosis. Only one of these patients had isolated aortic stenosis. The other three had associated moderate aortic regurgitation. Similarly a review of 25 pregnancies in 13 patients by Lao (22) included only five cases with aortic stenosis as the sole abnormality. Associated aortic regurgitation may not only artificially increase the aortic valve gradient but also tends to improve during conduction blockade.

The issue of regional versus general anesthesia for cesarean delivery was highlighted by two recent editorials (23,24) in relation to a case report of cesarean delivery performed by using a subarachnoid catheter technique (25). The patient reported had mild disease (pregnant transvalvar gradient of 57 mm Hg with good left ventricular function) and did well after incremental spinal anesthesia via a microcatheter, despite a transient predelivery decrease in systolic pressure to 70 mm Hg. The arguments for each method of anesthesia were clearly stated, with no definite conclusion. The most important elements to emerge were that patients should be identified early in pregnancy, assessed regularly throughout, and have a clearly documented management plan (23). Whereas symptomatic deterioration is an indication for intervention, symptoms alone cannot guide management (24).

Noninvasive monitoring is sufficient in mild cases, but for severe cases, we strongly recommend direct arterial pressure monitoring and a pulmonary artery catheter for perioperative fluid management. Avoid bolus injections of synthetic oxytocin. Use phenylephrine rather than ephedrine to treat hypotension that does not respond readily to volume. Whatever the method, the anesthesia should be conducted by an experienced anesthesiologist, well practiced in the techniques used.

Aortic Regurgitation

Any reduction in heart rate or increase in systemic vascular resistance can cause acute volume overload in a chronically distended left ventricle. The sympathetic block associated with epidural anesthesia reduces systemic vascular resistance and improves cardiac output. We recommend this technique for labor and cesarean delivery. If general anesthesia has to be used, consider a continuous vasodilator infusion. Avoid myocardial depression, and attempt to suppress the intubation response. Pulmonary artery catheters are not particularly useful for routine use because an increase in left atrial pressure occurs late in the disease process.

Hypertrophic Obstructive Cardiomyopathy (Idiopathic Hypertrophic Subaortic Stenosis)

This uncommon condition occurs in young people and may complicate pregnancy. Although it is hemodynamically and symptomatically similar to valvular aortic stenosis, the management is sufficiently different to warrant separate consideration. Like aortic stenosis, decreases in systemic vascular resistance are tolerated poorly. However, epinephrinergic stimulation (increased inotropy) and the Valsalva maneuver significantly increase the subvalvular obstruction. Pay close attention to maternal volume status. Use fluids to avoid decreases in left ventricular volume. Injudicious fluid therapy, however, may precipitate pulmonary edema. Tachycardia, which increases the obstruction, increases the risk of decompensation (26, 27). If hypotension develops, use a vasoconstrictor without inotropic activity (phenylephrine). As the obstruction to left ventricular outflow can increase rapidly, all patients should be monitored invasively, even if asymptomatic, with systemic and pulmonary artery catheters.

These patients benefit significantly from effective epidural analgesia for labor and delivery (28). Epidural block can prevent the effects of stress and pain on the outflow obstruction. Still, the extensive sympathetic block associated with epidural anesthesia for cesarean section is likely to prove hazardous. We prefer general anesthesia for abdominal delivery. Because most of these patients already will be receiving β-blockers, the addition of alfentanil to the induction sequence should successfully obtund the intubation response. Halothane is the most appropriate inhalational agent for maintenance of anesthesia. If the left ventricle fails, treat hypotension and tachycardia by using a vasopressor and propranolol. Inotropic therapy worsens the obstruction and is contraindicated.

Peripartum Cardiomyopathy

Peripartum cardiomyopathy is defined as the onset of left ventricular dilatation and congestive cardiac failure during the third trimester of pregnancy or in the first 6 months postpartum without obvious cause or prior evidence of cardiac disease (29). It has an incidence of between 1 in 3,000 (30) and 1 in 30,000 deliveries (31).

Although peripartum cardiomyopathy most commonly is seen in the second postpartum month, it may arise during cesarean section (32,33) or any time in the last trimester or first 6 months postpartum. Epidural analgesia is strongly indicated for labor and delivery. Decreased systemic vascular resistance improves cardiac output. For cesarean delivery, we also choose epidural anesthesia. Although opinions differ as to the optimal method of providing anesthesia, we recommend incremental lumbar epidural injection of local anesthetic with opioids (34).

These women need little or no additional volume before induction of regional block. If the cardiomyopathy is asymptomatic, a central venous pressure catheter is adequate with noninvasive blood pressure monitoring, but we suggest using a percutaneous catheter introducer to allow rapid insertion of a pulmonary artery catheter if needed (35). If cardiomyopathy is symptomatic or echocardiographic findings show severe left ventricular dysfunction, then a pulmonary artery catheter and arterial line should be inserted.

Some patients are taking anticoagulants because of the possibility of mural thrombosis. For general anesthesia, avoid increases in afterload and negative inotropic agents. Use invasive monitors. Isoflurane or desflurane would be the inhalational agents of choice. Consider the use of a vasodilator infusion, and have inotropic support available.

Two recent articles discussed specific problems associated with peripartum cardiomyopathy. Connelly et al. (37) described a case of pregnancy and delivery in a patient with recent peripartum cardiomyopathy, and Hawthorne and Lyons (34) described a case of cardiac arrest complicating spinal anesthesia for cesarean section in a women with undiagnosed dilated cardiomyopathy. The availability of cardiac transplantation has improved the outlook for those with persistent dysfunction (38–40).

ARRHYTHMIAS

Any disturbance of cardiac rhythm should be treated promptly. Supraventricular arrhythmias are particularly problematic in patients with rheumatic heart disease and occur commonly in mitral valve disease. Atrial fibrillation occurring during pregnancy may increase the maternal mortality rate to as high as 19% (41). Patients with chronic atrial fibrillation should be taking digoxin or propranolol to control ventricular rate. They also may be using anticoagulants to prevent thromboembolic complications.

Sudden onset of atrial fibrillation or supraventricular tachycardia with severe cardiac compromise should be treated by direct-current cardioversion. This therapy often is best done in the operating room under general anesthesia, with the usual precautions. Energy discharges of approximately 1 watt/s/kg usually suffice. Although transient fetal arrhythmias may occur, cardioversion during pregnancy does not adversely affect mother or child (42).

PREVIOUS VALVE REPLACEMENT

Increasing numbers of patients are seen in pregnancy with a history of valve replacement. Usually, these patients are hemodynamically corrected and do not cause many problems if the valve prosthesis is working properly. However, pulmonary hypertension and atrial fibrillation may persist after mitral valve replacement. Stenosis of tissue valves and perivalvular regurgitation should be excluded, and ventricular function should be assessed before anesthesia.

Anticoagulant Therapy

The use of anticoagulants is the most common problem in patients with mechanical prostheses. This therapy may contraindicate epidural anesthesia. The practice in our unit is to use intravenous heparin during the first trimester (when possible) and during the 2 weeks before delivery, with oral warfarin during the intervening weeks. Planned vaginal or operative delivery allows heparin therapy to be stopped the evening before and recommenced 3 to 24 hours after delivery (43,44). A 12-hour delay after the last heparin dose usually ensures normal coagulation. Even so, check partial thromboplastin time and platelet count before beginning a major conduction anesthetic. Patients receiving low-molecular-weight heparin (LMWH) may be at greater risk of bleeding complications. Here, LMWH should be stopped 24 hours before planned delivery and not restarted until 24 hours postpartum.

Antiplatelet agents alone are ineffective anticoagulants (45). But they are occasionally used as an adjunct to subcutaneous heparin. If this is the case, platelet function also should be assessed.

Although the exact safety margin is uncertain, the epidural catheter should be removed as soon as it is no longer needed and well before restarting the anticoagulant therapy. Epidural hematoma has been described after catheter removal in a patient receiving anticoagulant therapy (46).

If a patient is in labor while receiving anticoagulant therapy, protamine can reverse the effects of heparin. The patient taking warfarin should receive fresh frozen plasma to prevent hemorrhagic complications. However, the baby will remain anticoagulated and often is delivered by urgent cesarean section to avoid the trauma of vaginal delivery. This operation should be done under general anesthesia if time does not permit confirmation of anticoagulant reversal in the mother and induction of regional block. Remember, however, that maternal blood loss can be managed as it occurs, whereas there are limited options for a thrombosed valve or thromboembolism.

PREVIOUS HEART TRANSPLANTATION

There have been a number of successful pregnancies after heart or heart–lung transplantation. The main issues relate to immunosuppression, which may need to be adjusted during pregnancy because of increased drug clearance, and the problems of the denervated heart. Resting heart rate is increased because of absent vagal tone, and indirectly acting agents will have no effect on heart rate. Upregulation of β-adrenergic receptors may increase sensitivity to directly acting agents (39). As the heart-rate effects of anesthetics are sympathetically mediated, they will not occur in the denervated heart. Direct myocardial-depressant effects will dominate.

Pregnancies tend to be complicated, with a high incidence of premature labor and pregnancy-associated hypertension (47). Epidural analgesia is not contraindicated, but preload must be maintained.

PRIMARY PULMONARY HYPERTENSION

Primary pulmonary hypertension in combination with pregnancy carries an extremely high maternal mortality rate of 60% (48). Wherever possible, these patients should be advised not to become pregnant. Management includes early admission and hospitalization beginning around 28 weeks of gestation. A team approach is essential.

Evaluation

Assessment of the severity of the disease includes a history, clinical examination, EKG, and chest radiograph to determine the presence of right ventricular dysfunction. Definitive assessment must be made by pulmonary artery catheter. A cardiac index less than 4.0 L/min/m^2, right atrial pressure greater than 10 mm Hg, or pulmonary vascular resistance greater than 1,000 dyne/s/cm^{-5} suggest an extremely poor prognosis. At the time of pulmonary artery catheterization, estimate the pharmacologic reversibility of the increased pulmonary vascular resistance (49,50). Drugs used to assess pulmonary vascular reactivity include prostacyclin (10 ng/kg/h), diltiazem (20 mg/h), and isoproterenol (0.4 mg/h). These drugs may decrease pulmonary vascular resistance and pulmonary artery pressure and increase cardiac output (50). However, a marked reduction in pulmonary vascular resistance is not the most common response, and the efficacy of pulmonary vasodilation appears to decrease as the pregnancy progresses.

After the initial hemodynamic assessment, the echocardiogram provides an ongoing estimate of systolic pulmonary artery pressure and atrial and ventricular size. Increasing right ventricular failure must be managed by bed rest, digitalis, and diuretics. Avoid hypoxia by the continuous administration of oxygen. Prophylactic low-dose heparin, 10,000 units twice a day, should be administered in the face of low cardiac output and bed rest.

Labor and Delivery

Vaginal delivery is preferable to cesarean section because the latter appears to lead to a poorer maternal outcome. Regardless of the mode of delivery, these women require intensive monitoring. Systemic and pulmonary artery catheters and continuous estimation of oxygen delivery by oximetry are essential. Associated tricuspid incompetence may make difficult the insertion of the pulmonary artery catheter. Anticipate the potential for severe bradycardia. Have atropine, isoproterenol, and transvenous pacing facilities available. Pay meticulous attention to blood loss to avoid hypovolemia. Any decrease in venous return to the heart aggravates the reduced right ventricular output owing to the obstruction presented by the pulmonary circulation. A decrease in right ventricular output, in turn, leads to hypoxia, which further increases pulmonary vascular resistance, creating a vicious cycle. Unless broken, this cycle leads to progressive ventricular failure, hypoxemia, and acidosis in both mother and fetus. Death ultimately follows.

Labor Analgesia

Epidural block, by using reduced doses of 3 to 5 mL 0.25% bupivacaine, provides first-stage analgesia. Using 5 mL of 0.5% bupivacaine in the sitting position ensures perineal second-stage anesthesia. Alternate techniques include the sole use of intrathecal morphine (51); however, such a technique may not be suitable for primipara or oxytocin-augmented labor. (Oxytocin causes severe increases in pulmonary vascular resistance and should be avoided, if possible.) Other techniques used include epidural infusion of dilute local anesthetic/opioid mixtures (52). Caudal analgesia, pudendal blocks, and dual epidural catheter techniques with one catheter directed caudally also have been used to provide second-stage analgesia (50).

Cesarean Delivery

For operative delivery, the balance of risk lies between the extensive sympathetic blockade associated with epidural anesthesia and the marked increase in pulmonary vascular resistance associated with laryngoscopy and tracheal intubation. Epidural anesthesia has been used successfully for cesarean section (53). The alternative would be balanced anesthesia by using etomidate for induction, vecuronium for muscle relaxation, and early intubation with fentanyl, 10 μg/kg, to modify the hemodynamic response. Isoflurane is the volatile agent of choice because it is associated with the least myocardial depression. Avoid hypoxia, hypercarbia, high intrathoracic pressures, and acidosis. Maintain maternal hypocapnia. Patients should be ventilated postoperatively with continued invasive monitoring.

Drugs to be avoided include ergometrine, oxytocin, prostaglandin $F_{2\alpha}$, ketamine, and nitrous oxide. If needed, use pulmonary vasodilators (sodium nitroprusside, nitroglycerin, prostaglandin E, isoproterenol), but monitor for systemic hypotension and arterial hypoxemia, negative inotropism, and fetal and uterine side effects. Use oxygen delivery as the therapeutic end point. Inotropic support (dopamine, up to 10 μg/kg/min, or dobutamine) may be required to improve right ventricular function. Increasing preload with volume loading is usually unsuccessful and may precipitate right ventricular ischemia.

MYOCARDIAL INFARCTION

Myocardial infarction is rare during pregnancy, with an estimated incidence of 1 in 10,000. The greatest frequency is in the third trimester in women older than 35 years (54). Overall maternal mortality approximates 37% to 50%. Mortality is increased if the infarct occurs in the third trimester, if the patient is younger than 35 years, if she delivers within 2 weeks of her infarct, and if she has a cesarean section. Recently, Webber et al. (55) reviewed the literature on myocardial infarction in pregnancy and presented a case with all four prognostically poor factors in whom emergency treatment in a cardiac catheterization laboratory with intracoronary thrombolysis and primary percutaneous transluminal coronary angioplasty (PTCA) of an occluded left anterior descending (LAD) coronary artery was successful. Intravenous tissue plasminogen activator also has been successfully used for acute myocardial infarction complicating the second trimester of pregnancy (56).

Pregnancy after myocardial infarction and coronary artery bypass grafting has been reported (57), as has coronary artery bypass surgery during pregnancy (58). In many cases, risk factors for coronary artery disease are obvious and angiography positive (59). However, not all cases of acute myocardial infarction have abnormal coronary angiography or positive pharmacologic provocation of coronary spasm (60). Because myocardial infarction is rare, clinicians should suspect associated disease, especially if hypertension is present (i.e., underlying pheochromocytoma) (61).

Normal electrocardiographic findings in pregnancy include reversible ST-, T-, and Q-wave changes. These aberrations can be differentiated from those indicating heart disease by echocardiographic assessment of ventricular wall motion. Peripartum EKG changes were recently reviewed (62,63).

There is no convincing argument for either cesarean or vaginal delivery in parturients with recent myocardial infarction (64). Vaginal delivery with epidural analgesia eliminates stress, reduces blood loss, provides hemodynamic stability, and allows early ambulation. However, we have to deal with the unpredictable course of labor and delivery. Cesarean delivery under epidural anesthesia eliminates the capriciousness of vaginal delivery, yet may be associated with greater blood loss and increased cardiopulmonary and metabolic demands. A two-catheter epidural technique for labor and vaginal delivery has been used successfully by using the upper catheter for the first stage of labor and the lower catheter for second-stage pain (65).

Predelivery assessment of the patient with previous or recent myocardial infarction should include Holter monitoring and exercise testing, if appropriate. In addition, two-dimensional echocardiography and radionuclide ventriculography can assess left ventricular function.

Patients with poor ventricular function require insertion of a pulmonary artery catheter to monitor cardiac function during labor and delivery. Nitroglycerin (0.5 μg/kg/min) may help provide coronary artery vasodilation. Carefully maintain diastolic pressure to allow subendocardial perfusion.

Use phenylephrine to treat hypotension associated with regional block. Ephedrine increases myocardial work owing to β-stimulation, and metaraminol is a potent coronary vasoconstrictor. Keep these patients in the lateral position. The reduction in uterine blood flow associated with any degree of aortocaval compression may release uterine renin. The subsequent production of angiotensin can yield coronary artery spasm (66).

CONGENITAL HEART DISEASE

Congenital heart disease is now more common in pregnancy because of the prolonged survival of children with these lesions (19).

Important factors to consider when planning to care for these women are that pediatric and adult cardiology have become increasingly subspecialized, and adult cardiologists may not be familiar with congenital heart disease. Patients who have had surgery to correct congenital heart disease may be asymptomatic and consider themselves cured. Pregnant women often prefer local care where experience is limited.

Most patients who are asymptomatic or barely symptomatic before pregnancy will be fine. The ability to tolerate pregnancy successfully depends primarily on the ability to increase stroke volume or to tolerate a reflex increase in heart rate. Women at particular risk are outlined in Table 1. Remember, the presence of congenital heart disease does not preclude superimposed preeclampsia or peripartum cardiomyopathy.

Initial diagnosis of a congenital lesion may sometimes occur at the antenatal clinic when a murmur, produced by the increased cardiac output, is heard. Most commonly, echocardiography will reveal an atrial septal defect, although restrictive ventricular septal defects, patent ductus arteriosus, pulmonary stenosis, and acyanotic Ebstein's anomaly may be found.

In general, if the patient wants children, pregnancy should not be delayed unless corrective surgery is planned. The heart disease can only get worse and the risks increase. Optimal management requires a team effort, and planning for delivery should include the anesthesiologist as an integral member of the team. The risk of pregnancy and the likelihood of a successful outcome must be determined individually. The literature does not provide categorical answers. Common sense and applied hemodynamic principles are most useful.

TABLE 1. *Pregnancy and congenital heart disease: women at particular risk*

Left-sided obstructive lesions
Pulmonary hypertension
Poor ventricular function
Potentially fragile aortas
Valve prostheses
Cyanosis

From ref. 19, with permission.

Left-to-Right Shunt

Atrial Septal Defect

Serious clinical manifestations do not usually occur until the fourth or fifth decade. Patients with an atrial septal defect who become pregnant and are asymptomatic without evidence of pulmonary hypertension or right ventricular failure require little additional management.

Use epidural analgesia for labor, vaginal delivery, and cesarean section. This technique avoids increases in systemic vascular resistance, which could increase left-to-right shunting. If a general anesthetic is required, take care to avoid exacerbating preexisting pulmonary hypertension. Patients with atrial septal defect are prone to supraventricular arrhythmias, which are poorly tolerated. Acute onset of supraventricular tachycardia in association with either hypotension or right ventricular failure should be managed with direct-current cardioversion or intravenous β-blockers. In less acute situations, patients should be digitalized. Usually, however, most patients with uncorrected atrial septal defect do not develop supraventricular arrhythmias until they are past child-bearing age.

In patients with repaired defects, blood loss can force left-to-right shunting, to the sudden detriment of left ventricular and coronary flow.

Ventricular Septal Defect

Patients with a small ventricular septal defect, no evidence of pulmonary hypertension, and who are asymptomatic tolerate pregnancy well and require no intervention. Examine those with a large ventricular septal defect to exclude respiratory infection, pulmonary hypertension, bacterial endocarditis, and ventricular failure.

Continuous lumbar epidural analgesia prevents marked increases in systemic vascular resistance due to pain. This technique is optimal for labor and vaginal delivery. Epidural anesthesia also is preferred for operative delivery. These patients do not tolerate increases in heart rate associated with endotracheal intubation. If using general anesthesia, we favor a balanced technique with opioids and inhalation agents.

Marked increases in systemic vascular resistance may require low-dose vasodilator therapy with either sodium nitroprusside or phentolamine. To counteract the development of a right-to-left shunt and hypoxemia, treat significant decreases in systemic vascular resistance with small doses of vasopressor.

Either of two mechanisms may incite peripheral cyanosis. An increase in the left-to-right shunt (due to increased systemic vascular resistance) may cause pulmonary edema. Volume overload, however, is an uncommon cause of pulmonary edema in the adult. More likely, the increased right ventricular workload leads to right ventricular failure and, ultimately, biventricular failure and pulmonary edema with a low cardiac output. Alternatively, an increase in pulmonary vascular resistance or a decrease in systemic vascular resistance may reverse interventricular flow (right-to-left shunt), increasing left ventricular output.

- If the patient becomes hypotensive and cyanosed with signs of increased cardiac output (warm peripheries, full pulse), she should be managed with 100% oxygen, lightening of depth of anesthesia, and small doses of a vasopressor until the blood pressure increases and the shunt reverts to left-to-right.
- Cyanosis accompanied by low cardiac output (poor peripheral perfusion, decreased urine output, increased central venous pressure) should be treated with 100% oxygen, inotropic support, and vasodilation.

Patent Ductus Arteriosus

This lesion is serious only if the patent ductus arteriosus is large and surgically uncorrected. Look for signs and symptoms of left or right ventricular failure, pulmonary hypertension, and shunt reversal. Treat asymptomatic patients with no evidence of ventricular dysfunction as normal. Use continuous epidural analgesia for labor and vaginal and operative delivery, but take care to avoid excessive reduction of systemic vascular resistance. When using general anesthesia, avoid changes in systemic vascular resistance and myocardial depressants.

Corrected Lesions

Successful pregnancy is possible after the Fontan operation (67). Increasing systemic venous pressure during pregnancy causes discomfort due to hepatic congestion and edema of the lower extremities. Atrial thrombosis is a major threat and some patients may need continuous anticoagulant therapy.

Ventricular function needs careful assessment after the Mustard and Senning operation for transposition, as eventually the right ventricle, which handles the systemic circulation, will fail. Successful pregnancy has been reported (68). The development of atrial arrhythmias, particularly flutter, can be a major problem.

Right-to-Left Shunt

Tetralogy of Fallot

Uncorrected tetralogy is associated with high maternal and fetal mortality. After surgical correction, only fetal mortality remains increased. For uncorrected women, the immediate postpartum period has the greatest risk of complications. Avoid decreases in systemic vascular resistance, blood volume, venous return, and myocardial depression. If possible, avoid epidural and spinal local anesthetics. However, epidural or spinal opioids may be useful. Alternatively, use a low-dose intravenous infusion of opioid. Manage any decline in systemic vascular resistance that exacerbates the right-to-left shunt with increased left lateral tilt and fluids. Vasopressors that increase pulmonary vascular resistance should be used judiciously.

General anesthesia is recommended for cesarean section. Maintain a slightly increased central venous pressure. An opioid-based technique avoids the myocardial depression caused by volatile agents. Patients with infundibular obstruction may decompensate in response to a decrease in right ventricular filling, a faster heart rate, or depressed myocardial contractility. Increased peripheral cyanosis usually indicates right ventricular outflow obstruction with increased right-to-left shunt. Give 100% oxygen and fluids, deepen the anesthetic, and eliminate any tachycardia with β-blockade.

Eisenmenger's Syndrome

Pulmonary hypertension threatens a pregnant woman's life whether associated with a central shunt in the Eisenmenger syndrome or when solitary as after previous closure of a nonrestrictive ventricular septal defect or arterial duct. Nothing has changed over the past thirty years (69,70), and laparoscopic sterilization under general anesthesia should be advised in all young women with Eisenmenger's syndrome (19). Patients who are first seen when pregnant should be told the risks and therapeutic abortion advised. Those who decide to continue their pregnancy should be admitted as soon as the resting oxygen saturation decreases, definitely before the end of the second trimester (19). Treatment includes bed rest, which minimizes right-to-left shunting and maximizes fetal growth, prophylactic heparin, nasal oxygen, continuous pulse oximetry, and careful fetal monitoring.

Maternal and fetal progress depend on the severity of the pulmonary hypertension. Maternal mortality ranges between 12% and 33%. The right-to-left shunt may be at the atrial, ventricular, or aortopulmonary level. Increases in pulmonary vascular resistance must be avoided (see section on primary pulmonary hypertension). Oxygen may reduce the peripheral vascular resistance as well as right-to-left shunt. Assess oxygen saturation both before and after oxygen therapy.

Decreases in systemic vascular resistance will result in a marked increase in right-to-left shunt and must be avoided. Sympathetic blockade with local anesthetics is contraindicated; however, first-stage analgesia can be provided by neuraxial opioids. Pollack (71) used 1.5 mg of subarachnoid morphine and carefully monitored for respiratory depression and apnea. Pudendal block provided second-stage analgesia. Because of the high incidence of thromboembolism, some patients may require a low-dose (45 IU/h) intravenous infusion of heparin throughout labor, precluding use of an epidural catheter.

Although first-stage analgesia has been provided by neuraxial opioids and second-stage analgesia by pudendal block, the most prudent method of delivery may be by cesarean section under general anesthesia with generous hydration, avoidance of systemic vasodilatation, and prompt replacement of blood loss.

Sadly, sudden death occurs all too often, and postmortem examination reveals no cause. Systemic vasodilation, bradycardia, and increasing right-to-left shunt usually precede cardiac arrest.

Monitoring should include EKG, S_aO_2, and central venous pressure. Avoid decreases in central venous pressure by administering fluids. Give supplementary oxygen. The use of a pulmonary artery catheter is controversial. The high risk of arrhythmias, thrombi, paradoxical emboli, pulmonary artery rupture, patent ductus arteriosus occlusion, and misleading data contraindicate its use. A decrease in oxygen saturation equates with an increase in right-to-left shunt. In the presence of a patent ductus arteriosus, right hand and foot saturations can be used simultaneously to monitor the degree of shunt, because blood flow to the right arm is predominantly preductal (71). Increases in heart rate and stroke volume increase right ventricular oxygen consumption. Right ventricular failure should be treated with inotropic support.

Potentially Fragile Aortas

Women with Marfan or Ehlers–Danlos syndromes face an increased risk of aortic dissection or rupture during pregnancy. β-Blockade should continue throughout pregnancy. Women with Marfan syndrome, whose aortic root is already dilated, or who have a family history of aortic rupture should be advised to delay pregnancy until after aortic root replacement. Resuspension of the aortic valve is usually possible and avoids the need for long-term anticoagulant treatment (72).

Coarctation of the Aorta

Coarctation of the aorta is a rare congenital vascular defect occurring in approximately one per 2,000 to 3,000 women. Only 2% of these cases involve the abdominal aorta, and maternal mortality approaches 4%, with death usually due to aortic rupture or dissection. Hypertension is a common associated feature, usually requiring β-blockade for control. Magnetic resonance imaging has been used as a safe and reliable means of confirming a clinically suspected coarctation during pregnancy (73). Echocardiography also should be performed to exclude bicuspid aortic valve and other cardiac lesions.

Maternal and fetal mortality and morbidity are not increased after surgical correction. Asymptomatic patients require no additional care. In uncorrected patients, avoid decreases in systemic vascular resistance, heart rate, and left ventricular filling, although survival to term pregnancy implies well-developed collateral flow.

Epidural anesthesia has not been recommended in the past because of the potential for bleeding into the epidural space as a result of enlarged collaterals. However, hard clinical evidence to support this stance is lacking. Neuraxial opioids can provide adequate analgesia and allow rapid detection of any compromise from an expanding hematoma. Alternatives include intravenous opioid infusion or inhalation analgesia.

For cesarean section, we currently recommend general anesthesia. Maintain heart rate, myocardial contractility, and vascular resistance. Manage maternal bradycardia by removing the precipitating cause and giving atropine or isoproterenol.

Congenital Aortic Stenosis

Anesthetic and hemodynamic considerations are similar to those for acquired aortic stenosis. In the developed world, the majority of cases of aortic stenosis are congenital in origin. Investigations should look for other associated lesions.

Congenital Pulmonary Stenosis

Asymptomatic patients with little right ventricular dysfunction require no additional intervention. In other women, avoid changes in right ventricular filling pressure, decreased heart rate, decreased systemic vascular resistance, and myocardial depressants. Epidural analgesia with local anesthetics should be used cautiously. Neuraxial or systemic opioids, inhalation agents, and pudendal blocks can be used for labor and vaginal delivery. If using epidural local anesthetics, carefully monitor central venous pressure and maintain systemic vascular resistance with ephedrine. General anesthesia is recommended for cesarean section. Sustain vascular resistance, heart rate, and myocardial contractility. Withdraw volatile agents, and give inotropic support for any evidence of right ventricular failure.

REFERENCES

1. Mangano DT. Anesthesia for the pregnant cardiac patient. In: Shnider SM, Levinson G, eds. *Anesthesia for obstetrics.* 2nd ed. Baltimore: Williams & Wilkins, 1987:345.

2. *Report on confidential enquiries into maternal deaths in the United Kingdom 1991-1993.* London: HMSO, 1996.
3. Alderson JD. Cardiovascular collapse following epidural anaesthesia for caesarean section in a patient with aortic incompetence. *Anaesthesia* 1987;42:643.
4. Renou P, Newman W, Wood C. Autonomic control of fetal heart rate. *Am J Obstet Gynecol* 1969;105:949.
5. Al Kasab SM, Sabag T, Al Zaibag M, et al. β-Adrenergic receptor blockade in the management of pregnant women with mitral stenosis. *Am J Obstet Gynecol* 1990;163:37.
6. Szekely P, Snaith L. Atrial fibrillation and pregnancy. *Br Med J* 1961;1:1407.
7. Oakley CM. Valvular disease in pregnancy. *Curr Opin Cardiol* 1996; 11:155.
8. Bahl VK, Chandra S, Mishra S. Concurrent balloon dilatation of mitral and tricuspid stenosis during pregnancy using an Inoue balloon. *Int J Cardiol* 1997;59:199.
9. Poirier P, Champagne J, Alain P, et al. Mitral balloon valvuloplasty in pregnancy: limiting radiation and procedure time by using transesophageal echocardiography. *Can J Cardiol* 1997;13:843.
10. Ben Farhat MB, Gamra H, Betbout F, et al. Percutaneous balloon mitral commissurotomy during pregnancy. *Heart* 1997;77:564.
11. Oto MA, Kabukcu M, Ovunc K, et al. Percutaneous balloon valvuloplasty for severe mitral stenosis in pregnancy: four case reports. *Angiology* 1997;48:463.
12. Dommisse J, Commerford PJ, Levetan B. Balloon valvuloplasty for severe mitral valve stenosis in pregnancy: a report of 11 cases. *S Afr Med J* 1996;86:1194.
13. Lau KW, Ding ZP, Lee CY, Koh TH, Gao W, Johan A. Technically demanding Inoue-balloon mitral commissurotomy: broadened indications for the procedure. *Singapore Med J* 1996;37:34.
14. Yaryura RA, Carpenter RJ Jr, Duncan JM, Wilansky S. Management of mitral valve stenosis in pregnancy: case presentation and review of the literature. *J Heart Valve Dis* 1996;5:16.
15. Presbitero P, Prever SB, Brusca A. Interventional cardiology in pregnancy. *Eur Heart J* 1996;17:182.
16. Onderoglu L, Tuncer ZS, Oto A, Durukan T. Balloon valvuloplasty during pregnancy. *Int J Gynaecol Obstet* 1995;49:181.
17. Gorlin R, Gorlin SG. Hydraulic formula for calculation of the area of the stenotic mitral valve, other cardiac valves and central circulatory shunts. *Am Heart J* 1951;41:1.
18. Sharma SK, Gambling DR, Gajraj NM, Truong C, Sidawi EJ. Anesthetic management of a parturient with mixed mitral valve disease and uncontrolled atrial fibrillation. *Int J Obstet Anesth* 1994;3:157.
19. Oakley CM. Pregnancy and congenital heart disease. *Heart* 1997; 78:12.
20. Banning AP, Pearson JF, Hall RJC. Role of balloon dilatation of the aortic valve in pregnant patients with severe aortic stenosis. *Br Heart J* 1993;70:544.
21. Easterling TR, Chadwick HS, Otto CM, Benedetti TJ. Aortic stenosis in pregnancy. *Obstet Gynecol* 1988;72:113.
22. Lao TT, Sermer M, MaGee L, Farine D, Colman JM. Congenital aortic stenosis and pregnancy—a reappraisal. *Am J Obstet Gynecol* 1993; 169:540.
23. Brighouse D. Anaesthesia for caesarean section in patients with aortic stenosis: the case for regional anaesthesia. *Anaesthesia* 1998;53:107.
24. Whitfield A, Holdcroft A. Anaesthesia for caesarean section in patients with aortic stenosis: the case for general anaesthesia. *Anaesthesia* 1998;53:109.
25. Pittard A, Vucevic M. Regional anaesthesia with a spinal microcatheter for caesarean section in a parturient with aortic stenosis. *Anaesthesia* 1998;53:169.
26. Tessler MJ, Hudson R, Naugler-Colville M, Biehl DR. Pulmonary oedema in two parturients with hypertrophic obstructive cardiomyopathy (HOCM). *Can J Anaesth* 1990;37:469.
27. Boccio RV, Chung JH, Harrison DM. Anesthetic management of cesarean section in a patient with idiopathic hypertrophic subaortic stenosis. *Anesthesiology* 1986;65:663.
29. Minnich ME, Quirk JG, Clark RB. Epidural anesthesia for vaginal delivery in a patient with idiopathic hypertrophic subaortic stenosis. *Anesthesiology* 1987;67:590.
30. Veille JC. Peripartum cardiomyopathies: a review. *Am J Obstet Gynecol* 1984;148:805.
31. Homans DC. Peripartum cardiomyopathy. *N Engl J Med* 1985;312:1432.
32. Lee W. Clinical management of gravid women with peripartum cardiomyopathy. *Obstet Gynecol Clin North Am* 1991;18:257.
33. Malinow AM, Butterworth JF IV, Johnson MD, et al. Peripartum cardiomyopathy presenting at cesarean delivery. *Anesthesiology* 1985; 63:545.
34. Hawthorne L, Lyons G. Cardiac arrest complicating spinal anaesthesia for caesarean section. *Int J Obstet Anesth* 1997;6:126.
35. Breen TW, Janzen JA. Pulmonary hypertension and cardiomyopathy: anaesthetic management for caesarean section. *Can J Anaesth* 1991; 38:895.
36. Gambling DR, Flanagan ML, Huckell VF, Lucas SB, Kim JH. Anaesthetic management and non-invasive monitoring for caesarean section in a patient with cardiomyopathy. *Can J Anaesth* 1987;34:505.
37. Connelly NR, Chin MT, Parker RK, Moran T, Fitzpatrick T. Pregnancy and delivery in a patient with recent peripartum cardiomyopathy. *Int J Obstet Anesth* 1998;7:38.
38. Ladwig P, Fischer E. Peripartum cardiomyopathy. *Aust N Z J Obstet Gynaecol* 1997;37:156.
39. Camann WR, Goldman GA, Johnson MD, Moore J, Greene M. Cesarean delivery of a patient with a transplanted heart. *Anesthesiology* 1989;71:618.
40. Carvalho AC, Almeida D, Cohen M, et al. Successful pregnancy, delivery and puerperium in a heart transplant patient with previous peripartum cardiomyopathy. *Eur Heart J* 1992;13:1589.
41. Mendelson CL. Disorders of the heartbeat during pregnancy. *Am J Obstet Gynecol* 1956;72:1268.
42. Klepper I. Cardioversion in late pregnancy. *Anaesthesia* 1981;36:611.
43. Gothard JWW. Heart disease in pregnancy. *Anaesthesia* 1978;33:523.
44. Saka DM, Marx GF. Management of a parturient with cardiac valve prosthesis. *Anesth Analg* 1976;55:214.
45. Oakley C. Valve prostheses and pregnancy. *Br Heart J* 1987;58:303.
46. Varkey GP, Brindle GF. Peridural anaesthesia and anticoagulant therapy. *Can Anaesth Soc J* 1974;21:106.
47. Wagoner LE, Taylor DO, Olsen SL, et al. Immunosuppressive therapy, management, and outcome of heart transplant recipients during pregnancy. *J Heart Lung Transplant* 1993;12:993.
48. Roberts NV, Keast PJ. Pulmonary hypertension and pregnancy—a lethal combination. *Anaesth Intens Care* 1990;18:366.
49. Simonneau G, Herve P, Escouttou P, Baudriun C, Nebout T, Durouz P. Short- and long-term effects of vasodilators in primary pulmonary hypertension: predictive value of prostacyclin acute infusion [Abstract]. *J Crit Care* 1986;1:117.
50. Slomka F, Salmeron S, Zetlaoui P, Cohen H, Simonneau G, Samii K. Primary pulmonary hypertension and pregnancy: anesthetic management for delivery. *Anesthesiology* 1988;69:959.
51. Abboud TK, Raya J, Noueihed R, Daniel J. Intrathecal morphine for relief of labor pain in a parturient with severe pulmonary hypertension. *Anesthesiology* 1983;59:477.
52. Robinson DE, Leicht CH. Epidural analgesia with low-dose bupivacaine and fentanyl for labor and delivery in a parturient with severe pulmonary hypertension. *Anesthesiology* 1988;68:285.
53. Roessler P, Lambert TF. Anaesthesia for caesarean section in the presence of primary pulmonary hypertension. *Anaesth Intens Care* 1986; 14:317.
54. Hankins GD, Wendel GDV Jr, Leveno KJ, Stoneham J. Myocardial infarction during pregnancy: a review. *Obstet Gynecol* 1985;65:139.
55. Webber MD, Halligan RE, Schumacher JA. Acute infarction, intracoronary thrombolysis, and primary PTCA in pregnancy. *Cathet Cardiovasc Diagn* 1997;42:38.
56. Schumacher B, Belfort MA, Card RJ. Successful treatment of acute myocardial infarction during pregnancy with tissue plasminogen activator. *Am J Obstet Gynecol* 1997;176:716.
57. Dufour P, Berard J, Vinatier D, et al. Pregnancy after myocardial infarction and a coronary artery bypass graft. *Arch Gynecol Obstet* 1997; 259:209.
58. Silberman S, Fink D, Berko RS, Mendzelevski B, Bitran D. Coronary artery bypass surgery during pregnancy. *Eur J Cardiothorac Surg* 1996; 10:925.
59. Makkonen M, Hietakorpi S, Orden MR, Saarikoski S. Myocardial infarction during pregnancy. *Eur J Obstet Gynecol Reprod Biol* 1995; 58:81.
60. Fujito T, Inoue T, Mizoguchi K, et al. Acute myocardial infarction during pregnancy. *Cardiology* 1996;87:361.
61. Hamada S, Hinokio K, Naka O, Higuchi K, Takahashi H, Sumitani H.

Myocardial infarction as a complication of pheochromocytoma in a pregnant woman. *Eur J Obstet Gynecol Reprod Biol* 1996;70:197.

62. Palmer CM. Maternal electrocardiographic changes in the peripartum period. *Int J Obstet Anesth* 1994;3:63.
63. Burton A, Camann W. Electrocardiographic changes during cesarean section: a review. *Int J Obstet Anesth* 1996;5:47.
64. Aglio LS, Johnson MD. Anaesthetic management of myocardial infarction in a parturient. *Br J Anaesth* 1990;65:258.
65. Laughlin MP, From RF, Choi W. Recent myocardial infarction in a parturient: discussion of risk, delivery alternative, and choice of anesthesia. *Anesthesiol Rev* 1986;13:43.
66. Sasse L, Wagner R, Murray FE. Transmural myocardial infarction during pregnancy. *Am J Cardiol* 1975;35:448.
67. Canobbio MM, Mair D. Pregnancy outcome following Fontan operation. *Circulation* 1993;88:1.
68. Clarkson PM, Wilson NJ, Neutze JM, North RA, Calder AL, Barratt-Boyes BG. Outcome of pregnancy after the mustard operation for transposition of the great arteries with intact ventricular septum. *J Am Coll Cardiol* 1994;24:190.
69. Morgan Jones A, Howitt G. Eisenmenger syndrome in pregnancy. *BMJ* 1965;I:1627.
70. Avila WS, Grinberg M, Snitcowsky R, et al. Maternal and fetal outcome in pregnant women with Eisenmenger's syndrome. *Eur Heart J* 1995;16:460.
71. Pollack KL, Chestnut DH, Wenstrom KD. Anesthetic management of a parturient with Eisenmenger's syndrome. *Anesth Analg* 1990;70:212.
72. Child A. Management of pregnancy in Marfan syndrome, Ehlers-Danlos syndrome and the other heritable connective tissue diseases. In: Oakley C, ed. *Heart disease in pregnancy.* London: BMJ Publishing Group, 1997:153.
73. Dizon-Townson D, Magee KP, Twickler DM, Cox SM. Coarctation of the abdominal aorta in pregnancy: diagnosis by magnetic resonance imaging. *Obstet Gynaecol* 1995;85:817.

Obstetric Anesthesia, second edition,
edited by Mark C. Norris.
Lippincott Williams & Wilkins, Philadelphia © 1999.

CHAPTER 24

Anesthesia and Hematologic Disease

C. E. P. Orlikowski and David Anthony Rocke

Hematologic problems facing the obstetric anesthesiologist are most commonly those of anemia and coagulation defects. In the woman with chronic anemia, we must understand the physiologic consequences of decreased oxygen delivery and the effects of her underlying disease. As the risks of transfusion are increasingly recognized, blood must only be offered after careful consideration of the needs of the individual, rather than based solely on laboratory values.

Problems of coagulation usually involve the amount or function of platelets and clotting factors. The greatest, and yet unresolved, problem is the relation between platelet count and the safe use of regional anesthesia.

The purpose of this chapter is to provide some guidelines for the clinician faced with providing anesthetic care for these complicated parturients.

PATHOLOGIC ANEMIA IN PREGNANCY

Anemia, defined as a hemoglobin (Hb) concentration less than 11.0 g/dL, is due to an absolute reduction in red cell mass rather than a dilutional effect and is very common in pregnancy (Table 1). In pregnancy, maternal 2,3-diphosphoglycerate (2,3-DPG) increases, and the oxygen hemoglobin dissociation curve shifts to the right to increase oxygen availability to the fetus (1). Mild anemia poses little risk to mother and fetus (2). Fetal oxygen consumption is reduced only in severe anemia or in the presence of placental problems.

Indications and Risks of Blood Transfusion

There is no set minimum Hb concentration for labor, vaginal delivery, or cesarean section. In a retrospective analysis of 1,166 patients undergoing cesarean section, only 1.1% were transfused (3). This number would be halved if the Red Cross recommended minimum Hb of 7 g/dL were used to assess transfusion requirements.

Indications for the transfusion of red blood cells should be based on the clinical condition of the patient, not the use of a transfusion trigger, based on an arbitrary Hb level. A higher Hb may be required in hypermetabolic states such as sepsis or poor oxygen-delivery states such as heart failure or myocardial ischemia. Animal studies and observation in postoperative patients indicate that tissue repair is not adversely affected until a Hb of 5 g/dL or less (4). We do not transfuse patients with a hemoglobin concentration greater than 7 g/dL without cardiorespiratory symptoms. This hemoglobin concentration easily provides the oxygen needs of the body (5).

Transfusion of blood and blood products carries a small but definite risk of disease transmission (Table 2). Concern has been raised about the possibility of transmission of Creutzfeldt–Jakob disease (CJD). Buffy coat cells from the peripheral blood of patients with CJD inoculated into the brains of rodents resulted in spongiform degeneration (6). The absence of any documented cases in humans may reflect the long incubation period.

Anesthetic Concerns in the Anemic Patient

During anesthesia, always maintain plasma volume. Regional anesthesia is associated with sympathetic block-

TABLE 1. *Differential diagnosis of anemia in pregnancy*

Dilutional
Iron deficiency
Folate and/or B_{12} deficiency
Hemoglobinopathies
HELLP syndrome
Aplastic anemia or pure red cell aplasia
Paroxysmal nocturnal hemoglobinuria
Hematologic malignancies

From ref. 2, with permission.

C. E. P. Orlikowski: Department of Anesthesiology, King Edward Memorial Hospital for Women, Perth, Australia.
D. A. Rocke: Department of Anesthesiology, University of Natal, Durban, South Africa.

TABLE 2. *Current risk of transfusion-transmitted infections (per unit infused)*

Disease	Risk
Hepatitis A	Rare
Hepatitis B	1/66,000–1/200,000
Hepatitis C	1/120,000
Hepatitis G	Unknown
HIV-1	1/563,000–1/825,000
Bacterial contamination	
Platelets	1/2,400
RBC	?–1/1,000,000
Malaria	1/4,000,000
Cytomegalovirus	Variable

From ref. 102, with permission.

ade and vasodilation. Epidural block, with a more gradual onset of sympathetic blockade than spinal anesthesia, allows easier control of blood pressure with fluids and vasopressors. Transfusion is indicated in patients receiving general anesthesia with preoperative hemoglobins of less than 7 g/dL (7). Monitor both end-tidal carbon dioxide, to prevent respiratory alkalosis, and temperature, to avoid hypothermia.

Postoperative management of the severely anemic patient includes oxygen and prevention of shivering. Shivering can increase oxygen consumption by 35% to 40% (8). Adequate oxygen-carrying capacity to maintain cardiopulmonary function can be met by a hemoglobin of 7 g/dL (equivalent to a hematocrit of 21%) when intravascular volume is adequate (9). Despite a lower hematocrit (23%), nontransfused patients have similar lengths of hospital stay and incidences of postoperative infection and wound complications compared with transfused patients with higher hematocrits (28%) (10). It is acceptable to discharge asymptomatic patients to home with Hb of 7 g/dL and adequate oral therapy (1).

Erythropoietin (EPO)

Maternal EPO increases substantially during normal pregnancy, and at term, plasma concentration is 2 to 4 times higher than in nonpregnant and nonanemic controls (11). In the fetus, EPO also is the major regulator of erythropoiesis, but regulation of erythropoiesis takes place independently in the two circulations because the placenta forms a barrier to both endogenous and recombinant EPO.

The use of recombinant human EPO (rHuEPO) has been described to treat effectively the anemia associated with renal failure in pregnancy (12). rHuEPO with intravenous iron also has been used to treat iron-deficiency anemia during pregnancy (11). Treatment with rHuEPO may be associated with some serious side effects:

- Seizures in a small percentage of patients,
- A tendency to thrombotic events associated with increased fibrinogen and improved platelet function, and
- Development or worsening of hypertension (12).

However, erythropoietin therapy for the treatment of long-term anemia or to avoid recurrent transfusions is probably a viable alternative in pregnant patients.

Autologous blood transfusion may be safely used during pregnancy (4). No serious fetal effects were noted during autologous blood donation in 272 pregnant blood donors (13). Indications might include the management of placenta previa or accreta or elective cesarean hysterectomy. However, the low rate of transfusion seen in cesarean section patients (1.1%) makes it hard to justify a routine policy of autologous donation (3).

Iron-deficiency Anemia in Pregnancy

Iron deficiency is the commonest cause of anemia in pregnancy (1). It is characterized by hypochromic and microcytic red cells with a blunted reticulocyte response (2). Treatment in most cases is with oral iron, and early treatment may reduce the need for later transfusion (1). Rarely, with severe deficiency, intramuscular or intravenous iron may be necessary. Intravenous iron may cause anaphylaxis (2).

Megaloblastic Anemia Due to Folate Deficiency in Pregnancy

Folate deficiency is the most common cause of macrocytic anemia in pregnancy (2). Folate deficiency may be associated with premature births, and severe and prolonged deficiency may lead to neural tube defects and development of cleft palate in the fetus (2). Folate deficiency is easily diagnosed by a peripheral smear, which usually shows large hypersegmented polymorphonuclear leukocytes. Folate is usually supplemented routinely during pregnancy, but the dose may need to be increased in the setting of exaggerated folate consumption such as sickle cell disease (2). Severe vitamin B_{12} deficiency is very rare, as it leads to sterility, and the needs of pregnancy are easily met by the large body stores of this vitamin.

Sickle Cell Anemia

This is an inherited disorder with a structurally abnormal β-globin chain of the hemoglobin molecule. Sickle hemoglobinopathies can be classified into major or minor disorders (Table 3). The most common sickle cell disorder is the heterozygous form of hemoglobin S (HbAS), which occurs in one in 12 adult African Americans (14). The most common major sickle hemoglobinopathy is the homozygous form, hemoglobin S (HbSS), with an incidence of one in 625 African Americans (14). Individuals who are heterozygous for hemoglobin C and hemoglobin S (HbSC) manifest a major clinical syndrome similar to HbSS and have a similar incidence (14). HbS, when combined with β-thalassemia, is called HbS β-thal and may be clinically significant. HbSS, HbSC, and HbS β-thal account for the majority of sickle cell disease (SCD) (14).

TABLE 3. *Classification of sickle hemaglobinopathies*

Minor disorders
Sickle cell trait (Hb AS)
Hemoglobin C trait (Hb AC)
Hemoglobin C disease (Hb CC)
Hemoglobin SE disease (Hb SE)
Hemoglobin SD disease (Hb SD)
Hemoglobin S-Memphis (Hb S-Memphis)
Major disorders
Sickle cell anemia (Hb SS)
Hemoglobin SC disease (Hb SC)
Hemoglobin S β-thalassemia (HB S β-Thal)

From ref. 14, with permission.

The additional physiologic demands of pregnancy increase the frequency of complications of SCD (Table 4). Perinatal mortality rates in the United Kingdom are 4 to 6 times those of women with SCD, and the maternal mortality rate is estimated at 2.5% (15).

Sickle Cell Crisis

Almost all the signs and symptoms of sickle cell anemia are the result of hemolysis, vasooclusive crisis, and increased susceptibility to infection (14). The sudden onset of the clinical manifestations associated with SCD is known as sickle cell crisis, which is most often caused by vasooclusive disease. Symptoms of vasooclusive crisis include recurring attacks of pain involving the skeleton, chest, and abdomen and occur as a result of sickling in the microcirculation. Antenatal crises have been reported in 35% of affected parturients (16), with an increased incidence later in pregnancy (14). Treatment involves fast and adequate pain relief, fluid replacement, and antibiotic treatment if infection is suspected (15). Intravenous fluids correct dehydration and reduce viscosity. We should use systemic opioids, if necessary, to treat pain. Analgesia can be maintained by continuous infusions or patient-controlled analgesia (PCA). A good outcome by using epidural analgesia for labor pain in a patient in crisis has been described (17). Partial-exchange transfusions are an important therapeutic maneuver (18). Simple additive transfusions are not indicated in patients whose Hb has not decreased by at least 2 g/dL below the stable state and is more than 5 g/dL (19).

TABLE 4. *Pregnancy complications in sickle cell disease*

Miscarriage
Intrauterine growth retardation
Premature labor
Proteinuric hypertension
Fetal distress in labor
Increased risk of cesarean section
Increased maternal mortality rates
Increased perinatal mortality rates
Puerperal sepsis and thrombosis

From ref. 15, with permission.

Preoperative Preparation

The role of prophylactic transfusion during pregnancy is controversial. One study compared prophylactic transfusion to maintain an Hb greater than 10 g/dL with indicated transfusion (Hb less than 6.0 g/dL, hemolysis due to ongoing crisis, before cesarean section if Hb less than 8.0 g/dL and postpartum hemorrhage) (20). There were no differences in preterm labor, intrauterine growth retardation, or perinatal or maternal mortality. In a large, multicenter study, nonpregnant patients with SCD were randomized to receive either an aggressive transfusion regimen designed to decrease the HbS level to less than 30% or a conservative regimen designed to increase the Hb level to 10 g/dL (21). Apart from an increased incidence of transfusion-related complications in the aggressive transfusion group, there were no differences in serious complications between the groups. A conservative approach to preanesthetic preparation of these patients is appropriate.

Anesthetic Care

Rigorously avoid hypoxemia, cold, acidosis, and dehydration in both homozygous and heterozygous parturients. Provide a warm operating suite (or labor room), warming blanket, humidified inspired gases, and avoid hypoventilation. Measure arterial blood gases for evidence of metabolic acidosis (22). Choice of anesthetic technique is less important than avoidance of precipitating factors and careful attention to detail (23). In a review of 1,079 surgical procedures in 717 patients with SCD, mortality was 1.1% (24). SCD-related complications after surgery were more frequent in HbSS patients who received regional compared with general anesthesia ($p = 0.058$).

Wrap the legs in elasticized bandages to reduce stasis in the lower extremities. Use lateral tilt and avoid aortocaval compression, because massive sickling can occur in the lower limbs, even in those with sickle cell trait. Monitor lower-limb oxygen saturation with a pulse oximeter on the foot to assess the adequacy of uterine displacement. We recommend epidural blockade, with careful attention to proper prehydration and gradual onset of sensory blockade for these women. Spinal anesthesia may result in sudden hypotension and the subsequent need for vasopressors. Treat hypotension during regional anesthesia initially with fluids and then ephedrine.

Complications can continue to arise postoperatively. Pay persistent attention to a warm environment, fluid intake, oxygen, and analgesia. Epidural opioid analgesia, with careful monitoring for respiratory depression, is ideal. Encourage early mobilization and vigorous chest physiotherapy.

Thalassemia

The thalassemias are a family of inherited disorders that result in decreased synthesis of β-globulin or α-globulin, leading to reduced hemoglobin concentration (25). The thalassemia syndromes are named by the type of chain that is inadequately represented. The two major groups are the α- and β-thalassemias, which affect the synthesis of HbA, which is made up of 2 α and 2 β chains. The globin chains in thalassemia are structurally normal. It is the quantity that is reduced.

The most severe form of α-thalassemia is Bart's hemoglobinopathy or homozygous α-thalassemia, with all four genes absent and no α chains produced. This disease is incompatible with life. However, mothers whose babies have Bart's hemoglobinopathy have an increased incidence of pregnancy-induced hypertension, antepartum and postpartum hemorrhage, and retained placenta (26). Hemoglobin H disease is associated with three deleted genes. In α-thalassemia minor, the heterozygous state (α-thalassemia-1), the absence of two genes causes a mild anemia, and a single gene deletion is undetectable (α-thalassemia-2) (25).

β-Thalassemia is due to a relative or absolute lack of formation of the β-globulin chains of hemoglobin. As a result, normal adult hemoglobin is not formed. β-Thalassemia is categorized as minor, intermedia, or major (Cooley's anemia). Patients with β-thalassemia intermedia may have increased hemolysis. If hemolysis induces significant anemia, these women may need preoperative transfusion. Patients with thalassemia major will have severe anemia and will require frequent transfusions. Strategies to ensure maximal effectiveness of transfusion include availability of safe blood, leukocyte-depleted red blood cell (RBC) transfusion, and intensive iron chelation with subcutaneous desferrioxamine (27).

Thalassemia minor and intermedia do not present many peripartum anesthetic problems. Women with thalassemia major rarely become pregnant. If they do, they may require up to 6 L of washed packed cells during the antenatal period to maintain an adequate hemoglobin. Women with hemosiderosis (from hemolysis and multiple transfusions) may have significant hepatic damage and lack clotting factors. Splenomegaly may lead to increased hemolysis and thrombocytopenia. Cardiac hemosiderosis leads to left ventricular mechanical dysfunction and, eventually, arrhythmias (28). Evaluate cardiac function with an electrocardiogram and echocardiography. Examine the airway closely. Maxillary overgrowth secondary to extramedullary erythropoiesis can make visualization of the glottis difficult.

During labor, correct severe anemia early. Monitor volume status carefully. Women with severe left ventricular dysfunction will need a pulmonary artery catheter. For pain relief, we advocate continuous-infusion epidural analgesia. Induce blockade slowly. Treat hypotension with phenylephrine, 20 to 40 μg, intravenously. This drug corrects hypotension more readily than does ephedrine without increasing the heart rate. For cesarean section, we prefer epidural anesthesia. Provide postoperative analgesia with epidural opioids. Avoid spinal anesthesia in women with significant myocardial compromise.

Aplastic Anemia

Patients with profound pancytopenia in pregnancy have a high mortality (33%) and a poor prognosis (29). Others, with less stem-cell depression, recover between pregnancies. Steroids often are used. Treatment with antilymphocyte globulin also has been reported (30).

At term, transfuse the symptomatic, severely anemic parturient. If the platelet count is adequate, major conduction anesthesia is safe. Avoid unnecessary urinary and central venous catheters because of the risk of infection.

Hemolytic Anemia

Patients with hereditary spherocytosis and hereditary elliptocytosis usually have a mild anemia. In patients with glucose-6-phosphate dehydrogenase deficiency, drugs such as aspirin, penicillin, sulfonamides, antimalarials, vitamin K, and methylene blue can induce intravascular hemolysis (31).

Hematologic Malignancies

Although neoplasms do not directly interfere with pregnancy, indirect effects may be important. The most common malignancies in women of reproductive age are shown in Table 5 (32). Pregnancy does not appear to affect outcome in women with leukemia or lymphoma (32). Cytotoxic treatment should not be postponed because of pregnancy, but antifolic or alkylating agents and radiotherapy should be avoided (33).

TABLE 5. *The frequency of malignancies diagnosed in women of reproductive age*

15–24 yr	25–34 yr	35–44 yr
Hodgkin's lymphoma	Breast carcinoma	Breast carcinoma
Thyroid carcinoma	Cervical carcinoma	Cervical carcinoma
Melanoma	Thyroid carcinoma, melanoma	Melanoma

From ref. 32, with permission.

Fanconi's Anemia

Pregnancy is rare and usually happens only in women with mild disease (34). The use of regional analgesia is based on the platelet count. These patients have an increased incidence of hypertensive disorders. Platelet transfusion is usually required at delivery. Significant bleeding, very low platelet counts, and the need for blood and platelet transfusion may complicate the postoperative course.

COAGULATION DISORDERS

Vascular Purpuras

Systemic Lupus Erythematosus (SLE)

About a third of patients with SLE have thrombocytopenia, although fewer than 5% have a platelet count less than 30,000/mm^3 (35). Occasionally a more severe and abrupt-onset thrombocytopenia may be seen with platelet-associated immunoglobulin G (IgG). High-dose corticosteroids may occasionally be indicated. Treatment of thrombocytopenia is difficult, and the response to corticosteroids may be poor, although aspirin occasionally increases the platelet count.

Henoch–Schonlein Purpura

This usually benign vasculitis occurs in children and young adults. Despite the purpura, prothrombin time (PT), activated partial thromboplastin time (aPTT), platelets, and bleeding time are often normal, and regional anesthesia is not contraindicated.

Platelet Disorders

Spurious (Laboratory-Induced) Thrombocytopenia

Any unexpected low platelet count should be checked manually, as platelet clumping, which may not be detected by automated counters, may occur under certain laboratory conditions. Spurious thrombocytopenia has been reported in 0.85% to 1.9% of processed samples (36).

Incidental Thrombocytopenia

Routine platelet count before regional anesthesia in healthy patients is not indicated. Of 15,471 consecutive women who had platelet counts measured at delivery, 6.6% had counts less than 150,000/mm^3 and 1.2% less than 100,000/mm^3 (37). Of those with platelet counts less than 150,000/mm^3, 74% had incidental thrombocytopenia, 21%, hypertensive disease of pregnancy, and 4%, an immunologic disorder such as SLE or autoimmune thrombocytopenia.

In another series of 1,621 healthy parturients, 6.4% had platelet counts less than 150,000/mm^3, and 0.4%, less than 100,000/mm^3 (38). Among the parturients with less than 150,000/mm^3 platelets, 61 (three with platelet counts of 50,000 to 99,000/mm^3) received epidural analgesia without neurological complications. The authors estimated that in the last 30 years, more than 80,000 epidural catheters had been inserted in their hospital. Assuming that the distribution of platelet counts had not changed, more than 5,000 women with a platelet count less than 150,000/mm^3 and more than 300 women with fewer than 100,000/mm^3 platelets had received epidural anesthesia without a single epidural hematoma (38). A chart review of 2,929 consecutive parturients identified 10 patients (0.3%) with platelet counts less than 100,000/mm^3 before delivery (39). Of these 10 parturients, two received an epidural and one a spinal block, without any complications. Uneventful epidural analgesia followed by a vacuum-assisted vaginal delivery was reported in a patient with a platelet count of between 2,000 and 4,000/mm^3 (40). In a patient with idiopathic thrombocytopenia (platelet count, 73,000/mm^3), the use of thromboelastography and sonoclot analysis to confirm adequate clotting before epidural anesthesia was described (41).

Autoimmune or Idiopathic Thrombocytopenic Purpura

Autoimmune thrombocytopenic purpura (ATP) is the most common autoimmune disease in childbearing women. Practice guidelines in pregnancy are available (42). ATP is characterized by the presence of antibodies, usually IgG, directed against the platelet membrane (43). Multiple episodes of relapse and remission are a feature of this disorder. ATP cannot be distinguished from gestational thrombocytopenia with certainty because both diagnoses are based on low platelets without an apparent cause (42). Platelet-associated antibody (PA-IgG) is not always present and may not correlate with the clinical disease.

Although symptoms may worsen, the risk of severe exacerbation of ATP does not increase during pregnancy (43). Pregnant women with more than 50,000/mm^3 platelets do not require treatment and should not receive steroids or immunoglobulin (42). Women with platelet counts between 30 and 50,000/mm^3 in the first and second trimester also do not require treatment. Oral corticosteroids are the initial treatment of choice and are started if clinical manifestations develop (36). Between 70% and 90% of patients will respond within 3 weeks (35). High-dose intravenous immunoglobulin is appropriate initial treatment for women with fewer than 10,000/mm^3 platelets in the third trimester and for those with platelet counts between 10 and 30,000/mm^3 who are bleeding (42). Splenectomy is very rarely indicated but may be safely performed during the second trimester. It is usually reserved for women for whom medical treatment fails (43). Platelet transfusion is of limited benefit because of rapid consumption by circulating antibodies and should be reserved for life-threatening hemorrhage (35,43).

Maternal antibodies may cross the placenta and affect the fetus. Infants with low platelet counts are theoretically at an increased risk of intracranial hemorrhage if delivered vaginally. Maternal platelet count, steroid therapy, or previous splenectomy are of limited use in predicting neonatal thrombocytopenia. The correlation of either maternal platelet count or circulating antiplatelet antibodies with neonatal thrombocytopenia is uncertain (44). The only reliable predictor of risk is a fetal platelet count. Before labor, this can be ascertained from a percutaneous umbilical blood sample, although this test confers some risk to the fetus. A scalp sample during labor requires adequate cervical dilatation, and accuracy may be affected by dilution with amniotic fluid or by clotting of the sample. At this stage, there is no convincing evidence that mode of delivery affects the rate of intracranial hemorrhage, and it has been recommended that patients with ATP be managed according to obstetric indications (44).

Maternal mortality is exceptionally rare, and postpartum hemorrhage is the most common complication. The incidence of postpartum hemorrhage appears to correlate with the severity of thrombocytopenia and is more frequently associated with cervical or vaginal lacerations or episiotomies than with uterine atony (36,43). A maternal platelet count greater than 50,000/mm^3 is considered sufficient to prevent excessive maternal bleeding at vaginal delivery or cesarean section (42).

Thromboelastography may have a place in the assessment of the overall clotting (41). Because of the increase in marrow turnover in ATP, platelets tend to be younger and larger, and therefore more efficient. As a result, regional anesthesia, in particular spinal, may be considered in asymptomatic women with platelet counts as low as 50,000/mm^3. Platelet transfusion to cover regional techniques is not recommended because the life span of the transfused platelets is indeterminable and may be very short because of circulating antibodies. General anesthesia, especially intubation, also requires care.

Postoperatively patients should be nursed in a high-care area and be carefully monitored for any bleeding or respiratory obstruction secondary to airway trauma after intubation. Neonatal platelet counts should be measured daily for at least 7 days, because they may decrease over the first week of life to less than 50,000/mm^3.

Thrombotic Thrombocytopenic Purpura

Thrombotic thrombocytopenia purpura (TTP) is a rare, severe disease characterized by thrombocytopenia, microangiopathic hemolytic anemia, transient neurological abnormalities, fever, and renal failure (45). Diffuse intravascular thrombosis occludes capillaries and arterioles throughout the body. Prognosis of TTP in pregnancy is poor for both the mother and fetus. Unlike ATP, damage to maternal organs and placenta indirectly injures the fetus. The condition may be confused with severe preeclampsia or abruption. Disseminated intravascular coagulation (DIC) is absent in most cases (35). In the acute phase, plasma infusion or plasma-exchange therapy results in improvement in 90% of cases. This treatment may enhance maternal and fetal survival (46). Steroids, aspirin, and dipyridamole are commonly used.

Postpartum Hemolytic Uremic Syndrome

This syndrome resembles TTP, but it is characterized by acute renal failure associated with microangiopathic hemolytic anemia. Maternal mortality and long-term morbidity are high, and preterm delivery and intrauterine fetal deaths are frequent complications (47). Treatment is as for TTP, but dialysis is often required.

Drug-Induced Platelet Disorders

Thrombocytopenia

Many drugs can induce thrombocytopenia. The most common pathway is through the formation of an immune complex, a mechanism that often involves IgG, which can cross the placenta and affect the fetus. Generalized bone-marrow depression (e.g., chloramphenicol) or a selective effect involving only the megakaryocytes (e.g., thiazides, tolbutamide) may occur.

Thrombopathy

Many commonly used drugs can inhibit platelet life span and function. Dipyridamole inhibits primary aggregation (48). Penicillin, in high doses, but more commonly ticarcillin and carbenicillin, epsilon aminocaproic acid in high doses, and ethanol can interfere with platelet function (48). Heparin-associated thrombocytopenia occurs in 5% of patients receiving heparin therapy. This problem usually arises after 6 to 12 days. Diazepam, chlordiazepoxide, propranolol, and phentolamine also may decrease platelet function. Phenothiazines may alter platelet numbers and function. After stopping the offending drug, platelets should recover within 1 to 2 weeks.

Aspirin and other nonsteroidal antiinflammatory drugs impair platelet aggregation by inhibiting the formation of platelet thromboxane after binding with cyclooxygenase. Low-dose aspirin reduces the incidence of pregnancy-induced hypertension in high-risk patients (49). A single dose of aspirin prolongs the bleeding time for 48 to 72 hours, and the duration of effect on platelet aggregation may be longer.

The clinical dilemma posed by aspirin is whether its platelet effect translates into a significant risk of increased bleeding and therefore spinal hematoma. In a prospective study of spinal or epidural anesthesia for 1,000 procedures in 924 orthopedic patients, blood was detected in the spinal or epidural needle or catheter in 22% of cases, but no patient developed any signs or symptoms of epidural hematoma (50). Although 39% of these patients were receiving antiplatelet medication, such as aspirin, other nonsteroidal antiinflammatory drug (NSAID), or combination, this therapy was not associated with an increase in minor hemorrhagic complications. Anesthetic factors that were significantly associated with a higher incidence of minor hemorrhagic complications included:

- Continuous spinal or epidural techniques as compared with single-injection epidural anesthesia,
- Increasing needle gauge, and
- Increased number of needle passes.

There was no difference in risk of bleeding between midline and paramedian approaches. A total of 239 epidural and seven spinal anesthetics was performed in patients receiving aspirin without any evidence of spinal cord compression (51).

Aspirin, 600 mg, does not alter any thromboelastogram (TEG) parameters in either pregnant or nonpregnant subjects (52). TEG also is not affected in pregnant patients at risk for preeclampsia treated with low-dose aspirin (53). In a large, blinded, randomized study comparing aspirin, 60 mg daily, vs placebo, 2,783 women (1,422 aspirin-allocated vs 1,361 placebo-allocated) underwent epidural analgesia (54). There were no differences in adverse events between the two groups and no hemorrhagic complications. In a similar randomized study, 451 women taking daily aspirin, 60 mg, received epidural analgesia with no bleeding complications (55).

There are only three reported cases of spinal hematoma in which an NSAID has been associated with epidural anesthesia (56). Although the overall risk of epidural hematoma after regional anesthesia in patients taking aspirin is unknown, it must be considered extremely rare (56,57). There is no good evidence that regional anesthesia should be denied to patients currently receiving aspirin in the absence of other risk factors.

Preeclampsia and Eclampsia

Preeclampsia is the most common cause of thrombocytopenia in pregnancy (58). Thrombocytopenia associated with preeclampsia is probably due to increased platelet consumption (59). Thirty-four percent of parturients with preeclampsia have fewer than 150,000 platelets/mm^3 (60), and 7.5% have platelet counts less than 100,000/mm^3 (61). There also may be a defect in platelet function despite adequate platelet numbers (62).

In preeclampsia, abnormalities of coagulation occur only in conjunction with reduced platelet counts. In a prospective study of 100 women with severe preeclampsia or chronic hypertension with superimposed preeclampsia, no patient had reduced fibrinogen or prolonged PT or aPTT if the platelet count was greater than 100,000/mm^3 (63). Therefore platelet counts are useful screening tests, and other coagulation tests should be reserved in the presence of thrombocytopenia.

The lowest platelet count compatible with safe regional anesthesia in the presence of normal clotting tests is unknown and controversial. Platelet counts between 60,000 and 100,000/mm^3 have been suggested, but these recommendations are not evidence based. Uneventful epidural analgesia has been described in 30 parturients with platelet counts between 69,000 and 98,000/mm^3 (64).

Thromboelastography

A small study in 19 patients with mild preeclampsia and eight with severe preeclampsia suggested that TEG may be useful in assessing platelet function in patients with thrombocytopenia (65). The MA (maximum amplitude) of the TEG tracing (Fig. 1) is a measure of maximum clot strength and depends on fibrinogen concentration and the number and function of platelets. Figure 2 shows the relation between the MA and platelet count in patients with severe preeclampsia and eclampsia. In women with platelet counts less than 100,000/mm^3, there is a strong correlation between the MA of the TEG and platelet count (r = 0.78; p = 0.04) (66). The lower limit of MA in normal pregnancy (MA, 53 mm) correlated with a platelet count of 54,000/mm^3 (95% CI, 40 to 75,000/mm^3). The authors suggested that a platelet count of 75,000/mm^3 should be adequate for neuraxial blocks in preeclamptic patients. The use of the TEG before regional anesthesia in three nonobstetric patients with potential hemostatic abnormalities was described (67). The TEG may provide useful information about overall hemostasis before regional anesthesia (Figs. 3 and 4).

Bleeding Time

There is no evidence that:

- The bleeding time is a specific in vivo indicator of platelet function,

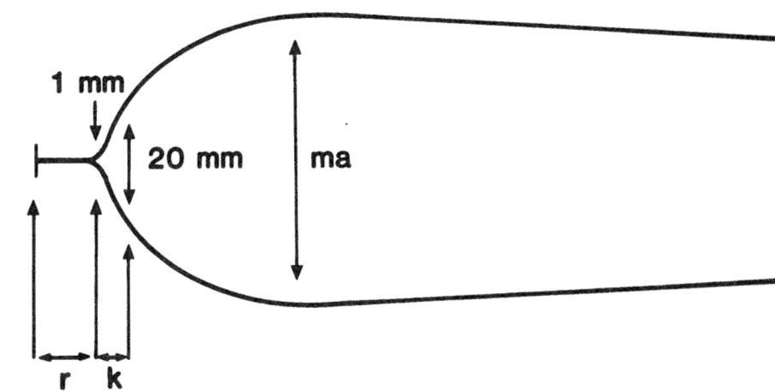

FIG. 1. Normal thromboelastogram tracing showing the measurement of *r, k,* and maximal amplitude *(MA).* In the term parturient, normal mean (±SD) values include r = 7.6 ± 0.9 min; k = 3.4 ± 0.7 min; and MA = 59.7 ± 3.5 min.

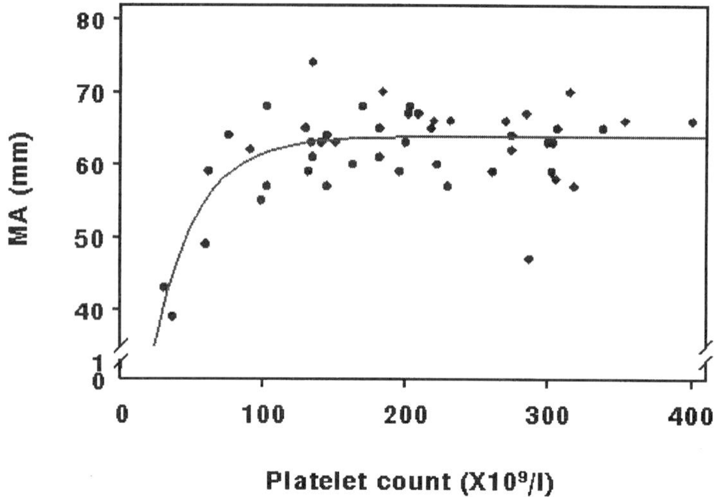

FIG. 2. Scattergram of maximal amplitude (*MA*) of the thromboelastograph vs platelet count. The equation MA = 63.9 × [1 – exp (–0.033 platelets)] describes a negative exponential curve or best fit that has been calculated by using a nonlinear regression procedure. (Reprinted from ref. 66, with permission.)

- The bleeding time can predict the risk of hemorrhage, or
- The degree of bleeding from the skin accurately reflects the risk of bleeding elsewhere in the body (68).

The bleeding time provides no useful information about the risk of bleeding within the spinal canal.

HELLP Syndrome

Between 4% and 12% of women with severe preeclampsia may have hemolysis, increased liver enzymes, and low platelets (HELLP syndrome) (69). In 33 such patients, the incidence of cesarean section was 94%; 23 patients received general anesthetic, and eight, epidural anesthesia (70). Complications included postpartum hemorrhage, excessive bleeding, DIC, and wound hematoma.

In a patient with HELLP syndrome, who after delivery developed hepatic, renal, and respiratory failure, TEG was used to detect a heparin effect, reversed with protamine on one occasion, and fibrinolysis, treated with aprotinin on another (69).

Platelet counts continue to decrease after delivery, and in one series, 17 of 19 patients with HELLP syndrome, who had not been transfused, reached the nadir of platelet count 29 hours (SD, 15 hours) after delivery (58). The average time from delivery to reach a platelet count more than 100,000/mm^3 was 60 hours (range, 36 to 95 hours). Always check the platelet count in these parturients, before removing an epidural catheter, as the risk of epidural hematoma is probably as great at time of removal as that at insertion (71).

Primary Thrombocythemia

This disease is a rare myeloproliferative disorder with increased platelet counts and increased marrow megakaryocytes (72). Symptoms may relate to either thrombosis or hemorrhage. Treatment may include aspirin, low-dose subcutaneous heparin, plateletpheresis, and, rarely, antiproliferative drugs, such as busulfan. Regional anesthetics are usually contraindicated.

Clotting Disorders

Lupus Anticoagulant

The lupus anticoagulant (LA) is an antibody of the IgG, or occasionally IgM, class, and its presence prolongs the aPTT and very rarely the PT (73). Paradoxically these patients are at risk for thrombosis, not bleeding. Treatment is often with aspirin, prednisone, and heparin.

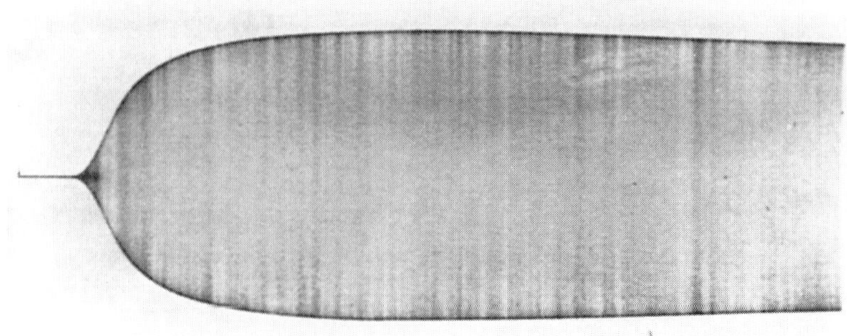

FIG. 3. Thromboelastogram (TEG) of a patient with severe preeclampsia. Platelet count was 219,000/mm^3; bleeding time, 13 min. This TEG is normal for pregnancy.

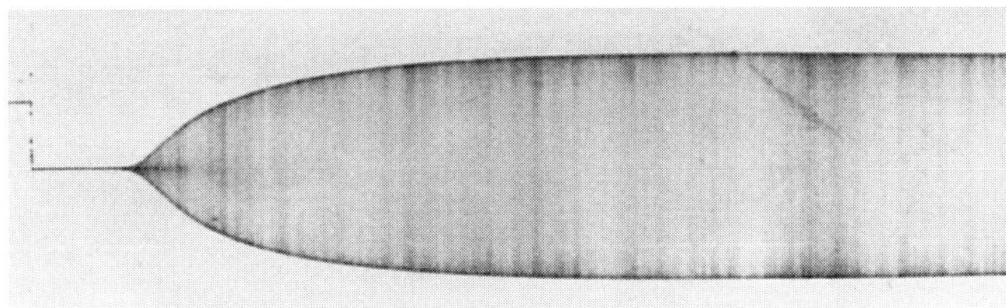

FIG. 4. Thromboelastogram (TEG) from a patient with severe preeclampsia. Platelet count was 30,000/mm^3; bleeding time was 7 min. On TEG the maximal amplitude (MA) is reduced to 43 mm. Other TEG measurements are r = 7.0 min, and k = 6.0 min.

An isolated increase of the aPTT secondary to the presence of LA and not associated with thrombocytopenia is not a contraindication to regional anesthesia (74). However, first exclude other causes of prolonged aPTT. Laboratory testing may be time consuming and require more than one confirmatory test (73). Although the TEG readily diagnoses hypercoagulability, it does not consistently detect LA abnormalities (75).

von Willebrand's Disease

von Willebrand's disease (vWD) is the most commonly inherited disorder of hemostasis in women, with an incidence of up to 1% (76). However, the incidence of severe disease is much lower, about 1:10,000, which is similar to the frequency of hemophilia (77). The factor (vWF) circulates in plasma as a complex with factor VIII and is responsible for platelet adhesion to exposed collagen after vessel injury. Any abnormality or quantitative decrease of vWF may be associated with a factor VIII decrease (78).

The most common form of the disease, type 1, occurs in about 75% of patients and is characterized by a reduction in all forms of vWF (76). Type 2A (10% of patients with vWD) is characterized by the absence of the large and intermediate-size multimers and by the absence of ristocetin-induced platelet agglutination. Bleeding episodes are more common and severe than those in type 1. In type 2B (7% of patients with vWD), only large multimers are absent, and ristocetin agglutination is increased (76,79). Type 3 vWD is least common (1%) and clinically the most severe (77). The entire vWF molecule is undetectable in plasma, platelets, or endothelial cells, and as a result, factor VIII also is absent (77).

The most sensitive test for vWD is ristocetin cofactor activity, which measures the ability of vWF to bind to the platelet membrane (80). The bleeding time is still used, even though its prolongation does not invariably predict a more severe bleeding tendency. Ristocetin-induced platelet agglutination allows identification of type 2B disease (80). The aPTT is prolonged only with marked reductions in factor VIII.

Desmopressin, which releases vWF from endothelial cells, may be useful in the bleeding patient (78). In type 1 disease, desmopressin produces a median 3.1- to 8.8-fold increase of factor VIII, with return to baseline within 4 to 6 hours (78). In the different subtypes of type 2, responsiveness to desmopressin is variable, and type 3 patients usually have no response. In the past, some antihemophilic factor (AHF) preparations have lacked ristocetin cofactor activity and have been associated with failures in the treatment of bleeding in patients with vWD (81). However, purified viral inactivated plasma-derived products (AHF-vWF) are as effective as cryoprecipitate. They are preferred to cryoprecipitate, which involves the infective risks of blood transfusion (81).

The vWF and factor VIII increase during normal pregnancy (82,83). Most women with vWD have a variable increase in vWF and factor VIII during pregnancy, which depends in part on the severity of the disease (76).

Preoperative evaluation should include hemoglobin, PT, aPPT, bleeding time, and, if possible, factor VIII, vWF, ristocetin cofactor activity, and determination of type of disease. Response to desmopressin is variable, and a test infusion a few weeks before surgery or delivery is recommended.

The most important determinant of abnormal hemorrhage at delivery is low factor VIII (84). In patients with type 1 disease, factor VIII concentrations greater than 50% appear sufficient for vaginal delivery. Bleeding may occur postpartum, as factor VIII and vWF concentrations decrease after delivery.

Anesthetic management is guided by the preoperative test results. Regional anesthesia is considered safe in mild disease, and there is a case report of uneventful epidural analgesia in pregnancy (85). However, in those with type 2 disease, because the vWF is abnormal, blood products are usually required, even though factor VIII concentration may increase in pregnancy. This precaution is especially important if cesarean section is required (82).

Hemophilia A (Classic Hemophilia)

Hemophilia A is the result of decreased factor VIII activity. Because it is an X-linked recessive disorder, women are usually only carriers, but one tenth of these women may experience excessive bleeding (82). Bleeding may occur if the patient develops lyonization (suppression of normal gene expression), is homozygous, or has a spontaneous gene mutation (86). vWF concentration and activity are not affected. Diagnosis is made by history, prolonged aPTT, normal PT, and low factor VIII activity. Factor VIII activity increases in pregnancy (83) and also may increase in hemophilic patients (86).

The safety of regional anesthesia depends on the severity of the factor VIII decrease. In carriers with normal aPTT (76,86), regional anesthesia is not contraindicated. Avoid regional anesthesia in patients with reduced factor VIII activity and prolonged aPTT. Hemostasis after vaginal delivery requires factor VIII concentrations greater than 40% for at least 3 to 4 days. After cesarean section, levels greater than 50% for 4 to 5 days are needed (76). Factor VIII concentrate (AHF) is the treatment of choice to increase levels of factor VIII, with cryoprecipitate or fresh-frozen plasma reserved for emergencies (86).

The half-life of factor VIII is about 8 hours. Factor VIII concentration may decrease dramatically within hours of delivery and should be monitored closely (86). Check aPTT before removing any epidural catheter. If bleeding occurs, desmopressin may increase factor VIII activity. Serious bleeding should be treated with AHF.

Hemophilia B (Christmas Disease)

This disease is diagnosed by low factor IX and prolonged aPTT in the presence of normal factor VIII activity. Management is similar to that for hemophilia A. In general, during normal pregnancy, factor IX activity does not increase as much as factor VIII. Female carriers of hemophilia B, who have low factor IX activity, are more likely to require specific factor replacement to raise their factor IX activity to safe levels for vaginal delivery (40%) or cesarean section (50%) (76).

Factor XI Deficiency

This problem occurs only occasionally in pregnancy. It is usually a mild defect, although serious deficiencies may occur. Treatment is with virally inactivated factor XI. Fresh-frozen plasma may be used if factor XI is not available (86).

Fibrinogen

Congenital abnormalities of fibrinogen include afibrinogenemia, dysfibrinogenemia, and hypofibrinogenemia (87). Dysfibrinogenemia is less severe, many patients are asymptomatic, and in one series, only seven of 83 patients had mild to moderate bleeding (88). If bleeding is a problem, cryoprecipitate or fresh-frozen plasma may be required. The PT and aPTT may be normal with low concentrations of fibrinogen, but thrombin and reptilase times will be prolonged (87).

Antithrombin III Deficiency

Antithrombin III (ATIII) is the major inhibitor of thrombin Xa and other serine proteases, and deficiency is associated with a high risk of venous thrombosis (40% to 70%) and pulmonary embolism. These risks are markedly increased in pregnancy. Measuring low plasma ATIII activity makes the diagnosis.

High doses of heparin may be required because ATIII concentrations are low (heparin exerts its anticoagulant effect by binding and activating ATIII). Try to prolong the aPTT by 5 to 10 seconds.

ANTICOAGULANTS IN PREGNANCY

Anticoagulation during gestation may be necessary for the treatment of acute thromboembolic disease or for prophylaxis. Unfortunately no large randomized trials have examined the efficacy of thromboembolism prophylaxis in pregnancy with definitive results (89,90). Most of the current clinical recommendations are not supported by good evidence.

Warfarin is contraindicated in the first trimester in pregnancy because of embryopathy and is best avoided in the second and third trimesters because of risks of chondrodysplasia punctata and fetal cerebral hemorrhage (89). However, the frequency of these fetal risks may have been overstated in the past, and warfarin may still have a place during pregnancy (90).

Heparin does not cross the placenta because of its relatively large molecular weight. Heparin-induced thrombocytopenia is rare (2.4% for therapeutic heparin and 0.3% for prophylactic heparin), and platelet count should be checked 5 to 14 days after starting therapy (89).

Although heparin is the anticoagulant of choice in pregnancy, its pharmacokinetics are significantly altered (89,91). As pregnancy progresses, patients require increasing doses of heparin (90). The aPTT is used to monitor heparin therapy, and the suggested target aPTT varies between 1.5 and 2.5 times normal. The risk of bleeding complications with higher aPTT must be balanced against the risk of thrombosis at lower levels (90).

Regional techniques are contraindicated in patients who are anticoagulated with either heparin or oral anticoagulants. A recent comprehensive review discovered 61 spinal hematomas after either spinal (25%) or epidural (75%) blocks (71). Some form of heparin therapy was identified in 49% of these cases. This review also emphasized the hazards of removal of the epidural catheter in anticoagulated patients.

Nevertheless, there is evidence that regional anesthesia can be safely performed in the presence of abnormal coagulation, although the numbers of patients involved are still quite small. For the control of chronic pain, 336 caudal blocks of morphine and bupivacaine have been described in 37 anticoagulated patients (PT or aPTT more than 1.5 times control) and 19 patients with profound thrombocytopenia (platelet count less than 50,000/mm^3) without any problems (80). In a series of 1,000 epidural blocks in partially anticoagulated patients,

42% had a thrombotest of 15% or less (equivalent to an INR of 2.1 or more) and 73%, a thrombotest of 20 or less (equivalent to an INR of 1.8 or more) (92,93). Heparin was used intraoperatively, and catheters were removed at 48 hours. No neurological sequelae were reported.

Low-molecular-weight heparin (LMWH) has been shown to be effective in preventing venous thrombosis in pregnancy (94). LMWH was not associated with increased bleeding at delivery, and anti-Xa activity in the babies was undetectable. Its use in obstetrics is increasing.

More controversial is the risk of regional anesthesia in patients receiving prophylactic subcutaneous doses of heparin. A questionnaire survey of anesthetic departments in Denmark showed that 60% of departments used spinal and epidural techniques in these patients, and no side effects were reported (95). Heparin prophylaxis was not identified as a risk factor for epidural hematoma in a recent review (56). No epidural hematoma were reported in several series totaling 9,013 patients receiving either spinal or epidural blocks while receiving LMWH (96). In contrast, the manufacturer of enoxaparin (an LMWH compound) has received 14 reports worldwide of epidural hematoma. Almost all these cases involved postoperative indwelling epidural catheters (97). In most of these cases, patients had the epidural catheter inserted within a few hours of receiving enoxaparin. In November, 1997, the United States of America Food and Drug Administration (FDA) issued an "Alert" that reported 30 patients have developed an epidural or spinal hematoma with concurrent use of enoxaparin and spinal/epidural anaesthesia or spinal puncture (98). Many of these patients had neurological injury, including long-term or permanent paralysis. Approximately 75% of these patients were elderly women undergoing orthopedic surgery. No information was provided about the timing of the LMWH and the procedure.

The response to subcutaneous heparin is very unpredictable. Fifty percent of nonpregnant patients who receive 5,000 units of unfractionated heparin subcutaneously will have therapeutic heparin blood concentrations for up to 4 hours. Many patients who are receiving heparin prophylaxis would benefit from epidural anesthesia or analgesia. However, the risks and benefits of this procedure must be assessed in each patient. Some experts recommend delaying regional block for 4 to 6 hours after the last dose of unfractionated heparin (57). In patients receiving LMWH, 12 to 24 hours should elapse before attempting regional block (57,98). If the block needs to be done sooner, measure the aPTT in patients receiving unfractionated heparin or anti-Xa for those taking LMWH. Remove the epidural catheter just before heparin is restarted after delivery.

Anticoagulation with heparin after lumbar puncture has been shown to be associated with an increased risk of spinal hematoma (99). The risk was particularly increased if heparin was started within 1 hour of the lumbar puncture, if the procedure was traumatic, or if there was concurrent treatment with aspirin. Consider these factors before starting heparin therapy after a central neuraxial block.

REGIONAL ANESTHESIA IN THE PRESENCE OF COAGULOPATHY OR PLATELET DYSFUNCTION

Regional anesthesia is contraindicated in the presence of marked thrombocytopenia or coagulopathy as manifested by abnormal coagulation tests. Most published reports of spinal hematoma after epidural injection have been in patients with bleeding diatheses (57).

However, a more common situation for the obstetric anesthesiologist is a pressing indication for spinal or epidural analgesia or anesthesia in a patient with borderline coagulation status. The indication for regional block will need to be balanced against the risks involved with an alternative choice. Unfortunately, excessive concern about the risk of bleeding may dissuade anesthesiologists from offering spinal or epidural block. As a result, patients may be denied the benefits of these techniques for uncertain reasons.

A thorough history is essential to determine whether any bleeding problems are present in the patient or her family. Direct questions to prolonged bleeding or rebleeding after tooth extraction, recurrent epistaxis, or excessive bleeding in connection with previous surgery (100). Pay particular attention to medications taken within the last 10 days. Examine the patient for signs of bruising or bleeding from mucous membranes and venipuncture sites. Absence of evidence of bleeding elsewhere is often the most important and reassuring sign that regional anesthesia may be safe.

The risk of vessel damage during insertion of an epidural catheter in the parturient is higher than the approximately 10% incidence reported in surgical patients. When 16- or 18-gauge Tuohy needles are used, 18% of parturients have detectable bleeding (101). Attempts to minimize the risk of bleeding at time of induction of neuraxial block include:

- Spinal instead of epidural block: the lowest incidence of minor bleeding at the time of insertion is associated with the smallest needles (50);
- Avoid using a catheter: either spinal or epidural single-injection techniques are associated with less risk of minor hemorrhage than are spinal or epidural catheters (50). Insertion of an epidural catheter has been shown to be important in the genesis of an epidural hematoma (71);
- Limited insertion of catheter: if an epidural catheter is used, insertion should be limited ideally to 3 cm and a maximum of 5 cm in the epidural space;
- The left lateral position: this position is associated with less epidural vein distention and may theoretically offer some advantages. However, in obese women, it is eas-

ier to identify the epidural or subarachnoid space in the sitting position. This effect may be more important in reducing risk of bleeding as number of passes or difficulty identifying the epidural space is a risk factor for minor hemorrhage (50) and for epidural hematoma (71); and

- Midline approach: theoretically this choice should be safer as the epidural veins are located laterally in the space. However, no difference in the incidence of minor venous bleeding was shown between paramedian and midline approaches (50).

In early labor, opioids alone can be used by spinal or epidural routes. Later in labor, use only dilute local anesthetic/opioid mixtures. Assess motor function regularly. Postoperatively, monitor patients closely for symptoms or signs of cord compression. Here, a well-educated nursing staff is essential. For postoperative pain management, avoid local anesthetics and use only neuraxial opioids. Remove the epidural catheter only when laboratory tests confirm normal hemostasis.

REFERENCES

1. Ekeroma AJ, Ansari A, Stirrat GM. Blood transfusion in obstetrics and gynaecology. *Br J Obstet Gynaecol* 1997;104:278.
2. Mani S, Duffy TP. Anemia of pregnancy. *Clin Perinatol* 1995;22:593.
3. Ross A, Malkoutzis E. Blood transfusion practice in obstetric and gynaecological anaesthesia. *Anaesth Intens Care* 1995;23:645.
4. Santoso JT, Lin DW, Miller DS. Transfusion medicine in obstetrics and gynecology. *Obstet Gynecol Surv* 1995;50:470.
5. Kowalyshyn J, Prager D, Young J. A review of the present status of preoperative hemoglobin requirements. *Anesth Analg* 1972;51:75.
6. Lee CA. Transfusion-transmitted disease. *Baillieres Clin Haematol* 1996;9:369.
7. Rosen NR, Bates LH, Herod G. Transfusion therapy: improved patient care and resource utilization. *Transfusion* 1993;33:341.
8. Lichtenstein A, Eckhart WF, Swanson KJ, et al. Unplanned intraoperative and postoperative hemodilution: oxygen transport and consumption during severe anemia. *Anesthesiology* 1988;69:119.
9. U.S. Report of Health and Human Services. *Indications for the use of red blood cells, platelets and fresh frozen plasma.* Washington, DC: U.S. Department of Health and Human Services, 1989.
10. Naef RW III, Washburne JF, Martin RW, et al. Hemorrhage associated with cesarean delivery: when is transfusion needed? *J Perinatol* 1995; 15:32.
11. Huch R, Huch A. Erythropoietin in obstetrics. *Hematol Oncol Clin North Am* 1994;8:1021.
12. Scott DB, Hibbard BM. Serious non-fatal complications associated with extradural block in obstetric practice. *Br J Anaesth* 1990;64:537.
13. O'Dwyer G, Mylotte M, Sweeney M. Experience of autologous blood transfusion in an obstetrics and gynaecology department. *Br J Obstet Gynaecol* 1993;100:571.
14. Rust OA, Perry KG Jr. Pregnancy complicated by sickle hemoglobinopathy. *Clin Obstet Gynecol* 1995;38:472.
15. Howard RJ. Management of sickling conditions in pregnancy. *Br J Hosp Med* 1996;56:7.
16. Howard RJ, Tuck SM, Pearson TC. Pregnancy in sickle cell disease in the UK: results of a multicentre survey of the effect of prophylactic blood transfusion on maternal and fetal outcome. *Br J Obstet Gynaecol* 1995;102:947.
17. Finer P, Blair J, Rowe P. Epidural analgesia in the management of labor pain and sickle cell crisis—a case report. *Anesthesiology* 1988;68:799.
18. Martin J Jr, Martin RW, Morrison JC. Acute management of sickle cell crisis in pregnancy. *Clin Perinatol* 1986;13:853.
19. Davies SC. Blood transfusion in sickle cell disease. *Vox Sang* 1995; 68:145.
20. El-Shafei AM, Dhaliwal JK, Sandhu AK, et al. Indications for blood transfusion in pregnancy with sickle cell disease. *Aust N Z J Obstet Gynaecol* 1995;35:405.
21. Vichinsky EP, Haberkern CM, Neumayr L, et al. A comparison of conservative and aggressive transfusion regimens in the perioperative management of sickle cell disease. *N Engl J Med* 1995;333:206.
22. Esseltine DW, Baxter MR, Bevan JC. Sickle cell states and the anaesthetist. *Can J Anaesth* 1988;35:385.
23. Maduska AL, Guinee WS, Heaton JA, et al. Sickling dynamics of red blood cells and other physiologic studies during anesthesia. *Anesth Analg* 1975;54:361.
24. Koshy M, Weiner SJ, Miller ST, et al. Surgery and anesthesia in sickle cell disease. *Blood* 1995;86:3676.
25. Kilpatrick SJ, Laros RK. Thalassemia in pregnancy. *Clin Obstet Gynecol* 1995;38:485.
26. Liang ST, Wong VC, So WW, et al. Homozygous alpha-thalassaemia: clinical presentation, diagnosis and management: a review of 46 cases. *Br J Obstet Gynaecol* 1985;92:680.
27. Rebulla P. Blood transfusion in beta thalassaemia major. *Transf Med* 1995;5:247.
28. Leon MB, Borer JS, Bacharach SL, et al. Detection of early cardiac dysfunction in patients with severe beta-thalassemia and chronic iron overload. *N Engl J Med* 1979;301:1143.
29. Snyder TE, Lee LP, Lynch S. Pregnancy-associated hypoplastic anemia: a review. *Obstet Gynecol Surv* 1991;46:264.
30. Aitchison RGM, Marsh JCW, Hows JM, et al. Pregnancy associated aplastic anaemia: a report of five cases and review of current management. *Br J Haematol* 1989;73:541.
31. Stoelting RK, Dierdorf S, McCammon RL. *Anesthesia and co-existing disease.* 2nd ed. New York: Churchill Livingstone, 1988:557.
32. Sadural E, Smith LG Jr. Hematologic malignancies during pregnancy. *Clin Obstet Gynecol* 1995;38:535.
33. Zuazu J, Julia A, Sierra J, et al. Pregnancy outcome in hematologic malignancies. *Cancer* 1991;67:703.
34. Alter BP, Frissora CL, Halpérin DS, et al. Fanconi's anaemia and pregnancy. *Br J Haematol* 1991;77:410.
35. Biswas A, Arulkumaran S, Ratnam SS. Disorders of platelets in pregnancy. *Obstet Gynecol Surv* 1994;49:585.
36. Sullivan CA, Martin JN Jr. Management of the obstetric patient with thrombocytopenia. *Clin Obstet Gynecol* 1995;38:521.
37. Burrows RF, Kelton JG. Fetal thrombocytopenia and its relation to maternal thrombocytopenia. *N Engl J Med* 1993;329:1463.
38. Rolbin SH, Abbott D, Musclow E, et al. Epidural anaesthesia in pregnant patients with low platelet counts. *Obstet Gynecol* 1988;71:918.
39. Rasmus KT, Rottman RL, Kotelko DM, et al. Unrecognized thrombocytopenia and regional anesthesia in parturients: a retrospective review. *Obstet Gynecol* 1989;73:943.
40. Hew-Wing P, Rolbin SH, Hew E, et al. Epidural anaesthesia and thrombocytopenia. *Anaesthesia* 1989;44:775.
41. Steer PL. Anaesthetic management of a parturient with thrombocytopenia using thrombelastography and sonoclot analysis. *Can J Anaesth* 1993;40:84.
42. George JN, Woolf SH, Raskob GE, et al. Idiopathic thrombocytopenic purpura: a practice guideline developed by explicit methods for The American Society of Hematology. *Blood* 1996;88:3.
43. Perry KG Jr, Morrison JC. Hematologic disorders in pregnancy. *Obstet Gynecol Clin North Am* 1992;19:783.
44. Cook RL, Miller RC, Katz VL, et al. Immune thrombocytopenic purpura in pregnancy: a reappraisal of management. *Obstet Gynecol* 1991;78:578.
45. Ruggenenti P, Remuzzi G. The pathophysiology and management of thrombotic thrombocytopenic purpura. *Eur J Haematol* 1996;56:191.
46. Maina A, Donvito V, Giachino O, et al. Thrombotic thrombocytopenic purpura in pregnancy with maternal and fetal survival. *Br J Obstet Gynaecol* 1990;97:443.
47. Egerman RS, Witlin AG, Friedman SA, et al. Thrombotic thrombocytopenic purpura and hemolytic uremic syndrome in pregnancy review of 11 cases. *Am J Obstet Gynecol* 1996;175:950.
48. George JN, Shattil SJ. The clinical importance of acquired abnormalities of platelet function. *N Engl J Med* 1991;324:27.
49. Sibai BM, Caritis SN, Thom E, et al. Prevention of preeclampsia with

low-dose aspirin in healthy, nulliparous pregnant women. *N Engl J Med* 1993;329:1213.
50. Horlocker TT, Wedel DJ, Schroeder DR, et al. Preoperative antiplatelet therapy does not increase the risk of spinal hematoma associated with regional anesthesia. *Anesth Analg* 1995;80:303.
51. Benzon HT, Brunner EA, Vaisrub N. Bleeding time and nerve blocks after aspirin. *Reg Anesth* 1983;9:86.
52. Orlikowski CEP, Payne AJ, Moodley J, et al. Thrombelastography after aspirin ingestion in pregnant and non-pregnant subjects. *Br J Anaesth* 1992;69:159.
53. Payne AJ, Orlikowski CEP, Moodley J, et al. Thrombelastography as a measure of coagulation in high risk pregnant patients receiving low dose aspirin. *J Obstet Gynaecol* 1993;13:222.
54. CLASP Collaborative Group. CLASP: a randomised trial of low-dose aspirin for the prevention and treatment of pre-eclampsia among 9364 pregnant women. *Lancet* 1994;343:619.
55. Sibai BM, Caritis SN, Thom E, et al. Low-dose aspirin in nulliparous women: safety of continuous epidural block and correlation between bleeding time and maternal-neonatal bleeding complications. *Am J Obstet Gynecol* 1995;172:1553.
56. Wulf H. Epidural anaesthesia and spinal haematoma. *Can J Anaesth* 1996;43:1260.
57. Stafford-Smith M. Impaired haemostasis and regional anaesthesia. *Can J Anaesth* 1996;43:R129.
58. Neiger R, Contag SA, Coustan DR. The resolution of preeclampsia-related thrombocytopenia. *Obstet Gynecol* 1991;77:692.
59. Redman CWG, Bonnar J, Beilin L. Early platelet consumption in pre-eclampsia. *BMJ* 1978;1:467.
60. Kelton JG, Hunter DJS, Neame PB. A platelet function defect in preeclampsia. *Obstet Gynecol* 1985;65:107.
61. Ramanathan J, Sibai BM, Vu T, et al. Correlation between bleeding times and platelet counts in women with preeclampsia undergoing cesarean section. *Anesthesiology* 1989;71:188.
62. Whigham KAE, Howie PW, Drummond AH, et al. Abnormal platelet function in pre-eclampsia. *Br J Obstet Gynaecol* 1978;85:28.
63. Leduc L, Wheeler JM, Kirshon B, et al. Coagulation profile in severe preeclampsia. *Obstet Gynecol* 1992;79:14.
64. Beilin Y, Zahn J, Comerford M. Safe epidural analgesia in thirty parturients with platelet counts between 69,000 and 98,000 mm^{-3}. *Anesth Analg* 1997;85:385.
65. Wong CA, Liu S, Glassenberg R. Comparison of thrombelastography with common coagulation tests in preeclamptic and healthy parturients. *Reg Anesth* 1995;20:521.
66. Orlikowski CEP, Rocke DA, Murray WB, et al. Thrombelastography changes in pre-eclampsia and eclampsia. *Br J Anaesth* 1996;77:157.
67. Bigeleisen PE, Kang Y. Thrombelastography as an aid to regional anesthesia: preliminary communication. *Reg Anesth* 1991;16:59.
68. Rodgers RPC, Levin J. A critical reappraisal of the bleeding time. *Semin Thromb Hemost* 1990;16:1.
69. Whitta RKS, Cox DJA, Mallett SV. Thrombelastography reveals two causes of haemorrhage in HELLP syndrome. *Br J Anaesth* 1995;74:464.
70. Crosby ET. Obstetrical anaesthesia for patients with the syndrome of haemolysis, elevated liver enzymes and low platelets. *Can J Anaesth* 1991;38:227.
71. Vandermeulen EP, Van Aken H, Vermylen J. Anticoagulants and spinal-epidural anesthesia. *Anesth Analg* 1994;79:1165.
72. Beard J, Hillmen P, Anderson CC, et al. Primary thrombocythaemia in pregnancy. *Obstet Gynecol* 1991;77:371.
73. Davies SR. Systemic lupus erythematosus and the obstetrical patient—implications for the anaesthetist. *Can J Anaesth* 1991;38:790.
74. Madan R, Khoursheed M, Kukla R, et al. The anaesthetist and the antiphospholipid syndrome. *Anaesthesia* 1997;52:72.
75. Confino E, El-Roeiy A, Friberg J, et al. The thrombelastogram and circulating lupus anticoagulant. *J Reprod Med* 1989;34:289.
76. Walker ID, Walker JJ, Colvin BT, et al. Investigation and management of haemorrhagic disorders in pregnancy. *J Clin Pathol* 1994;47:100.
77. Cameron CB, Kobrinsky N. Perioperative management of patients with von Willebrand's disease. *Can J Anaesth* 1990;37:341.
78. Castaman G, Rodeghiero F. Current management of von Willebrand's disease. *Drugs* 1995;50:602.
79. Conti M, Mari D, Conti E, et al. Pregnancy in women with different types of von Willebrand disease. *Obstet Gynecol* 1986;68:282.
80. Waldman SD, Feldstein GS, Waldman HJ, et al. Caudal administration of morphine sulfate in anticoagulated and thrombocytopenic patients. *Anesth Analg* 1987;66:267.
81. Menache D, Aronson DL. New treatments of von Willebrand disease: plasma derived von Willebrand Factor concentrates. *Thromb Hemost* 1997;78:566.
82. Greer IA, Lowe GDO, Walker JJ, et al. Haemorrhagic problems in obstetrics and gynaecology in patients with congenital coagulopathies. *Br J Obstet Gynaecol* 1991;98:909.
83. Stirling Y, Woolf L, North WRS, et al. Haemostasis in normal pregnancy. *Thromb Hemost* 1984;52:176.
84. Letsky EA. Haemostasis and epidural anaesthesia. *Int J Obstet Anaesth* 1991;1:51.
85. Cohen S, Daitch JS, Amar D, et al. Epidural analgesia for labor and delivery in a patient with von Willebrand's disease. *Reg Anesth* 1989;14:95.
86. Gatt S. Haematological disorders responsible for maternal bleeding in late pregnancy. *Anaesth Intens Care* 1990;18:335.
87. Goodwin TM. Congenital hypofibrinogenemia in pregnancy. *Obstet Gynecol Surv* 1989;44:157.
88. Mammen EF. Fibrinogen abnormalities. *Semin Thromb Hemost* 1983;9:1.
89. Barbour LA, Pickard J. Controversies in thromboembolic disease during pregnancy: a critical review. *Obstet Gynecol* 1995;86:621.
90. Oakley CM. Anticoagulation and pregnancy. *Eur Heart J* 1995;16:1317.
91. Brancazio LR, Roperti KA, Stierer R, et al. Pharmacokinetics and pharmacodynamics of subcutaneous heparin during the early third trimester of pregnancy. *Am J Obstet Gynecol* 1995;173:1240.
92. Odoom JA, Sih IL. Epidural analgesia and anticoagulant therapy. *Anaesthesia* 1983;38:254.
93. Molnar LI, Rø JS. Epidural analgesia and anticoagulant therapy. *Anaesthesia* 1984;39:602.
94. Rasmussen C, Wadt J, Jacobsen B. Thromboembolic prophylaxis with low molecular weight heparin during pregnancy. *Int J Gynaecol Obstet* 1994;47:121.
95. Wille-Jørgensen P, Jørgensen LN, Rasmussen LS. Lumbar regional anaesthesia and prophylactic anticoagulant therapy. *Anaesthesia* 1991;46:623.
96. Bergqvist D, Lindblad B, Mätzsch T. Low molecular weight heparin for thromboprophylaxis and epidural/spinal anaesthesia—is there a risk? *Acta Anaesthesiol Scand* 1992;36:605.
97. Weitz SR, Chan V. Enoxaparin and epidural analgesia. *Anesthesiology* 1996;85:432.
98. Food and Drug Administration. *FDA Alert: reports of epidural or spinal hematomas with the concurrent use of low molecular weight heparin and spinal/epidural anesthesia or spinal puncture.* Rockville, MD: US Department of Health and Human Services, Public Health Service, Food and Drug Administration.
99. Ruff RL, Dougherty JH Jr. Complications of lumbar puncture followed by anticoagulation. *Stroke* 1981;12:879.
100. Haljamae H. Thromboprophylaxis, coagulation disorders, and regional anaesthesia. *Acta Anaesthesiol Scand* 1996;40:1024.
101. McNeill MJ, Thorburn J. Cannulation of the epidural space: a comparison of 18- and 16-gauge needles. *Anaesthesia* 1988;43:154.
102. Menitove JE. Transfusion-transmitted infections: update. *Semin Hematol* 1996;33:290.

Obstetric Anesthesia, second edition,
edited by Mark C. Norris.
Lippincott Williams & Wilkins, Philadelphia © 1999.

CHAPTER 25

Anesthesia and Coexisting Maternal Disease

Diabetes Mellitus, Obesity, Pulmonary, and Neurological Disease

Beth Glosten and Holly C. Gunn

Anesthesiologists often assist with the management of labor and vaginal or cesarean delivery in parturients with significant medical problems. These medical conditions can alter choice and conduct of anesthesia. This chapter reviews the impact of some common medical problems on anesthetic management. Some relatively uncommon medical problems that significantly alter anesthetic care also are discussed. Specific problems covered include diabetes mellitus, obesity, pulmonary disease (asthma, cigarette use), and neurological disorders (seizure disorders, multiple sclerosis, myasthenia gravis, paraplegia, and intracranial vascular abnormalities).

ANESTHETIC MANAGEMENT OF THE DIABETIC PARTURIENT

Maternal glucose homeostasis, the potential for impaired uteroplacental perfusion, and the high likelihood of cesarean delivery are important features for the anesthesiologist to consider when caring for the diabetic parturient.

Preoperative Evaluation

Preoperative evaluation of the diabetic parturient includes assessment of the severity of maternal diabetes and the presence of renal, cardiac, neurological, or vascular disease or preeclampsia (Table 1). Preoperative evaluation also should include careful assessment of the airway. Diabetic patients with "stiff-joint" syndrome may have reduced neck and jaw mobility, which predisposes them to airway difficulties (1). Evaluation also includes a review of fetal well-being [fetal heart-rate tracing, biophysical profile (see Chapter 7)] (2) as well as fetal maturity, and estimated fetal weight. Review the maternal insulin requirements during pregnancy.

Glucose Control

Maintaining normal maternal glucose is very important throughout gestation, and the anesthesiologist is

TABLE 1. *The diabetic parturient and anesthesia*

Maternal considerations
Glucose control
Concomitant organ dysfunction
Renal
Cardiovascular (ischemic heart disease)
Vascular (hypertension, peripheral vascular disease)
Neuropathy
Retinopathy
Preeclampsia
Need for operative intervention
Cesarean section
Forceps delivery
Shoulder dystocia
Fetal/Neonatal considerations
Lung maturity
Uteroplacental insufficiency
Macrosomia
Acidosis
Hypoglycemia after birth
Birth trauma

B. Glosten and H. C. Gunn: Department of Anesthesiology, University of Washington, Seattle, Washington 98195-6540.

often involved with this task in the peripartum period. Patients in labor can be managed with slow infusions of insulin (1 U/10 mL normal saline) and glucose (such as 125 mL/h of D_5LR or D_5 normal saline; Table 2) (3,4). Monitor blood glucose closely and adjust glucose and insulin infusions accordingly. Most obstetricians try to keep maternal glucose below 90 to 110 mg/dL. Avoid maternal hyperglycemia. Do not use glucose-containing solutions for intravenous hydration before induction of regional anesthesia (5,6).

Studies in animals and humans suggest that maternal hyperglycemia (and consequent fetal hyperglycemia and hyperinsulinemia) contributes to fetal hypercarbia and acidemia (Fig. 1) (7,8). The placenta metabolizes maternal glucose to lactate (9), contributing to neonatal acidosis. Increased hydrogen ion concentration displaces oxygen from hemoglobin, limiting the oxygen-carrying capacity of fetal blood and decreasing blood oxygen content (Haldane effect) (Fig. 1). Glucose in the maternal circulation crosses the placenta via facilitated diffusion and produces fetal hyperglycemia. By stimulating fetal secretion of insulin, fetal hyperglycemia also can cause fetal hypoxemia. Animal studies have shown that fetal insulin infusion increases fetal glucose uptake and reduces fetal oxygen content, presumably by increasing fetal oxygen consumption (10).

Maternal hyperglycemia at delivery also can cause neonatal hypoglycemia. Increased maternal glucose just before delivery causes high umbilical venous concentrations of glucose (Fig. 2) (11). This hyperglycemia stimulates fetal hyperinsulinemia. After delivery, hyperinsulinemia leads to neonatal hypoglycemia (Fig. 3). The neonate cannot readily mobilize glucose stores to maintain a normal serum glucose concentration. The higher the umbilical cord glucose at birth, the more likely neonatal hypoglycemia (11).

Diabetes further worsens fetal condition by hindering placental function and uteroplacental perfusion. Pathologic examinations of the diabetic placenta reveal enlarged villi that reduce the surface area over which gas exchange can occur (12). Maternal vascular disease impairs placental perfusion and the delivery of oxygen and substrates to the fetus. These changes result in intrauterine growth retardation and a fetus at risk for hypoxemia and acidosis during the stress of labor.

TABLE 2. *Suggested insulin and glucose infusion rates based on finger-stick glucose measurements*

Glucose (mg/100 mL)	Insulin dose (units/h)	Intravenous fluids (125 mL/h)
<100	0	D_5LR
100–140	1.0	D_5LR
141–180	1.5	Normal saline
181–220	2.0	Normal saline
>220	2.5	Normal saline

From ref. 4, with permission.

For both metabolic and placental reasons, the fetus of a diabetic parturient has less reserve than the fetus of a normal gestation. Concern about fetal well-being may lead to urgent or emergency operative delivery. The anesthesiologist must recognize the potential for limited fetal reserve when inducing anesthesia in these patients.

Often the fetus of a diabetic mother has macrosomia. Large fetal size increases the likelihood of cephalopelvic disproportion and need for cesarean delivery (13). Further, vaginal delivery of a macrosomic fetus may require the use of forceps or result in shoulder dystocia. The large uterus of a diabetic parturient may not contract well after delivery, resulting in uterine atony and postpartum hemorrhage. These problems must be anticipated.

Analgesia for Labor and Delivery

Systemic opioids and sedatives can provide analgesia during early labor. Consider the effects of placental transfer of these medications. If birth occurs shortly after their administration, the neonate of the diabetic patient may be particularly sensitive to depression from sedatives. Prematurity further increases the susceptibility to central nervous depression from opioids and sedatives.

Regional analgesia is a very useful and effective technique for providing pain relief for labor and delivery in diabetic parturients. In nondiabetic laboring parturients, epidural analgesia reduces circulating maternal plasma catecholamines and 11-hydroxycorticosteroids (14,15). This effect has two potential benefits for diabetic patients. First, epinephrine and cortisol stimulate hyperglycemia and may contribute to difficulties with maternal glucose control. Further, reducing circulating maternal catecholamines should improve placental perfusion.

Before inducing regional analgesia in diabetic parturients, establish normal intravascular volume status with a glucose-free solution. Remember the potential for impaired uteroplacental perfusion. Pay close attention to fetal monitoring and proper maternal positioning. Avoid aortocaval compression.

Juvenile-onset diabetic parturients may have lower epidural local anesthetic dose requirements. For unclear reasons, these patients respond as if older than their chronologic age (16). Therefore dose their epidural catheters judiciously.

Spinal administration of opioids or local anesthetics can be used for labor and vaginal delivery. A saddle block is appropriate should forceps delivery be necessary in a patient without a functioning epidural catheter. Be attentive to the clinical situation and communicate with the obstetrician. Be prepared to proceed to cesarean delivery should the attempted forceps delivery fail.

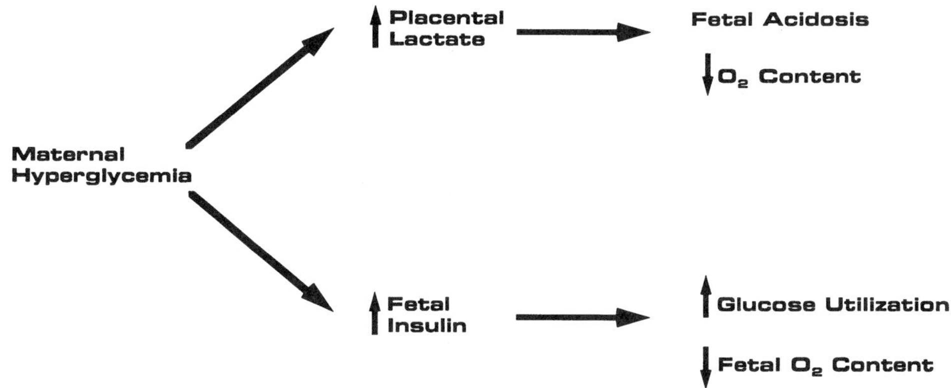

FIG. 1. Maternal hyperglycemia contributes to fetal acidosis and reduced fetal oxygen content.

Anesthesia for Cesarean Delivery

Patient Preparation

Several conditions may lead to the need for elective or urgent cesarean delivery in the diabetic parturient, including fetal macrosomia or a nonreassuring fetal status. Do not use glucose-containing fluids for prehydration or volume replacement.

Insulin and glucose therapy after the nothing-by-mouth (NPO) period before elective cesarean delivery depends on the severity of the patient's disease. If admitted the morning of surgery, many patients can be managed by maintaining an overnight fast, coming into the hospital early on the morning of surgery and withholding the usual morning insulin. On admission, measure maternal glucose by finger-stick. Start an intravenous infusion of insulin (1 U/10 mL normal saline) and glucose (such as 125 mL/h of D_5LR or D_5 normal saline) (Table 2). Thereafter, measure blood glucose frequently.

After delivery, maternal insulin requirements decrease (17). The loss of insulin resistance conferred by the placenta stimulates this change in insulin sensitivity. Patients receiving insulin before delivery may develop hypoglycemia. Carefully monitor maternal plasma glucose before and after delivery and adjust glucose/insulin therapy as indicated.

Anesthetic Technique

The specific anesthetic technique chosen depends on the patient's preference and the clinical situation. Good maternal and fetal outcome follows both regional and general anesthesia provided the earlier issues are considered.

Clinical studies of acid–base status of neonates born of normal or diabetic parturients who received general anesthesia for cesarean delivery have shown no major differences between the two patient groups (18). However, neonatal depression (defined as Apgar scores less than 7 at 1

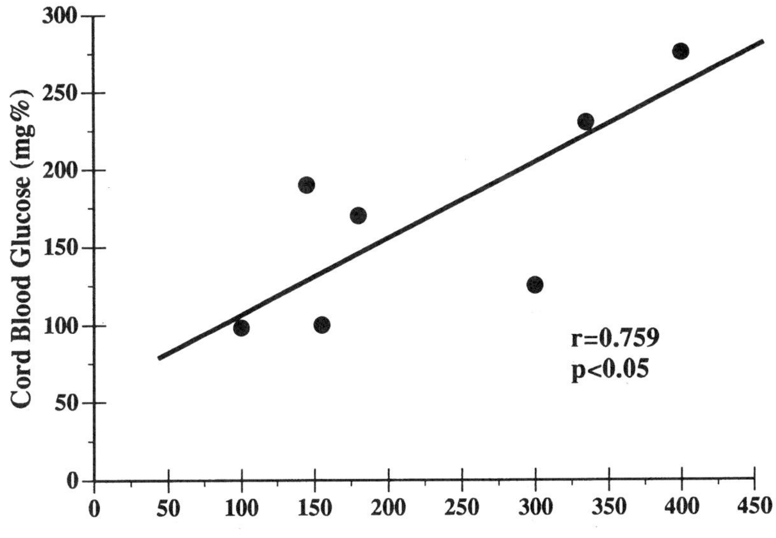

FIG. 2. Cord blood glucose reflects maternal glucose before delivery. The amount of antenatal maternal intravenous glucose is directly related to the umbilical cord blood glucose. (Redrawn from ref. 11, with permission.)

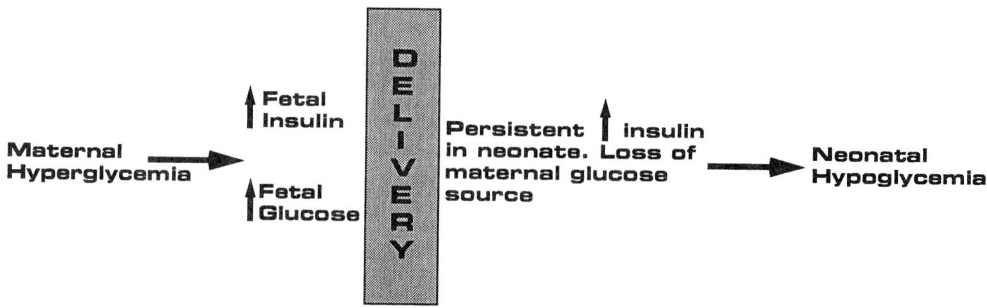

FIG. 3. Maternal hyperglycemia results in neonatal hypoglycemia.

minute) occurs more commonly in the infants of diabetic mothers. The increased likelihood of immaturity and prematurity in neonates of diabetic mothers may explain this higher risk of depression.

Spinal anesthesia is appropriate for cesarean delivery provided that hypotension is avoided. Early studies suggested infants of diabetic pregnancies developed more severe acidosis after spinal anesthesia–induced hypotension than do infants of normal pregnancies (18). However, these patients received glucose-containing solutions for prehydration; therefore maternal hyperglycemia likely contributed to the fetal acidosis. Later studies found that avoiding maternal hyperglycemia and treating hypotension aggressively (ephedrine, 10 to 20 mg, i.v., when systolic blood pressure decreases 10 mm Hg), ensures comparable neonatal outcome in normal and diabetic pregnancies receiving spinal anesthesia for cesarean delivery (19).

Epidural anesthesia is another reasonable choice of anesthesia for cesarean delivery in diabetic patients. As with spinal anesthesia, maternal hypotension may cause neonatal acidosis, particularly if the maternal diabetes is severe (20). Use care when giving large doses of epidural local anesthetics to a potentially acidotic fetus of a diabetic parturient. Local anesthetic ion-trapping may occur in these fetuses, resulting in accumulation of the anesthetic in the neonate (20). The rapid metabolism of 2-chloroprocaine may make it useful in this setting. Still, its rapid onset, greater incidence of hypotension (21), and short duration also must be considered.

Be certain that the person responsible for neonatal resuscitation is aware that they are receiving an infant of a diabetic mother. Measure glucose in the neonate after delivery and watch for signs of hypoglycemia (blood glucose less than 35 mg/dL in term infants). These signs include poor tone, poor color, apnea, respiratory distress, lethargy, hypothermia, or seizures (22).

ANESTHETIC MANAGEMENT OF THE OBESE PARTURIENT

The obese parturient (weighing more than 90 kg) can pose considerable physiologic and technical challenges to the anesthesiologist (Table 3). Obesity complicates 6% to 10% of pregnancies and is more common in older patients of greater parity (23–25). The impact of obesity on obstetric outcome is difficult to determine because of varied definitions of obesity and the presence of concomitant medical problems. Obese parturients develop preeclampsia, hypertension, and diabetes more commonly than do nonobese parturients (23,24,26–28), and these disorders affect obstetric care. Obese women also may have hypertriglyceridemia and coronary artery disease (29,30). Obesity is a risk factor for a long and difficult labor and has been associated with a high cesarean-delivery rate (23,25–28). Associated fetal problems include macrosomia, shoulder dystocia, and birth trauma.

Obesity affects pulmonary (Table 4) and cardiac function. During normal pregnancy, functional residual capacity (FRC) decreases (because of a reduction in expiratory reserve volume), and oxygen consumption increases (31).

TABLE 3. *The obese parturient and anesthesia*

- Concomitant medical problems
  - Pulmonary dysfunction
  - Hypertension
  - Diabetes
  - Cardiovascular disease
- Fetal complications
  - Macrosomia
  - Abnormal presentation
- Anesthetic difficulties
  - Maternal and fetal monitoring problematic
  - Regional anesthesia
    - Landmarks difficult to palpate
    - Gravid uterus and abdominal fat pad contribute to hypotension
    - Epidural/spinal local anesthetic dose requirements reduced/unpredictable
  - General anesthesia
    - Difficult intubation
    - Pulmonary aspiration of gastric contents
    - Hypoxemia
    - Unpredictable drug dose requirements
- Postoperative problems
  - Hypoxia, hypoventilation
  - Thromboembolism

TABLE 4. *Pulmonary changes in the obese parturient*

↓ Functional residual capacity
↓ Chest wall compliance
Small-airway closure
Ventilation/perfusion mismatch
↓ Ventilatory response to CO_2
↑ Minute ventilation
↑ Work of breathing

Pulmonary changes from obesity include decreased lung and chest-wall compliance due to chest-wall and abdominal fat, increased work of breathing, increased minute ventilation, and, possibly, a further reduction in total lung capacity and FRC (32,33). Pulmonary-function studies in obese nonpregnant patients show a restrictive ventilatory defect. Further, in volunteer subjects, obesity imposes a diminished ventilatory response to hypercarbia when compared with that of nonobese volunteers (33). The pulmonary changes resulting from pregnancy plus obesity lead to the potential for ventilation/perfusion mismatching. Closing capacity may be within the range of tidal ventilation in obese parturients, particularly when supine. Airway closure causes ventilation/perfusion defects and hypoxemia. Hypoventilation from sedatives or residual anesthetics further increases the risk of hypoxemia.

The cardiovascular system is stressed during obesity and pregnancy; both conditions contribute to increased cardiac work. This combination may produce symptoms of myocardial failure during pregnancy. If a patient gives a history of orthopnea or severe dyspnea on exertion, seek a cardiac evaluation to clarify cardiac function. Further, obstructive sleep apnea can occur in obese patients, causing pulmonary hypertension and right heart failure. Hypertensive disorders of pregnancy also are common in these patients.

Obese parturients often require anesthetic care because of a long labor or operative vaginal or cesarean delivery. Preanesthetic evaluation must include careful assessment of the patient's cardiac and pulmonary function. Look for evidence of preeclampsia and diabetes. Check that intravenous access is adequate. Pay particular attention to the airway, and assess the advisability of performing a rapid induction of anesthesia. Know the obstetric plan and share any anesthetic concerns with the obstetricians.

Analgesia for Labor and Delivery

Use systemic medications with caution. The sedative effects of systemic opioids can contribute to hypoventilation, resulting in hypoxemia. The effective dose of opioids for labor analgesia in the obese patient may be unpredictable. Therefore give opioids in small incrementals, titrating to the desired effect. Should somnolence occur, use a pulse oximeter to assess adequacy of oxygenation and to guide treatment with supplemental oxygen.

Regional analgesia can be very helpful in obese parturients. Adequate analgesia will diminish ventilatory requirements during labor, a beneficial effect in these women with already stressed cardiopulmonary systems (34). Regional analgesia can help maintain good oxygenation by preventing the cycle of hyperventilation with painful contractions and hypoventilation in the rest period between contractions (35). Hypoxemia may occur during this period of hypoventilation because of airway closure, high oxygen consumption, and altered ventilatory drive. Finally, a continuous epidural block provides a means of anesthetizing the patient should cesarean or operative vaginal delivery become necessary.

Monitoring

Monitoring of both mother and fetus while establishing regional anesthesia can prove difficult in obese parturients. The fetal heart rate may be difficult to trace with an external monitor, and having the patient sit for epidural placement can exacerbate this problem. Nonetheless, try to monitor fetal heart rate continuously, particularly when administering an anesthetic. Accurately measuring maternal blood pressure is another challenge. An appropriately sized blood pressure cuff should be 20% to 30% as wide as the arm circumference. A thigh cuff on the upper arm or a large blood pressure cuff on the forearm may be necessary. Pulse oximetry can be very helpful in guiding the use of supplemental oxygen in these patients with potentially reduced pulmonary reserve.

Epidural Technique

Identifying the epidural space, inserting a catheter, and successfully providing labor analgesia can prove a daunting task in obese parturients (26). Feeling landmarks for epidural needle placement is often impossible in obese patients. It is helpful to place the epidural catheter with the patient in the sitting position, and recent clinical studies suggested that this position is more comfortable for these patients (36). The sitting position allows identification of the midline of the patient by drawing a line between the often easily palpated C_7 spinous process and the gluteal fold (37). Marks at the waist from undergarments or the fetal heart-rate monitor belt can approximate the level of the L_{3-4} or L_{4-5} interspaces (Fig. 4). The spinous processes above and below the interspace used can be identified, after local infiltration, by probing with a long 26-gauge spinal needle. An extra long epidural needle may be needed to reach the epidural space. If reaching the epidural space necessitates indenting the skin or subcutaneous tissue of the back, be sure the needle stays in a stable position while inserting the epidural catheter to prevent the indented skin from displacing the needle.

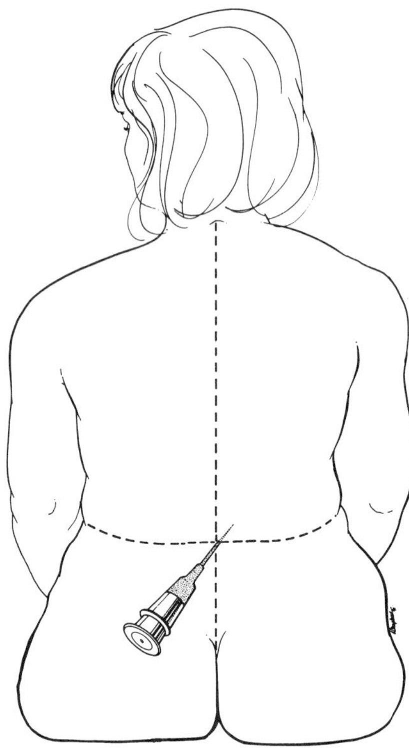

FIG. 4. Landmarks for regional anesthesia in the obese patient. Midline is estimated by drawing a line from the prominence of the C_7 vertebra to the gluteal fold. The lower lumbar interspaces are estimated from skin creases left by undergarments or the fetal heart-rate monitor belt.

Initial labor analgesia can be provided with either intrathecal opioids (with or without local anesthetic) or epidural opioid and local anesthetic. The rapid onset of analgesia with intrathecal opioids and the relative certainty of proper placement of intrathecal opioids [by observing cerebrospinal fluid (CSF) flow] are beneficial features of this technique in the obese parturient. However, I prefer to place and test an epidural catheter for proper function with local anesthetics as soon as possible. I want to know whether the epidural catheter will provide a reliable block. Not uncommonly, the epidural catheter needs replacement or repositioning to achieve and maintain continuous pain relief (38). Hood and Dewan (26) reported the need to repeat epidural catheter placement in 42% of morbidly obese (more than 300 lb) parturients receiving epidural analgesia compared with 6% of normal-weight parturients.

Placing an epidural catheter early in labor allows time to assure proper function. In addition, the patient may be more cooperative in early labor than in the more painful active phase. Hood and Dewan (26) stated: "Performing successful epidural anesthesia in morbidly obese parturients proved to be difficult. Misidentification of appropriate landmarks and anatomic distortion contributed to our high initial epidural anesthetic failure rate. However, we believe that critical evaluation of the quality of epidural anesthesia, and replacement of questionable epidural catheters, produced our high regional anesthesia success rate for morbidly obese parturients. Early placement and evaluation of the epidural catheter function is essential to allow enough time to replace failed epidural catheters."

Dilute local anesthetic/opioid solutions are useful in obese patients to both confirm proper catheter location (by demonstration of a bilateral block) and minimize motor block (to allow the patient to move and assist with transfer, if needed).

Be careful dosing the epidural catheter for labor analgesia. Both the gravid uterus and the obese abdomen contribute to aortocaval compression. Dose the catheter slowly to avoid sudden hypotension and fetal compromise, which could lead to the need for an emergency delivery. In addition, epidural local anesthetics may spread farther in obese parturients, increasing the level of sensory blockade achieved with a given dose of drug (Fig. 5) (39,40). Although Milligan et al. (41) did not observe any differences in extent of epidural block in obese (more than 100 kg) compared with control (less than 80 kg) parturients after injection of 12 mL of 0.25% bupivacaine.

If dural puncture occurs while attempting to identify the epidural space, consider taking advantage of the situation by threading a catheter into the intrathecal space and conducting a continuous spinal anesthetic. Either opioids or a combination of opioids and local anesthetics can be used for effective labor analgesia (see Chapter 16).

Anesthesia for Cesarean Section

Anesthesia for the obese parturient undergoing cesarean delivery is challenging. Patient positioning is difficult. The operating table may be narrow or unstable. The addition of extra arm boards along the side can increase the width of the table. The supine position may exacerbate dyspnea, airway closure, and inadequate alveolar ventilation, leading to hypoxemia and hypercarbia. A modified "lawn chair" position (42) with both head and legs slightly elevated may help maintain FRC and, at the same time, preserve venous return and patient comfort. Positioning the patient in a proper "sniffing" position also should help (Fig. 6).

Surgical Technique

The type of skin incision used for cesarean delivery can affect the patient's ventilatory status. The Pfannenstiel incision may produce less postoperative pain and allow earlier ambulation (43,44). However, the abdominal fat pad needs to be displaced cephalad to provide good surgical exposure. Doing so may compromise the patient's pulmonary status and contribute to caval compression and diminished venous return. Hodgkinson and

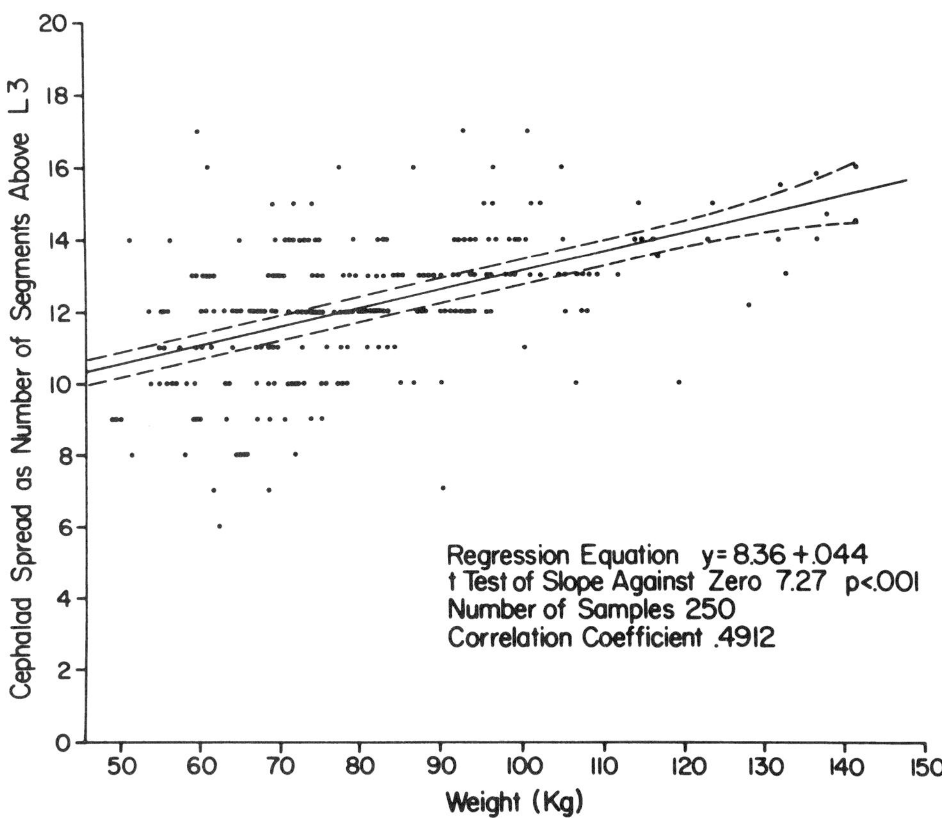

FIG. 5. Relation of parturient's weight to highest point of cephalad spread of epidural analgesia as determined by pin-prick after single injection at $L_{3\text{-}4}$ of 20 mL of 0.75% bupivacaine. The three lines on the graph represent the regression line with the 95% confidence limits drawn on either side. (Reprinted from ref. 40, with permission.)

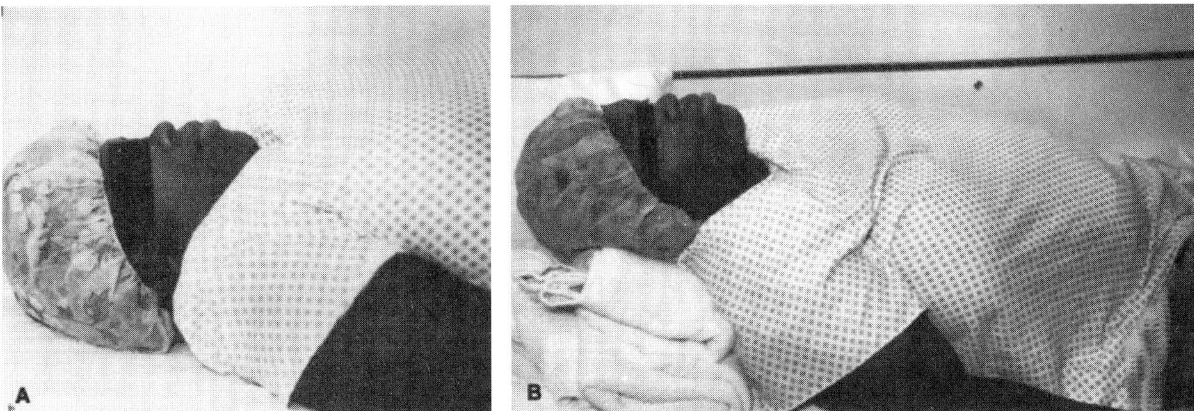

FIG. 6. A: An obese pregnant woman in the supine position. The inability to extend the head on the atlantooccipital joint prevents alignment of oral, pharyngeal, and laryngeal axes and limits access to the airway with the laryngoscope. **B:** Proper positioning includes elevation of the shoulders, flexion of the cervical spine, and extension of the head on the atlantooccipital joint (the "sniffing" position). The sniffing position helps align the oral, pharyngeal, and laryngeal axes and improves access to the airway. (Photographs courtesy of Dr. B. Leighton, Philadelphia, PA, with permission.)

Husain (45) reported a case of an obese parturient undergoing cesarean section with epidural anesthesia and a Pfannenstiel incision in whom refractory hypotension due to cephalad retraction of the panniculus resulted in fetal demise. Carefully evaluate the hemodynamic and pulmonary affects of the patient's position.

Monitoring

Maternal monitoring may be difficult. Use a properly sized blood pressure cuff. If noninvasive blood pressure monitoring is unreliable, consider an arterial catheter for measuring blood pressure and maternal blood gas tensions. Older obese parturients with severe hypertension or cardiac disease may require hemodynamic monitoring with central venous or pulmonary artery catheters. Pulse oximetry is necessary to assess maternal oxygenation. During general anesthesia, the immediate ability to measure end-tidal CO_2 is crucial to determine proper placement of an endotracheal tube. Monitor the fetus during positioning and induction of anesthesia when at all possible.

Anesthetic Technique

Epidural Anesthesia

Regional anesthesia, especially epidural block, has significant advantages over general anesthesia in obese patients, provided the patient can maintain adequate alveolar ventilation when lying supine. With epidural anesthesia, the level of sensory blockade can be extended slowly and in a relatively controlled fashion. The slower onset of sympathetic block improves hemodynamic stability. Because of the risk of aortocaval compression by the uterus and abdominal fat pad, the slower onset of sympathetic blockade will provide additional time to alter maternal position and volume status should hypotension occur. Given the possibility of reduced epidural local anesthetic requirements associated with obesity (39,40), inject local anesthetic in small (5-mL) increments until an adequate level of blockade is achieved. An epidural catheter can provide anesthesia for as long as needed. The catheter also can be used for postoperative analgesia.

Spinal Anesthesia

Spinal anesthesia also can prove useful in the obese parturient. However, the rapid onset of a relatively unpredictable block height is a disadvantage. Norris (46) studied the affect of patient weight on the spread of 12 mg of intrathecal hyperbaric bupivacaine and did not find a correlation between increased maternal weight and the level of sensory blockade (Fig. 7). However, the patients studied weighed between 57 and 94 kg. The obese population per se has not been carefully evaluated. Most likely, the spread of spinal anesthesia in obese parturients, as in all parturients, is unpredictable. The anesthesiologist must be prepared for the challenge of managing extensive spread of sensory and motor blockade in the morbidly obese parturient.

Another disadvantage of a single-injection technique is that surgery may be technically difficult and outlast the anesthetic. Perlow and Morgan (38) found that 21 of 43 (49%) cesarean sections in massively obese (more than 300 lb) patients had operative times longer than 60 min, compared with four of 43 (9.3%) control patients. In one series of obese cesarean patients, spinal anesthesia was used less often than epidural anesthesia (Table 5) (26). Successful use of single-injection spinal anesthesia in the obese parturient requires an understanding of the predicted operative time and skill of the obstetricians (26).

The limited duration of single-injection spinal anesthesia can be overcome by using a continuous spinal technique. As with a continuous epidural block, local anesthetic can be titrated to effect, and the duration of anesthesia can be extended rather than having to resort to intraoperative general anesthesia. Milligan and Carp (47)

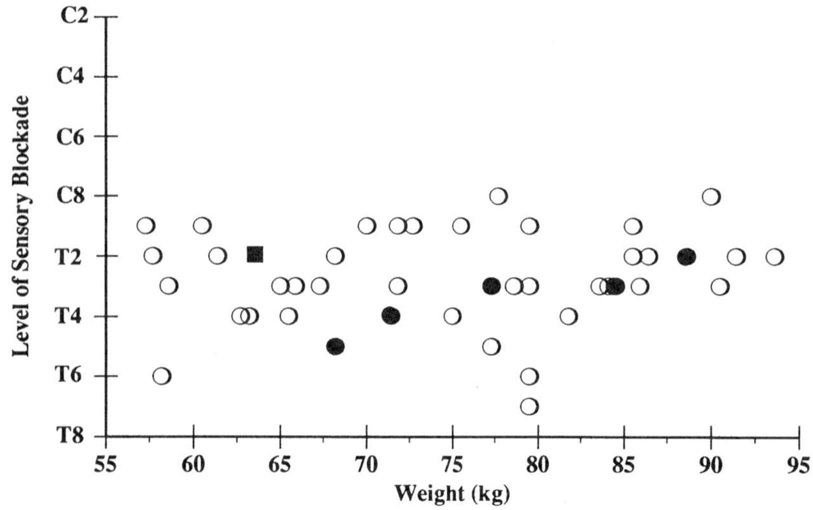

FIG. 7. Relation between weight of parturient and maximal cephalad spread of anesthesia after intrathecal injection of 12 mg hyperbaric bupivacaine in 50 term parturients. (Redrawn from ref. 46, with permission.

TABLE 5. *Anesthesia for cesarean delivery in morbidly obese (>300 lb) vs normal-weight parturients*

	Morbidly obese	Normal weight
General anesthesia	17/72 (24%)	8/28 (29%)
Difficult intubation	6/17 (35%)	0/8 (0%)
Epidural anesthesia	51/72 (71%)	13/28 (46%)
Spinal anesthesia	4/72 (5%)	7/28 (25%)

Adapted from ref. 26, with permission.

described three cases of morbidly obese (180 to 230 kg) parturients managed with continuous spinal anesthesia (a 20-gauge epidural catheter was threaded into the subarachnoid space via a 17-gauge epidural needle). Surgical anesthesia was accomplished and maintained with 0.5- to 1.0-mL injections of hyperbaric 0.75% spinal bupivacaine.

General Anesthesia

General anesthesia presents significant risks to the obese parturient. The inability to secure an airway is a leading cause of maternal mortality (48,49), and obesity is an important risk factor for difficult intubation (50). Hood and Dewan (26) reported that six of the 17 morbidly obese patients who required general anesthesia for cesarean section were difficult to intubate (Table 5). Beware that general anesthesia may be needed to rescue failed regional anesthesia in obese parturients.

Thorough preoperative airway evaluation is essential. If this examination suggests a potentially difficult intubation, inform the obstetric staff that a rapid induction of general anesthesia could jeopardize maternal safety. If general anesthesia is necessary, allow time for either awake fiberoptic intubation or awake direct laryngoscopy.

Rocke et al. (51) examined preoperatively identifiable factors that could predict a difficult intubation in the parturient. Although obesity per se was not an independent risk factor, other factors, which occur in obese patients, did correlate with airway-management difficulties (Mallampati class airway greater than I, short neck, receding mandible).

Other factors contribute to airway difficulties in the obese parturient. A short neck with limited mobility may make it difficult to insert the laryngoscope into the mouth. A short-handled laryngoscope is helpful in this situation (52). Redundant tissue in the airway may be difficult to displace with any laryngoscope blade. Use of the Bullard laryngoscope with an intubating stylet was reported to be useful in this situation (53).

To optimize the chances of a successful intubation, pay close attention to maternal position before inducing anesthesia. Have the patient in the "sniffing" position. This position includes flexion of the cervical spine with extension of the head on the atlantooccipital joint. However, because of the generous fat pad behind the shoulders, many obese parturients have difficulty assuming this position with only a small pillow under their heads. Support the patient's shoulders on blankets and further support the base of her skull with additional towels (Fig. 6). This support helps the breasts to fall forward, increases the space between the neck and the chest, and allows proper alignment of the oral, pharyngeal, and laryngeal axes. Finally, confirm proper endotracheal placement with capnography.

Even with the best of preoperative evaluations, unpredicted difficult intubation may arise. Always be prepared to manage a difficult airway. Set your priorities in advance. Know ahead of time the steps you will take if intubation proves difficult or impossible (see Chapter 32). Have appropriate (and familiar) equipment available and have practiced a "failed intubation drill." As soon as you identify a difficult airway, call for help. Have small endotracheal tubes and a variety of laryngoscope blades readily available. Mask ventilation may be particularly difficult in the obese patient because of airway edema and redundant pharyngeal tissue. The laryngeal mask airway (LMA) may be quite useful in such a situation to assist with maternal oxygenation. Remember, the LMA does not protect against aspiration of gastric contents.

The physiologic changes of pregnancy place all obstetric patients at increased risk for gastric acid aspiration, and obese patients have even larger gastric volumes and lower gastric pH values (54). Furthermore, difficulties with intubation and the potential for multiple manipulations of the airway predispose these patients to regurgitate gastric contents. For these reasons, use a rapid-sequence induction with cricoid pressure and endotracheal intubation when inducing general anesthesia in parturients.

Before induction, use pharmacologic measures to reduce intragastric volume and increase intragastric pH. Give clear antacids within 30 minutes of the planned surgery. H_2 blockers will increase intragastric pH (55,56). Metoclopramide may help reduce gastric volume in these patients. Because of the increased risk in obese patients, I recommend using several pharmacologic measures to help minimize the chance of pulmonary damage should aspiration occur.

Obese parturients are at high risk for developing hypoxemia during the induction of anesthesia. As a result of both a reduced FRC (57) and a high oxygen consumption, parturients of normal weight have a more rapid decrease in P_aO_2 during apnea than do nonpregnant patients (Fig. 8) (58). Obesity further reduces FRC. Significant airway closure occurs during tidal ventilation in the supine position (33,57). General anesthesia exacerbates this problem, causing mismatch of ventilation and perfusion, increasing the risk of hypoxemia (57,59). Oxygen consumption is higher in obese versus nonobese parturients (33). Consequently, obese parturients rapidly deplete their already low oxygen stores.

Preoxygenation is essential before the induction of anesthesia. In nonobese parturients, clinical studies have shown that either 3 to 5 minutes of tidal breathing or four deep

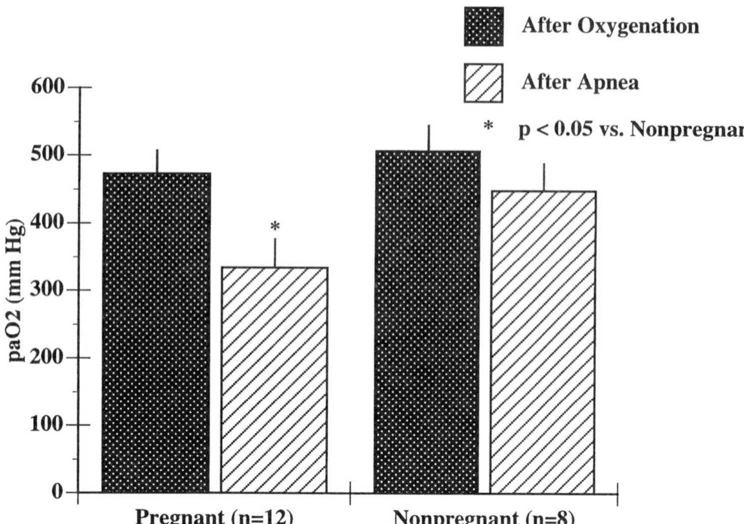

FIG. 8. The decrease in p_aO_2 after 60 seconds of apnea is greater in pregnant than in nonpregnant women. (Data from ref. 58, with permission.)

breaths of 100% oxygen provide adequate preoxygenation before the induction of anesthesia (60). Both techniques also provide effective preoxygenation in nonpregnant obese patients (61). In addition, obese patients taking four deep breaths do not experience the same increase in p_aCO_2 as when they breath quietly into a facemask for 3 minutes. This factor may help avoid hypercarbia during airway management. Remember, with any technique of preoxygenation, use high fresh gas flows (8 to 10 L/min) to prevent rebreathing of exhaled nitrogen, and maintain a tight mask fit to avoid entrainment of room air.

Intraoperatively, pulse oximetry and capnometry provide important information to guide mechanical ventilation. Because of the changes in pulmonary function during general anesthesia, obese patients may need a high F_IO_2 to maintain adequate maternal oxygenation. Large tidal volumes or positive end-expiratory pressure (PEEP) will help maintain maternal oxygenation. However, if using PEEP, watch for adverse effects on cardiac output and blood pressure (62).

Obese parturients have altered pharmacokinetics. Obese nonpregnant patients metabolize halothane more than do nonobese patients (63). They also may respond unpredictably to muscle relaxants. Weinstein et al. (64) studied the pharmacodynamics of vecuronium and atracurium in nonpregnant surgical patients and found prolonged recovery times for vecuronium in obese patients. They concluded that obesity most likely alters hepatic clearance. Therefore carefully titrate vecuronium and other drugs dependent on hepatic metabolism in obese patients.

After completion of surgery, carefully evaluate the adequacy of ventilation, oxygenation, and airway reflexes

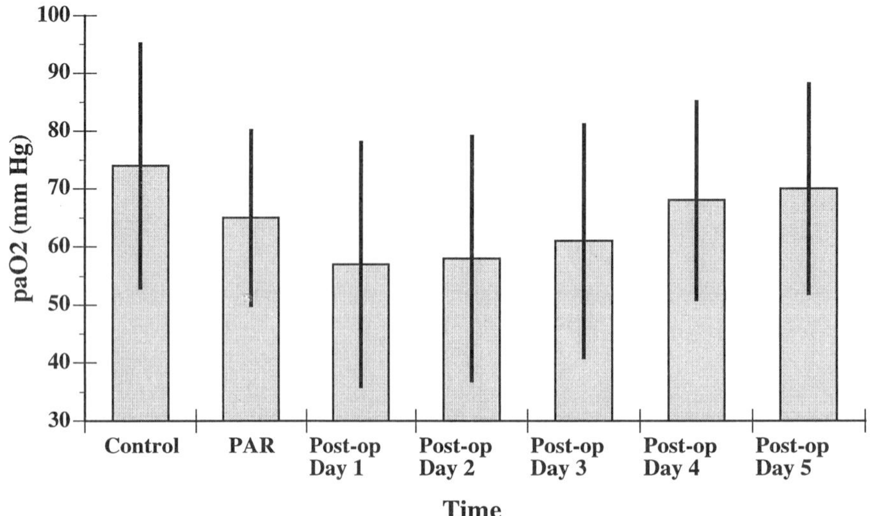

FIG. 9. Graphic representation of the decrease in p_aO_2 (mm Hg) with time postoperatively in obese patients who have undergone major abdominal surgery. (Data from ref. 66, with permission.)

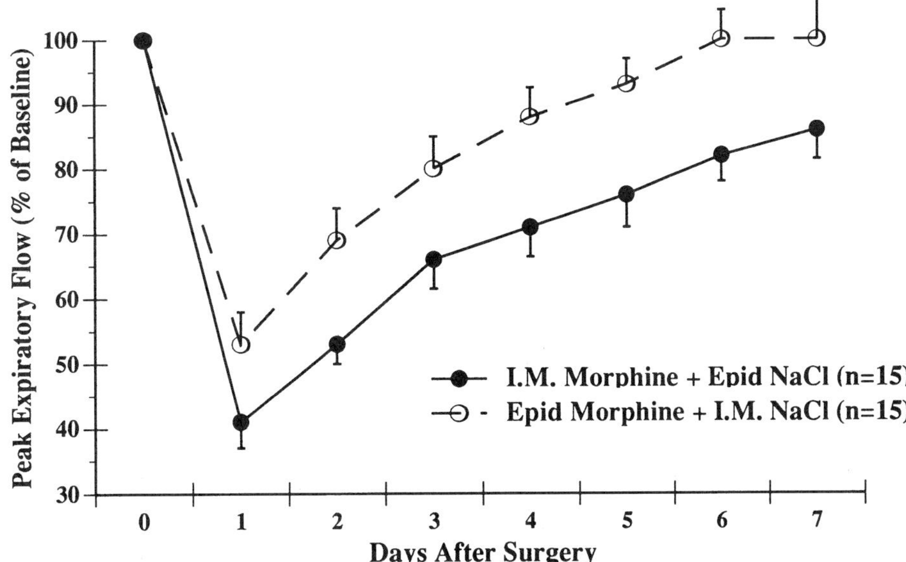

FIG. 10. Peak expiratory flow pre- and postoperatively in obese patients who received either intramuscular or epidural morphine for postoperative analgesia. (Redrawn from ref. 67, with permission.)

before extubating the trachea. Assist ventilation in the early postoperative period as needed.

Cesarean delivery in the obese parturient also can pose significant risks for the neonate. Because of technical difficulties during surgery, the time from induction of anesthesia to delivery of the infant may be prolonged (38). With general anesthesia, placental passage of anesthetic drugs for a prolonged time (greater than 10 to 15 minutes) can contribute to neonatal depression. The time from uterine incision to delivery also may be prolonged in the obese patient. When this time exceeds 3 minutes, fetal acidosis can develop (65). Diabetes is common in the obese parturient, and these infants may be hypoglycemic after delivery (23). The person responsible for resuscitation of the newborn must be aware of these risks.

Postoperative Care

Significant problems continue to occur after cesarean delivery in obese patients. Pulmonary-function abnormalities persist. In nonpregnant obese patients undergoing abdominal surgery, oxygenation remains poor up to postoperative day 4 (Fig. 9) (66). Possible etiologies for this hypoxemia include pain and inadequate ventilation, excessive sedation from analgesics, and diaphragmatic dysfunction. Good postoperative analgesia should promote early ambulation and good pulmonary toilet. Spinal or epidural opioids are helpful by providing good analgesia without excessive maternal sedation. They can help promote early ambulation, coughing and deep breathing, and good alveolar ventilation. In nonobstetric obese patients, the use of epidural opioids for postoperative pain relief after abdominal surgery improves early postoperative pulmonary function (Fig. 10) (67).

Cardiac function may be stressed in the early postoperative period. Cardiac demands are highest immediately postpartum because of delivery of the placenta, the loss of the low-resistance placental bed, and autotransfusion of blood from the contracted uterus. Volume overload is possible during this time in patients with borderline cardiac function. Resolution of regional anesthesia-induced sympathetic blockade will contribute to this volume load, as will mobilization of interstitial edema in the preeclamptic patient. The obese parturient with hypertension, preeclampsia, or other evidence of myocardial dysfunction must be monitored carefully after delivery.

Obese patients are at risk for venous stasis and thrombosis in the postoperative period. Thromboembolic disease is a leading cause of mortality in obese parturients (Table 6) (68). Early ambulation, compression stockings, and subcutaneous heparin may help prevent venous thrombosis.

TABLE 6. *Causes of death in obstetric patients weighing >175 pounds*

Cause	No. of patients
Pulmonary embolism	7
Hemorrhage	6
Infection (obstetric)	2
Meningitis	1
Toxemia	1
Amniotic fluid embolism	1
Anesthesia	1
Intracranial hemorrhage	1
Pneumonia	1
Hemorrhagic pancreatitis	1
Acute fatty metamorphosis of liver	1
Total	23

Adapted from ref. 68, with permission.

ANESTHETIC MANAGEMENT OF THE PARTURIENT WITH PULMONARY DISEASE

Asthma

Preoperative Evaluation

Preoperative evaluation of the patient with asthma (Table 7) includes assessment of the severity of asthma during pregnancy, symptoms (shortness of breath, cough, wheezing, chest tightness), medications (inhaled β-agonists, cromolyn sodium, corticosteroids, systemic corticosteroids, oral theophylline), and events that precipitate asthma (stress, exercise, allergens, infections). Examine the patient for evidence of bronchospasm. Remember, in severe bronchospasm, auscultation may not detect wheezing because of limited air movement (69). Spirometry, and if necessary, arterial blood gases provide more information when evaluating the current status of the patient's disease (Table 8) (69,70). When interpreting arterial blood gases, remember that a normal p_aCO_2 during pregnancy ranges from 32 to 34 mm Hg (71). Try to optimize maternal pulmonary status before induction of labor or cesarean delivery. Maternal hypoxia and hypocapnia will impair fetal oxygenation. Good control of asthma is important to minimize adverse effects of the disease on pregnancy outcome (72).

Important goals for the anesthesiologist caring for the parturient with asthma include avoiding events or agents that would precipitate bronchoconstriction and minimizing the work of breathing during labor or cesarean section. Continue bronchodilator therapy throughout labor.

Acute asthma occurs fairly uncommonly during labor and delivery. Schatz et al. (73) studied 336 pregnancies in asthmatic patients and found that asthma symptoms occurred during labor in only 10% of these women. If bronchospasm develops during labor and delivery, give supplemental oxygen, make sure the patient is well hydrated, and look for an inciting cause (such as upper respiratory infection, exposure to allergens) (Table 9). Treat the bronchospasm initially with inhaled β_2-adrenergic agonists such as metoproterenol or albuterol (69,74–77). Alternatively, terbutaline, 0.25 mg, can be given subcutaneously. Parenteral corticosteroid therapy may be necessary if inhaled β-agonists do not relieve bronchospasm (76,77). Patients who have taken oral steroids to manage asthma during the previous year should receive steroid coverage during labor and delivery with intravenous hydrocortisone, 100 mg, every 6 hours (69). Note that patients receiving corticosteroids may have concomitant diabetes (78).

The methylxanthines (aminophylline or theophylline) are not commonly used for the treatment of asthma. Some patients may take oral preparations to supplement inhaled β-agonists. Intravenous aminophylline for the treatment of acute asthma can be used if symptoms have not improved with inhaled β-agonists and corticosteroids (72,75–77). Aminophylline may predispose a patient to dysrhythmias during halothane general anesthesia (79–81).

TABLE 7. *The asthmatic parturient and anesthesia*

Optimize pulmonary status before delivery, if possible
Give supplemental oxygen
Avoid events that precipitate asthma (hyperventilation, hypocarbia, airway manipulation)
Continue bronchodilator therapy during labor and delivery or perioperative period
Monitor the fetus for evidence of compromise due to maternal asthma
Regional analgesia for labor diminishes ventilatory work
General anesthesia via endotracheal tube may precipitate bronchospasm
Avoid 15-methyl $PGF_{2\alpha}$

PGF, prostaglandin F.

TABLE 8. *Clinical classification of impairment of pulmonary function in asthma*

	VC, FVC, FEV_1, MVV	$FEF_{25\%-75\%}$
Normal	>80	>75
Mild	65–80	60–75
Moderate	50–64	45–59
Severe	35–49	30–44
Very severe	<35	<30

From ref. 70, with permission.
Values expressed as percentage of predicted value.
VC, vital capacity; FVC, forced vital capacity; FEV_1, forced expiratory volume in 1 sec; MVV, maximal voluntary ventilation; $FEF_{25\%-75\%}$, maximal midexpiratory flow rate.

Anesthesia for Labor and Delivery

Systemic medications can provide analgesia and sedation in the early phases of labor. However, in more active and painful labor, epidural analgesia has distinct advantages. In patients without analgesia, the pain of active labor increases minute ventilation and oxygen consumption (34). In the asthmatic patient, this hyperventilation and hypocarbia may precipitate bronchospasm. Epidural analgesia blunts these effects (34). For patients who do not receive epidural analgesia for labor, spinal anesthesia may be used for spontaneous or assisted vaginal delivery.

TABLE 9. *Peripartum bronchospasm: treatment*

Oxygen
Hydration
Inhaled bronchodilators
Metoproterenol
Albuterol
Subcutaneous terbutaline
Intravenous corticosteroids

Anesthesia for Cesarean Section

If at all possible, optimize a patient's pulmonary status before surgery begins. Continue asthma medications up to the time of surgery. Monitor pulmonary status during surgery. In most patients, this task requires only verbal communication and pulse oximetry. In unstable patients, sample arterial blood gases as needed.

Epidural Anesthesia

Regional anesthesia offers significant advantages in asthmatic patients. Avoiding general anesthesia and endotracheal intubation may decrease the incidence of bronchospasm. In an awake patient, continuous verbal contact will elicit signs of respiratory difficulty. Tanaka et al. (82) compared the incidence of bronchospasm in nonpregnant, asthmatic patients undergoing nonthoracic surgery with either epidural or general anesthesia. The incidence of bronchospasm was significantly lower in patients with epidural anesthesia (2.9%) compared with general anesthesia (5.6%). In the Closed Claims analysis of adverse respiratory events, Cheney et al. (83) reported eight cases of obstetric patients who experienced bronchospasm of a degree sufficient to result in patient injury and lawsuit. Seven of the cases involved administration of general anesthesia (two were patients who required conversion from regional to general anesthesia because of failed block and high block).

The motor block accompanying the high levels of regional anesthesia necessary for abdominal delivery can impair pulmonary function. However, the level of motor blockade is usually four to five segments below the level of sensory blockade, and resting pulmonary ventilation is not significantly affected (84). Ramanathan et al. (85) assessed arterial blood gases in 24 asthmatic parturients during cesarean delivery with epidural anesthesia (T_2 to T_4 sensory block) and found no evidence of respiratory insufficiency. None of the patients experienced bronchospasm. High levels of epidural anesthesia can, however, reduce peak expiratory flow rates and may interfere with the ability to cough (86). Assess the patient's ventilatory function continuously. Reassure the patient should the loss of sensation in the chest wall contribute to a feeling of shortness of breath. If coughing is impaired, avoid sedatives that may further suppress coughing, and watch for problems with oral secretions or regurgitation.

Epinephrine (1:200,000) in epidural local anesthetics may aid in bronchodilation. However, no documentation exists that this small amount of absorbed epinephrine produces significant bronchodilation. This technique, however, is probably not harmful.

Spinal Anesthesia

Spinal anesthesia also is appropriate for cesarean delivery in asthmatic parturients. One case report of intraoperative bronchospasm in an asthmatic patient with a T_5 level of spinal blockade raised the concern that loss of circulating epinephrine from the sympathetic blockade (leaving unbalanced parasympathetic tone) could precipitate bronchospasm (87). This single case of bronchospasm should not discourage the use of spinal anesthesia in the asthmatic parturient. Most other data suggest that extensive sensory and sympathetic blockade lack effect on respiratory function in these patients (85). As with epidural anesthesia, reductions in peak expiratory flow rates have been reported under spinal anesthesia for cesarean delivery (88).

General Anesthesia

General anesthesia carries significant risks for the parturient with asthma. The rapid induction and intubation sequence used for cesarean delivery can precipitate bronchospasm (89). Provide as deep a plane of anesthesia as possible to help prevent bronchospasm during intubation.

Ketamine, even in low doses (less than 0.5 mg/kg), causes bronchodilation in nonpregnant patients with pulmonary disorders (90). Bronchodilation begins within 1.5 minutes, and lasts for 6 to 8 minutes (90). Animal studies confirmed the bronchodilatory characteristics of ketamine (91). This feature makes ketamine a good induction agent in asthmatic parturients. Minimal neonatal depression occurs if the induction dose remains less than 1.5 mg/kg (92). Ketamine also causes sympathetic stimulation, increasing maternal blood pressure and heart rate (92). This effect makes ketamine a less favorable induction agent in hypertensive parturients.

Another option is propofol, 2.5 mg/kg. As an induction agent at cesarean section, it produces less maternal hypertension but similar neonatal outcome as thiopental 4 to 5 mg/kg (93). Further, in nonpregnant asthmatic (94) and nonasthmatic (94,95) patients, propofol reduces the incidence of bronchospasm (94) and incites smaller increases in airway resistance (95) after intubation compared with thiobarbiturates (94,95) and etomidate (95).

Other techniques to prevent intubation-related bronchospasm include intravenous lidocaine (96) or small doses of opioid (such as fentanyl). Because coughing and straining can trigger bronchospasm, avoid manipulation of the airway until full skeletal-muscle relaxation has been achieved.

If endotracheal intubation is complicated by severe bronchospasm or if bronchospasm occurs any time during general anesthesia, give high concentrations of oxygen. Inhaled bronchodilators can be given via the endotracheal tube. Volatile anesthetics are potent bronchodilators and should be used to maintain anesthesia and promote bronchodilation (97,98). Halothane and isoflurane provide equivalent bronchodilation at high doses, but animal data suggest that halothane is a better bronchodilator at lower doses [0.6 and 1.1 minimal alveolar concentration (MAC); such as are usually used during cesarean delivery] (99). If high concentrations of inhaled anesthetics are used before delivery, neonatal depression may occur. Alert the physician responsible for newborn resuscitation of the potential for volatile anesthetic-induced depression and the need to provide ventilatory support to the infant. High concentrations of these anesthetics also may contribute to uterine atony and increase blood loss (100).

As in all parturients, take the usual precautions to minimize the chance of pulmonary aspiration of gastric contents. Asthmatic patients tolerate irritation of the airways and any intrapulmonary process very poorly.

Extubation is a tricky time in asthmatic parturients. An awake extubation will minimize the chance of pulmonary aspiration of gastric contents. However, the endotracheal tube may prompt bronchospasm as the level of anesthesia wanes. Inhaled bronchodilators and small doses of intravenous fentanyl or lidocaine before emergence can help minimize airway reactivity during extubation.

Uterine Atony

Asthmatic patients are sensitive to the bronchoconstricting effects of the prostaglandin, $PGF_{2\alpha}$ (101). Therefore avoid the synthetic analogue of this prostaglandin, 15-methyl $PGF_{2\alpha}$, carboprost-tromethamine (Hemabate), when treating uterine atony in these women. As well, three cases of bronchospasm after the administration of ergot preparations (two patients received the medication intravenously, and all three patients had a history of asthma) were reported. The role of the ergot derivatives in these cases is a bit unclear. Use vigorous uterine massage and intravenous infusions of oxytocin as first treatment of uterine atony in the asthmatic patient. Resort to the ergot preparations only if necessary.

CIGARETTE USE

Cigarette use is common and can significantly affect pregnancy outcome. In a dose-dependent fashion, cigarette smoking decreases birth weight, increases perinatal mortality (102), and increases the risk of abruptio placenta, placenta previa, and bleeding during pregnancy (103). Premature and prolonged rupture of membranes also occurs more commonly in smokers (103). Cigarette smoking contributes to fetal hypoxemia by increasing maternal carbon monoxide. Carbon monoxide competes with oxygen for binding sites on hemoglobin in both the mother and the fetus. Increased carbon monoxide decreases fetal oxygen content. This chronic hypoxemia alters both fetal and placental development. The fetus redirects perfusion to priority organs (brain, heart, and adrenal glands) at the expense of overall growth. The placenta increases in size, surface area, and vascularity to optimize fetal oxygenation. These changes predispose the mother to hemorrhagic complications.

Regional anesthetic techniques are appropriate for labor and vaginal or cesarean delivery. However, during induction of either spinal or epidural anesthesia, take care to avoid reductions in uteroplacental blood flow with adequate maternal prehydration, left uterine displacement, and careful monitoring of blood pressure. Monitor the fetus during induction to assess any potential anesthetic effects on fetal well-being.

General anesthesia for cesarean delivery has significant disadvantages for parturients who smoke. Airway reactivity increases in patients who smoke regularly (104). Therefore the induction of general anesthesia may provoke bronchospasm. The induction techniques and treatments for intraoperative bronchospasm described in the section on patients with asthma are appropriate in smokers. General anesthesia also has adverse effects on mucociliary clearance and macrophage function in patients who smoke cigarettes (105). This action may increase the risk of postoperative pulmonary problems.

Regional anesthesia, in contrast, avoids airway manipulation and suppression of mucociliary clearance. However, the motor blockade that accompanies the high sensory level of blockade necessary for cesarean delivery may interfere with the ability of some parturients to cough intra- and immediately postoperatively (86,88).

Cigarette smokers produce more airway secretions than do nonsmokers. Encourage aggressive postoperative pulmonary toilet with incentive spirometry and deep breathing and coughing. Avoid drugs that cause cough suppression (systemic opioids and sedatives) as much as possible. Postoperative analgesia with intraspinal opioids can minimize cough suppression and help maintain optimal pulmonary function.

ANESTHETIC MANAGEMENT OF THE PARTURIENT WITH NEUROLOGICAL DISEASE

Anesthetic care of the parturient with preexisting neurological disease must be individualized. It should take into consideration the natural history of the patient's disease and the likelihood that a specific anesthetic technique or drug will alter the course of that disease. Some anesthesiologists hesitate, for example, to do a regional anesthetic in a patient with a neuropathy. If the patient's condition worsens after the anesthetic, they fear their anesthetic will be blamed for the problem. Others believe it is unfair to consider all patients with neurological disease ineligible for the potential benefits of regional anesthesia for labor, delivery, or cesarean section (106,107). Consider each case individually. Consult with the patient, her neurologist, and her obstetrician to design a reasonable and safe anesthetic plan. Understand the pathophysiology of the neurological problem, and consider the potential affects of anesthesia on the disease. Come to an agreement with the patient regarding anesthetic management before labor begins. The following sections outline the information available concerning the effects of anesthetics on patients with seizure disorders, multiple sclerosis, myasthenia gravis, paraplegia, and intracranial vascular abnormalities.

Seizure Disorder

Possible causes of seizures during pregnancy include eclampsia, intracranial tumor or vascular abnormality, subarachnoid hemorrhage, metabolic disturbances, drug or alcohol withdrawal, trauma, and idiopathic. Be aware of the etiology of seizures in a given parturient. Review the medications taken by the patient with a preexisting seizure disorder. Check the blood concentration of the patient's medication and give supplemental drug if needed. Avoid situations that could lower seizure threshold.

Labor epidural analgesia can significantly benefit these patients. Hypocarbia, which develops when labor pain causes maternal hyperventilation, lowers seizure threshold. Epidural analgesia limits this maternal hyperventilation in response to pain (35). Similarly, regional anesthesia is quite suitable for anesthesia for cesarean delivery.

Two anesthetic agents, enflurane and ketamine, can cause seizures. High concentrations (2.5% to 3%) of enflurane in the presence of hypocarbia lower the seizure threshold and cause convulsions (108). However, at lower doses and with normocarbia, Oshima et al. (109) found enflurane to have anticonvulsant properties in cats. These authors concluded that enflurane carries little risk of exacerbating a preexisting epileptic focus. The presence of a seizure disorder probably does not contraindicate the use of enflurane in low doses during cesarean delivery. Ketamine incites electroencephalogram (EEG) seizure activity when given to patients with preexisting seizure disorders (110,111). Ferrer-Allado (111) found electrical seizure activity in all six patients with epilepsy who received 2 or 4 mg/kg ketamine. It seems reasonable to avoid ketamine as an induction agent in parturients with epilepsy. It also is reasonable to avoid repeated doses of meperidine for labor or postoperative analgesia. Accumulation of the metabolite normeperidine has been reported to cause seizures (112).

Some seizure medications may alter anesthetic requirements. Phenytoin and carbamazepine reportedly antagonize the action of nondepolarizing muscle relaxants (113,114). Monitor neuromuscular function carefully in patients receiving these medications. Phenobarbital increases hepatic metabolism of anesthetics by inducing hepatic enzyme function. I suggest using only the minimally metabolized volatile anesthetics.

Multiple Sclerosis

Multiple sclerosis is a disease of the central nervous system characterized by nerve demyelination with intermittent exacerbations and improvements in symptoms (Table 10). Hyperpyrexia, infection, electrolyte imbalance, emotional and physical stress, and fatigue can worsen symptoms or trigger relapses. Parturients with multiple sclerosis who relapse tend to do so in the 3 months after delivery rather than during pregnancy (115).

There are theoretical concerns about the use of regional anesthesia in patients with multiple sclerosis. Local anesthetics may be neurotoxic when injected close to demyelinated nerves. They could contribute to or be associated with exacerbations of the disease. Currently available prospective longitudinal studies of pregnancy and multiple sclerosis have not included data about anesthesia for delivery (115,116). Still, individual case reports (107, 117) and a case series document safe use of epidural block for labor analgesia and cesarean delivery (118).

There is, though, an association between the use of high concentrations of epidural local anesthetics and the incidence of postpartum relapse of multiple sclerosis (Table 11) (118). The number of patients in this series was small, and other factors, such as a long, difficult labor, fetal malpresentation, difficult delivery, and so on, may both fuel the need for high concentrations of local anesthetics and magnify the risk of relapse of multiple sclerosis. Nevertheless, in light of these findings, we should probably use as little local anesthetic as possible in these women.

Hyperpyrexia has been shown to exacerbate multiple sclerosis and even increases in body temperature of 0.5° to 1.0°C may reversibly block conduction in marginally functional demyelinated neurons and worsen symptoms (119). This effect is worrisome in light of recent reports

TABLE 10. *Signs and symptoms of multiple sclerosis*

Classic signs
Optic neuritis
Internuclear ophthalmoplegia
Lhermitte's sign (neck flexion produces sharp sensation down back and into legs)
Motor
Weakness (ultimately paralysis)
Stiffness
Clumsiness
Spasticity (contractures can develop)
Sensory
Paresthesias
Girdle-like pressure
Trigeminal neuralgia
Impaired two-point discrimination
Cerebellar
Lack of coordination
Loss of position and vibration sense
Other
Cognitive losses
Dysarthria
Dysphagia
Neurgenic bladder
Seizures

TABLE 11. *Relapse of multiple sclerosis in the first 3 months postpartum*

Type of anesthetic	No.	Relapse number
Cesarean delivery		
Epidural	5	1
General	3	1
Vaginal delivery		
Epidural	9	4
Local	13	2
General	2	1

From ref. 118, with permission.

of increases in maternal core temperature associated with labor epidural analgesia (120–122). Maternal temperature is most notable when room temperature is warm (121). It may be prudent to monitor carefully maternal and room temperature throughout labor and delivery.

No data exist concerning the use of spinal anesthesia in these women. It is generally not recommended because of the theoretic concern of neurotoxicity from injecting the local anesthetic close to demyelinated nerves. Regardless of the type of neuraxial anesthesia selected, discuss the possibility of relapse with the patient preoperatively.

General anesthesia with a variety of agents has been used in nonpregnant patients with multiple sclerosis without consistent alterations in relapse rate (123). There is one case report of hyperkalemia after succinylcholine administration (124). The absence of other reports suggests a low incidence of this problem in these patients (125). Routine general anesthetic techniques are probably appropriate.

Myasthenia Gravis

Myasthenia gravis (Table 12) is a disease characterized by a lack of responsiveness of the postsynaptic acetylcholine receptor, probably due to antibodies to the receptor. Symptoms include weakness and easy fatigability associated with repetitive use of voluntary muscles. Symptoms usually improve with anticholinesterase therapy, although other treatments including corticosteroids, immunosuppressives, and plasmapheresis may be required (126,127). This disease affects mostly women and becomes symptomatic usually around age 20 years. Pregnancy has a variable effect on the course of the disease. Not uncommonly, postpartum exacerbations arise (128). Preoperative evaluation of the parturient with myasthenia gravis must include knowledge of the muscles involved (respiratory, bulbar), current symptoms, ventilatory status assessed by serial spirometric measurements, and knowledge of anticholinesterase therapy. Continue anticholinesterase medications throughout the peripartum period to preserve muscle strength during the work of labor and delivery.

TABLE 12. *Anesthesia and myasthenia gravis*

Preoperative evaluation
Muscles involved
Ventilatory status, serial spirometry
Anticholinesterase medications
Avoid fatigue
Continue anticholinesterase medications
Use minimal systemic sedatives
Avoid aminoglycoside antibiotics and magnesium therapy
Response to muscle relaxants unpredictable
Avoid ester local anesthetics in patients receiving anticholinesterase medications

Labor Analgesia

Systemic medications may be used to provide labor analgesia to myasthenic patients, but give only small doses to avoid ventilatory depression (126). Epidural analgesia will reduce the ventilatory work associated with painful labor without interfering with the muscles of respiration (84).

Anesthesia for Cesarean Section

Parturients with myasthenia gravis present a more difficult anesthetic challenge should they require cesarean delivery. Anesthetic choice depends on the patient's ventilatory status and muscle strength. Although regional anesthesia may be used in these patients, excessively high levels of spinal anesthesia can further impair ventilatory function. An epidural anesthetic may prove advantageous. In contrast to spinal anesthesia, the anesthetic level can be carefully titrated. The level of motor blockade is lower and less profound than that seen with a comparable sensory level of spinal anesthesia (84). These effects minimize the interference with ventilatory function (84). With any regional anesthetic technique, be prepared to intubate and support ventilation should muscle weakness and ventilatory failure develop.

Regional anesthesia also offers the option of using neuraxial opioids for postoperative pain relief, minimizing the need for systemic opioids and sedative medications. Anticholinesterase medications may impede the metabolism of ester local anesthetics (i.e., 2-chloroprocaine). Use only amide local anesthetics in women taking these drugs.

Because of either maternal or fetal concerns, general anesthesia may be appropriate for a patient with myasthenia gravis. Parturients unable to maintain satisfactory ventilation during labor are unlikely to tolerate the stress of surgery under regional anesthesia. However, when contemplating general anesthesia for such a patient, consider her unpredictable response to muscle relaxants (125,126).

Patients with myasthenia gravis respond erratically to succinylcholine, with both resistance and early onset of phase II block reported. Long-term anticholinesterase therapy may decrease plasma cholinesterase activity and prolong the duration of succinylcholine (127). Baraka et al. (129) reported the response to 1.5 mg/kg succinylcholine in three myasthenic patients (two had their anticholinesterase medications discontinued the evening before surgery, but one did not). Complete neuromuscular blockade occurred in 60 seconds and lasted for 10 to 15 minutes (129).

Because of the decreased number of functional acetylcholine receptors, myasthenic patients are very sensitive to nondepolarizing muscle relaxants. In nonpregnant patients, without the risk of pulmonary aspiration of gastric contents or neonatal depression, adequate conditions for tracheal intubation can be obtained with sedative agents or volatile anesthetics alone. Others recommend small amounts of nondepolarizing muscle relaxants (125) or intermediate-acting nondepolarizing muscle relaxants (130). The short-acting muscle relaxant, mivacurium, will have a substantially prolonged action in patients receiving long-term anticholinesterase therapy because of decreased plasma cholinesterase (131). Rocuronium may be another alternative to rapid-sequence intubation (132).

In pregnancy, in which aspiration is a risk, I recommend either awake intubation with topical anesthesia, or a rapid-sequence induction of anesthesia by using 1.5 mg/kg succinylcholine or 0.6 mg/kg rocuronium. Closely monitor neuromuscular function throughout the procedure. Before extubation, look for clinical evidence of full recovery of neuromuscular function. As the bulbar muscles exhibit greater sensitivity to neuromuscular blockers than do peripheral muscles, I insist on a negative inspiratory force of -40 cm H_2O and a sustained head lift of greater than 5 seconds before extubation. Finally, prepare for the possibility of postoperative mechanical ventilation. Four risk factors predicting the need for postoperative mechanical ventilation in myasthenic patients have been identified (133):

- Duration of myasthenia gravis for longer than 6 years,
- A history of chronic respiratory disease other than myasthenia gravis,
- A dose of pyridostigmine greater than 750 mg per day, and
- A preoperative vital capacity less than 2.9 L.

Paraplegia and Quadriplegia

Proper anesthetic management is crucial to the safe conduct of labor and delivery in the patient with chronic spinal cord injury. Paraplegic and quadriplegic patients are at risk for a variety of medical complications including anemia, urinary tract infections, decubitus ulcers, thromboembolic phenomena, respiratory compromise, and autonomic hyperreflexia, which may be exacerbated by pregnancy (134,135). Preoperative evaluation of these patients must include assessment of the level of spinal cord injury, symptoms of autonomic hyperreflexia, ventilatory function, and hemoglobin.

Autonomic Hyperreflexia

Autonomic hyperreflexia is a syndrome seen in 85% of patients with spinal cord lesions at or above T_6, although it has been described in parturients with lesions below T_6 (136,137). Symptoms include flushing and sweating above the level of injury, severe hypertension, bradycardia, headache, and anxiety. Reflex sympathetic discharge, not modified or inhibited by supraspinal centers, follows distention or contraction of a viscus below the level of spinal cord injury. The vasculature in the region below the level of injury is very sensitive to catecholamines and responds with pronounced vasoconstriction. The resulting severe hypertension, via afferents from the carotid and aortic arch baroreceptors, stimulates vagally mediated bradycardia (Fig. 11).

Uterine contractions can induce autonomic hyperreflexia (136,138–141), and paroxysmal hypertension may be the only sign of labor in patients with complete spinal cord transection (142,143). Indeed, labor is a particularly potent trigger of autonomic hyperreflexia, and previously asymptomatic patients may first experience this problem during labor (135).

Other triggers described during pregnancy include skin incision, perineal manipulation, suprapubic pressure, and distention of the bladder or rectum. The more caudal the spinal segment receiving the afferent stimulation, the more potent the stimulus, and the greater the autonomic response. Maximal reaction occurs with stimuli to the anogenital area innervated by S_2 to S_4 nerve roots. Therefore autonomic hyperreflexia may be seen in the late first stage or early second stage of labor with stretching of the perineum, despite a previously uneventful labor. Autonomic hyperreflexia also may be triggered postpartum by abdominal or perineal pain caused by cesarean or vaginal delivery.

If undiagnosed or untreated, the extreme hypertension during labor can lead to convulsions or cerebral hemorrhage (144,145). Measure blood pressure and heart rate frequently in patients at risk for autonomic hyperreflexia throughout labor, delivery, and after birth. Consider invasive blood pressure monitoring with a radial artery catheter in these patients.

Labor Analgesia

Epidural analgesia can block autonomic hyperreflexia during labor (Fig. 12) (135,136,138,140–143). In patients with known histories of autonomic hyperreflexia, placement of the epidural catheter before elective induction of labor has been recommended (135, 143). An epidural anesthetic allows continuous adminis-

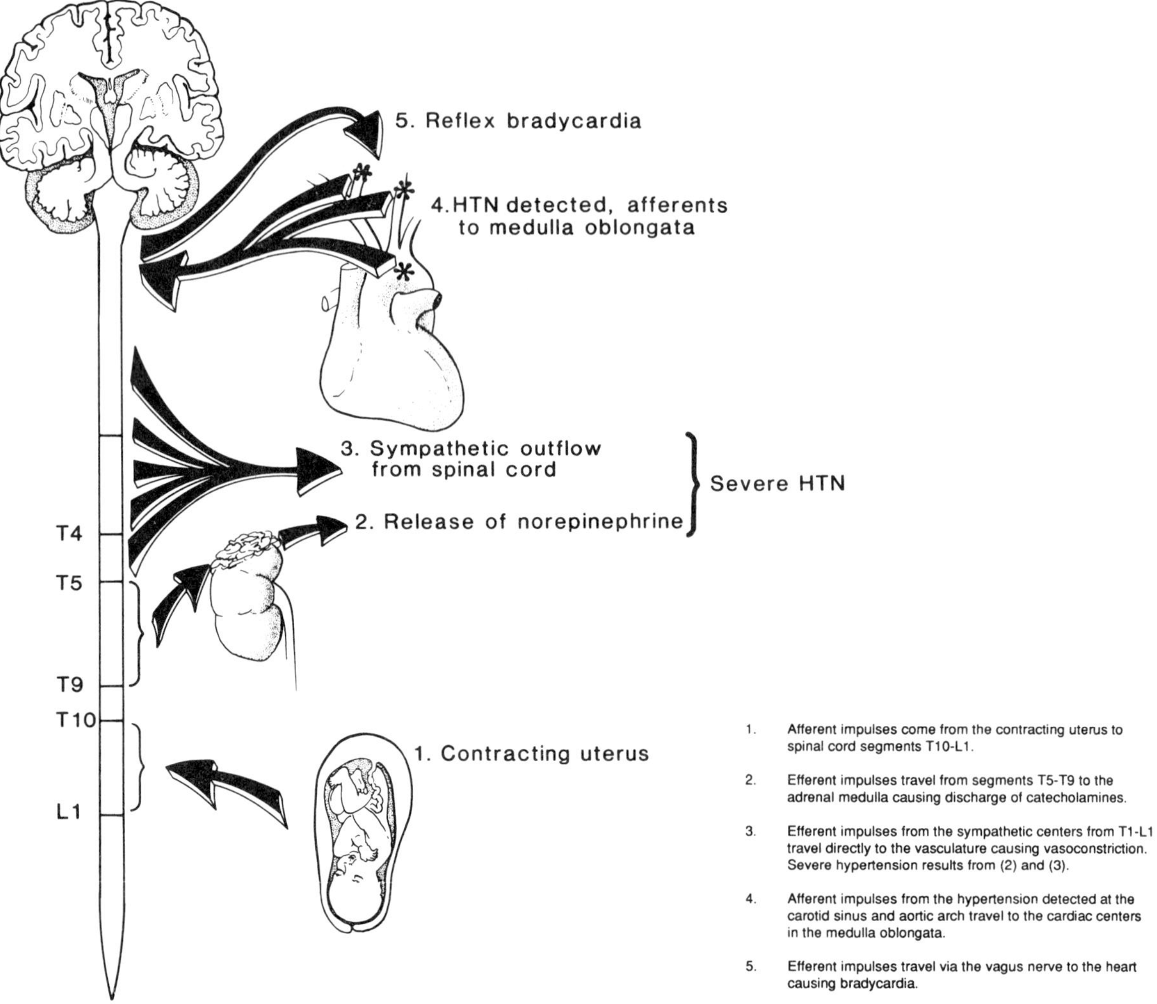

FIG. 11. Mechanism of cardiovascular changes in autonomic hyperreflexia. (Redrawn from ref. 140, with permission.)

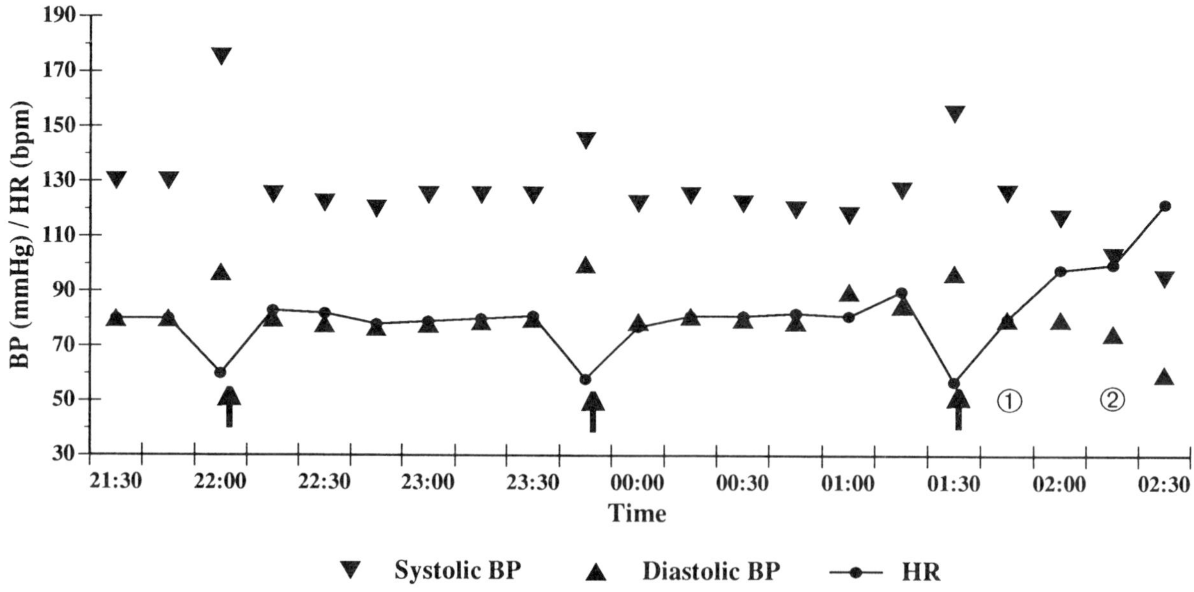

FIG. 12. Vital signs in a paraplegic parturient during labor. Autonomic hyperreflexia was managed with epidural anesthesia. Note the severe hypertension responsive to repeated dosing of the epidural catheter with bupivacaine. *1,* delivery of 1st twin; *2,* delivery of 2nd twin. (Redrawn from ref. 138, with permission.)

tration of local anesthetic throughout labor with supplementation for delivery.

Several practical problems must be considered when providing epidural analgesia for these women. Catheter placement may be difficult because of the presence of scoliosis, spinal instrumentation, or reflex muscle spasms. Assistance with patient positioning is useful. In a patient with complete spinal cord transection, unintentional intrathecal injection of local anesthetic may be difficult to detect. Proceed cautiously with initial dosing of an epidural catheter. Testing for intravascular injection should be done according to usual practice. There is no evidence that epinephrine-containing test doses are contraindicated in this population.

Choice of anesthetic is important. Epidural fentanyl or morphine alone do not block autonomic hyperreflexia beyond the very earliest stages of labor (140,142). In contrast, epidural meperidine, probably via its local anesthetic effect, can (139). As the level and adequacy of neural blockade cannot be assessed with the usual techniques in these patients, epidural local anesthetic should be given in concentrations suitable to block completely the pain of labor in normal patients. Boluses of 0.25% bupivacaine and infusions of 0.125% bupivacaine with and without fentanyl have been reported to block autonomic hyperreflexia successfully during labor (135,142, 143,146). Continuous epidural infusion may offer advantages over bolus administration to avoid the emergence of autonomic hyperreflexia symptoms between doses (Fig. 12).

In all cases, strict vigilance is essential to detect evidence of inadequate analgesia or block failure, which may result in the rapid onset of dangerous hypertension (146). Intravenous vasodilators should be immediately available to treat severe hypertension. Finally, it is reasonable to leave the epidural catheter in for 24 to 48 hours after delivery, as autonomic hyperreflexia triggered by postpartum pain may occur (143).

Anesthesia for Cesarean Section

Epidural anesthesia also should work nicely for cesarean delivery. In patients with high spinal cord injury, ventilatory function and the ability to lie flat should be thoroughly evaluated before induction.

If general anesthesia is necessary in the paraplegic parturient, beware of the potential for difficult intubation in patients with cervical injuries. Awake intubation may be indicated (147).

Succinylcholine may cause hyperkalemia (124,148). This complication has been reported to occur up to a year after the injury (124). Alternatively, intubation can be facilitated with a nondepolarizing muscle relaxant. Vecuronium has been studied for rapid-sequence intubation in healthy parturients seen for cesarean delivery. A bolus dose of 0.2 mg/kg or divided doses of 0.01 mg/kg followed 4 to 6 min later with 0.1 mg/kg produced good to excellent intubating conditions about 2.5 minutes after injection (149). Duration of neuromuscular blockade was 115 minutes after the single bolus dose and 73 minutes after the divided doses of vecuronium. The newer neuromuscular blocking agent, rocuronium, provided good to excellent intubating conditions in 90% of patients for cesarean delivery, 90 seconds after injection of an intubating dose of 0.6 mg/kg with thiopental, 6 mg/kg (132). Neuromuscular blockade lasted about 35 minutes.

Once the airway is secured, maintain an adequate depth of general anesthesia to prevent autonomic hyperreflexia during surgery (137). Again, monitor blood pressure carefully. As autonomic hyperreflexia also can occur postoperatively, adequate analgesia is important. Epidural (and presumably spinal) morphine appears to help limit postoperative sympathetic discharge due to pain (150).

Intracranial Vascular Lesions

Subarachnoid hemorrhage complicates one of every 10,000 pregnancies, a rate 5 times that of nonpregnant women of the same age (151). Most intracranial bleeding follows rupture of either a berry (sacular) aneurysm or an arteriovenous malformation. A review of 154 patients found an average gestational age of 30 weeks at the time of rupture for both aneurysms and arteriovenous malformations (152). Unlike earlier reports (153), this review found no correlation between type of lesion and incidence of rupture during the labor and delivery process (152). Events that may increase the risk of subarachnoid hemorrhage include coughing, straining, emotional stress, lifting, or any sudden cardiovascular stress (153,154). Anesthetic management of these patients must limit those situations that could magnify the risk of hemorrhage while preserving a healthy environment for the fetus.

Preoperative Evaluation

Preoperative evaluation of patients with intracranial vascular lesions must examine several factors. What is the intracranial pathology? What surgical intervention, if any, has been performed? Has the lesion bled in the past? Does the patient currently have symptoms attributable to intracranial blood (meningismus, headache) or increased intracranial pressure (ICP; headache, nausea, vomiting, altered sensorium)? What is the obstetrical plan (labor vs. cesarean delivery)? For patients whose lesions have been obliterated surgically, obstetric and anesthetic management proceed as usual. For patients with uncorrected lesions, mode of delivery may depend on the timing of the subarachnoid hemorrhage during the gestation and the degree of maternal morbidity from the hemorrhage (151,152).

Labor Analgesia

Continuous lumbar epidural or caudal anesthesia has been used for labor and vaginal delivery in patients with intracranial vascular lesions. This type of anesthesia can limit the hypertensive response to the pain of uterine contractions, prevent "bearing down" during the late stage of labor, and provide anesthesia for forceps delivery (155–158). All these effects potentially benefit the patient with intracranial lesions.

Direct measurements in normal parturients have shown that CSF pressure increases markedly during a painful uterine contraction associated with maternal pushing efforts. It then decreases quickly when the Valsalva is released. Blood pressure increases simultaneously because of improved venous return (159). This reaction increases transmural stress on intracranial vessels (Fig. 13). Avoiding pain and bearing down is a priority in the laboring patient with an intracranial vascular lesion.

Anesthetic management differs after acute intracerebral hemorrhage if the patient has increased ICP. When increased ICP is suspected, careful neurological examination must be performed. As in the patient with an intact lesion, avoid events that can increase ICP. In these women, however, epidural anesthesia may not be the best way to accomplish this end. First, cerebellar herniation may follow accidental dural puncture in a patient with increased ICP. Injecting fluid into the epidural space also may increase CSF pressure. In patients with abnormal intracranial compliance after head trauma, lumbar epidural injection of 10 mL of bupivacaine or saline transiently increased ICP (160) (Fig. 14). Smaller increments in ICP followed injection of 5 mL of fluid.

Proceed cautiously when injecting an epidural catheter in someone who may have reduced intracranial compliance. Inject the anesthetic in small increments, and observe the patient carefully for signs of increased ICP or decreasing blood pressure.

Murthy et al. (161) recently reported an eclamptic patient who developed severe headaches with each 10 mL top-up dose injected into her epidural catheter during labor. These headaches lasted approximately 20 minutes and were presumed to be due to decreased intracranial compliance.

Systemic medications may be used in patients in whom regional anesthesia is thought to be contraindicated because of high ICP (162). Use opioids sparingly to avoid hypoventilation, hypercarbia, and cerebral venodilation. Nitrous oxide and oxygen analgesia may help during labor and avoid the ventilatory depressant effects of systemic medications. Minimize the hemodynamic effects of uterine contractions (hypertension, tachycardia) in these patients with appropriate antihypertensive therapy. Pudendal block can provide pain relief during delivery.

Anesthesia for Cesarean Section

If cesarean delivery is indicated, minimizing hemodynamic disturbances and preventing ICP increases are essential. With strict attention to hemodynamic stability, epidural anesthesia has been used successfully in patients with intracranial vascular lesions for cesarean delivery (163,164). Invasive arterial blood pressure monitoring may be useful. Prophylactic antiemetics, such as metoclopramide or droperidol, are recommended to limit nausea and vomiting.

Certain situations (coma, high ICP, emergency surgery, simultaneous aneurysm clipping) may necessitate general anesthesia for cesarean delivery (165–167). In addition to invasive arterial pressure monitoring, central venous pressure monitoring may be useful in these situations to guide therapy directed at blood pressure control and maintenance of normal intravascular volume.

Maternal hypertension develops commonly during the usual rapid-sequence induction of general anesthesia. This hypertension can rupture an aneurysm or arteriovenous malformation and will contribute to increases in ICP. Deep anesthesia, accomplished by giving small doses of fentanyl and generous induction dose of thiopental (4 to 6 mg/kg) is essential before attempting laryn-

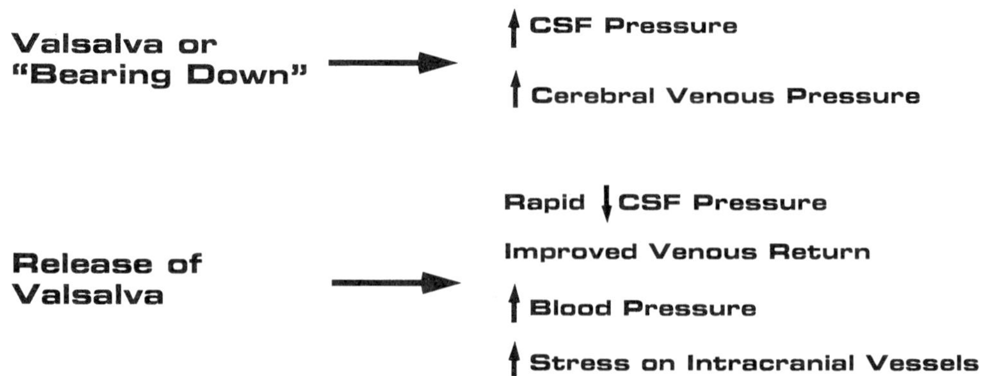

FIG. 13. The effects of a Valsalva maneuver, or "pushing" on cerebrospinal fluid (CSF) and intravascular pressures.

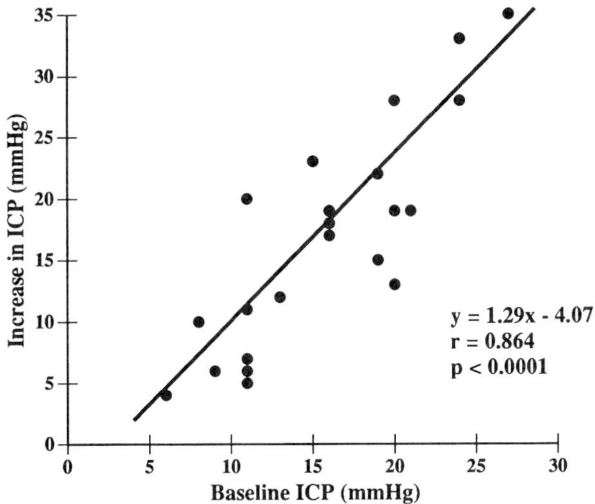

FIG. 14. Increases in intracranial pressure *(ICP)* seen after injection of 10 mL of bupivacaine or saline into the lumbar epidural space of two patients with abnormal intracranial compliance. (Redrawn from ref. 160, with permission.)

goscopy and intubation. Intravenous lidocaine and voluntary hyperventilation before the induction of anesthesia also will help blunt changes in ICP.

Pretreat with a small dose of nondepolarizing muscle relaxant to blunt fasciculations due to succinylcholine. Avoid airway manipulation until anesthesia and complete muscle relaxation has occurred.

Treat any increases in blood pressure aggressively. Infusions of nitroprusside or trimethaphan are helpful. Nitroprusside should be used only with direct arterial pressure monitoring to avoid precipitate hypotension.

When the risk of hemodynamic perturbations from a rapid-sequence induction is greater than the likelihood of aspiration, a slower induction of anesthesia may be indicated. The parturient with acutely increased ICP or recent bleed from an aneurysm would probably be in this category (165,166). After preoxygenation, apply cricoid pressure and slowly induce anesthesia with barbiturate, opioid, and a nondepolarizing muscle relaxant. Manually hyperventilate the patient via bag and mask. Control blood pressure with antihypertensive medications or additional anesthetic. Secure the airway only after the onset of complete paralysis. Neonatal depression is predictable with this technique. Communicate with the pediatrician and be prepared to resuscitate the newborn as needed.

With any techniques, consider the potential for adverse effects on uteroplacental perfusion and the fetus. Maternal positioning must avoid aortocaval compression and hypotension. Whereas hyperventilation may decrease maternal ICP, it may have adverse effects on the fetus. Positive-pressure ventilation reduces uterine blood flow, and hypocarbia reduces fetal blood oxygen content (168).

After delivery, do not use ergot derivatives to treat uterine atony; they cause hypertension via α-receptor stimulation. Oxytocin has been used after delivery in these patients without a problem.

SUMMARY

Proper anesthetic management of the parturient with medical problems requires knowledge of:

- The patient's disease,
- The impact of her pregnancy on her disease,
- The impact of her disease on the pregnancy and fetus, and
- The impact of an anesthetic on both the patient and the fetus.

Consult the patient's internist, endocrinologist, pulmonologist, or neurologist to learn the extent and management of the medical problem. Discuss the delivery plan with patient's obstetrician. Consider the side effects of the available anesthetic techniques and what specific agents are best used or avoided. Finally, spend time discussing these concerns with the patient. This is not always possible in the labor and delivery suite, where management plans change frequently. Talking to these patients in advance of delivery will allow time to gather information from the patient's primary physicians, discuss anesthetic options with the patient, and formulate an anesthetic plan.

REFERENCES

1. Reissell E, Orko R, Maunuksela EL, Lindgren L. Predictability of difficult laryngoscopy in patients with long-term diabetes mellitus. *Anaesthesia* 1990;45:1024.
2. Landon MB, Gabbe SG. Fetal surveillance and timing of delivery in pregnancy complicated by diabetes mellitus. *Obstet Gynecol Clin North Am* 1996;23:109.
3. West TET, Lowy C. Control of blood glucose during labour in diabetic women with combined glucose and low-dose insulin infusion. *Br Med J* 1977;1:1252.
4. American College of Obstetricians and Gynecologists. *Diabetes and pregnancy,* technical bulletin 200. Washington, DC: American College of Obstetricians and Gynecologists, 1994.
5. Kenepp NB, Shelley WC, Kumar S, Gutsche BB, Gabbe S, Delivoria-Papadopoulos M. Effects on newborn of hydration with glucose in patients undergoing caesarean section with regional anesthesia. *Lancet* 1980;1:645.
6. Kenepp NB, Kumar L, Shelley WC, Stanley CA, Gabbe SG, Gutsche BB. Fetal and neonatal hazards of maternal hydration with 5% dextrose before caesarean section. *Lancet* 1982;1:1150.
7. Lawrence GF, Brown VA, Parsons RJ, Cooke ID. Feto-maternal consequences of high-dose glucose infusion during labour. *Br J Obstet Gynecol* 1982;89:272.
8. Robillard JE, Sessions C, Kennedy RL, Smith FG. Metabolic effects of constant hypertonic glucose infusion in well-oxygenated fetuses. *Am J Obstet Gynecol* 1978;130:199.
9. Hauguel S, Desmaizieres V, Challier JC. Glucose uptake, utilization, and transfer by the human placenta as functions of maternal glucose concentration. *Pediatr Res* 1986;20:269.
10. Carson BS, Phillips AF, Simmons MA, Battaglis FC, Meschia G. Effects of a sustained insulin infusion upon glucose uptake and oxygenation of the ovine fetus. *Pediatr Res* 1980;14:147.
11. Light IJ, Keenan WJ, Sutherland JM. Maternal intravenous glucose administration as a cause of hypoglycemia in the infant of the diabetic mother. *Am J Obstet Gynecol* 1972;113:345.

12. Jones CJP, Fox H. Placental changes in gestational diabetes: an ultrastructural study. *Obstet Gynecol* 1976;48:274.
13. Cousins L. Pregnancy complications among diabetic women: review 1965–1985. *Obstet Gynecol Surg* 1987;42:140.
14. Shnider SM, Abboud TK, Artal R, Henriksen EH, Stefani SJ, Levinson G. Maternal catetcholamines decrease during labor after lumbar epidural anesthesia. *Am J Obstet Gynecol* 1983;147:13.
15. Buchan PC, Milne MK, Browning MCK. The effect of continuous epidural blockade on plasma 11-hydroxycorticosteroid concentrations. *J Obstet Gynaecol Br Commonw* 1973;80:974.
16. Bromage PR. Physiology and pharmacology of epidural analgesia. *Anesthesiology* 1967;28:592.
17. Lev-Ran A. Sharp temporary drop in insulin requirement after cesarean section in diabetic patients. *Am J Obstet Gynecol* 1974;120:905.
18. Datta S, Brown WU. Acid-base status in diabetic mothers and their infants following general or spinal anesthesia for cesarean section. *Anesthesiology* 1977;47:272.
19. Datta S, Kitzmiller JL, Naulty JS, Ostheimer GW, Weiss JB. Acid-base status of diabetic mothers and their infants following spinal anesthesia for cesarean section. *Anesth Analg* 1982;61:662.
20. Datta S, Brown WU, Ostheimer GW, Weiss JB, Alper MH. Epidural anesthesia for cesarean section in diabetic parturients: maternal and neonatal acid-base status and bupivacaine concentration. *Anesth Analg* 1981;60:574.
21. James FM, Dewan DM, Floyd HM, et al. Chloroprocaine vs. bupivacaine for lumbar epidural analgesia for elective cesarean section. *Anesthesiology* 1980;52:488.
22. Tyrala EE. The infant of the diabetic mother. *Obstet Gynecol Clin North Am* 1996;23:221.
23. Kliegman RM, Gross T. Perinatal problems of the obese mother and her infant. *Obstet Gynecol* 1985;66:299.
24. Gross T, Sokol RJ, King KC. Obesity in pregnancy: risks and outcome. *Obstet Gynecol* 1980;56:446.
25. Thomson M, Hanley J. Factors predisposing to difficult labor in primiparas. *Am J Obstet Gynecol* 1988;158:1074.
26. Hood DD, Dewan DM. Anesthetic and obstetric outcome in morbidly obese parturients. *Anesthesiology* 1993;79:1210.
27. Garbaciak JA, Richter M, Miller S, Barton JJ. Maternal weight and pregnancy complications. *Obstet Gynecol* 1985;152:238.
28. Perlow JH, Morgan MA, Montgomery D, Towers CV, Porto M. Perinatal outcome in pregnancy complicated by massive obesity. *Am J Obstet Gynecol* 1992;167:958.
29. Manson JE, Colditz GA, Stampfer MJ, et al. A prospective study of obesity and risk of coronary heart disease in women. *N Engl J Med* 1990;322:882.
30. Douglas MJ, Flanagan ML, McMorland GH. Anaesthetic management of a complex morbidly obese parturient. *Can J Anaesth* 1991;38:900.
31. Bevan DR, Holdcroft A, Loh L, MacGregor WG, O'Sullivan JC, Sykes MK. Closing volume and pregnancy. *Br Med J* 1974;1:13.
32. Eng M, Butler J, Bonica JJ. Respiratory function in pregnant obese women. *Am J Obstet Gynecol* 1975;123:241.
33. Burki NK, Baker RW. Ventilatory regulation in eucapnic morbid obesity. *Am Rev Respir Dis* 1984;129:538.
34. Hgerdal M, Morgan CW, Sumner AE, Gutsche BB. Minute ventilation and oxygen consumption during labor with epidural analgesia. *Anesthesiology* 1983;59:425.
35. Peabody JL. Transcutaneous oxygen measurement to evaluate drug effects. *Clin Perinatol* 1979;6:109.
36. Vincent RD, Chestnut DH. Which position is more comfortable for the parturient during identification of the epidural space? *Int J Obstet Anesth* 1991;1:9.
37. Maitra AM, Palmer SK, Bachhuber SR, Abram SE. Continuous epidural analgesia for cesarean section in a patient with morbid obesity. *Anesth Analg* 1979;58:348.
38. Perlow JH, Morgan MA. Massive maternal obesity and perioperative cesarean morbidity. *Am J Obstet Gynecol* 1994;170:560.
39. Hodgkinson R, Husain FJ. Obesity and the cephalad spread of analgesia following epidural administration of bupivacaine for cesarean section. *Anesth Analg* 1980;59:89.
40. Hodgkinson R, Husain FJ. Obesity, gravity, and spread of epidural anesthesia. *Anesth Analg* 1981;60:421.
41. Milligan KR, Cramp P, Schatz L, Johnston D, Carp H. The effect of patient position and obesity on the spread of epidural analgesia. *Int J Obstet Anesth* 1993;2:134.
42. Martin JT. The lawn chair (contoured supine) position. In: Martin JT, ed. *Positioning in anesthesia and surgery.* Philadelphia: WB Saunders, 1987:37.
43. Ahern JK, Goodlin RC. Cesarean section in the massively obese. *Obstet Gynecol* 1978;51:509.
44. Wolfe HM, Gross TL, Sokol RJ, Bottoms SF, Thompson KL. Determinants of morbidity in obese women delivered by cesarean. *Obstet Gynecol* 1988;71:691.
45. Hodgkinson R, Husain FJ. Caesarean section associated with gross obesity. *Br J Anaesth* 1980;52:919.
46. Norris MC. Height, weight, and the spread of subarachnoid hyperbaric bupivacaine in the term parturient. *Anesth Analg* 1988;67:555.
47. Milligan KR, Carp H. Continuous spinal anaesthesia for caesarean section in the morbidly obese. *Int J Obstet Anesth* 1992;1:111.
48. Hibbard BM, Anderson MM, Drife JO, et al. *Deaths associated with anaesthesia: report on confidential enquiries into maternal deaths in the United Kingdom, 1988-1990.* London: HMSO, 1994:80.
49. Hibbard BM, Anderson MM, Drife JO, et al. *Deaths associated with anaesthesia: report on confidential enquiries into maternal deaths in the United Kingdom, 1991-1993.* London: HMSO, 1997.
50. Endler GC, Mariona FG, Sokol RJ, Stevenson LB. Anesthesia-related maternal mortality in Michigan, 1972 to 1984. *Am J Obstet Gynecol* 1988;159:187.
51. Rocke DA, Murray WB, Rout CC, Gouws E. Relative risk analysis of factors associated with difficult intubation in obstetric anesthesia. *Anesthesiology* 1992;77:67.
52. Datta S. Modified laryngoscope for endotracheal intubation of obese patients. *Anesth Analg* 1981;60:120.
53. Cohn AI, Hart RT, McGraw SR, Blass NH. The Bullard laryngoscope for emergency airway management in a morbidly obese parturient. *Anesth Analg* 1995;81:872.
54. Vaughan RW, Bauer S, Wise L. Volume and pH of gastric juice in obese patients. *Anesthesiology* 1975;43:686.
55. Colman RD, Frank M, Loughnan BA, Cohen DG, Cattermole R. Use of i.m. rantidine for the prophylaxis of aspiration pneumonitis in obstetrics. *Br J Anaesth* 1988;61:720.
56. Hodgkinson R, Glassenberg R, Joyce THI, Coombs DW, Ostheimer GW, Gibbs CP. Comparison of cimetidine (Tagamet) with antacid for safety and effectiveness in reducing gastric acidity before elective cesarean section. *Anesthesiology* 1983;59:86.
57. Hedenstierna G, Santesson J, Norlander O. Airway closure and distribution of inspired gas in the extremely obese, breathing spontaneously and during anaesthesia with intermittent positive pressure ventilation. *Acta Anaesthesiol Scand* 1976;20:334.
58. Archer GW Jr, Marx GF. Arterial oxygen tension during apnoea in parturient women. *Br J Anaesth* 1974;46:358.
59. Vaughan RW, Wise L. Intraoperative arterial oxygenation in obese patients. *Ann Surg* 1976;184:35.
60. Norris MC, Dewan DM. Preoxygenation for cesarean section: a comparison of two techniques. *Anesthesiology* 1985;62:827.
61. Goldberg ME, Norris MC, Larijani GE, Marr AT, Seltzer JL. Preoxygenation in the morbidly obese: a comparison of two techniques. *Anesth Analg* 1989;68:520.
62. Eriksen J, Andersen J, Rasmussen JP, Sorensen B. Effects of ventilation with large tidal volumes or positive end-expiratory pressure on cardiorespiratory function in anesthetized obese patients. *Acta Anaesthesiol Scand* 1978;22:241.
63. Bentley JB, Vaughan RW, Gandolfi AJ, Cork RC. Halothane biotransformation in obese and nonobese patients. *Anesthesiology* 1982; 57:94.
64. Weinstein JA, Matteo RS, Ornstein E, Schwartz AE, Goldstoff M, Thal G. Pharmacodynamics of vecuronium and atracurium in the obese surgical patient. *Anesth Analg* 1988;67:1149.
65. Datta S, Ostheimer GW, Weiss JB, Brown WJ Jr, Alper MH. Neonatal effect of prolonged anesthetic induction for cesarean section. *Obstet Gynecol* 1981;58:331.
66. Vaughan RW, Engelhardt RC, Wise L. Postoperative hypoxemia in obese patients. *Ann Surg* 1974;180:877.
67. Rawal N, Sjostrand U, Christoffersson E, Dahlstrom B, Arvill A, Rydman H. Comparison of intramuscular and epidural morphine for postoperative analgesia in the grossly obese: influence on postoperative ambulation and pulmonary function. *Anesth Analg* 1984;63:583.
68. Maeder EC Jr, Barno A, Mecklenburg F. Obesity: a maternal high-risk factor. *Obstet Gynecol* 1975;45:669.
69. Schmidt GA, Hall JB. Pulmonary disease. In: Baron WM, Lindheimer

MD, eds. *Medical disorders during pregnancy.* St. Louis: Mosby Year Book, 1991:197.
70. Kingston HGG, Hirshman CA. Perioperative management of the patient with asthma. *Anesth Analg* 1984;63:844.
71. Prowse CM, Gaensler EA. Respiratory and acid-base changes during pregnancy. *Anesthesiology* 1965;26:381.
72. Clark SL. Asthma in pregnancy. *Obstet Gynecol* 1993;82:1036.
73. Schatz M, Harden K, Forsythe A, et al. The course of asthma during pregnancy, postpartum, and with successive pregnancies: a prospective analysis. *J Allergy Clin Immunol* 1988;81:509.
74. Schatz M, Zeiger RS, Harden KM, et al. The safety of inhaled β-agonist bronchodilators during pregnancy. *J Allergy Clin Immunol* 1988; 82:686.
75. Siegel D, Sheppard D, Gelb A, Weinberg PF. Aminophylline increases the toxicity but not the efficacy of an inhaled beta-adrenergic agonist in the treatment of acute exacerbations of asthma. *Am Rev Respir Dis* 1985;132:283.
76. Barnes PJ. A new approach to the treatment of asthma. *N Engl J Med* 1989;321:1517.
77. American College of Obstetrics and Gynecology. *Pulmonary disease in pregnancy,* technical bulletin 224. Washington, DC: American College of Obstetrics and Gynecology, 1996.
78. Perlow JH, Montgomery D, Morgan MA, Towers CV, Porto M. Severity of asthma and perinatal outcome. *Am J Obstet Gynecol* 1992;167:963.
79. Roizen MF, Stevens WC. Multiform ventricular tachycardia due to the interaction of aminophylline and halothane. *Anesth Analg* 1978;57:738.
80. Stirt JA, Berger JM, Roe SD, Ricker SM, Sullivan SF. Safety of enflurane following administration of aminophylline in experimental animals. *Anesth Analg* 1981;60:871.
81. Stirt JA, Berger JM, Sullivan SF. Lack of arrhythmogenicity of isoflurane following administration of aminophylline in dogs. *Anesth Analg* 1983;62:568.
82. Tanaka K, Shono S, Watanabe R, Dan K. Incidence of asthmatic attack is not increased during high epidural anesthesia (abstract). *Anesthesiology* 1992;77:A1090.
83. Cheney FW, Posner KL, Caplan RA. Adverse respiratory events infrequently leading to malpractice suits. *Anesthesiology* 1991;75:932.
84. Freund FG, Bonica JJ, Ward RJ, Akamatsu TJ, Kennedy WF Jr. Ventilatory reserve and level of motor block during high spinal and epidural anesthesia. *Anesthesiology* 1967;28:834.
85. Ramanathan J, Osborne B, Sibai B. Epidural anesthesia in asthmatic parturients [Abstract]. *Anesth Analg* 1990;70:S317.
86. Gamil M. Serial peak expiratory flow rates in mothers during caesarean section under extradural anaesthesia. *Br J Anaesth* 1989;62:415.
87. Mallampati R. Bronchospasm during spinal anesthesia. *Anesth Analg* 1981;60:839.
88. Kelly MC, Fitzpatrick KTJ, Hill DA. Respiratory effects of spinal anesthesia for caesarean section. *Anaesthesia* 1996;51:1120.
89. Gal TJ. Pulmonary mechanics in normal subjects following endotracheal intubation. *Anesthesiology* 1980;52:27.
90. Huber FC Jr, Reves JG, Gutierrez J, Corssen G. Ketamine: its effect on airway resistance in man. *South Med J* 1972;65:1176.
91. Hirshman CA, Downes H, Farbood A, Bergman NA. Ketamine block of bronchospasm in experimental canine asthma. *Br J Anaesth* 1979; 51:713.
92. Dich-Nielsen J, Holasek J. Ketamine as induction agent for caesarean section. *Acta Anaesthesiol Scand* 1982;26:139.
93. Abboud TK, Zhu J, Richardson M, Peres Da Silva E, Donovan M. Intravenous propofol vs thiamylal-isoflurane for caesarean section: comparative maternal and neonatal effects. *Acta Anaesthesiol Scand* 1995;39:205.
94. Pizov R, Brown RH, Weiss YS, et al. Wheezing during induction of general anesthesia in patients with and without asthma. *Anesthesiology* 1995;82:1111.
95. Eames WO, Rooke GA, Wu RS, Bishop MJ. Comparison of the effects of etomidate, propofol, and thiopental on respiratory resistance after tracheal intubation. *Anesthesiology* 1996;84:1307.
96. Yukioka H, Hayashi M, Terai T, Fujimori M. Intravenous lidocaine as a suppressant of coughing during tracheal intubation in elderly patients. *Anesth Analg* 1993;77:309.
97. Hirshman CA, Berman NA. Halothane and enflurane protect against bronchospasm in an asthma dog model. *Anesth Analg* 1978;57:629.
98. Hirshman CA, Edelstein G, Peetz S, Wayne R, Downes H. Mechanism of action of inhalational anesthesia on airways. *Anesthesiology* 1982;56:107.
99. Brown RH, Zerhouni EA, Hirshman CA. Comparison of low concentrations of halothane and isoflurane as bronchodilators. *Anesthesiology* 1993;78:1097.
100. Marx GF, Kim YI, Lin C-C, Halevy S, Schulman H. Postpartum uterine pressures under halothane or enflurane anesthesia. *Obstet Gynecol* 1978;51:695.
101. Mathe AA, Hedqvist P, Holmgren A, Svanborg N. Bronchial hyperreactivity to prostaglandin $F_{2\alpha}$ and histamine in patients with asthma. *Br Med J* 1973;27:193.
102. Kleinman JC, Peirre MB, Madans JH, Land GH, Schramm WF. The effects of maternal smoking on fetal and infant mortality. *Am J Epidemiol* 1988;127:274.
103. Meyer B, Tonascia JA. Maternal smoking, pregnancy complications, and perinatal mortality. *Am J Obstet Gynecol* 1977;128:494.
104. Gerrard JW, Cockcroft DW, Mink JT, Cotton DJ, Poonawala R, Dosman JA. Increased nonspecific bronchial reactivity in cigarette smokers with normal lung function. *Am Rev Respir Dis* 1980;122:577.
105. Hegab E-S, Matulionis DH. Pulmonary macrophage mobilization in cigarette smoke-exposed mice after halothane anesthesia. *Anesth Analg* 1986;65:37.
106. Crawford JS, James FM III, Nolte H, Van Steenberge A, Shah JL. Regional analgesia for patients with chronic neurological disease and similar conditions. *Anaesthesia* 1981;35:821.
107. Crawford JS. Epidural analgesia for patients with chronic neurological disease. *Anesth Analg* 1983;62:620.
108. Neigh JL, Garman JK, Harp JR. The electroencephalographic pattern during anesthesia with ethrane: effects of depth of anesthesia, P_aCO_2 and nitrous oxide. *Anesthesiology* 1971;35:482.
109. Oshima E, Urabe N, Shingu K, Mori K. Anticonvulsant actions of enflurane on epilepsy models in cats. *Anesthesiology* 1985;63:29.
110. Bennett DR, Madsen JA, Jordan WS, Wiser WC. Ketamine anesthesia in brain-damaged epileptics: electroencephalographic and clinical observations. *Neurology* 1973;23:449.
111. Ferrer-Allado T, Brechner VL, Dymond A, Cozen H, Crandall P. Ketamine-induced electroconvulsive phenomena in the human limbic and thalamic regions. *Anesthesiology* 1973;38:333.
112. Modica PA, Tempelhoff R, White PF. Pro- and anticonvulsant effects of anesthetics (Part I). *Anesth Analg* 1990;70:303.
113. Ornstein E, Matteo RS, Young WL, Diaz J. Resistance to metocurine-induced neuromuscular blockade in patients receiving phenytoin. *Anesthesiology* 1985;63:294.
114. Roth S, Ebrahim ZY. Resistance to pancuronium in patients receiving carbamazepine. *Anesthesiology* 1987;68:691.
115. Roullet E, Verdier-Taillefer M-H, Amarenco P, Gharbi G, Alperovitch A, Marteau R. Pregnancy and multiple sclerosis: a longitudinal study of 125 remittent patients. *J Neurol Neurosurg Psychiatry* 1993;56:1062.
116. Worthington J, Jones R, Crawford M, Forti A. Pregnancy and multiple sclerosis: a 3 year prospective study. *J Neurol* 1994;241:228.
117. Warren TM, Datta S, Ostheimer GW. Lumbar epidural anesthesia in a patient with multiple sclerosis. *Anesth Analg* 1982;61:1022.
118. Bader AM, Hunt CO, Datta S, Naulty JS, Ostheimer GW. Anesthesia for the obstetric patient with multiple sclerosis. *J Clin Anesth* 1988;1:21.
119. Davis FA, Michael JA, Neer D. Serial hyperthermia testing in multiple sclerosis: a method for monitoring subclinical fluctuation. *Acta Neurol Scand* 1973;49:63.
120. Camann WR, Hortvet LA, Hughes N, Bader AM, Datta S. Maternal temperature regulation during extradural analgesia for labour. *Br J Anaesth* 1991;67:565.
121. Macaulay JH, Bond K, Steer PJ. Epidural analgesia in labor and fetal hyperthermia. *Obstet Gynecol* 1992;80:665.
122. Fusi L, Steer PJ, Maresh MJA, Beard RW. Maternal pyrexia associated with the use of epidural analgesia in labour. *Lancet* 1989;1:1250.
123. Bamford C, Sibley W, Laguna J. Anesthesia in multiple sclerosis. *Can J Neurol Sci* 1978;5:41.
124. Cooperman LH. Succinylcholine-induced hyperkalemia in neuromuscular disease. *JAMA* 1970;213:1867.
125. Azar I. The response of patients with neuromuscular disorders to muscle relaxants: a review. *Anesthesiology* 1984;61:173.
126. Foldes FF, McNall PG. Myasthenia gravis: a guide for anesthesiologists. *Anesthesiology* 1962;23:837.
127. Baraka A. Anaesthesia and myasthenia gravis. *Can J Anaesth* 1992; 39:476.
128. Rolbin SH, Levinson G, Shnider SM, Wright RG. Anesthetic considerations for myasthenia gravis and pregnancy. *Anesth Analg* 1978; 57:441.

129. Baraka A, Tabboush Z. Neuromuscular response to succinylcholine-vecuronium sequence in three myasthenic patients undergoing thymectomy. *Anesth Analg* 1991;72:827.
130. Chan KH, Yang MW, Huang MH, et al. A comparison between vecuronium and atracurium in myasthenia gravis. *Acta Anaesthesiol Scand* 1993;37:679.
131. Seigne RD, Scott RPF. Mivacurium chloride and myasthenia gravis. *Br J Anaesth* 1994;72:468.
132. Abouleish E, Abboud T, Lechevalier J, Zhu AC, Alford K. Rocuronium (Org 9426) for caesarean section. *Br J Anaesth* 1994;73:336.
133. Leventhal SR, Orkin FK, Hirsh RA. Prediction of the need for postoperative mechanical ventilation in myasthenia gravis. *Anesthesiology* 1980;53:26.
134. Baker ER, Cardenas DD. Pregnancy in spinal cord injured women. *Arch Phys Med Rehabil* 1996;77:501.
135. Crosby E, St-Jean B, Reid D, Elliott RD. Obstetrical anaesthesia and analgesia in chronic spinal cord-injured women. *Can J Anaesth* 1992; 39:487.
136. Katz VL, Thorp JM, Cefalo RC. Epidural analgesia and autonomic hyperreflexia: a case report. *Am J Obstet Gynecol* 1990;162:471.
137. Schonwald G, Fish KJ, Perkash I. Cardiovascular complications during anesthesia in chronic spinal cord injured patients. *Anesthesiology* 1981;55:550.
138. Watson DW, Downey GO. Epidural anesthesia for labor and delivery of twins of a paraplegic mother. *Anesthesiology* 1980;52:259.
139. Baraka A. Epidural meperidine for control of autonomic hyperreflexia in a paraplegic parturient. *Anesthesiology* 1985;62:688.
140. Abouleish EI, Hanley ES, Palmer SM. Can epidural fentanyl control autonomic hyperreflexia in a quadriplegic parturient? *Anesth Analg* 1989;68:523.
141. Stirt JA, Marco A, Conklin KA. Obstetric anesthesia for a quadriplegic patient with autonomic hyperreflexia. *Anesthesiology* 1979; 51:560.
142. Pauzner D, Wolman IDN, Menachem PD. Epidural morphine bupivacaine combination for the control of autonomic hyperreflexia during labor. *Gynecol Obstet Invest* 1994;37:215.
143. Kobayashi A, Mizobe T, Tojo H, Hashimoto S. Autonomic hyperreflexia during labour. *Can J Anaesth* 1995;42:1134.
144. McGregor JA, Meeuwsen J. Autonomic hyperreflexia: a mortal danger for spinal cord-damaged women in labor. *Am J Obstet Gynecol* 1985;151:330.
145. Abouleish E. Hypertension in a paraplegic parturient. *Anesthesiology* 1980;53:348.
146. Owen MD, Stiles MM, Opper SE, McNitt JD, Fibuch EE. Autonomic hyperreflexia in a pregnant paraplegic patient. *Reg Anesth* 1994;19:415.
147. Litman RS, Voisine R. Obstetric anaesthesia and spinal cord injury [Letter]. *Can J Anaesth* 1992;39:1117.
148. Cooperman LH, Strobel GE, Kennell EM. Massive hyperkalemia after administration of succinylcholine. *Anesthesiology* 1970;32:161.
149. Hawkins JL. Vecuronium for rapid-sequence intubation for cesarean section. *Anesth Analg* 1990;71:185.
150. Breslow MJ, Jordan DA, Christopherson R, et al. Epidural morphine decreases postoperative hypertension by attenuating sympathetic nervous system hyperactivity. *JAMA* 1989;261:3577.
151. Fox MW, Harms RW, Davis DH. Selected neurologic complications of pregnancy. *Mayo Clin Proc* 1990;65:1595.
152. Dias MS, Sekhar LN. Intracranial hemorrhage from aneurysms and arteriovenous malformations during pregnancy and the puerperium. *Neurosurgery* 1990;27:855.
153. Robinson JL, Hall CS, Sedzimir CB. Arteriovenous malformations, aneurysms, and pregnancy. *J Neurosurg* 1974;41:63.
154. Yau G, Lee TL. Repeat epidural caesarean section in a patient with cerebral arteriovenous malformation. *Ann Acad Med Singapore* 1994; 23:579.
155. Tuttleman RM, Gleicher N. Central nervous system hemorrhage complicating pregnancy. *Obstet Gynecol* 1981;58:651.
156. Young DC, Leveno KJ, Whalley PJ. Induced delivery prior to surgery for ruptured cerebral aneurysm. *Obstet Gynecol* 1983;61:749.
157. Dunn JM, Raskind R. Rupture of a cerebral arteriovenous malformation during pregnancy. *Obstet Gynecol* 1967;30:423.
158. Hunt HB, Schifrin BS, Suzuki K. Ruptured berry aneurysms and pregnancy. *Obstet Gynecol* 1974;43:827.
159. Marx GF, Zemaitis MT, Orkin LR. Cerebrospinal fluid pressures during labor and obstetrical anesthesia. *Anesthesiology* 1961;22:348.
160. Hilt H, Gramm JH, Ling K. Changes in intracranial pressure associated with extradural anaesthesia. *Br J Anaesth* 1986;58:676.
161. Murthy BVS, Fogarty DJ, Fitzpatrick K, Brady MM. Headache during epidural top-ups in labour: a sign of reduced intracranial compliance. *Anaesth Intens Care* 1995;23:744.
162. Baker JW. Subarachnoid haemorrhage associated with pregnancy. *Aust N Z J Obstet Gynaecol* 1969;9:12.
163. Laidler JA, Jackson KU, Redfern N. The management of caesarean section in a patient with an intracranial arteriovenous malformation. *Anaesthesia* 1989;44:490.
164. Sharma SK, Herrera ER, Sidawi JE, Leveno KJ. The pregnant patient with an intracranial arteriovenous malformation: cesarean or vaginal delivery using regional or general anesthesia? *Reg Anesth* 1995; 20:455.
165. Kofke WA, Wuest HP, McGinnis LA. Cesarean section following ruptured cerebral aneurysm and neuroresuscitation. *Anesthesiology* 1984; 60:242.
166. Lennon RL, Sundt TM Jr, Gronert GA. Combined cesarean section and clipping of intracerebral aneurysm. *Anesthesiology* 1984;60:240.
167. Whitburn RH, Laishley RS, Jewkes DA. Anaesthesia for simultaneous caesarean section and clipping of intracerebral aneurysm. *Br J Anaesth* 1990;64:642.
168. Levinson G, Shnider SM, deLorimier AA, Steffenson JL. Effects of maternal hyperventilation on uterine blood flow and fetal oxygenation and acid-base status. *Anesthesiology* 1974;40:340.

Obstetric Anesthesia, second edition,
edited by Mark C. Norris.
Lippincott Williams & Wilkins, Philadelphia © 1999.

CHAPTER 26

Anesthesia and Maternal Substance Abuse

David J. Birnbach

Substance abuse is a major public health problem in our society (1). With illicit drug use reaching epidemic proportions in some communities, many physicians are being confronted with these patients and their numerous medical problems. Drug use crosses geographic and socioeconomic boundaries; patients under the influence of these substances are being seen not only in "inner cities" but also in small communities and private hospitals (2). Substance abuse during pregnancy is no longer a rare event. Many women of child-bearing age are currently abusing at least one illicit substance. Almost 15% of pregnant women delivering at a hospital in Florida had a positive urine toxicology screen for cocaine, marijuana, alcohol, or heroin (3). Reports from numerous locations including Italy (4), Amsterdam (5), Spain (6), and Eastern Europe (7) suggest that illicit drug use is an international problem.

Anesthesiologists may need to provide care for an abusing parturient requesting labor analgesia, requiring cesarean section, or requiring nonobstetric surgery, often related to trauma. In New York City, recent substance abuse can be documented in 48% of parturients with trauma-related deaths (8).

Perinatal substance abuse has been linked to numerous maternal and neonatal complications and may alter the anticipated response to commonly administered anesthetics. The unusual and clinically challenging situations that may arise in this patient population have been attributed to many factors, including:

- The direct and indirect effects of illicit drugs and contaminants,
- Failure of many of drug-abusing patients to receive antenatal care,
- Poor diet, and
- The presence of untreated coexisting diseases.

D.J. Birnbach: Department of Obstetric Anesthesiology, St. Luke's–Roosevelt Hospital Center, New York, New York 10019.

Of all the causative factors, prenatal care has the greatest impact on outcome (9).

Because of the increase in perinatal substance abuse, obstetricians, pediatricians, and anesthesiologists encounter a growing number of pregnant patients who use illicit substances. This chapter reviews the maternal and neonatal consequences of the commonly abused substances including cocaine, opiates, amphetamines, alcohol, and tobacco. In addition, this chapter addresses the anesthetic management of the substance-abusing pregnant patient.

Multiple drug use is common (10). A recent study examined drug-use patterns of pregnant women in two inner-city sites. Women who used cocaine were much more likely to use other drugs (11). Although all patients should be questioned regarding the use of illicit drugs, self-reporting of drug abuse by pregnant patients underestimates actual use (12). Risk factors for substance abuse include lack of prenatal care, preterm labor, and cigarette smoking (13,14).

COCAINE

The prevalence of cocaine abuse in pregnant women dramatically increased during the past decade and resulted in a variety of maternal and perinatal complications (15). Positive cocaine toxicology results were reported in pregnant patients from many geographic, socioeconomic, and cultural groups (16). Although the exact extent of perinatal cocaine use is unknown, the epidemic of drug use has far-reaching effects (17).

Cocaine (benzoylmethylecgonine) is a naturally occurring alkaloid derived from the *Erythroxylon coca* plant, which is indigenous to Peru, Bolivia, and Ecuador (18). The drug is readily absorbed through mucous membranes and metabolized rapidly by the liver and plasma cholinesterases to water-soluble products that are excreted in the urine. Cocaine is highly lipid soluble and has a low molecular weight and ionization, thus allowing easy transplacental diffusion. The alkalinized form of cocaine can be smoked and is known as "crack." It is inexpensive and the most widely used form of cocaine in the United States (19). The pharmacologic effects of cocaine are mediated via the norepinephrine, dopamine, and serotonin neurotransmitter systems (20). Because of inhibition of neuronal reuptake, extracellular norepinephrine accumulates, producing hypertension, tachycardia, and vasoconstriction (21).

Maternal Risks

Perinatal cocaine abuse has been linked to many maternal complications (Table 1) including:

- Placental abruption (22,23),
- Pneumothorax (24),
- Uterine rupture (25,26),
- Preterm labor (27,28),
- Myocardial ischemia and infarction (29,30),
- Renal failure (31),
- Hyperthermia (32),
- Stroke (33),
- Bowel ischemia (34),
- Hepatic rupture (35),
- Thrombocytopenia (36), and
- Sexually transmitted diseases and human immunodeficiency virus (HIV) (37,38).

Cardiovascular Effects

The effects of maternal cocaine use are incremental and cumulative, although erratic use of cocaine in pregnancy results in complications that may be as severe as those occurring with daily binging (39). Pregnancy may increase the sensitivity to the cardiovascular effects of cocaine (Fig. 1) (40). Studies in pregnant and progesterone-treated nonpregnant animals suggested that pregnancy alters the metabolism of cocaine (41). Pregnancy may stress the heart so that cocaine produces abnormalities that would not have occurred in a healthy nonpregnant patient. Cocaine can cause lethal cardiovascular events in pregnant patients without preexisting cardiac disease (42). Cocaine can decrease the caliber of coronary arteries and may impair myocardial blood flow (43).

TABLE 1. *Common obstetric complications of cocaine abuse*

Preterm labor
Abruptio placentae
Preeclampsia
Fetal distress

Cocaine can reduce the diameter of the left anterior descending coronary artery and increase the coronary vascular resistance while increasing the heart rate, blood pressure, and cardiac output (43).

Cocaine is a potent dysrhythmogenic agent (44). Atrial extrasystoles, atrial tachycardia, and ventricular extrasystoles are common sequelae of cocaine use. Sinus tachycardia, ventricular premature contraction, ventricular tachycardia, ventricular fibrillation, and asystole also may occur (45). Electrocardiographic changes that may occur after cocaine use include prolongation of the PR, QRS, and QT intervals, increased QRS voltage, ST-T wave changes, and pathologic Q waves (45,46). Both direct drug effects and indirect effects of catecholamine release produce these dysrhythmias. The exact mechanism by which cocaine-induced catecholamine release causes ventricular arrhythmias is unknown. Catecholamines may bind to membrane receptors and evoke a cascade of intracellular responses (47). The combination of the anesthetic properties of cocaine with its adrenergic properties may explain the arrhythmias and cardiac dysfunction that can occur after cocaine administration (Fig. 1).

The true incidence of cocaine-induced myocardial infarction is unknown, but it can occur after cocaine use in young, healthy women (48). The time from cocaine use to infarction is variable, ranging from minutes to hours (49). Both Q wave and non-Q wave infarcts were reported (50). Many patients with cocaine-related myocardial infarctions have normal coronary arteries. These infarcts are due to coronary artery spasm, thrombus, or a combination (51). Although thrombi are not the only cause of cocaine-induced myocardial infarction, thrombolytic therapy has been used successfully to dissolve intraluminal coronary thrombi in patients with acute infarction temporally related to cocaine use (52).

Coronary ischemia and angina without myocardial infarction also can follow cocaine use, as can silent ischemia (53). Frequent episodes of transient ST elevation, similar to that seen in patients with Prinzmetal's angina, are seen in chronic users (54). In addition, recent evidence suggests that chronic cocaine use may cause an acceleration of atherosclerosis and lead to ventricular hypertrophy (55,56).

Cocaine may have a direct negative inotropic effect (57). Left ventricular (LV) dysfunction has been temporally related to cocaine use. Severe global LV hypokinesis and greatly reduced ejection fractions have been reported (58). Reports of pulmonary edema and cardiomyopathy were associated with cocaine abuse (59).

Recognition of the cocaine user can be difficult (60). Most deny drug use when interviewed by physicians (61). Physical examination may be misleading due to difficulty in differentiating between preeclampsia and cocaine use (62). As with other illicit drugs, lack of prenatal care and cigarette smoking are of predictive value

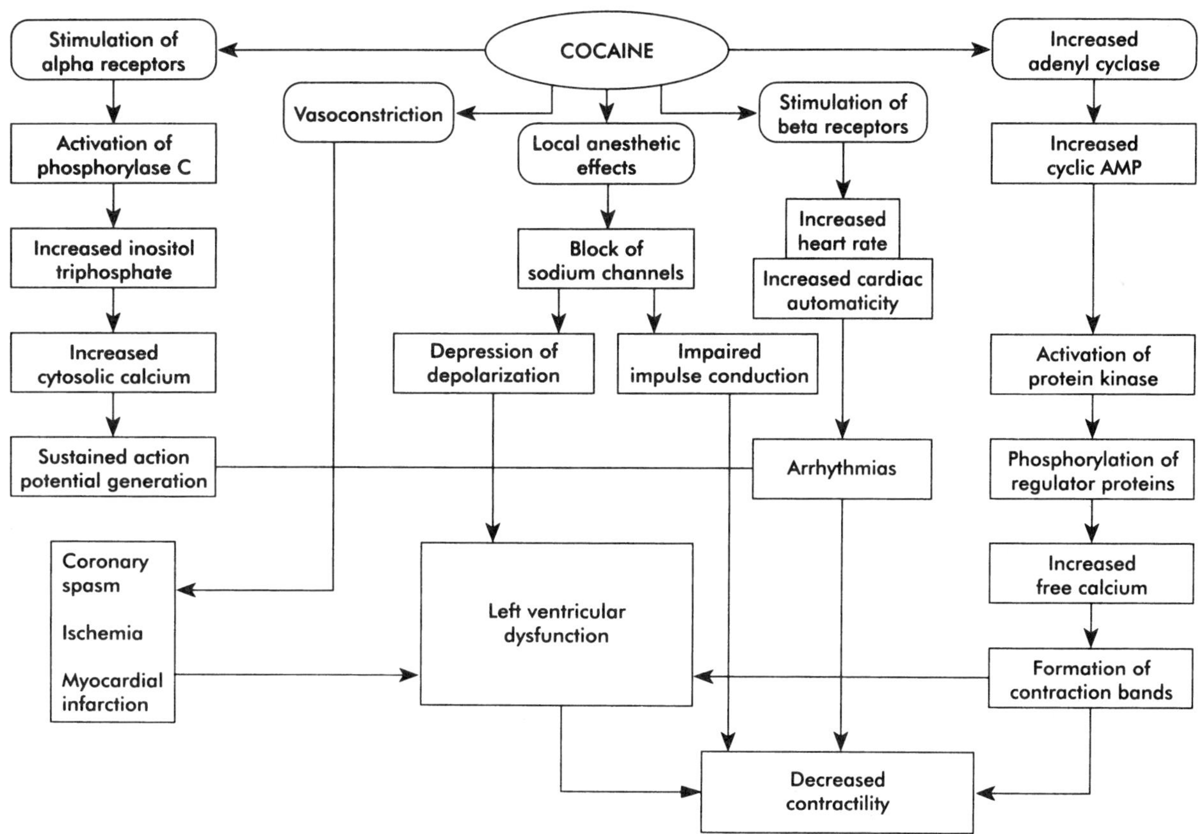

FIG. 1. Mechanisms of cocaine-induced myocardial dysfunction. (From Birnbach DJ. Substance abuse. In: Chestnut DH, ed. *Obstetric anesthesia.* St. Louis: Mosby, 1994:984, with permission.

in the recognition of a cocaine abuser (63). At St. Luke's–Roosevelt Hospital Center, in New York City, approximately 60% of parturients without prenatal care seen in the labor suite tested positive for cocaine (63). Some of the fetal effects of cocaine may be due, at least in part, to other factors, such as cigarettes, alcohol, and poor nutrition.

Fetal Risks

Cocaine use in pregnancy imperils both mother and fetus (64,65). Neonatal and fetal complications of maternal cocaine abuse are numerous and include:

- Intrauterine fetal death (66),
- Congenital abnormalities (67,68),
- Cerebral infarction (69),
- Central nervous system (CNS) irritability (70),
- Increased incidence of fetal desaturation (71), and
- Fetal myocardial ischemia (72).

The risk of these complications remains high even after accounting for confounding variables such as age, race, alcohol abuse, and smoking. Cocaine may increase fetal risk by inducing vasoconstriction of uterine and umbilical vessels (73). The drug may alter the balance of placental prostaglandin production, favoring thromboxane, which may cause vasoconstriction and decreased uteroplacental blood flow (74). There also is evidence that cocaine may have direct effect on several biochemical processes within the placenta (75). The interaction of cocaine with the human placental serotonin transporter has been investigated. It appears that the function of the placental serotonin transporter may be severely impaired by cocaine use during pregnancy (76).

The American College of Obstetricians and Gynecologists (ACOG) recognized that cocaine use has become a major public health concern and published a Committee Opinion reviewing the ramifications of cocaine abuse in pregnancy (77). They make several suggestions:

- A drug history should be taken on all patients,
- A woman acknowledging cocaine use should be counseled and offered support mechanisms to aid in her abstinence,

- Periodic urine testing should be considered to encourage abstinence, and
- Testing the mother and neonate may be useful in some clinical situations, such as unexplained fetal growth retardation, prematurity, or abruptio placenta.

Detecting Cocaine Abuse

Current laboratory screening methods for cocaine metabolites include gas chromatography, mass spectrometry, and radioimmunoassay. The difficulty with some of these tests is the lag between sending the sample and reporting of results. For example, in some hospitals, it may take several days to receive mass spectrometry toxicology results. Instant latex agglutination tests for cocaine metabolites in maternal urine can provide an accurate result within several minutes. One of these tests (OnTrak; Roche Diagnostics, Branchburg, NJ) is highly sensitive and specific when used by anesthesiologists to determine cocaine use by parturients (63). Recent studies also evaluated the use of hair and meconium testing and found that they can greatly improve detection of cocaine use in pregnancy (78,79).

Legal Implications

Legal controversies surrounding maternal rights and the status of the fetus are complex and vary among states. Since 1985, at least 200 women in 30 states have been criminally prosecuted for using illicit drugs or alcohol during pregnancy. In most of these cases, the prosecutors lacked both established precedent and clear statutory authority.

Confusion regarding antenatal toxicology testing arose after a 1993 lawsuit against the Medical University of South Carolina (80). This lawsuit was brought by three women who were incarcerated after positive urine toxicologic tests and refusal to attend substance-abuse and prenatal-care clinics. The suit claimed that the University had violated the patients' rights to privacy and liberty and their rights to refuse medical treatment and to procreate. This case demonstrates the importance of assessing the ethical and legal standing of drug-testing policies. Toxicologic testing of parturients, per se, should not be abandoned when it is considered clinically important for the safe treatment of mother or fetus. However, safeguards to avoid bias and to protect patients' rights must be considered. Many public health organizations, including the AMA and ACOG, suggest that the imposition of criminal sanctions is inappropriate to the caregiver's role, which should focus on treatment. At St. Luke's–Roosevelt Hospital Center, urine toxicology testing is performed on all "high risk" patients after consent, and the results are considered to be an essential piece of information used in the patient's obstetric and anesthetic management. Any patient who refuses to give consent for toxicology testing is treated as if positive.

Anesthetic Considerations

Because cocaine-abusing patients have a higher incidence of cesarean section for "fetal jeopardy," anesthesiologists may meet these women in an emergency setting. Severe hypertension often occurs as a result of the generalized vasoconstriction. Severe hypotension, however, may occur because of cocaine-related hemorrhage.

General endotracheal anesthesia is usually selected for the hemodynamically compromised parturient (Table 2), for example, the patient with acute hemorrhage due to abruptio placenta. Although abruptio placenta after cocaine use has been well described, there is now evidence that placenta previa also may be related to cocaine use and may be another cause of bleeding in the cocaine-abusing patient (81).

In more controlled situations, the anesthesiologist must weigh the risks and benefits of regional and general anesthesia for each patient (Table 3). Epidural or spinal anesthesia have been used successfully to anesthetize the cocaine-abusing patient for cesarean section (82), although hemodynamic perturbations and ephedrine resistance may occur (83).

General Anesthesia

Stimulation, as with laryngoscopy during induction of general anesthesia, can produce severe hypertension in the cocaine-abusing patient. To limit the risks of this complication, blood pressure should be pharmacologically controlled before induction and intubation (Table 4). β-Blockade with propranolol is contraindicated in the cocaine-abusing patient, as it may cause unopposed α-adrenergic stimulation and therefore worsen the hypertension (84). In addition, β-blockade has been reported to enhance cocaine-induced coronary vasoconstriction (85). Hydralazine has been used to treat hypertension in the cocaine-abusing parturient but may produce profound maternal tachycardia and does not restore uterine blood flow.

Hughes et al. (86) compared hydralazine with labetalol in gravid ewes and concluded that labetalol may be preferable to hydralazine for treatment of the acutely cocaine-intoxicated parturient. Pearce and Wallin (87) similarly reported that, unlike pure β-blockers, labetalol could successfully be used to treat cocaine-induced catecholamine crises. Hollander (88), however, suggested caution because the β-antagonistic effects of labetalol are

TABLE 2. *Indications for general anesthesia for cesarean section in the cocaine-abusing parturient*

Massive hemorrhage/hemodynamic instability
Clinically significant thrombocytopenia
Disseminated intravascular coagulation (DIC)
Sepsis
Patient refusal

TABLE 3. *Associated conditions that do not necessarily preclude the use of regional anesthesia*

Mild thrombocytopenia
Abruptio placentae with hemodynamic stability
HIV positivity
Hypertension

HIV, human immunodeficiency virus.

more potent than its α-blocking effects and may thus produce a paradoxic hypertensive response.

Metabolic and respiratory acid–base abnormalities often accompany cocaine toxicity, and sodium bicarbonate may have an important role in the short-term treatment of the cocaine-abusing patient (89). Calcium channel blockers have been considered to be ineffective for prevention or treatment of cocaine toxicity; however, they were recently advocated (88,90).

Because the cocaine-abusing patient is at high risk for cardiac arrhythmias, avoid halothane and other drugs that may sensitize the myocardium to catecholamines (18). Although isoflurane was administered to cocaine-abusing patients without incident (91), it was reported that cocaine toxicity during isoflurane anesthesia is associated with a marked increase in systemic vascular resistance and a tendency to produce cardiac arrhythmias (92). Ketamine may potentiate the cardiac effects of cocaine by further increasing catecholamine concentrations (93). It may, however, precipitate hypotension due to myocardial depression, if the patient is unable to mount a further catecholamine release.

There was a report of a prolonged block from succinylcholine in a cocaine-abusing patient, presumably due to a depletion of cholinesterases involved in cocaine metabolism (94). Succinylcholine can be safely used in standard doses if general anesthesia becomes necessary in the cocaine-abusing parturient, because even if cholinesterase deficiency occurs, the ensuing neuromuscular block should not last as long as the surgery. Use a nerve stimulator to ensure that the effect of the succinylcholine has terminated before giving nondepolarizing muscle relaxants to these patients.

TABLE 4. *Treatment of cocaine intoxication*

Hypertension
Calcium channel blocker
Intravenous nitroglycerin
Benzodiazepines
Labetolol
Angina
Nitroglycerin
Benzodiazepines
Calcium channel blockers
Lidocaine
CNS agitation
Benzodiazepines

CNS, central nervous system.

Regional Anesthesia

Problems also can occur during regional anesthesia in a cocaine-abusing parturient. Profound hypotension may follow sympathetic blockade, and the cocaine-abusing patient may not respond as expected to ephedrine. Apparently these women cannot develop a tachycardia in response to this indirect-acting agent (83). Should these patients develop ephedrine-resistant hypotension, they do respond to small doses of phenylephrine. Although not seen in all studies, thrombocytopenia was reported to be associated with cocaine abuse. If no other conditions, such as HIV disease exist, these patients are not at greater risk for epidural hematoma. Even in the cases in which thrombocytopenia occurs, platelet counts remain clinically adequate (95).

Postoperative Care

Vigilant postoperative monitoring is essential, as signs and symptoms of cocaine toxicity may arise until hours after the drug exposure (96,97). In addition, cocaine users may have silent myocardial ischemia with episodes of ST elevation during the first weeks of withdrawal (98).

AMPHETAMINES

The amphetamines are sympathomimetic agents that cause profound CNS stimulation. These drugs may be abused individually or in conjunction with other substances such as cocaine. Acute ingestion produces signs and symptoms that mimic cocaine abuse (99) and also may be mistaken for preeclampsia (100). As with cocaine, amphetamines may cause uteroplacental vasoconstriction and precipitate worrisome fetal conditions.

As with other illicit drugs, patients abusing amphetamines often receive little or no prenatal care. Amphetamine use has been associated with intrauterine growth retardation, intrauterine fetal death, and abruptio placenta (101).

The acute ingestion of amphetamines has been reported to increase the dose requirement (maximal allowable concentration; MAC) for general anesthetics, whereas the chronic ingestion decreases MAC (102). Because amphetamines produce an accumulation of norepinephrine, halothane and other potentially arrhythmogenic agents should not be used. Reports have described cardiac arrest in amphetamine-abusing patients undergoing cesarean section under regional (103) and general (104) anesthesia.

OPIOIDS

Although the number of pregnant patients who abuse opioids appears to be decreasing in New York City, this problem still exists. Approximately 250,000 women in the United States are intravenous drug abusers, with 90% of child-bearing age (105). Perinatal abuse of opioids is associated with numerous medical problems including HIV/acquired immunodeficiency syndrome (AIDS), hepatitis, endocarditis, and pulmonary, renal, and cardiac disease (106). Acute withdrawal syndrome also may occur, producing tremors, anxiety, muscle pains, nausea, vomiting, anorexia, gastrointestinal pain, tachycardia, hypertension, and mydriasis. These signs peak 48 to 72 hours after the last drug exposure. Opioid antagonists or agonist–antagonists can precipitate acute withdrawal and therefore should be avoided in known or suspected addicts (107).

Pregnant opioid abusers may be seen with overdose, identified by coma, miosis, or respiratory depression. These women can be at risk of regurgitation and aspiration. If in doubt about the patient's ability to protect her airway, secure it with a cuffed endotracheal tube.

Methadone

Methadone is currently used for the treatment of pregnant opioid addicts. Although infants born to mothers taking methadone weigh more than infants of heroin-abusing mothers, methadone has been associated with its own problems including newborn withdrawal, neurobehavioral depression, and death (108). Methadone-maintained pregnancies are associated with a higher incidence of nonreactive nonstress tests (NSTs) and lower NST scores compared with nonopiate controls (109). Methadone may alter fetal CNS neurotransmitters and change fetal behavior. Regardless of side effects, methadone maintenance poses far fewer hazards, both to mother and fetus, than continued use of intravenous heroin (38,110). Maternal intravenous drug use is associated with maternal HIV culture positivity at delivery and perinatal HIV transmission (38).

When a pregnant patient is receiving methadone maintenance, it is important to monitor the dose carefully, especially late in pregnancy when metabolism may be altered. Maintenance methadone is traditionally given once daily; however, this may not be adequate in pregnant patients. Pond et al. (111) showed that methadone concentrations decrease more rapidly during the later stages of pregnancy. Wittman and Sewgal (112) suggested that dividing the dose of methadone and giving it twice a day reduces fetal stress. Selecting the optimal methadone dose is a complex problem in which the favorable neurobehavioral outcome must be weighed against the risks associated with neonatal withdrawal. Hagopian et al. (110) suggested that higher methadone doses may improve long-term neonatal outcome. Regardless of drug or regimen, to avoid maternal withdrawal, daily opioid administration must continue during labor and postpartum.

Acute Withdrawal

Although not recommended, intentional withdrawal has occasionally been undertaken during pregnancy. Reasons for withdrawal during pregnancy include patient refusal to take methadone, lack of methadone maintenance program in the patient's vicinity, patient request, and the patient who is so disruptive to the treatment setting that other patients are jeopardized. It has been long suggested that women should only be withdrawn in the second trimester of pregnancy, because first-trimester withdrawal may result in spontaneous abortion, and third-trimester withdrawal may cause premature labor. There is little evidence, however, to support these claims.

The Neonate

The anesthesiologist is occasionally called on to resuscitate or assist in the management of a neonate who has symptoms of acute withdrawal syndrome. The Committee on Drugs of the American Academy of Pediatrics recommends that thoughtful consideration be given to the need for the administration of pharmacologic agents to newborn infants who have symptoms of drug withdrawal (113).

Anesthetic Considerations

Regional anesthetic techniques offer many advantages in the management of the opioid-addicted parturient. Spinal and epidural analgesia can provide pain relief without opioids. The opioid-abusing patient may be intolerant to pain because of decreased endogenous opioid peptides. In the rehabilitated abuser, the use of a regional anesthetic provides pain relief without opioids, which many rehabilitated addicts fear may precipitate readdiction. If a catheter technique is chosen, local anesthetics also can be used for postoperative pain management.

ETHANOL

There are an estimated 15 million alcoholics in the United States; approximately one fourth of them are women (114). Alcohol abuse has been associated with numerous maternal abnormalities including cardiomyopathy, decreased albumin concentration, coagulopathy, liver disease, ascites, and electrolyte abnormalities (115,116).

Alcohol is a known teratogen, and alcohol use during pregnancy is associated with the fetal alcohol syndrome (117). Signs and symptoms of this syndrome include craniofacial, cardiac, renal, and musculocutaneous abnormalities. Children with complete fetal alcohol syndrome are usually born to mothers who consume large amounts of alcohol throughout pregnancy. However, because a safe level of alcohol intake in pregnancy has not been established, total abstinence is considered the safest course (118).

In the absence of coagulopathy or neuropathy, both of which have been associated with end-stage disease, alcoholics can safely receive a regional anesthetic. Occasionally, regional techniques may fail because of psychotic or combative behavior. Should these patients require a general anesthetic, a major consideration is prevention of aspiration, because alcohol both increases gastric acid secretion and decreases protective reflexes. Because these women may have severe hypoalbuminemia or cardiac manifestations of alcohol abuse, they may be sensitive to the effects of myocardial depressant anesthetics. Because of tolerance and an expanded plasma volume, however, many alcoholics will require larger than normal doses of induction agents (119).

CIGARETTES

Tobacco is still the most commonly abused drug during pregnancy. It has been suggested that 15% of low birth weight in infants could be prevented if no women smoked during pregnancy (120). In 1990, it was estimated that 29% of American women of child-bearing age smoked cigarettes (121). Despite the clear evidence that cigarette smoking has adverse effects on mother and fetus, only 20% of cigarette-smoking women in the United States quit during pregnancy (122). Cigarette smoking during pregnancy has been associated with intrauterine growth retardation, spontaneous abortion, premature rupture of membranes, preterm birth, placenta previa, abruptio placentae, congenital anomalies, and sudden infant death syndrome (123,124). It has been suggested that cigarette smoking be abandoned during pregnancy and that if necessary, nicotine-replacement therapy be considered for pregnant smokers (125). Although passive cigarette smoke is a risk to pregnant and nonpregnant patients, a recent case-controlled study found that passive smoking during pregnancy was not associated with an increased risk of term small-for-gestational-age (SGA) infants (126).

Cigarette smoke is composed of more than 1,000 components, many of which affect the respiratory, cardiovascular, and immune systems (127). The respiratory effects of cigarette smoke include abnormalities in mucus secretion, ciliary transport, and small airway function (128). Postoperative respiratory morbidity is therefore a risk of general anesthesia in cigarette-smoking patients. Although 4 to 6 weeks of abstinence are required to decrease the risk of postoperative respiratory complications, after as little as 48 hours of abstinence, carboxyhemoglobin concentrations decrease and oxygen delivery increases. In addition, a few days of abstinence will improve mucociliary transport. The use of regional anesthesia is particularly beneficial to the cigarette-smoking patient undergoing cesarean section, by allowing an alternative to general anesthesia and the risk of bronchospasm that may accompany endotracheal intubation.

REFERENCES

1. Slutsker L, Smith R, Higginson G, Fleming D. Recognizing illicit drug use by pregnant women: reports from Oregon birth attendants. *Am J Public Health* 1993;83:61.
2. Bendrsky M, Alessandri S, Gilbert P, Lewis M. Characteristics of pregnant substance abusers in two cities in the northeast. *Am J Drug Alcohol Abuse* 1996;22:349.
3. Chasnoff IJ, Landress HJ, Barrett ME. The prevalence of illicit drug or alcohol use during pregnancy and discrepancies in mandatory reporting in Pinellas County, Florida. *N Engl J Med* 1990;322:1202.
4. Offidani C, Pomini F, Caruso A, et al. Cocaine during pregnancy: a critical review of the literature. *Minerva Ginecol* 1995;47:381.
5. Smit BJ, Boer K, van Huis AM, et al. Cocaine use in pregnancy in Amsterdam. *Acta Paediatr* 1994;404:32.
6. Martrinez Crespo JM, Antolin E, Comas C, et al. The prevalence of cocaine abuse during pregnancy in Barcelona. *Eur J Obstet Gynecol Reprod Biol* 1994;56:165.
7. Davis RB. Drug and alcohol use in the former Soviet Union: selected factors and future considerations. *Int J Addictions* 1994;29:303.
8. Dannenberg AL, Carter DM, Lawson HW, et al. Homicide and other injuries as causes of maternal death in New York City, 1987-1991. *Am J Obstet Gynecol* 1995;172:1557.
9. Chazotte C, Youcah J, Freda MC. Cocaine using during pregnancy and low birth weight: the impact of prenatal care and drug treatment. *Semin Perinatol* 1995;19:293.
10. Matera C, Warren WB, Moomjy M, et al. Prevalence of use of cocaine and other substances in an obstetric population. *Am J Obstet Gynecol* 1990;63:797.
11. Bendersky M, Alessandri S, Gilbert P, Lewis M. Characteristics of pregnant substance abusers in two cities in the northeast. *Am J Drug Alcohol Abuse* 1996;2:349.
12. Frank DA, Zuckerman BS, Amaro H, et al. Cocaine use during pregnancy: prevalence and correlates. *Pediatrics* 1988;2:888.
13. McCalla S, Minkoff HL, Feldman J, et al. Predictors of cocaine use in pregnancy. *Obstet Gynecol* 1992;79:641.
14. Spence MR, Williams R, Digregorio JG, et al. The relationship between recent cocaine use and pregnancy outcome. *Obstet Gynecol* 1991;78:326.
15. Kain ZN, Rimar S, Barash PG. Cocaine abuse in the parturient and effects on the fetus and neonate. *Anesth Analg* 1993;77:835.
16. Hawthorne JL, Maier RC. Drug abuse in an obstetric population of a midsized city. *South Med J* 1993;86:1334.
17. Rosenak D, Diamant YZ, Yaffe H, Hornstein E. Cocaine: maternal use during pregnancy and its effect on the mother, the fetus and the infant. *Obstet Gynecol Surv* 1990;45:348.
18. Fleming JA, Byck R, Barash PG. Pharmacology and therapeutic applications of cocaine. *Anesthesiology* 1990;73:518.
19. Cone EJ. Pharmacokinetics and pharmacodynamics of cocaine. *J Analyt Toxicol* 1995;19:459.
20. Gold MS, Washton AM, Dackis CA. Cocaine abuse: neurochemistry phenomenology, and treatment. *Nat Inst Drug Abuse Res Monogr Ser* 1985;61:13.
21. Pitts DK, Marwah J. Autonomic actions of cocaine. *Can J Physiol Pharmacol* 1989;67:1168.
22. Dombrowski MP, Wolfe HM, Welch RA, et al. Cocaine abuse is associated with abruptio placentae and decreased birth weight, but not shorter labor. *Obstet Gynecol* 1991;77:139.
23. MacGregor SN, Keith LG, Chasnoff IJ. Cocaine use during pregnancy: adverse perinatal outcome. *Am J Obstet Gynecol* 1987;157:686.
24. Chan L, Pham H, Reece EA. Pneumothorax in pregnancy associated with cocaine use. *Am J Perinatol* 1997;14:385.
25. Iriye BK, Bristow RE, Hsu CD, Bruni R, Johnson TR. Uterine rupture associated with recent antepartum cocaine abuse. *Obstet Gynecol* 1994;83:840.
26. Mishra A, Landzberg BR, Parente JT. Uterine rupture in association with alkaloidal cocaine use. *Am J Obstet Gynecol* 1995;173:243.
27. Chasnoff IJ, Burns WJ, Schnoll SH, Burns KA. Cocaine use in pregnancy. *N Engl J Med* 1985;313:666.
28. Chouteau M, Mamerow PB, Leppert P. The effect of cocaine use on birth weight and gestational age. *Obstet Gynecol* 1988;72:351.
29. Chao CR. Cardiovascular effects of cocaine during pregnancy. *Semin Perinatol* 1996;20:107.
30. Kloner RA, Hale S, Aiker K, Rezkalla S. The effect of acute and chronic cocaine use on the heart. *Circulation* 1992;85:4079.
31. Lampley EC, Williams S, Myers SA. Cocaine-associated rhabdomyolysis causing renal failure in pregnancy. *Obstet Gynecol* 1996;87:804.
32. Calaway CW, Clark RF. Hyperthermia in psychostimulant overdose. *Ann Emerg Med* 1994;24:68.

33. Quereshi AI, Akbar MS, Czander E, Safdar K, Janssen RS, Frankel MR. Crack cocaine use and stroke in young patients. *Neurology* 1997; 48:341.
34. Nalbandian H, Sheth N, Dietrich R, Geogiou J. Intestinal ischemia caused by cocaine ingestion: report of two cases. *Surgery* 1985; 97:374.
35. Moen MD, Caliendo MJ, Marshall W, Uhler ML. Hepatic rupture in pregnancy associated with cocaine use. *Obstet Gynecol* 1993;82:687.
36. Orser B. Thrombocytopenia and cocaine abuse. *Anesthesiology* 1991; 74:195.
37. Minkoff HL, McCalla S, Delke I, et al. The relationship of cocaine use to syphilis and human immunodeficiency virus infections among inner city parturient women. *Am J Obstet Gynecol* 1990;163:521.
38. Rodriguez EM, Mofenson LM, Chang BH, et al. Association of maternal drug use during pregnancy with maternal HIV culture positivity and perinatal HIV transmission. *AIDS* 1996;10:273.
39. Burkett G, Yasin SY, Palow D, LaVoie L, Martinez M. Patterns of cocaine binging: effect on pregnancy. *Am J Obstet Gynecol* 1994; 171:372.
40. Woods JR, Scott KJ, Plessinger MA. Pregnancy enhances cocaine's actions on the heart and within the peripheral circulation. *Am J Obstet Gynecol* 1994;170:1027.
41. Woods JR Jr, Plessinger MA. Pregnancy increases cardiovascular toxicity to cocaine. *Am J Obstet Gynecol* 1990;162:529.
42. Burkett G, Bandstra ES, Cohen J, et al. Cocaine related maternal death. *Am J Obstet Gynecol* 1990;163:40.
43. Lange RA, Cigarroa RG, Yancy CW, et al. Cocaine-induced coronary-artery vasoconstriction. *N Engl J Med* 1989;321:1557.
44. Nanji AA, Filipenko JD. Asystole and ventricular fibrillation associated with cocaine intoxication. *Chest* 1994;85:132.
45. Chakko S, Myerburg RJ. Cardiac complications of cocaine abuse. *Clin Cardiol* 1995;18:67.
46. Perera R, Kraebber A, Schwartz MJ. Prolonged QT interval and cocaine use. *J Electrocardiol* 1997;30:337.
47. Billman GE. Mechanisms responsible for the cardiotoxic effects of cocaine. *FASEB J* 1990;4:2469.
48. Liu S, Forrester RM, Murphy GS, et al. Anesthetic management of a parturient with myocardial infarction related to cocaine use. *Can J Anaesth* 1992;39:858.
49. Isner JM, Estes M, Thompson PD, et al. Acute cardiac events temporally related to cocaine abuse. *N Engl J Med* 1986:315;1438.
50. Kossowsky WA, Lyon AF, Chou SY. Acute non-Q wave cocaine-related myocardial infarction. *Chest* 1989;96:617.
51. Rezjakka SH, Hale S, Kloner RA. Cocaine-induced heart diseases. *Am Heart J* 1990;120:1403.
52. Yao SS, Spindola-Franco H, Menegus M, et al. Successful intracoronary thrombolysis in cocaine-associated acute myocardial infarction. *Cathet Cardiovasc Diagn* 1997;42:294.
53. Nadamanee K, Gorelick DA, Josephson MA, et al. Myocardial ischemia during cocaine withdrawal. *Ann Intern Med* 1989;111:876.
54. Clarkson CW, Chang C, Stolfi A, et al. Electrophysiological effects of high cocaine concentrations on intact canine heart. *Circulation* 1993; 87:950.
55. Dressler FA, Malekzadeh S, Roberts WC. Quantitative analysis of amounts of coronary arterial narrowing in cocaine addicts. *Am J Cardiol* 1990;65:303.
56. Brickner ME, Willard JE, Eichhorn EJ, et al. Left ventricular hypertrophy associated with chronic cocaine abuse. *Circulation* 191;84:1130.
57. Hale SL, Alker KJ, Rezkalla S, Figurs G, Kloner RA. Adverse effects of cocaine in cardiovascular dynamics, myocardial blood flow, and coronary artery diameter in an experimental model. *Am Heart J* 1989;188:927.
58. Chokshi SK, Moore R, Pandian NG, Isner JM. Reversible cardiomyopathy associated with cocaine intoxication. *Ann Intern Med* 1989; 111:1039.
59. Weiner RS, Lockhart JT, Schwartz RG. Dilated cardiomyopathy and cocaine abuse: report of two cases. *Am J Med* 1986;81:699.
60. Campbell D, Parr MJA, Shutt LE. Unrecognized "crack" cocaine abuse in pregnancy. *Br J Anaesth* 1996;77:553.
61. Zuckerman B, Amaro H, Cabral H. Validity of self reporting of marijuana and cocaine use among pregnant adolescents. *J Pediatr* 1989; 115:812.
62. Towers CV, Pircon RA, Nageotte MP, Porto M, Garite TJ. Cocaine intoxication presenting as preeclampsia and eclampsia. *Obstet Gynecol* 1993;81:545.
63. Birnbach DJ, Stein DJ, Grunebaum A, Danzer BI, Thys DM. Cocaine screening of parturients without prenatal care: an evaluation of a rapid screening assay. *Anesth Analg* 1997;84:76.
64. Snodgrass SR. Cocaine babies: a result of multiple teratogenic influences. *J Child Neurol* 1994;9:227.
65. Little BB, Snell LM, Klein VR, et al. Cocaine abuse during pregnancy: maternal and fetal implications. *Obstet Gynecol* 1989;73:157.
66. Martinez A, Larabee K, Monga M. Cocaine is associated with intrauterine fetal death in women with suspected preterm labor. *Am J Perinatol* 1996;13:163.
67. Jasnosx KM, Hermansen MC, Snider C, Sang K. Congenital complete absence of the diaphragm: a rare variant of congenital diaphragmatic hernia. *Am J Perinatol* 1994;11:340.
68. Chavez GF, Mulinare J, Cordero JF. Maternal cocaine use during early pregnancy as a risk factor for congenital urogenital anomalies. *JAMA* 1989;262:795.
69. Chasnoff IJ, Bussey ME, Savich R, Stack CM. Perinatal cerebral infarction and maternal cocaine use. *J Pediatr* 1986;108:456.
70. Chasnoff IJ, Burns KA, Burns WJ. Cocaine use in pregnancy: perinatal morbidity and mortality. *Neurotoxicol Teratol* 1987;9:291.
71. Woods JR, Plessinger MA, Clark KE. Effect of cocaine on uterine blood flow and fetal oxygenation. *JAMA* 1987;257:957.
72. Mehta SK, Finkelhor RS, Anderson RL, et al. Transient myocardial ischemia in infants prenatally exposed to cocaine. *J Pediatr* 1993; 122:945.
73. Van Allen MI. Fetal vascular disruption: mechanisms and some resulting birth defects. *Pediatr Ann* 1981;10:219.
74. Togna G, Grazianin M, Sorrentino C, Caprino L. Prostanoid production in the presence of platelet activation in hypoxic cocaine-treated rats. *Haemostasis* 1996;26:311.
75. Ganapathy V, Ramamoorthy S, Leibach FH. Transport and metabolism of monoamines in the human placenta. *Trophoblast Res* 1998;7:35.
76. Prasad PD, Leibach FH, Mahesh VB, Ganapathy V. Human placenta as a target organ for cocaine action: interaction of cocaine with the placental serotonin transporter. *Placenta* 1994;15:267.
77. ACOG. Committee opinion: Committee on obstetrics: maternal and fetal medicine: number 114. *Int J Gynecol Obstet* 1998;41:102.
78. Oyler J, Darwin WD, Preston KL, et al. Cocaine disposition in meconium from newborns of cocaine-abusing mothers and urine of adult drug users. *J Analyt Toxicol* 1996;20:453.
79. Kline J, Ng SK, Schittini M, et al. Cocaine use during pregnancy: sensitive detection by hair assay. *Am J Public Health* 1997;87:352.
80. Jos PH, Marshall MF, Perlmutter M. The Charleston policy on cocaine use during pregnancy: a cautionary tale. *J Law Med Ethics* 1995; 23:120.
81. Macones GA, Sehdev HM, Parry S, Organ MA, Berlin JA. The association between maternal cocaine use and placenta previa. *Am J Obstet Gynecol* 1997;177:1097.
82. Kain ZN, Mayes LC, Ferris CA, Pakes J, Scottenfeld R. Cocaine-abusing parturients undergoing cesarean section: a cohort study. *Anesthesiology* 1995;85:1028.
83. Birnbach DJ, Stein DJ, Danzer BI, Hartman JK, Thys DM. Ephedrine resistance in the cocaine-positive parturient: prevalence and treatment. *Anesthesiology* 1996;85:A892.
84. Ramoska E, Sacchetti A. Propranolol induced hypertension in the treatment of cocaine intoxication. *Ann Emerg Med* 1985;14:1112.
85. Lange RA, Cigarroa RG, Flores ED, et al. Potentiation of cocaine-induced coronary vasoconstriction by beta-adrenergic blockade. *Ann Intern Med* 1990;112:897.
86. Hughes SC, Vertommen JD, Rosen MA, et al. Cocaine induced hypertension in the ewe and response to treatment with labetalol. *Anesthesiology* 1991;77:A1075.
87. Pearce CJ, Wallin JD. Labetalol and other agents that block both alpha- and beta-adrenergic receptors. *Cleveland Clin J Med* 1994;61:59.
88. Hollander JE. The management of cocaine-associated myocardial ischemia. *N Engl J Med* 1995;333:1267.
89. Williams RG, Kavanagh KM, Teo KK. Pathophysiology and treatment of cocaine toxicity: implications for the heart and cardiovascular system. *Can J Cardiol* 1996;12:1295.
90. Derlet RW, Tseng CC, Albertson TE. Cocaine toxicity and the calcium channel blockers nifedipine and nimodipine in rats. *J Emerg Med* 1994;12:1.
91. Bernards CM, Kern C, Cullen BF. Chronic cocaine administration does not modify haemodynamic responses to isoflurane anaesthesia in sheep. *Can J Anaesth* 1997;44:202.

92. Boylan JF, Cheng DC, Sandler AN, et al. Cocaine toxicity and isoflurane anesthesia: hemodynamic, myocardial metabolic, and regional blood flow effects in swine. *J Cardiothorac Vasc Anesth* 1996;10:772.
93. Murphy JL. Hypertension and pulmonary oedema associated with ketamine administration in a patient with a history of substance abuse. *Can J Anaesth* 1993;40:160.
94. Jatlow P, Barash PG, Van Dyke C, et al. Cocaine and succinylcholine sensitivity: a new caution. *Anesth Analg* 1979;58:235.
95. Gershon RY, Fisher AJ, Graves WL. The cocaine-abusing parturient is not at increased risk for thrombocytopenia. *Anesth Analg* 1996;82:865.
96. Cooke JE, Vila H, Kaplan R. Anesthetic complications 14 hours after the use of crack cocaine. *Anesth Analg* 1993;76:676.
97. Bird DJ, Markey JR. Massive pulmonary edema in a habitual crack cocaine smoker not chemically positive for cocaine at the time of surgery. *Anesth Analg* 1997;84:1157.
98. Schindler CW, Tella SR, Erzouki HK, Goldberg SR. Pharmacological mechanisms in cocaine's cardiovascular effects. *Drug Alcohol Depend* 1995;37:183.
99. Ong BH. Hazards to health: dextroamphetamine poisoning. *N Engl J Med* 1962;266:1321.
100. Eliot RH, Rees GB. Amphetamine ingestion presenting as eclampsia. *Can J Anaesth* 1990;37:130.
101. Oro AS, Dixon SD. Perinatal cocaine and methamphetamine exposure: maternal and neonatal correlates. *J Pediatr* 1987;111:571.
102. Johnston RR, Way WL, Miller RD. Alteration of anesthetic requirement by amphetamine. *Anesthesiology* 1972;36:357.
103. Smith DS, Gutsche BB. Amphetamine abuse and obstetrical anesthesia. *Anesth Analg* 1980;59:710.
104. Samuels SI, Maze A, Albright A. Cardiac arrest during cesarean section in a chronic amphetamine abuser. *Anesth Analg* 1979;58:528.
105. Little BB, Snell LM, Klein VR, et al. Maternal and fetal effects of heroin addiction during pregnancy. *J Reprod Med* 1990;35:159.
106. Kliman L. Drug dependence and pregnancy: antenatal and intrapartum problems. *Anaesth Intens Care* 1990;18:358.
107. Weintraub SJ, Naulty JS. Acute abstinence syndrome after epidural injection of butorphanol. *Anesth Analg* 1985;64:452.
108. Jarvis MA, Schnoll SH. Methadone use during pregnancy. *NIDA Res Monogr* 1995;149:58.
109. Anyaegbunam A, Tran T, Jadali D, et al. Assessment of fetal well-being in methadone-maintained pregnancies: abnormal stress tests. *Gynecol Obstet Invest* 1997;43:25.
110. Hagopian GS, Wolfe HM, Sokol RJ, et al. Neonatal outcome following methadone exposure in utero. *J Matern Fetal Med* 1996;5:348.
111. Pond SM, Kreek MJ, Tong TG, et al. Altered methadone pharmacokinetics in methadone-maintained pregnant women. *J Pharmacol Exp Ther* 1985;2231:1.
112. Wittman BK, Sewgal SA. A comparison of the effects of single and split dose methadone administration on the fetus: ultrasound evaluation. *Int J Addict* 1991;26:213.
113. Committee on Drugs. Neonatal drug withdrawal. *Pediatrics* 1983; 72:895.
114. Pietrantoni M, Knupel RA. Alcohol use in pregnancy. *Clin Perinatol* 1991;18:93.
115. Bruce DL. Alcoholism and anesthesia. *Anesth Analg* 1983;62:84.
116. Wolfson B, Freed B. Influence of alcohol on anesthetic requirements and acute toxicity. *Anesth Analg* 1980;59:826.
117. Lemoine P, Harroussean H, Borteyrn JP. Les enfans de partents alcoolques: anomalies observees. *Quest Med* 1968;25:477.
118. Council on Scientific Affairs, American Medical Association. Fetal effects of maternal alcohol use. *JAMA* 1983;249:2517.
119. Edwards R. Anaesthesia and alcohol. *Br Med J* 1985;291:423.
120. Shiono PH, Klebanoff MA, Nugent RP, et al. The impact of cocaine and marijuana use on low birth weight and preterm birth: a multicenter study. *Am J Obstet Gynecol* 1995;172:19.
121. U.S. Department of Health and Human Services, Public Health Service. *National household survey on drug abuse*. Washington, DC: U.S. Department of Health and Human Services, Public Health Service, 1991.
122. Prager K, Malin H, Spiegler D, et al. Smoking and drinking behavior before and during pregnancy of married mothers of live-born infants and stillborn infants. *Public Health Rep* 1984;99:117.
123. Feng T. Substance abuse in pregnancy. *Current Opin Obstet Gynecol* 1993;5:16.
124. Kistin N, Handler A, Davis F, Ferre C. Cocaine and cigarettes: a comparison of risks. *Paediatr Perinat Epidemiol* 1996;10:269.
125. Benowitz NL. Nicotine replacement therapy during pregnancy. *JAMA* 1991;266:3174.
126. Chen LH, Petitti DB. Case control study of passive smoking and the risk of small for gestational-age at term. *Am J Epidemiol* 1995;142:158.
127. Stedman RL. The chemical composition of tobacco and tobacco smole. *Chem Rev* 1968;68:153.
128. Pearce AC, Jones RM. Smoking and anesthesia: preoperative abstinence and perioperative morbidity. *Anesthesiology* 1984;61:576.

Obstetric Anesthesia, second edition,
edited by Mark C. Norris.
Lippincott Williams & Wilkins, Philadelphia © 1999.

CHAPTER 27

Anesthesia and Preeclampsia/Eclampsia

Joy Hawkins

Hypertensive disorders are the third leading cause of pregnancy-related mortality. Death is primarily due to cerebrovascular or other central nervous system (CNS) event (1). Pregnancy-induced hypertension (PIH), or preeclampsia, alters function in many organ systems. The physiologic changes of a pregnancy complicated by preeclampsia may differ markedly from those of a healthy gestation. Recognition of these differences allows anesthesiologists to modify their routine practice to provide optimal care for these high-risk parturients.

Although mild preeclampsia may have few anesthetic implications, severe disease requires special consideration (2). Preoperative evaluation of these women requires additional and more frequent laboratory evaluation. They may need invasive hemodynamic monitoring. Control of blood pressure assumes a high priority. A safe anesthetic requires careful planning. We must:

- Understand the pathophysiology of preeclampsia,
- Assess the extent and severity of the disease, and
- Tailor the anesthetic to the needs of the patient and the obstetric situation (3).

In obstetric anesthesia, several plans must be developed for each patient. A patient seen for a trial of labor and vaginal delivery may eventually require cesarean section. Although some indications for cesarean delivery can be managed semielectively, others may be true emergencies. The anesthetic plan must cover all of these possibilities. Be flexible. Plan ahead. Communicate actively with the obstetrician.

PREOPERATIVE ASSESSMENT

The parturient with preeclampsia requires thorough evaluation to assess the extent of organ-system involvement. Baseline laboratory studies should include a complete blood count, platelet count, blood urea nitrogen (BUN), creatinine, and liver-function tests. Additional tests should be ordered as clinically indicated. Patients with severe preeclampsia will require more extensive and frequent laboratory evaluation than those with mild disease.

Hemoglobin and Hematocrit

The hematocrit provides an initial estimation of volume status. The "physiologic anemia of pregnancy" rarely permits a hematocrit greater than 36% at sea level. Attribute higher values to intravascular volume contraction. In 10% of patients with severe preeclampsia, a microangiopathic hemolytic anemia associated with thrombocytopenia and increased liver enzymes (HELLP syndrome) may develop.

Even in milder forms of preeclampsia, endothelial cell damage and vasospasm cause destruction of red cells. Increased heme catabolism increases production of carboxyhemoglobin and causes a leftward shift of the oxyhemoglobin dissociation curve (4). Normally, pregnancy shifts half-saturation pressure (p_{50}) rightward to approximately 30 mm Hg. In preeclampsia, p_{50} is 24.4 mm Hg, to the left of even the nonpregnant value (Fig. 1). This leftward shift decreases the release of oxygen to the fetus at the placenta, perhaps increasing the risk of intrauterine growth retardation and fetal distress.

Coagulation

Laboratory Evaluation

Disseminated intravascular coagulation is rare in the preeclamptic patient. It occurs most commonly in association with placental abruption or fetal death. In the absence of thrombocytopenia (less than 100,000/mm^3), it is extremely unlikely that a woman with severe preeclampsia will have an abnormal fibrinogen or prolonged prothrom-

J. Hawkins: Department of Anesthesiology, University of Colorado Health Sciences Center, Denver, Colorado 80262.

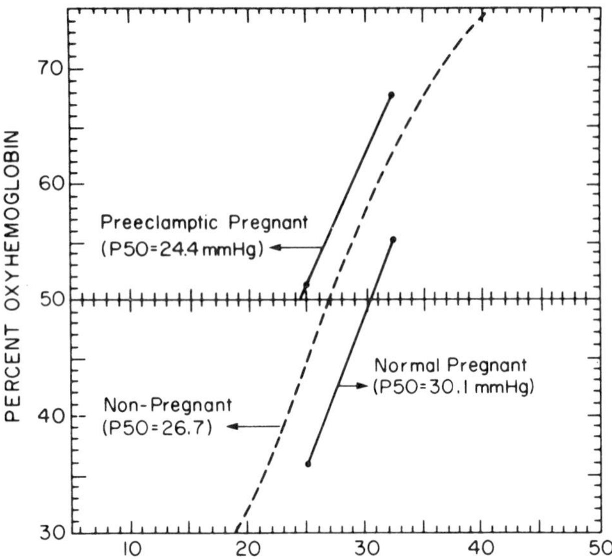

FIG. 1. Effect of normal and preeclamptic pregnancies on p_{50}. The rightward shift in normal pregnancy encourages oxygen release to the fetus. The leftward shift in preeclamptic pregnancies inhibits oxygen release and contributes to fetal hypoxemia. (Reprinted from ref. 4, with permission.)

bin time (PT) or partial thromboplastin time (PTT) (5). Thus we can safely monitor only the platelet count during admission in most patients. In another study of preeclamptic patients without evidence of abruption or hemorrhage but with platelet counts less than 100,000/mm^3, there were no abnormal PT or PTT values, and no patient had a fibrinogen concentration less than 200 mg/dL (6). These additional tests can probably be reserved for patients with abruption, hemorrhage, fetal death, or severe liver dysfunction.

The D-dimer assay uses monoclonal anti-D dimer antibody to detect degradation products of stable (cross-linked) fibrin rather than fibrinogen. The test specifically detects in vivo clot dissolution. Presence of D-dimer in preeclamptic women correlates consistently with increased fibrin-degradation products and platelet counts less than 100,000/mm^3 (7). This test may help to define a subset of patients with severe disease. When compared with preeclamptic women who were negative for the D-dimer, positive women had higher blood pressures, greater proteinuria, higher serum creatinine, and more abnormal liver-function tests. They also had a higher incidence of cesarean section and premature delivery. Their infants often had low birth weights and Apgar scores (7).

Thrombocytopenia is the most common coagulopathy in preeclampsia; it occurs in about 20% of cases (8). Two studies documented platelet abnormalities in patients with preeclampsia despite platelet counts greater than 100,000/mm^3. Kelton et al. (9) reported that 25% of preeclamptic patients with a platelet count greater than 150,000/mm^3 had a bleeding time longer than 10 minutes. Likewise, Ramanathan et al. (10) found that 34% of patients with severe preeclampsia and 13% of those with mild preeclampsia had prolonged bleeding times despite platelet counts more than 100,000/mm^3. Of note, 2% of normotensive parturients, with normal platelet counts, also had abnormal bleeding times. Overall, patients with preeclampsia had lower platelet counts and longer bleeding times than did healthy controls. These two studies caused tremendous controversy among obstetric anesthesiologists.

Despite the concerns about abnormal platelet function, there are no definitive reports of epidural hematoma in preeclamptic patients after epidural anesthesia (11). Indeed, several anesthesiologists reported performing epidural anesthesia in parturients with unrecognized thrombocytopenia without complications (12–14). Given the 6% to 8% incidence of thrombocytopenia in normal parturients (15), many patients have probably received regional anesthesia while thrombocytopenic without incident.

Clinical Evaluation

Routine use of bleeding time to make clinical judgements is, at best, inconvenient. Laboratory personnel are rarely available to perform the test during evenings and nights. Although anesthesiologists can be trained to perform accurate and reproducible bleeding times (16), the test may provide little useful information. A recent extensive review of the literature on the bleeding time concluded that no existing data support its use to predict adequacy of hemostasis, nor do any data show that bleeding from the skin can predict bleeding elsewhere in the body. In addition, there is no evidence the bleeding time will prolong sufficiently in advance of serious bleeding to allow intervention or a change in management (17). Many institutions no longer offer or use the bleeding-time test.

Aspirin

Recently two large multicenter trials evaluated the use of low-dose aspirin in pregnancy to prevent and treat preeclampsia (18,19). Neither supported routine use of aspirin for prevention of preeclampsia, but both found some benefit for women at increased risk of the disease or for those who have early increases of systolic blood pressure. Aspirin inhibits thromboxane synthesis and corrects the imbalance of thromboxane and prostacyclin production seen in preeclampsia.

Because aspirin impairs platelet function, anesthesiologists have been concerned about the use of regional anesthesia in these patients. Benigni et al. (20) reported that the ingestion of 60 mg of aspirin per day from 12 weeks' gestation until term did not abnormally prolong bleeding times performed at 28 weeks (20). Williams et al. (21) also found no difference in bleeding times between parturients on low-dose aspirin and controls. In the absence of other indications of coagulopathy, bleeding times are not necessary in women taking low-dose aspirin.

Guidelines

What then should we use as criteria for performing regional anesthesia in these patients? A recent survey found some differences in practice among academic and private anesthesiologists (22). The standard of practice seems reasonably consistent, although private practitioners often require more laboratory tests. When questioned about coagulation and preeclampsia, most practitioners in both groups:

- Would place an epidural anesthetic in a parturient taking one aspirin a day,
- Would require only a platelet count in mild preeclampsia, but
- Also require a PT and PTT in severe preeclampsia.

More private practitioners would require a fibrinogen level in severe preeclampsia and a bleeding time if the woman had a low platelet count.

The thromboelastogram (TEG) has not found widespread use in obstetric anesthesia. Orlikowski et al. (23) correlated platelet count, bleeding time, and TEG in preeclamptic and eclamptic patients (Table 1). All women with platelet counts greater than 100,000/mm^3 but an abnormal bleeding time had a normal TEG, suggesting that they had adequate coagulation. A maximal amplitude of 53 mm, the lower limit of normal for pregnancy, correlated with a platelet count of 54,000/mm^3, and they concluded that a platelet count of 75,000/mm^3 should provide adequate hemostasis.

I require a screening platelet count on all women with the diagnosis of preeclampsia. If the initial value is greater than 150,000/mm^3, no further workup is required. If less than 150,000/mm^3, I repeat the value to rule out a rapid downward trend, which would indicate a worsening of the disease process. A level of 100,000/mm^3 is an arbitrary cut-off and has no supporting outcome data. The actual safe lower limit for platelet count before epidural placement is unknown. If regional anesthesia, in preference to parenteral medications or general anesthesia, offers an overwhelming therapeutic advantage to the parturient (e.g., suspected inability to intubate, prolonged induction of labor), I proceed after evaluating the patient for any clinical signs of bleeding. Modifications of technique that may decrease the risk of bleeding include midline placement, use of the smallest possible needle and catheter, and administration of saline or local anesthetic through the needle before inserting the epidural catheter. Use of spinal analgesia for labor also might be considered. Motor block should be minimized to allow hourly neurological examination. Ultimately, the decision rests on the facts of the case at hand and the anesthesiologist's clinical judgement.

What about the patient who develops thrombocytopenia or other coagulopathy with an epidural catheter in place? The literature offers no definite guidelines for the management of this situation. It seems prudent to allow the platelet count to normalize before removing the catheter; however, the longer a catheter is left in place, the greater the chance that the catheter will damage or migrate into a blood vessel. In patients with HELLP syndrome, the nadir of the platelet count often occurs 1 to 3 days after delivery. Recovery to a concentration greater than 100,000/mm^3 may require 5 to 6 days (24). Few practitioners would transfuse patients to correct thrombocytopenia for catheter removal, but it also is difficult to justify leaving a catheter in place for 3 to 6 days. If the catheter is removed while the patient is thrombocytopenic, frequent neurological examinations must be performed to detect potential spinal cord compression from an epidural hematoma.

Renal Function

Intravascular volume depletion and renal artery vasospasm can decrease creatinine clearance and cause oliguria. Maternal urine output is probably the best way to assess volume status in the absence of invasive hemodynamic monitoring. When creatinine values exceed 1.0 mg/dL in the parturient, significant renal dysfunction is present, and the excretion of drugs like magnesium sulfate will be compromised. To prevent toxicity, reduce the dose of magnesium if creatinine is increased. Check deep tendon reflexes and serum magnesium concentrations frequently.

Liver Function

Laboratory examination may reveal increased liver enzymes due to vasospasm and ischemia. Patients with

TABLE 1. *Abnormalities in bleeding time (BT) and thrombolelastogram in parturients with preeclampsia or eclampsia*

	No. patients	MA <53 mm[a]	BT >9.5 min
Platelets <50,000/mm^3	2	2	1
Platelets 50–100,000/mm^3	5	1	2
Platelets 100–150,000/mm^3	11	0	5

[a]Maximal amplitude (53 mm is lower limit of normal during pregnancy).
From ref. 23, with permission.

preeclampsia may complain of right upper quadrant or epigastric pain due to stretching of the liver capsule. Subcapsular hemorrhage, hematoma, or liver rupture can occur. This catastrophic event, characterized by acute maternal and fetal deterioration, requires immediate cesarean section and exploratory laparotomy (25). Maternal mortality approaches 75%. When associated with HELLP syndrome, coagulopathy and hemolysis increase maternal morbidity. Assure large-bore intravenous access and blood, fresh-frozen plasma, and platelet availability if hepatic involvement is suspected.

Nervous System

Complete a neurological examination before any anesthetic intervention. Deficits due to cerebral edema, cerebral hemorrhage, or a postictal state already may exist. Headaches, visual disturbances, including cortical blindness, and seizures characterize CNS involvement. Although the etiology of eclampsia is unknown, histopathologic examination of the brain reveals numerous hemorrhages, capillary thrombi, and small infarcts. Eclamptic patients have lower arterial blood pressure, systemic vascular resistance (SVR), and colloid osmotic pressure than do parturients with severe preeclampsia who do not seize (26,27). Computed tomography (CT) in the eclamptic patient with recurrent seizures may reveal structural lesions. Changes seen resemble those found in hypertensive encephalopathy in nonpregnant patients: cerebral edema, cerebral vein thrombosis, and low-density white matter (28). The indications for CT or magnetic resonance imaging (MRI) in the eclamptic patient are controversial. Patients who have focal signs, decreasing level of consciousness, or recurrent seizures despite therapeutic concentrations of magnesium or phenytoin need further evaluation.

Evaluation of the Fetus

In addition to fetal heart-rate monitoring, other parameters of fetal well-being help predict the eventual mode of delivery. Intrauterine growth retardation, oligohydramnios, extreme prematurity, and uteroplacental insufficiency can contribute to fetal intolerance of labor. Fetal evaluation includes documentation of fetal presentation, estimated weight, biophysical profile, and possibly an oxytocin contraction test. Hypertensive parturients are much more likely than normotensive women to develop ominous fetal heart-rate patterns during labor (20.5% vs 7.6%) (29). Therefore early and continuous fetal monitoring is a necessity.

Other preparation should include large-bore intravenous access for rapid infusion of fluid or blood products. I recommend early aspiration prophylaxis with some combination of a histamine-2 receptor-blocking agent, metoclopramide, and a nonparticulate antacid. Early administration may assure a therapeutic effect should seizures or operative delivery occur.

MONITORING

Basic intrapartum monitoring of a parturient with preeclampsia should include:

- Automated noninvasive blood pressure,
- Accurate intake and output measurements (usually requiring a urinary bladder catheter),
- Hourly examination of deep tendon reflexes,
- Fetal scalp electrode as soon as the cervix is adequately dilated, and
- An intrauterine pressure catheter to monitor strength and frequency of contractions and timing of any decelerations.

I do not continuously monitor maternal electrocardiogram (ECG) unless I also am monitoring cardiac filling pressures; however, continuous ECG monitoring of 21 patients with hypertensive crises during pregnancy found that 13 had episodes of ventricular tachycardia within 24 hours (30). These women were screened to assure normal serum potassium but had central venous catheters in place. The authors suggested that dysrhythmia might play a role in the pathogenesis of pulmonary edema and sudden death in these patients.

Invasive Hemodynamic Monitoring

General Considerations

When and how to use invasive hemodynamic monitoring in the parturient with preeclampsia is controversial. Most obstetric patients are young and healthy. Many hospitals hesitate to provide labor and delivery units with the expertise and equipment needed to care for critically ill parturients. Nursing issues are a primary concern. Without nurses trained in critical care and comfortable with invasive monitoring, attempts to treat these patients aggressively in the labor unit will not succeed and could be dangerous. Likewise, placing a laboring patient with a fetal monitor in a medical or surgical intensive care unit (ICU) does not allow optimal monitoring of the fetus and disrupts the unit's normal routine. Ideally, the labor and delivery unit should have an ICU bed staffed by nurses comfortable with invasive monitoring and knowledgeable about critical care issues. As an alternative, the patient could be co-nursed by both an ICU and labor and delivery nurse. The anesthesiologist becomes an important and necessary source of information and support for the nursing service in this situation.

Arterial Catheter

Possible indications for intraarterial blood pressure monitoring include:

- Sustained diastolic blood pressure greater than 90 mm Hg,

- Use of parenteral vasodilators such as nitroprusside or nitroglycerin,
- Induction of regional or general anesthesia with the potential for rapid blood pressure changes,
- Inability to obtain accurate blood pressure measurements by cuff in a morbidly obese patient,
- The need for repeated sampling for arterial blood gas tensions or other laboratory studies (especially if venipuncture is difficult because of edema, obesity, or intravenous drug abuse), and
- The patient with a coagulopathy (avoids repeated venipuncture).

Pulmonary Artery Catheter

Patients with severe preeclampsia may have profound hemodynamic derangements and benefit from a pulmonary artery (PA) catheter. However, there are no controlled clinical-outcome studies of this issue (31,32). Presently accepted indications for use of a PA catheter in the parturient with severe preeclampsia include:

- Severe hypertension unresponsive to conventional antihypertensive therapy,
- Pulmonary edema, and
- Persistent oliguria unresponsive to fluid challenge (33).

Pulmonary artery catheters can be used safely in a labor and delivery suite and may offer useful clinical information (34). Advantages of this approach include:

- Consolidation of care when the pathophysiology is unique to pregnancy (such as severe preeclampsia),
- Fetal monitoring, and
- The ability to provide immediate medical and surgical management.

However, the "establishment of such a service requires an ICU with properly trained nurses, appropriate equipment, and physicians with the necessary clinical skill to place and troubleshoot central lines" (34). It would also require a large number of deliveries to maintain nursing and physician skills in this area.

Central Venous Pressure or Pulmonary Artery Catheter?

The choice of a central venous pressure (CVP) catheter versus a PA catheter has been controversial (35). The CVP alone may provide misleading information. Several studies showed that CVP cannot reliably predict pulmonary artery occlusion pressure (PAOP). Cotton et al. (36) compared 208 CVP and PAOP measurements in 18 patients with severe preeclampsia. They found no linear relation between the CVP and PAOP in 39% of their patients. In the 56% of women in whom the two measurements correlated, the gradient between PAOP and CVP varied too widely to have any predictive value. The relation between CVP and PAOP becomes discordant when SVR increases and acutely increases left ventricular afterload. The CVP may be the more accurate index of true intravascular volume, especially when the value is low. The PAOP reflects the risk of pulmonary edema and the amount of left ventricular dysfunction. Although CVP is rarely low in the presence of an increased PAOP, higher CVP values are difficult to interpret.

The PA catheter provides far more information than volume status. The CVP gives no indication of cardiac output, and unfortunately there is no good noninvasive substitute for the thermodilution technique. Impedance cardiography is inaccurate in pregnancy when compared with thermodilution ($r = 0.17$) (37), although software updates may have improved the correlation (38). Although the Doppler technique correlates well with thermodilution ($r = 0.91$) (39), it provides little assessment of filling pressures.

Colloid osmotic pressure (COP) is lower in patients with preeclampsia than in normal parturients, perhaps due to proteinuria. One of the mechanisms thought responsible for pulmonary edema in severe preeclampsia is an imbalance of Starling forces across the pulmonary capillary membrane. A PAOP/COP gradient of less than 4 mm Hg may allow excessive fluid flux out of the pulmonary vasculature (26,40). The COP reaches its nadir postpartum, whereas filling pressures often increase before the onset of postpartum diuresis. Cotton et al. (26) noted that the two women they saw with pulmonary edema also were the only two with a negative COP-to-PAOP gradient (26). If COP measurements are used, they can be combined with PAOP measurements to guide fluid therapy and use of diuretics. Again, this information is not available with only a CVP catheter.

Finally, there is the issue of risk. Most of the risks of central monitoring (i.e., carotid or subclavian artery puncture, pneumothorax, dysrhythmias, hematoma, or infection) are related to obtaining central venous access and are common to both CVP and PA catheter placement. The additional risks of placing the PA catheter, such as pulmonary infarction and rupture of the PA, are very rare in this patient population. Because the risks of access are similar, the more comprehensive information obtained from the PA catheter provides a favorable risk/benefit ratio. If we are concerned about central venous access in a patient with abnormal coagulation studies, we can insert the CVP catheter or PA catheter sheath through the antecubital basilic vein or external jugular vein. If needed, we can easily apply pressure to bleeding at these sites. Also consider central access via an antecubital vein in the uncooperative (postictal or actively laboring) patient, as well as the obese or edematous patient with obscured landmarks.

Hemodynamic Profile

There is now more than a decade's worth of literature on hemodynamic findings in severe preeclampsia. Early

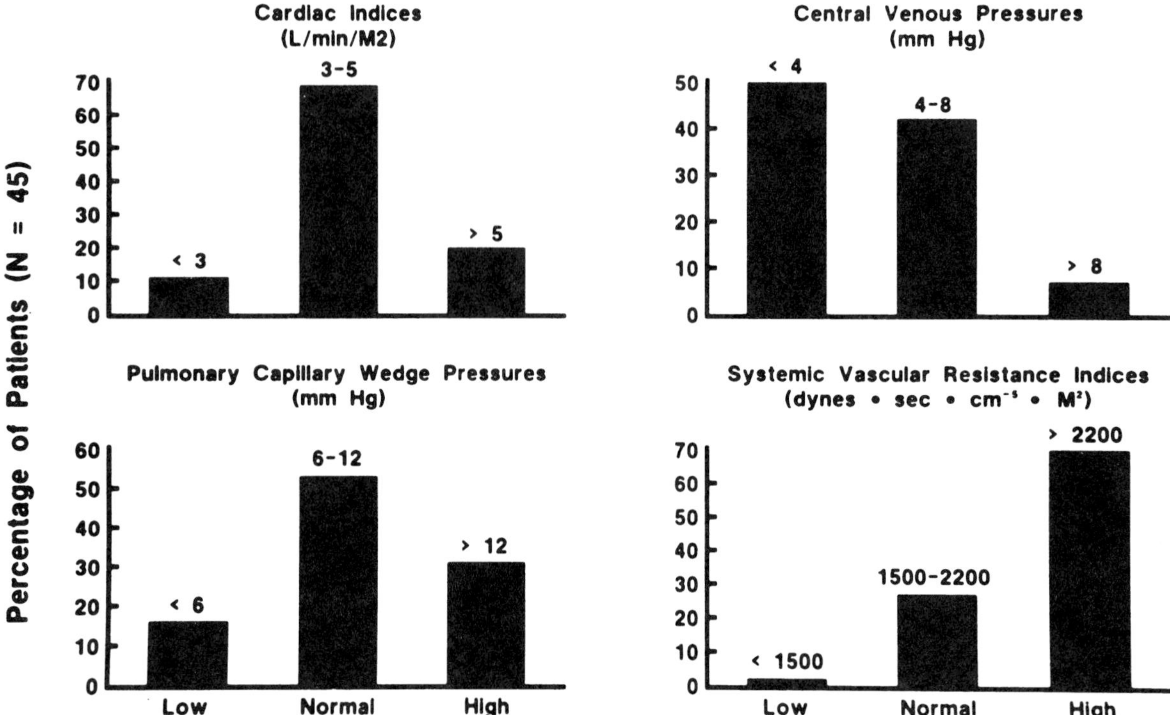

FIG. 2. Hemodynamic subsets associated with severe pregnancy-induced hypertension. These women have a wide range of initial findings. (Reprinted from ref. 26, with permission.)

studies revealed a hyperdynamic state with increased cardiac output and low-to-normal filling pressures in the face of high SVR (41–43). Others, however, found a depressed cardiac index with low filling pressures and high vascular resistance (44). In a group of 45 women with severe preeclampsia or eclampsia, Cotton et al. (26) found a wide range of hemodynamic patterns that could not be easily classified (Fig. 2). When investigating persistent oliguria in severe preeclampsia, Clark et al. (45) described three distinct hemodynamic subsets requiring markedly different therapies. Yang et al. (46) used Doppler velocimetry to group parturients with severe preeclampsia by SVR (Table 2). They found marked differences in maternal cardiac index, left ventricular stroke-work index, mode of delivery, and newborn size and pH between the groups. Thus no single hemodynamic profile describes all parturients with preeclampsia.

Easterling et al. (47) monitored 120 women throughout their pregnancies and measured cardiac output by using a Doppler technique (Fig. 3). Women destined to develop preeclampsia had significantly higher cardiac outputs and lower SVR from early gestation compared with parturients who remained normotensive. These differences persisted after delivery. The authors suggested that vasodilation of terminal arterioles increases the risk of end-organ damage by exposing capillary beds, especially the renal glomeruli, to systemic pressures (48). The resultant endothelial damage incites platelet adherence, vasospasm, and the clinically overt disease we see in patients with severe preeclampsia. Thus women with preeclampsia present a

TABLE 2. *Maternal and neonatal parameters based on maternal systemic vascular resistance before treatment in severe preeclampsia*

	Vascular Resistance (dyne/s/cm^2)		
Parameter	Low <800	Normal 800–1,500	High >1,500
CI (L/min/m^2)	6.0	5.0	2.0
LVSWI (g/m/m^2)	83.3	50.5	20.5
Birth weight (g)	3,591	2,645	1,740
Incidence of emergency delivery (%)	0	50	66.7
Incidence of newborn pH <7.2 (%)	0	33.3	50

CI, cardiac index; LVSWI, left ventricular stroke work index.
From ref. 46, with permission.

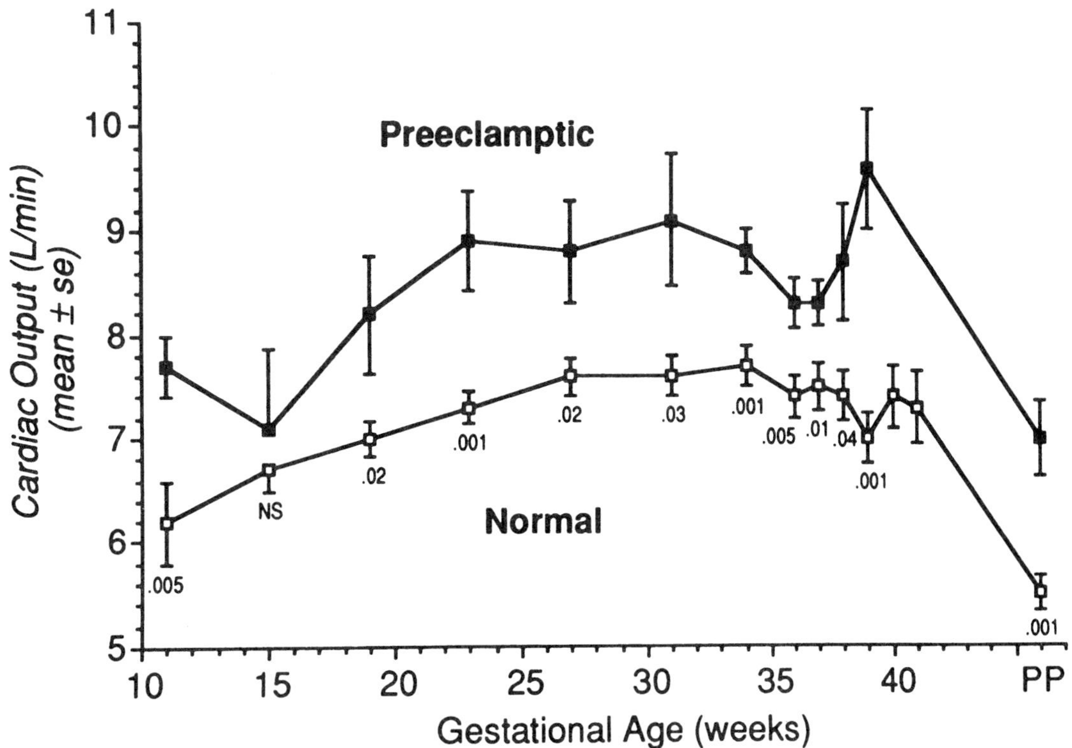

FIG. 3. Mean ± standard error of cardiac output in normotensive (normal) and preeclamptic patients throughout pregnancy. NS, not significant; PP, postpartum. (Reprinted from ref. 47, with permission.)

spectrum of hemodynamic patterns reflecting the variable extent of endothelial and end-organ damage.

Wheeler et al. (49) found that a base deficit exceeding −8.0 mEq/L in the mother consistently predicted fetal acidosis, fetal death, and maternal end-organ ischemic injury. They viewed severe preeclampsia as another form of distributive shock resulting in multisystem organ failure.

PERIOPERATIVE MANAGEMENT OF SPECIAL PROBLEMS

Eclampsia

Convulsions occur in the antepartum or intrapartum periods in 63% of cases of eclampsia (50). The obstetric anesthesiologist may have to evaluate or manage the seizing or postictal parturient. Manage the eclamptic woman initially with airway support, oxygen by mask, left uterine displacement, and cricoid pressure. Do not force an oral airway or tongue blade into her mouth; this action may cause vomiting or break teeth. A simple jaw lift should suffice. Intubate if the seizure is prolonged, if regurgitation occurs, or if ventilation cannot be maintained. If necessary, treat the seizure with thiopental, 75 mg, instead of a long-acting sedative such as diazepam. Thiopental will rapidly end the seizure, yet allow faster awakening for neurological assessment. Magnesium is the treatment of choice for prevention of seizures in preeclampsia, but a nontherapeutic serum concentration may permit recurrent seizures. Infuse magnesium sulfate as a bolus dose of 4 to 6 grams over a 20-minute period, and repeat once if seizures recur. Focal seizures, or seizures in the presence of a therapeutic magnesium concentration, should raise the suspicion of a structural lesion or intracerebral hemorrhage. In that situation, give an additional parenteral anticonvulsant such as phenytoin. Consider further neurological workup such as CT or MRI scans.

In a large series of eclamptic patients, magnesium sulfate successfully prevented recurrent seizures (51). It remains the anticonvulsant of choice for preeclampsia in North America (Table 3) (52). Its mechanism of action is

TABLE 3. *Reported effects of magnesium sulfate in preeclampsia*

Beneficial
Vasodilation in vascular beds
Increased uterine blood flow
Increased prostacyclin release by endothelial cells
Decreased plasma renin activity
Decreased angiotension-converting enzyme levels
Attenuation of vascular response to pressor substances
Bronchodilation
Reduced platelet aggregation
Detrimental
Decreased uterine activity and prolonged labor
Decreased fetal heart-rate variability
Excessive blood loss after vaginal delivery
Neonatal neuromuscular and respiratory depression
Low Apgar scores

unclear; however, magnesium enhances production of prostacyclin by vascular endothelium, thereby promoting vasodilation and inhibiting platelet aggregation. This effect on the cerebral vasculature may account for its antiseizure effects (53). Doppler ultrasonography of the middle cerebral artery in preeclamptic patients receiving magnesium suggests that magnesium dilates the smaller-diameter intracranial vessels, thereby relieving cerebral ischemia (54). A randomized trial comparing magnesium sulfate with phenytoin for prevention of eclamptic seizures found a significant reduction in the incidence of seizures in the magnesium group and concluded that magnesium sulfate is superior for the prevention of eclampsia in hypertensive pregnant women (55). Unfortunately, when compared with phenytoin, magnesium, because of its tocolytic effects, also slows cervical dilation and increases blood loss at delivery (56).

Eclampsia is rarely an indication for immediate delivery. Give precedence to stabilization, monitoring, and neurological evaluation of the mother to avoid unnecessary maternal obstetric and anesthetic risks. Once seizure activity stops, continue to give the mother supplemental oxygen. Fetal decelerations occur commonly during a seizure because of maternal hypoxia and acidosis. Unless placental abruption has occurred, fetal acidosis will improve more quickly in utero than if delivery occurs during or immediately after the seizure. Induction of labor should be attempted if the cervix is favorable. Begin aspiration prophylaxis early in labor because seizures may recur, and these women are more likely to need urgent or emergency cesarean section.

Oliguria

Oliguria is a common complication of severe preeclampsia. Although postpartum renal failure rarely occurs, most physicians become anxious when urine output decreases below 0.5 ml/kg/hr for several hours. Because magnesium sulfate is cleared only by glomerular filtration, oliguria also can increase the risk of magnesium toxicity. Begin treating oliguria with a fluid challenge of 500 mL of crystalloid over a 20-minute period. If urine output remains unchanged or declines, I recommend central venous or pulmonary artery catheterization before further fluid therapy. Clark et al. (45) found three distinctly different hemodynamic profiles in parturients with persistent oliguria (Table 4). Most commonly, patients had low filling pressures, hyperdynamic ventricular function, and moderate increase of vascular resistance, reflecting intravascular volume depletion. These women responded to further volume infusion with an increase in PAOP, a decrease in SVR, and no change in blood pressure. Patients in the second group also had hyperdynamic ventricular function, but with higher filling pressures (9 to 18 mm Hg) and normal SVR. In these women, the authors suspected renal artery vasospasm as the cause of oliguria. Women with preeclampsia may have selective vasospasm. Selective renal artery vasospasm would decrease renal blood flow in the presence of normal filling pressures and cardiac output. In this group of patients, urine production increased after vasodilator therapy with hydralazine and cautious fluid administration. A single patient had depressed left ventricular function, increased PAOP, and marked increase of SVR. She responded to afterload reduction to relieve vasospasm and improve cardiac output. Again, this report underscored the importance of evaluating the patient's hemodynamic status to avoid overly aggressive and inappropriate use of fluid or diuretic therapy.

Kirshon et al. (57) used another approach to renal artery vasospasm (Table 3). They gave low-dose dopamine (1 to 5 μg/kg/min) to patients who were oliguric with PAOP greater than 8 mm Hg. Dopamine selectively dilates splanchnic vessels and increases renal blood flow,

TABLE 4. *Hemodynamic subsets associated with oliguria in preeclampsia and their therapy*

	Group I (Clark)	Group II (Clark)	Group III (Clark)	Kirshon
Before therapy				
MAP	111	125	140	114
CVP	2	8	3	6
PCWP	4	12	18	12
CI	3.9	5.4	2.6	4.0 (estimated)
SVR	1,330	1,019	2,790	1,371
	Volume	Vasodilator and volume	Vasodilator and fluid restriction	Dopamine (1–5 μg/kg/h)
After therapy				
MAP	115	107	104	116
CVP	7	9	—	8
PCWP	10	9	8	11
CI	4.5	5.4	4.0	4.7 (estimated)
SVR	1,150	879	1,867	1,157

From refs. 45 and 57.

sodium excretion, and glomerular filtration rate. Without changing blood pressure, PAOP, or CVP, dopamine significantly increased urine production and cardiac output. Fractional excretion of sodium and osmolar clearance also tended to increase. No nonreassuring fetal heart-rate patterns developed, implying that dopamine did not compromise placental perfusion.

Pulmonary Edema

Pulmonary edema is a significant cause of maternal and perinatal morbidity and mortality. In one large series, 70% of cases occurred in the postpartum period (58). Most patients had a medical, surgical, or obstetric complication that required large-volume crystalloid or colloid infusions. These complications included sepsis, abruption, disseminated intravascular coagulation, aspiration, and ruptured liver. The incidence of pulmonary edema also was higher in older multigravidae and in those with chronic hypertension. Volume infusion for regional anesthesia did not contribute to pulmonary edema in any case. These authors emphasized the need to monitor severely preeclamptic patients for 72 hours after delivery.

Pulmonary edema normally occurs at a PAOP of 20 to 25 mm Hg, but if the patient also has a low COP, clinical symptoms may manifest earlier. Preeclampsia reduces COP, but antepartum correction of COP with albumin leads to much higher filling pressures after delivery. These women then often need diuretic therapy (59).

Pulmonary artery catheterization helps to determine the cause of pulmonary edema and to guide therapy. In addition to oxygen and diuresis, nitroglycerin can reduce preload and correct the hemodynamic derangements associated with pulmonary edema (60). However, nitroglycerin inhibits hypoxic pulmonary vasoconstriction, and in preeclampsia, hypoxemia does not improve (60).

ANTIHYPERTENSIVE THERAPY

The purpose of antihypertensive therapy is to prevent cerebral hemorrhage, pulmonary edema, and other complications of acute hypertension in the mother, while preserving or improving uteroplacental circulation. To this end, strive to reduce mean maternal blood pressure to 105 to 110 mm Hg, but by no more than 30%. The fetus with uteroplacental insufficiency is an exquisitely sensitive monitor of perfusion during reduction of maternal blood pressure. Fetal decelerations may limit the degree of blood pressure reduction. If hemodynamic monitoring is available, use these values to guide your choice of antihypertensive therapy. For example, the parturient with hyperdynamic left ventricular function and normal SVR may respond well to a negative inotrope (i.e., labetalol), whereas a vasodilating agent would best correct an increased vascular resistance in the presence of high filling pressures.

Although each has its pros and cons, a number of antihypertensive drugs can be used in obstetrics (61). The anesthesiologist should be aware of the safety and any potential harmful effects of the drugs chosen to control blood pressure (Table 5). These agents can be divided based on their mechanism of action:

- Direct-acting vasodilators,
- Ganglionic blocking drugs,
- Competitive β-receptor–blocking agents,
- Sympatholytic agents,
- Calcium channel blocking drugs, and
- Angiotensin-converting enzyme inhibitors.

Magnesium sulfate is not an antihypertensive agent, although it attenuates the hyperreactive vascular responses in preeclampsia and has other beneficial effects (Table 3). Magnesium bolus and infusion produce a rapid, sustained decrease in SVR and an increase in cardiac index in preeclamptic patients (62). Patients receiving magnesium for preterm labor do not show the same effects.

Direct-Acting Vasodilators

Hydralazine

Hydralazine remains a popular drug for use in PIH. It causes direct dilation of arteriolar smooth muscle while improving renal and uterine blood flow (63). Its onset is relatively slow (15 to 20 minutes); its effects last hours. Parturients given a bolus dose of 10 mg hydralazine while monitored with a PA catheter had a significant increase in heart rate and cardiac index and a decrease in SVR. The peak effect and duration varied considerably (64). In the presence of unrecognized hypovolemia, hydralazine can produce acute hypotension and fetal heart-rate changes. Its unpredictable onset and duration make dose titration difficult.

TABLE 5. *Reported adverse effects of antihypertensive therapy during pregnancy*

Drug	Adverse effect
Esmolol (Brevibloc)	Decreased in fetal arterial pO_2 Equivalent maternal and fetal β-blockade Prolonged fetal β-blockade ? decreased fetal tolerance to asphyxia
Clonidine (Catapres)	Fetal hypoxemia Increased uterine tone Decreased uterine blood flow
Nifedipine (Adalat, Procardia)	Tocolysis Additive myocardial depression with magnesium Additive neuromuscular blockade with magnesium ? fetal hypoxemia with nicardipine infusion
ACE inhibitors (Enalapril)	Neonatal hypotension Neonatal renal failure Teratogenicity

ACE, angiotensin-converting enzyme.

Nitroprusside

Nitroprusside causes arterial and venous dilation. Its fast onset, short duration, and rapid metabolism (plasma half-life of 12 seconds) make it titratable as an infusion. Patients are rarely resistant to its effect, and it preserves uterine blood flow (65). Like all vasodilators, it can cause severe hypotension when the patient is hypovolemic, and heart rate will increase in response to the decrease in SVR. Concern about its use in obstetrics arose when Naulty et al. (66) reported extensive placental transfer of nitroprusside in pregnant ewes. In addition, when ewes exhibited tachyphylaxis to the drug, fetuses died of cyanide toxicity. However, these sheep had two different responses to the drug. When infusion rates required to control blood pressure were low (less than 1 μg/kg/min), mothers and fetuses did well. When animals exhibited tachyphylaxis to nitroprusside and required a mean dose of 25 μg/kg/min to control blood pressure, all fetuses died. In both groups, uterine blood flow did not change. Cyanide caused all the toxicity seen. Keep in mind, however, that the maximum acceptable dose of nitroprusside is 8.0 μg/kg/min or 0.5 mg/kg/hr. If exceeding this amount to achieve adequate blood pressure control, use another hypotensive agent. Many obstetricians and obstetric anesthesiologists have used nitroprusside safely and effectively within these guidelines (67). Nitroprusside is a cerebral and pulmonary vasodilator. Potential increases in intracranial pressure (ICP) may be detrimental in a postictal patient if the neurological examination is equivocal, or a structural intracerebral lesion is suspected. Pulmonary vasodilation decreases hypoxic pulmonary vasoconstriction and could cause hypoxemia.

Nitroglycerin

Nitroglycerin has venous and arterial vasodilating properties. Its short duration makes it easily titratable. In animals, it partially restores uterine blood flow diminished by phenylephrine infusion (68). Its low molecular weight allows rapid placental transfer. In untreated preeclamptics, nitroglycerin reduces blood pressure, PAOP, and cardiac output. Volume expansion prevents the decrease in filling pressures and cardiac index. After volume expansion, however, patients can develop a marked resistance to nitroglycerin's hypotensive effects (69). Fetal heart-rate variability also diminishes, possibly as a result of loss of cerebral autoregulation and increased ICP in the fetus. The decrease in filling pressures may help correct the hemodynamic abnormalities associated with pulmonary edema. Increased ICP and decreased hypoxic pulmonary vasoconstriction are concerns.

Ganglionic Blocking Agents

Trimethaphan exerts its hypotensive effect by ganglionic blockade of sympathetic nerve impulses. It can be used as an infusion or in bolus doses without causing reflex tachycardia. However, tachyphylaxis can develop during prolonged infusion. Of the vasodilating agents, it has the largest molecular weight (597 Dalton), which should limit its placental transfer. Although it is not a direct cerebral vasodilator, ICP increases transiently during the induction stage of hypotension in animals (70). The risk seems greatest when blood pressure decreases rapidly (less than 1 minute) to a mean below 60 mm Hg or in patients who already have critically increased ICP (71). Pupillary dilation due to ganglionic blockade can be expected and should not cause concern. Trimethaphan inhibits plasma cholinesterase (72) and can prolong the duration of succinylcholine (73). However, that patient had received 1,700 mg of trimethaphan over a 2-hour period, suggesting that tachyphylaxis had developed. In the usual clinical doses, trimethaphan might double the normal duration of succinylcholine.

β-Receptor Blocking Agents

Labetalol

Labetalol has achieved great popularity in obstetrics. It has nonselective β- and α_1-blocking properties in a ratio of about 7:1 when given intravenously. It decreases SVR and blood pressure without changing heart rate or cardiac index (74). Despite this decrease in maternal blood pressure, uteroplacental flow does not change, suggesting that labetalol reduces placental vascular resistance (75,76). In pregnant ewes, labetalol can completely reverse norepinephrine-induced hypertension. At the same time, uterine blood flow, markedly diminished by the norepinephrine, returns toward normal (77). Labetalol does not produce significant adrenergic blockade in the fetus or newborn (78), an important finding because cardiac output in the newborn is rate dependent. Peak effect after parenteral use occurs within 10 minutes, but the dose–response is variable. A study comparing labetalol and hydralazine for control of hypertension in PIH found that labetalol acted more rapidly but failed to reduce blood pressure in 10% of patients. The dose of intravenous labetalol required varied considerably from patient to patient, ranging from 20 to 300 mg (79). Those women requiring the largest doses also had the shortest duration of effect. In an urgent situation, the unpredictability in dose could be a problem.

Esmolol

Esmolol is an ultra–short-acting β_1 selective blocking agent with an elimination half-life of 9 minutes. Metabolism occurs by hydrolysis by red blood cell esterases. Initial animal studies showed rapid maternal and fetal elimination, with minimal placental transfer or effect on fetal hemodynamics [maximal decreases in fetal mean arterial pressure (MAP) and heart rate were 7% and 12%] (80). However, further animal studies found adverse fetal effects. Fetal arterial pO_2 decreased significantly, and isoproterenol challenge testing revealed fetal β-blockade that persisted for 30 minutes after completion of the esmolol infusion (81). In contrast to labetalol, which produced minimal fetal adrenergic blockade, esmolol produced equivalent degrees of β-blockade in the fetus and ewe. Other animal work showed that maternal β_1-blockade with metoprolol reduced fetal tolerance to asphyxia. In addition, fetal neural function, as assessed by somatosensory evoked potentials, recovered more slowly than in the control group (82). These studies suggest that the fetus requires intact adrenergic function to respond to stress.

There are no human studies of esmolol in pregnancy. When given to a parturient at 22 weeks' gestation undergoing resection of a cerebral arteriovenous malformation, esmolol infusion (50 μg/kg/min) had no significant effect on fetal heart rate (83). However, in a similar situation at 30 weeks' gestation, esmolol (100 μg) was associated with a decrease of 30 beats per minute in fetal heart rate (84). Both women later delivered healthy babies. In contrast, its use at 38 weeks' gestation to correct maternal supraventricular tachycardia resulted in severe fetal distress necessitating emergency cesarean section (85). It is unclear whether a decrease in maternal cardiac output or fetal β-blockade was the precipitating factor.

Sympatholytic Agents

Sympatholytic drugs gradually reduce blood pressure without reflex tachycardia. α-Methyldopa is a centrally acting α_2-receptor agonist with a long history of safe use in obstetrics. It provides a peripheral sympathectomy and has both parenteral and oral forms. Its main drawbacks are its long latency (6 hours) and only moderate efficacy. Additionally, it is contraindicated in patients with liver dysfunction, not uncommon in severe PIH.

Clonidine acts by the same mechanism as α-methyldopa, but it is not available in a parenteral form. Although it seems to be safe in long-term use in parturients with chronic hypertension (86), intravenous use in animals caused fetal hypoxemia, increased uterine tone, and decreased uterine blood flow (87). The patch formulation has been used for long-term postpartum control of blood pressure, but hypertensive crises can be precipitated if patients develop rebound hypertension after removing the patch.

Calcium Channel Blocking Drugs

Calcium-antagonist drugs exert their hypotensive effects mostly by vasodilation. Verapamil is available in oral and intravenous forms, whereas nifedipine can be given orally or sublingually. Animal studies showed verapamil and nifedipine to be effective antihypertensive agents in pregnancy, although neither improved the decrease in uterine blood flow induced by norepinephrine (88). Unlike nifedipine, verapamil does not produce a maternal tachycardia. In severely preeclamptic parturients, verapamil infusion after volume expansion with colloid allowed effective control of maternal blood pressure. Cardiac index increased significantly, whereas SVR decreased (89). Doppler ultrasound studies found no change in impedance in the uterine or umbilical arteries and no change in uteroplacental blood flow (90). Oral nimodipine has been used for acute antepartum control of hypertension (91), and nicardipine has been used both orally and intravenously for long-term antepartum blood pressure control with good maternal and fetal outcomes (92). However, these agents produce significant uterine relaxation, not a desirable feature in the patient undergoing induction of labor. Oral nifedipine has been successfully used to treat acute hypertensive episodes during pregnancy and in the postpartum period (93). Nifedipine-treated patients also had significantly higher urine output in the postpartum period than did control patients. At present, it is unclear whether the antepartum use of these "tocolytic" drugs will slow the progress of labor or increase the risk of postpartum hemorrhage.

Another problem with calcium channel blocking drugs is the potential interaction with magnesium, another calcium antagonist. This combination could potentiate the neuromuscular effects of magnesium and increase the risk of cardiac or respiratory toxicity. In isolated, perfused hearts, the combination of magnesium sulfate and nifedipine produced additive myocardial depression and decreased heart rate, left ventricular contractility, and left ventricular systolic pressure (94). Progressive degrees of heart block and even asystole occurred with increasing doses of nifedipine. Acute respiratory insufficiency was reported when magnesium was given to patients receiving nifedipine for tocolysis or blood pressure control, indicating that neuromuscular blockade may be potentiated when these drugs are combined (95,96).

Angiotensin-Converting Enzyme Inhibitors

There are numerous case reports associating angiotensin-converting enzyme (ACE) inhibitors during pregnancy with neonatal hypotension, neonatal renal failure, and teratogenicity (97). Avoid these drugs in the parturient.

ANALGESIA FOR LABOR AND VAGINAL DELIVERY

After initial stabilization of the mother and fetus, the obstetrician must decide on the most appropriate mode of delivery. The anesthesiologist needs time for thorough preoperative preparation of these high-risk patients. Obstetricians must understand that these women deserve no less attention than a seriously ill patient having surgery in the main operating suite. Lack of sufficient time to prepare the patient is almost always the result of a failure in communication.

Epidural Analgesia

Advantages and Disadvantages

Pritchard et al. (51) reported excellent maternal outcome in a large series of eclamptic patients. Pritchard advocated magnesium sulfate by intramuscular injection, hydralazine to reduce diastolic blood pressure to less than 110 mm Hg, fluid restriction, and rapid delivery (usually by the vaginal route) after convulsions have stopped. He avoided regional anesthesia for fear of inducing precipitate maternal hypotension. Because the maternal and perinatal results are very good despite the serious nature of the disease, Pritchard's regimen is the standard with which others are compared. However, the strong bias against fluid administration and regional anesthesia led to conflicts between anesthesiologists and their obstetric colleagues.

Most centers consider epidural blockade for labor and vaginal delivery or cesarean section the best anesthetic for parturients with preeclampsia (98). Besides providing better patient comfort than the alternatives, epidural analgesia offers numerous benefits to the woman with preeclampsia. The preeclamptic patient is more sensitive to catecholamines than is the healthy parturient. Catecholamines, secreted in response to pain and stress, can increase blood pressure and compromise uteroplacental blood flow. Epidural analgesia during labor reduces circulating catecholamine concentrations. Preeclamptic patients have higher baseline serum concentrations of epinephrine than do normal parturients. The serum concentration of epinephrine decreases significantly after induction of epidural anesthesia (Fig. 4) (99). The resultant improvement in uteroplacental blood flow might prove beneficial.

Other investigators showed that epidural blockade improves intervillous blood flow during labor in women with severe preeclampsia. Jouppila et al. (100,101) published the results of two studies on this issue. They gave epidural local anesthetics to laboring women with preeclampsia. All of their patients received 500 mL of crystalloid before blockade and were lying in a 15-degree left-lateral tilt position. Providing a narrow band of analgesia, between T_{10} and T_{12}, produced a small but statistically insignificant 34% increase in intervillous blood flow (100). Providing a wider band of sympathetic blockade, with 10 mL of 0.25% bupivacaine, significantly increased intervillous blood flow by 77% (101). No patient in either series became hypotensive.

Epidural analgesia also furnishes the obstetrician and anesthesiologist with considerable flexibility. Once in place, the epidural catheter can provide effective anesthesia for labor and vaginal delivery or cesarean section. Early placement can avoid inducing general anesthesia if an urgent cesarean section is required. If the need arises for extensive episiotomy repair or cesarean section, epidural opioids can provide excellent postoperative analgesia. Finally, sympathectomy can be maintained in the postpartum period if desired to buffer intravascular volume changes during fluid mobilization.

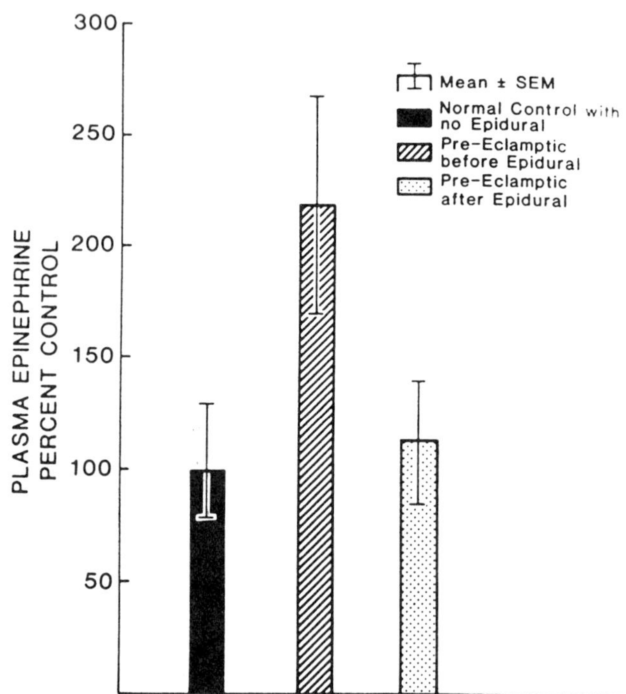

FIG. 4. Plasma concentration of epinephrine in normal and preeclamptic parturients. Epinephrine concentration decreases significantly after induction of epidural anesthesia in preeclamptic women. (Reprinted from ref. 49, with permission.)

Hemodynamic Effects

A retrospective study of 185 women with PIH who delivered vaginally found no harmful effects of epidural blockade. The incidence of maternal hypotension (6% vs 7%), abnormal fetal heart-rate tracings, low Apgar scores, and neonatal ICU admissions did not differ whether or not women received epidural anesthesia (102). These authors concluded that the technique of epidural anesthesia was safe and effective in this patient population. Epidural blockade provokes little hemodynamic change in women with severe preeclampsia. Neither PAOP, CVP, nor cardiac index changed after epidural local anesthetic injection in women hydrated to a PAOP of 8 to 12 mm Hg (103). Prudent use of fluids guided by clinical judgement and invasive monitoring when indicated will minimize risk of precipitous hypotension when using regional anesthesia in the preeclamptic patient. Obstetric or medical complications, not fluids given before epidural placement, predispose to pulmonary edema. In experienced hands, epidural anesthesia is a safe and beneficial technique for the preeclamptic patient that allows maximal flexibility for the obstetrician and anesthesiologist.

Magnesium and Epidural Anesthesia

In North America, essentially all patients with PIH receive magnesium sulfate. Because of its vasodilating properties, magnesium could increase the incidence or severity of hypotension after concomitant epidural anesthesia. In pregnant sheep, intravenous magnesium is associated with slightly lower blood pressure during epidural anesthesia compared with controls (18% below baseline vs 5% below baseline) (104). Maternal cardiac output, uterine blood flow, and fetal oxygenation did not change in either group. Additional animal work compared ephedrine and phenylephrine as vasopressors to correct hypotension after epidural anesthesia in the presence of a therapeutic magnesium concentration. Ephedrine restored both maternal blood pressure and uterine blood flow to baseline, whereas phenylephrine corrected maternal blood pressure but failed to improve uterine blood flow (105).

Some Technical Issues

Epinephrine

Controversy surrounds the use of epinephrine-containing local-anesthetic solutions in women with preeclampsia. Normal parturients have attenuated responses to endogenous and exogenous catecholamines. Isolated uterine arteries from pregnant animals are less sensitive to vasoconstrictive drugs than are vessels from nonpregnant animals (106). Norepinephrine infusion increases blood pressure in normal parturients not by vasoconstriction but by increasing cardiac output (107). Parturients also become resistant to the chronotropic effects of isoproterenol. Pregnancy reduces the response to this synthetic catecholamine by fivefold (108). Women who develop preeclampsia do not make these adaptations (Fig. 5) (109). Preeclamptic patients have an exaggerated hypertensive response to norepinephrine infusion. As in nonpregnant women, SVR increases, but cardiac output does not change. Accidental intravascular injection or excessive systemic absorption of epinephrine might cause an exaggerated heart-rate or blood-pressure response in a woman with preeclampsia.

Epidural epinephrine also may impair uteroplacental blood flow. Early studies reported no change in intervillous blood flow after epidural injection of 2-chloroprocaine with 50 μg of epinephrine. Because blood pressure decreased significantly, these authors postulated that the placental bed undergoes vasodilation when perfusion pressure decreases. They concluded that epinephrine had no deleterious effect on placental perfusion (110). Epinephrine-containing local anesthetics caused no apparent complications in four preeclamptic mothers during vaginal or cesarean delivery (111). These authors concluded that the use of epinephrine did not exacerbate preexisting hypertension.

More recent work contradicts these conclusions. With dynamic placental scintigraphy, one group of investigators found a 34% decrease in placental blood flow when patients underwent cesarean section with epidural anesthesia by using 0.5% bupivacaine with 2.5 μg/mL epinephrine (1:400,000) (112). These authors noted a negative correlation between changes in maternal blood pressure and placental flow. They speculated that maternal blood pressure was maintained at the expense of pla-

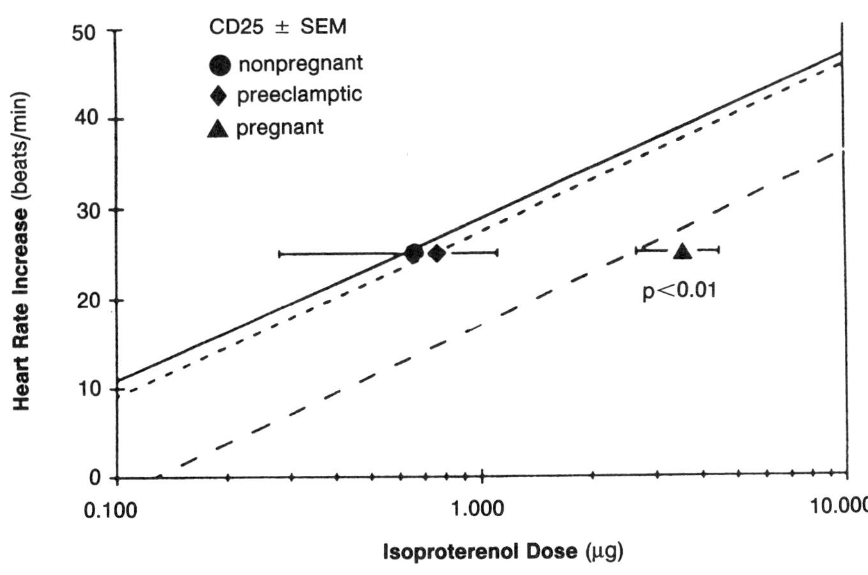

FIG. 5. The chronotropic response to isoproterenol in preeclamptic, healthy pregnant and nonpregnant women. The heart-rate response is significantly attenuated in healthy pregnant patients but not in preeclamptic women. (Reprinted from ref. 109, with permission.)

cental blood flow. Unfortunately, this study had no control group, and the women received a relatively small bolus of fluid (10 mL/kg) during induction. All infants had normal Apgar scores and umbilical artery pH values.

Doppler ultrasound can measure uterine artery resistance. In healthy primigravidae, umbilical arterial resistance decreased after induction of labor epidural analgesia using plain lidocaine. In contrast, patients receiving epidural lidocaine with epinephrine (40 μg) fell into two groups. Those with an initially normal umbilical arterial resistance also responded with a decline in uterine artery resistance. In contrast, those with a high initial resistance had a further increase; one third developed fetal heart-rate decelerations (113). Thus in a subgroup of normal parturients, the addition of epinephrine to epidural local anesthetic may have adverse consequences.

The risks of epinephrine might be even greater in preeclamptic patients with generalized arteriolar vasospasm. Alahuhta et al. (114) studied epidural anesthesia with and without epinephrine during cesarean section in hypertensive parturients. After local anesthetic with epinephrine, vascular resistance increased in the uteroplacental circulation, including the fetal renal and middle cerebral arteries. Hadzic et al. (115) reported a case of a hypertensive crisis in a preeclamptic parturient after successful placement of an epidural anesthetic containing 150 μg of epinephrine. She required treatment with sodium nitroprusside despite an adequate level of anesthesia for the procedure. Lower concentrations of epinephrine (1:400,000) still improve the quality of epidural lidocaine, but may have fewer hemodynamic consequences (116).

Although lower concentrations of epinephrine can be used, we cannot predict what amount of epinephrine is "safe" for a particular mother and fetus. Because of the increased responsiveness to vasopressors in women with preeclampsia, maternal and fetal sequelae could be disastrous should unintentional intravenous injection or systemic absorption of epinephrine occur. If you decide to include epinephrine in your local-anesthetic solution, use the lowest concentration possible, and use small incremental doses and meticulous technique to avoid intravascular injection.

Patient Preparation

Several points must be addressed before placing an epidural catheter in a patient with preeclampsia. First, check a recent coagulation profile, at least a platelet count. Look at sequential values to evaluate whether or not a downward trend exists. Do not routinely measure bleeding time. If the platelet count is 70,000 to 100,000/mm^3 but stable, and there are no clinical signs of coagulopathy, then proceed with epidural anesthesia. If ultrasound examination suggests abruption or fetal death, or if the patient has liver dysfunction associated with the HELLP syndrome, check the PT and PTTs and fibrinogen concentration.

Next, evaluate volume status. A hematocrit greater than 36% or a urine output less than 0.5 mL/kg/h suggests significant volume contraction. Patients who are not severely volume contracted need only 500 mL of crystalloid before induction of epidural block. In seriously ill patients requiring invasive hemodynamic monitoring, increase the CVP to a positive value or the PAOP to 5 to 10 mm Hg. Some would increase COP to at least 17 mm Hg by using albumin or other colloid; however, colloid infusion correlates with increased filling pressures after delivery. These women then require diuretics to prevent pulmonary edema. Whatever the preload, give the local anesthetic slowly. This precaution allows adequate time to respond if hypotension develops as the level of blockade rises.

Suggested Technique

A parturient with preeclampsia may receive epidural analgesia whenever the obstetrician has committed her to delivery and she feels discomfort. While continuously monitoring the fetus, give the mother oxygen by face mask, have her assume the lateral or sitting position, and insert the epidural catheter. Then position the patient comfortably while ensuring good uterine displacement and provide pain relief with incremental doses of 3 to 5 mL of 0.125% bupivacaine with or without 0.0002% fentanyl (2 μg/mL). The issue of an appropriate test dose for obstetric patients is controversial. I prefer to use incremental doses of local anesthetic to avoid problems due to unrecognized intravascular or subarachnoid injection. Monitor blood pressure by arterial catheter or at least every 2 minutes by automated cuff for 20 minutes after the initial dose. A continuous infusion of 0.1% bupivacaine with 2 μg/mL fentanyl at a rate of 10 mL/h helps to maintain pain relief. I avoid lidocaine for infusion because preeclampsia significantly prolongs its clearance (117). If mean arterial pressure decreases more than 30% from baseline or if nonreassuring fetal heart-rate patterns develop, use further left uterine displacement, a fluid bolus, and intravenous ephedrine, 2.5 to 5.0 mg. In severely ill patients, evaluate filling pressures and SVR repeatedly as the level of sympathetic blockade rises. Monitoring trends in these measurements will help to guide fluid and vasopressor therapy.

Intrathecal Opioids

Intrathecal opioids are becoming increasingly popular for labor pain relief. They may offer some advantages to women with preeclampsia. Opioids can be given by single injection, as a combined spinal–epidural technique followed by an epidural infusion, or via a subarachnoid catheter. Intrathecal injection of morphine (0.25 mg), fentanyl (25 μg), sufentanil (5 to 10 μg), or meperidine (10 to 20 mg) can provide analgesia for the first stage of labor

(118,119).* This technique may minimize sympathectomy and the need for volume loading (120). Supplemental analgesia will usually be required for the second stage of labor and certainly for instrumental delivery. Either a pudendal block, a low "saddle" block with local anesthetic, or a top-up dose through a previously placed epidural catheter can be effective. As with epidural anesthesia, consider coagulation status before placement.

Other Choices

Other anesthetic options must be considered for the parturient who cannot have or does not want regional anesthesia. Although traditionally obstetricians or labor and delivery personnel have administered narcotics and tranquilizers for labor analgesia, anesthesiologists have much to offer in their knowledge of the pharmacokinetics, efficacy, and side effects of the available drugs (121). Patient-controlled analgesia with fentanyl, nalbuphine, or meperidine can provide better labor analgesia than intermittent bolus injection by nursing personnel. Total drug required and side effects are less with patient-controlled analgesia; neonatal outcomes are similar. This technique will likely continue to gain popularity (122).

ANESTHESIA FOR CESAREAN DELIVERY

Always be prepared to provide an anesthetic for operative delivery. Both maternal and fetal complications increase the incidence of cesarean section in the parturient with preeclampsia. Because parturients may experience a rapid decrease in blood pressure during induction of spinal anesthesia, many experts recommended epidural rather than spinal anesthesia in these women. However, recent studies showed spinal anesthesia to be a safe and acceptable technique in preeclamptic patients (123,124). There is no reliable way to completely prevent hypotension, but spinal anesthesia may be a better alternative than general anesthesia in some women. A spinal catheter allows slower titration of dose, but the onset of sympathetic block will still be more rapid than that with epidural blockade.

Epidural Anesthesia

Advantages

Stress Response

Epidural anesthesia provides a number of advantages over general anesthesia. Epidural blockade markedly blunts the hormonal and hemodynamic responses to surgery. Extensive epidural blockade prevents adrenocortical and hyperglycemic responses to stress in women undergoing hysterectomy (125). In women undergoing elective cesarean section, epidural anesthesia correlates with lower maternal plasma cortisol, glucose, insulin, and adrenocorticotropic hormone (ACTH) concentrations. These women also have lower mean blood pressures and heart rates, and their infants have higher Apgar scores when compared with parturients having general anesthesia (126,127). Epinephrine and norepinephrine concentrations increase markedly in patients given a general anesthetic, whereas the amounts of these compounds decrease in patients given an epidural anesthetic. Severely preeclamptic patients undergoing cesarean section have similar responses. Although plasma concentrations of epinephrine, norepinephrine, ACTH, and β-endorphin increase with general anesthesia, they remain unchanged in preeclamptic parturients having an epidural anesthetic (128).

Hemodynamic Changes

Because the stress response is so well controlled in patients receiving epidural anesthesia, it is not surprising that their hemodynamic course also is smoother. Hodgkinson et al. (129) monitored the MAP, PA pressure (PAP), PAOP, and CVP in patients with severe preeclampsia undergoing cesarean delivery (Fig. 6). Those who had a general anesthetic experienced significant increases in MAP, PAP, and PAOP at intubation and extubation. The hemodynamic measurements in the group receiving epidural anesthesia remained unchanged.

Uteroplacental Blood Flow

The effects of epidural anesthesia for cesarean section on uteroplacental blood flow in women with preeclampsia are unclear. Two studies found inconsistent effects with both pronounced increases and decreases in placental blood flow. The overall effect in both studies was a small but insignificant decrease in flow (130,131). Apgar scores and umbilical cord blood gases were normal in all infants regardless of changes in uteroplacental perfusion. On the other hand, induction of general anesthesia with 4 mg/kg thiopental and succinylcholine consistently decreased intervillous blood flow by 35% (Fig. 7) (132).

Miscellaneous Advantages

In addition to blunting maternal stress responses during surgery and avoiding excessive hypertension during intubation and extubation, epidural anesthesia maintains maternal consciousness and decreases the risk of aspiration. When the patient is awake, neurological status can be monitored if there is concern about changing level of consciousness or recovery after an eclamptic seizure.

*Editor's note: I have abandoned both intrathecal morphine and intrathecal meperidine in my current clinical practice. Intrathecal morphine, 0.25 mg, combined with sufentanil, 10 μg, provides only an additional 20 minutes of analgesia but causes significant, prolonged itching and nausea. Whereas intrathecal meperidine, 10 to 20 mg, does afford both visceral and somatic analgesia, it induces vomiting in 30% of parturients. In its place, I use sufentanil and bupivacaine as a part of a combined spinal–epidural technique.

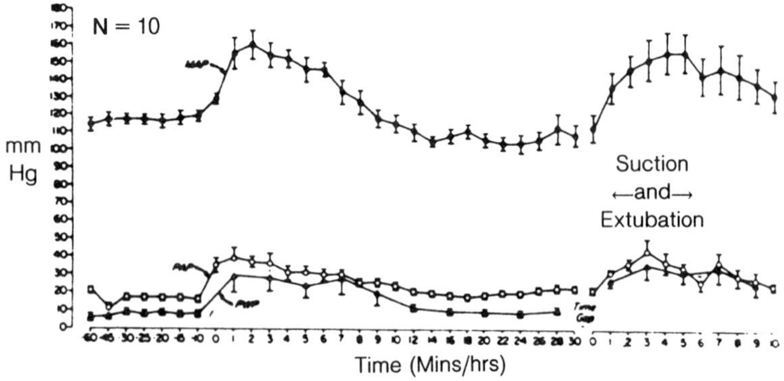

Mean and SE of MAP, PAP, and PwP of Pre-Eclamptic Patients Undergoing Caesarean Section Under Epidural Anesthesia

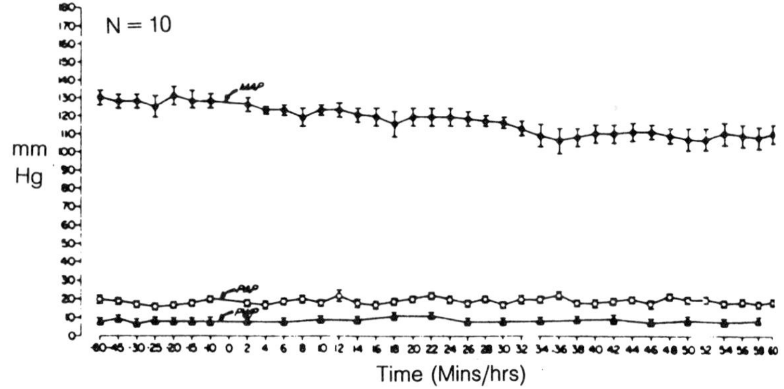

FIG. 6. A comparison of systemic and pulmonary pressures during cesarean section under general or epidural anesthesia in preeclamptic parturients. General anesthesia consisted of thiopental, 3 mg/kg; succinylcholine, 100 mg; nitrous oxide, 40%; halothane, 0.5%; and a succinylcholine, 0.2%, infusion. Epidural block was established by using 0.75% bupivacaine injected at time 0. (Reprinted from ref. 129, with permission.)

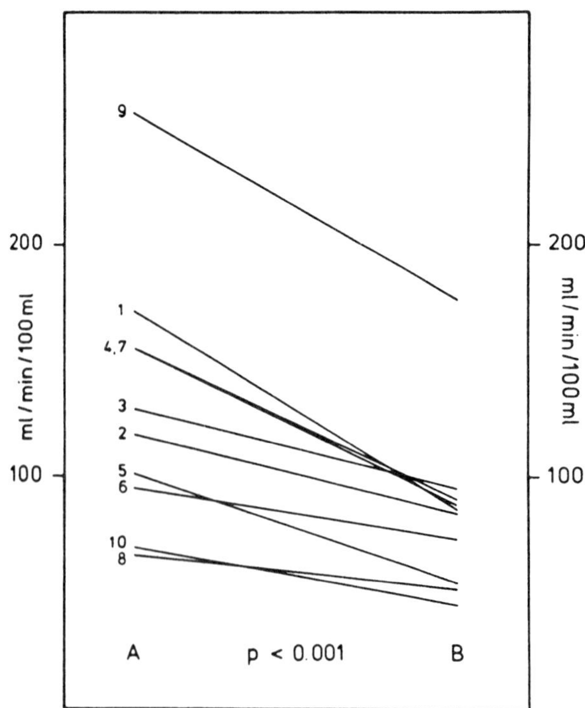

FIG. 7. The individual intervillous blood-flow (IVBF) changes. **A:** Before anesthesia (mean IVBF, 131 ± 57 mL/min/100 mL). **B:** During induction of general anesthesia (mean IVBF, 84 ± 37 mL/min/100 mL). (Reprinted from ref. 132, with permission.)

Epidural blockade avoids the increases in ICP associated with a rapid-sequence induction of general anesthesia. Regional anesthesia also exposes the premature neonate to less drug than does general anesthesia.

Some Technical Issues

When planning an epidural anesthetic for cesarean delivery, the issues of coagulopathy and the safety of epinephrine remain. Fluid management becomes more difficult. These women may require large volumes of crystalloid to maintain hemodynamic stability. There will be rapid volume shifts of 1,000 mL or more at the time of delivery. For these reasons, careful monitoring of volume status can help to avoid sudden and potentially dangerous changes in blood pressure.

You will need large-bore intravenous access because:

- Hemodynamic changes during induction of epidural anesthesia may require treatment with rapid fluid infusion,
- Magnesium therapy may cause some degree of tocolysis and can contribute to uterine atony and blood loss, and
- Patients with HELLP syndrome or liver injury may require blood products.

The optimal choice of local anesthetic for cesarean delivery is not clear. 2-Chloroprocaine has the most rapid onset but timely intervention to correct hypotension may be more difficult. Slow titration to increase the anesthetic level is difficult with 2-chloroprocaine. Dosing at intervals of more than a few minutes will often fail to increase the anesthetic level. Finally, redosing will have to be done about every 30 minutes, so you may be faced with giving a bolus of drug just after delivery when the incidence of hypotension is already high.

Lidocaine is metabolized less efficiently in the preeclamptic patient, but this should not be of concern with a single dose for cesarean section. A more difficult problem is the maximal allowable dose of lidocaine. If the toxic dose of plain lidocaine is assumed to be 5 mg/kg and the average-size woman is 60 kg, her maximal dose of 2% lidocaine is only 15 mL. This volume may fail to produce sensory block to T_4.

Finally, although 0.5% bupivacaine is best for slow titration of anesthetic level, it is not as potent as 3% chloroprocaine or 2% lidocaine. Because bupivacaine provides less dense motor and sensory blockade, the mother may require supplemental analgesia. Adding 100 μg fentanyl to the local-anesthetic solution will improve intraoperative analgesia. Injecting the epidural catheter several times during labor before extending the block for cesarean section will significantly improve the quality of blockade. In animals, magnesium had no effect on the plasma concentration of bupivacaine at which seizures or cardiovascular collapse occurred. Magnesium did prevent bupivacaine-induced cardiac dysrhythmias (133). Ropivacaine may have similar characteristics and benefits but less potential for cardiotoxicity.

TABLE 6. *A suggested technique for elective cesarean section in a severely preeclamptic parturient under epidural anesthesia*

1. Assess coagulation status
2. Assess volume status and determine need for invasive hemodynamic monitoring
3. Administer aspiration prophylaxis
4. Insert additional 16-gauge i.v. catheter, separate from medication infusions. Hydrate with 20 mL/kg or until CVP is positive or PAOP is 5–10 mm Hg
5. After identifying the epidural space, administer 0.5% bupivacaine, 10–15 mL, with fentanyl, 100 μg, in incremental doses
6. Assess hemodynamic changes before each additional increment of drug, and give additional intravenous fluids or vasopressor as needed
7. When hemodynamics are stable, proceed to the operating room and administer an additional 10 mL of 2% plain lidocaine in increments as needed to raise sensory level to T_4
8. Treat hypotension at delivery as dictated by hemodynamic changes (i.e., volume vs pressor vs inotropic support)
9. Administer 4 mg of preservative-free morphine through the epidural catheter after the umbilical cord is clamped

CVP, central venous pressure; PAOP, pulmonary artery occlusion pressure.

Suggested Technique (Table 6)

Give oral sodium citrate just before going to the operating room. Use invasive monitoring to guide fluid and vasopressor therapy. Treat hypotension with additional fluids and small doses of a vasopressor (ephedrine before delivery and phenylephrine after delivery). Maintain adequate uterine displacement at all times. If time allows, I initiate the block in a labor room with 10 to 15 mL of 0.5% bupivacaine plus 100 μg fentanyl. This dose of bupivacaine usually provides a sensory level of T_8 to T_{10}. After each dose, reassess hemodynamic values to determine the need for additional fluids or vasopressor. Slow titration of local anesthetic and continuous assessment of hemodynamics should avoid or allow rapid correction of hypotension. Once the sympathectomy has stabilized (in about 20 minutes), move the patient to the operating room and raise the level of sensory block to T_4 with an additional 10 mL of plain 2% lidocaine in incremental doses.

Within a few minutes of delivery, a short period of moderate to severe hypotension often occurs. Air or amniotic fluid embolus or the sudden loss of a significant amount of blood in a relatively vasoconstricted patient may contribute to this decrease in blood pressure. Treat with fluid replacement and vasopressors if the mother is symptomatic. In the presence of maternal tachycardia, phenylephrine will improve vascular tone while reducing heart rate. Choose an appropriate vasopressor based on the patient's hemodynamics.

A functioning epidural catheter also often proves effective for urgent cesarean delivery. Use 2% lidocaine or 3% 2-chloroprocaine to provide more rapid sensory blockade. Infuse additional fluids simultaneously to maintain stable blood pressure. During labor, be certain that the epidural catheter is working effectively should cesarean delivery be needed. Good communication with the obstetric service should provide adequate warning of an impending operative procedure.

General Anesthesia

The anesthesiologist may have to resort to general anesthesia in some instances. Patients may refuse regional block or have a significant coagulopathy. General anesthesia may be the only choice for an emergency cesarean delivery in a woman without an epidural catheter. Several important issues must be considered when preparing a woman with preeclampsia for general anesthesia.

Airway

The generalized edema seen in preeclampsia may produce glottic swelling, which can make endotracheal intubation extremely difficult (134,135). Be prepared for a potential airway problem if you note marked facial edema or the patient complains of hoarseness, difficulty swallowing, or respiratory distress (136). Glottic edema cannot be adequately assessed on routine airway examination. If you anticipate difficulty, consider gentle awake laryngoscopy under topical anesthesia to visualize the glottis.

Awake Intubation

The vascularity of the pregnant airway and our reluctance to premedicate parturients heavily just before delivery can make awake nasal or oral intubation traumatic for all involved. A simple, comfortable method of anesthetizing the airway involves nebulizing 4 mL 4% lidocaine and 1 mL 1% phenylephrine by face-mask (137). If desired, this step can be preceded by phenylephrine nasal drops to facilitate nasal breathing and a small amount of intravenous fentanyl to prevent coughing. A lubricated nasal airway is then placed and removed gently to dilate the nares, and an appropriate-size endotracheal tube is introduced over the fiberoptic bronchoscope. This technique can obtund protective airway reflexes; aspiration prophylaxis should be given beforehand if possible. The technique is rapid, minimally uncomfortable for the patient, and provides reliable anesthesia for nasotracheal or oral intubation. Whatever technique is used for induction, a variety of smaller endotracheal tubes and a difficult airway box should be immediately available in the delivery room.

Blood Pressure

Dramatic and dangerous hypertension can complicate intubation and cause pulmonary edema or cerebral hemorrhage (138). Numerous approaches can obtund this hypertensive response. In some settings, nitroglycerin can reduce blood pressure before induction and limit the hypertensive response to intubation (139). Because nitroglycerin primarily affects venous capacitance and ventricular preload, it will be less effective in the volume-expanded patient. Longmire et al. (140) used nitroglycerin after volume loading to a PAOP of 10 to 15 mm Hg. At intubation, despite very high infusion rates of nitroglycerin, heart rate, MAP (from 134 to 164 mm Hg), and SVR increased significantly.

Labetalol in doses up to 1 mg/kg may prove effective (141). In some patients, this dose of labetalol will not produce a 20% reduction in MAP. Even in these women, however, some decrease in blood pressure occurs without reflex tachycardia. Sublingual nifedipine also attenuates the hypertensive response to laryngoscopy and intubation, but does not prevent maternal tachycardia (142).

Opioids also can blunt the hemodynamic response to intubation. They are often avoided in parturients because of the risk of neonatal respiratory depression. In healthy parturients, alfentanil (10 μg/kg) given just before induction effectively controls the pressor response to intubation without adversely affecting Apgar scores (143). Alfentanil readily crosses the placenta with a transfer ratio of 0.35. Although there are no data yet, remifentanil might provide similar hemodynamic control at induction.

A comparison of lidocaine (1.5 mg/kg), magnesium sulfate (40 mg/kg), and alfentanil (10 μg/kg) given intravenously just before induction favored alfentanil and magnesium for controlling the cardiovascular responses to intubation, but alfentanil caused significant neonatal respiratory depression (144). These patients had moderate to severe preeclampsia, and mean birth weight was 1,726 g. These compromised neonates might have been more sensitive than healthy babies to the depressant effects of alfentanil. There was no indication of neonatal depression in the magnesium group, and neonatal magnesium concentration did not correlate with Apgar scores or ventilatory status. Recent work varying the time interval between intravenous lidocaine administration and tracheal intubation found that 1.5 mg/kg of lidocaine helped to control the hemodynamic response to intubation only if administered more than 2 minutes in advance (145).

Maintenance

The choice of an inhalation agent for maintenance of the parturient with severe preeclampsia is not critical. Neither renal toxicity with enflurane nor liver dysfunction with halothane have been reported in preeclamptic parturients (146). Isoflurane, sevoflurane, or desflurane may be the agents of choice, however. All avoid the issue of hepatic dysfunction (common in preeclampsia) and halothane. Enflurane may lower the seizure threshold, not a desirable feature in this patient population.

Remember that p_{50} shifts to the left in preeclampsia. Mechanical hyperventilation will shift the oxyhemoglobin-dissociation curve even farther to the left. Mechanical ventilation also decreases venous return and cardiac output. Both events decrease oxygen delivery to an already compromised fetus.

Magnesium and Muscle Relaxants

Therapeutic serum magnesium concentrations significantly potentiate nondepolarizing muscle relaxants (Fig. 8). Neuromuscular-transmission studies of preeclamptic women receiving magnesium therapy show a defect in neuromuscular transmission that increases in severity with increasing magnesium exposure (147). Train-of-four demonstrates fade, with T_4/T_1 ratios ranging from 0.72 to 0.92, at clinically relevant doses of magnesium (148). Magnesium decreases neuromuscular transmission at multiple sites. Magnesium:

- Decreases presynaptic release of acetylcholine,
- Reduces the sensitivity of the postjunctional muscle end-plate, and

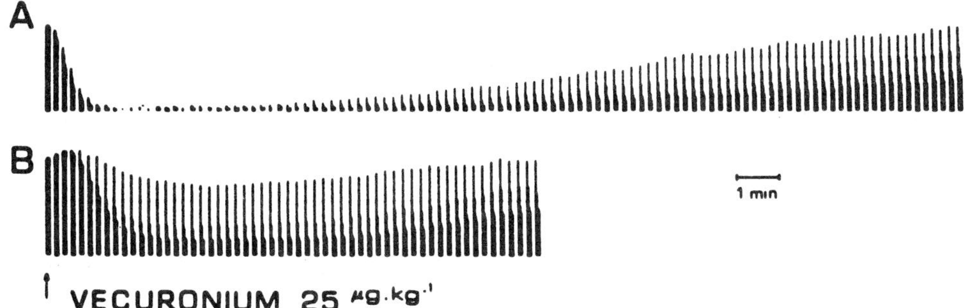

FIG. 8. Electromyographic tracing comparing the neuromuscular blockade achieved by vecuronium, 25 µg/kg, in an eclamptic patient (receiving intravenous magnesium sulphate at 2 g/h) **(A)**, with that achieved in a control parturient **(B)**. (Reprinted from ref. 151, with permission.)

- Depresses the excitability of the muscle fiber membrane.

Both animal and human studies showed that magnesium increases the density and duration of nondepolarizing neuromuscular blockade (Fig. 6) (149–153).

The interaction of magnesium with depolarizing relaxants is more complicated. The neuromuscular effects of magnesium should antagonize succinylcholine. (Succinylcholine mimics acetylcholine at the nerve terminal. Magnesium inhibits the action of acetylcholine.) However, patients treated with magnesium require less succinylcholine by infusion than do normal parturients (4.73 mg/kg/hr vs 7.39 mg/kg/hr) during uncomplicated cesarean section (154). Likewise, in an isolated-nerve preparation, magnesium doubles the potency of succinylcholine (155). Preparation of the isolated-nerve model, however, involved multiple washings to remove plasma cholinesterase. Therefore these results probably represent the direct neuromuscular effect of succinylcholine or phase 2 block. The prolongation of succinylcholine after repeated doses or continuous infusion also may represent development of phase 2 block potentiated by magnesium.

Human studies have failed to document any prolongation of onset or duration of a single intubating dose of succinylcholine in patients receiving magnesium (Fig. 9) (151,156). Clinically, parturients receiving magnesium respond normally to a single bolus injection of succinylcholine. Recovery after repeated doses or continuous infusion may be prolonged. Carefully monitor neuromuscular function with a nerve stimulator when giving any muscle relaxant to a woman with preeclampsia who has received magnesium.

Suggested Technique

The following is a suggested technique for general anesthesia for cesarean section in a woman with preeclampsia (Table 7). Before beginning, give appropriate aspiration prophylaxis. Thoroughly assess the patient's airway. Place any needed monitors. During preoxygenation in the left-tilt position, carefully control maternal blood pressure. Aim for a blood pressure of 140/90 mm Hg, but do not allow it to decrease by more than 20%. Stop if a nonreassuring fetal heart-rate pattern develops. I recommend either trimethaphan, in doses of 1 to 2 mg or as an infusion, nitroprusside by infusion, or labetalol in 5- to 10-mg increments. Once you have reduced maternal blood pressure adequately, begin a rapid-sequence induction of general anesthesia. I use 1.5 mg/kg lidocaine, 4 mg/kg of thiopental, and 1.0 mg/kg of succinylcholine. In severely hypertensive mothers, or if I am concerned about rapid increases in ICP, I add alfentanil, 10 µg/kg, to the induction sequence. I then advise the pediatricians that the neonate may be narcotized.

If fetal intolerance to labor is the indication for delivery, maintain anesthesia with 100% oxygen and 1.0% to 1.5% isoflurane to assure maternal amnesia. If the fetus appears healthy, a lower oxygen concentration with 50% nitrous oxide can be used with 0.75% isoflurane. After

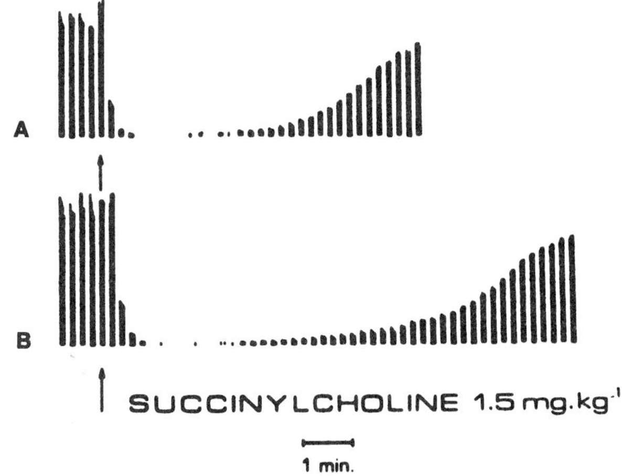

FIG. 9. Electromyographic tracing comparing the neuromuscular blockade achieved by succinylcholine, 1.5 mg/kg, in an eclamptic patient (receiving intravenous magnesium sulphate at 2 g/h) **(A)**, with that achieved in a control parturient **(B)**. (Reprinted from ref. 151, with permission.)

TABLE 7. *A suggested technique for cesarean section in a severely preeclamptic parturient under general anesthesia*

1. Administer aspiration prophylaxis
2. Determine need for invasive hemodynamic monitoring
3. Insert additional 16-gauge i.v. catheter, separate from medication infusions
4. Evaluate the airway. Have smaller endotracheal tubes (5.5, 6.0 mm) available in the operating room
5. In the operating room, place the patient in the left-tilt position and begin preoxygenation with 100% oxygen
6. Lower blood pressure to a mean of ~105–110 mm Hg or as the fetus tolerates by using labetalol or vasodilators depending on the patient's hemodynamic status
7. Induction sequence
   Lidocaine, 1.5 mg/kg
   Alfentanil, 10 μg/kg
   Thiopental, 4 mg/kg
   Succinylcholine, 1 mg/kg
8. Maintain anesthesia before delivery with 50% nitrous oxide in oxygen and 0.75% isoflurane. Maintain normocarbia. If there is fetal distress, consider using 100% oxygen and 1.0%–1.5% isoflurane
9. After delivery, increase nitrous oxide to 60%–70% as tolerated and titrate morphine, 0.2–0.3 mg/kg intravenously. Decrease isoflurane. Treat hypotension at delivery based on hemodynamic changes (i.e., volume vs pressor vs inotropic support)
10. By using a neuromuscular blockade monitor, titrate atracurium in 10-mg increments to maintain 80%–90% blockade, if relaxation is required
11. At emergence, reverse neuromuscular blockade if a nondepolarizing relaxant was used. Discontinue nitrous oxide. Treat emergence hypertension with agents used at induction. Extubate when patient is awake and can maintain 5-s head lift.

delivery, increase the concentration of nitrous oxide, give incremental doses of morphine (total dose, 0.2 to 0.3 mg/kg), and a muscle relaxant as needed. I find the vasodilating properties of morphine helpful in controlling blood pressure after stopping the halogenated agent. Morphine also provides longer postoperative analgesia than fentanyl.

If the surgery lasts less than 1 hour, a succinylcholine infusion can be used. I prefer to avoid nondepolarizing muscle relaxants, which are more difficult to titrate and reverse completely in the presence of magnesium sulfate.* If the procedure is expected to require more than 1 hour, however, atracurium may be preferable to rocuronium because it is not dependent on hepatic metabolism.

Oxytocin infusion must begin immediately at delivery to counteract the tocolytic effects of magnesium. Be prepared for hypotension. Treat significant hypotension with vasopressors and additional fluids as appropriate. Vasodilators will probably be needed during emergence to control hypertension until the patient is fully awake and ready to be extubated.

*Editor's note: I find succinylcholine infusions difficult to use even under normal circumstances. In this setting, I carefully titrate small increments of atracurium or cisatracurium. I strongly agree on the need to monitor neuromuscular function.

POSTPARTUM CONSIDERATIONS

Care of the preeclamptic patient does not end with emergence and extubation. Monitoring should continue for at least 24 hours after delivery, or until diuresis begins. Mobilization of fluid should begin by 24 hours, and if a spontaneous diuresis does not occur, cardiac filling pressures will increase. If the patient had an epidural anesthetic, resolution of the sympathectomy with return of vascular tone may cause central pressures to increase as well. Increased filling pressures put the patient at risk for pulmonary edema. If invasive monitoring is in place, monitor CVP and PAOP carefully, and if they begin to rise without diuresis, small doses of diuretics or low-dose dopamine may help.

In HELLP syndrome, thrombocytopenia may not reach its nadir until 2 to 3 days after delivery. An upward trend in platelet count should be apparent by postpartum day 3. Resolution to a count above 100,000/mm^3 may require 5 to 6 days. Fourteen percent to 27% of eclamptic seizures occur after delivery. Women with HELLP syndrome are at especially high risk of postpartum eclampsia (157).

Patients will need to be changed from short-term (parenteral) to long-term (oral) blood pressure medications. Most patients will need treatment of their hypertension for up to 6 weeks after delivery. Oral medications may include nifedipine, α-methyldopa, labetalol, or clonidine. Their efficacy and the patient's compliance should be documented before she is discharged from the hospital.

CONCLUSION

The preeclamptic patient requires the same meticulous attention from the anesthesiologist as a seriously ill patient in the general operating room, and perhaps more, because only in the obstetric patient can mortality be 200%! This attention includes detailed preoperative preparation, selection of appropriate monitors, development of anesthetic plans for all possible modes of delivery, and close postoperative follow-up. A good working relationship with our obstetrical colleagues and the development of open lines of communication for consultation and planning will best serve the parturient in our care.

REFERENCES

1. Berg CJ, Atrash HK, Koonin LM, Tucker M. Pregnancy-related mortality in the United States, 1987-1990. *Obstet Gynecol* 1996;88:161.
2. American College of Obstetricians and Gynecologists. *Hypertension in pregnancy.* ACOG technical bulletin 219. Washington, DC: ACOG, 1996.
3. Mushambi MC, Halligan AW, Williamson K. Recent developments in the pathophysiology and management of pre-eclampsia. *Br J Anaesth* 1996;76:133.

4. Kambam JR, Entman S, Mouton S, Smith BE. Effect of preeclampsia on carboxyhemoglobin levels: a mechanism for a decrease in p50. *Anesthesiology* 1988;68:433.
5. Leduc L, Wheeler JM, Kirshon B, Mitchell P, Cotton DB. Coagulation profile in severe preeclampsia. *Obstet Gynecol* 1992;79:14.
6. Prieto JA, Mastrobattista JM, Blanco JD. Coagulation studies in patients with marked thrombocytopenia due to severe preeclampsia. *Am J Perinatol* 1995;12:220.
7. Trofatter KF, Howell ML, Greenberg CS, Hage ML. Use of the fibrin D-dimer in screening for coagulation abnormalities in preeclampsia. *Obstet Gynecol* 1989;73:435.
8. Pritchard JA, Cunningham FG, Mason RA. Coagulation changes in eclampsia: their frequency and pathogenesis. *Am J Obstet Gynecol* 1976;124:855.
9. Kelton JG, Hunter DJS, Neame PB. A platelet function defect in preeclampsia. *Obstet Gynecol* 1985;65:107.
10. Ramanathan J, Sibai BM, Vu T, Chauhan D. Correlation between bleeding times and platelet counts in women with preeclampsia undergoing cesarean section. *Anesthesiology* 1989;71:188.
11. Lao TT, Halpern SH, MacDonald D. Spinal subdural haematoma in a parturient after attempted epidural anaesthesia. *Can J Anaesth* 1993; 40:340.
12. Rolbin SH, Abbott D, Musclow E, Papsin F, Lie LM, Freedman J. Epidural anesthesia in pregnant patients with low platelet counts. *Obstet Gynecol* 1988;71:918.
13. Rasmus KT, Rottman RL, Kotelko DM, Wright WC, Stone JJ, Rosenblatt RM. Unrecognized thrombocytopenia and regional anesthesia in parturients: a retrospective review. *Obstet Gynecol* 1989;73:943.
14. Hew-Wing P, Rolbin SH, Hew E, Amato D. Epidural anaesthesia and thrombocytopenia. *Anaesthesia* 1989;44:775.
15. Burrows RF, Kelton JG. Incidentally detected thrombocytopenia in healthy mothers and their infants. *N Engl J Med* 1988;319:142.
16. Kopacz DJ, Gibbs CP. Training anesthesia residents to perform bleeding times. *Reg Anesth* 1991;161:16.
17. Rodgers RPC, Levin J. A critical reappraisal of the bleeding time. *Semin Thromb Hemost* 1990;16:1.
18. Sibai BM, Caritis SN, Thom E, et al. Prevention of preeclampsia with low-dose aspirin in healthy, nulliparous pregnant women. *N Engl J Med* 1993;329:1213.
19. Collaborative Low-Dose Aspirin Study in Pregnancy Collaborative Group. CLASP: a randomized trial of low-dose aspirin for the prevention and treatment of pre-eclampsia among 9364 pregnant women. *Lancet* 1994;343:619.
20. Benigni A, Gregorini G, Frusca T, et al. Effect of low-dose aspirin on fetal and maternal generation of thromboxane by platelets in women at risk for pregnancy-induced hypertension. *N Engl J Med* 1989; 321:357.
21. Williams HD, Howard R, O'Donnell N, Findley I. The effect of low dose aspirin on bleeding times. *Anaesthesia* 1993;48:331.
22. Beilin Y, Bodian CA, Haddad EM, Leibowitz AB. Practice patterns of anesthesiologists regarding situations in obstetric anesthesia where clinical management is controversial. *Anesth Analg* 1996;83:735.
23. Orlikowski CEP, Rocke DA, Murray WB, et al. Thrombelastography changes in pre-eclampsia and eclampsia. *Br J Anaesth* 1996;77:157.
24. Maltin JN, Blake PG, Lowry SL, Perry KG, Files JC, Morrison JC. Pregnancy complicated by preeclampsia-eclampsia with the syndrome of hemolysis, elevated liver enzymes, and low platelet count: how rapid is postpartum recovery? *Obstet Gynecol* 1990;76:737.
25. Smith LG, Moise KJ, Dildy GA, Carpenter RJ. Spontaneous rupture of liver during pregnancy: current therapy. *Obstet Gynecol* 1991;77:171.
26. Cotton DB, Lee W, Huhta JC, Dorman KF. Hemodynamic profile of severe pregnancy-induced hypertension. *Am J Obstet Gynecol* 1988; 158:523.
27. Clark SL, Divon MY, Phelan JP. Preeclampsia/eclampsia: hemodynamic and neurologic correlations. *Obstet Gynecol* 1985;66:337.
28. Milliez J, Dahoun A, Boudraa M. Computed tomography of the brain in eclampsia. *Obstet Gynecol* 1990;75:975.
29. Montan S, Ingemarsson I. Intrapartum fetal heart rate patterns in pregnancies complicated by hypertension. *Am J Obstet Gynecol* 1989; 160:283.
30. Naidoo DP, Bhorat I, Moodley J, Naidoo JK, Mitha AS. Continuous electrocardiographic monitoring in hypertensive crises in pregnancy. *Am J Obstet Gynecol* 1991;164:530.
31. American Society of Anesthesiologists Task Force on Pulmonary Artery Catheterization. Practice guidelines for pulmonary artery catheterization. *Anesthesiology* 1993;78:380.
32. Fox DB, Troiano NH, Graves CR. Use of the pulmonary artery catheter in severe preeclampsia: a review. *Obstet Gynecol Surv* 1996;51:684.
33. Clark SL, Cotton DB. Clinical indications for pulmonary artery catheterization in the patient with severe preeclampsia. *Am J Obstet Gynecol* 1988;158:453.
34. Clark SL, Horenstein JM, Phelan JP, Montag TW, Paul RH. Experience with the pulmonary artery catheter in obstetrics and gynecology. *Am J Obstet Gynecol* 1985;152:374.
35. Woodward DG, Romanoff ME. Is central venous pressure monitoring contraindicated in patients with severe preeclampsia? *Am J Obstet Gynecol* 1989;161:837.
36. Cotton DB, Gonik B, Dorman K, Harrist R. Cardiovascular alterations in severe pregnancy-induced hypertension: relationship of central venous pressure to pulmonary capillary wedge pressure. *Am J Obstet Gynecol* 1985;151:762.
37. Easterling TR, Benedetti TJ, Carlson KL, Watts DH. Measurement of cardiac output in pregnancy by thermodilution and impedance techniques. *Br J Obstet Gynaecol* 1989;96:67.
38. Masaki DI, Greenspoon JS, Ouzounian JG. Measurement of cardiac output in pregnancy by thoracic electrical bioimpedance and thermodilution. *Am J Obstet Gynecol* 1989;161:680.
39. Easterling TR, Watts DH, Schmucker BC, Benedetti TJ. Measurement of cardiac output during pregnancy: validation of Doppler technique and clinical observations in preeclampsia. *Obstet Gynecol* 1987;69:845.
40. Benedetti TJ, Carlson RW. Studies of colloid osmotic pressure in pregnancy-induced hypertension. *Am J Obstet Gynecol* 1979;135:308.
41. Benedetti TJ, Cotton DB, Read JC, Miller FC. Hemodynamic observations in severe preeclampsia with a flow-directed pulmonary artery catheter. *Am J Obstet Gynecol* 1980;136:465.
42. Rafferty TD, Berkowitz RL. Hemodynamics in patients with severe toxemia during labor and delivery. *Am J Obstet Gynecol* 1980;138:263.
43. Phelan JP, Yurth DA. Severe preeclampsia: peripartum hemodynamic observations. *Am J Obstet Gynecol* 1982;144:17.
44. Groenendijk R, Trimbos JBMJ, Wallenburg JCS. Hemodynamic measurements in preeclampsia: preliminary observations. *Am J Obstet Gynecol* 1984;150:232.
45. Clark SL, Greenspoon JS, Aldahl D, Phelan JP. Severe preeclampsia with persistent oliguria: management of hemodynamic subsets. *Am J Obstet Gynecol* 1986;154:490.
46. Yang JM, Yang YC, Wang KG. Central and peripheral hemodynamics in severe preeclampsia. *Acta Obstet Gynecol Scand* 1996;75:120.
47. Easterling TR, Benedetti TJ, Schmucker BC, Millard SP. Maternal hemodynamics in normal and preeclamptic pregnancies: a longitudinal study. *Obstet Gynecol* 1990;76:1061.
48. Easterling TR, Benedetti TJ. Preeclampsia: a hyperdynamic disease model. *Am J Obstet Gynecol* 1989;160:1447.
49. Wheeler TC, Graves CR, Troiano NH, Reed GW. Base deficit and oxygen transport in severe preeclampsia. *Obstet Gynecol* 1996;87:375.
50. Sibai BM, McCubbin JH, Anderson GD, Lipshitz J, Dilts PV. Eclampsia. I. Observations from 67 recent cases. *Obstet Gynecol* 1981; 58:609.
51. Pritchard JA, Cunningham FG, Pritchard SA. The Parkland Memorial Hospital protocol for treatment of eclampsia: evaluation of 245 cases. *Am J Obstet Gynecol* 1984;148:951.
52. Sibai BM. Magnesium sulfate is the ideal anticonvulsant in preeclampsia-eclampsia. *Am J Obstet Gynecol* 1990;162:1141.
53. Watson KV, Moldow CF, Ogburn PL, Jacob HS. Magnesium sulfate: rationale for its use in preeclampsia. *Proc Natl Acad Sci U S A* 1986; 83:1075.
54. Belfort MA, Moise KJ. Effect of magnesium sulfate on maternal brain blood flow in preeclampsia: a randomized, placebo-controlled study. *Am J Obstet Gynecol* 1992;167:661.
55. Lucas MJ, Leveno KJ, Cunningham FG. A comparison of magnesium sulfate with phenytoin for the prevention of eclampsia. *N Engl J Med* 1995;333:201.
56. Friedman SA, Lim KH, Baker CA, Repke JT. A comparison of phenytoin infusion versus magnesium sulfate infusion in preeclampsia [Abstract]. *Soc Perinat Obstet* 1990;10:12.
57. Kirshon B, Lee W, Mauer MB, Cotton DB. Effects of low-dose dopamine therapy in the oliguric patient with preeclampsia. *Am J Obstet Gynecol* 1988;159:604.
58. Sibai BM, Mabie BC, Harvey CJ, Gonzalez AR. Pulmonary edema in

severe preeclampsia-eclampsia: analysis of thirty-seven consecutive cases. *Am J Obstet Gynecol* 1987;156:1174.
59. Kirshon B, Moise KJ, Cotton DB, et al. Role of volume expansion in severe preeclampsia. *Surg Gynecol Obstet* 1988;167:367.
60. Cotton DB, Jones MM, Longmire S, Dorman KF, Tessem J, Joyce TH. Role of intravenous nitroglycerin in the treatment of severe pregnancy-induced hypertension complicated by pulmonary edema. *Am J Obstet Gynecol* 1986;154:91.
61. Sibai BM. Treatment of hypertension in pregnant women. *N Engl J Med* 1996;335:257.
62. Scardo JA, Hogg BB, Newman RB. Favorable hemodynamic effects of magnesium sulfate in preeclampsia. *Am J Obstet Gynecol* 1995; 173:1249.
63. Ring G, Krames E, Shnider SM, Wallis KL, Levinson G. Comparison of nitroprusside and hydralazine in hypertensive ewes. *Obstet Gynecol* 1977;50:598.
64. Cotton DB, Gonik B, Dorman KF. Cardiovascular alterations in severe pregnancy-induced hypertension seen with an intravenously given hydralazine bolus. *Surg Gynecol Obstet* 1985;161:240.
65. Wheeler AS, James FM, Meis PJ, et al. Effects of nitroglycerin and nitroprusside on the uterine vasculature of gravid ewes. *Anesthesiology* 1980;52:390.
66. Naulty J, Cefalo RC, Lewis PE. Fetal toxicity of nitroprusside in the pregnant ewe. *Am J Obstet Gynecol* 1981;139:708.
67. Stempel JE, O'Grady JP, Morton MJ, Johnson KA. Use of sodium nitroprusside in complications of gestational hypertension. *Obstet Gynecol* 1982;60:533.
68. Craft JB, Co EG, Yonekura ML, Gilman RM. Nitroglycerin therapy for phenylephrine induced hypertension in pregnant ewes. *Anesth Analg* 1980;59:494.
69. Cotton DB, Longmire S, Jones MM, Dorman KF, Tessem J, Joyce TH. Cardiovascular alterations in severe pregnancy-induced hypertension: effects of intravenous nitroglycerin coupled with blood volume expansion. *Am J Obstet Gynecol* 1986;154:1053.
70. Ishikawa T, Funatsu N, Okamoto K, Takeshita H, McDowall DG. Cerebral and systemic effects of hypotension induced by trimethaphan or nitroprusside in dogs. *Acta Anaesth Scand* 1982;26:643.
71. Karlin A, Hartung J, Cottrell JE. Rate of induction of hypotension with trimethaphan modifies the intracranial pressure response in cats. *Br J Anaesth* 1988;60:161.
72. Sklar GS, Lanks KW. Effects of trimethaphan and sodium nitroprusside on hydrolysis of succinylcholine in vitro. *Anesthesiology* 1977;47:31.
73. Poulton TJ, James FM III, Lockridge O. Prolonged apnea following trimethaphan and succinylcholine. *Anesthesiology* 1979;50:54.
74. MacCarthy EP, Bloomfield SS. Labetalol: a review of its pharmacology, pharmacokinetics, clinical uses and adverse effects. *Pharmacotherapy* 1983;3:193.
75. Nylund L, Lunell NO, Lewander R, Sarby B, Thornstrom S. Labetalol for the treatment of hypertension in pregnancy. *Acta Obstet Gynecol Scand Suppl* 1984;118:71.
76. Jouppila P, Kirkinen P, Koivula A, Ylikorkala O. Labetalol does not alter the placental and fetal blood flow or maternal prostanoids in preeclampsia. *Br J Obstet Gynaecol* 1986;93:543.
77. Eisenach JC, Mandell G, Dewan DM. Maternal and fetal effects of labetalol in pregnant ewes. *Anesthesiology* 1991;74:292.
78. MacPherson M, Pipkin FB, Ruker N. The effect of maternal labetalol on the newborn infant. *Br J Obstet Gynaecol* 1986;93:539.
79. Mabie WC, Gonzalez AR, Sibai BM, Amon E. A comparative trial of labetalol and hydralazine in the acute management of severe hypertension complicating pregnancy. *Obstet Gynecol* 1987;70:328.
80. Ostman PL, Chestnut DH, Robillard JE, Weiner CP, Hdez MJ. Transplacental passage and hemodynamic effects of esmolol in the gravid ewe. *Anesthesiology* 1988;69:738.
81. Eisenach JC, Castro MI. Maternally administered esmolol produces fetal beta-adrenergic blockade and hypoxemia in sheep. *Anesthesiology* 1989;71:718.
82. Kjellmer I, Dagbjartsson A, Hrbek A, Karlsson K, Rosen KG. Maternal beta-adrenoceptor blockade reduces fetal tolerance to asphyxia. *Acta Obstet Gynecol Scand Suppl* 1984;118:75.
83. Losasso TJ, Muzzi DA, Cucciara RF. Response of fetal heart rate to maternal administration of esmolol. *Anesthesiology* 1991;74:782.
84. Larson CP Jr, Shuer LM, Cohen SE. Maternally administered esmolol decreases fetal as well as maternal heart rate. *J Clin Anesth* 1990;427:2.
85. Ducey JP, Knape KG. Maternal esmolol administration resulting in fetal distress and cesarean section in a term pregnancy. *Anesthesiology* 1992;77:829.
86. Horvath JS, Phippard A, Korda A, Henderson-Smart DJ, Child A, Tiller DJ. Clonidine hydrochloride: a safe and effective antihypertensive agent in pregnancy. *Obstet Gynecol* 1985;66:634.
87. Eisenach JC, Castro MI, Dewan DM, Rose JC, Grice SC. Intravenous clonidine hydrochloride toxicity in pregnant ewes. *Am J Obstet Gynecol* 1988;160:471.
88. Norris MC, Rose JC, Dewan DM. Nifedipine or verapamil counteracts hypertension in gravid ewes. *Anesthesiology* 1986;65:254.
89. Belfort M, Anthony J, Buccimazza A, Davey DA. Hemodynamic changes associated with intravenous infusion of the calcium antagonist verapamil in the treatment of severe gestational proteinuric hypertension. *Obstet Gynecol* 1990;75:970.
90. Belfort M, Anthony J, Kirshon B. Respiratory function in severe gestational proteinuric hypertension: the effects of rapid volume expansion and subsequent vasodilatation with verapamil. *Br J Obstet Gynaecol* 1991;98:964.
91. Belfort MA, Saade GR, Moise KJ, et al. Nimodipine in the management of preeclampsia: maternal and fetal effects. *Am J Obstet Gynecol* 1994;171:417.
92. Carbonne B, Jannet D, Touboul C, Khelifati Y, Milliez J. Nicardipine treatment of hypertension during pregnancy. *Obstet Gynecol* 1993; 81:908.
93. Scardo JA, Vermillion ST, Hogg BB, Newman RB. Hemodynamic effects of oral nifedipine in preeclamptic hypertensive emergencies. *Am J Obstet Gynecol* 1996;175:336.
94. Thorp JM, Spielman FJ, Valea FA, Payne FG, Mueller RA, Cefalo RC. Nifedipine enhances the cardiac toxicity of magnesium sulfate in the isolated perfused Sprague-Dawley rat heart. *Am J Obstet Gynecol* 1990;163:655.
95. Snyder SW, Cardwell MS. Neuromuscular blockade with magnesium sulfate and nifedipine. *Am J Obstet Gynecol* 1989;161:35.
96. Ben-Ami M, Giladi Y, Shalev E. The combination of magnesium sulphate and nifedipine: a cause of neuromuscular blockade. *Br J Obstet Gynaecol* 1994;101:262.
97. Mehta N, Modi N. ACE inhibitors in pregnancy. *Lancet* 1989;2:96.
98. Gutsche B. Is epidural block for labor and delivery and for cesarean section a safe form of analgesia in severe preeclampsia or eclampsia? *Surv Anesthesiol* 1986;30:304.
99. Abboud T, Artal R, Sarkis F, Henriksen EH, Kammula RK. Sympathoadrenal activity, maternal, fetal, and neonatal responses after epidural anesthesia in the preeclamptic patient. *Am J Obstet Gynecol* 1982;144:915.
100. Jouppila R, Jouppila P, Hollmen A, Koivula A. Epidural analgesia and placental blood flow during labour in pregnancies complicated by hypertension. *Br J Obstet Gynaecol* 1979;86:969.
101. Jouppila P, Jouppila R, Hollmen A, Koivula A. Lumbar epidural analgesia to improve intervillous blood flow during labor in severe preeclampsia. *Obstet Gynecol* 1982;59:158.
102. Moore TR, Key TC, Reisner LS, Resnik R. Evaluation of the use of continuous lumbar epidural anesthesia for hypertensive pregnant women in labor. *Am J Obstet Gynecol* 1985;152:404.
103. Newsome LR, Bramwell RS, Curling PE. Severe preeclampsia: hemodynamic effects of lumbar epidural anesthesia. *Anesth Analg* 1986; 65:31.
104. Vincent RD, Chestnut DH, Sipes SL, Weiner CP, DeBruyn CS, Bleuer SA. Magnesium sulfate decreases maternal blood pressure but not uterine blood flow during epidural anesthesia in gravid ewes. *Anesthesiology* 1991;74:77.
105. Sipes SL, Chestnut DH, Vincent RD, DeBruyn CS, Bleuer SA, Chatterjee P. Which vasopressor should be used to treat hypotension during magnesium sulfate infusion and epidural anesthesia? *Anesthesiology* 1992;77:101.
106. Weiner CP, Martinez E, Chestnut DH, Ghodsi A. Effect of pregnancy on uterine and carotid artery response to norepinephrine, epinephrine, and phenylephrine in vessels with documented functional endothelium. *Am J Obstet Gynecol* 1989;161:1605.
107. Nisell H, Hjemdahl P, Linde B. Cardiovascular responses to circulating catecholamines in normal pregnancy and in pregnancy-induced hypertension. *Clin Physiol* 1985;5:479.
108. DeSimone CA, Leighton BL, Norris MC, Chayen B, Menduke H. The chronotropic effect of isoproterenol is reduced in term pregnant women. *Anesthesiology* 1988;69:626.

109. Leighton BL, Norris MC, DeSimone CA, Darby MJ, Menduke H. Preeclamptic and healthy term pregnant patients have different chronotropic responses to isoproterenol. *Anesthesiology* 1990;72:392.
110. Albright GA, Jouppila R, Hollmen AI, Jouppila P, Vierola H, Koivula A. Epinephrine does not alter human intervillous blood flow during epidural anesthesia. *Anesthesiology* 1981;54:131.
111. Heller PJ, Goodman C. Use of local anesthetics with epinephrine for epidural anesthesia in preeclampsia. *Anesthesiology* 1986;65:224.
112. Skjoldebrand A, Eklund J, Lunell N-O, Nylund L, Sarby B, Thronstrom S. The effects on uteroplacental blood flow of epidural anaesthesia containing adrenaline for caesarean section. *Acta Anaesthesiol Scand* 1990;34:85.
113. Marx GF, Elstein ID, Schuss M, Anyaegbunam A, Fleischer A. Effects of epidural block with lignocaine and lignocaine-adrenaline on umbilical artery velocity wave ratios. *Br J Obstet Gynaecol* 1990;97:517.
114. Alahuhta S, Rasanen J, Jouppila P, Jouppila R, Hollmen AI. Uteroplacental and fetal circulation during extradural bupivacaine-adrenaline and bupivacaine for caesarean section in hypertensive pregnancies with chronic fetal asphyxia. *Br J Anaesth* 1993;71:348.
115. Hadzic A, Vloka J, Patel N, Birnbach D. Hypertensive crisis after a successful placement of an epidural anesthetic in a hypertensive parturient. *Reg Anesth* 1995;20:156.
116. Brose WG, Cohen SE. Epidural lidocaine for cesarean section: effect of varying epinephrine concentration. *Anesthesiology* 1988;69:936.
117. Ramanathan J, Bottorff M, Jeter JN, Khalil M, Sibai BM. The pharmacokinetics and maternal and neonatal effects of epidural lidocaine in preeclampsia. *Anesth Analg* 1986;65:120.
118. Leighton BL, DeSimone CA, Norris MC, Ben-David B. Intrathecal narcotics for labor revisited: the combination of fentanyl and morphine intrathecally provides rapid onset of profound, prolonged analgesia. *Anesth Analg* 1989;69:122.
119. Honet JE, Arkoosh VA, Norris MC, Huffnagle HJ, Silverman NS, Leighton BL. Comparison among intrathecal fentanyl, meperidine, and sufentanil for labor analgesia. *Anesth Analg* 1992;75:734.
120. Cohen SE, Cherry CC, Holbrook RH Jr, El-Sayed YY, Gibson RN, Jaffe RA. Intrathecal sufentanil for labor analgesia: sensory changes, side effects, and fetal heart rate changes. *Anesth Analg* 1993;77:1155.
121. Heyman HJ. Systemic analgesia in labor: still a viable option? *Anesth Clin North Am* 1990;8:43.
122. McIntosh DG, Rayburn WF. Patient-controlled analgesia in obstetrics and gynecology. *Obstet Gynecol* 1991;78:1129.
123. Karinen J, Rasanen J, Alahuhta S, Jouppila R, Jouppila P. Maternal and uteroplacental haemodynamic state in pre-eclamptic patients during spinal anaesthesia for caesarean section. *Br J Anaesth* 1996;76:616.
124. Wallace DH, Leveno KJ, Cunningham FG, Giesecke AH, Shearer VE, Sidawi JE. Randomized comparison of general and regional anesthesia for cesarean delivery in pregnancies complicated by severe preeclampsia. *Obstet Gynecol* 1995;86:193.
125. Engquist A, Brandt MR, Fernandes A, Kehlet H. The blocking effect of epidural analgesia on the adrenocortical and hyperglycemic responses to surgery. *Acta Anaesth Scand* 1977;21:330.
126. Lindahl S, Norden N, Nybell-Lindahl G, Westgren M. Endocrine stress response during general and epidural anaesthesia for elective caesarean sections. *Acta Anaesthesiol Scand* 1983;27:50.
127. Loughran PG, Moore J, Dundee JW. Maternal stress response associated with caesarean delivery under general and epidural anaesthesia. *Br J Obstet Gynaecol* 1986;93:943.
128. Ramanathan J, Sibai B. Maternal stress response during cesarean delivery in severe preeclampsia [Abstract]. *Soc Obstet Anesth Perinatol* 1988;20:G28.
129. Hodgkinson R, Husain FJ, Hayashi RH. Systemic and pulmonary blood pressure during caesarean section in parturients with gestational hypertension. *Can Anaesth Soc J* 1980;27:389.
130. Jouppila R, Jouppila P, Kuikka J, Hollmen A. Placental blood flow during caesarean section under lumbar extradural analgesia. *Br J Anaesth* 1978;50:275.
131. Skjolderbrand A, Eklund J, Johansson H, et al. Uteroplacental blood flow measured by placental scintigraphy during epidural anaesthesia for caesarean section. *Acta Anaesthesiol Scand* 1990;34:79.
132. Jouppila P, Kuikka J, Jouppila R, Hollmen A. Effect of induction of general anesthesia for cesarean section on intervillous blood flow. *Acta Obstet Gynaecol Scand* 1979;58:249.
133. Solomon D, Bunegin L, Albin M. The effect of magnesium sulfate administration on cerebral and cardiac toxicity of bupivacaine in dogs. *Anesthesiology* 1990;72:341.
134. Jouppila R, Jouppila P, Hollmen A. Laryngeal oedema as an obstetric anaesthesia complication. *Acta Anaesthesiol Scand* 1980;24:97.
135. Rocke DA, Scoones GP. Rapidly progressive laryngeal oedema associated with pregnancy-aggravated hypertension. *Anaesthesia* 1992; 47:141.
136. Heller PJ, Scheider EP, Marx GF. Pharyngolaryngeal edema as a presenting symptom in preeclampsia. *Obstet Gynecol* 1983;62:523.
137. Bourke DL, Katz J, Tonneson A. Nebulized anesthesia for awake endotracheal intubation. *Anesthesiology* 1985;63:690.
138. Fox EJ, Sklar GS, Hill CH, Villanueva R, King BD. Complications related to the pressor response to endotracheal intubation. *Anesthesiology* 1977;47:524.
139. Hood DD, Dewan DM, James FM, Floyd HM, Bogard TD. The use of nitroglycerin in preventing the hypertensive response to tracheal intubation in severe preeclampsia. *Anesthesiology* 1985;63:329.
140. Longmire S, Leduc L, Jones MM, Hawkins JL, Joyce TH, Cotton DB. The hemodynamic effects of intubation during nitroglycerin infusion in severe preeclampsia. *Am J Obstet Gynecol* 1991;164:551.
141. Ramanathan J, Sibai BM, Mabie WC, Chauham D, Ruiz AG. The use of labetalol for attenuation of the hypertensive response to endotracheal intubation in preeclampsia. *Am J Obstet Gynecol* 1988;159:650.
142. Kumar N, Batra YK, Bala I, Gopalan S. Nifedipine attenuates the hypertensive response to tracheal intubation in pregnancy-induced hypertension. *Can J Anaesth* 1993;40:329.
143. Cartwright DP, Dann WL, Hutchinson A. Placental transfer of alfentanil at caesarean section. *Eur J Anaesthesiol* 1989;6:103.
144. Allen RW, James MFM, Uys PC. Attenuation of the pressor response to tracheal intubation in hypertensive proteinuric pregnant patients by lignocaine, alfentanil and magnesium sulphate. *Br J Anaesth* 1991;66:216.
145. Wilson IG, Meiklejohn BH, Smith G. Intravenous lignocaine and sympathoadrenal responses to laryngoscopy and intubation. *Anaesthesia* 1991;46:177.
146. Crowhurst JA, Rosen M. General anaesthesia for caesarean section in severe preeclampsia. *Br J Anaesth* 1984;587:56.
147. Ramanathan J, Sibai BM, Pillai R, Angel JL. Neuromuscular transmission studies in preeclamptic women receiving magnesium sulfate. *Am J Obstet Gynecol* 1988;158:40.
148. Ross RM, Baker T. An effect of magnesium on neuromuscular function in parturients. *J Clin Anesth* 1996;8:202.
149. Giesecke AH, Morris RE, Dalton MD, Stephen CR. Of magnesium, muscle relaxants, toxemic parturients, and cats. *Anesth Analg* 1968; 47:689.
150. Sinatra RS, Philip BK, Naulty JS, Ostheimer GW. Prolonged neuromuscular blockade with vecuronium in a patient treated with magnesium sulfate. *Anesth Analg* 1985;64:1220.
151. Baraka A, Yazigi A. Neuromuscular interaction of magnesium with succinylcholine vecuronium sequence in the eclamptic parturient. *Anesthesiology* 1987;67:806.
152. Hodgson RE, Rout CC, Louw NJ, Rocke DA. Mivacurium for cesarean section with concurrent magnesium therapy [Abstract]. *Anesthesiology* 1995;83:A953.
153. Gaiser RR, Seem EH. Use of rocuronium in a pregnant patient with an open eye injury, receiving magnesium medication, for preterm labour. *Br J Anaesth* 1996;77:669.
154. Morris R, Giesecke AH. Potentiation of muscle relaxants by magnesium sulfate therapy in toxemia of pregnancy. *South Med J* 1968;61:25.
155. Ghoneim MM, Long JP. The interaction between magnesium and other neuromuscular blocking agents. *Anesthesiology* 1970;32:23.
156. James MFM, Cork RC, Dennett JE. Succinylcholine pretreatment with magnesium sulfate. *Anesth Analg* 1986;65:373.
157. Miles JF, Martin JN, Blake PG, Perry KG, Martin RW, Meeks GR. Postpartum eclampsia: a recurring perinatal dilemma. *Obstet Gynecol* 1990;76:328.

Obstetric Anesthesia, second edition,
edited by Mark C. Norris.
Lippincott Williams & Wilkins, Philadelphia © 1999.

CHAPTER 28

Vaginal Birth after Cesarean Section

Divina Juson Santos

The use of cesarean delivery in the United States more than quadrupled from 5.5% in 1970 to 24% in 1986 (Fig. 1). The rate increased by approximately 1% per year until its peak at nearly 25% in 1988 (1). The almost 900,000 cesarean sections per year (2) exceeded the combined yearly total of tonsillectomies, appendectomies, and mastectomies (1). It was extrapolated that, if this trend continued, the cesarean section rate would reach 40% by the year 2000 (1). The practice of automatic repeat cesarean section was primarily responsible for this increase. Part of a nationwide attempt to reduce the cesarean section rate included informing physicians that, in the absence of a contraindication to vaginal delivery, patients with prior cesarean scar should be encouraged to attempt vaginal delivery by undergoing a trial of labor (TOL) (3).

In 1985, Leveno et al. (4) estimated that for every 100 women with prior cesarean scar who deliver vaginally, the cesarean section rate at the Parkland Hospital would fall by 1% (Fig. 2). Fortunately, as evidence for the safety of vaginal birth after cesarean (VBAC) mounted, the national rate of cesarean birth gradually declined from 24.7% in 1988 to 20.8% in 1995 (Table 1) (5). During this time, the frequency of VBAC has risen from 12.6% to 35.5%. While the national health objective for the year 2000 of a 35% VBAC rate had been met in 1995, the similar goal of 15% total cesarean and 12% primary cesarean rates are off target by 39% and 29%, respectively (2,5). The experience at Columbia Hospital for Women in Washington, DC, reflects these trends (Fig. 3).

BACKGROUND

Before the late nineteenth century, when antiseptic surgical technique and suturing of the uterine wound became common, too few mothers survived the cesarean delivery to even worry about subsequent pregnancies. Then, the fundal vertical or classic incision in the thick upper uterine segment was the most common way to deliver the baby (Fig. 4A) (6).

As maternal mortality from cesarean section decreased and patients became pregnant again, the question arose as to how to manage these subsequent deliveries. As early as 1903, Williams recognized the dangers of rupture of the previous uterine scar. At that time, uterine rupture was associated with a 50% to 75% maternal mortality and was invariably fatal to the fetus. Because of these conditions, Cragin's 1916 recommendation of "once a cesarean, always a cesarean" was well received (7). The cesarean section rate at the time was 1% to 2%, all using the classic uterine incision.

In contrast, as early as 1917, Williams thought that the fear of uterine rupture following cesarean section was greatly exaggerated. He argued that this complication occurred only if the uterus was not properly sutured or its healing was complicated by infection (6).

In 1921, because catastrophic rupture of the classic uterine incision occurred in 4% of patients, Kerr revived the use of the transverse lower uterine segment incision proposed by Kehrer in 1882 (Fig. 4B). The use of this incision rapidly gained in popularity and comprised 90% of uterine incisions in 1976 (6).

In subsequent pregnancies, a low transverse incision behaves differently than a classic one (Table 2) (8). The classic scar is more than four times as likely to rupture as is the low transverse scar. It also is more likely to rupture before labor, with sudden severe symptoms. Rupture of the classic incision carries a higher fetal and maternal mortality.

In 1957, after analyzing the British literature, Dewhurst (8) concluded that vaginal birth after a previous cesarean section could be undertaken with considerable safety. Indeed, "trial of scar" was common in Europe but rarely practiced in the United States or Canada.

To allow time for the lower uterine segment to develop, Riva and Teich (9) intentionally delayed repeat cesarean

D. J. Santos: Department of Anesthesiology, Columbia Hospital for Women, Washington, DC 20037.

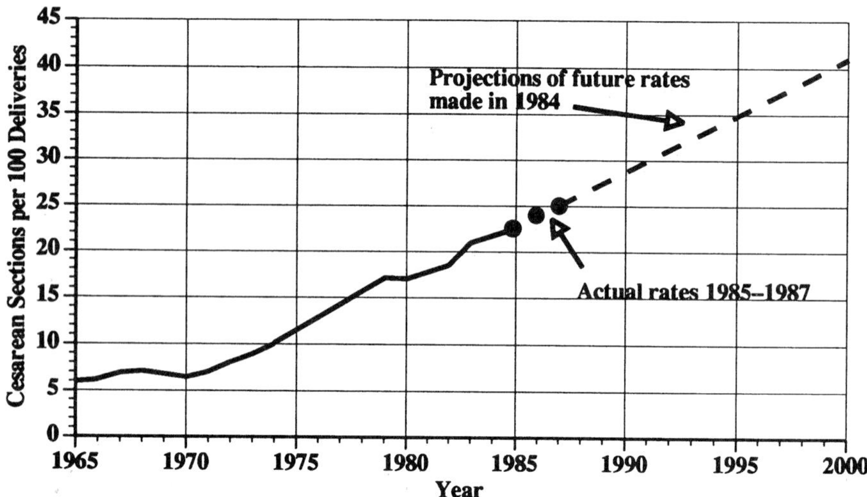

FIG. 1. Cesarean delivery rate in the United States, 1965 to 1987. *Dashed line* represents projected growth to the year 2000 if earlier trends had not abated. (Redrawn from ref. 1, with permission.)

section until after the onset of labor. In some patients, labor progressed rapidly to vaginal delivery before the repeat operation could be done. Because they found few uterine defects after delivery, by serendipity, the practice of deliberate TOL after previous cesarean section for selected patients began to evolve. From 1953 to 1960, 158 of 214 patients with prior uterine scar attempted vaginal delivery and 74% succeeded. These women awaited labor in the hospital for the last 2 weeks of their pregnancy. Neither uterine rupture nor maternal death occurred in the women who delivered vaginally.

In 1968, Sloan (10) asked a group of obstetricians if they would permit labor in patients with a previous low transverse cesarean scar if overwhelming evidence of the safety of such practice existed. Eighty percent said "No!" (10). Despite reports of the relative safety of VBAC, by 1978, 99% of eligible patients had an automatic repeat cesarean section (6).

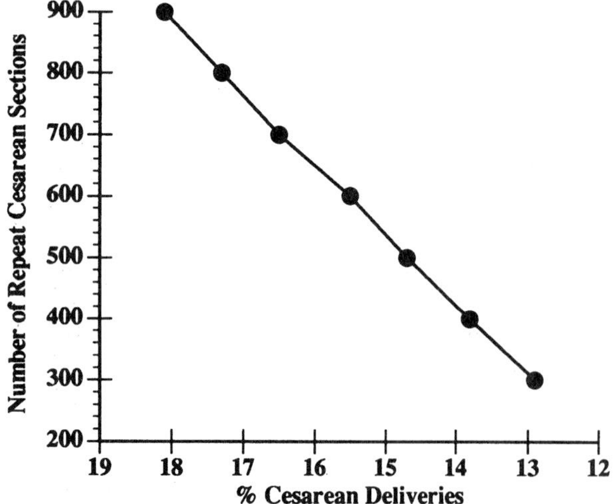

FIG. 2. Projected impact of increased vaginal births in patients with prior cesarean section on the overall cesarean section rate at Parkland Hospital in Houston. Projections are based on 1983 data. (Redrawn from ref. 4, with permission.)

Concerned about the rising cesarean delivery rate, the National Institutes of Health (NIH) Consensus Development Conference on Cesarean Section met in 1980. They recommended revoking the practice of automatic repeat cesarean section (11). The American College of Obstetricians and Gynecologists (ACOG) published and revised guidelines for VBAC in 1982 and in 1985. Despite these recommendations and reports of the low risk and successful outcomes of TOL, obstetricians in North America responded very slowly. While TOL increased fourfold, from 2.1% to 8% between 1979 and 1984, only a fraction of eligible gravidae were offered a choice other than automatic repeat cesarean section (12).

In October 1988, the ACOG Committee on Obstetrics: Maternal and Fetal Medicine (12) published "Guidelines for Vaginal Delivery After a Previous Cesarean Birth." They suggested that repeat cesarean section should no longer be automatic; instead, VBAC should be the norm. Any obstetric service should be able to do an emergency cesarean section within 30 minutes of making the decision and should be able to offer VBAC. The report emphasized the data collected in the previous 10 years and extolled the virtues and safety of a TOL.

An updated ACOG Committee Opinion was published in October 1994 (13). The available evidence regarding the relative safety of VBAC was compelling. The incidence of transverse lower uterine scar interruption was not increased by TOL. Symptomatic uterine rupture requiring

TABLE 1. *Changes in cesarean delivery in the United States*

Year	Total C/S rate	Primary C/S Rate	Repeat C/S	VBAC rate
1988	24.7%	17.5%	36.3%	12.6%
1993	22.8%	16.3%	36.5%	25.4%
1994	22.0%	15.9%		29.7%
1995	20.8%	15.5%		35.5%

C/S, cesarean section; VBAC, vaginal birth after cesarean. Data from refs. 2 and 5.

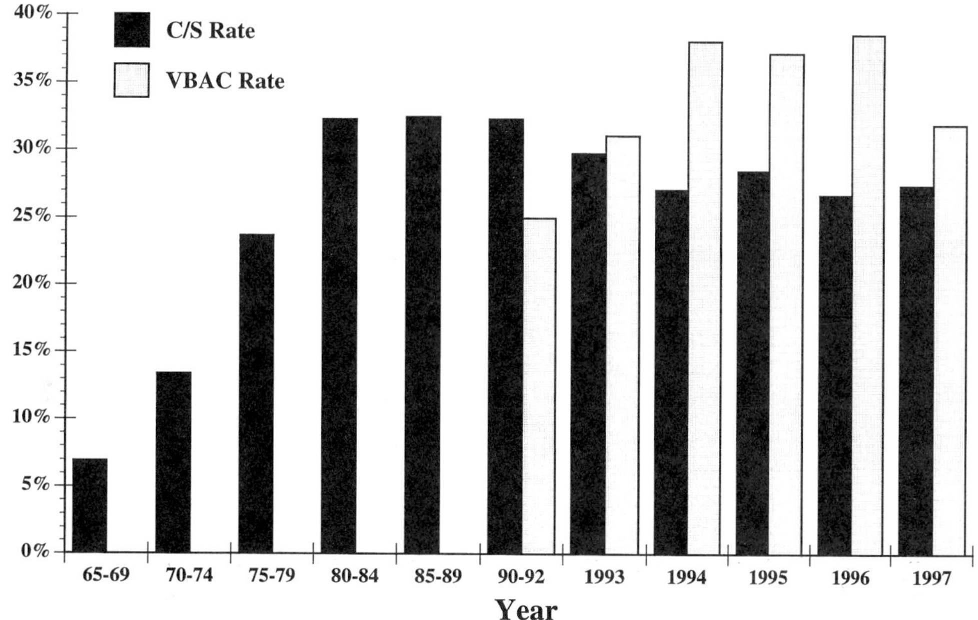

FIG. 3. Frequency of cesarean section (C/S) and vaginal birth after cesarean section (VBAC) at Columbia Hospital for Women in Washington, DC.

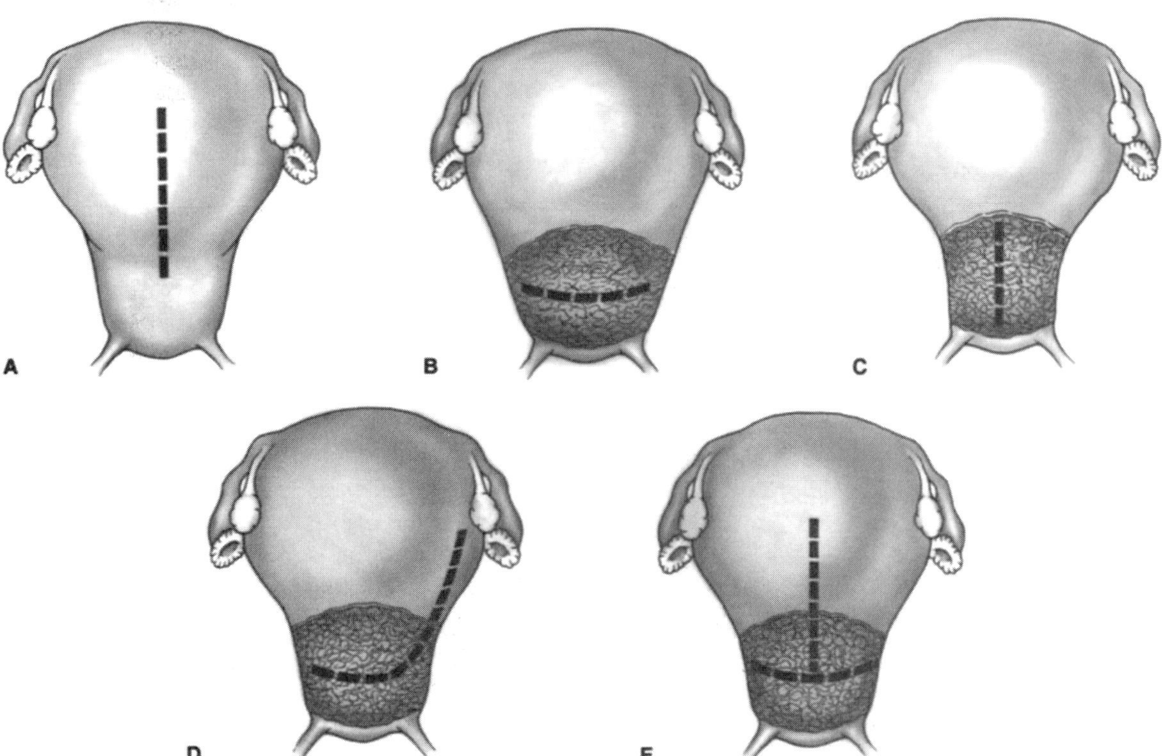

FIG. 4. Types of cesarean section scars: *A*, classic incision; *B*, transverse incision in the lower uterine segment; *C*, vertical incision in the lower uterine segment; *D*, "J" incision, extension of a low transverse incision curvilinearly into the upper uterine segment; *E*, "T" incision, a combined low transverse with a low vertical incision. (Courtesy Res Medica, St. John's Mercy Medical Center, St. Louis, MO.)

TABLE 2. *Differences in behavior of classic and low transverse scars*

	Classic scar	Low transverse scar
Incidence of rupture	2.2%	0.5%
Maternal mortality	5%	0%
Fetal mortality	73%	12.5%
Time of scar rupture		
Before labor	57%	24%
During labor	43%	76%
Clinical rupture before labor		
Symptomatic rupture	84%	18%
Incidental finding	16%	82%
Severity of symptoms		
No symptoms	13%	47%
Symptoms but no collapse	21%	43%
Collapse	66%	8%

Clinical features

Classic scar	Low transverse scar
Sudden severe pain	Pain may be absent
Contractions may cease	Contractions may continue
Abnormal uterine shape	Bulging lower uterine segment
Readily palpable fetus	Recession of fetal presenting part
Absent fetal heart tones	Fetal distress
Explosive, sudden collapse	Slower progression of symptoms,
Diffuse tenderness	suprapubic tenderness

Data from Dewhurst CJ. The ruptured cæsarean section scar. *J Obstet Gynæcol* 1957;64:113.

emergency operative intervention occurred in less than 1% of patients. Serious maternal and fetal consequences seemed to be minimized by appropriate intrapartum surveillance. Hospitals were encouraged to develop protocols for counseling and managing patients who attempt a TOL after a cesarean birth. In the absence of contraindication to vaginal delivery, a woman with one previous cesarean scar should be counseled and encouraged to undertake a TOL.

In 1995, ACOG published clinical practice guidelines under the heading of "ACOG Practice Patterns" (14), which were based on an extensive review and evaluation of the available literature on VBAC. The review gave priority to published studies involving more than 50 subjects. It categorized available data as follows:

I: Evidence obtained from at least one properly designed randomized controlled trial.

II-1: Evidence obtained from well-designed controlled trials without randomization.

II-2: Evidence obtained from well-designed cohort or case control analytic studies, preferably from more than one center or research group.

II-3: Evidence obtained from multiple time series with or without intervention. Dramatic results from uncontrolled experiments could also be regarded as this type of evidence.

III: Opinions of respected authorities, based on clinical experience, descriptive studies, or reports of expert committees.

Then, based on the highest level of evidence found in the literature, ACOG provided graded recommendations according to the following categories:

A. There is good evidence to support the recommendation.

B. There is fair evidence to support the recommendation.

C. There is insufficient evidence to support the recommendation; however, the recommendation can be made on other grounds.

For TOL and VBAC, ACOG made the following recommendations:

- *Success Rates of TOL*

Success rates for VBAC range from 60% to 80% (A:II-2).

- *Risks and Benefits*

The benefits of a TOL outweigh the risks (A:II-2).

- *Candidates for VBAC*

In the absence of contraindications, a woman with one previous low-segment transverse uterine incision is a candidate for VBAC and should be counseled and encouraged to undergo TOL (A:II-2).

A woman who has two or more previous low-segment transverse uterine incisions, who has no contraindications, and who desires TOL should not be discouraged from doing so (B:II-B).

When confronted with a pregnant patient with a previous uterine scar, the ACOG recommends a self-explanatory clinical pathway (Fig. 5).

- *Contraindications*

A previous classic uterine incision is a contraindication for TOL (C:III).

Epidural analgesia is not a contraindication for TOL (A:II-2).

Oxytocin use for induction or augmentation of labor is not contraindicated (B:II-3).

Suspicion of macrosomia in a nondiabetic should not disqualify the patient from attempting VBAC (B:II-2).

Available data are insufficient to determine the risks and benefits of TOL for patients with multiple gestation, breech presentation, or for use of prostaglandin gel (C:II-3;II-2).

- *Management of VBAC*

VBAC should not be limited to large subspecialty hospitals. Well-equipped basic and specialist hospitals with the capacity to respond to intrapartum emergencies can be appropriate settings for TOL (A:II-3) (14).

WHY DOES THE ANESTHESIOLOGIST NEED TO KNOW ABOUT VAGINAL BIRTH AFTER CESAREAN SECTION?

Today's patient is a well-informed consumer who can ask intelligent questions about health care. She questions the effect of epidural analgesia on the progress of labor, pushing efforts, and is aware of the literature suggesting that epidural analgesia, especially in early labor, may increase the incidence of cesarean section due to dystocia or failure to progress. The patient also may ask about the safety of epidural analgesia for TOL and the possibility of its masking the signs and symptoms of impending uterine rupture. The anesthesiologist should be well prepared to answer these questions.

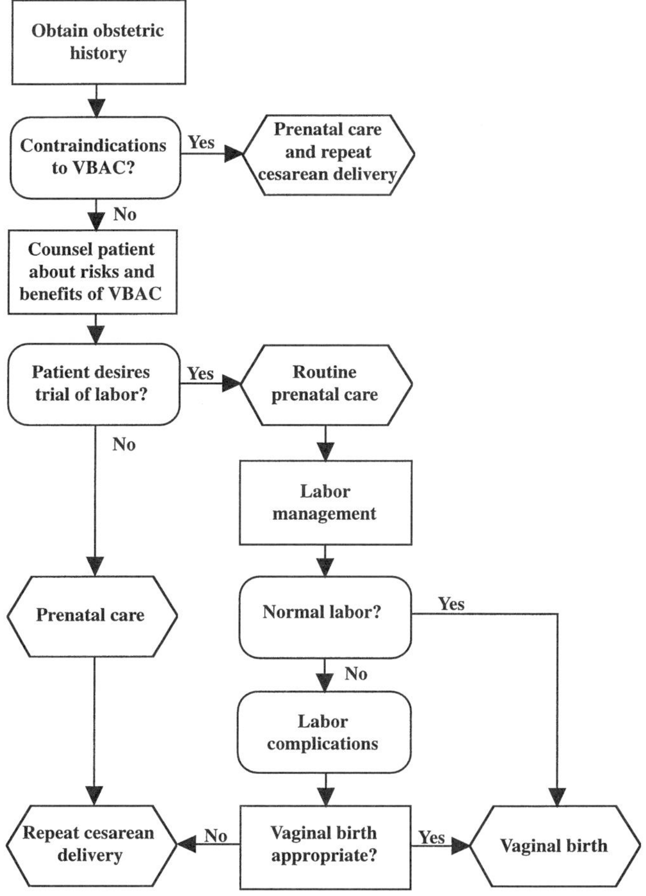

FIG. 5. Clinical algorithm for vaginal birth after cesarean delivery (VBAC). (Modified from ref. 14.)

In a labor suite, the anesthesiologist is often the first physician called upon to evaluate a patient's complaint of pain. In patients undergoing TOL, atypical pain may herald an obstetric complication rather than failure of the epidural catheter (15).

Fetal heart rate changes can follow the induction of neuraxial labor analgesia. These changes must be distinguished from those suggestive of uterine rupture. Early detection of impending uterine rupture requires a high index of suspicion. During TOL, a fetal bradycardia to 90 beats/min or less, lasting longer than 1 minute, is often the first warning of uterine rupture. When rupture occurs, every minute counts and the infant must be delivered immediately. A large study on uterine rupture related to VBAC found no significant perinatal morbidity when the fetus was delivered within 17 minutes (7).

Knowledge of available data about the risks, benefits, safety, and dangers associated with labor following a previous cesarean section should enable the clinician to confidently care for the patient attempting VBAC (15). Attempting VBAC is low risk, but clearly not risk-free. Uterine rupture can complicate 0.5% to 0.8% of cases. Prompt intervention usually results in good maternal outcome. However, hysterectomy due to irreparable uterine rupture may be required in 1 of 2,000 TOL. Despite electronic fetal monitoring and careful observation, rupture-related birth asphyxia with neurological sequelae may occur in 1 of 5,000 TOL. These rare and serious complications must be weighed against the maternal and neonatal complications associated with repeat cesarean delivery. The 125 to 200 elective repeat cesarean sections that would have to be performed to avoid one uterine rupture also are not risk-free. "The only definitive way to eliminate these risks is to avoid the operation that originally scars the uterus. This point must be considered when pondering the decision to perform the *first* cesarean" (16).

The physician and other health care providers must examine their own knowledge and beliefs toward VBAC and cesarean birth because patients are sensitive to the verbal and nonverbal cues given to them. Health care providers are the most influential source of information for both VBAC and repeat cesarean section (17). They must be prepared to provide accurate information. The ACOG 1995 Practice Patterns (see previous) can serve as a useful guide (14).

Ninety percent of patients consider themselves the primary decision maker about the method of delivery after a previous cesarean section. By the fourth month of the current pregnancy, 70% of patients who will attempt VBAC have made that decision, whereas only 42% of patients who will have an elective repeat cesarean section have made up their minds. Thirty-six percent of patients make their decision on VBAC before they get pregnant again, whereas patients rarely choose to have a repeat cesarean section before the current pregnancy. With preparation, knowledge of options, and realistic expectations, a positive outlook can lay the groundwork for a satisfactory experience with either VBAC or repeat cesarean. Childbirth classes for couples desiring VBAC need to address those concerns that differ from the ones encountered in the conventional prepared childbirth series (18).

The integration process after birth can be longer and more difficult after cesarean section compared with vaginal delivery. Childbirth is a developmental crisis. Cesarean birth, especially when it occurs unexpectedly, creates a situational crisis for a woman already under stress. The combination of developmental and situational crises may overwhelm the patient and delay the resolution of her feelings for months or years. Unresolved feelings related to the primary cesarean delivery may interfere with the psychological well-being during a subsequent pregnancy (17). The patient's unresolved emotional reactions to a prior cesarean section often cause grief and negative feelings (19), which must be addressed, preferably before or early in a subsequent pregnancy to reduce anxiety and promote well-being. Anxiety can inhibit oxytocin release (17,19) and increase release of catecholamines. Both effects may slow labor.

Patients and obstetricians also may express concerns about the effects of labor epidural analgesia on the progress of labor and the need for cesarean delivery (see Chapter 18). The obstetric anesthesiologist should be cognizant of these issues and able to participate in reasoned discussions with patients and other health care providers. Patients contemplating VBAC who have questions or concerns about earlier anesthetic experiences should seek early consultation to relieve anxiety and apprehension.

Collected studies from 1950 to 1985 show that 60% to 80% of patients with a single previous cesarean section can deliver vaginally (20,21). Patients with two or more prior cesarean sections can achieve up to 69% VBAC rate (21). Attempted VBAC will have a high rate of success regardless of the indication for the original operation (Table 3) (21). It appears that, given a chance, almost four of five patients can deliver vaginally and avoid repeat cesarean birth. By adopting a liberal VBAC program, a group of university obstetricians successfully reduced their repeat cesarean section rate by 54% (20). At the University of Chicago, routine VBAC stabilized the cesarean delivery rate at 16% to 17% between 1985 and 1988, despite a continuing increase in the primary cesarean rate. In 1982, women with a previous cesarean delivery were ten times as likely to deliver abdominally after a previous cesarean birth. By 1988, the relative risk of repeat cesarean section had fallen to five times that of nonoperated women (22).

During the past 8 years, VBAC at Kaiser Hospitals increased from 36% to 70%. Several of the participating medical centers have adopted a policy of performing repeat cesarean sections only for specific medical indications and over 80% of patients have a TOL (16).

TABLE 3. *Success of vaginal delivery following cesarean section and the original indications for cesarean section*

Indication for prior cesarean section	Trial of labor	Vaginal delivery
Cephalopelvic disproportion/ failure to progress	774	509 (66%)
Fetal distress	317	238 (75%)
Breech	467	391 (84%)
Other	584	426 (73%)

Modified from Davies JA, Spencer JAD. Trial of scar. *Br J Hosp Med* 1988;40:379, with permission.

A TOL after cesarean section should be encouraged in virtually all women who are willing to attempt it, regardless of the indication for the prior operation, provided that there is no contraindication to a vaginal birth (23).

BENEFITS OF VAGINAL BIRTH AFTER CESAREAN

Maternal

The practice of allowing patients to attempt VBAC offers many distinct advantages over automatic repeat cesarean section (Table 4). It is safer for the mother. Women are five to ten times more likely to die after cesarean than vaginal birth (24,25). Patients delivering abdominally are more likely to die of sepsis, pulmonary embolism, hemorrhage, and complications from anesthesia. On the other hand, there has been no reported maternal death from uterine rupture during VBAC in more than 11,000 patients over the past 30 years (3).

Women who fail VBAC have good chance of developing infection, but their risk is no more than women undergoing primary cesarean section in labor. Because about 70% of VBAC patients succeed in delivering vaginally, the total febrile morbidity of VBAC patients is lower than patients delivering by elective repeat cesarean section (26,27). Endometritis and urinary tract infection are the usual causes of fever in the puerperium. Febrile morbidity is 10.8 times more common following cesarean section than vaginal delivery (23). VBAC avoids operative complications (13), such as injury to vital organs, blood transfusions, anesthetic complications, postoperative adhesions, and wound infections (25). Patients delivering vaginally experience less discomfort and require less analgesia and nursing care (28). They also recover more quickly, care for their infants, and return to work sooner (29). The hospital stay is 2 to 3 days shorter (26). The psychological benefits of shared labor and delivery experience for the patient and her spouse are immeasurable (17). Fetal–maternal bonding is more readily established (27,30).

Shunning elective repeat cesarean section saves from $2,000 to $3,000 per delivery (31,32); avoiding 200,000 elective repeat procedures would save approximately

TABLE 4. *Maternal benefits of vaginal birth after cesarean*

Maternal benefits (reference)	Vaginal delivery	Cesarean section
Maternal mortality	1.7/10,000 0–2.7/100,000	10.8/10,000[24] 0–10/100,000[25]
Febrile morbidity (24,26,27)	0.6%–3.6%	27%–35% (1° C/S) 13%–18% (Repeat C/S)
Overall morbidity (24)	3.2%	48% (1° C/S) 27% (Repeat C/S)
Discomfort (28)	Less	More
Recovery (29)	Quicker	Slower
Hospital stay (26,31)	1–3 days	5–6 days
Cost (32,33)	Less	$2,000–$3,000 more
Number of pregnancies (35)	No limit	More limited

Overall morbidity includes endometritis, mastitis, thrombophlebitis, infected wound, peritonitis, septicemia, pyelonephritis, urinary retention, oliguria/anuria, thrombosis/emboli, psychosis, respiratory diseases, abdominal wound dehiscence, postspinal symptoms, and neurological events.
C/S, cesarean section; 1° C/S, primary cesarean section.

$600,000,000! (33,34). About 1.2 million hospital days could be saved if half the nearly 1 million women undergoing repeat cesarean section could have delivered vaginally (34). In emerging countries with large families, successful VBAC allows the patient to have more pregnancies (35). Even a failed VBAC ending in repeat abdominal delivery offers the advantage of shorter operating time compared to elective repeat cesarean section (36).

Fetal

Vaginal delivery avoids certain fetal risks associated with cesarean section (Table 5) (37). Elective cesarean section increases the risk of iatrogenic prematurity and neonatal respiratory morbidity (38). In the term newborn, the absence of labor before abdominal delivery can result in the syndrome of transient tachypnea or "neonatal wet lung." Final fetal lung adaptation to extrauterine respiration may require a few hours of labor (37,38). Transient tachypnea may require admission to the intensive care nursery (39). Occasionally, this syndrome leads to pulmonary hypertension (40). Of 12 cases of persistent pulmonary hypertension in one report, only two had any labor. Unexplained respiratory distress occurred in four infants by 1 hour of age and in the rest by 8 hours. By 12 hours, all infants required mechanical ventilation. Three of 12 infants died (40). The absence of labor may prevent fluid reabsorption, lung maturation, and surfactant release (40).

TABLE 5. *Fetal risks from cesarean delivery*

Fetal asphyxia due to anesthesia or maternal supine hypotension
Increased neonatal respiratory morbidity due to:
Iatrogenic prematurity
Transient tachypnea of the newborn or "wet lung"
Persistent pulmonary hypertension
Accidental fetal scalpel lacerations
Uterine rupture and abnormalities of placentation with subsequent pregnancies

Accidental scalpel lacerations can occur when the lower uterine segment thins and the surgeon is relatively inexperienced (37,41). Subsequent pregnancies in patients with previous cesarean section present high risk to the fetus owing to the likelihood of abnormal placentation or possible catastrophic uterine rupture (37).

RISK OF VAGINAL BIRTH AFTER CESAREAN

Uterine Rupture

The danger of rupture of a previous uterine scar is the greatest concern when considering TOL and VBAC. There are two types of uterine rupture (Table 2).

Complete or true rupture involves the entire thickness of the uterine wall, usually with extrusion of uterine contents. Symptoms occur suddenly and explosively. There usually is pain, hemorrhage, shock, and significant fetal and maternal morbidity and mortality. A classic uterine scar usually splits this way. The unscarred uterus also may suffer true rupture following trauma. Complete rupture is rarely seen in low transverse uterine scars (33).

Incomplete uterine rupture does not involve the entire thickness of the uterine wall; there usually is overlying peritoneum, which prevents extraperitoneal extrusion. There may be extension to the retroperitoneum or broad ligament (22,33). Because there frequently is no associated bleeding or extrusion of uterine contents, symptoms may be absent, atypical, or nonspecific. Except when diagnosis is markedly delayed, fetal and material morbidity or mortality are rare. This is the usual type of uterine rupture seen in the low transverse uterine scar. Synonyms include occult, silent, window, or dehiscence (33).

The risk of uterine rupture depends largely on the location of the uterine scar. A classic incision is a vertical cut in the thicker, more contractile upper uterine segment (Fig. 4A). Classic cesarean section rarely is performed today (specific indications can include anterior placenta previa, transverse lie with the fetal back down, or dense scarring in the lower uterine segment) (41).

Most uterine incisions (90%) are transverse in the passive, less contractile lower uterine segment (Fig. 4B). This portion of the uterus is thinner, less vascular, and only becomes fully formed during labor. Uterine contractions originate from a "pacemaker" region near the uterotubal junctions. The muscle fibers of the myometrium are uniquely arranged in a spiral fashion from the outer layer inward and from the fundus toward the lower uterine segment. Such an arrangement pulls on the circumferentially arranged muscles of the lower uterine segment. The contracting upper portion of the uterus thickens after each contraction because the muscle fibers do not relax to their original length. To maintain normal tension, the lower uterine segment thins and expands as it is pulled upward. Meanwhile, it becomes distended as the presenting part of the fetus is pushed toward the birth canal (42). This gradual stretching may explain why the transverse lower uterine scar is more prone to dehisce rather than to complete rupture. In addition, peritoneal signs may be absent because the loose bladder peritoneum covering the lower uterine segment prevents peritoneal soiling during uterine rupture (43).

If the lower uterine segment is not well developed, the obstetrician may choose to do a low vertical incision (Fig. 4C). Because the incision may not remain confined in the lower uterine segment, a low vertical scar may rupture more often than the transverse scar.

The "J" (Fig. 4D) incision also may be more prone to rupture than the uncomplicated low transverse scar because the incision extends into the thicker upper segment. The "T" (Fig. 4E) could be a dangerous incision, because a weak junction is created where the low transverse meets the low vertical incision.

Uterine rupture also can occur in the intact or unscarred uterus, before or during labor. Most ruptures of the intact uterus follow accidents, traumatic obstetric maneuvers (i.e, version and extraction, forceps delivery), obstructed labor, or oxytocin use in the grand multipara. Following rupture of the intact uterus, maternal mortality is 14% and fetal mortality is 76%. In contrast, fetal mortality falls to 35% and maternal death rarely occurs with rupture of previous cesarean scars (44).

The most common cause of uterine rupture is reportedly the separation of prior cesarean section scar (45). However, a review of reports of uterine rupture during pregnancy shows that 70% occurred in the unscarred uterus (Table 6) (45–47). Shy et al. (48) estimated 73 uterine ruptures during labor per 10,000 planned VBACs. Although uterine rupture and dehiscence of the transverse scar do occur during TOL, this complication does not present a greater risk of maternal or fetal mortality than elective repeat cesarean section (29,48).

VBAC is not completely risk-free. Chazotte and Cohen (49) presented 17 cases of catastrophic complications in patients with one or more cesarean section scars. These complications included:

- Fetal or maternal death,
- Hemorrhage requiring transfusion of 5 U or more of blood,
- Hysterectomy or major artery ligation, and
- Uterine rupture requiring emergent surgery, associated with fetal extrusion or neonatal depression.

Ten of 17 cases involved a low-segment transverse scar (four after preterm primary cesarean section). Six cases involved an unknown type of scar, and one involved a vertical scar. Eight patients had more than one scar. Twelve infants were born preterm; eight required admission to the neonatal intensive care unit. Two mothers died. One suffered intractable hemorrhage from placenta previa/percreta. The other succumbed to pulmonary embolism 4 weeks after cesarean hysterectomy.

There were three fetal deaths. Two died after uterine rupture with fetal extrusion. One infant, at 22 weeks of gestation, died of exsanguinating maternal hemorrhage from a placenta previa. These maternal and fetal deaths were not related to TOL.

Serious hemorrhage occurred in 11 patients, resulting in eight hysterectomies. Of seven elective repeat cesarean sections, five had placenta previa with varying degrees of accreta. In three patients, uterine rupture caused the hemorrhage. Only two of the hemorrhages occurred during VBAC.

TABLE 6. *Incidence of rupture of the pregnant uterus*

		Scarred uterus			
Year	Total ruptures	Vertical	Low transverse	Other	Intact Uterus
1976	335	10	50	15	260
1978	47	15	9	1	22
1979	15	2	5	0	8
1980	93	6	23	3	61
1983	23	8	4	2	9
1986	24	3	2	0	19
1987	15	1	6	9	8
Total	552	45 (8%)	99 (18%)	21 (4%)	387 (70%)

Data from refs. 44, 46, 47.

Nine of 17 patients had serious uterine rupture. Five of the ruptures were associated with VBAC (1.4% of patients allowed a TOL). Three of five patients who had a rupture during labor received oxytocin. In one rupture, the fetus, and in another, the umbilical cord, extruded through the rupture. One fetus was severely depressed after rupture of unknown scar in a patient with severe preeclampsia, late decelerations, and clinical diagnosis of abruptio placentae. All three patients who received epidural anesthesia complained of pain. All five low transverse scar ruptures were repaired.

Rupture of the low transverse scar is not always benign. Scott (50) reports 14 serious uterine ruptures during the TOL: three from the University of Utah, and nine from four community hospitals in Salt Lake City. These ruptures were symptomatic and endangered the life of the fetus or mother

Ten of these patients had spontaneous labor, whereas two patients were induced at 38 and 42 weeks. Oxytocin was used in four patients and epidural anesthesia in three. Fetal distress was seen in nine (64%) cases. Four patients had surgery less than 1 hour after admission to the hospital. Six patients (43%) experienced abdominal pain. Three patients (21%) had vaginal bleeding. Three patients had recession of the presenting part. At laparotomy, there was partial to complete extrusion through the uterine rupture in nine patients. The estimated blood loss was 1,000 to 4,000 mL, with four patients requiring blood transfusion. There was one hysterectomy and one internal iliac ligation. Thirteen cases were amenable to repair of the uterine rupture.

Six infants were severely depressed at birth. There were three perinatal deaths, all of which occurred when the fetal monitor tracing was not under direct observation of the physician. One infant was severely damaged owing to delay in diagnosis of uterine rupture with fetal extrusion. One infant died within 1 year after suffering severe perinatal asphyxia and neurological damage. Another infant continues to show neurological damage.

Jones et al. (51) also reported eight cases of rupture of the low-segment scar during TOL (Table 7). These cases occurred in five hospitals in the Denver metropolitan area over a 13-month period. All patients had electronic fetal monitoring, and seven patients had an intrauterine pressure catheter. All but one patient (case 2) received oxytocin: four for induction (three had earlier cervical ripening with prostaglandin E_2 and three for augmentation). There were two instances of uterine hyperstimulation. Of four who received both epidural anesthesia and oxytocin, two experienced pain during rupture. The diagnosis of uterine rupture was not always immediately apparent. Four patients had severe variable decelerations before the fetal head receded. The most frequent finding was sudden deterioration of the fetal heart rate tracing. Recession of the fetal head (50%) and suprapubic bulging were associated with pain or suprapubic tenderness. All eight parturients underwent emergency exploratory laparotomy. Rupture of the uterus was an incidental finding at surgery in two patients. Uterine repair was possible in seven. Three cases of bladder perforation were repaired. Estimated blood loss ranged from minimal to 1,900 mL. There was one neonatal death due to fetal extrusion and abruptio placentae. Two infants with perinatal asphyxia were normal at discharge. Although the use of oxytocin during VBAC is safe, this study serves as a reminder that it may not be used with impunity. Oxytocin must be carefully titrated, and any evidence of fetal distress must be viewed with a high index of suspicion.

Risk factors associated with uterine rupture during TOL were studied by Leung et al. (52). Excessive oxytocin, dysfunctional labor (primarily active-phase arrest disorders, failure of dilation and descent), and history of two or more cesarean sections were associated with increased risk of rupture. Epidural anesthesia, macrosomia, history of previous vaginal delivery after cesarean section, unknown uterine scar, and prior cesarean section for cephalopelvic disproportion (CPD) were not associated with uterine rupture (52).

Diagnosis of Uterine Rupture

Because of its rarity and protean manifestations, early diagnosis of uterine rupture is not easy. The clinician

TABLE 7. *Details of eight uterine ruptures during trial of labor*

Case No.	Weeks Gestation	OB management	Fetal findings (extrusion)	Apgar scores	UA pH	Outcome
1	37	PGE_2 oxy, epid	Head	8/9	—	Normal
2	37	Expectant (three previous C/S)	Complete	7/9	7.2,4	Normal
3	41	Oxy, epidural	Head	8/8	—	Normal
4	41	Oxy induction	Head	1/2	6.7,6	Asphyxia, normal
5	40	PGE_2, oxy ind	Complete	1/3	6.9,0	Asphyxia, normal
6	40	Oxy aug, epid	Complete	0/0	—	Neonatal death
7	40	Oxy aug, epid	Umbilical cord	2/7	7.1,5	Normal
8	41	PGE_2, oxy ind	Head and shoulder	8/9	7.1,4	Normal

Aug, augmentation; epid, epidural anesthesia; ind, induction; oxy, oxytocin; PGE_2, prostaglandin E_2.
Data from ref. 51.

must maintain a high index of suspicion in any patient with a uterine scar. The few premonitory signs may be indistinguishable from the normal aches, pains, and "bloody show" of labor. The classic symptoms of uterine rupture arise in only 17% of cases (Table 8) (46). Even when suprapubic pain is present, uterine rupture was confirmed at operation in only one of 20 cases (53).

Abdominal pain is an inconsistent finding that is neither sensitive nor specific (46,54–56). If present, pain usually is described as severe suprapubic shearing or tearing (57,58). Some physicians fear that epidural labor analgesia may mask the pain of uterine rupture. However, there is a growing consensus that this apprehension is not valid (3,59–61). Properly administered labor epidural analgesia will allow the patients to perceive the so-called "breakthrough pain" associated with abruptio placenta or complete uterine rupture (60,62).

A case reported by Eckstein et al. (15) illustrates how the pain of uterine rupture can "break through" analgesic concentrations of epidural local anesthetics. This woman received epidural labor analgesia with 10 mL of 2% 2-chloroprocaine. Another 6 mL of 2% 2-chloroprocaine 30 minutes later maintained satisfactory analgesia. However, 15 minutes after this dose, the patient became restless and complained of diffuse abdominal pain, which was exaggerated during uterine contractions. Her vital signs were stable. The catheter was repositioned, and she was given two additional 8-mL injections of 2% 2-chloroprocaine without relief despite absence of sensation to pinprick. Labor progressed quickly. When the cervix was completely dilated, the fetal heart rate slowed repeatedly and mid forceps extraction was performed. The newborn had Apgar scores of 6 and 9 at 1 and 5 minutes, respectively. Following spontaneous placental delivery, the patient became hypotensive and unresponsive. Uterine exploration revealed a defect at the old uterine scar that was confirmed at laparotomy. Other authors have reported similar cases (63,64).

Pain is not always present in uterine rupture. The clinical manifestations of uterine rupture depend on:

- Location of the rupture,
- Completeness of the tear,
- Degree of hemorrhage (58), and
- Presence of communication with the peritoneal cavity (15).

TABLE 8. *Signs and symptoms of uterine rupture of the gravid uterus (scarred or unscarred)*

Signs and symptoms of uterine rupture	Incidence
Pain	0 to 50%–80%
Fetal distress	50%–75%
Vaginal bleeding	17%–67%
Recession of presenting part	25%–50%
Shock	0%–50%
Readily palpable fetal parts	17%
Peritoneal signs	17%

Complete ruptures that communicate with the peritoneal cavity can extrude blood and other irritants intraabdominally. Subsequent irritation of the diaphragm can cause referred shoulder pain. Complete ruptures may be sudden and explosive, associated with severe pain and shock. Incomplete ruptures may develop more gradually. The pain may be less intense, with abdominal tenderness instead of cardiovascular collapse. If blood distends the broad ligament, the pain may be felt down the leg. If the bleeding is retroperitoneal, the patient may complain of back pain and there may not be peritoneal signs. Pain resulting from uterine rupture may resemble that associated with bladder perforation during urologic procedures under regional anesthesia. The urologic patient usually complains of sudden abdominal pain, which may be diffuse or localized in the paraumbilical, suprapubic, or epigastric region; occasionally it is referred to the shoulder or precordium. The anesthesiologist may be the first physician to diagnose uterine rupture provided that unusual pain is recognized as a symptom of obstetric complication rather than a failure of an epidural block (15).

Fetal distress signals uterine rupture in 20% to 60% of monitored patients (50,51,56). There may be fetal bradycardia or severe variable decelerations. Baseline intrauterine pressure rises progressively up to 35 mm Hg in association with severe variable decelerations (Fig. 6) (65). Or a sudden loss of uterine tone may accompany fetal heart rate changes (Fig. 7) (66). When pain, vaginal bleeding, and fetal distress are present, abruptio placentae is a more common diagnosis than uterine rupture. Placental abruption and uterine rupture can coexist, as sudden uterine decompression with rupture can extrude its contents. Recession of the fetal presenting part, readily palpable fetal parts, peritoneal signs, and shock are late signs (50).

Treatment of Uterine Rupture

Early diagnosis is the key to minimizing maternal and fetal morbidity and mortality. Resuscitation of the mother must start simultaneously with preparations for immediate surgical intervention. Procrastination may be devastating: 13 of 20 patients with uterine rupture associated with severe hemorrhage died when treated medically. Shock does not contraindicate surgery when intraperitoneal hemorrhage is suspected (67). Repair of the uterine rent should be the operative goal, especially if the woman desires future pregnancy or if she is hemodynamically unstable. However, if hemostasis cannot be achieved by internal iliac ligation, hysterectomy should be done. Total hysterectomy is preferred if the patient can tolerate the procedure; otherwise, subtotal hysterectomy should suffice (68).

Fetal outcome depends largely on the timeliness of the operation. As soon as the diagnosis of uterine rupture is suspected, it is important to proceed with cesarean

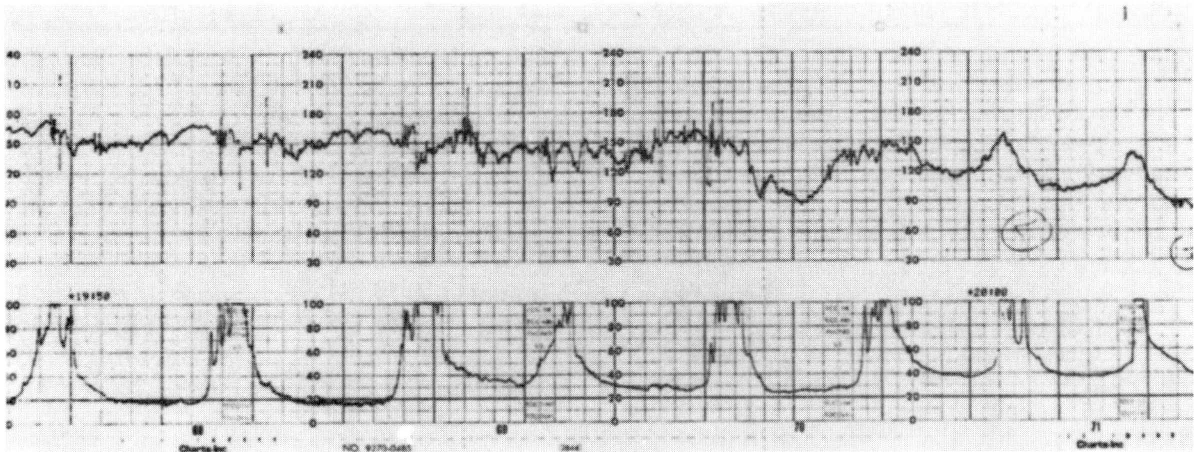

FIG. 6. The monitor tracing shows fetal heart rate decelerations associated with an increase in intrauterine pressure of up to 35 to 40 mm Hg in a patient with uterine rupture during a trial of labor. (Reprinted from ref. 65, with permission.)

section immediately. No infants had significant perinatal morbidity when delivered within 17 minutes of the onset of prolonged bradycardia (7).

Failed Vaginal Birth after Cesarean

Patients who fail a TOL have higher likelihood of febrile morbidity following repeat cesarean section compared with women who have an elective operation. This risk is greater than that seen in patients undergoing primary cesarean section during labor (14). Indications for repeat cesarean section in these patients include arrest disorders or failure to progress (72%) and fetal distress (15%) (14). Despite the failure and accompanying disappointment, most patients do not seem to regret having tried to delivery vaginally (69,70).

Increased Perineal Lacerations

The risk of significant perineal lacerations in VBAC patients who delivered spontaneously was higher than in control group of nulliparae (18% vs 13%) (71). The incidence of lacerations increased when babies weighed more than 3,600 g.

Fetal Risk

For patients awaiting labor, Gibbs (27) and Phelan et al. (26) have reported a few cases of unexplained stillbirth

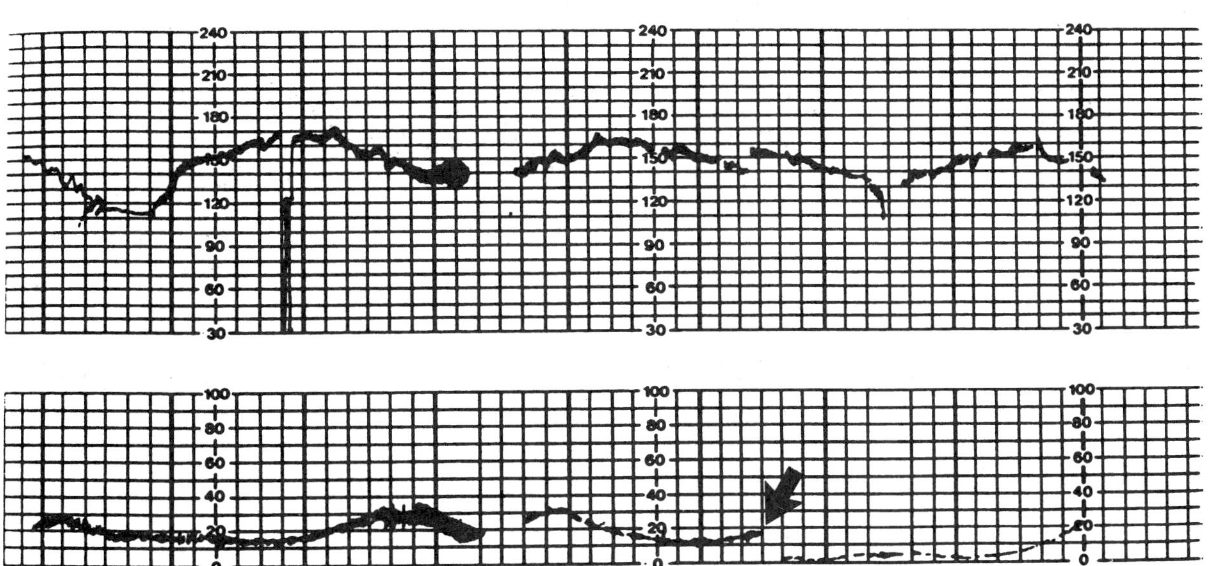

FIG. 7. Monitor tracing of a patient with uterine rupture of a low transverse scar during trial of labor. There are late decelerations of the fetal heart associated with an abrupt decrease in intrauterine pressure indicated by the *arrow*. (Reprinted from ref. 66, with permission.)

after 38 weeks of gestation that might have been averted by an elective repeat cesarean section. Whether the VBAC patient is at greater risk for late fetal demise than her unscarred counterpart is unknown. Nevertheless, Phelan et al. (26) recommend routine antepartum fetal surveillance beginning at or around 38 weeks of gestation.

Although the low transverse scar is more likely to dehisce than rupture, delayed diagnosis of complete rupture is associated with poor perinatal outcome. In one series of eight cases of uterine rupture of the low-segment transverse incision, there was one neonatal death and two cases of severe perinatal asphyxia (51). Scott (50) presented two stillbirths, two neonatal deaths, and three severely depressed infants (two have persistent neurologic deficits) in 14 VBAC patients.

Medicolegal Risks

Patients are increasingly aware of the option of VBAC from a variety of sources. Some women choose a particular physician or hospital because of the availability of this alternative. Review of the operative note and counseling must begin early in the pregnancy. Analysis, perception, and acceptance of risk must be faced by patients and obstetricians alike (72).

Medicolegal problems can arise if there is an adverse result from TOL. Scott (50) mentions that litigation has been initiated in four cases of uterine rupture with poor perinatal outcome. All cases he presented appear to have followed the ACOG guidelines. The media coverage regarding VBAC may be partly responsible for the cavalier attitude of a few patients. One patient at 43 weeks of gestation tried to deliver at home with a lay midwife; this resulted in fetal death from uterine rupture. The patient claimed that she had read that VBAC was safe (50). It is important to involve the patient actively in the decision process. She must be aware that there are risks associated with both VBAC and repeat cesarean section. The mere presence of a prior scar puts her at a higher risk for uterine rupture. The patient must be aware of the risk and behavior of the different types of uterine scars. As patients seek greater control of their health care, they also must begin to assume some of the responsibilities. For instance, she should know the details of her prior operation, keep a copy of the operative report, obtain early and regular prenatal care, be familiar with the signs of labor, and promptly report anything unusual.

Obstetricians and courts have questioned the ACOG guideline suggesting that only 30 minutes pass from decision to delivery (7). In one case, the court considered this ACOG "30-minute rule" to mean the maximum time, and it ruled that delivery within 30 minutes may not be adequate in certain situations (7). Because of this verdict, Flamm (7) proposed that the consent form for VBAC include the statement: "I understand that if my uterus ruptures during my VBAC, there may not be sufficient time to operate and prevent the death or permanent brain injury to my baby." Clearly, few women would sign such a form (7).

At least one major malpractice insurance company (Cooperative of American Physicians, Inc., Mutual Protection Trust) has incorporated a modification of the proposed statement in the consent form they want their members to use. An additional statement is included that the risk of fetal death or permanent infant brain damage may be as high as 50% after uterine rupture. In addition, the patient is required to initial the following statement: "maternal risks of uterine rupture include, though not limited to, hysterectomy, blood transfusion, injury to internal organs (bowel, bladder, ureter), blood coagulation problems and death." Risks for elective repeat cesarean are not listed (7).

Although thousands of patients have undergone VBAC with generally good outcomes, most published experience took place in hospitals where obstetricians, anesthesiologists, and operating room personnel were immediately available and could perform "crash" cesarean sections within 10 to 15 minutes. In many obstetric suites, this response time from the onset of ominous fetal heart tracing to delivery may be impossible. Although patients can be referred to centers with immediate cesarean capabilities, it does not seem logical to mandate such referrals (7).

Predicting the Integrity of the Uterine Scar

When considering VBAC, it would be helpful to know if there are defects in uterine scar. Michaels et al. (73) used ultrasound to prospectively study 70 patients with a low-segment scar and compared them to 12 nulliparous controls. They found a 21% incidence of scar defects that were confirmed at repeat cesarean section. It appears that the optimum time to study the lower uterine segment is between 26 and 36 weeks. At this time, the lower uterine segment has begun to develop, the presenting part is not too deep in the pelvis, and amniotic fluid volume is still copious.

Rozenberg et al. (74) conducted ultrasonographic measurement of the lower uterine segment of 642 patients with a history of previous cesarean section. The ultrasound examination was carried out transabdominally at 35 to 38 weeks' gestation. The lowest value measured was used to describe the thickness of the lower uterine segment. The obstetrician then assessed the status of the uterine scar at the time of cesarean section or by digital palpation after vaginal delivery. There were 15 (2.5%) uterine ruptures and 10 (1.5%) uterine dehiscences. Two infants died: one was dead on arrival to the hospital due to uterine rupture at home. One distressed fetus died despite emergency cesarean. The thickness of the lower uterine segment ranged from 1.9 to 12.3 mm. The proportion of defects rose with decreasing thickness. In the

3.6- to 4.5-mm group of 177 patients, there were two dehiscences and one rupture; in the 2.6- to 3.5-mm group of 136 patients, there were five dehiscences and nine ruptures; and in the 1.6- to 2.5-mm group of 51 patients, there were three dehiscences and five ruptures. Using the cutoff point of 3.5 mm or less as pathologic, the authors found that 71% of patients were at low risk for uterine rupture. This threshold value allows excellent sensitivity (88%) and negative predictive value (99.3%). The positive predictive value of the study was low, suggesting that all thin uterine segments are not abnormal. On the other hand, the strong negative predictive value confirms that a thick lower uterine segment usually is strong.

Another more direct method to assess the integrity of a uterine scar before TOL is by use of a fiberscope (75). In this study, patients with an anterior placenta on ultrasound examination were excluded. In late pregnancy or early labor, after spontaneous or artificial rupture of membranes, a sterilized fiberscope was introduced into the uterine cavity to visualize the lower uterine segment. The fiberscope was 65 cm long, 5.8 cm thick, and had an angle of vision of 75 degrees. Insertion, similar to inserting an intrauterine pressure catheter, was tolerated by patients without anesthesia. The procedure lasted less than 15 minutes. At endoscopy, the presumed scar site in 45 patients was indistinguishable from the rest of the lower uterine segment. Forty-one of these patients delivered spontaneously, and all had competent scars on postpartum manual exploration; one patient had a repeat cesarean for fetal distress and the lower uterine scar was intact. Seven women had abnormal endoscopic findings. Four patients whose scar was unknown had a vertical scar from the lower to the upper uterine segment. Two had dehiscence of two-thirds of the transverse scar with bleeding edges and visualization of loops of small bowel. One had a large "window" in the central portion of the transverse scar. None of these patients had any clinical signs of uterine rupture. All seven had repeat cesarean section, at which time the endoscopic findings were confirmed (75,76).

OBSTETRIC CONSIDERATIONS FOR VAGINAL BIRTH AFTER CESAREAN SECTION

In October 1994, the ACOG published its Committee Opinion on "Vaginal Delivery After a Previous Cesarean Birth" (13), in which it noted that the success rate of VBAC was 60% to 80%. Moreover, nearly 70% of patients with a primary cesarean delivery for CPD could deliver vaginally. Each hospital was encouraged to develop its own protocol for counseling and managing patients who attempt TOL. The protocol should include the following:

- Women with one previous cesarean scar, in the absence of contraindication to vaginal delivery, should be counseled and encouraged to undergo TOL.
- Those with more than one uterine scar who wish to attempt VBAC and in whom no contraindication to vaginal birth exists should not be discouraged.
- Reasonable effort must be made to document the type of uterine incision during the primary cesarean, but, if unsuccessful, clinical judgment can be used as to the advisability of permitting TOL. Bear in mind, however, that although classic cesarean sections rarely are performed today, it may still be used in certain geographic areas and for extreme prematurity or transverse line.
- A previous low vertical scar and an estimated fetal weight greater than 4,000 g are not contraindications to TOL.
- TOL should occur in a hospital setting where trained professionals can respond to acute intrapartum emergencies.
- A physician capable of evaluating labor and performing a cesarean section should be readily available.
- Patients need not be restricted to a labor bed until they are in active labor.
- Oxytocin is contraindicated in patients with a classic uterine scar. The use of oxytocin for augmentation of labor does not appear to increase the risks in patients undergoing a TOL or to increase perinatal mortality. Less is known about the safety of oxytocin for induction of labor in this population, including the use of prostaglandin gel for cervical ripening. However, judicious use of these agents appears safe.
- Epidural analgesia does not decrease the likelihood of success of TOL, neither does it delay the diagnosis of uterine rupture in patients undergoing VBAC. The primary signs of uterine rupture, including abrupt change in the fetal heart tracing, uterine activity or pressure; vaginal bleeding; or loss of fetal station, can be detected despite diminution of the patient's ability to perceive pain. The availability and use of epidural analgesia may encourage more women to attempt TOL (13).

Predicting the Success of a Trial of Labor

Many authors have attempted to predict successful VBAC in specific patients. In 1986, Thurnau et al. (77) introduced the concept of fetal–pelvic index as a way to identify fetal–pelvic disproportion. This method compares fetal head and abdominal circumference (passenger) obtained by ultrasound with the respective maternal pelvic inlet and mid-pelvic circumference (passage) measured by standard x-ray pelvimetry. Despite four reports from this group showing good predictive value, fetal–pelvic index has not gained in popularity.

Troyer and Parisi (78) developed a scoring system to predict success of VBAC based on an analysis of their experience in Houston, Texas. They found their overall success of TOL was 72.7%. One or more of the following parameters decreased the likelihood of success: previous dysfunctional labor, no prior vaginal delivery, nonreassuring fetal heart rate tracing on admission, and labor induction.

Weinstein et al. (79) also proposed a scoring system for the prediction of successful VBAC. The maximum score is 12, which gives an estimated success rate for VBAC equal to or greater than 88%.

More recently, Flamm and Geiger (80) prospectively evaluated a scoring system based on admission characteristics (Table 9). This admission VBAC scoring system may help in the counseling of patients who are vacillating about whether or not to proceed with TOL. The higher the score, the better the chances of success (Table 10).

Use of Oxytocin for Induction or Augmentation of Labor

Some investigators fear that use of oxytocin increases the risk of uterine rupture during TOL. There seems to be no reason to believe that a given uterine pressure achieved by oxytocin administration is any more dangerous to the uterine scar than the same pressure produced during natural labor. A uterus strong enough to withstand spontaneous labor should be able to withstand a properly induced labor as well (33). In properly selected cases, with careful surveillance and precisely controlled administration, the use of oxytocin for induction or augmentation of labor in patient with a prior low-segment cesarean section appears safe (81,82). As is true in any patient with dysfunctional labor, if oxytocin is required to augment labor, the incidence of repeat operative delivery increases (65,82). In studies in which oxytocin was withheld because of fear of uterine rupture, the success rate for vaginal delivery was lower than in those studies in which oxytocin was used to treat uterine inertia (57,62,66,70, 81,83–86). More recent studies find no difference in success rates in patients with or without oxytocin (57,83). This trend may suggest increased confidence in the safety of oxytocin in these patients. There does appear to be a difference in successful outcome when using oxytocin for induction (58%) compared to using it for augmentation of labor (88%) (87).

Multiple Prior Cesarean Section Scars

The success rate of VBAC in women after multiple previous cesarean deliveries varies between 45% and 81%. The largest available study of 501 patients reported a 69% success rate (88). Thirty percent of patients received epidural analgesia without problems. The number of previous scars did not affect the dehiscence rate. The VBAC group had a 1.8% dehiscence rate versus 4.6% in patients undergoing elective repeat cesarean section (89). Even patients with more than one previous cesarean section can safely and often successfully attempt VBAC (Table 11) (9,57,88,90–97).

Previous Low-segment Vertical Incision

The incidence of rupture of the low vertical scar is 1.3% compared to 2.2% for the classic and 0.7% for the low transverse scar (98). Most studies exclude patients that have this scar (57). However, available data suggest that VBAC is safe in patients with one or more low vertical scars (27,66,91,92,99,100).

Unknown Type of Uterine Scar

VBAC in women with an unknown uterine scar is a highly controversial issue. At the Women's Hospital in Los Angeles County, Beall et al. (101) could document the type of uterine scar in only 48% of their patients. Ninety-two percent had a low transverse scar, and 8% had vertical scars. There was no difference in the success of VBAC in patients with unknown and low transverse scars

TABLE 9. *Admission characteristics and assigned score points predicting successful vaginal birth after cesarean (score development group)*

Characteristic	β Coefficient	Odds ratio	95% CI	Score points[a]
Age under 40 years	0.95	2.58	1.5–4.3	2
Vaginal birth history				
Before and after first cesarean section	2.21	9.11	2.18–38.04	4
After first cesarean section	1.22	3.39	2.25–5.11	2
Before first cesarean section	0.43	1.53	1.12–2.10	1
None	Referent			0
Reason other than FTP for first cesarean section	0.66	1.93	1.58–2.35	1
Cervical effacement at admission				
>75%	1.00	2.72	2.00–3.71	2
25%–75%	0.58	1.79	1.31–2.44	1
<25%	Referent			0
Cervical dilation 4 cm or more at admission	0.77	2.16	1.66–2.82	1

CI, confidence interval; FTP, failure to progress.
[a]Select one value, which may be zero, from each of the five categories.
From ref. 80.

TABLE 10. *Performance of admission score*

Score	Score, development group		Score, testing group	
	Number with score	% VBAC	Number with score	%VBAC
0–2	120	41.7	114	49.1
3	346	59.2	329	59.9
4	605	64.3	595	66.7
5	664	79.1	660	77.0
6	354	87.6	360	88.6
7	183	93.4	189	92.6
8–10	142	99.3	158	94.9
Total	**2,414**	**74.2%**	**2,405**	**74.9%**

VBAC, vaginal birth after cesarean.
From ref. 80.

(86% vs 72%). Pruett et al. (95) found more unknown uterine incisions (76%) in their patients at Jefferson Davis Hospital in Houston, Texas. VBAC succeeded in 62% of patients with unknown scars and 52% of patients with low transverse scars. The uterine dehiscence rate was 3.4% for the low transverse and 2.6% for the unknown scars (95). Oxytocin was used in about 35% of patients in both series. A total of 397 patients with unknown uterine scars from both studies attempted VBAC. The authors concluded that patients with an unknown uterine scar can attempt labor without risk to them or the fetus, provided intensive maternal and fetal monitoring are carried out and facilities are available to perform emergency operation.

Previous Cesarean Section for Failure to Progress

Patients with a history of cesarean section for failure to progress or CPD should not be automatically excluded from considering a TOL. Sixty-eight percent of these women can deliver vaginally (102). Two studies (82,98) of a total of 208 patients showed no significant difference in the success rate of TOL if the primary cesarean section was done for arrest of labor in the latent, active, or second stage of labor. Nor did there appear to be a relationship between the maximum cervical dilatation obtained in the earlier labor and the likelihood of success in achieving vaginal delivery in the subsequent delivery.

Others, however, have found a much higher failure rate in patients who got to complete cervical dilatation before the original cesarean delivery. In a recent study, only 13% of these women delivered vaginally (103). In this retrospective review of 1,917 patients, the original indications for cesarean delivery included arrest disorders (80%), fetal distress (14.9%), and malpresentation (5.1%). The overall success of VBAC was 63.6% and did not differ if the initial cesarean section was for fetal distress, malpresentation, or arrest of labor at ≤9 cm cervical dilation. But, only 13% of women whose primary cesarean section was performed by arrest of labor at 10-cm cervical dilation had a subsequent vaginal delivery (103).

Macrosomic Fetus

Some investigators recommend cesarean delivery for macrosomic (more than 4,000 g) infants to avoid traumatic birth injuries, including shoulder dystocia (104). There is even greater concern about delivering these babies in the presence of uterine scar. Phelan et al. (105) attempted VBAC in 140 patients whose babies were esti-

TABLE 11. *Success rate of trial of labor in patients with two or more low segment transverse scars*

Authors (reference)	Year	Vaginal Delivery (n)	Vaginal Delivery (%)	Repeat cesarean section (n)	Repeat cesarean section (%)	Total (n)
Riva and Teich (9)	1961	50	66	26	34	76
Saldana et al. (90)	1979	22	58	16	42	38
Martin et al. (91)	1983	12	63	7	37	19
Porreco and Meier (92)	1983	17	81	4	19	21
Farmakides et al. (93)	1987	44	77	13	33	57
Pruett et al. (95)	1988	25	45	30	55	55
Phelan et al. (88)	1989	346	69	155	31	501
Novas et al. (94)	1989	29	80	7	20	36
Flamm et al. (57)	1990	1376	75	451	25	1827
Asakura and Myers (97)	1995	194	64	108	36	302
Total		**2,115**	**72%**	**817**	**28%**	**2,932**

mated to weigh more than 4,000 g. Sixty-seven percent delivered vaginally. Eighty-three percent of women whose babies weighed less than 4,000 g had a successful VBAC. Patients who had an intervening vaginal delivery after the first cesarean section and did not have the primary cesarean section for CPD were more likely to succeed. Eighty-nine percent of babies delivered spontaneously. The most serious complication was shoulder dystocia, which occurred in three patients (3.2%). In patients without a uterine scar, the frequency of shoulder dystocia is quoted as 1.7% for babies weighing more than 4,000 g and 10% for babies weighing more than 4,500 g (42). Ollendorf et al. (106) achieved an 81% successful VBAC rate when infants weighed less than 4,000 g but only 40% if the infant weighed more than 4,000 g. Flamm and Goings (107) studied a total of 301 macrosomic babies. Fifty-eight percent and 43% of babies weighing between 4,000 and 4,499 g and more than 4,500 g, respectively, were delivered vaginally (107).

Postterm Pregnancy

Seven to 12% of pregnancies are postterm (more than 42 weeks' gestation) (108). The fetal dangers associated with prolonged pregnancy include oligohydramnios and possible cord accidents, macrosomia and birth trauma, meconium passage and aspiration, placental insufficiency, perinatal hypoxia, and death (109). Elective repeat cesarean section, usually scheduled shortly after completion of 38 weeks, theoretically should avoid these problems. MacKenzie (110) induced labor in 143 postterm patients who wanted to attempt VBAC with vaginal prostaglandins and achieved a 76% success rate. This series included 77 patients with unfavorable cervix, 68% of whom delivered vaginally. Meehan (111) induced 38% of his postterm VBAC patients with good success. Yeh et al. (112) followed 78 postterm patients who attempted VBAC and reported 73% success rate with no increase in morbidity.

Multiple Gestation

Gravidae with twin gestations and previous cesarean section generally are excluded from attempting VBAC because of concern that the uterus may not withstand the stress of overdistention. However, Strong et al. (113) reported a 72% success rate in 25 patients who tried to deliver vaginally. The dehiscence rate of 4% was twice that seen in singleton pregnancies. The authors concluded that TOL is reasonable in properly motivated and monitored patients.

Breech Presentation

The incidence of cesarean delivery for breech presentation has increased fourfold, from 22% in 1963 to 94% in 1978, with no perceptible improvement in fetal outcome (114). The increased number of cesarean sections done for breech presentation has increased maternal operative morbidity (115). Ophir et al. (116) studied patients with a uterine scar and breech presentation in the current pregnancy. Of the 47 patients who chose TOL, 79% delivered vaginally without an increase in neonatal morbidity. A smaller study of 13 patients reported 48% vaginal deliveries, also with no increase in fetal or maternal morbidity (117). Vaginal birth seems reasonable in carefully selected cases of breech presentation after a previous cesarean section.

One of the proposed methods of decreasing cesarean sections in the presence of breech presentation is to attempt external cephalic version near term (118). Flamm et al. (119) performed external cephalic version in 56 patients with a uterine scar. Version attempts were successful in 82% of patients, 65% of whom went on to deliver vaginally. They conclude that external cephalic version is a reasonable option in patients with prior low transverse scar.

ANESTHETIC CONSIDERATIONS

The anesthesiologist must be involved in the formulation of the hospital protocol for patients planning a TOL after previous cesarean section. When planning the anesthetic for these women, consider a variety of issues.

What Is the Incidence of Emergent Cesarean Section in Patients Attempting Vaginal Birth after Cesarean?

Finley and Gibbs (120) studied this question by reviewing their 5-year experience with 1,156 patients electing a TOL after cesarean delivery. Eighteen patients required emergent operation (1.56%). This rate did not differ from patients laboring without a uterine scar (Table 12).

In another group of 751 women attempting VBAC, 7 (0.9%) needed emergent cesarean section. In contrast, 2 of 458 (0.4%) patients who were planning an elective repeat cesarean section required emergent abdominal delivery for fetal distress (121).

What Is the Risk of Epidural Labor Analgesia in Vaginal Birth after Cesarean Patients?

A previous cesarean section is not a contraindication to the use of epidural labor analgesia. However, some worry that labor epidural analgesia may mask pain and delay diagnosis of uterine rupture. Maternal hypotension and compensatory tachycardia caused by hemorrhage from uterine rupture may be mistaken for sympathetic blockade. Another possible hazard is the reduced ability of these women to vasoconstrict in the presence of hypovolemia. In addition, the cessation of uterine contractions

TABLE 12. *Emergent cesarean section during trial of labor*

Preoperative diagnosis	n	Percent of VBAC patients (n = 1,156)	General incidence (%)
Uterine scar complication	3	0.26	
Abruptio placenta	3	0.26	0.49–1.3
Cord prolapse	4	0.35	0.2–0.5
Fetal distress	8	0.69	0.32–1.9
Total	18	1.56	

Data from ref. 120.

after fetal extrusion may be misinterpreted as the temporary decrease in uterine activity sometimes seen after induction of epidural analgesia.

Table 13 compiles the results of 21 studies in which epidural analgesia was used during TOL. Among the 13,408 patients attempting VBAC, 2,504 received epidural labor analgesia. The incidence of uterine rupture for the entire group was 0.37%.

Table 14 compares the clinical presentation of uterine rupture in 14 patients with and 29 without labor epidural analgesia (131). Abdominal pain alone (19%) was not a prominent symptom. Fetal distress alone (51%) was the most common symptom. The incidence of uterine rupture was higher in the group receiving epidural labor analgesia (0.76% vs 0.28%), but the presenting symptoms did not differ between the two groups. Nineteen percent received both epidural analgesia and a uterine stimulant (18 oxytocin, one prostaglandin), 28% had oxytocin alone, and 34% received neither epidural analgesia nor oxytocin. Half of the patients with uterine rupture (47%) received some form of uterine stimulant.

The diagnosis of uterine rupture may be simplified in the presence of epidural analgesia. View any pain that "breaks through" a functioning epidural block with suspicion. At low anesthetic concentrations used to relieve labor pain, axons are exposed to just slightly more than minimal blocking concentration of drug. More intense stimuli, such as uterine rupture, abruptio placentae, or acute bladder distention, can provoke an impulse that may be conducted through the "blocked" segment of the axon. Crawford (60) called this phenomenon "epidural sieve." Similarly, peritoneal irritation from blood or amniotic fluid underneath the diaphragm can cause referred pain in the shoulder. A recent case report described a patient who complained of shoulder pain after epidural injection of 2% lidocaine for cesarean section. Complete uterine rupture was found at operation (61).

When providing epidural analgesia during a TOL, limit the concentration and dose of the local anesthesia to maintain analgesic levels not much above T_{10}. A small amount of opioid may further decrease the dose of local anesthetic (125). Establish good bilateral neural blockade. Monitor the anesthetic level frequently. Continuous epidural infusion allows the maintenance of analgesia. The level of sensory blockade usually can be rapidly extended if immediate operative intervention is required. Three percent 2-chloroprocaine or 2% lidocaine are equally useful for this purpose.

TABLE 13. *Trial of labor and epidural analgesia*

Study	Year	Total	Epidural (n)	No epidural (n)	Ruptured uterus (n)	Ruptured uterus (%)
Carlsson et al. (62)	1980	119	77	42	2	1.7
Demianczuk et al. (122)	1982	92	41	51	2	2.2
Meier and Porreco (70)	1982	207	19	188	0	0
Martin et al. (91)	1983	717	98	619	3	0.42
Uppington (125)	1983	222	71	151	4	1.8
Rudick et al. (126)	1984	115	115	0	1	0.87
Flamm et al. (85)	1984	230	73	157	0	0
Horenstein et al. (81)	1985	732	0	732	2	0.27
Stovall et al. (66)	1987	272	153	119	1	0.37
Molloy et al. (83)	1987	1,781	85	1,696	8	0.45
Phelan et al. (26)	1987	1,796	178	1,618	5	0.28
Flamm et al. (3)	1988	1,776	181	1,595	3	0.17
Ollendorf et al. (106)	1988	229	64	165	1	0.4
Meehan et al. (127)	1989	1,498	187	1,311	4	0.27
Meehan and Magani (55)	1989	1,350	345	1,005	6	0.44
Nielsen et al. (56)	1989	1,008	205	803	6	0.6
Veridiano et al. (130)	1989	194	30	164	0	0
Sakala et al. (128)	1991	237	87	150	0	0
Johnson et al. (129)	1991	110	51	59	2	1.8
Chelmow and Laros (123)	1992	510	293	217	0	0
Hanley et al. (124)	1996	213	151	62	0	0
Total		**13,408**	**2,504**	**10,904**	**50**	**0.37%**

TABLE 14. *Presenting signs and symptoms of uterine rupture during trial of labor in women with and without epidural blockade*

Presenting signs and symptoms of rupture	No. of ruptures	Epidural anaglesia (n = 1,828)	No epidural analgesia (n = 10,147)
Abdominal pain	8 (19%)	3 (21%)	5 (17%)
Fetal distress	22 (51%)	7 (50%)	15 (52%)
Incidental finding at cesarean section	3 (7%)	1 (2%)	2 (5%)
Fetal distress and abdominal pain	6 (14%)	2 (14%)	4 (14%)
Postpartum bleeding	4 (9%)	1 (7%)	3 (10%)
Total rupture incidence	43	14 (0.76%)	29 (0.28%)

Modified from ref. 131, with permission.

Tehan (63) recently raised the possibility that addition of fentanyl to bupivacaine may abolish the "epidural sieve" and delay the diagnosis of uterine rupture. In this report, a patient's repeated complaints of atypical pain were treated with intermittent injections of 0.25% bupivacaine and occasionally fentanyl. Eventually, persistent fetal bradycardia, irregular uterine contour, and bloody amniotic fluid prompted delivery by forceps after another ineffective dose of 0.25% bupivacaine. Delivery was followed by brisk postpartum hemorrhage and shock. At laparotomy, complete rupture of the lower uterine segment scar with right lateral extension was found and repaired. The baby, weighing 3,200 g, had Apgar scores of 1 and 1 at 1 and 5 minutes, respectively, and died after several days. Here, the use of epidural fentanyl did *not* mask the signs of uterine rupture. Instead, these signs were ignored.

Does the Use of Epidural Anesthesia Decrease the Likelihood of Successful Vaginal Birth after Cesarean?

Stovall et al. (66) noted a 25.5% repeat cesarean section rate in patients receiving epidural labor analgesia compared to 14.3% in unmedicated patients. Of the 39 patients who received epidural labor analgesia and subsequently required a repeat section, 28 (72%) had history of labor dystocia in their primary cesarean section. Twenty-three of these same 28 patients (82%) were given oxytocin during the TOL. Epidural analgesia correlated with the use of oxytocin. Seventy-seven percent of patients receiving oxytocin (103 of 133) also used epidural labor analgesia. In contrast, only 36% (50 of 136) patients not receiving oxytocin received epidural labor analgesia. The estimated risk of cesarean section in patients receiving both oxytocin and epidural labor analgesia was 31% compared with 14% in patients who received only epidural labor analgesia (66). Sakala et al. (128) reported similar findings in 87 patients who received epidural block for labor analgesia and 150 patients who did not. When the oxytocin subjects were excluded from the data analysis, both epidural and nonepidural groups had the same high rates of successful outcome (94% and 92%) and spontaneous vaginal delivery (70% and 76%) (85).

Does Sitting for Induction of Epidural Analgesia Increase Risk of Uterine Rupture?

Golan et al. (68) reported five cases of uterine rupture (four intact, one scarred) occurring during epidural placement in the sitting position. Plauche et al. (44) also reported two cases of uterine rupture of low transverse scar under similar circumstances. Both groups of investigators suggest that the uterus may have ruptured because of marked increase in intraabdominal pressure caused by acute anteflexion of the torso. It is difficult to imagine that sitting could cause a greater rise in intraabdominal pressure than the same degree of flexion in the lateral decubitus position.

CASE REPORTS

Uterine rupture in a patient with previous cesarean section can present in many different ways. The following are illustrative cases.

Case 1

A woman with no prenatal care presented with the complaint of abdominal pain. On examination, she was noted to be about 32 weeks pregnant, with a mid-line suprapubic scar, abdominal tenderness, and absent fetal heart tones. She admitted a previous cesarean section for placenta previa but did not know the type of scar. On admission, blood pressure was 105/70 and pulse was 96 per minute. While evaluation progressed, her vital signs deteriorated. An exploratory laparotomy was performed under general anesthesia. A stillborn fetus AND placenta inside intact membranes floating free in the abdomen (Fig. 8) and completely ruptured classical scar (Fig. 9) were found. Although this patient was not attempting VBAC, this case underscores the dangers of a cesarean section scar. A classical scar usually ruptures catastrophically before the onset of labor. A lower uterine scar can rupture similarly, albeit less frequently (D. Santos and R. Lachica, unpublished data, 1988).

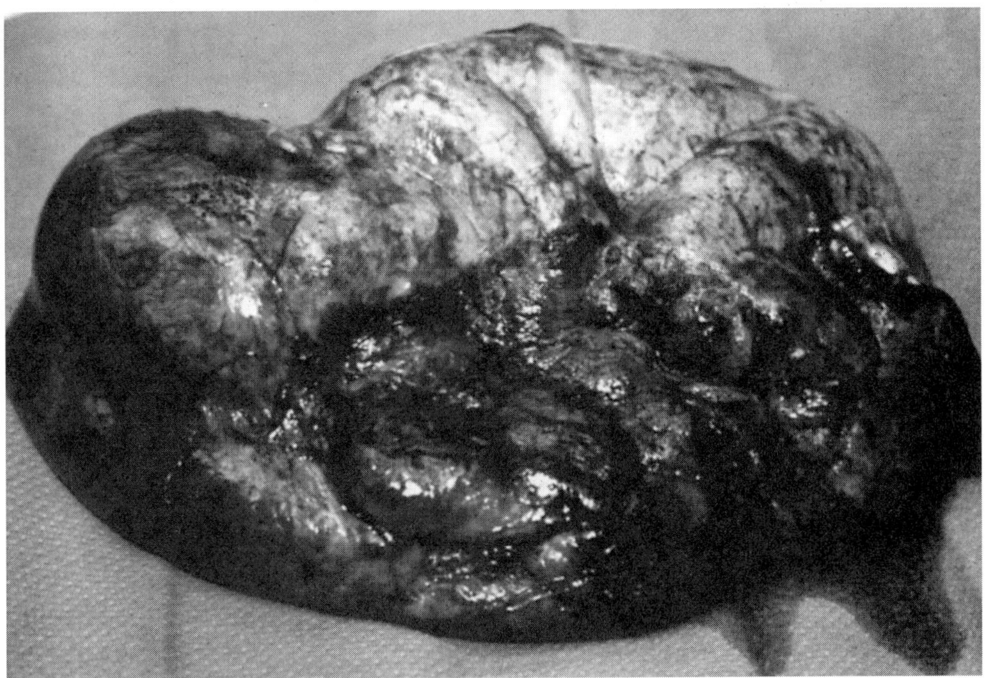

FIG. 8. A free-floating dead 32-week fetus complete with placenta inside an intact sac seen during exploratory laparotomy of a patient with an unknown uterine scar who developed deterioration of vital signs.

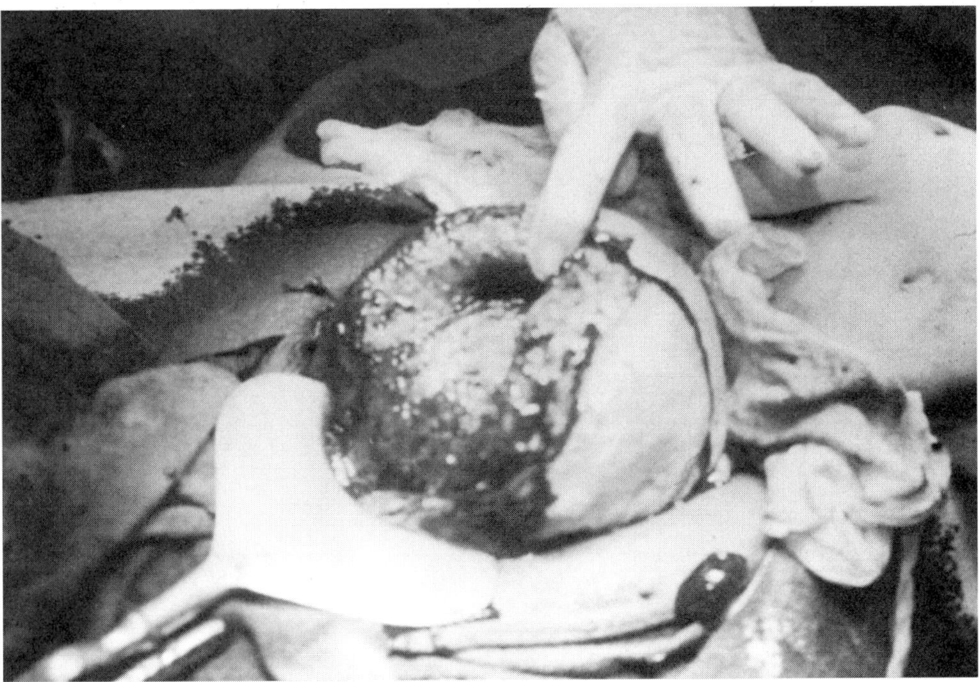

FIG. 9. Ruptured classic uterine scar.

Case 2

A gravida 2, para 1 patient with one previous low transverse cesarean section was attempting VBAC. At 4 cm of cervical dilation, she received epidural labor analgesia. A bilateral T_9 sensory level developed within 30 minutes of injection of 3 mL of 2% lidocaine and 10 mL of 0.25% bupivacaine. Analgesia was maintained with a continuous infusion of 0.125% bupivacaine at 10 mL/h. When the patient was comfortable, oxytocin augmentation was begun. After excellent labor analgesia for 4 hours, the patient suddenly complained of severe suprabupic pain. Anesthetic level to pinprick was T_{10} bilaterally. Severe variable fetal heart rate decelerations were noted. Because the cervix had not changed despite good uterine activity, a decision was made to proceed with a repeat cesarean section. The suprapubic pain lessened after administration of 18 mL of 2% lidocaine with 1:200,000 epinephrine. At cesarean section, a meconium-stained fetal elbow was seen protruding through the rupture low-segment scar. The bladder peritoneum was still intact. Apgar scores were 8 and 9 at 1 and 5 minutes, respectively. The uterus was repaired in the usual fashion. Both mother and baby did well. In this case, epidural labor analgesia did not mask the pain of uterine rupture. However, surgical anesthesia did (R. Lachica and C. Koh, personal communication, 1991).

Case 3

A 31-year-old gravida 2, para 1, with a history of low transverse cesarean section presented at 40+ weeks of gestation in early labor. Several hours after admission, membranes were ruptured artificially, and internal fetal and uterine pressure monitors were placed. Dilute oxytocin was administrated to improve labor pattern. Intermittent variable decelerations occurred. Epidural labor analgesia was initiated when the patient was 4 cm dilated. The cervix was completely dilated 6 hours after epidural placement. When the patient started to push, severe repetitive variable decelerations in fetal heart rate began (Fig. 10). She was given supplemental oxygen, and the vacuum extractor was used to deliver a 3,500-g baby with Apgar scores of 7 and 8 at 1 and 5 minutes, respectively. The anterior placenta was removed manually with no difficulty, and the lower uterine segment was noted to be intact.

Postpartum, the patient did well until 1.5 hours later, when her blood pressure fell to 90/60 mm Hg. The uterus was firm, and vaginal bleeding was minimal. Her blood pressure did not respond to fluid infusion. She had postural hypotension. Her abdomen was diffusely tender with rebound. Her hemoglobin and hematocrit dropped to 8.2 g/dL and 25.3%, from 11.9 g/dL and 36.3%, respectively. An exploratomy laparotomy was performed under general anesthesia. Upon entering the peritoneal cavity, about 500 mL of blood was seen coming from the completely ruptured lower segment transverse scar. The defect was repaired, and the hemostasis was secured. The patient did well postoperatively. This case emphasizes the need to continue to be vigilant into the postpartum period (D. Santos and C. Ahlering, unpublished data, 1992).

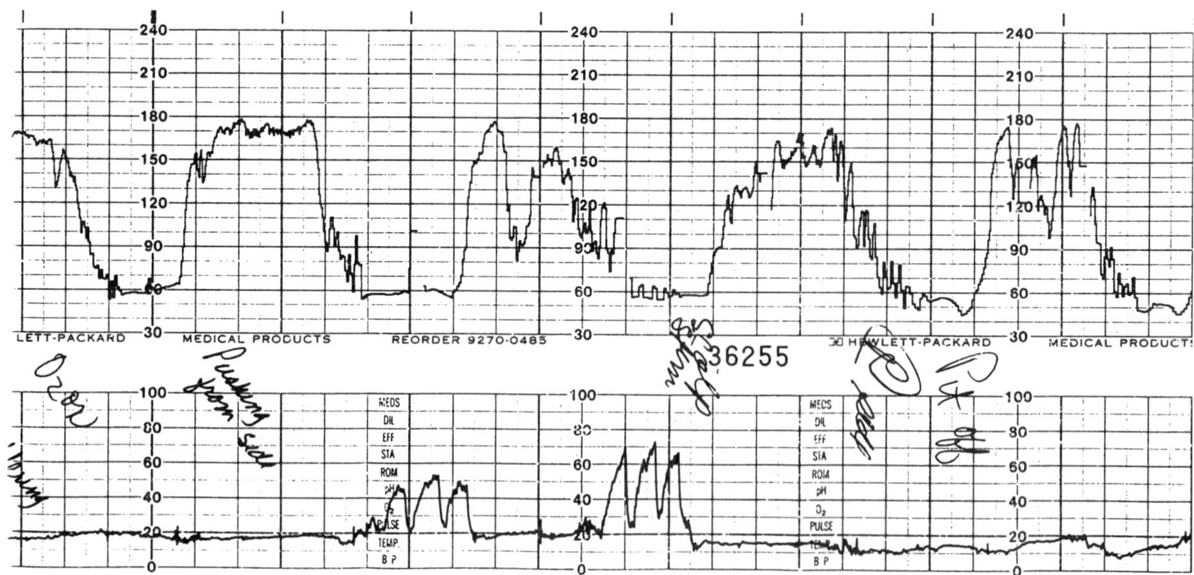

FIG. 10. Fetal and uterine monitor tracing just before vacuum-assisted delivery of a patient with a previous cesarean section undergoing a trial of labor. The fetal heart rate shows repetitive deep variable decelerations with quick return to the baseline and good beat-to-beat variability. There is no notable change in uterine tone. The infant's Apgar scores were 7 and 8 at 1 and 5 minutes, respectively.

TABLE 15. *Incidence of uterine rupture at Columbia Hospital for Women, Washington, DC, from 1991–1997*

Year	Ruptured uterus	Rupture with VBAC	VBAC rate (%)	Vaginal delivery after TOL	Repeat C/S
1991	4	0	15.8	114	608
1992	8	2	25.0	187	562
1993	4	3	31.1	239	529
1994	5	5	38.1	281	456
1995	4	1	37.2	263	444
1996	4	2	38.6	257	409
1997	5	3	31.9	165	352
Total	**34 (1.5%)**	**16 (0.7%)**	**40.4**	**2,277**	**3,360**

C/S, cesarean section; TOL, trial of labor; VBAC, vaginal birth after cesarean.

REVIEW OF VAGINAL BIRTH AFTER CESAREAN AND CASES OF UTERINE RUPTURE AT COLUMBIA HOSPITAL FOR WOMEN, WASHINGTON, DC

At Columbia Hospital for Women, VBAC began in the early 1980s. Data were collected from 1988, but formal analysis and yearly reporting did not start until 1990. The material presented comprises data from 1991 to 1997 (Table 15).

All charts that included the diagnosis of uterine rupture or dehiscence were reviewed for true uterine ruptures related to TOL. There were 15 complete ruptures. There was one serious rupture that must be considered incomplete by strict definition, because no uterine contents were extruded. [Different authors use different definitions of the various types of uterine rupture (8,11,31,43, 46,47). Differing definitions make it difficult to compare various reports.] The incidence of all types of uterine rupture was 1.5%. The incidence of complete rupture associated with TOL was 0.7%.

Of these 16 cases, two patients had a hysterectomy. Three patients received blood transfusion: one patient, whose uterus was repaired, received 4 U of blood; one patient who had a subtotal hysterectomy received 2 U; and a patient who had a modified radical hysterectomy and bladder repair received 23 U of blood and other blood products. Three patients required bladder repair. Two infants developed respiratory problems, one recovered completely but one of the infants continues to have difficulty. These cases emphasize the need for vigilance and caution in taking care of these patients, because transverse lower uterine segment scars *can rupture catastrophically*.

Further analysis show that four physicians had three uterine ruptures, whereas six physicians had two each. These physicians continue to allow patients to attempt VBAC but are very cautious.

All 16 patients received epidural labor analgesia. Three patients received epidural analgesia only, 10 patients received oxytocin, and three patients received oxytocin and prostaglandin (Table 16). Nearly all patients (87.5%) had a nonreassuring fetal heart tracing, and in almost all instances this was the primary or contributory diagnosis that led to the repeat cesarean section.

CONCLUSION

The literature about VBAC must be viewed in proper perspective. Most studies are nonrandomized and retrospective. They usually were conducted in teaching institutions with continuous obstetric and anesthesia coverage. The frequently quoted incidence of uterine rupture of 0.7% to 2.2% (44,46,47) is many times higher than the overall rate of rupture of both scarred and unscarred uteri. It is a mistake to think that VBAC patients are so low risk that they can be managed as if they did not have a uterine scar. The mere presence of a uterine scar places a woman at greater risk for uterine rupture than her unscarred counterpart. Low-segment incision scars are safer than scars after classic incision. The slower progress of the tear in a low-segment scar allows the clinician more time to make the diagnosis and act before catastrophe occurs. However, the signs and symptoms of rupture are less definite and may be atypical. Recent reports should serve as reminders that rupture of the low-segment scar may occur with serious consequences for the fetus and mother if the diagnosis is not made early and managed promptly (7,49–51).

TABLE 16. *Uterine rupture during trial of labor at Columbia Hospital For Women, Washington, DC, from 1991–1997, related to the use of epidural labor analgesia and uterine stimulants*

Presentation	Epidural analgesia	Epidural and oxy	Epid, oxy, PGE_2	Total
Severe fetal heart rate changes	2	10 (see also*)	2	14 (87.5%)
Failure to descend, suprapubic bulging			1	1 (6%)
Bronchospasm		1*		1 (6.%)
Uterine tetany and tenderness	1			1 (6%)
Vaginal bleeding		1*		1 (6%)

Oxy, oxytocin; PGE_2, prostaglandin E_2.

REFERENCES

1. Cesarean section in America: Dramatic trends, 1970 to 1987. *Stat Bull* 1989;70:2.
2. Clarke SC, Taffel S. Changes in cesarean delivery in the United States, 1988 and 1993. *Birth* 1995;22:63.
3. Flamm BL, Lim OW, Jones C, Fallon D, Newman LA, Mantis JK. Vaginal birth after cesarean section: results of multicenter study. *Am J Obstet Gynecol* 1988;158:1079.
4. Leveno KJ, Cunningham FG, Pritchard JA. Cesarean section: an answer to the House of Horne. *Am J Obstet Gynecol* 1985;153:838.
5. Curtin SC, Kozak LJ. Cesarean delivery rates in 1995 continue to decline in the United States. *Birth* 1997;24:194.
6. Enkin M. Labour and delivery following previous cesarean section. In: Chalmers I, Enkin M, Keirse MJNC, eds. *Effective care in pregnancy and childbirth.* Oxford: Oxford University Press, 1989:1196.
7. Flamm BL. Once a cesarean, always a controversy. *Obstet Gynecol* 1997;90:312.
8. Dewhurst CJ. The ruptured cesarean section scar. *J Obstet Gynaecol* 1957;64:113.
9. Riva HL, Teich JC. Vaginal delivery after cesarean section. *Am J Obstet Gynecol* 1961;81:501.
10. Sloan D. Inconclusive conclusion. *Am J Obstet Gynecol* 1968;101:133.
11. The Cesarean Birth Task Force. NIH consensus development statement on cesarean childbirth. *Obstet Gynecol* 1981;57:537.
12. Committee on obstetrics, maternal and fetal medicine: Guidelines for vaginal birth after previous cesarean birth, ACOG committee opinion No. 64, Washington, DC, American Colleges of Obstetricians and Gynecologists, 1988.
13. ACOG. Vaginal delivery after a previous cesarean birth. ACOG Committee Opinion. October 1994.
14. ACOG. Vaginal delivery after previous cesarean birth. ACOG Practice Patterns. August 1995.
15. Eckstein KL, Oberlander SG, Marx GF. Uterine rupture during extradural block. *Can Anaesth Soc J* 1973;20:566.
16. Flamm BL, Goings JR, Liu Y, Wolde-Tsadik G. Elective repeat cesarean delivery versus trial of labor: a prospective multicenter study. *Obstet Gynecol* 1994;83:927.
17. Lipson JG. Repeat cesarean births: social and psychological issues. *JOGN Nurs* 1984;13:157.
18. Austin SEJ. Childbirth classes for couples desiring VBAC. *Mat Child Nurs* 1986;11:250.
19. Catanese ML. Vaginal birth after cesarean: recommendations, risks, realities, and the client's right to know. *Holistic Nurs Pract* 1987;2:35.
20. Martin JN, Morrison JC, Wiser WL. Vaginal birth after cesarean section: the demise of routine repeat abdominal delivery. *Obstet Gynecol Clin North Am* 1988;15:719.
21. Davies JA, Spencer JAD. Trial of scar. *Br J Hosp Med* 1988;40:379.
22. Pridjian G, Hibbard JU, Moawad AH. Cesarean: changing trends. *Obstet Gynecol* 1991;77:195.
23. Weinstein D, Benshushan A, Ezra Y, Rojansky N. Vaginal birth after cesarean: current opinion. *Int J Obstet Gynecol* 1996;53:1.
24. Minkoff HL, Schwarz RH. The rising cesarean section rate: can it be safely reversed? *Am J Obstet Gynecol* 1980;56:135.
25. Canady C, Goldstein PJ. Elective repeat cesarean section: old controversy, new concepts. *MMJ* 1988;37:133.
26. Phelan JP, Clark SL, Diaz D, Paul RH. Vaginal birth after cesarean section. *Am J Obstet Gynecol* 1987;157:1510.
27. Gibbs CE. Planned vaginal delivery following cesarean section. *Clin Obstet Gynecol* 1980;23:507.
28. Graham AR. Trial labor following previous cesarean section. *Am J Obstet Gynecol* 1984;149:35.
29. Rosen MG, Dickinson JC, Westhoff CL. Vaginal birth after cesarean: a meta-analysis of morbidity and mortality. *Obstet Gynecol* 1991;77:465.
30. Petitti DB. Maternal mortality and morbidity in cesarean section. *Clin Obstet Gynecol* 1985;28:763.
31. Costs of normal births: regional variation, 1986. *Stat Bull* 1988;69:25.
32. Birth by cesarean: cost changes, 1982–83 to 1986. *Stat Bull* 1988;69:18.
33. Flamm BL. Vaginal birth after cesarean section: controversies old and new. *Clin Obstet Gynecol* 1985;28:735.
34. Placek PJ, Taffel SM. Vaginal birth after cesarean (VBAC) in the 1980s. *Am J Public Health* 1988;78:512.
35. De Jong P. Trial of labor following cesarean section—study of 212 patients. *Int J Gynaecol Obstet* 1987;25:405.
36. Boucher M, Tahilramaney MP, Eglinton GS, Phelan JP. Maternal morbidity as related to trial of labor after previous cesarean section delivery: a quantitative analysis. *J Reprod Med* 1984;29:12.
37. Minton SD. Resuscitation of the newborn infant. In: Phelan JP, Clark SL, eds. *Cesarean delivery.* New York: Elsevier, 1988:320.
38. Bowes WA Jr. Clinical aspects of normal and abnormal labor. In: Creasy RK, Resnik R, eds. *Maternal-fetal medicine: principles and practice,* 2nd ed. Philadelphia: WB Saunders, 1989:530.
39. Faranoff AA, Martin RJ, Miller MJ. Other pulmonary problems. In: Fanaroff AA, Martin RJ, eds. *Neonatal-perinatal medicine: diseases of the fetus and infant,* 4th ed. St. Louis: CV Mosby, 1987:608.
40. Heritage CK, Cunningham MD. Association of the elective repeat cesarean delivery and persistent pulmonary hypertension of the newborn. *Am J Obstet Gynecol* 1985;152:627.
41. Hibbard LT. Cesarean section and other surgical procedures. In: Gabbe SGI, Neibyl JR, Simpson JL, eds. *Obstetrics: normal and problem pregnancies.* New York: Churchill Livingstone, 1986:517.
42. Sokol RJ, Brindley BA. Practical diagnosis and management of abnormal labor. In: Scott JR, DiSaia PJ, Hammond CB, Spellacy WN, eds. *Danforth's obstetrics and gynecology*, 6th ed. Philadelphia: JB Lippincott, 1990:602.
43. Pedowitz P, Schwartz RM. The true incidence of silent rupture of cesarean section scars: a prospective analysis of 403 cases. *Am J Obstet Gynecol* 1957;74:1071.
44. Plauche WC, Von Almen W, Muller R. Catastrophic uterine ruptures. *Obstet Gynecol* 1984;64:792.
45. Injuries to the birth canal. In: Cunningham FG, MacDonald PC, Grant HF, eds. *Williams obstetrics*, 18th ed. Norwalk: Appleton and Lange, 1989:406.
46. Eden RD, Parker RT, Gall SA. Rupture of the pregnant uterus: a 53-year review. *Obstet Gynecol* 1986;68:671.
47. Fedorkov DM, Nimrod CA, Taylor PJ. Ruptured uterus in pregnancy: a Canadian hospital's experience. *Can Med Assoc J* 1987;137:27.
48. Shy KK, LoGerfo JP, Karp LE. Evaluation of the elective repeat cesarean section as a standard of care: an application of decision analysis. *Am J Obstet Gynecol* 1981;139:123.
49. Chazotte C, Cohen WR. Catastrophic complications of previous cesarean section. *Am J Obstet Gynecol* 1990;163:738.
50. Scott JR. Mandatory trial of labor after cesarean delivery: an alternative viewpoint. *Obstet Gynecol* 1991;77:811.
51. Jones RO, Nagashima AW, Hartnett-Goodman MM, Goodlin RC. Rupture of low transverse cesarean scars during trial of labor. *Obstet Gynecol* 1991;77:815.
52. Leung AS, Farmer RM, Leung EK, Madearis AL, Paul RH. Risk factors associated with uterine rupture during trial of labor after cesarean delivery: a case-control study. *Am J Obstet Gynecol* 1993:168:1358.
53. Case BD, Corcoran R, Jeffcoate N, Randle GH. Cesarean section and its modern obstetric practice. *J Obstet Gynaecol Br Cmnwlth* 1971;78:203.
54. Horenstein J, Clark SL. Epidural anesthesia in patients undergoing trial of labor after previous cesarean birth. In: Phelan JP, Clark SL, eds. *Cesarean delivery.* New York: Elsevier, 1988:497.
55. Meehan FP, Magani IM. True rupture of the cesarean section scar (a 15-year review, 1972–1987). *Eur J Obstet Gynecol Reprod Biol* 1989;30:129.
56. Nielsen TF, Ljungblad UI, Hagberg H. Rupture and dehiscence of cesarean section scar during pregnancy and delivery. *Am J Obstet Gynecol* 1989;160:569.
57. Flamm BL, Newman LA, Thomas SJ, Fallon D, Yoshida MJ. Vaginal birth after cesarean delivery: results of a 5-year multicenter collaborative study. *Obstet Gynecol* 1990;76:750.
58. Lavin JP, Stevens RJ, Miodovnik M, Barden TP. Vaginal delivery in patients with a prior cesarean section. *Am J Obstet Gynecol* 1982;59:135.
59. Chestnut DH. Anesthetic considerations for vaginal birth after previous cesarean section [Lecture]. Obstetric Anesthesia 1991, San Francisco, March 15, 1991.
60. Crawford JS. The epidural sieve and MBC (minimum blocking concentration): an hypothesis. *Anaesthesia* 1976;31:1277.
61. Shin YK. Shoulder pain in a trial of labor after cesarean delivery. *South Med J* 1989;82:1320.

61a. Rowbottom SJ, Tabrizian I. Epidural analgesia and uterine rupture during labour. *Anaesth Intens Care* 1994;22:79.

62. Carlsson C, Nybell-Lindhal, Ingemarsson I. Extradural block in patients who have previously undergone cesarean section. *Br J Anaesth* 1980;52:827.
63. Tehan B. Abolition of the extradural sieve by addition of fentanyl to extradural bupivacaine. *Br J Anaesth* 1992;69:620.
64. Rashiq S, Huston LJ. Fentanyl and the extradural sieve. *Br J Anaesth* 1993;71:920.
65. Rodriguez MH, Masaki DI, Phelan JP, Diaz FG. Uterine rupture: are intrauterine pressure catheters useful in the diagnosis? *Am J Obstet Gynecol* 1989;161:666.
66. Stovall TG, Shaver DC, Solomon SK, Anderson GD. Trial of labor in previous cesarean section patients, excluding classical cesarean sections. *Obstet Gynecol* 1987;70:713.
67. Schrinsky DC, Benson RC. Rupture of the pregnant uterus: a review. *Obstet Gynecol Surv* 1978;33:217.
68. Golan A, Sandbank O, Rubin A. Rupture of the pregnant uterus. *Obstet Gynecol* 1980;56:549.
69. Roumen FJME, Janssen AAJM, Vrouenraets FPJM. The course of delivery after previous cesarean section. *Eur J Obstet Gynecol Reprod Med* 1990;34:15.
70. Meier PR, Porreco RP. Trial of labor following cesarean section: a two-year experience. *Am J Obstet Gynecol* 1982;144:671.
71. Yetman TJ, Nolan TE. Vaginal birth after cesarean section: a reappraisal of risk. *Am J Obstet Gynecol* 1989;161:1119.
72. Mariona FG. Discussion of Martin et al. paper on vaginal birth following previous cesarean birth. *Am J Obstet Gynecol* 1983;161:261.
73. Michaels WH, Thompson HO, Boutt A, Scheiber FR, Michaels SL, Karo J. Ultrasound diagnosis of defects in the scarred lower uterine segment during pregnancy. *Obstet Gynecol* 1988;71:112.
74. Rozenberg P, Goffinet F, Philippe HJ, Nisand I. Ultrasonographic measurement of lower uterine segment to assess the defects of scarred uterus. *Lancet* 1996;347:281.
75. Petrikovsky BM. Endoscopic assessment of the integrity of the post-cesarean uterine wall before a trial of labor. *J Reprod Med* 1994;39:464.
76. Petrikovsky BM. Rupture of the scarred uterus: prediction and diagnosis. *Lancet* 1996;347:838.
77. Thurnau GR, Scates DH, Morgan MA. The fetal-pelvic index: a method of identifying fetal-pelvic disproportion in women attempting vaginal birth after previous cesarean delivery. *Am J Obstet Gynecol* 1991;165:353.
78. Troyer LR, Parisi VM. Obstetric parameters affecting success in trial of labor: designation of a scoring system. *Am J Obstet Gynecol* 1992; 167:1099.
79. Weinstein D, Benshushan A, Tanos V, Zilberstein R, Rojansky N. Predictive score for vaginal birth after cesarean section. *Am J Obstet Gynecol* 1996;174:192.
80. Flamm BL, Geiger AM. Vaginal birth after cesarean delivery: an admission scoring system. *Obstet Gynecol* 1997;90:907.
81. Horenstein JM, Eglinton GS, Tahilramaney MP, Boucher M, Phelan JP. Oxytocin use during a trial of labor in patients with previous cesarean section. *J Reprod Med* 1984;29:26.
82. Horenstein JM, Phelan JP. Previous cesarean section: the risk and benefits of oxytocin usage in a trial of labor. *Am J Obstet Gynecol* 1985; 151:564.
83. Molloy BG, Sheil O, Duignan NM. Delivery after cesarean section: a review of 2176 consecutive cases. *Br Med J* 1987;294:1645.
84. Lao TT, Leung BFH. Labor induction for planned vaginal delivery in patients with previous cesarean section. *Acta Obstet Gynecol Scand* 1987;66:413.
85. Flamm BL, Dunnett C, Fisherman E, Quilligan EJ. Vaginal delivery following cesarean section: use of oxytocin augmentation and epidural anesthesia with internal tocodynamic and internal fetal monitoring. *Am J Obstet Gynecol* 1984;148:759.
85a. Flamm BL, Goings JR, Fuelberth N, Fishermann E, Jones C, Hersh E. Oxytocin during labor after previous cesarean section: results of a multicenter study. *Obstet Gynecol* 1987;70:709.
86. Silver RK, Gibbs RS. Predictors of vaginal delivery in patients with previous cesarean section who require oxytocin. *Am J Obstet Gynecol* 1987;156:57.
87. Sakala EP, Kaye S, Murray RD, Munson LJ. Oxytocin use after previous cesarean: why a higher rate of failed labor trial? *Obstet Gynecol* 1990;75:356.
88. Phelan JP, Ahn MC, Diaz F, Brar H, Rodriguez MH. Twice a cesarean, always a cesarean? *Obstet Gynecol* 1989;73:161.
89. Targett C. Cesarean section and trial of scar. *Aust N Z Obstet Gynaecol* 1988;28:249.
90. Saldana LR, Schulman H, Reuss L. Management of pregnancy after cesarean section. *Am J Gynecol* 1979;135:555.
91. Martin JN, Harris BA, Huddleston JF, et al. Vaginal delivery following previous cesarean birth. *Am J Obstet Gynecol* 1983;146:255.
92. Porreco RP, Meier PR. Trial of labor in patients with multiple previous cesarean section. *J Reprod Med* 1983;28:770.
93. Farmakides G, Duvivier R, Schulman H. Vaginal birth after two or more cesarean sections. *Am J Obstet Gynecol* 1987;156:565.
94. Novas J, Myers SA, Gleicher N. Obstetric outcome of patients with more than one previous cesarean section. *Am J Obstet Gynecol* 1989; 160:364.
95. Pruett KM, Kirson B, Cotton DB. Unknown uterine scar and trial of labor. *Am J Obstet Gynecol* 1988;159:807.
96. Cowan RK, Kinch RAH, Ellis B, Anderson R. Trial of labor following cesarean delivery. *Obstet Gynecol* 1994;83:933.
97. Asakura H, Myers SA. More than one previous cesarean delivery: a 5-year experience with 435 patients. *Obstet Gynecol* 1995;85:924.
98. Palerme GR, Friedman EA. Rupture of the gravid uterus in the third trimester. *Am J Obstet Gynecol* 1966;94:571.
99. Naef RW, Ray MA, Chauhan SP, Roach H, Blake PG, Martin JN Jr. Trial of labor after cesarean delivery with a lower-segment, vertical uterine incision: is it safe? *Am J Obstet Gynecol* 1995;172:1666.
100. Adair CD, Sanchez-Ramos L, Whitaker D, McDyer DC, Farah L, Briones D. Trial of labor in patients with a previous lower uterine vertical cesarean section. *Am J Obstet Gynecol* 1996;174:966.
101. Beall M, Eglinton GS, Clark SL, Phelan JP. Vaginal delivery after cesarean section in women with unknown types of uterine scar. *J Reprod Med* 1984;29:31.
102. Duff P, Southmayd K, Read JA. Outcome labor in patients with a single previous low transverse cesarean section for dystocia. *Obstet Gynecol* 1988;71:380.
103. Hoskins IA, Gomez JL. Correlation between maximum cervical dilatation at cesarean delivery and subsequent vaginal birth after cesarean delivery. *Obstet Gynecol* 1997;89:591.
104. Hollingsworth D, Moore TR. Diabetes and pregnancy. In: Creasy RK, Resnik R, eds. *Maternal-fetal medicine: principles and practice,* 2nd ed. Philadelphia: WB Saunders, 1989:970.
105. Phelan JP, Eglinton GS, Horenstein JM, Clark SL, Yeh S. Previous cesarean birth: trial of labor in women with macrosomic infants. *J Reprod Med* 1984;29:36.
106. Ollendorf DA, Goldberg JM, Minogue JP, Socol ML. Vaginal birth after cesarean section for arrest of labor: is the success determined by maximum cervical dilatation during prior labor? *Am J Obstet Gynecol* 1988;159:636.
107. Flamm BL, Goings JR. Vaginal birth after cesarean section: is suspected fetal macrosomia a contraindication? *Obstet Gynecol* 1989; 74:694.
108. Resnik R. Post-term pregnancy. In: Creasy RK, Resnik R. *Maternal-fetal medicine: principles and practice,* 2nd ed. Philadelphia: WB Saunders, 1989:505.
109. Spellacy WN. The postdate pregnancy. In: Scott JR, DiSaia PJ, Spellacy WN, eds. *Danforth's obstetrics and gynecology*, 6th ed. Philadelphia: JB Lippincott, 1990:375.
110. MacKenzie IZ. Vaginal prostaglandins and labour induction for patients previously delivered by cesarean section. *Br J Obstet Gynaecol* 1984;91:7.
111. Meehan FP. Trial of scar with induction/oxytocin in delivery following prior section. *Clin Exp Obstet Gynecol* 1988;15:117.
112. Yeh S, Huang X, Phelan JP. Postterm pregnancy after previous cesarean section. *J Reprod Med* 1984;29:41.
113. Strong TH, Phelan JP, Ahn MO, Sarno AP Jr. Vaginal birth after cesarean delivery in twin gestation. *Am J Obstet Gynecol* 1989;161:29.
114. Gifford DS, Morton SC, Fiske M, Kahn K. A meta-analysis of infant outcomes after breech delivery. *Obstet Gynecol* 1995;85:1047.
115. Cruikshank DP. Malpresentations and umbilical cord complications. In: Scott JR, DiSaia PJ, Spellacy WN. *Danforth's obstetrics and gynecology*, 6th ed. Philadelphia: JB Lippincott, 1990:570.
116. Ophir E, Oettinger M, Yagoda A, et al. Breech presentation after cesarean section: always a section? *Am J Obstet Gynecol* 1989;161:25.
117. Sarno MP Jr, Phelan JP, Ahn MO, Strong TH Jr. Vaginal birth after cesarean delivery: trial of labor in women with breech presentation. *J Reprod Med* 1989;34:831.

118. Laros RK, Flanagan TA, Kilpatrick SJ. Management of term breech presentation: a protocol of external cephalic version and selective trial of labor. *Am J Obstet Gynecol* 1995;172:1916.
119. Flamm BL, Fried MW, Lonky NM, Saurenman W. External cephalic version after previous cesarean section. *Am J Obstet Gynecol* 1991; 165:370.
120. Finley BE, Gibbs CE. Emergent cesarean delivery in patients undergoing trial of labor with a transverse lower segment scar. *Am J Obstet Gynecol* 1986;155:936.
121. Paul RP, Phelan JP, Yeh S. Trial of labor in the patient with a prior cesarean birth. *Am J Obstet Gynecol* 1985;151:297.
122. Demianczuk NN, Hunter DJS, Taylor DW. Trial of labor after previous cesarean section: prognostic indicators of outcome. *Am J Obstet Gynecol* 1982;142:640.
123. Chelmow D, Laros RK. Maternal and neonatal outcomes after oxytocin augmentation in patients undergoing a trial of labor after prior cesarean delivery. *Obstet Gynecol* 1992;80:966.
124. Hanley ML, Smulian JC, Lake MF, McLean DA, Vintzileos AM. Analysis of repeat cesarean delivery indications: implications of heterogeneity. *Am J Obstet Gynecol* 1996;175:883.
125. Uppington J. Epidural analgesia and previous cesarean section. *Anesthesia* 1983;38:336.
126. Rudick V, Niv D, Hetman-Peri M, Geller E, Avni A, Golan A. Epidural analgesia for planned vaginal delivery following previous cesarean section. *Obstet Gynecol* 1984;64:621.
127. Meehan FP, Burke G, Casey C, Sheil JG. Delivery following cesarean section and perinatal mortality. *Am J Perinatol* 1989;6:90.
128. Sakala EP, Kaye S, Murray RD, Munson LJ. Epidural analgesia: effect on the likelihood of successful trial of labor after cesarean section. *J Reprod Med* 1990;35:886.
129. Johnson C, Oriol N, Flood K. Trial of labor: a study of 110 patients. *J Clin Anesth* 1991;3:216.
130. Veridiano NP, Thorner NS, Ducey J. Vaginal delivery after cesarean section. *Int J Gynecol Obstet* 1989;29:307.
131. Johnson C, Oriol N. The role of epidural anesthesia in trial of labor. *Reg Anesth* 1990;15:304.
132. Meehan FP, Moolgaoker AS, Stallworthy J. Vaginal delivery under caudal analgesia after cesarean section and other major uterine surgery. *Br Med J* 1972;2:740.
133. Phelan JP, Clark SL. Reply to Jakobi et al. *Am J Obstet Gynecol* 1989;160:1539.
134. Jakobi P, Zimmer EZ, Weissman A. Oxytocin administration and uterine exploration in the management of vaginal birth after cesarean—not a routine procedure. *Am J Obstet Gynecol* 1989;160:1538.

Obstetric Anesthesia, second edition,
edited by Mark C. Norris.
Lippincott Williams & Wilkins, Philadelphia © 1999.

CHAPTER 29

Intraamniotic Infection

Evan Goodman

Infection within the uterus, a common cause of morbidity during pregnancy, can complicate anesthetic management. This condition has been termed chorioamnionitis, amniotic fluid infection, and intrapartum fever; however, the term intraamniotic infection (IAI) alludes to both the site and symptoms of the disease (1). IAI is the term used by the original authors (2). The term amniotic infection syndrome is used less commonly. It denotes the combination of fetal infection (e.g., acute congenital pneumonia) and histologic chorioamnionitis (3).

Although various authors use differing criteria, IAI occurs in as many as 10% of parturients (4). Many authors (5–7) base the diagnosis on the combination of a fever ≥37.8°C (≥100°F) plus two or more of the following:

- Maternal tachycardia (greater than 100 beats/min),
- Fetal tachycardia (greater than 160 beats/min),
- Maternal leukocytosis (white blood cell count ≥15,000),
- Uterine tenderness, and/or
- Foul-smelling amniotic fluid.

Others (8,9) base the diagnosis primarily on a maternal temperature exceeding 38°C with no other apparent source of infection.

FEVER AND THE ACUTE PHASE RESPONSE

The parturient must be febrile to have clinically significant IAI. This elevation in the patient's body temperature is merely one facet of the cascade of events, termed the acute phase response, that occurs after exposure to pathogenic organisms. Initially, endothelial cells and cells of the immune system are activated to produce cytokines, such as interleukin-1 and tumor necrosis factor (10). These compounds, in turn, affect the functioning of almost every organ system (Fig. 1) and lead to the production of other acute phase reactants, including C-reactive protein, serum amyloid A protein, α-1 acid glycoprotein, and fibrinogen (11). Together, these compounds bolster the host's defenses and enable the body to rid itself of the infectious threat.

Fever is caused by the effects of endogenous pyrogens (from the acute phase response) and of exogenous (bacterial) pyrogens on temperature regulating centers, such as the hypothalamus and its lamina terminalis (12). The change in body temperature triggers both behavioral and autonomic responses. For example, a warm person is inclined to seek a cooler environment, change to cooler clothing, and adjust the temperature of the room. Activation of the autonomic nervous system leads to increased sweating and peripheral vasodilatation to increase evaporative heat loss.

TEMPERATURE REGULATION IN THE PARTURIENT AND FETUS

The many forces competing to raise or lower the temperature of a pregnant woman, especially during active labor, make defining the normal temperature range for this population exceedingly difficult. While the merits of the long-held normal body temperature of 37.0°C can be debated (13), the situation during pregnancy is even more complicated, as heat is produced and dissipated by additional factors (Table 1).

By the fifteenth week of gestation, a pregnant woman's basal metabolic rate has started to increase. Oxygen uptake and heart rate continue to increase until after delivery (14). Eventually, these sources of heat production are coupled with heat from muscular exertion during labor. Uterine contractions play a significant part in this process, comprising a constant and important source of heat at term. Lymphatic and vascular engorgement also may contribute to a rise in the mother's temperature, although this effect should last less than 24 hours (15).

E. Goodman: Department of Anesthesia, Case Western Reserve University/University Hospitals of Cleveland, Cleveland, Ohio 44106.

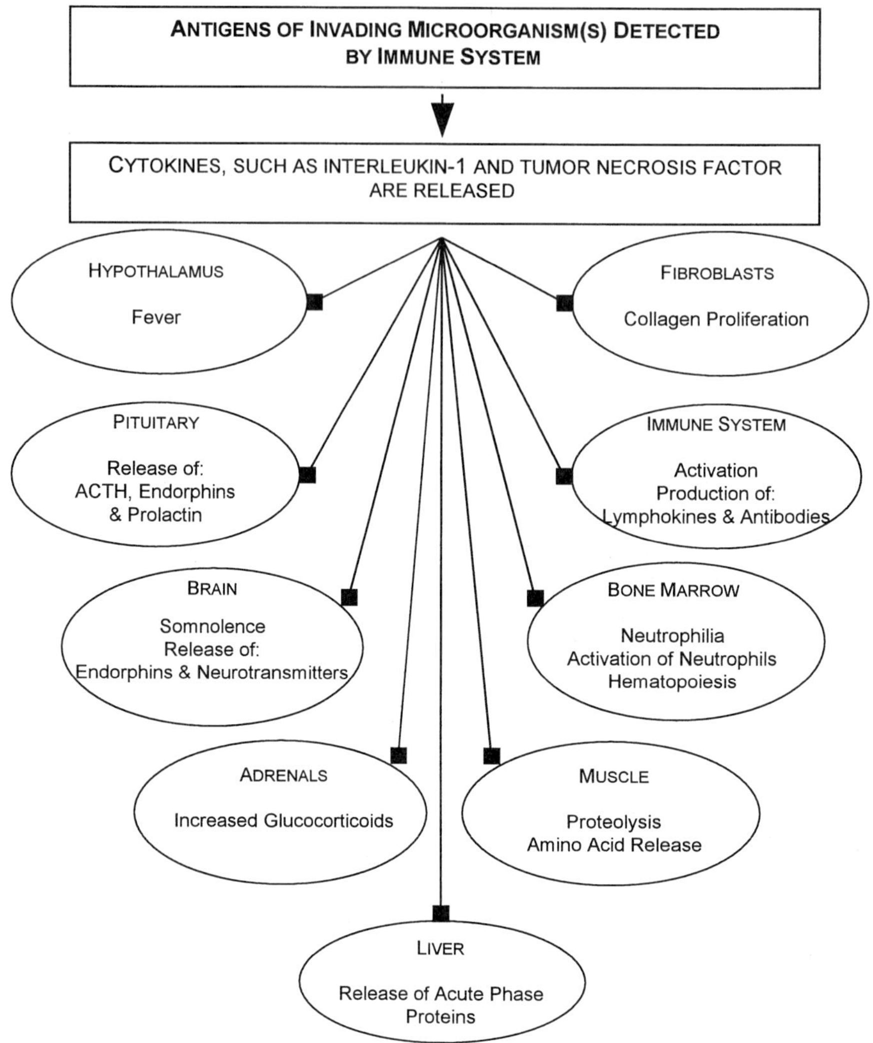

FIG. 1. The cascade of the acute phase response, which affects many organ systems through intermediate compounds.

The active metabolism of the developing fetus produces large quantities of heat (16). The fetus has two available methods to eliminate heat. The uteroplacental circulation can rapidly regulate fetal temperature. In addition, the amniotic fluid provides a reservoir for heat that crosses fetal skin. Sheep studies (17) have shown that the uteroplacental circulation is the more important pathway of heat elimination, accounting for 85% of maternal—fetal heat exchange. The human fetus generally remains 0.4°C warmer than the mother (18).

Effects of Labor

The pain of labor causes the parturient to hyperventilate well above the level of increased respiration seen

TABLE 1. *Competing forces in temperature regulation in the parturient*

	Heat gain	Heat loss
Without conduction anesthesia	↑ Basal metabolic rate Uterine contractions Vascular and lymphatic engorgement	Hyperventilation Perspiration
After conduction anesthesia	Vasoconstriction above block ↓ Hyperventilation ↓ Sweating with sympathetic block	Vasodilatation within block ↓ Muscle activity Transfer of heat from core to periphery Central effects of medications in the epidural and spinal spaces

throughout pregnancy. The hyperventilation, along with the accompanying perspiration, leads to compensatory heat loss.

Effects of Analgesia

Neuraxial analgesia provides invaluable relief from the agony of labor pains. However, at the same time, it upsets the balance between heat producing and eliminating mechanisms. Once contraction pain is relieved, labored breathing subsides. Local anesthetic-induced sympathectomy produces vasodilatation within the blocked area. Heat transfers from the core compartment to the periphery. Both sympathectomy and analgesia also decrease sweating.

Less well understood are the central effects of spinal and epidural anesthesia. Unblocked areas have a delayed vasoconstriction response. Shivering and vasoconstriction in these regions occur 1°C lower than in nonanesthetized individuals (19,20). This reduction in the shivering and vasoconstriction thresholds is seen equally with spinal and epidural anesthetics (21), although the effect may be more pronounced with higher blocks (22).

As all of these forces come into play, maternal body temperature fluctuates widely, depending on the intensity of the labor pains and the extent to which they are felt (23,24). Without regional anesthesia, heat dissipating mechanisms predominate, and maternal temperature slowly decreases until delivery. Relief of labor pains leads to a stabilization of the core temperature. Occasionally, the parturients' temperature rises slowly throughout labor, possibly dependent on the degree of heat loss before placement of the regional anesthetic.

Most studies of temperature changes during labor have found that labor epidural analgesia either does not cause much increase in maternal temperature (25) or causes only mild elevation that should not be confused with fever (38°C) (26–29). Marx et al. (23) found a rise in maternal tympanic temperature of about 1.5°C throughout labor, whether or not the parturients received epidural analgesia. They noted that temperatures of primigravidae rose faster than those of multigravidae. The relatively greater effort expended by an inexperienced uterus to expel the fetus could explain this observation.

Some studies, however, have reported more significant elevations in temperature among parturients who benefited from labor epidural analgesia (27,28). Here, the women's temperature did not begin to rise until 4 to 6 hours after induction of analgesia (Fig. 2). Presumably, this time span was necessary for the changes in blood flow and temperature flux caused by the epidural local anesthetics to make a difference.

Despite the many reassuring reports, some more worrisome findings have surfaced. For example, Macaulay et al. (30) reported that the fetal skin temperatures were above 38°C in 17% of laboring patients who received epidural analgesia, but in none of the patients who labored without the benefit of an epidural block. The high ambient temperatures (24° to 28°C) may have exaggerated the effect of epidural analgesia on temperature balance in these women. Another study (31) found that intrapartum fevers (greater than 38°C) occurred in 14.5% of parturients who had epidural analgesia and in only 1% of the women who labored without it. Neonatal sepsis evaluations also were performed more frequently in the group of women who had epidural blocks. However, their practice of performing a neonatal sepsis evaluation whenever the maternal temperature rose above 38°C differs from the custom of many institutions, including my own.

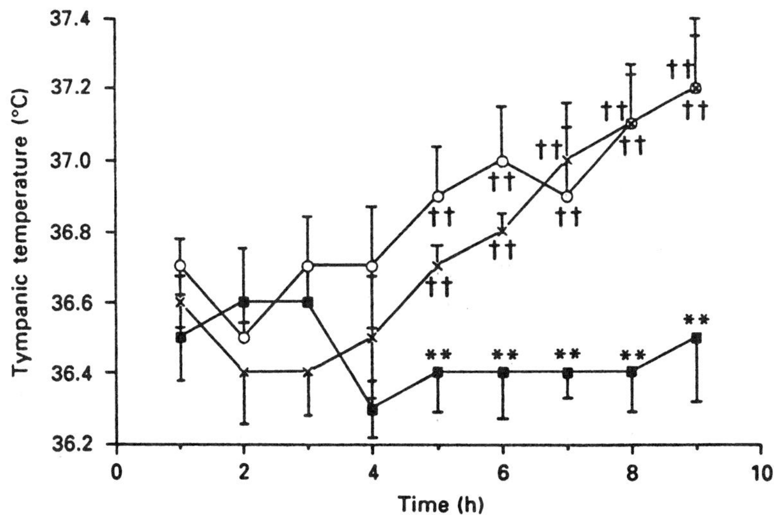

FIG. 2. Mean (SE) tympanic temperatures during labor in women receiving parenteral opioids only *(squares)*, epidural infusions of 0.25% bupivacaine alone *(Xs)*, or epidural infusions of 0.25% bupivacaine with 2 μg/mL fentanyl *(open circles)*. *Double stars* indicate $p < 0.01$ compared with the groups receiving epidural medications, and *double crosses* indicate $p < 0.01$ compared with the preanesthetic temperature. (Reprinted from ref. 28, with permission.)

Effects of Maternal Fever

The elevation of body temperature that occurs during the acute phase response assists the host in the fight against the invading organism (32). Heart rate and cardiac output increase while peripheral resistance decreases, helping immune system cells and proteins reach their targets. Higher temperatures at target sites improve the performance of these protective factors. The more efficient circulation also delivers oxygen and nutrients to satisfy the increased demand.

Changes in the mother's body temperature alter fetal metabolism. With mild elevations in maternal temperature (1°C), fetal temperatures also rise to maintain the fetal—maternal gradient. As in the mother, fetal heart rate increases with higher temperature. The fetus copes well with the demands of increased temperature. Mean blood pressure, arterial pH, pO_2 and pCO_2 remain unchanged (33).

With marked increases in maternal body temperature (1.5° to 2°C), compensatory mechanisms show signs of failure (34,35). The fetus finds it increasingly difficult to dispose of its heat, and the fetal—maternal gradient widens. There is an increase in uterine activity. Uterine and umbilical blood flow decreases. Fetal cardiac output declines, and fetal blood pressure may fall. When fetal heart rate cannot increase further, dysrhythmias begin to appear. The fetus may become hypoxemic, but often the fetal p_aO_2 is maintained. As the fetal p_aCO_2 rises, pH declines. The pH change may have both a respiratory component from the fetus and a metabolic contribution from fixed acids, such as lactic acid, coming from the mother. If left untreated, the worsening fetal hypoxemia and acidosis eventually can lead to fetal injury or even death.

ETIOLOGY OF INTRAAMNIOTIC INFECTION

The organisms that give rise to IAI can gain entry to the uterus in various ways (Fig. 3). Most commonly, pathogenic bacteria ascend from the lower genital tract. For example, parturients with bacterial vaginosis are more likely to develop IAI (37,38). A polymicrobial infection

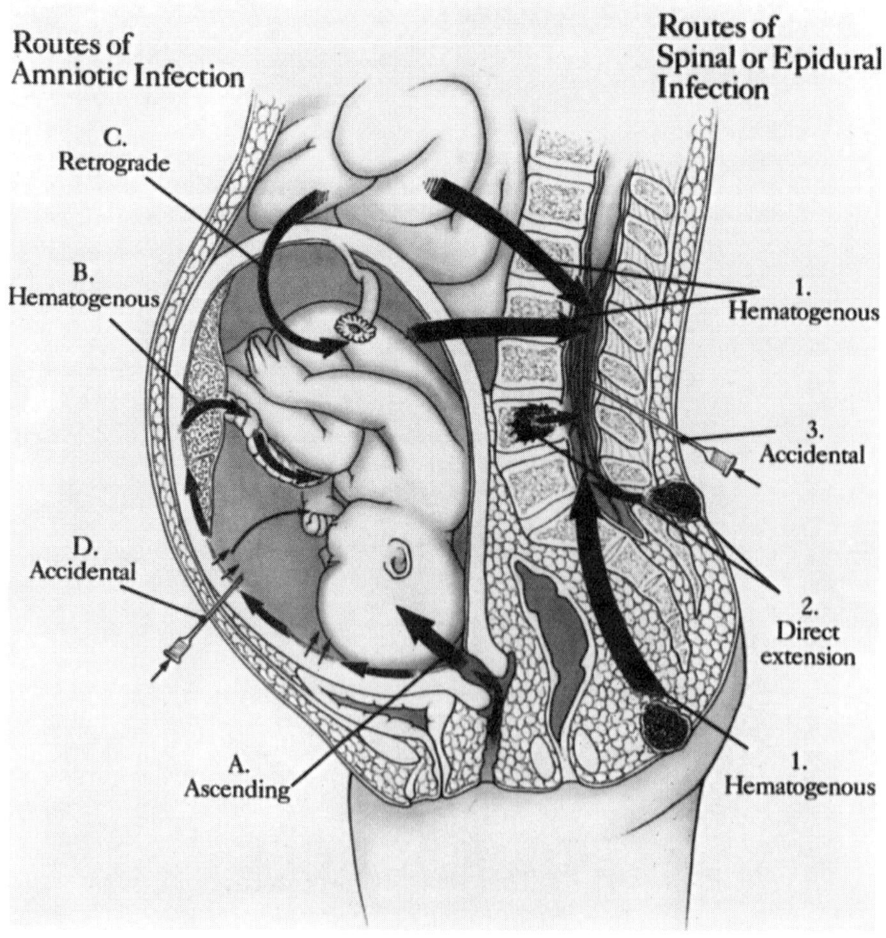

FIG. 3. Routes of intraamniotic infection (depicted on the *right*) and of infection from spinal or epidural anesthetics. (Reprinted from ref. 36, with permission.)

of the vagina, bacterial vaginosis depletes the normal population of lactobacilli species that maintains the protective acidic pH of the vaginal wall (39). Frequent vaginal examinations and the placement of internal fetal monitors are other ways that bacteria are introduced through the cervix (40,41). Coitus during pregnancy is unlikely to increase the likelihood of IAI (42).

When barriers to invasion by pathogens are removed, such as when the amniotic membranes are ruptured, infection of the uterus is much more likely (43). Although amniotic fluid may inhibit the growth of certain bacteria (44), its alkaline nature can raise the vaginal pH and allow other pathogens to proliferate (45). Because premature rupture of membranes exposes the woman to the risk of infection for a longer time, the incidence of IAI with preterm deliveries is greater (Fig. 4). IAI occurs in over 20% of parturients whose membranes have been ruptured for more than 24 hours (46). For each hour of ruptured membranes or internal monitoring, the probability of IAI increases by approximately 2% in both nulliparae and multiparae (47). Conversely, IAI may predispose to premature rupture of membranes (48). The inflammatory response and the neutrophils that it attracts can lead to the release of proteolytic enzymes that may weaken the amniotic membrane.

Other routes for infection to reach the uterus include hematogenous spread from a distant site, retrograde seeding from the peritoneal cavity through the fallopian tubes, and iatrogenic introduction of organisms during invasive procedures (49). IAI can occur with intact membranes. Fluid specimens collected by amniotomy can grown bacteria. Although the risk of acute IAI with diagnostic amniocentesis is low (1 in 1,000), the frequency of infection increases to 1% to 5% after an intrauterine transfusion, percutaneous umbilical blood sampling, or cervical cerclage.

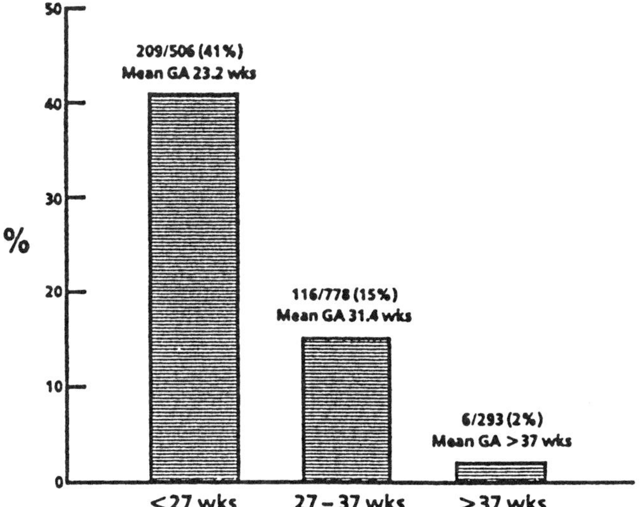

FIG. 4. Incidence of intraamniotic infection by gestational age at delivery. (Reprinted from ref. 1, with permission.)

The bacteria isolated from amniotic fluid samples may indicate the origin of the IAI (50). The constellation of *Gardnerella vaginalis, M. hominis,* and anaerobes suggests bacterial vaginosis as the source. On the other hand, enterococci, *E. coli,* and other aerobic gram-negative rods point to hematogenous spread as the vehicle for these gut-associated organisms.

INTRAAMNIOTIC INFECTION AND PRETERM LABOR

Efforts have been made to link the inflammatory response associated with IAI with preterm labor (45,51,52). However, the paucity of knowledge about the factors that trigger the onset of labor in normal pregnancies has hampered these studies. At term, concentrations of prostaglandins (PGs) and their precursors increase in both amniotic fluid and maternal plasma. PGs, especially PGE_2, can mediate cervical ripening and induce labor. PG inhibitors can arrest preterm labor. Inflammation stimulates the production of PGs (53). Placental inflammation induces extremely high PGE production by amniotic epithelium (54). Furthermore, some species of bacteria, such as *Clostridium,* produce phospholipase, which can cleave arachidonic acid and increase the amount of PG present in the infected area. Bacterial endotoxins produced by gram-negative bacteria also can directly stimulate PG production (51). These bacteria, in concert with the inflammatory response they initiate, can impair placental membrane integrity and predispose it to premature rupture (55). The precise role that these changes play in the initiation of labor has yet to be elucidated.

DIAGNOSIS OF INTRAAMNIOTIC INFECTION

Clinical IAI is diagnosed on the basis of multiple nonspecific signs and symptoms (Table 2). An elevated temperature usually must be present for the diagnosis to be entertained. Foul-smelling amniotic fluid and uterine tenderness are infrequent, despite their close association with the problem. Increases in the maternal and fetal

TABLE 2. *Criteria used in the diagnosis of intraamniotic infection*

Criteria	Frequency (%)
Fever (>37.8°C)	100
Maternal tachycardia (>100 beats/min)	20–80
Leukocytosis (>15,000 cells/mm^3)	36–90
Fetal tachycardia (>160 beats/min)	40–70
Foul amniotic fluid	4–22
Uterine tenderness	4–25
Fetal distress	<5

From refs. 1 and 6.

heart rates are variable and simply may reflect the effects of the fever on their joined physiologies. The degree of leukocytosis required to diagnose IAI also is unclear. Noninfected women can have a white blood cell count well above 15,000/mL, especially postpartum (56,57). Other factors, such as exogenous steroids, also elevate the white blood cell count.

Laboratory tests have played a limited role in the diagnosis of IAI because of their disappointing predictive values (1). Serum concentration of C-reactive protein, an acute phase reactant, can be measured, and samples of amniotic fluid can be gram stained and cultured. Amniotic fluid also can be assayed for leukocyte esterase, glucose, cytokines, ceramide lactoside, short-chain organic acids, and fetal fibronectin.

MATERNAL COMPLICATIONS

Pregnancies complicated by IAI often are associated with dysfunctional labor (8). However, a cause-and-effect relationship is unclear. Abnormal labor patterns usually appear at least 2 hours before clinical IAI is diagnosed, and they may be well established before the infection ever reaches the uterus. However, subclinical infections may be present well before symptoms are seen. A low-grade infection in the uterus may be detrimental to uterine contractility and yet not be extensive enough to cause overt symptoms.

The dystocia seen in IAI leads to a higher than usual percentage of patients requiring oxytocin augmentation. The amount of oxytocin required to increase uterine contractility and induce in cervical change may be increased as well (8). Abnormal labor often continues in these patients, and they often fail to make adequate progress. This failure to progress combined with the increased incidence of nonreassuring fetal heart patterns in pregnancies complicated by IAI increases the cesarean section rate by two- to threefold (26% to 53%) (5,50).

Infectious processes that begin before delivery increase the risk of postpartum infection. The additional care that these women require tends to prolong their hospital stay (7). Intrauterine infection also may weaken the uterine wall and increase the chances of uterine rupture and postpartum hemorrhage (58).

MATERNAL SEPTICEMIA

The bacteria involved with IAI can enter the blood stream and produce symptoms of septicemia in 8% to 12% of patients (5,7). However, bacteremia *per se* is not unusual, and can be documented in 1% of all obstetric admissions (59). Furthermore, approximately 20% of patients having a cesarean section have a transient bacteremia after surgery (60). Remember, 8% of patients who undergo urethral catheterization alone experience bacteremia (61).

The appearance of symptoms of sepsis in the parturient with IAI marks a significant turning point in the clinical course (Table 3). The condition of both mother and fetus may deteriorate more rapidly, and delivery of the fetus becomes more urgent. Unfortunately, the diagnosis of sepsis often is not obvious, especially in the early stages, and requires a high index of suspicion. Even documenting bacteremia alone may present a challenge. Results of blood cultures, the definitive test, are not available for days after they are drawn. The degree of leukocytosis may not be helpful, because elevated white blood counts (up to 18,000/mL) are expected in the peripartum period (56). Similarly, the presence of tachycardia, tachypnea, or hypocarbia may represent normal variations seen in pregnancy, especially during labor. Finally, even fever may not be significant. Bader et al. (65) and Goodman et al. (66) found no significant difference between the temperatures of bacteremic and nonbacteremic patients. Blanco et al. (59) found elevated temperatures in patients with documented bacteremia, although half had peak temperatures below 38.8°C.

Untreated septic patients can develop pronounced and life-threatening signs of shock. Blood pressure, central venous pressure, and systemic vascular resistance all decrease, while the heart rate and cardiac index gradually rise (60). These women require fluid resuscitation and cardiovascular support with inotropes and vasopressors. Close monitoring in an intensive care setting is appropriate, because other conditions, such as disseminated intravascular coagulation, pneumonia, and lung abscess (67), may develop (Table 4).

TABLE 3. *Sepsis syndrome: signs and symptoms*

Fever or hypothermia
Organ hypoperfusion and failure
Lungs: Ventilation-perfusion mismatching, increased alveolar capillary permeability, pulmonary edema, arterial hypoxemia, cyanosis, acidosis, tachypnea, hypoxemia, hypercapnia, adult respiratory distress syndrome
Heart: Myocardial depression, congestive heart failure, increased or decreased cardiac index, decreased ejection fraction, tachycardia
Kidney: Acute renal failure, oliguria/anuria, proteinuria, azotemia, lactic acidemia, acidosis
Liver: Cholestatic jaundice, elevated liver function tests
Bowel: Ischemic necrosis, diarrhea/ileus, nausea/vomiting
Cardiovascular system: Decreased systemic vascular resistance, hypotension
Central nervous system: Disorientation/confusion, obtundation, polyneuropathy with distal motor weakness
Skin: Various lesions (e.g., erythroderma, ecthyma gangrenosum), ischemic necrosis in peripheral regions (e.g., digits)
Blood: Leukocytosis or leukocytopenia, thrombocytopenia, disseminated intravascular coagulation, bleeding
Metabolism: Hypoglycemia

From refs. 62–64.

TABLE 4. *Complications of intraamniotic infection*

Maternal	Fetal
Dystocia	Fetal distress
Higher rate of cesarean section	Preterm birth
Postpartum infection	Intrauterine death
Postpartum hemorrhage (?)	Intraventricular hemorrhage
Sepsis	Infections manifesting at birth:
Shock	Pneumonia/respiratory distress syndrome
Disseminated intravascular coagulation	
Respiratory distress syndrome	Meningitis/ meningoencephalitis sepsis
Pulmonary edema	Otitis media/sinusitis
Pneumonia	Gastroenteritis
Lung abscess	Osteomyelitis
Septic pulmonary emboli	Pyelonephritis
Death	Dermatitis

From refs. 2, 7, 67, 68, 127.

FETAL COMPLICATIONS

The fetus is protected from harmful effects of puerperal infection by its location in the mother (68). The placenta acts as a natural barrier to invasion by pathogens, and maternal immunoglobulin G (IgG) is able to assist on both sides of the placenta. Amniotic fluid also inhibits bacterial growth (44). The ability of the fetus, especially if preterm, to defend itself is limited. However, it can synthesize immunoglobulins (mainly IgM) and recruit its sluggish leukocytes into action.

Infecting organisms can reach the fetus by hematogenous spread or through the amniotic fluid. Fetal bacteremia may follow infection and inflammation of the placenta and umbilical cord. The fetus may swallow or aspirate pathogens in the amniotic fluid.

Fetal well-being may be jeopardized within a short time of membrane rupture. More than 10% of neonates born more than 24 hours after rupture of membranes may be bacteremic (69). Perinatal mortality doubles if more than 24 hours elapse between membrane rupture and delivery. It doubles again if more than 48 hours elapse (70). Infants born prematurely after infection-induced preterm labor are exposed to the risks of survival with immature organ systems. At birth, fetuses who survive prolonged exposure to intrauterine infection are at increased risk for infection of almost every major organ system (Table 4).

OBSTETRIC MANAGEMENT OF INTRAAMNIOTIC INFECTION

The timing of antibiotic administration in the presence of IAI was controversial until approximately a decade ago. Early administration had the obvious advantage of early eradication of the infection and avoidance of the feared consequences in mother and fetus. The argument for delaying treatment centered around concerns that newborn blood culture results might be obscured and that diagnosis of neonatal sepsis delayed (71). Furthermore, intrapartum treatment could encourage growth of resistant organisms and prolong the hospital stay of the neonate. These fears proved unjustified. Early administration of antimicrobials decreases the incidence of neonatal sepsis and shortens the length of the neonates' hospital stay (9,71–73).

Giving antibiotics to women whose membranes have ruptured prematurely not only reduces maternal and fetal morbidity, but it can safely prolong pregnancy (74,75). In these women, it is even more critical to avoid or strictly limit those maneuvers that increase the risk of IAI. Vaginal examinations should be performed only if very necessary. Fetal heart rate and uterine contraction monitoring should be done externally as long as the fetus appears healthy.

ANESTHETIC CONSIDERATIONS

Before inducing regional anesthesia in a febrile parturient, the risk–benefit ratio of either proceeding with or withholding the anesthetic must be considered. Regional anesthesia provides needed labor pain relief. At the same time, the procedure could expose the patient to infectious risks that may not arise for weeks or even months. Withholding treatment is not without risk. Should the patient need a cesarean section, difficulty with the intubation caused by infection-induced airway edema could prove to be life threatening (76). The two main infectious complications associated with neuraxial analgesia are spinal epidural abscess and meningitis. Both occur rarely, but can have devastating effects if not diagnosed and treated promptly and effectively.

Abscess

Risk

The incidence of spinal epidural abscess is surprisingly low, given the popularity of regional anesthesia for a wide variety of surgical procedures. It occurs 0.2 to 1.2 times per 10,000 hospital admissions (77,78). It is probably even rarer among obstetric patients, as only ten cases have been reported in the literature (79–88). Two of these cases (79,85) occurred in the absence of anesthesia. However, an accurate estimate of the frequency of this complication cannot be made based on the appearance of case reports. A survey of anesthesia personnel from 245 hospitals around the world suggested that the true incidence of abscess following regional anesthesia is much greater, as 22% of the respondents were aware of a case of meningitis or epidural abscess after a spinal or epidural technique (89).

Source of Infection

Infecting organisms may reach the epidural space by several routes (84,90). During needle or catheter insertion, microbes can be transferred from the person performing the anesthetic to the patient. Poor aseptic technique can be involved, or organisms from the nasopharynx of the anesthesia provider can reach the epidural needle (91). Anesthetic medications can become contaminated, especially if drawn from multidose vials. Luckily, contamination of local anesthetics is rare, probably due to the bacteriostatic nature of these solutions (92).

The source of the infection may be within the patient's own body. During a regional technique, organisms can be brought from more superficial areas of the back to the vicinity of the spinal canal. If a catheter is left in place, a path is available for the infection to continue its spread. The catheter can act as a nidus for infection. Hematogenous spread from a distant site is a danger in bacteremic patients. Disruption of small vessels in the epidural space occurs in 8% of epidural placements (93,94). Blood from these vessels can introduce pathogenic organisms into the epidural space.

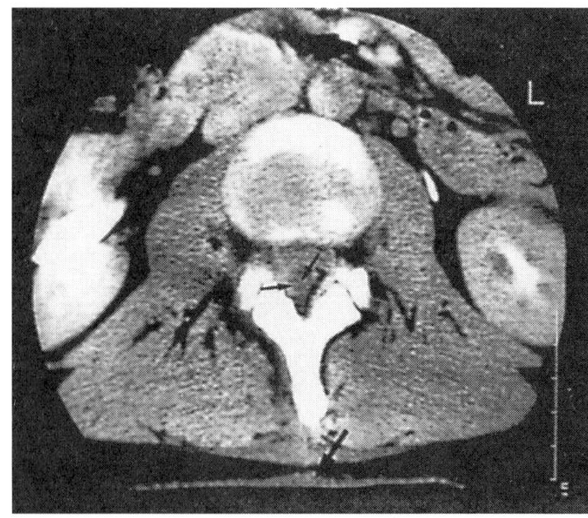

FIG. 5. Axial scan at the L_2 level. The *upper arrows* show the anterior displacement of the dural sac and its contents by an abscess in the posterior epidural space of the spinal canal. Inflamed subcutaneous tissue around the previous puncture site is shown by the *lower arrow.* (Reprinted from ref. 87, with permission.)

Symptoms

Days to months can pass before symptoms of spinal epidural abscess appear. Then, a typical progression classically occurs (95). First there are complaints of fever and backache. Complaints due to radiculopathy follow shortly. Sensory deficits and muscle and sphincter weakness eventually are found and progress finally to paralysis. The rate of neurological deterioration varies from hours to weeks (77). On presentation, most patients complain of deep back pain, and the majority are febrile (96). Leukocytosis and an elevated erythrocyte sedimentation rate are common.

Diagnosis

Definitive diagnosis of spinal epidural abscess involves radiologic imaging. Using computed tomography (CT) scanning (Fig. 5), most of the important structures can be visualized (97). Myelography can be helpful in addition to visualize the soft tissue. However, myelography adds to the infectious risk of the diagnostic process, but some abscess lesions cannot be diagnosed with CT imaging alone (98).

Magnetic resonance imaging (MRI) (Fig. 6) is as sensitive as CT scanning in diagnosing these lesions (99). It has the advantage of being able to identify other associated conditions, such as disc herniation or cord infarct (77). It also is more helpful in demarcating the extent of the lesion. Unfortunately, MRI may not distinguish between frank pus, granulation tissue, and hematoma. It also may not differentiate between epidural and subdural lesions. These deficiencies of MRI may be corrected by enhancing the signal intensity with gandolinium (86). Lastly, MRI also is more susceptible to motion artifacts than CT scanning.

Treatment

Once the diagnosis is made, management usually involves surgical exploration and drainage, followed by antibiotic therapy for at least 2 to 4 weeks. Medical therapy alone has been used successfully in some cases (100),

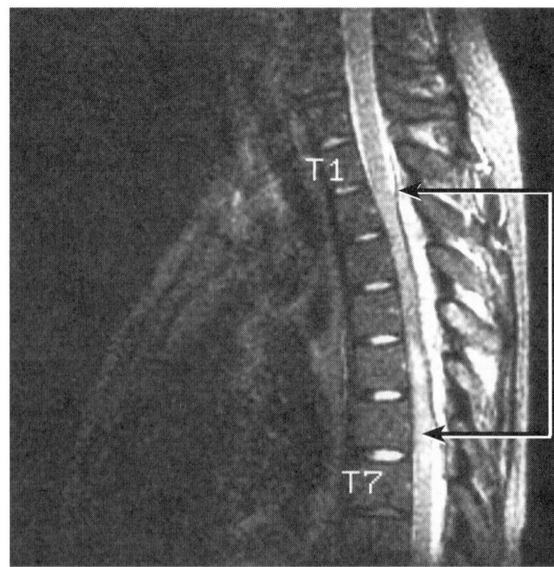

FIG. 6. Magnetic resonance image of the spine of a 27-year-old pregnant woman, showing epidural abscess from T_1 to T_6 *(bracketed area).* (Reprinted from ref. 83, with permission.)

but it increases the risk of further neurological deterioration. Outcome depends on the degree of neurological impairment at the time of diagnosis and the length of time it has been present before surgery is performed (101).

Meningitis

Infection of the subarachnoid space is very rare following regional anesthesia. Studies that include tens of thousands of patients do not report a single case (102,103). No cases were found among 14,000 spinal blocks for obstetrics (104). However, meningitis after the dural barrier has been breached by a spinal needle is well documented. Focusing on patients in a meningitis ward, Kilpatrick and Giris (105) identified 17 who had recent spinal anesthesia. Likewise, isolated cases have been reported of obstetric patients who developed meningitis after spinal (106,107) or epidural (108) anesthesia.

The causes of septic meningitis—contamination of equipment of anesthetics, nonsterile techniques, or bacteremia or infection at the site of injection—are similar to those of abscess formation (109). In addition, detergent residues on needles or syringes and coring of tissues by the spinal needle can produce aseptic meningitis (107).

The onset of symptoms can vary from days to weeks. Once the characteristic fever, headache, and stiff neck appear, the infection must be treated aggressively with antibiotic therapy to prevent further deterioration.

Risk of Dural Puncture

Whether introducing a needle into the subarachnoid space of bacteremic patients increases the risk for developing meningitis has been debated for decades. Interestingly, the diagnosis of meningitis is made routinely by lumbar puncture (LP) in patients suspected of having the condition. However, some researchers have long warned that this diagnostic maneuver may initiate the disease. In 1919, Wegeforth and Latham (110) reported that LPs are associated with subsequent meningitis. Later, Teele et al. (111) repeated the warning when they reported that bacteremic babies were more likely to develop meningitis if they had a diagnostic LP. However, in both studies, the clinicians may have performed the LPs in individuals who were in the early stages of the progression of meningitis and who would have developed the infection anyway. For example, Wegeforth and Latham performed their study during a meningitis epidemic.

In contrast, other studies of both bacteremic and nonbacteremic individuals concluded that performing diagnostic LPs does not increase the risk of contracting meningitis (112–115). Given the frequent use of diagnostic LPs, if they posed a significant risk of meningitis, unequivocal data to that effect probably would be available (116).

RISK OF REGIONAL ANESTHESIA IN INTRAAMNIOTIC INFECTION

Only three retrospective studies have examined the risk of epidural or spinal anesthesia in patients with clinical IAI.

Ramanathan et al. (117) reviewed records of 115 parturients with IAI symptoms who received epidural or spinal anesthetics. They found no anesthetic-associated infectious complications. However, none of these women had blood cultures done, and only 39 were symptomatic at the time of anesthetic induction. All of these women had first received antibiotic therapy. Although this study included only a small number of patients, it suggested that regional anesthesia was safe in patients who had received antibiotics.

A larger study by Bader et al. (65) found no infectious complications related to 279 regional anesthetics in women with clinically diagnosed IAI. Although 84% of the patients had not received antibiotics before the anesthetic, it was unclear if these women were symptomatic at the time. None of the bacteremic patients received antibiotics before their anesthetic. However, only three patients fell into this subgroup, and their bacteremia may not have occurred until after the anesthetic. This study did show that the diagnosis of IAI did not make it imperative that a patient receive antibiotics before anesthetic induction.

Taking a different approach, Goodman et al. (66) started with a list of patients whose placentas were positive for chorioamnionitis on pathologic examination after delivery. Here, too, no infectious complications were found among 531 such women who received regional anesthetics. In this study, the temporal relationship between the symptoms of IAI and the placement of the regional anesthetic was more carefully documented. One-fourth of the patients with fever and three-fourths of those with leukocytosis just before anesthetic induction did not receive previous antibiotic therapy (Fig. 7). Also, the epidural catheter was left in place for at least 24 hours after delivery in dozens of women who were febrile and who had elevated white blood counts without complications.

The association of histologic chorioamnionitis and clinical infection is controversial (118,119). Histologic chorioamnionitis is defined as the infiltration of the chorioamnion by polymorphonuclear leukocytes and can be found three times as often as clinical signs of IAI. Conversely, clinical IAI may be seen occasionally when histologic chorioamnionitis is absent. The assumption that the presence of histologic chorioamnionitis will predict all cases of IAI therefore may be erroneous.

Our group confirmed the safety of regional anesthesia in patients with IAI (66). Neither the presence of symptoms nor the absence of antibiotics contraindicates regional anesthesia. Furthermore, the presence of fever or leukocytosis does not mandate removal of an epidural catheter.

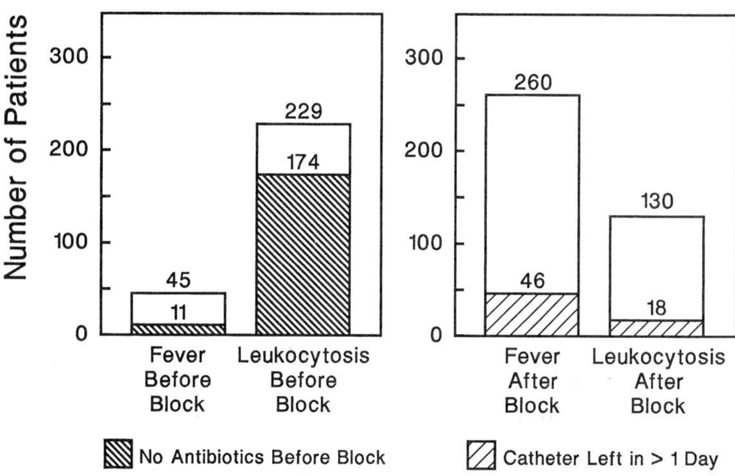

FIG. 7. *Left:* Frequency of regional block placement despite the presence of fever or leukocytosis with and without prior antibiotic administration. *Right:* Fraction of parturients who had fever or leukocytosis after their epidural anesthetic and whose epidural catheter was left in place for at least 24 hours. (Reprinted from ref. 66, with permission.)

Unfortunately, all of these studies may be skewed by the fact that sicker patients may not have been offered the option of regional anesthesia. These studies may have only established the safety of regional techniques if the infectious symptoms have not advanced past a certain point.

Animal Studies

The link between diagnostic LP and meningitis also has been studied in animals. In both cats and dogs, trauma to the meninges (lumbar or cisternal puncture) after inducing bacteremia increases the incidence of meningitis (120,121). Unfortunately, the bacterial inoculum used in these studies may have been too large to have clinical relevance. In contrast, spinal puncture after inducing pneumococcal bacteremia in rabbits and dogs did not cause leukocyte infiltration of the meninges and cerebrospinal fluid (CSF) (122).

More recently, Carp and Bailey (123) performed a similar protocol in rats. Twenty-four hours after dural puncture, cisternal CSF was sampled and cultured. Twelve of 40 animals with a clinically relevant *E. coli* bacteremia had positive CSF cultures. Bacteremic animals not having dural puncture always had sterile CSF. Nonbacteremic animals undergoing dural puncture also had sterile CSF. Giving a single dose of gentamycin before dural puncture prevented meningitis (Fig. 8). The investigators concluded that previous antibiotic therapy may eliminate the risk of meningitis after dural puncture in septic animals.

The clinical implications of the study by Carp and Bailey are unclear (116). Although *E. coli* is a common cause of bacteremia in humans, it is an unusual cause of meningitis. Their method of using a cisternal site of dural puncture differed from clinical practice too. The 26-gauge needle that they used in the rats would translate to a very large dural tear in humans. Finally, they knew the identification of the organism and its susceptibility to gentamycin from the start.

Recommendations

- Parturients at risk for IAI but who currently are asymptomatic can be given a regional anesthetic without hesitation. No prior administration of antibiotics is needed.
- Parturients who are febrile, but show no other signs or symptoms of infection, also may receive a regional anesthetic. If no antibiotic is administered before the anesthetic induction, these women most likely will follow an uneventful course. In the absence of signs of an infection elsewhere, their IAI can be assumed to be confined to the uterus. However, lacking prospective and conclusive proof of the safety of regional block in women with untreated IAI, the prudent course may be to give at least one dose of antibiotic before the anesthetic.

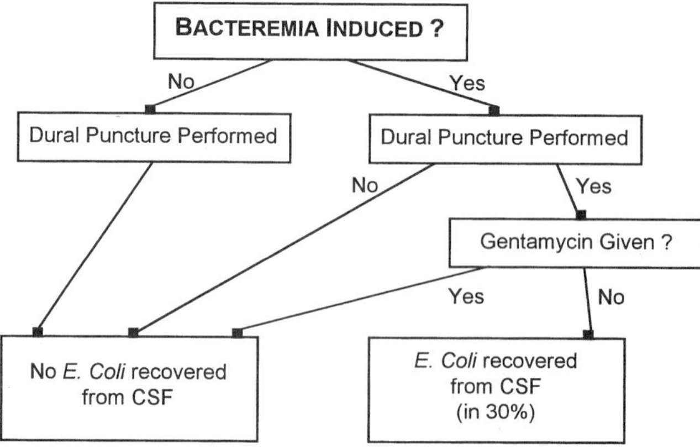

FIG. 8. Experiment by Carp and Bailey (123) in bacteremic rats, which showed that *E. coli* could be isolated from the spinal fluid only if no gentamycin was administered before the dural puncture.

- Febrile parturients with foul-smelling amniotic fluid or other signs and symptoms of IAI should be treated as described previously. Their infection in all likelihood is confined to the uterus, and they probably are not bacteremic. However, here too, in the absence of conclusive evidence to the contrary, antibiotics should be given before regional anesthesia.
- Parturients who are overtly septic need antipyretic analgesics and antibiotic therapy before regional anesthesia can be considered. Here, the risk of spreading the infection while placing the regional block may be too high unless the patient shows signs of responding to the antimicrobial medication. However, even in these women, the risk of spinal or epidural infection after neuraxial analgesia may be less than the risks of alternative therapies. For instance, at cesarean section, the minute risk of an infectious complication from a regional block in a septic patient on appropriate antibiotic therapy may be dwarfed by the significant risk of general anesthesia, failed intubation, and aspiration (116).
- If an epidural catheter had been placed before signs of sepsis are noted, the catheter need not be removed (124,125). An epidural catheter in a properly treated patient would not be expected to serve as a nidus for infection. As always, vigilance is the key to safe practice, and a discharge at the insertion site (but not erythema alone) should dictate immediate removal of the catheter (126).

SUMMARY

- Intraamniotic infection complicates up to 10% of pregnancies and is associated with significant maternal and fetal morbidity. Most infections ascend from vaginal flora, but bacteria also can arrive from the blood stream.
- Mild infection is well tolerated by mother and fetus, but more serious cases can lead to maternal and fetal acidosis and fetal distress.
- Diagnosis of IAI must be made from multiple insensitive and nonspecific signs and symptoms.
- Regional anesthesia can upset the temperature balance and cause a mild elevation in core temperature in parturients.
- Risks of regional anesthesia include spinal epidural abscess and meningitis. These complications occur infrequently and must be balanced against the benefits of the procedure.

REFERENCES

1. Newton ER. Chorioamnionitis and intraamniotic Infection. *Clin Obstet Gynecol* 1993;36:795.
2. Gibbs RS, Duff P. Progress in pathogenesis and management of clinical intraamniotic infection. *Am J Obstet Gynecol* 1991;164:1317.
3. Fiscella K. Race, perinatal outcome, and amniotic infection. *Obstet Gynecol Surv* 1995;51:60.
4. Soper DE, Mayhall CG, Dalton HP. Risk factors for intraamniotic infection: a prospective epidemiologic study. *Am J Obstet Gynecol* 1989;161:562.
5. Gibbs RS, Castillo MS, Rodgers PJ. Management of acute chorioamnionitis. *Am J Obstet Gynecol* 1980;136:709.
6. Gibbs RS, Blanco JD, St. Clair PJ, Castaneda YS. Quantitative bacteriology of amniotic fluid from women with clinical intraamniotic infection at term. *J Infect Dis* 1982;145:1.
7. Yoder PR, Gibbs RS, Blanco JD, Castaneda YS, St. Clair PJ. A prospective, controlled study of maternal and perinatal outcome after intra-amniotic infection at term. *Am J Obstet Gynecol* 1983; 145:695.
8. Duff P, Sanders R, Gibbs RS. The course of labor in term patients with chorioamnionitis. *Am J Obstet Gynecol* 1983;147:391.
9. Gilstrap LC, Leveno KJ, Cox SM, et al. Intrapartum treatment of acute chorioamnionitis: impact on neonatal sepsis. *Am J Obstet Gynecol* 1988;159:579.
10. Tramount EC, Hoover DL. General or nonspecific host defense mechanisms. In: Mandell GL, Bennett JE, Dolin R, eds. *Principles and practice of infectious disease,* 4th ed. New York: Churchill Livingstone, 1995:30.
11. Hoeprich PD, O'Grady LF. Manifestations of infectious diseases. In: Hoeprich PD, Jordan MC, Ronald AR, eds. 5th ed. Philadelphia: JB Lippincott, 1994:102.
12. Cooper KE. *Fever and antipyresis.* Cambridge: Cambridge University Press, 1995:36.
13. Mackowiak PA, Wasserman SS, Levine MM. A critical appraisal of 98.6°F, the upper limit of the normal body temperature, and other legacies of Carl Reinhold August Wunderlich. *JAMA* 1992;268:1578.
14. McMurray RG, Katz VL, Berry MJ, Cefalo RC. The effect of pregnancy on metabolic responses during rest, immersion, and aerobic exercise in the water. *Am J Obstet Gynecol* 1988;158:481.
15. Cunningham FG, MacDonald PC, Gant NF, eds. *Williams' obstetrics,* 18th ed. Norwalk: Appleton & Lange, 1989:251.
16. Gilbert RS, Power GG. Fetal and uteroplacental heat production in sheep. *J Appl Physiol* 1986;61:2018.
17. Gilbert RD, Schroder H, Kawamura T, Dale PS, Power GG. Heat transfer pathways between fetal lamb and ewe. *J Appl Physiol* 1985;59:634.
18. Walker DW, Wood C. Temperature relationship of the mother and fetus during labor. *Am J Obstet Gynecol* 1970;107:83.
19. Joris J, Ozaki M, Sessler DI, et al. Epidural anesthesia impairs both central and peripheral thermoregulatory control during general anesthesia. *Anesthesiology* 1994;80:268.
20. Emerick TH, Ozaki M, Sessler DI, Walters K, Schroeder M. Epidural anesthesia increases apparent leg temperature and decreases the shivering threshold. *Anesthesiology* 1994;81:289.
21. Ozaki M, Kurz A, Sessler DI, et al. Thermoregulatory thresholds during epidural and spinal anesthesia. *Anesthesiology* 1994;81:282.
22. Leslie K, Sessler DI. Reduction in the shivering threshold is proportional to spinal block height. *Anesthesiology* 1996;84:1327.
23. Marx GF, Loew DAY. Tympanic temperature during labour and parturition. *Br J Anaesth* 1975;47:600.
24. Goodlin RC, Chapin JW. Determinants of maternal temperature during labor. *Am J Obstet Gynecol* 1982;143:97.
25. Birnbach DJ, Stein DJ, Hartman JK, Danzer BI, Grunebaum A. Is maternal fever associated with the administration of regional anesthesia in laboring patients? *Anesthesiology* 1996;85:A899.
26. Kapusta L, Confino E, Ismajovich Y, David M. The effect of epidural analgesia on maternal thermoregulation in labor. *Int J Gynaecol Obstet* 1985;23:185.
27. Fusi L, Maresh MJ, Steer PJ, Beard RW. Maternal pyrexia associated with the use of epidural analgesia in labour. *Lancet* 1989;1:1250.
28. Camann WR, Hortvet LA, Hughes N, Bader AM, Datta S. Maternal temperature regulation during extradural analgesia for labour. *Br J Anaesth* 1991;67:565.
29. Mercier FJ, Benhamou D. Hyperthermia related to epidural analgesia during labor. *Int J Obstet Anesth* 1997;6:19.
30. Macaulay JH, Bond K, Steer PJ. Epidural analgesia in labor and fetal hyperthermia. *Obstet Gynecol* 1992;80:665.
31. Lieberman E, Lang JM, Frigoletto F, Richardson DK, Ringer SA, Cohen A. Epidural analgesia, intrapartum fever, and neonatal sepsis evaluation. *Pediatrics* 1997;99:415.

32. Dinarello CA, Wolff SM. Pathogenesis of fever and the acute phase response. In: Mandell GL, Bennett JE, Dolin R, eds. *Principles and practice of infectious disease,* 4th ed. New York: Churchill Livingstone. 1995:530.
33. Harris WH, Pittman QJ, Veale WL, Cooper KE, Van Petten GR. Cardiovascular effects of fever in the ewe and fetal lamb. *Am J Obstet Gynecol* 1977;128:262.
34. Cefalo RC, Hellegers AE. The effects of maternal hyperthermia on maternal and fetal cardiovascular and respiratory function. *J Obstet Gynecol* 1978;131:687.
35. Morishima HO, Glaser B, Niemann WH, James LS. Increased uterine activity and fetal deterioration during maternal hyperthermia. *Am J Obstet Gynecol* 1975;121:531.
36. Santos DJ. Intra-amniotic infection. In: Norris MC, ed. *Obstetric anesthesia.* Philadelphia: JB Lippincott, 1993:559.
37. Gibbs RS. Chorioamnionitis and bacterial vaginosis. *Am J Obstet Gynecol* 1993;169:460.
38. Krohn MA, Hillier SL, Nugent RP, et al. The genital flora of women with amniotic infection. *J Infect Dis* 1995;171:1475.
39. Eschenbach DA, Hillier S, Critchlow C, Stevens C, DeRouen T, Holmes KK. Diagnosis and clinical manifestations of bacterial vaginosis. *Am J Obstet Gynecol* 1988;158:819.
40. Soper DE, Mayhall CG, Froggatt JW. Characterization and control of intraamniotic infection in an urban teaching hospital. *Am J Obstet Gynecol* 1996;175:304.
41. Ledger WJ, Norman M, Gee C, Lewis W. Bacteremia on an obstetric-gynecologic service. *Am J Obstet Gynecol* 1975;121:205.
42. Mills JL, Harlap S, Harley EE. Should coitus late in pregnancy be discouraged? *Lancet* 1981;2:136.
43. Soper DE, Mayhall CG, Dalton HP. Risk factors for intraamniotic infection: a prospective epidemiologic study. *Am J Obstet Gynecol* 1989;161:562.
44. Galask RP, Snyder IS. Bacterial inhibition by amniotic fluid. *Am J Obstet Gynecol* 1968;102:949.
45. MacVicar J. Chorioamnionitis. In: Charles D, Finland M, eds: *Obstetric and perinatal infections.* Philadelphia: Lea & Febiger, 1973:479.
46. Lanier LR, Scarbrough RW, Fillingim DW, Baker RE. Incidence of maternal and fetal complications associated with rupture of the membranes before onset of labor. *Am J Obstet Gynecol* 1965;93:398.
47. Newton ER, Prihoda TJ, Gibbs RS. Logistic regression analysis of risk factors for intra-amniotic infection. *Obstet Gynecol* 1989;73:571.
48. Shubert PJ, Diss E, Iams JD. Etiology of preterm rupture of membranes. *Obstet Gynecol Clin North Am* 1992;19:251.
49. Romero R, Mazor M. Infection and preterm labor. *Clin Obstet Gynecol* 1988;31:553.
50. Gibbs RS, Duff P. Progress in pathogenesis and management of clinical intraamniotic infection. *Am J Obstet Gynecol* 1991;164:1317.
51. Gibbs RS, Romero R, Hillier SL, Eschenbach DA, Sweet RL. A review of premature birth and subclinical infection. *Am J Obstet Gynecol* 1992;166:1515.
52. Bennett P, Fisk N. Chorioamnionitis and pre-term delivery. *Baillieres Clin Obstet Gynaecol* 1993;7:25.
53. Bernal AL, Watson SP, Phaneuf S, Europe-Finner GN. Biochemistry and physiology of preterm labour and delivery. *Baillieres Clin Obstet Gynaecol* 1993;7:523.
54. Lopez Bernal A, Hansell DJ, Khong TY, Keeling JW, Turnbull AC. Prostaglandin E production by the fetal membranes in unexplained preterm labour and preterm labour associated with chorioamnionitis. *Br J Obstet Gynaecol* 1989;96:1133.
55. Schoonmaker JN, Lawellin DW, Lunt B, McGregor JA. Bacteria and inflammatory cells reduce chorioamniotic membrane integrity and tensile strength. *Obstet Gynecol* 1989;74:590.
56. Efrati P, Presentey B, Margalith M, Rozenszajn L. Leukocytes of normal pregnant women. *Obstet Gynecol* 1964;23:429.
57. Taylor DJ, Lind T. Puerperal haematological indices. *Br J Obstet Gynaecol* 1981;88:601.
58. Webb GA. Maternal death associated with premature rupture of membranes. *Am J Obstet Gynecol* 1967;98:594.
59. Blanco JD, Gibbs RS, Castaneda YS. Bacteremia in obstetrics: clinical course. *Obstet Gynecol* 1981;58:621.
60. Lee W, Clark SL, Cotton DB, et al. Septic shock during pregnancy. *Am J Obstet Gynecol* 1988;159:410.
61. Sullivan NM, Sutter VL, Mims MM, Marsh VH, Finegold SM. Clinical aspects of bacteremia after manipulation of the genitourinary tract. *J Infect Dis* 1973;127:49.
62. Munford RS. Sepsis and septic shock. In: Fauci AS, Braunwald E, Isselbacher KJ, et al., eds. *Harrison's principles of internal medicine*, 14th ed. New York: McGraw-Hill, 1998:776.
63. Parrilo JE. Shock syndromes related to sepsis. In: Bennett JC, Plum F, eds. *Cecil textbook of medicine*, 20th ed. Philadelphia: WB Saunders, 1996:496.
64. Young LS. Sepsis syndrome. In: Mandell GL, Benett JE, Dolin R, eds. *Principles and practices of infectious diseases*, 4th ed. New York: Churchill Livingstone, 1995:690.
65. Bader AM, Gilbertson L, Kirz L, Datta S. Regional anesthesia in women with chorioamnionitis. *Reg Anesth* 1992;17:84.
66. Goodman EJ, DeHorta E, Taguiam JM. Safety of spinal and epidural anesthesia in parturients with chorioamnionitis. *Reg Anesth* 1996; 21:436.
67. Malhotra M, Gupta HL, Mondal A. Pulmonary complications of septicaemia in women. *J Ind Med Assoc* 1990;88:131.
68. Gamsu H. Intrauterine bacterial infections. In: *Intrauterine infections—CIBA Foundation symposium.* New York: Associated Scientific Publishers, 1973:135.
69. Wolf RL, Olinsky A. Prolonged rupture of fetal membranes and neonatal infections. *S Afr Med J* 1976;50:574.
70. Burchell RC. Premature spontaneous rupture of the membranes. *Am J Obstet Gynecol* 1964;88:251.
71. Sperling RS, Ramamurthy RS, Gibbs RS. A comparison of intrapartum versus immediate postpartum treatment of intra-amniotic infection. *Obstet Gynecol* 1987;70:861.
72. Gibbs RS, Dinsmoor MJ, Newton ER, Ramamurthy RS. A randomized trial of intrapartum versus immediate postpartum treatment of women with intra-amniotic infection. *Obstet Gynecol* 1988;72:823.
73. Kirschbaum T. Antibiotics in the treatment of preterm labor. *Am J Obstet Gynecol* 1993;168:1239.
74. Zlatnik FJ. Management of premature rupture of membranes at term. *Obstet Gynecol Clin North Am* 1992;19:353.
75. Mercer BM, Arheart KL. Antimicrobial therapy in expectant management of preterm premature rupture of the membranes. *Lancet* 1995; 346:1271.
76. Thomas DG. Epidural analgesia in the presence of fever [Letter]. *Anaesthesia* 1986;41:553.
77. Hlavin ML, Kaminski HJ, Ross JS, Ganz E. Spinal epidural abscess: a ten-year perspective. *Neurosurgery* 1990;27:177.
78. Crawford JS. Some maternal complications of epidural analgesia for labour. *Anaesthesia* 1985;40:1219.
79. Mail CG, Martin R. Puerperal spinal epidural abscess. *Lancet* 1973;1:608.
80. Crawford JS. Pathology in the epidural space. *Br J Anaesth* 1975;47: 412.
81. Usubiaga JE. Neurological complications following epidural anesthesia. *Int Anesth Clin* 1975;13:33.
82. Scott DB, Hibbard BM. Serious non-fatal complications associated with extradural block in obstetric practice. *Br J Anaesth* 1990;64:537.
83. Van Winter JT, Nielsen SNJ, Ogburn PL. Epidural abscess associated with intravenous drug abuse in a pregnant patient. *Mayo Clin Proc* 1991;66:1036.
84. Ngan Kee WD, Jones MR, Thomas P, Worth RJ. Extradural abscess complicating extradural anaesthesia for caesarean section. *Br J Anaesth* 1992;69:647.
85. Kitching AJ, Rice ASC. Extradural abscess in the postpartum period. *Br J Anaesth* 1993;70:703.
86. Borum SE, McLeskey CH, Williamson JB, Harris FS, Knight AB. Epidural abscess after obstetric epidural analgesia. *Anesthesiology* 1995;82:1523.
87. Kindler C, Seeberger M, Siegemund M, Schneider M. Extradural abscess complicating lumbar extradural anaesthesia in an obstetric patient. *Acta Anaesthesiol Scand* 1996;40:858.
88. Dhillon AR, Russell IF. Epidural abscess in association with obstetric epidural analgesia. *Int J Obstet Anesth* 1997;6:118.
89. Pue A, Ng M, Poelter D. Complications in Ob anesthesia—a survey of occurrence and related patterns of practice. *S.O.A.P. Abstracts* 1997:69.
90. Carson D, Wildsmith JAW. The risk of extradural abscess. *Br J Anaesth* 1995;75:520.
91. North JB, Brophy BP. Epidural abscess: a hazard of spinal epidural anaesthesia. *Aust N Z J Surg* 1979;49:484.
92. Schmidt RM, Rosenkranz HS. Antimicrobial activity of local anesthetics: lidocaine and prilocaine. *J Infect Dis* 1970;121:597.

93. Beilin Y, Bernstein HH, Zucher-Pinchoff B. The optimal distance that a multiorifice epidural catheter should be threaded into the epidural space. *Anesth Analg* 1995;81:301.
94. D'Angelo R, Berkibile BL, Gerancher JC. Prospective examination of epidural catheter insertion. *Anesthesiology* 1996;84:88.
95. Heusner AP. Nontuberculous spinal epidural infections. *N Engl J Med* 1948;239:845.
96. Curling OD, Gower DJ, McWhorter JM. Changing concepts in spinal epidural abscess: a report of 29 cases. *Neurosurgery* 1990;27:185.
97. Leys D, Lesoin F, Viaud C, et al. Decreased morbidity from acute bacterial spinal epidural abscess using computed tomography and nonsurgical treatment in selected patients. *Ann Neurol* 1985;17:350.
98. Erntell M, Holtas S, Norlin K, Dahlquist E, Nilsson-Ehle I. *Scand J Infect Dis* 1988;20:323.
99. Donovan Post MJ, Quencer RM, Montalvo BM, Katz BH, Eismont FJ, Green BA. Spinal infection: evaluation with MR imaging and intraoperative US. *Radiology* 1988;169:765.
100. Mampalam TJ, Rosegay H, Andrews BT, Rosenblum ML, Pitts LH. Nonoperative treatment of spinal epidural infections. *J Neurosurg* 1989;71:208.
101. Verner EF, Musher DM. Spinal epidural abscess. *Med Clin North Am* 1985;69:375.
102. Phillips OC, Ebner H, Nelson AT, Black MH. Neurologic complications following spinal anesthesia with lidocaine: a prospective review of 10,440 cases. *Anesthesiology* 1969;30:284.
103. Dripps RD, Vandam LD. Long-term follow-up of patients who received 10,098 spinal anesthetics. *JAMA* 1954;156:1486.
104. Scott BD, Tunstall ME. Serious complications associated with epidural/spinal blockade in obstetrics: a two-year prospective study. *Int J Obstet Anesth* 1995;4:133.
105. Kilpatrick ME, Giris NI. Meningitis—a complication of spinal anesthesia. *Anesth Analg* 1983;62:513.
106. Berga S, Trierweiler MW. Bacterial meningitis following epidural anesthesia for vaginal delivery: a case report. *Obstet Gynecol* 1989;74:437.
107. Roberts SP, Petts HV. Meningitis after obstetric spinal anaesthesia. *Anaesthesia* 1990;45:376.
108. Ready LB, Helfer D. Bacterial meningitis in parturients after epidural anesthesia. *Anesthesiology* 1989;71:988.
109. Berman RS, Eisele JH. Bacteremia, spinal anesthesia, and development of meningitis. *Anesthesiology* 1978;48:376.
110. Wegeforth P, Latham JR. Lumbar puncture as a factor in the causation of meningitis. *Am J Med Sci* 1919;158:183.
111. Teele DW, Dashefsky B, Rakusan T, Klein JO. Meningitis after lumbar puncture in children with bacteremia. *N Engl J Med* 1981; 305:1079.
112. Pray LG. Lumbar puncture as a factor in the pathogenesis of meningitis. *Am J Dis Child* 1941;62:295.
113. Eng RHK, Seligman SJ. Lumbar puncture-induced meningitis. *JAMA* 1981;245:1456.
114. Shapiro ED, Aaron NH, Wald ER, Chiponis D. Risk factors for development of bacterial meningitis among children with occult bacteremia. *J Pediatr* 1986;109:15.
115. Smith KM, Deddish RB, Ogata ES. Meningitis associated with serial lumbar punctures and post-hemorrhagic hydrocephalus. *J Pediatr* 1986;109:1057.
116. Chestnut DH. Spinal anesthesia in the febrile patient. *Anesthesiology* 1992;76:667.
117. Ramanathan J, Vaddadi A, Mercer BM, Sibai B, Angel JJ. Epidural anesthesia in women with chorioamnionitis. *Anesth Rev* 1992;19:35.
118. Dong Y, St. Clair PJ, Ramzy I, Kagan-Hallet KS, Gibbs RS. A microbiologic and clinical study of placental inflammation at term. *Obstet Gynecol* 1987;70:175.
119. Zlatnik FJ, Gellhaus TM, Benda JA, Koontz FP, Burmeister LF. Histologic chorioamnionitis, microbial infection, and prematurity. *Obstet Gynecol* 1990;76:355.
120. Weed LH, Wegeforth P, Ayer JB, Felton LD. The production of meningitis by release of cerebrospinal fluid. *JAMA* 1919;72:190.
121. Petersdorf RG, Swarner DR, Garcia M. Studies on the pathogenesis of meningitis. II. Development of meningitis during pneumococcal bacteremia. *J Clin Invest* 1962;41:320.
122. Idzumi G. Experimental pneumoccocus meningitis in rabbits and dogs. *J Infect Dis* 1920;26:373.
123. Carp H, Bailey S. The association between meningitis and dural puncture in bacteremic rats. *Anesthesiology* 1992;76:739.
124. Behl S. Epidural analgesia in the presence of fever. *Anaesthesia* 1985;40:1240.
125. Jakobsen KB, Christensen MK, Carlsson PS. Extradural anaesthesia for repeated surgical treatment in the presence of infection. *Br J Anaesth* 1995;75:536.
126. Darchy B, Forceville X, Bavoux E, Soriot F, Domart Y. Clinical and bacteriologic survey of epidural analgesia in patients in the intensive care unit. *Anesthesiology* 1996;85:988.
127. Greenberg LR, Moore TR. Staphylococcal septicemia and adult respiratory distress syndrome in pregnancy treated with extracorporeal carbon dioxide removal. *Obstet Gynecol* 1995;86:657.

Obstetric Anesthesia, second edition,
edited by Mark C. Norris.
Lippincott Williams & Wilkins, Philadelphia © 1999.

CHAPTER 30

Peripartum Hemorrhage and Maternal Resuscitation

Fazeela Ferouz

Despite advances in both obstetric and anesthetic care, peripartum hemorrhage remains a leading cause of maternal morbidity and mortality (1). Although decreasing in frequency, maternal mortality from peripartum hemorrhage occurs in 10 to 2,000 per 100,000 live births (2). In less developed countries, peripartum hemorrhage is among the leading causes of death in women of childbearing age.

Excessive bleeding occurs in 5% to 8% of pregnancies (2). Minimizing the maternal risks of peripartum hemorrhage first requires recognition of patients at increased risk. This chapter will detail the multiple risk factors for maternal bleeding. Advances in antepartum and intrapartum care have decreased the frequency of maternal death from antepartum hemorrhage. Along with obstetric intervention, prompt management by the anesthesia care team is vital in reducing maternal mortality and morbidity.

INITIAL EVALUATION

Preanesthetic evaluation of any obstetric patient involves a directed history and physical examination. Look for medical illnesses, prior surgeries, and obstetric complications that can increase the risk of maternal hemorrhage (Table 1). On physical examination, look for signs and symptoms of abnormal coagulation or hypovolemia (Table 2). Patients at high risk for peripartum hemorrhage may need additional laboratory evaluation (Table 3).

If a parturient presents with vaginal bleeding, assess the nature and quantity of blood loss. It can be difficult to quantitate the exact amount of hemorrhage. During pregnancy, blood volume expands 40% to 50%; thus, hemodynamic changes may not be apparent until significant bleeding has already occurred. Measurement of orthostatic changes blood pressure and heart rate can give an indication of volume status (Table 4).

General considerations for the parturient predisposed to hemorrhage include preparation for surgical delivery of the fetus, volume resuscitation, and transfusion of blood and blood products as indicated by clinical status.

F. Ferouz: Department of Anesthesiology, St. Luke's–Roosevelt Hospital Center, College of Physicians & Surgeons of Columbia University, New York, New York 10019.

TABLE 1. *Maternal conditions that can increase the risk of peripartum hemorrhage*

Bleeding disorders
von Willebrand's
Coagulation abnormalities
Anemia, history of uterine myoma, polyps
Pregnancy-related disorders
Pregnancy-induced thrombocytopenia
Preeclampsia
HELLP syndrome
Chorioamnionitis
Abnormal fetal presentation
Placenta previa
Previous uterine surgery
Low transverse cesarean section
Myomectomy
Grand multiparity
Multiple gestation, macrosomia
Maternal trauma
Medications
NSAIDs
Warfarin
Heparin
Illicit drug use (cocaine)

HELLP, hemolysis, elevated liver enzymes, and low platelet count; NSAIDs, nonsteroidal antiinflammatory drugs.

TABLE 2. *Physical findings suggesting increased risk of maternal hemorrhage*

Signs of abnormal coagulation
Bruises
Petechiae
Bleeding gingiva
Bleeding from IV sites
Hematoma at IM injection sites
Signs of hypovolemia or anemia
Skin turgor
Pale conjunctiva
Syncope
Mental status changes
Nausea
Abdominal pain unrelated to contractions
Vital signs changes
Hypotension
Tachycardia
Orthostatic hypotension

TABLE 3. *Laboratory evaluation of the parturient at risk of hemorrhage*

Hemoglobin/hematocrit
Prothrombin time
Partial thromboplastin time
Fibrinogen
Platelet count

The potential for rapid fluid administration requires at least one, preferably two, large-bore intravenous catheters. An indwelling urinary catheter can give a rough guide to adequacy of volume replacement and renal perfusion. In some cases, central access and an intraarterial catheter may be indicated.

In patients at risk for obstetric hemorrhage, a blood sample should be sent for type and screen. For those identified as being at significant risk for blood loss where transfusion is likely, a blood sample should be typed and cross-matched, with 2 to 4 U of packed red blood cells readily available. Equipment for rapid transfusion and fluid warming should be prepared. In addition to the anesthesiologist and obstetrician, key personnel, such as operating room staff and blood bank and laboratory technicians, should be alerted to the situation.

ANTEPARTUM HEMORRHAGE

Vaginal bleeding in early pregnancy may be due to:

- Ectopic pregnancy,
- Spontaneous abortion,
- Trophoblastic disorders,
- Local vaginal and cervical lesions,
- Malignancy, or
- Coagulation disorder.

TABLE 4. *Classification of hemorrhage in the 60-kg gravida at 30 weeks' gestation*

Class	Volume lost	Clinical findings
Modest bleeding	≤15% of blood volume (≤900 ml)	Mild tachycardia Variable pallor Normal blood pressure Normal respirations Negative capillary blanching test Negative tilt test Normal urine output
Moderate bleeding	20%–25% of blood volume (1,200–1,500 mL)	Tachycardia (heart rate 110–130) Diastolic hypertension, decreased pulse pressure Moderate tachypnea Positive capillary blanching test Positive tilt test Urine output 25–40 mL/h
Severe bleeding	30%–35% of blood volume (1,800–2,100 mL)	Marked tachycardia (heart rate 120–160) Cold, clammy, pallid skin Hypotension Tachypnea (respirations 30–50/min) Oliguria
Massive bleeding	≥40% of blood volume (≥2,400 mL)	Profound shock No peripheral blood pressure discernible (systolic blood pressure <80 mm Hg) Peripheral pulses absent Marked tachycardia Circulatory collapse Oliguria or anuria

After Baker RN. Evaluation and management of critically ill patients. In: Wynn RM, ed. *Obstetrics and gynecology annual: 1977,* vol. 6. New York: Appleton-Century-Crofts, 1977:295; and Beneditti TJ. Obstetric hemorrhage. In: Gabbe SG, Niebyl JR, Simpson JL, eds. *Obstetrics: normal and problem pregnancies,* 2nd ed. New York: Churchill Livingstone, 1991:573.

The most common causes of bleeding during mid-pregnancy include:

- Abnormalities of placental implantation (i.e., placenta previa),
- Placental abruption, and
- Preterm labor.

Placenta Previa

The placenta usually implants well away from the lower uterine segment and high in the body or fundus of the uterus. Placenta previa is positioning of the placenta over or very near the cervical os. The proximity of the placenta to the cervical os risks its disruption during cervical dilation. Or, a placenta previa could block the passage of the fetus through the birth canal. Placenta previa can be total (20% to 43% of cases), partial (31%), or marginal (Fig. 1) (3). Premature placental separation also can contribute to bleeding seen with a partial placenta previa.

Incidence

Placenta previa is the leading cause of third trimester maternal hemorrhage (4,5). This condition is responsible for one-third of antepartum hemorrhages. It occurs in approximately 5 per 1,000 deliveries, with death occurring in 0.03% of cases in the United States (4). Two major causes of maternal death in women with placenta previa are severe hemorrhage and complications of disseminated intravascular coagulation (DIC) (1). Fetal mortality is 4% to 8%. As most of these deliveries occur before 36 weeks' gestation, fetal immaturity is a major problem (5).

Risk Factors and Pathophysiology

Although the specific cause of placenta previa is unknown, there are several associated risk factors (Table 5) (3,6–10). Both uterine and placental factors may increase the risk of placenta previa. The mechanisms by which these factors increase the risk of placenta previa often are speculative.

Maternal age and parity increase the risk of placenta previa. Women over 30 years of age are three times more likely to have placenta previa than women less than 20 years (4). This finding may be related more to parity than age (11). Both placental and uterine factors may be involved in this risk. Gross and microscopic examination of placentas from older women often reveal infarcts, defective vascularization, and significant areas of decreased uteroplacental perfusion, which may be involved in the pathogenesis of placenta previa and abruption (11,12). The underlying cause of placenta previa may relate to atrophy or inflammation of placental blood vessels leading to abnormal decidual vascularization (13). Uterine vasculature is altered and endometrial blood flow is decreased to areas of previous placental implantation (i.e., previous pregnancies, abortions) (14). To maintain adequate perfusion in a subsequent pregnancy, the placenta implants over a larger surface, increasing the risk that it will encroach upon the cervical os (8).

Chronic mild hypoxemia due to exposure to nicotine and carbon monoxide from maternal cigarette smoking may cause compensatory placental hypertrophy (15). The larger placenta may be more likely to cover the cervical os.

Previous uterine surgery (especially low transverse uterine incision at cesarean delivery) is the greatest single risk factor for placenta previa. Here, the placenta may be more likely to implant over the uterine scar, or the scarred area of the uterus may not grow normally during a subsequent gestation.

More than 90% of ultrasonographically diagnosed placenta previas will resolve by term (16). This phenomenon, often called "placental migration," does not represent separation and reattachment of the placenta at a more cephalad site. Instead, proportionally greater development of the fundus and body of the uterus during the second and third trimester pulls the placenta away from the

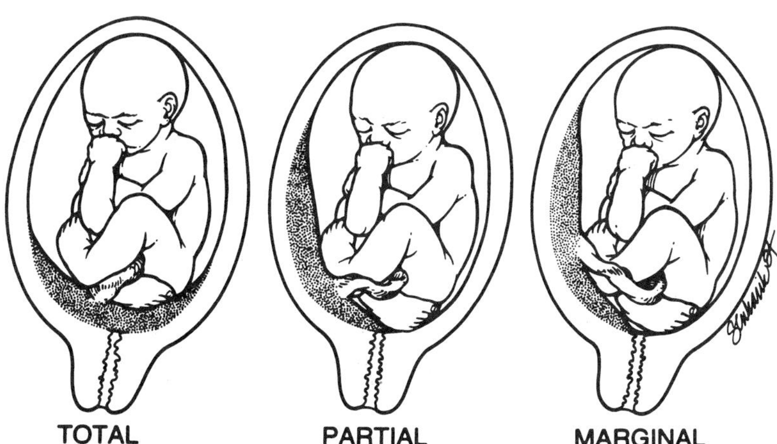

FIG. 1. Three types of placenta previa. (Reprinted from ref. 111, with permission.)

TABLE 5. *Maternal conditions associated with placenta previa*

	Relative Risk
Multiparity	2.0
Previous cesarean delivery	5.8
Prior uterine surgery: dilatation and curettage, myomectomy	2.0
Cigarette smoking	3.6
Age >34 y	4.7
Previous placenta previa	
Large placenta, multiple gestation	

cervical os. A scarred lower uterine segment will not grow normally, which may impair "migration" of a low-lying placenta (13). This phenomenon may explain the increased risks of placenta previa after cesarean section.

Diagnosis

Placenta previa often is identified early in gestation by ultrasound. Transabdominal ultrasound examination aids in confirming the diagnosis and defining the location of the placental margins. Placenta previa is seen in 6% to 45% of second trimester ultrasounds. Approximately 95% of these resolve by the end of the third trimester (4). Ultrasound may miss 7% of cases of placenta previa (17).

Transvaginal ultrasound provides greater resolution and can accurately diagnose placenta previa without increasing the risk of hemorrhage (18).Transperineal sonography also is better at identifying abnormal placental location than the transabdominal technique (19). Finally, magnetic resonance imaging (MRI) provides superior picture quality compared to ultrasound. It is useful in differentiating a low-lying placenta from partial previa and determining the margins of a posterior placenta (20). Presently, MRI is reserved for situations where sonographic examination is limited because of technical difficulty (21).

Obstetric Management

The management of a patient with placenta previa depends on several factors, including the gestational age and condition of the fetus, severity of hemorrhage, degree of placenta previa, and whether or not active labor is present. Ideally, delivery is postponed until the fetus is mature. However, fetal or maternal compromise may necessitate urgent intervention.

In cases of mild hemorrhage before fetal lung maturity, expectant management can promote the chances of fetal survival (22). Respiratory distress syndrome associated with prematurity is a significant cause of neonatal morbidity and mortality (5). Tocolysis, weekly ultrasonography, and blood transfusions as indicated may allow extension of pregnancy to at least 36 weeks. By then, the benefits of further fetal maturation must be weighed against the risk of maternal hemorrhage.

Manual examination of the cervix can precipitate severe bleeding. Obstetric experts recommend that cervical examination be performed only if imminent delivery is planned (12). Therefore, it should be done in the operating room where preparations for an emergent cesarean delivery and rapid treatment of hemorrhage have been made.

Women with placenta previa have a higher incidence of fetal malpresentation (4). Regardless of whether or not the previa is symptomatic, the combination of placenta previa and fetal malpresentation often precludes delivery by the vaginal route. Therefore, the majority of these patients are will undergo cesarean delivery.

Compared with other interventions such as blood transfusions and improved prenatal care, cesarean section has ultimately proven to be the most significant factor in reducing both maternal and perinatal mortality in cases of placenta previa (4,5).

Placenta Accreta, Increta, and Percreta

When the placenta abnormally attaches to or invades the myometrium in areas where the decidua basalis is absent or deficient, normal placental separation is impaired (23). Placenta accreta is the collective term for cases of abnormal placental adherence. Further classification is based on the degree to which the chorionic villi penetrate the myometrium (Fig. 2):

- Placenta accreta: villi adhere to the surface of the myometrium

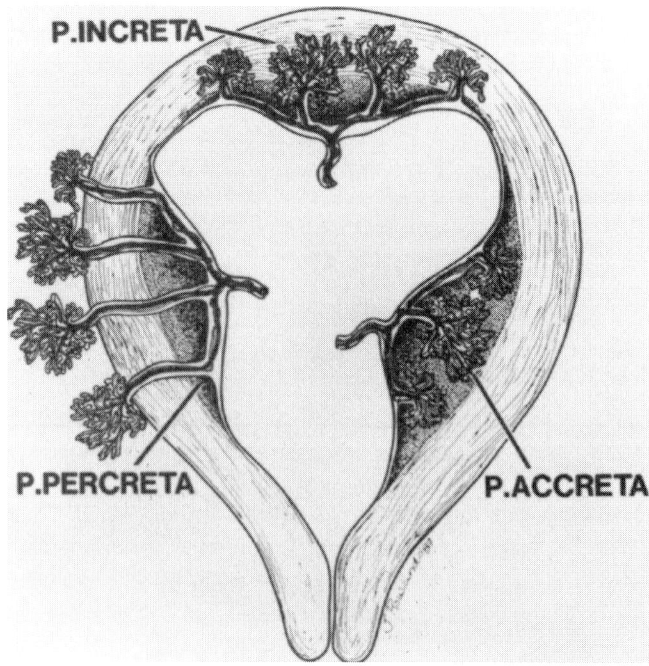

FIG. 2. Variations of abnormal placentation. (Reprinted from ref. 24, with permission.)

- Placenta increta: villi invade through the myometrial surface
- Placenta percreta: villi erode through the uterine wall.

The frequency of placenta accreta has increased in the past decade due to the rising number of cesarean deliveries (12,24). Placenta accreta is identified clinically in approximately 1 of 2,600 deliveries and is confirmed by histopathologic examination in about 1 of 4,000 (25,26).

Scarring of the uterus from previous cesarean delivery or dilatation and curettage decreases decidualization of the lower uterine segment (27). The risk of placenta accreta rises significantly in parturients with a history of both previous placenta previa and cesarean delivery (9). Other factors associated with placenta accreta include multiparity, leiomyomas, endometritis, manual removal of placenta, adenomyosis, and Asherman's syndrome (intrauterine adhesions and uterine synechiae) (Table 6) (23).

Placenta percreta, although rare (0.03 per 1,000 deliveries), risks significant morbidity (26) and severe hemorrhage. Placental invasion involving nearby organs, such as the bladder and bowel, can occur (28,29). Treatment involves surgical removal of areas of placental penetration.

In the past, placenta accreta was most often diagnosed immediately postpartum at the time of placental separation or intraoperatively during cesarean section (23). Currently, placental invasion in early pregnancy can be diagnosed by ultrasonography (30). In addition, transvaginal color Doppler sonography gives further evidence of the extent of placenta accreta (31). However, both of these sonographic modalities are associated with false-positives due to technical limitations. In such instances, MRI provides a definitive diagnosis in addition to accurate localization of the placenta in relation to the cervix (Fig. 3) (20).

Adherent placenta is the most common indication for peripartum hysterectomy (24,32,33). Hysterectomy usually is performed immediately following cesarean delivery. However, in one report, the adherent placenta was left in place and spontaneously reabsorbed (23). More recently, Matthews et al. (34) described a case of placenta accreta left in situ with bilateral internal iliac artery embolization performed 9 days postpartum to treat sudden bleeding. This patient remained stable and hysterectomy was performed 55 days postpartum. Leaving the placenta attached increases the risk of sepsis and hemorrhage. It is reserved for rare cases where there is a strong desire to preserve fertility (35).

TABLE 6. *Factors increasing the risk of placenta accreta*

Previous cesarean delivery
Dilatation and curettage
Manual removal of the placenta
Placenta previa in prior pregnancy
Multiparity
Endometritis
Asherman's syndrome
Leimyomas, adenomyosis

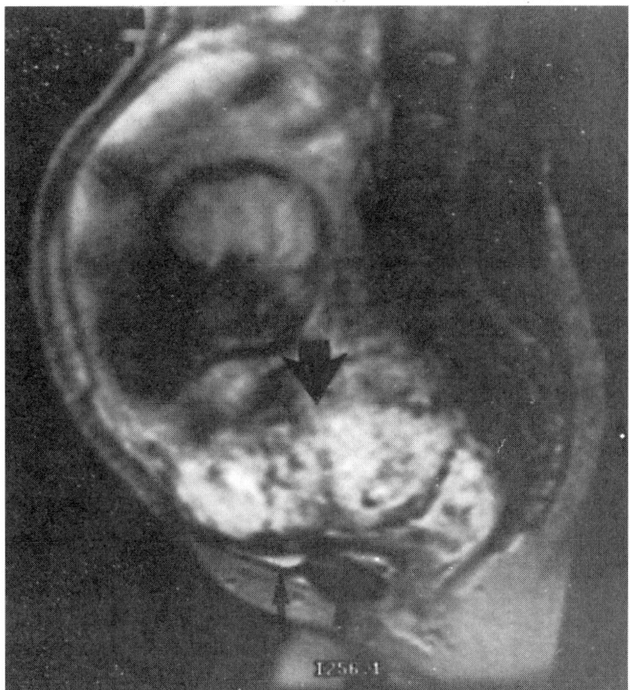

FIG. 3. Magnetic resonance imaging of pelvis with placenta percreta. *Large arrow,* placenta; *intermediate arrow,* symphysis pubis; *small arrow,* maternal bladder. Following the myometrial contour from the top, it disappears in the lower uterine segment, where it is obliterated by the adherent placenta. (Reprinted from ref. 20, with permission.)

Interventional Radiologic Approaches to Placenta Accreta

Interventional radiologic techniques are increasingly becoming instrumental in decreasing the morbidity and mortality in the parturient with massive hemorrhage (36,37). Selective embolization of pelvic vessels immediately after cesarean section can help control bleeding. If successful, selective embolization can eliminate the need for further surgery and, in some cases, preserve the uterus (36).

Angiographic procedures also are performed preoperatively. Paull et al. (38) described how balloon occlusion of the infrarenal aorta prevented rapid blood loss during hysterectomy in a patient with placenta percreta. A balloon catheter was placed via the right femoral artery preoperatively. After delivery, the catheter was inflated for 15 minutes while surgical removal of the uterus with adherent placenta was performed. The estimated blood loss was 1.5 L. The only blood product given was 275 mL of scavenged red blood cells. Compare this blood loss to the values reported for similar cases managed conventionally (6.5 to 20 L) (27).

At Thomas Jefferson University Hospital (Philadelphia, PA), several parturients with definitive sonographic evidence of placenta accreta/percreta underwent placement of percutaneous bilateral internal iliac artery balloon catheters under fluoroscopic guidance before elective cesarean delivery. After delivery, the catheters were intermittently inflated during cesarean hysterectomy. The entire procedure from placement of the groin catheters to hysterectomy was performed under epidural anesthesia. The average blood loss ranged from 4.5 to 6.2 L. Here, using bilateral internal iliac balloon catheters did not necessarily decrease total blood loss. Instead, inflating the catheters just before manipulation of the adherent placenta slowed blood loss and improved surgical conditions and hemodynamic stability.

Alvarez et al. (39) compared prophylactic versus emergent placement of arterial embolization catheters. Patients who underwent emergent embolization (i.e., catheters placed after both surgical and medical therapy failed) had a greater incidence of coagulopathy, transfusion requirements, and postpartum complications compared to those with prophylactic catheter placement. For parturients at significant risk for hemorrhage, selective embolization prior to major blood loss significantly improved hemodynamic stability and decreased morbidity.

Conservative Therapy

Nonsurgical management or "conservative treatment" is advocated by some practitioners for special cases (40). This approach involves leaving the placenta intact after cesarean delivery and delaying hysterectomy. In some instances, the placenta completely resorbs. This may be a preferable option when surgical excision may be technically difficult, such as a placenta percreta extending to the bowel and bladder.

In selected cases, "conservative management" with pharmacologic therapy can preserve fertility. Methotrexate has been used to promote involution of trophoblastic tissue that makes up the adherent placenta (41,42). In one report, the placenta was left in situ after cesarean delivery and resorbed completely after ten methotrexate injections (42).

Placental Abruption

Placental abruption (abruptio placentae) is the separation of a normally implanted placenta from the uterus before delivery of the infant. Separation allows bleeding into the layer between the placenta and myometrium (decidua basalis). The decidual hematoma that develops, isolates, compresses, and impairs the function of adjacent placental tissue. Continued bleeding from the decidual spiral arteries enlarges the hematoma. Maternal hemorrhage is varyingly concealed within the uterine cavity or passed per vagina (Fig. 4). Although abruption can occur at any time, it is most common in the third trimester.

Incidence

Placental abruption occurs in 0.6% to 1% of pregnancies (43,44). The exact frequency is unclear, because definitions and pathologic findings vary. In addition, incomplete records and selection bias may limit retrospective epidemiologic studies.

Placental abruption carries serious consequences for both mother and fetus. It is associated with 6% of all maternal deaths during pregnancy (1). Stillbirths, preterm delivery, and fetal death occur with increased frequency (45). Perinatal mortality may be as high as 50% (12,45).

Symptoms

The diagnosis of abruption is based primarily on clinical signs and symptoms of painful vaginal bleeding. Other signs and symptoms include uterine tenderness, uterine hypertonus, back pain, preterm labor, hypovolemia, shock, fetal heart rate abnormalities, and fetal demise (12). Milder cases of placental abruption may go unnoticed. Ultrasound may identify a retroplacental clot in the uterine cavity, yet the absence of clot does not exclude a severe abruption. The amount of blood loss, percentage of functioning placenta, and development of coagulopathy affect the severity of clinical presentation. Blood loss usually is underestimated. The amount of blood passed vaginally may often mislead. The uterus can

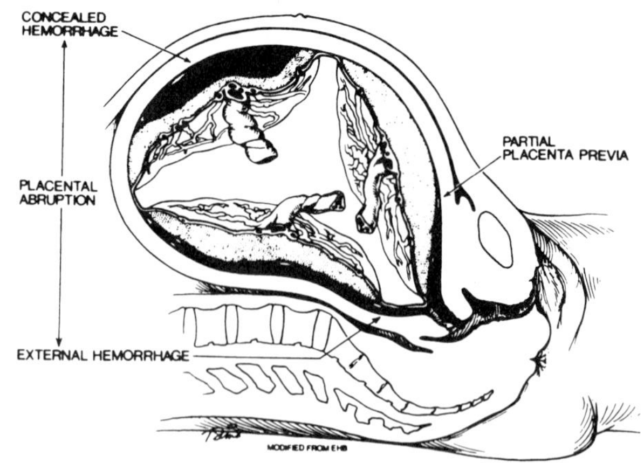

FIG. 4. Hemorrhage from premature placental separation. *Upper left:* Extensive placental abruption with the periphery of the placenta and the membranes still adherent to the endometrium. Hemorrhage is completely concealed. *Lower left:* Placental abruption with the placenta detached peripherally and with the membranes between the placenta and cervical canal stripped from the underlying decidua. External hemorrhage follows. *Right:* Partial placenta previa with placental separation and external hemorrhage. (Reprinted from ref. 112, with permission.)

hide significant blood loss without maternal evidence of hypotension or anemia. As much as 4,000 mL of blood may be concealed in the uterus. Here, fetal heart rate abnormalities may be the only indication of hemorrhage (14). The more concealed bleeding, the greater the risk of coagulopathy. Mild or moderate abruption comprises 85% to 90% of cases and correlates with good neonatal outcome. Maternal hypotension and coagulopathy are characteristics of severe abruption and are poor prognostic indicators. Continued blood loss with extravasation of blood, placental tissue, and amniotic fluid into the systemic circulation may cause systemic clotting abnormalities and consumptive coagulopathy. These problems complicate up to 50% of abruptions (46).

The coagulopathy that may accompany abruption is due to the consumption of clotting factors. The severity correlates with both the duration and amount of placental separation. Fetal death increases the risk of coagulopathy to 30% (47).

Pathology

Hemorrhage originates in the decidua basalis, possibly due to local vascular injury. Bleeding initiates separation of the placenta. The decidua divides and a thin layer adheres to the uterine wall. The expanding hematoma disrupts adjacent vasculature and its spread further separates the placenta. A retroplacental hematoma occurs with spiral artery rupture. Analysis of placental biopsies after abruption shows atypical vascularity, suggesting that separation is due to a preexisting structural defect (48). Entry of blood, amniotic fluid, placental tissue factor, and fetal debris into the maternal systemic circulation may precipitate coagulopathy and increase hemorrhage.

Risk Factors

Although a specific cause of placental abruption has not been identified, there are several known associations (Table 7). Hypertension, either chronic or pregnancy induced, is the most common (49). Prolonged premature rupture of membranes is a significant risk factor that results in increased preterm deliveries (50). The risk increases when gestational age is less than 34 weeks and when membranes have been ruptured more than 24 hours. Patients with a history of placental abruption are at increased risk of recurrence (5% to 17%) in a subsequent pregnancy (51,52).

Cigarette smoking, and alcohol and cocaine use have been implicated as etiologies of abruption (53,54). Increasing cocaine use among parturients over the past decade has been postulated as a contributing factor in the rise of cases. Transabdominal trauma, such as occurs with motor vehicle accidents, may precipitate abruption. Abruption also has been reported after percutaneous umbilical blood sampling (55). Finally, there is a weak association with male fetuses for unknown reasons (53).

TABLE 7. *Risk factors for placental abruption*

	Relative Risk
Maternal	
Age ≥35 y	1.5
Multiparity	
Coexisting diseases	
Diabetes mellitus	
Chronic renal disorders	
Preeclampsia	2.05
Chronic hypertension	1.77
Gestational hypertension	1.57
Fetal	
Short umbilical cord	
Male fetus	1.38
Obstetric	
Previous pregnancy with abruption	
Premature rupture of membranes (≥24 h)	2.38
Sudden decompression of uterus	
Chorioamnionitis	2.5
Other	
Transabdominal trauma	
Maternal drug use	
Cigarette smoking	1.4
Alcohol	
Cocaine	

Uterine Rupture

Uterine rupture is a rare, potentially catastrophic complication that occurs in approximately 0.05% to 0.09% of pregnancies (56,57). The risk increases with previous uterine surgery such as cesarean section (particularly classical incisions) and myomectomy (Table 8). Rupture of fundal scars from classical incisions may occur at any time and has been reported as early as 16 to 20 weeks (58). Rupture

TABLE 8. *Risk factors for uterine rupture*

Grand multiparity
Cocaine abuse
Trauma
Infection
Previous uterine surgery
Cesarean section
Myomectomy
Abnormal fetal presentation
Uterine distension
Macrosomia
Hydramnios
Mid-trimester termination using hypertonic solutions
Dysfunctional labor
Use of uterotonic agents
Oxytocin
Prostaglandins
Operative vaginal delivery
Forceps delivery
Vacuum delivery
Breech extraction
Internal podalic version
Manual removal of placenta

of lower segment scars are seen later in pregnancy (57). The highest maternal and fetal morbidities occur with rupture of an unscarred uterus (56). Patients with previous repair of a ruptured uterus are at increased risk of a second rupture in a subsequent pregnancy (59).

True uterine rupture (total separation of the wall of the uterus) is very rare. Spontaneous rupture occurs in areas of previous uterine surgery and uterine abnormalities, such as placental implantation over previous scarring (placenta accreta). Uterine scar dehiscence occurs with previous lower segment uterine incisions. Risk of rupture of an unscarred uterus is increased with vaginal instrumentation, uterine hyperstimulation from intravaginal prostaglandin E_1 (misoprostol) or E_2 gel (dinoprostone), chronic corticosteroid therapy, and placental abruption complicated by increased uterine tone (60–66).

Signs and symptoms vary but may include:

- Increasing atypical abdominal pain,
- Vaginal bleeding,
- Uterine tenderness,
- Loss of contractions,
- Uterine hypertonus, and
- Fetal heart rate abnormalities.
- Hypovolemia, shock, and loss of fetal heart tones are seen in more severe cases (63,64).

Because presenting signs are not always consistent, it may be difficult to differentiate rupture from other causes of antepartum hemorrhage. Abdominal pain is described as severe and continuous, occurring between contractions (67). However, Groves and Oriol report that abdominal pain is not a reliable symptom of uterine rupture.

Ultrasound may help with assessment of risk and early diagnosis of rupture of lower segment scars in parturients with previous cesarean sections (58,69). Rozenberg et al. (69) found that the risk of rupture of a defective scar relates to the amount of thinning of the lower uterine segment around 37 weeks' gestational age. Along with prompt diagnosis, management includes fluid resuscitation, delivery of fetus, and surgical repair of the ruptured uterus. Hysterectomy is common.

Some experts warn that labor epidural analgesia may mask the pain associated with uterine rupture (67,68,70, 71). Both high concentrations of local anesthetics and epidural opioids have been implicated (67,70,71). It is unlikely that dilute local anesthetic/opioid mixtures will mask the pain of uterine rupture. However, increased vigilance is appropriate.

Fetal Hemorrhage

Some causes of fetal hemorrhage include circumvallate placenta, vasa previa, fetal blood sampling, and percutaneous umbilical blood sampling.

Fetal hemorrhage is a rare event and poses no threat to the mother. However, a small amount of blood loss can be catastrophic to the fetus. The fetus at term has a blood volume of 78 mL/kg, or approximately 300 mL (72). A loss of 30 to 40 mL may produce evidence of fetal stress. A loss of 100 mL is life threatening. Fetal blood loss most often occurs into the maternal circulation. Although microscopic bleeding is common with delivery, more extensive loss is rare. Loss of up to 10 mL happens in 1 of 200 to 1 of 714 births (73). Life-threatening hemorrhage (greater than 150 mL) complicates 1 of 800 births (74). Causes of fetal hemorrhage include:

- Scalp sampling,
- Forceps delivery,
- Umbilical cord trauma,
- Medical conditions (von Willebrand's disease, idiopathic thrombocytopenic purpura),
- Velamentous insertion of the umbilical cord, and
- Vasa previa (75).

Umbilical cord trauma and vasa previa can lead to rapid exsanguination. Umbilical cord trauma can occur with a "velamentous insertion" of the umbilical cord. In this situation, umbilical vessels travel to the fetus from the placenta within the thin membrane of the amniotic sac instead of the cushioning, protective Wharton's jelly of the umbilical cord. The vessels are much more susceptible to trauma with labor and delivery. This abnormality is variable in its degree. It is more common in multiple gestations.

Vasa previa, "vessels going ahead," describes velamentous insertion of the umbilical cord in front of the presenting part of the fetus. The diagnosis is made upon palpation of pulsatile vessels in an unruptured sac during vaginal examination. The condition is most often diagnosed accidentally with elective rupture of the membranes. Tragically, perinatal mortality with rupture is 75% to 100% (76). Signs include fetal bradycardia and hemorrhage. Treatment involves immediate delivery, usually by emergent cesarean section. When the diagnosis is entertained in the setting of a less vigorous bleed, testing of vaginal blood will detect fetal hemoglobin (77). Fetal salvage requires a high index of suspicion with plans for infant volume resuscitation at delivery (75).

ANESTHETIC MANAGEMENT OF THE BLEEDING PARTURIENT

Normal Cesarean Section

In the past decade, the number of cesarean sections has increased steadily. In the United States, they now comprise 15% to 25% of all deliveries (1,78). The average blood loss during cesarean section is 900 to 1,100 mL (79). The physiologic changes of pregnancy allow parturients to tolerate up to 1,000 mL of blood loss without a change in hematocrit, blood pressure, or cardiac output (79–81). Factors associated with increased risk of hemorrhage during cesarean delivery include (82):

- General anesthesia,
- Chorioamnionitis,
- Preeclampsia,
- Prolonged active phase of labor,
- Second-stage arrest,
- Hispanic ethnicity, and
- Classic uterine incision.

Anesthesia for the Parturient at Risk for Hemorrhage

Assessment

The choice of anesthesia for cesarean section depends on several factors including, but not limited to, the urgency, amount of expected blood loss, and the volume and coagulation status of the parturient. Examine each patient to determine current volume status, potential for intraoperative blood loss, and risk of cesarean hysterectomy. Fetal status also will determine the urgency of the situation. The clinical presentation of placenta previa and placental abruption varies. A woman may present for elective cesarean section at term or, at the other extreme, a parturient may arrive with acute, severe bleeding carrying a gravely compromised premature fetus. Close communication with the obstetrician aids in initial assessment.

Careful assessment of blood loss and current volume status are important steps in formulating an anesthetic plan. Patients who are significantly hypovolemic or who are still bleeding are poor candidates for regional anesthesia. On the other hand, if the woman is stable, well hydrated, with little or no active bleeding, regional block may be an appropriate technique. Women with placental abruption also may have coagulation abnormalities.

Preparation

Check the availability of blood and blood products. When anesthetizing women with placenta previa or suspected placenta accreta, have 2 to 4 U of packed red blood cells immediately available. Even stable parturients presenting for elective cesarean delivery because of placenta previa can have significant, rapid hemorrhage. Insert two large-bore intravenous catheters to allow rapid fluid resuscitation. Prepare rapid transfusion and blood warming devices. Warming blood and intravenous fluids will help maintain temperature stability. Having extra personnel available to help may prove life saving.

Management

Either regional or general anesthesia are appropriate for elective or urgent cesarean delivery in a hemodynamically stable mother. Appreciate that sympathectomy induced by regional block impairs the mother's ability to cope with sudden hypovolemia. However, many experts consider regional anesthesia an appropriate choice for parturients with placenta previa or at high risk for placenta accreta (83). In a retrospective review, continuous epidural anesthesia for elective cesarean hysterectomy did not alter blood loss, transfusion requirements, or crystalloid replacement. In addition, no patient required intraoperative induction of general anesthesia. However, others advocate induction of general anesthesia at the beginning of the case (84) or after delivery of the fetus (24).

Although hemorrhage may lead to maternal hypotension, this problem usually is readily treated with intermittent boluses of ephedrine or phenylephrine. If blood loss and hypotension persist, a continuous infusion of epinephrine or norepinephrine can be titrated to maintain maternal blood pressure. Use maternal symptoms (i.e., nausea, light-headedness) to guide therapy. In addition, if cesarean hysterectomy becomes necessary, the operation may outlast a single injection spinal anesthetic. Plan ahead. If needed, induce general anesthesia in a calm, controlled manner. Do not wait until the block has regressed significantly and the patient is suffering severe pain. Continuous spinal, combined spinal–epidural, or continuous epidural block are appropriate alternatives if you suspect a prolonged procedure at the outset.

In some clinical situations, general anesthesia is the only safe choice. Actively bleeding, hypovolemic parturients can develop profound hypotension with regional anesthesia. Women with chronic abruption and significant coagulopathy should not receive regional block. If the maternal or fetal condition mandates immediate delivery (i.e., within 5 to 10 minutes) general anesthesia also may be the best choice.

The choice of induction agent depends on volume status. A reduced dose of thiopental (3 mg/kg) or ketamine 0.5 to 1.0 mg/kg is a safe choice in moderately hypovolemic women (85). In the severely compromised parturient, muscle relaxant alone may be the only safe choice. Ketamine causes central nervous system-mediated catecholamine release. In most hypovolemic patients, this effect supports heart rate and blood pressure. However, peripheral vasoconstriction may have reached its maximum in a severely volume-depleted patient. In this situation, ketamine cannot induce further vasoconstriction, and its cardiac depressant effects can result in hypotension and potential cardiac arrest (85). The remainder of a rapid-sequence induction, including application of cricoid pressure, succinylcholine 1 to 1.5 mg/kg intravenously, and endotracheal intubation proceeds as usual. After securing the airway, maintain anesthesia with 50% nitrous in oxygen and careful titration of volatile agent.

Central venous access may be a helpful to guide volume status; however, blood loss, urine output, and maternal hemodynamics usually provide enough information. An intraarterial catheter may be beneficial if multiple blood samples for hematocrit, coagulation studies, and acid–base analysis are needed.

POSTPARTUM HEMORRHAGE

Postpartum hemorrhage (PPH) is responsible for over 75% of complications after delivery (80). In the past, PPH was defined as more than 500 mL of blood loss with immediate PPH occurring within 24 hours of delivery and delayed PPH after 24 hours. However, this amount of blood loss is typical for uncomplicated vaginal deliveries (86). Moreover, blood loss in routine cesarean deliveries is about 900 to 1,100 mL (79). A more accurate definition of PPH after vaginal or cesarean delivery would be blood loss in excess of 1,000 mL (86).

Retained Placenta

After delivery, the placenta spontaneously separates from the uterus and is expelled within 5 minutes. Retention of the placenta in situ beyond 30 minutes after delivery is abnormal and occurs in 1 of 300 deliveries (12). If all or part of the placenta remains within the uterus, it prevents contraction of the uterus, inciting atony and ongoing blood loss. Retained placenta may be the first sign of placenta accreta.

Obstetric management consists of manual removal of the placenta with or without curettage. In a hemodynamically stable patient, analgesia for this procedure can be provided by paracervical block with intravenous sedation, extending a preexisting epidural anesthetic or spinal block. Inhalational analgesia with 50% nitrous in oxygen and intravenous opioid also is an option. General anesthesia rarely is necessary. In addition, the amount of volatile agent needed for uterine relaxation [≥2 minimum aleveolar concentration (MAC)] can aggravate hypotension.

Occasionally, uterine relaxation will be needed to allow the placenta to pass a tightly contracted lower uterine segment. Intravenous nitroglycerin 50 to 100 μg provides uterine relaxation within 30 seconds without significant hemodynamic effect (87). Uterine muscle tone returns within 1 minute of injection. Using nitroglycerin may avoid the need for general anesthesia if prompt relaxation is required (88). Once the placental fragments have been removed, intravenous oxytocin usually is sufficient to induce uterine contraction. Sometimes, methylergonovine 0.2 mg (intramuscular or intrauterine) or 15-methyl prostaglandin $F_{2\alpha}$ 0.25 mg (intramuscular or intrauterine) will be needed to increase uterine tone.

Vaginal and Cervical Lacerations

Cervical lacerations from delivery are a significant cause of PPH. Operative vaginal deliveries and cesarean section are risk factors. Bleeding also occurs from episiotomy sites and vaginal lacerations. A laceration, as opposed to uterine atony, should be suspected when bleeding persists despite good uterine tone.

For mild cases, anesthesia can be provided by the obstetrician: a paracervical block for cervical lacerations or a pudendal block for vaginal or perineal repair. Extending a previously placed epidural orand instituting a spinal anesthetic to a T_{10} sensory level are options in a hemodynamically stable patient.

Uterine Atony

Uterine atony is the most common cause of PPH occurring in 2%–5% of vaginal deliveries (Table 9) (56,89). The diagnosis is established by the presence of a flaccid uterus and steady uterine bleeding. Initial therapy consists of uterine massage and oxytocin infusion. Prostaglandins can further aid in increasing uterine tone. If these pharmacologic maneuvers are unsuccessful, surgical intervention may be necessary to prevent catastrophic hemorrhage.

Uterine Inversion

Uterine inversion occurs in about 1 of 3,600 vaginal deliveries (90). Although rare, uterine inversion has been reported during cesarean delivery (91). Fundal implantation of the placenta may be the underlying cause. Although it can occur spontaneously, uterine inversion usually arises when fundal pressure and traction on the umbilical cord are used to facilitate delivery of the placenta. Severe hemorrhage and immediate hypotension, often out of proportion to blood loss, occur rapidly.

Treatment involves forcing the everted fundus back through the cervical os. Uterine relaxation usually is required. Relaxation can be achieved by β-agonist tocolytics, intravenous nitroglycerin, or magnesium

TABLE 9. *Conditions associated with uterine atony*

Grand multiparity
Previous tocolysis
Uterine leiomyomas
Overdistended uterus
Multiple gestation
Macrosomia
Polyhydramnios
Molar pregnancy
Uterine rupture
Dysfunctional labor
Prolonged second stage
Secondary arrest of labor
Protracted active stage
Oxytocin
Prolonged induction of labor
Retained placenta/products of conception

sulfate. Nitroglycerin is an ideal agent as it provides rapid onset of relaxation of short duration. If these measures fail, general anesthesia at greater than 2 MAC via an endotracheal tube provides uterine relaxation but can worsen maternal hypotension. An epidural catheter can be used for analgesia but does not provide uterine relaxation (90). If the uterus cannot be replaced manually, laparotomy may be required. Once the uterus is repositioned, give intravenous oxytocin to increase uterine tone and prevent further blood loss.

Distant or Secondary Postpartum Hemorrhage

Late PPH occurs after 24 hours but within 6 weeks of delivery (86). A few causes of hemorrhage after delivery beyond 48 hours include infection, retained placenta, dislodgment of a hematoma, and coagulopathy (12).

Amniotic Fluid Embolism

Approximately 10% of maternal deaths during pregnancy are due to amniotic fluid embolism (1). In a review of 272 cases, only 39 (15%) patients survived (92). Clinical presentation includes restlessness, sudden dyspnea, cyanosis, hypotension, coagulopathy, and seizures (93,94). Severe coagulopathy and subsequent massive PPH are related to the presence of placental and fetal material in the maternal circulation. Treatment consists mainly of cardiorespiratory resuscitation, including transfusion of blood and blood products as needed. Diagnosis is confirmed by pathologic examination at autopsy demonstrating fetal squamous cells in the maternal pulmonary vasculature.

Amniotic fluid embolism has been reported in patients undergoing cesarean section with both epidural and spinal anesthesia (94,95). Major risk factors for amniotic fluid embolism include:

- Rapid labor with hypertonic contractions,
- Oxytocin induction,
- Placental abruption,
- Placenta previa,
- Placenta accreta, and
- Uterine rupture (96).

Obstetric Management of Postpartum Hemorrhage

Pharmacologic Management

Oxytocin infusion will decrease blood loss after most uncomplicated vaginal or cesarean deliveries. When oxytocin fails to correct uterine atony, other uterotonic drugs may be required (Table 10). Methylergonovine (Methergine) 0.20 mg intramuscularly produces intense uterine contraction and arterial constriction. The most worrisome side effect is severe hypertension. Alternatively, 15-methyl prostaglandin $F_{2\alpha}$ (Hemabate) is very effective in reducing PPH with uterine atony. Side effects of prostaglandins such as prostaglandin $F_{2\alpha}$ are due to its effects on smooth muscle and include an increase in pulmonary artery pressure and pulmonary vascular resistance, bronchoconstriction, and severe hypertension. Thus, this drug should be used with caution in parturients with cardiorespiratory disease. One report described profound arterial oxygen desaturation due to intrapulmonary shunting after prostaglandin administration (97). Douglas et al. (98) reported a case of an overdose of prostaglandin $F_{2\alpha}$ that produced cardiovascular collapse.

Surgical Management

Before surgical intervention, transvaginal and uterine packing with gauze can be a temporizing measure to control blood loss from placenta previa, placenta accreta, and uterine atony (99,100). This technique, described in older obstetric literature, recently has gained attention due to recent reports of its effectiveness in emergent situations (101,102). Surgical interventions before hysterectomy to control bleeding include ligation of pelvic vessels including the uterine, ovarian, and hypogastric arteries.

Angiography

Selective embolization of pelvic vessels is very effective in the treatment of PPH (36,37). After catheterization of the femoral artery, an aortogram can locate bleeding pelvic vessels. After selective embolization of the involved vessels, a repeat angiogram confirms adequate hemostasis (Fig. 5). Arterial catheters typically are left in situ for 24 to 48 hours in the event of continued hemorrhage.

TABLE 10. *Uterine contractile agents*

Drug	Dose	Contraindications	Side effects	Frequency	Total dose
Oxytocin	10 μ/min IV, 10 μ IM or intramyometrially	Hypotension	Hypotension, antidiuresis		
Ergonovine maleate	0.2 mg IM or intramyometrially	Hypersensitivity, hypertension, sepsis	Nausea, vomiting, hypertension, headache	q 2–4 h	1 mg
15-methyl prostaglandin $F_{2\alpha}$	250 μG IV, IM, or intramyometrially	Asthma	Nausea, vomiting, diarrhea, fever, hypotension	q 1.5–3.5 h	12 mg

Angiographic techniques are perhaps of greatest benefit to those patients in whom a significant risk of PPH is identified before actual hemorrhage occurs. Parturients with known placental abnormalities or bleeding disorders can have balloon catheters placed before delivery. These catheters subsequently can be used after delivery of the fetus to control bleeding before hypogastric artery ligation or hysterectomy (38).

Anesthetic Management of Maternal Hemorrhage

Transfusion

The American Society of Anesthesiologists (ASA) has published "evidence-based" recommendations for transfusion of blood and blood products (103). Transfusion rarely is necessary when the hemoglobin (Hgb) concentration is greater than 10 g/dL. In cases of acute blood loss where Hgb ≤ 6 g/dL, transfusion of red blood cells usually is indicated. When the Hgb falls between 6 and 10 g/dL, the decision to transfuse should be based on several factors, including adequacy of oxygen carrying capacity, hemodynamic signs, and potential for continuing blood loss.

Ideally, typed and cross-matched blood should be transfused. If only the blood type is known, type specific blood can be given in an emergency. When the blood type is unknown, type O-negative packed red blood cells should be used. Visual estimation of blood loss is inaccurate, especially when the blood loss is less that 150 mL or more than 500 mL (104). Moreover, blood loss during primary PPH often is underestimated. Hemodynamic signs and serial hematocrits are more accurate methods of determining the need for transfusion.

ASA recommendations for other blood products are summarized below.

Platelets

- Prophylactic transfusion is not warranted when thrombocytopenia is due to platelet destruction, such as in idiopathic thrombocytopenic purpura.
- Transfusion is not necessary when platelet count (PC) $\geq 100 \times 10^9$/L.
- Transfusion is indicated when PC $\leq 50 \times 10^9$/L.
- For PC between 50 and 100 $\times 10^9$/L, transfusion is determined by risk of bleeding.
- Transfusion is indicated if there is known platelet dysfunction and microvascular bleeding.

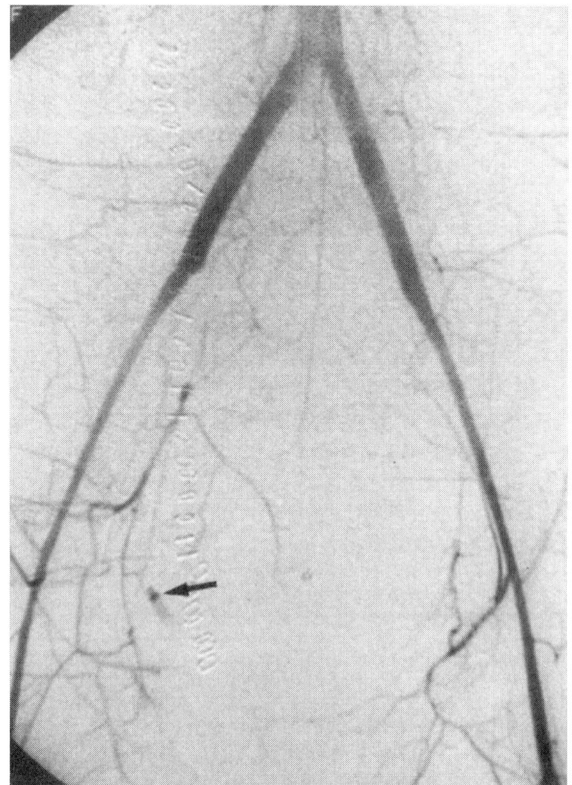
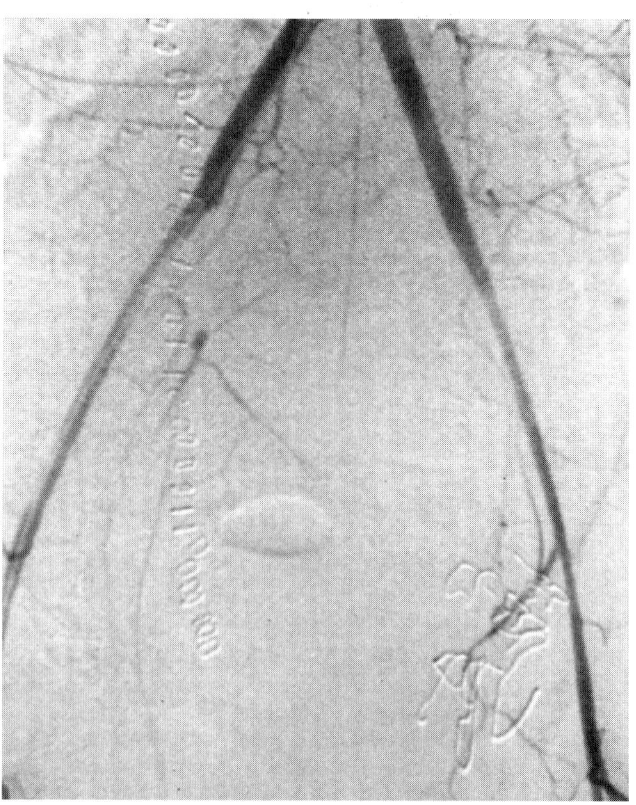

FIG. 5. A: Aortogram. Both internal iliac arteries are surgically ligated. *Arrow* points to an area of active bleeding where contrast medium has extravasated. **B:** Postembolization aortogram after occlusion of the branch of the right internal iliac artery where contrast had previously been seen. (Reprinted from ref. 30, with permission.)

Fresh Frozen Plasma

- Amount: 10 to 15 mL/kg or for a minimum of 30% of plasma factor level.
- Correction of specific factor deficits when concentrates are not available.
- Correction of microvascular bleeding with elevated prothrombin time (PT) and partial thromboplastin time (PTT) (greater than 1.5 × normal).
- In massive transfusion (more than one blood volume), when PT and PTT values cannot be obtained rapidly.
- Should not be used for increasing plasma volume or albumin concentration.

Cryoprecipitate

- Nonbleeding patients with congenital fibrinogen deficiencies or von Willebrand's disease that does not respond to desmopressin acetate.
- Patient with von Willebrand's disease who is bleeding.
- Massive transfusion to correct microvascular bleeding in patients with fibrinogen level less than 80 to 100 mg/dL or when fibrinogen level cannot be measured rapidly.

Autologous Blood Transfusion

Several studies have found autologous blood donation by pregnant women to be safe and effective (105–108). Transfusion of autologous blood decreases the risk of infectious complications, transfusion reactions, and incompatibilities (Table 11). Predonation is particularly beneficial in cases of known adherent placenta, elective cesarean hysterectomy, placenta previa, and parturients with documented antigens (106,108). Threshold for transfusion of autologous blood may be lower (103). However, it is important to recognize that autologous blood still carries risk, as blood can be mislabeled.

TABLE 11. *Transmissible disease testing of donor blood*

Syphilis	STS (serological test for syphilis); 1940s[a]
Hepatitis	HBsAg (hepatitis B surface antigen); 1971
	Anti-HBc (antibody to hepatitis B core antigen); 1987
	Anti-HCV (antibody to hepatitis C virus); 1990
HIV	Anti-HIV-1; 1985
	Anti-HIV-2; 1992
	HIV Ag (p24 antigen); 1996
HTLV-I/II	Anti-HTLV-1 (antibody to human T-cell lymphotrophic virus type I/II); 1988

[a]Year test instituted.

From American Society of Anesthesiologists. *Questions and answers about transfusion practices,* 3rd ed. 1998:8, with permission.

Intraoperative Blood Salvage

Blood collected from the operative field via suction can be collected, washed, and given back to the patient. This type of cell salvage system (Haemonetics Cell Saver 3, Haemonetics Inc., Braintree, MA) is capable of providing 225 mL of blood with a hematocrit of 50% in 3 minutes (109). The use of banked blood can be dramatically decreased in cases of massive transfusion. Concerns with the use of this procedure include intravascular transmission of amniotic fluid, air embolism, and infection. After delivery, amniotic fluid mixes with blood and contains tissue factor that can stimulate the coagulation system and precipitate DIC. Bernstein et al. (109) demonstrated that the cell saver system can be safely used to remove tissue factor from blood contaminated with amniotic fluid.

Disseminated Intravascular Coagulation

PPH and massive transfusion may be complicated by coagulopathy. Conditions associated with DIC include:

- Placental abruption,
- Amniotic fluid embolism,
- Prolonged fetal death in utero,
- Sepsis, and
- Preeclampsia/eclampsia.

DIC results from activation of the clotting cascade. There is increased production of thrombin, activation of the fibrinolytic system, and fibrin deposition in the microcirculation. Clotting factors are consumed. Laboratory test abnormalities reveal prolonged PT and PTT, low platelet counts and fibrinogen levels, and increased fibrin degradation products. Immediate treatment includes supportive care and administration of blood and coagulation products as indicated by clinical status and laboratory tests. However, elimination of the underlying cause of DIC is necessary for complete resolution of this syndrome (110).

REFERENCES

1. Atrash HK, Koonin LM, Lawson HW, Franks AL, Smith JC. Maternal mortality in the United States, 1979–1986. *Obstet Gynecol* 1990;76:155.
2. Hogber U. Maternal mortality: a worldwide problem. *Int J Gynecol Obstet* 1985;23:463.
3. Chelmow D, Andrew DE, Baker ER. Maternal cigarette smoking and placenta previa. *Obstet Gynecol* 1996;87:703.
4. Iyasu S, Saftlas AK, Rowley DL, et al. Epidemiology of placenta previa in the United States, 1979 through 1987. *Am J Obstet Gynecol* 1993;168:1424.
5. McShane PN, Heyl PS, Epstein MF. Maternal and perinatal morbidity resulting from placenta previa. *Obstet Gynecol* 1985;65:176.
6. Ananth CV, Wilcox AJ, Savitz DA, et al. Effect of maternal age and parity on risk of uteroplacental bleeding disorders in pregnancy. *Obstet Gynecol* 1996;88:511.
7. Taylor VM, Peacock S, Kramer MD, et al. Increased risk of placenta previa among women of Asian origin. *Obstet Gynecol* 1995;86:805.

8. Zhang J, Savitz DA. Maternal age and placenta previa: a population-based, case-control study. *Am J Obstet Gynecol* 1993;168:641.
9. To WWK, Leung WC. Placenta previa and previous cesarean section. *Int J Obstet Gynecol* 1995;51:25.
10. Taylor VM, Kramer MD, Vaughan TL, et al. Placenta previa and prior cesarean delivery: how strong is the association? *Obstet Gynecol* 1994;84:55.
11. Naeye RL. Maternal age, obstetric complications, and the outcome of pregnancy. *Obstet Gynecol* 1983;61:210.
12. Cunningham FG, MacDonald PC, Gant NF, et al., eds. *Williams' obstetrics,* 19th ed. Norwalk: Appleton & Lange, 1993:819.
13. Nielsen TF, Hagberg H, Ljunblad U. Placenta previa and antepartum hemorrhage after previous cesarean section. *Gynecol Obstet Invest* 1989;27:88.
14. Goplerud CP. Bleeding in late pregnancy. In: Danforth DN, Scott JR, eds. *Obstetrics and gynecology.* Philadelphia: JB Lippincott, 1986: 470.
15. Williams MA, Mittendorf R, Lieberman E, et al. Cigarette smoking during pregnancy in relation to placenta previa. *Am J Obstet Gynecol* 1991;165:28.
16. Rizos N, Doran T, Mikskin M, et al. Natural history of placenta previa ascertained by diagnostic ultrasound. *Am J Obstet Gynecol* 1979; 133:287.
17. Mabie WC. Placenta previa. *Clin Perinatol* 1992;19:425.
18. Leerentveld RA, Gilberts EC, Arnold MJ, et al. Accuracy and safety of transvaginal sonographic placental localization. *Obstet Gynecol* 1990;76:759.
19. Hertzberg BS, Bowie JD, Carroll BA, et al. Diagnosis of placenta previa: role of transperineal sonography. *AJR* 1992;159:83.
20. Thorp JM Jr, Councell RB, Sandrige DA, et al. Antepartum diagnosis of placenta percreta by magnetic resonance imaging. *Obstet Gynecol* 1992;80:506.
21. Powell MC, Buckley J, Price H, et al. Magnetic resonance imaging and placenta previa. *Am J Obstet Gynecol* 1986;154:565.
22. Mouer JR. Placenta previa: antepartum conservative management, inpatient versus outpatient. *Am J Obstet Gynecol* 1994;170:1683.
23. Breen JL, Neubecker R, Gregor CA, et al. Placenta accreta, increta and percreta. *Obstet Gynecol* 1977;49:43.
24. Kamani AAS, Gambling DR, Christilaw J, et al. Anaesthetic management of patients with placenta accreta. *Can J Anesth* 1987;34:613.
25. Read JA, Cotton DB, Miller FC. Placenta accreta: changing clinical aspects and outcome. *Obstet Gynecol* 1980;56:31.
26. Price FV, Resnik E, Heller KA, et al. Placenta previa percreta involving the urinary bladder: a report of two cases and a review of the literature. *Obstet Gynecol* 1991;87:508.
27. Clark SL, Koonings PP, Phelan JP. Placenta previa accreta and prior cesarean section. *Obstet Gynecol* 1985;66:890.
28. Srichrishanthan S, Fraser I. Successful pregnancy following placenta percreta with bladder invasion. *Aust N Z J Obstet Gynaecol* 1996;36:92.
29. Bakri YN, Sundin T, Mansi M, et al. Placenta percreta with bladder invasion: a report of three cases. *Am J Perinatol* 1993;10:468.
30. Wheeler TC, Anderson TL, Kelly J, et al. Placenta previa increta diagnosed at 18 weeks' gestation. *J Reprod Med* 1996;41:198.
31. Rosemund R, Kepple DM. Transvaginal color Doppler sonography in prenatal diagnosis of placenta accreta. *Obstet Gynecol* 1992;80:508.
32. Zelop CM, Harlow BL, Frigoletto FD, et al. Emergency peripartum hysterectomy. *Am J Obstet Gynecol* 1993;168:1443.
33. Manyonda IT, Varma TR. Massive obstetric hemorrhage due to placenta previa/accreta with prior cesarean section. *Int J Gynecol Obstet* 1990;43:183.
34. Matthews NM, McCowan LME, Patten P. Placenta praevia accreta with delayed hysterectomy. *Aust N Z J Obstet Gynaecol* 1996;36:476.
35. Davis JD, Cruz A. Persistent placenta increta. *Obstet Gynecol* 1996; 88:653.
36. Collins CD, Jackson JE. Pelvic arterial embolization following hysterectomy and bilateral internal iliac artery ligation for intractable primary post partum haemorrhage. *Clin Radiol* 1995;50:710.
37. Gilbert WM, Moore TR, Resnik R, et al. Angiographic embolization in the management of hemorrhagic complications of pregnancy. *Am J Obstet Gynecol* 1992;166:493.
38. Paul JD, Smith J, Williams L, et al. Balloon occlusion of the abdominal aorta during caesarean hysterectomy for placenta percreta. *Anesth Intens Care* 1995;23:731.
39. Alvarez M, Lockwood CJ, Ghidini A, et al. Prophylactic and emergent arterial catheterization for selective embolization in obstetric hemorrhage. *Am J Perinatol* 1992;9:441.
40. O'Brien JM, Barton JR, Donaldson ES. Management of placenta percreta: conservative and operative strategies. *Am J Obstet Gynecol* 1996;175:1632.
41. Arulkumaran S, Ingemarsson I, Ratman S. Medical treatment of placenta accreta with methotrexate. *Acta Obstet Gynecol Scand* 1986;65: 285.
42. Legro RS, Price FV, Hill LM, et al. Nonsurgical management of placenta percreta. *Obstet Gynecol* 1994;83:847.
43. Saftlas AF, Olson DR, Atrash HK, et al. National trends in the incidence of abruptio placentae, 1979–1987. *Obstet Gynecol* 1991;78: 1081.
44. Rasmussen S, Irgens LM, Bergsjo P, et al. Occurrence of placental abruption in Norway 1967–91. *Acta Obstet Gynecol Scand* 1996;75: 222.
45. Rasmussen S, Irgens LM, Bergsjo P, et al. Perinatal mortality and case fatality after placental abruption in Norway 1967–1991. *Acta Obstet Gynecol Scand* 1996;75:229.
46. Baker RN. Hemorrhage in obstetrics. *Obstet Gynecol Annu* 1977;6: 295.
47. Finely BE. Acute coagulopathy in pregnancy. *Med Clin North Am* 1989;73:723.
48. Dommisse J, Tiltman AJ. Placental bed biopsies in placental abruption. *Br J Obstet Gynecol* 1992;99:651.
49. Ananth CV, Savitz DA, Williams MA. Placental abruption and its association with hypertension and prolonged rupture of membranes: a methodologic review and meta-analysis. *Obstet Gynecol* 1996;88:309.
50. Spinillo A, Capuzzo E, Colonna L, et al. Factors associated with abruptio placentae in preterm deliveries. *Acta Obstet Gynecol Scand* 1994;73:307.
51. Crane S, Chun B, Acker D. Treatment of obstetrical hemorrhagic emergencies. *Curr Opin Obstet Gynecol* 1993;5:675.
52. Karegard M, Gennser G. Incidence and recurrence rate of abruptio placentae in Sweden. *Obstet Gynecol* 1986;67:523.
53. Kramer MS, Usher RH, Pollack R, et al. Etiologic determinants of abruptio placentae. *Obstet Gynecol* 1997;89:221.
54. Hoskins IA, Friedman DM, Freiden FJ, et al. Relationship between antepartum cocaine abuse, abnormal umbilical Doppler velocimetry, and placental abruption. *Obstet Gynecol* 1991;78:279.
55. Feinkind L, Nanda D, Delke I, et al. Abruptio placentae after percutaneous umbilical cord sampling: a case report. *Am J Obstet Gynecol* 1990;162:1203.
56. Lynch JC, Pardy JP. Uterine rupture and scar dehiscence. A five-year survey. *Anesth Intens Care* 1996;24:699.
57. Farmer RM, Kirschbaum T, Potter D, et al. Uterine rupture during trial of labour after previous caesarean section. *Am J Obstet Gynecol* 1991; 65:996.
58. Catanazarite VA, Mehalek KE, Wachtel T, et al. Sonographic diagnosis of traumatic and later recurrent uterine rupture. *Am J Perinatol* 1996;13:177.
59. Soltan MH, Khashoggi T, Adelusi B. Pregnancy following rupture of the pregnant uterus. *Int J Gynecol Obstet* 1996;52:37.
60. Miller DA, Goodwin TM, Gherman RB, et al. Intrapartum rupture of the unscarred uterus. *Obstet Gynecol* 1997;89:671.
61. Bennett BB. Uterine rupture during induction of labor at term with intravaginal misoprostol. *Obstet Gynecol* 1997;89:832.
62. Chin MMS, Harvey JA, Duffy BL. Uterine rupture during labour in a primigravida. *Aust N Z J Obstet Gynaecol* 1996;36:210.
63. Lynch JC, Pardy JP. Uterine rupture and scar dehiscence. A five-year survey. *Anesth Intens Care* 1996;24:699.
64. Petrikovsky B. Rupture of scarred uterus: prediction and diagnosis. *Lancet* 1996;347:838.
65. Mishra A, Landzberg BR, Parente JT. Uterine rupture associated with alkaloidal ("crack") cocaine abuse. *Am J Obstet Gynecol* 1995;173: 243.
66. Leung AS, Farmer RM, Leung EK, et al. Risk factors associated with uterine rupture during trial of labor after cesarean delivery: a case control study. *Am J Obstet Gynecol* 1993;168:1358.
67. Rowbottom SJ, Critchley LAH, Gin T. Uterine rupture and epidural analgesia during trial of labour. *Anaesthesia* 1997;52:483.
68. Groves PA, Oriol N. The extradural sieve. *Br J Anaesth* 1994;73:430.
69. Rozenberg P, Goffinet F, Nisand PI. Ultrasound measurement of lower uterine segment to assess risk of scarred uterus. *Lancet* 1996; 347:281.

70. Rashiq S, Huston LJ. Fentanyl and the extradural sieve. *Br J Anaesth* 1993;71:920.
71. Tehan B. Abolition of the extradural sieve by addition of fentanyl to extradural bupivacaine. *Br J Anaesth* 1992;69:520.
72. Usher R, Shephard M, Lind J. The blood volume of the newborn infant and placental transfusion. *Acta Paediatr* 1963;52:497.
73. Fay RA. Fetal maternal haemorrhage as a cause of fetal morbidity and mortality. *Br J Obstet Gynaecol* 1983;90:443.
74. Hoag RW. Fetomaternal hemorrhage associated with umbilical vein thrombosis: case report. *Am J Obstet Gynecol* 1986;154:1271.
75. Schellpfeffer MA. Improved neonatal outcome of vasa previa with aggressive intrapartum management. *J Reprod Med* 1995;40:327.
76. Antoine C, Young BK, Silverman F, Greco MA, Alvarez SP. Sinusoidal fetal heart rate pattern with vasa previa in twin pregnancy. *J Reprod Med* 1982;27:295.
77. Cunningham FG, MacDonald PC, Gant NF, eds. *Williams' obstetrics,* 18th ed. Norwalk: Appleton & Lange, 1989:538.
78. Hawkins JL, Koonin LM, Palmer SK, et al. Anesthesia-related deaths during obstetric delivery in the United States, 1979–1990. *Anesthesiology* 1997;86:277.
79. Naef RW, Chauhan SP, Chavalier SP. Prediction of hemorrhage at cesarean delivery. *Obstet Gynecol* 1994;83:923.
80. Pritchard JA, Baldwin RM, Dickey JC, et al. Blood volume changes in pregnancy and the puerperium. *Am J Obstet Gynecol* 1962;84:1271.
81. Robson SC, Boys RJ, Hunter S, et al. Maternal hemodynamics after normal delivery and delivery complicated by postpartum hemorrhage. *Obstet Gynecol* 1989;74:234.
82. Combs CA, Murphy EL, Laros RK. Factors associated with hemorrhage in cesarean deliveries. *Obstet Gynecol* 1991;77:77.
83. Chestnut DH, Dewan DM, Redick LF, et al. Anesthetic management of obstetric hysterectomy: a multi-institutional study. *Anesthesiology* 1989;70:607.
84. Hunter T, Kleiman S. Anaesthesia for caesarean hysterectomy in a patient with a preoperative diagnosis of placenta percreta with invasion of the urinary bladder. *Can J Anaesth* 1996;43:246.
85. Biehl DR. Anesthetic management of obstetric hemorrhage. *Int Anesthesiol Clin* 1990;20:52.
86. American College of Obstetricians and Gynecologists. Diagnosis and management of postpartum hemorrhage. *Int J Gynaecol Obstet* 1990; 36:159.
87. DeSimone CA, Norris MC, Leighton BL. Intravenous nitroglycerin aids manual extraction of a retained placenta. *Anesthesiology* 1990; 73:787.
88. Riley ET, Flanagan B, Cohen SE, et al. Intravenous nitroglycerin: a potent uterine relaxant for emergency obstetric procedures. Review of literature and report of three cases. *Int J Obstet Anesth* 1996;5:264.
89. George LS, Crandon AJ. Immediate postpartum complications. *Aust N Z J Obstet Gynaecol* 1990;30:52.
90. Abouleish E, Ali V, Joumaa B, et al. Anaesthetic management of acute puerperal uterine inversion. *Br J Anaesth* 1995;75:486.
91. Kriplani A, Relan S, Roy KK, et al. Complete inversion of the uterus during caesarean section: a case report. *Aust N Z Obstet Gynaecol* 1996;36:17.
92. Morgan M. Amniotic fluid embolism. *Anaesthesia* 1979;34:20.
93. Martin RW. Amniotic fluid embolism. *Clin Obstet Gynecol* 1996;39:101.
94. Noble WH, St-Amand J. Amniotic fluid embolus. *Can J Anaesth* 1993;40:971.
95. Margarson MP. Delayed amniotic fluid embolism following caesarean section under spinal anaesthesia. *Anaesthesia* 1995;50:804.
96. Joelsson UHI. Amniotic fluid embolism in Sweden, 1951–1980. *Gynecol Obstet Invest* 1985;20:130.
97. Hankins GDV, Berryman GK, Scott RT Jr, et al. Maternal arterial desaturation with 15-methyl prostaglandin F_2 alpha for uterine atony. *Obstet Gynecol* 1988;72:367.
98. Douglas MJ, Farquharson DF, Ross PLE, et al. Cardiovascular collapse following an overdose of prostaglandin F_2 alpha: a case report. *Can J Anaesth* 1989;36:466.
99. Jouppila P. Postpartum hemorrhage. *Curr Opin Obstet Gynecol* 1995; 7:446.
100. Maier RC. Control of postpartum hemorrhage with uterine packing. *Am J Obstet Gynecol* 1993;169:317.
101. Bobrowski RA, Jones TB. A thrombogenic uterine pack for postpartum hemorrhage. *Obstet Gynecol* 1995;5:836.
102. Hallak M, Dildy GA, Hurley TJ, et al. Transvaginal pressure pack for life-threatening pelvic hemorrhage secondary to placenta accreta. *Obstet Gynecol* 1991;78:938.
103. American Society of Anesthesiologists Task Force on Blood Component Therapy. Practice guidelines for blood component therapy. *Anesthesiology* 1996;84:732.
104. Razvi K, Chua S, Arulkumaran S, et al. A comparison between visual estimation and laboratory determination of blood loss during the third stage of labour. *Aust N Z J Obstet Gynaecol* 1996;36:152.
105. O'Dwyer G, Mylotte M, Sweeney M, et al. Experience of autologous blood transfusion in an obstetrics and gynaecology department. *Br J Obstet Gynaecol* 1993;100:571.
106. McVay PA, Hoag RW, Hoag MS, et al. Safety and use of autologous blood donation during third trimester of pregnancy. *Am J Obstet Gynecol* 1989;160:1479.
107. Santoso JT, Lin DW, Miller DS. Transfusion medicine in obstetrics and gynecology. *Obstet Gynecol Surv* 1995;50:470.
108. Dinsmoor MJ, Hogg BB. Autologous blood donation with placenta previa: is it feasible? *Am J Perinatol* 1995;12:382.
109. Bernstein HH, Rosenblatt MA, Gettes M, et al. The ability of the Haemonetics® 4 cell saver system to remove tissue factor from blood contaminated with amniotic fluid. *Anesth Analg* 1997;85:831.
110. Brandjes DPM, Schenk BE, Buller HR, et al. Management of disseminated intravascular coagulation in obstetrics. *Eur J Obstet Gynecol Reprod Biol* 1991;42:S87.
111. Gabbe SG, Niebyl JR, Simpson JL, eds. *Obstetrics: normal and problem pregnancies*, 2nd ed. New York: Churchill Livingstone, 1991:585.
112. Cunningham FG, MacDonald PC, Gant NF, eds. *Williams' obstetrics,* 18th ed. Norwalk, CT: Appleton & Lange, 1989:702.

Obstetric Anesthesia, second edition,
edited by Mark C. Norris.
Lippincott Williams & Wilkins, Philadelphia © 1999.

CHAPTER 31

Amniotic Fluid Embolism

Christopher M. Viscomi and Steven L. Clark

Amniotic fluid embolism (AFE) is an incompletely understood syndrome, which can be catastrophic for both mother and fetus. Classically, the syndrome presents with a triad of hypoxia, hypotension, and coagulopathy. The onset and lethality of the physiologic derangements induced by AFE are remarkable. As many as 86% of cases are fatal; death occurs within half an hour of symptom onset in more than 50% of cases (1,2). Although rare, AFE ranks among the leading causes of maternal death.

HISTORICAL DESCRIPTION

The first clinical report of AFE generally is credited to Meyer (3) in 1926; however, the syndrome may have been described more than 100 years earlier (4). In 1941, Steiner and Lushbaugh (5) described eight cases of peripartum cardiovascular collapse that they attributed to AFE. In all eight cases, fetal squamous cells and mucin were seen in the maternal pulmonary circulation on autopsy. Absence of this material in the lungs of parturients who died of other causes supported the diagnosis of AFE. A later series of 14 fatal AFE cases also reported fetal debris in the pulmonary circulation (6). Amniotic fluid components have been found in maternal brain, kidney, liver, spleen, and pancreas, although the route of access into the arterial circulation remains speculative.

For many years, antemortem diagnosis of AFE was based on clinical signs. Definitive diagnosis awaited autopsy. Central venous and pulmonary artery catheters provided a method of antemortem diagnosis by allowing detection of amniotic fluid components, mucin, and fetal squamous cells in central venous blood (Fig. 1) (7–9).

C.M. Viscomi: Department of Anesthesiology, University of Utah, Salt Lake City, Utah 84132.

S.L. Clark: Department of Obstetrics and Gynecology, University of Utah, Salt Lake City, UT 84132.

EPIDEMIOLOGY OF AMNIOTIC FLUID EMBOLISM

Based on their series of eight cases, Steiner and Lushbaugh (5) calculated an incidence for AFE of 1 in 8,000 deliveries. When they observed no additional cases in the next 26,000 deliveries, it appeared that this rate was an overestimate. Larger series have found frequencies as low as 1 in 92,000 (2). Most studies reported incidences that fall somewhere between these two extremes. A review of AFE cases in the United States reported an incidence of approximately 1 in 55,000 between 1968 and 1973 (7).

AFE carries a high risk of fatal outcome. One review of 272 cases reported a mortality rate of 86% (1). However, all but four reports in this review predate the use of central venous blood aspirations as an aid in antemortem diagnosis. Because the definitive diagnostic measure in this series was autopsy, nonfatal cases of AFE usually went undiagnosed and unreported. Recent literature supports a higher survival rate (10–12). This trend may reflect increased sensitivity of diagnosis, an improvement in treatment modalities, or the tendency of previous series to include only the most severe cases.

AFE causes 4.5% to 9% of peripartum maternal deaths (1,2,13). In the United States, AFE ranks behind preeclampsia/eclampsia, obstetric hemorrhage, pulmonary thromboembolism, and obstetric infection as a cause of death (Table 1). AFE causes nearly twice as many obstetric deaths as does anesthesia (13). The number of deaths due to hemorrhage, infection, and hypertensive disorders has declined with improved obstetric and anesthetic care. In contrast, the number of deaths of embolic origin has not decreased proportionately. This trend reflects the difficulty inherent in prevention, diagnosis, and treatment of embolic disease in the parturient.

Our understanding of the factors that predispose to AFE is largely anecdotal. Advanced maternal age, multi-

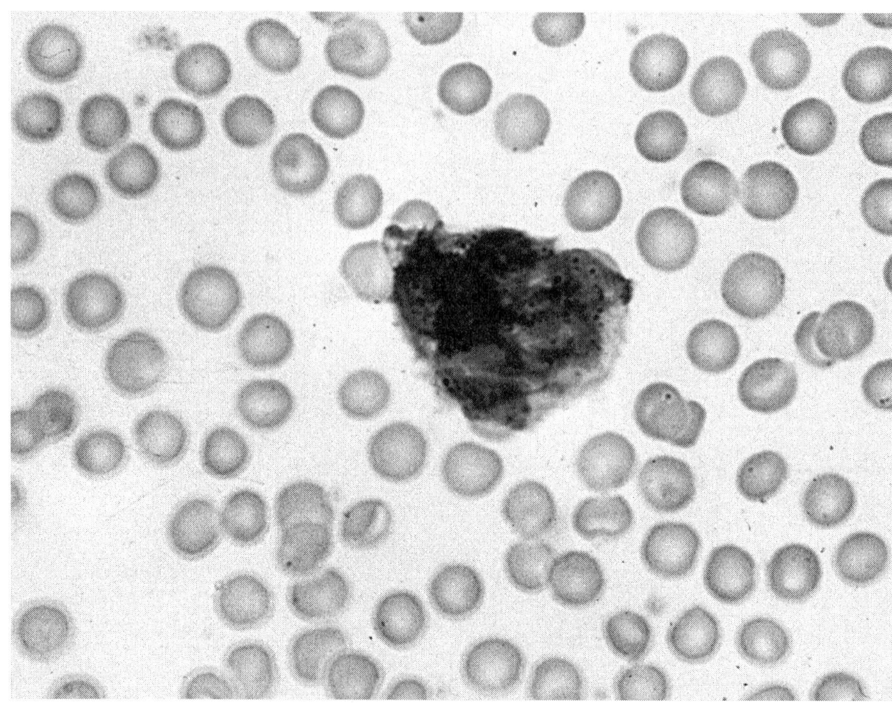

FIG. 1. Squamous cells present in aspirate of maternal central venous blood. Several studies have proposed this finding as diagnostic of amniotic fluid embolism. (Photomicrograph provided by Steven L. Clark, M.D.)

parity, large fetal size, rapid labor, and oxytocin augmentation may increase the risk. Most cases occur in older parturients, with a mean age of 32 years. One-third of cases in an Australian series occurred in patients older than 34 years (2). The incidence of AFE increases in multiparous patients; covariation of maternal age with increased parity may, at least partly, explain this association. Little evidence exists for macrosomia as a risk factor; the mean birth weight in a large series was 3.3 kg (1). Tumultuous labor was present in less than one-third of cases. Uterine stimulants were used in only 22%. To quote Morgan: "In view of the very wide use of accelerated labor and the rarity of AFE, it must be concluded that there is no direct association between the two" (1).

TABLE 1. *Principal causes of peripartum maternal death*

Source	Incidence[a]
Obstetric hemorrhage	28.7%
Preeclampsia/eclampsia	17.6%
Obstetric infection	13.1%
Pulmonary thromboembolism	10.9%
Amniotic fluid embolism	7.6%
Cardiomyopathy	5.6%
Anesthetic complications	2.5%

[a]Percent of maternal deaths (n = 1,453).

Data from Berg CJ, Atrash HK, Koonin LM, Tucker M. Pregnancy-related mortality in the United States, 1987–1990. *Obstet Gynecol* 1996;88:161.

Placental abruption occurs in up to 50% of AFE cases; fetal death precedes clinical presentation of AFE in 40% (14).

Most often, AFE presents during labor (90% of cases) (1). AFE also occurs during cesarean delivery, first- and second-trimester abortion, amniocentesis, and abdominal trauma (15–18). Some cases even present postpartum (19). An unusual AFE occurred spontaneously in the second trimester of a previously uncomplicated pregnancy (20).

The American Registry

In 1988, an Amniotic Fluid Embolism National Registry was created. A recent report detailed 46 cases that met the inclusion criteria (11). Although this series is much smaller than the 272 cases reported by Morgan (1), its strict inclusion criteria and systematic evaluation have yielded significant insights. AFE presented most often during labor (Table 2). There was no correlation with eth-

TABLE 2. *Time of diagnosis of amniotic fluid embolism*

Time	Percent of cases
Labor	70%
Cesarean delivery	19%
Postpartum	11%

Data from ref. 11.

nicity, age, oxytocin use, and rapidity or stage of labor. Maternal survival was 61%, although only 15% were neurologically intact. This intact survival rate is virtually identical to Morgan's earlier series (1). The improved overall survival likely reflects salvage of neurologically injured patients with more aggressive intensive care unit care. Neurologically intact neonatal survival was 39% and appeared to be related to expeditious delivery. In several patients, clinical signs of AFE had a striking temporal relationship to artificial rupture of membranes or placement of an intrauterine pressure catheter. This relationship between uterine instrumentation and AFE has been noted previously (21). Of interest, 41% of parturients had a history of atopy, and 67% of fetuses were male. In concert with the high incidence of bronchospasm and hypotension in the presentation of AFE, the authors suggested that the syndrome would be more appropriately termed anaphylactoid syndrome of pregnancy (11).

CLINICAL PRESENTATION

Presenting Symptoms

The clinical presentation of AFE syndrome often is dramatic. Shnider and Moya (22) offered the following description, which remains vivid 40 years later: "Suddenly and without warning, the signs of amniotic fluid infusion appear: hyperpnea or tachypnea, cyanosis and shock progressing into profound coma. In addition, there is often rigor, clonic-tonic convulsions and acute pulmonary edema. If the patient survives this initial phase, incoagulability of the blood develops with excessive bleeding from raw surfaces in the uterus, vagina, and perineum." Sometimes, nonspecific prodromal symptoms (nausea, vomiting, agitation, chills, apprehension, and restlessness) may precede overt evidence of AFE. The prevalence of these symptoms in the obstetric population renders them of limited use in predicting onset of AFE. Most cases continue to present as completely unheralded cardiorespiratory collapse.

Rapid onset of severe cardiopulmonary compromise characterizes the initial phase of AFE syndrome. In most cases, respiratory distress is the presenting symptom (Table 3), usually followed by severe hypotension and frequently, within minutes, cardiac arrest. Alternate initial presentations include cardiovascular collapse, uncontrolled hemorrhage, and seizures (1,2). More atypical presentations of AFE have included abdominal pain, chest pain, and ventricular tachycardia. Mortality is very high during the initial phase. In one review, over half the women died within 30 minutes of onset of symptoms. A later hemorrhagic phase develops in 40% to 50% of patients. Considering the very high immediate mortality, it is likely that this percentage underestimates the true incidence of coagulopathy (14).

TABLE 3. *Presenting symptoms in amniotic fluid embolism*

Respiratory distress	57%
Hypotension	37%
Coagulopathy	13%
Seizures	10%

Due to frequent overlap of presenting symptoms, percentages sum to >100%.
Data modified from refs. 1 and 2.

Cardiopulmonary Effects

The chief cardiovascular manifestation of AFE is severe hypotension, usually out of proportion to any blood loss. Tachycardia typically accompanies the rapid drop in blood pressure. Clinical and invasive monitoring data frequently suggest left ventricular dysfunction. Electrocardiographic findings are nondiagnostic. The electrocardiogram may be normal or show sinus tachycardia or other arrhythmias, with or without accompanying ST-segment changes. Usually, clinical evidence of pulmonary edema, such as rales, frothy pink sputum, and jugular venous distention, develops rapidly. In up to 70% of patients, chest radiograph reveals some degree of pulmonary edema. Although left ventricular filling pressures may increase, the degree of pulmonary edema often is out of proportion to this rise, suggesting involvement of both cardiogenic and noncardiogenic mechanisms. Adult respiratory distress syndrome frequently will develop in those who survive the acute event. Arterial blood gas tensions in AFE typically reveal severe hypoxemia and metabolic acidosis with incomplete respiratory compensation. Continuous pulse oximetry provided the initial evidence of AFE in one report (23). A patient's room air oxyhemoglobin saturation during cesarean section dropped abruptly without any other signs or symptoms. Within hours, she suffered a cardiac arrest and died. The autopsy findings suggested AFE.

Invasive Monitoring

At present, only a few published cases report data from early invasive central hemodynamic monitoring. In contrast to the pulmonary hypertension and elevated pulmonary vascular resistance of several animal models (5,24–27), left ventricular failure is the only consistent finding in humans (5,10,14,24–27). Several patients had elevations of pulmonary artery pressures that reflected elevated pulmonary artery occlusion pressures and left ventricular failure rather than intrinsic pulmonary artery vasospasm. These case reports consistently describe significant left ventricular dysfunction based on clinical criteria, nuclear scanning, or calculation of left ventricular stroke work index (Fig. 2).

Echocardiography also has shown severe left ventricular dysfunction in AFE (28). Diminished coronary artery

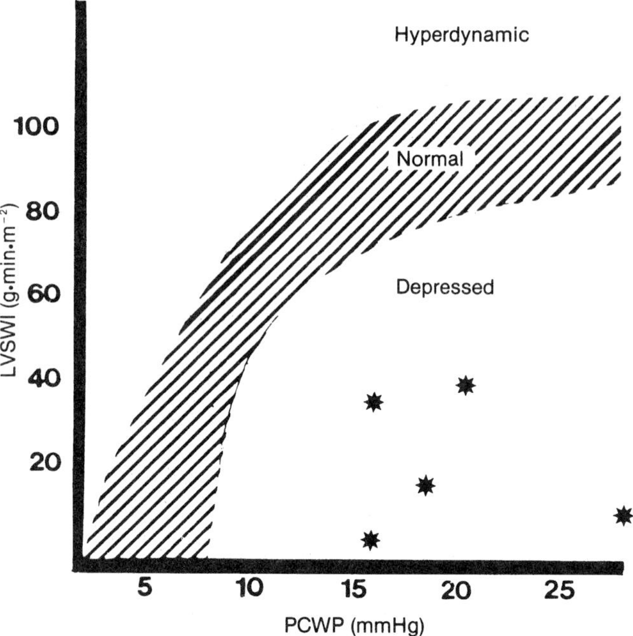

FIG. 2. Left ventricular performance in five amniotic embolism victims. (Reprinted from ref. 76, with permission.)

blood flow, as noted in an animal model of AFE (29), provides a possible basis for these observations. In addition to left ventricular failure, some patients have low calculated systemic vascular resistance (11).

Unfortunately, the earliest data from any of these patients was obtained 70 minutes after the onset of clinical symptoms. Much of the information reflects events occurring after vasoactive agents had been administered in efforts to stabilize the patient. Because mortality in excess of 65% occurs within 30 minutes of initial symptoms (2), invasive monitoring information from longer-term survivors may not represent all cases of AFE, especially those with more sudden and catastrophic presentations.

An additional report exists of a presumed AFE in a woman with a pulmonary artery catheter already in place (15). A 41-year-old patient with severe chronic hypertension and classic angina had invasive monitoring established for elective cesarean section. During delivery, under epidural anesthesia, left-sided chest pain developed, coincident with a rise in pulmonary artery pressures from 35/9 mm Hg to 38/16 mm Hg. Neither cardiac output nor pulmonary capillary occlusion pressure was measured. The chest pain did not respond to nitroglycerin infusion. The patient had several transient episodes of ventricular tachycardia. Examination of pulmonary artery catheter aspirate revealed squamous cells and fetal debris. No other signs of AFE (hypoxia, pulmonary edema, hypotension, or coagulopathy) developed. Unfortunately, the incomplete nature of the hemodynamic monitoring plus the patient's coexisting diseases and absence of classic signs of AFE render this case of little value in evaluating the hemodynamic course of AFE.

Coagulopathy

Some degree of coagulopathy will develop in 40% of patients who survive the immediate hemodynamic and pulmonary effects of AFE. Anything from subclinical coagulopathy with transient abnormalities in laboratory studies to fully developed disseminated intravascular coagulation with life-threatening hemorrhage may arise. Laboratory values will reflect consumption of clotting factors with decreased fibrinogen and platelet count, elevated fibrin split products, and prolonged prothrombin and partial thromboplastin times. Clinically, the patient will exhibit persistent vaginal or incisional bleeding and oozing from venipuncture sites. The simultaneous development of uterine atony, possibly secondary to direct inhibition of myometrial contractility by amniotic fluid, often complicates the coagulopathy (14). The underlying mechanism of AFE-associated disseminated intravascular coagulation is unclear. Amniotic fluid contains an activator of factor X, but in an amount that appears inadequate to initiate disseminated intravascular coagulation (30). Systemic release of trophoblastic material may play a significant role (14). Recent work suggests that the procoagulant property of amniotic fluid is due to tissue factor (31), which accounts for most of the procoagulant potential of amniotic fluid. Tissue factor concentration increases with gestational age.

Clinical signs of coagulopathy may precede other evidence of AFE. Rarely, coagulopathy has been reported as the sole manifestation of presumptive AFE (2). However, these cases might reflect a tendency to overdiagnose AFE in unexpected peripartum deaths (13).

Neurological and Other Manifestations

Seizures, likely secondary to cerebral hypoxia, occur in 10% to 20% of AFE cases. They may complicate management by increasing oxygen demand. Hypoxic brain injury, a potentially devastating complication of AFE, has caused severe disability in survivors (11,32). Acute renal failure due to prolonged hypoperfusion also may follow. AFE appears to have no permanent cardiac or pulmonary sequelae; survivors generally return to baseline cardiopulmonary function.

Fetal distress is inevitable following onset of AFE symptoms. Maternal hypoxemia and hypotension drastically reduce transplacental oxygen delivery. The fetus rarely survives unless delivered immediately. Fetal distress also may precede the development of maternal symptoms, reflecting the extreme sensitivity of the fetus to even asymptomatic maternal hypoxemia (33).

Differential Diagnosis

Clinically, it is difficult to differentiate AFE from other serious peripartum complications (Table 4). Pulmonary

TABLE 4. *Differential diagnosis of amniotic fluid embolism*

Condition	Symptom: Respiratory distress	Hypotension	Coagulopathy	Seizures
Pulmonary thromboembolism	+	+		
Venous air embolism	+	+		
Septic or hypovolemic shock		+	+	
Myocardial infarction		+		
Peripartum cardiomyopathy	+	+		
Decompensation of cardiac valvular disease	+	+		
Uterine rupture		+		
Supine hypotensive syndrome		+		
Preeclampsia/eclampsia			+	+
Local anesthetic toxicity				+
Placental abruption		+	+	
Cerebral vascular accident	+			+
Aspiration of gastric contents	+			

thromboembolism, venous air embolism, systemic sepsis, myocardial infarction, decompensation of significant valvular disease, and peripartum cardiomyopathy can cause acute cardiovascular collapse in the parturient. Venous air embolism, detectable by Doppler ultrasound in up to 65% of cesarean deliveries, often produces dyspnea and oxyhemoglobin desaturation (34). Both severe preeclampsia and placental abruption cause a coagulopathy that is clinically indistinguishable from that of AFE. Other complications to be considered in the differential diagnosis of AFE include eclampsia, cerebral hemorrhage, aspiration of gastric contents, severe supine hypotensive syndrome, uterine rupture, and systemic toxicity of local anesthetic agents.

AMNIOTIC FLUID IN THE MATERNAL CIRCULATION

Amniotic Fluid Composition

Amniotic fluid volume increases rapidly during pregnancy from approximately 50 mL at 12 weeks of gestation to a maximum of 1 L at term. In the first half of pregnancy, amniotic fluid has essentially the same electrolyte composition as maternal plasma. Particulate matter is nearly absent. As pregnancy progresses, fetal urine output makes the fluid hypotonic and increases its concentration of urea and creatinine. Varying amounts of particulate matter of fetal origin accumulate. This debris consists of desquamated fetal skin cells, lanugo and scalp hairs, vernix caseosa, mucin, and, occasionally, meconium. Amniotic fluid also contains prostaglandins and other arachidonic acid metabolites that may play an important role in the pathophysiology of AFE (35).

Entry into Maternal Circulation

Amniotic fluid entry into the maternal circulation requires communication between the amniotic sac and the maternal venous system. This interchange can occur through either the uteroplacental junction or uterine or cervical veins disrupted by incision or trauma. Endocervical veins are commonly lacerated during labor as the upper portion of the uterus becomes part of the lower uterine segment (36). Following membrane rupture, uterine contractions may force amniotic fluid into these vessels. Cervical veins frequently tear during normal labor, with no apparent ill effects on the parturient. This mechanism, therefore, most likely does not have a primary role in the onset of AFE syndrome. Placental abruption commonly occurs in cases of AFE. Possibly, premature separation of the placenta allows amniotic fluid entry through the placental implantation site. Disruption of the fetal membranes appears necessary for the development of AFE. The amniotic sac breaks before the onset of symptoms in most cases. When not apparent, concealed rupture has occurred, with intact membranes continuing to cover the cervical os.

Evidence exists for and against the routine entry of amniotic fluid into the maternal circulation. Sparr and Pritchard (37) examined this question in 1958 by injecting ^{51}Cr-labeled red blood cells into the amniotic fluid of parturients shortly before vaginal or cesarean delivery. They found only trace amounts of radioactivity in the maternal circulation after delivery and calculated the volume of amniotic fluid entry at less than 2 mL (37). A contrasting study found significant transfer of radiolabeled albumin from the amniotic fluid to the maternal circulation during hypertonic saline-induced abortion (38). Intraamniotic injection of hypertonic saline may raise intrauterine pressure well above that achieved during normal labor. Taken together, these two studies lend some support to the long-standing clinical impression that AFE occurs more frequently in cases of uterine tetany or a "hard" course of labor. Others believe that uterine tetany occurs after AFE and results from uterine ischemia (11).

Autopsy studies consistently report no evidence of amniotic fluid debris in maternal lungs without clinical signs of AFE. A study comparing lung biopsies from 20 AFE fatalities with samples from 20 parturients who died of complications of preeclampsia/eclampsia reported that 19 of 20 AFE patients had evidence of amniotic fluid debris on examination of a single tissue sample. The remaining case was positive in a second sample. None of the control samples contained evidence of amniotic fluid debris (39).

Unlike amniotic fluid, trophoblastic embolism is more common during pregnancy. A postmortem study found evidence of trophoblastic tissue in maternal lung in 96 of 220 cases (40). Between 30% and 80% of parturients have trophoblastic cells in their peripheral circulation (41). However, these findings are clouded by the histologic difficulty in distinguishing trophoblastic cells from maternal megakaryocytes. Reliable differentiation may require sophisticated immunohistochemical analysis techniques (42).

Significance of Fetal Debris

Pulmonary artery catheterization may allow rapid diagnosis of AFE and enable differentiation of AFE from other causes of peripartum cardiovascular compromise (9). Detection of fetal squamous cells in the maternal pulmonary circulation has been proposed as pathognomonic for AFE; however, reliable differentiation of fetal from adult squamous cells may not be possible. Recent evidence suggests that examination of mixed venous blood from patients with indwelling pulmonary artery catheters may commonly reveal squamous cells. Squamous cells were recovered from the central circulation in all 33 cases in a series of 16 pregnant and 17 nonpregnant patients who underwent pulmonary artery catheterization for a variety of indications (43). The cell count was slightly higher in the pregnant patients and tended to increase postpartum, suggesting that perhaps some cells were of fetal origin. Most were presumed to be contaminants introduced into the circulation during cannulation. Of interest, the series included one patient who eventually died of apparent AFE; her cell count was no higher than that of nonpregnant controls. A similar study examined pulmonary artery blood samples from a series of parturients without clinical signs of AFE (44). They compared these women to a nonpregnant patient and a parturient with clinical symptoms of AFE syndrome. Only the nonpregnant patient tested completely negative for amniotic fluid components. Although the patient with suspected AFE had the most fetal debris, all the other parturients also had squamous cells, lanugo hair, or mucin in their pulmonary artery blood. Therefore, the presence of squamous cells or other fetal debris in a parturient's central circulation is not pathognomonic for AFE. "In a critically ill obstetric patient, such a finding should not deter the clinician from a thorough search for other causes of hemodynamic instability" (43).

The lack of specificity of squamous cells in the maternal circulation has prompted a search for more sensitive markers of amniotic fluid in the maternal circulation. Recently, investigators reported high levels of zinc coproporphyrin in the serum of AFE patients (45). Zinc coproporphyrin is a characteristic component of meconium and can be identified by fluorometry after high-power liquid chromatography.

Animal Models of Amniotic Fluid Embolism

Although the clinical presentation of AFE is well described, the underlying mechanism of the maternal response to AFE remains elusive. Because AFE occurs so rarely and the early mortality is so high, controlled clinical trials of alternative therapeutic regimens are nearly impossible. Thus, we must rely heavily on animal models and in vitro experiments to explain the pathogenesis and evaluate treatment modalities for this vexing syndrome.

Unfortunately, no consensus exists for the proper animal model of AFE (Table 5). Rabbit, dog, sheep, monkey, cat, and calf models have been developed. A further complication is the use of heterologous (from another species) or autologous (same animal) amniotic fluid in the attempts to create experimental AFE. In addition, the amniotic fluid administered in these various models has varied from a particulate-free filtrate to highly meconium-enriched solutions.

Heterologous Models

Steiner and Lushbaugh (5) first studied AFE in animals. Rabbits and dogs received intravenous injection of either unaltered or meconium-enriched human amniotic fluid. Particulate-free human amniotic fluid was innocuous in rabbits. Thick, meconium-enriched, human amniotic fluid usually proved fatal in both rabbits and dogs.

At least 12 heterologous AFE studies exist, with widely varying findings (Table 4). Certain species, such as the rabbit, seem particularly sensitive to intravenous heterologous amniotic fluid (5). In contrast, calves (24), dogs (25), and sheep (26) suffer only transient alterations in pulmonary or systemic hemodynamics or temporary coagulopathy. A widely cited canine model of AFE evaluated both left- and right-sided cardiac function after intravenous injection of human amniotic fluid or suspended human meconium (28). Both substances transiently decreased blood pressure, cardiac output, and systemic vascular resistance while significantly elevat-

TABLE 5. *Animal models of amniotic fluid embolism*

Investigator	Year	Animal	Anesthetized	Pregnant	Filtered AF	Pathology with whole/ concentrated AF	AF species	Injection arterial	Injection venous	Hemodynamic changes	Coagulopathy	Autopsy
Steiner and Luschbaugh	1941	Rabbit/ dog	No	No	No	Yes	Human	NE	Yes	NE (death)	No	Debris in pulmonary artery
Gron	1952	Rabbit	No	No	NE	Yes	Human	No	Yes	NE (death)	No	Debris in pulmonary artery
Schneider	1953	Dog	No	No	NE	Yes	Human	NE	Yes	NE (death)	5 of 8	Debris in pulmonary artery
Jaques	1960	Dog	Yes	No	NE	Yes	Human/ dog	NE	Yes	↑PAP, NL BP	Fibrinogen 12 of 13	Debris in pulmonary artery
Halmagyi	1962	Sheep	Yes	No	No	Yes	Human	NE	Yes	↑PAP, NL SVR NL CO	No	NE
Attwood	1965	Dog	Yes	No	Yes (mild)	Yes	Human	Yes	Yes	↑PAP, ↑PVR, ↓SVR, NL to ↑LAP, BP	4 of 12	NE
Stolte	1967	Monkey	Yes	Yes	No	No	Human/ monkey	No	No	NL BP, NL P	1 of 12	NE
MacMillan	1968	Rabbit	No	No	No	Yes	Human	Yes	Yes	NE (death)	2 of 12	Minimal debris, hemorrhage
Reis	1969	Sheep	Yes	Yes	Yes	Yes	Sheep	Yes	Yes	↑PAP, ↑PVR, ↓SVR, ↓BP, NL LAP, NL PCWP	No	Normal
Dutta	1970	Rabbit	Yes	No	NE	Yes	Human	NE	Yes	NE (death)	No	Minimal debris, massive infarction
Adamsons	1971	Monkey	Yes	Yes	NE	No	Monkey	NE	No	NL BP, NL P, NL RR	No	NE
Kitzmiller	1972	Cat	Yes	No	No	Yes	Human	NE	Yes	↓BP, ↑P, ↑CVP	No	NE
Spence	1974	Rabbit	No	Yes	No	No	Rabbit	NE	No	NL BP, NL P, NL RR	No	NE
Reeves	1974	Calf	No	No	NE	Yes	Calf	NE	Yes	↓BP, ↑PAP, NL CO NL PCWP		
Azegami	1986	Rabbit	No	No	No	Yes	Human	NE	Yes	NE (death)	No	Pulmonary edema, debris in pulmonary vessels
Richards	1988	Rat*	Yes	No	Yes	NE	Human	NE	Yes	Coronary flow		
Hankins	1993	Goat	Yes	Yes	Yes	Yes	Goat	No	Yes	↑BP, ↑PAP, ↓CO with meconium	NE	NE

*Isolated heart preparation.

AF, amniotic fluid; BP, blood pressure; CO, cardiac output; CVP, central venous pressure; LAP, left atrial pressure; NE, not examined; NL, normal; P, pulse; PAP, pulmonary artery pressure; PCWP, pulmonary capillary wedge pressure; PVR, pulmonary vascular resistance; RR, respiratory rate; SVR, systemic vascular resistance.

From Clark SL, Phelan JP, Cotton DB. Amniotic fluid embolism. In: *Critical care obstetrics,* 2nd ed. Cambridge, MA: Blackwell Scientific Publications, 1991:318, with permission.

ing pulmonary vascular resistance. None of these animals developed hypofibrinogenemia or pulmonary edema. Although some clinicians accept these data as a valid basis for therapeutic recommendations, others claim that heterologous models of AFE only prove "that it is possible to kill animals by the systemic injection of large boluses of foreign material from another species" (14).

Autologous Models

Several groups have attempted to address some criticisms of heterologous AFE models by using autologous amniotic fluid. They have used both primate and lower animal models. In a highly invasive study of near-term ewes, Reis et al. (46) harvested amniotic fluid at the time of cesarean section (under local anesthesia). They then induced general anesthesia, did a median sternotomy, and placed flow probes and pressure sensors. Amniotic fluid was injected into the inferior vena cava or the left atrium. Transient decreases in blood pressure and systemic vascular resistance were accompanied by substantial increases in pulmonary artery pressures and pulmonary vascular resistance. Cardiac output did not change consistently. The absence of a difference in response between inferior vena caval and left atrial injections, or between filtered and particulate-rich amniotic fluid, suggests a humoral mechanism of AFE, rather than a mechanical-obstructive process (46). It is particularly interesting that, at necropsy, the lungs were normal, which is in strong contrast to the typical findings of amniotic fluid debris in the lungs of humans who succumb to AFE.

A more recent study of autologous AFE used gravid goats (47). The authors compared raw, filtered, filtered and boiled, and meconium-containing amniotic fluid. Transient increases in systemic arterial and pulmonary artery pressures were noted and were of the greatest magnitude in the meconium amniotic fluid group. Left ventricular dysfunction and hypoxemia were only seen in the meconium amniotic fluid group.

Reports of two primate models of autologous AFE are available (48,49). Nonpregnant, pregnant, and postpartum monkeys were injected with autologous amniotic fluid. These injections proved totally innocuous. The authors concluded that AFE syndrome is not caused by the introduction of "normal" amniotic fluid into the maternal vasculature.

The various animal models show inconsistent maternal responses to amniotic fluid injection. Studies of heterologous amniotic fluid in nonprimates usually find significant pathology; however, these models are probably the least relevant to human AFE. Autologous amniotic fluid injection in nonprimates produces transient hemodynamic effects. Most frequently, it causes pulmonary vasospasm and diminished systemic vascular resistance. Primate models, however, reveal few sequelae after amniotic fluid injection. These findings have led some to question the belief that "normal" amniotic fluid can account for the clinical picture of human AFE.

Several workers have attempted to reconcile animal and human data by postulating a "biphasic" pattern of pulmonary and cardiovascular response to AFE (10,50). They suggest an initial phase involving pulmonary hypertension and elevated pulmonary vascular resistance, as seen in several animal experiments. In this model, those surviving the initial insult experience a secondary phase or left-heart failure with normalization of pulmonary artery pressures. This hypothesis remains purely speculative; no evidence of the proposed initial phase exists in humans.

Models of Amniotic Fluid Embolism: Role of Prostaglandins and Leukotrienes

Amniotic fluid contains significant amounts of prostaglandins, leukotrienes, and other arachidonic acid metabolites (51). Figure 3 reviews the activation of arachidonic acids and the subsequent formation of prostaglandins and leukotrienes. Many arachidonic acid metabolites have hemodynamic and coagulation effects that mimic clinical AFE.

The amount and type of arachidonic acid metabolites in the amniotic fluid change throughout pregnancy. Early in gestation, only prostaglandins of the E series are found. With the onset of labor, prostaglandin $F_{2\alpha}$ becomes detectable and prostaglandin F_1 concentrations rise. Simultaneously, the concentration of prostaglandin E declines (52,53).

Kitzmiller and Lucas (54) first noted the increased toxicity of amniotic fluid obtained from laboring versus nonlaboring women. The changing prostaglandin content of amniotic fluid during labor may account for its increased toxicity. A lipid extract of amniotic fluid induces pulmonary hypertension in the bovine model of AFE (24). Furthermore, aspirin (a potent inhibitor of prostaglandin synthesis) totally prevents the occurrence of pulmonary hypertension. Leukotrienes also may play a role in the pathology of rabbit AFE (52). Prior administration of 5-lipoxygenase inhibitors, which block the formation of leukotrienes, prevents acute death in these animals (52).

Other vasoactive peptides have been implicated in the pathogenesis of AFE. Endothelin is a highly potent vasoconstrictor found in amniotic fluid, with significant effects on pulmonary and coronary vessels as well as on bronchial smooth muscle. Amniotic fluid concentration of endothelin increases with gestational age. These data are consistent with goat and human results (11,47) that suggest a pressor response to AFE, followed by ventricular dysfunction.

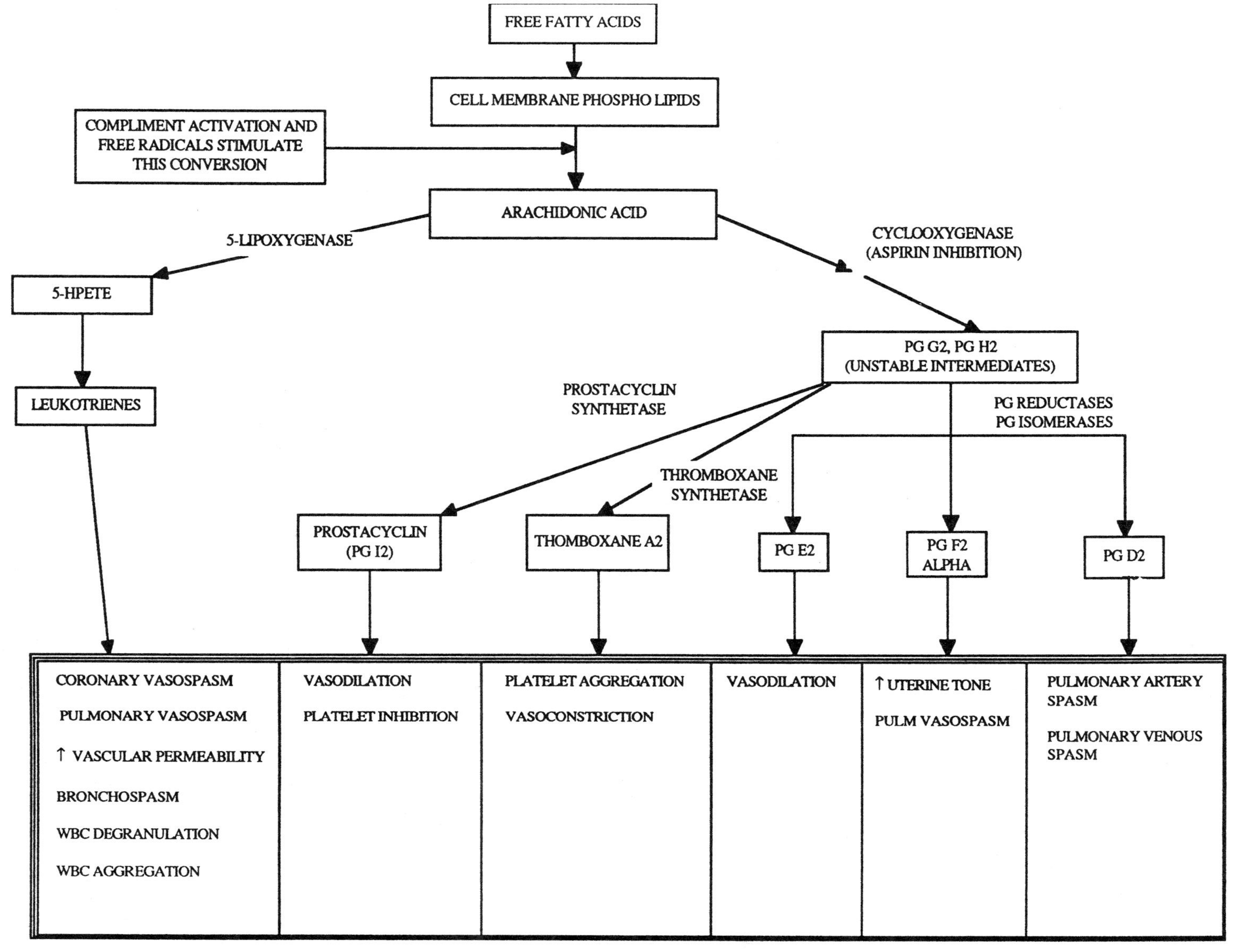

FIG. 3. Arachidonic acid synthesis, metabolites, and clinical effects.

Data from humans also indirectly implicate arachidonic acid metabolites in the genesis of AFE syndrome. Hankins et al. (55) reported a series of women who developed severe hypoxemia after intramuscular or intramyometrial injection of 15-methyl prostaglandin $F_{2\alpha}$. Intrapulmonary shunts of up to 28% developed. The authors suggest that this compound can induce severe bronchoconstriction and pulmonary vasospasm leading to V/Q mismatch. Douglas et al. (56) reported fulminant pulmonary edema and cardiovascular collapse in a parturient receiving high-dose intramyometrial prostaglandin $F_{2\alpha}$. Amniotic fluid from laboring parturients, which contains large amounts of prostaglandin $F_{2\alpha}$, could initiate similar pathology.

Hammerschmidt et al. (57) provide further evidence for a role of prostaglandins in AFE syndrome. They were stimulated by the finding of extensive leukostasis in pulmonary sections of human AFE victims. Leukostasis of this degree usually involves extensive complement and granulocyte activation and has been described in acute respiratory distress syndrome and extracorporeal circulation-induced pulmonary dysfunction. They showed that human amniotic fluid could activate complement, principally via the alternative pathway. Complement activation was more likely to occur in plasma samples from gravid women than in samples from nongravid women. Furthermore, the amniotic fluid of "stressed" pregnancies (stressors include toxemia, diabetes, amnionitis, and hydrops fetalis) was a more potent activator of complement than fluid from uncomplicated pregnancies. In response to complement activation, leukocytes produce toxic free radicals that stimulate the arachidonic acid pathway (58). Arachidonic acid in maternal serum and amniotic fluid during labor (59,60) provides a substrate for the production of thromboxanes and leukotrienes, which have potent vasoactive, leukocyte-aggregating, and platelet-stimulating action. Hammerschmidt et al. (57) proposed that a gravid woman is "primed" for an exaggerated cellular and vascular response in the event of complement activation (as in AFE). Clinical AFE occurs when a significant volume of amniotic fluid, rich in complement-activating property, enters the circulation of women unfortunate enough to have plasma that can be activated (57).

Other work complements these findings that amniotic fluid entry into the systemic circulation can trigger a maternal arachidonic acid metabolite response. Amniotic fluid surfactant injection into the systemic circulation is a potent stimulus of leukotriene synthesis (61). Leukotrienes are derived from arachidonic acid through activation of the enzyme 5-lipoxygenase. Amniotic fluid surfactant appears to stimulate 5-lipoxygenase activity in a dose-dependent manner. Leukotrienes then could induce the circulatory collapse and bronchoconstriction seen in AFE.

Taken as a whole, there is strong and evolving evidence that biochemical events, not pulmonary obstruction by fetal debris, are primarily responsible for clinical AFE.

TREATMENT

Historically, therapeutic recommendations have been based upon heterologous animal models of AFE. Efforts focused on relieving presumed pulmonary vasospasm with atropine, papaverine, aminophylline, steroids, and vasodilators (1,14,62–64). In light of more recent human invasive monitoring data, a more rational approach involves initial stabilization, consideration of the differential diagnosis, and the use of appropriate vasoactive drugs guided by invasive monitoring (Fig. 4).

Cardiopulmonary Resuscitation

With a potential first-hour mortality of 65%, considerable attention should be focused on the ABCs of cardiopulmonary resuscitation. Hypoxemia is a nearly universal finding in early AFE. Many patients have survived the initial insult, yet ultimately die of complications of cerebral hypoxia (14,65). Thus, early oxygen supplementation, preferably via an endotracheal tube, is imperative. AFE patients frequently need blood pressure support to provide acceptable perfusion pressures for maternal vital organs and the fetus. Ephedrine has long been the acute vasopressor of choice in obstetrics, as it usually preserves uterine blood flow (66). Left uterine displacement should accompany other resuscitative efforts.

Should full cardiac arrest occur, controversy surrounds the effectiveness of closed-chest cardiopulmonary resuscitation in parturients (67–69). Diminished venous return in the supine position impairs cardiopulmonary resuscitation in the antepartum patient. Lateral tilt introduces technical difficulty and mechanical disadvantage. Even optimal cardiopulmonary resuscitation produces only 30% of normal cardiac output (70). Thus, it is unlikely that adequate placental and fetal oxygen delivery can be sustained during cardiopulmonary resuscitation. Expeditious delivery correlated may improve maternal and neonatal outcome after cardiac arrest (71,72). To this end, immediate and rapid preparation for cesarean delivery must start once maternal cardiac arrest occurs. Of course, aggressive resuscitation and continuous cardiopulmonary resuscitation should continue during this time.

Once initial stabilization and appropriate noninvasive monitoring (electrocardiogram, pulse oximetry, blood pressure monitor) have been accomplished, attention should focus on the differential diagnosis. Clinical AFE syndrome is rare. Conditions that easily mimic AFE include complications of preeclampsia (severe cerebral hemorrhage, hepatic rupture, eclamptic seizure with aspiration), overwhelming sepsis, concealed abruptio placenta, and intravenous or cerebrospinal fluid-mediated local anesthetic toxicity (Table 4).

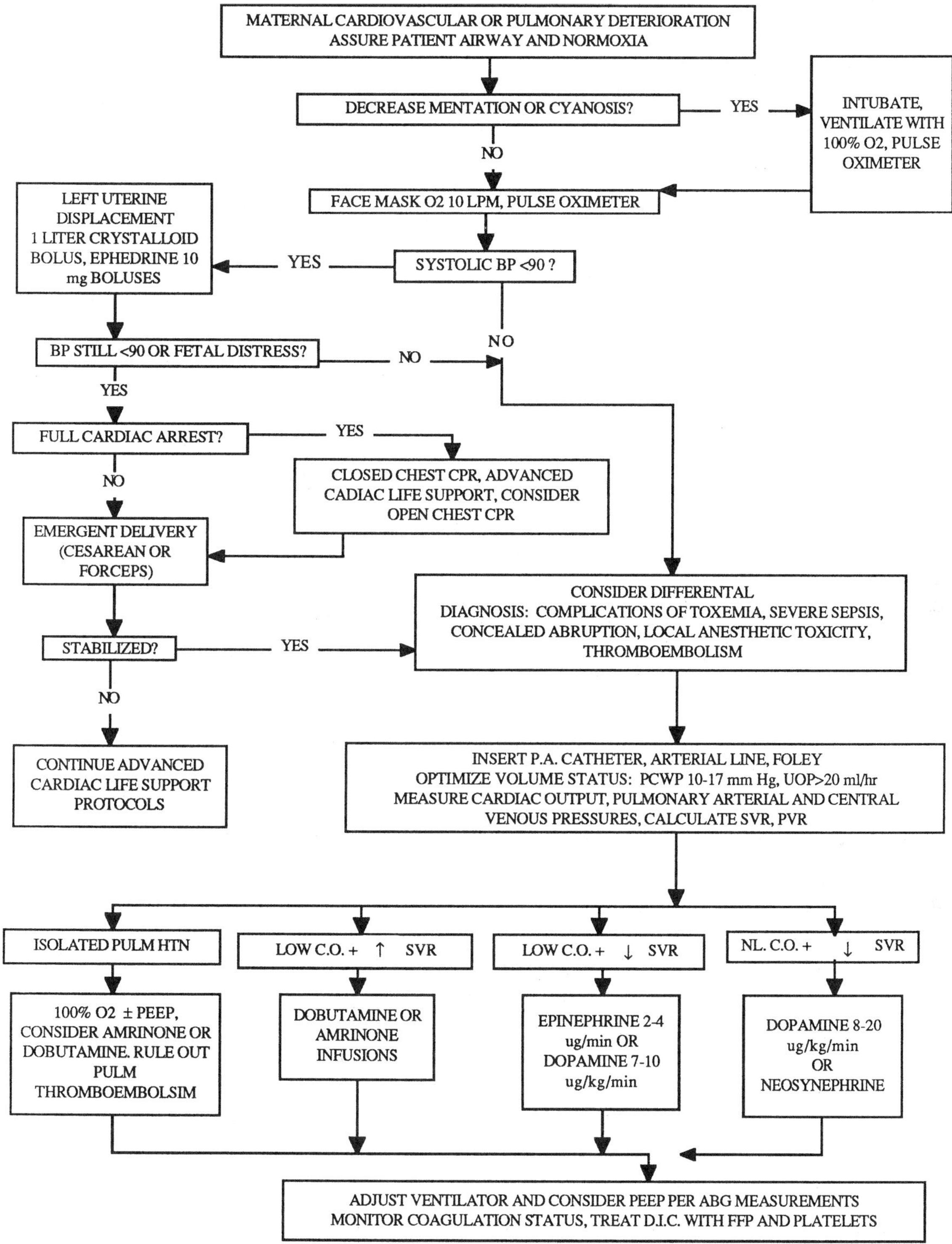

FIG. 4. A therapeutic algorithm for amniotic fluid embolism syndrome.

If AFE appears likely and severe sepsis has been excluded, some clinicians advocate administering a very large bolus of steroids, possibly combined with H_1 and H_2 blockers (11). This therapy is based upon the similarities of AFE to anaphylaxis and the data linking inflammatory mediators to the clinical manifestations of AFE. If available, zinc coproporphyrin concentrations may rapidly help diagnose or exclude AFE (45).

Invasive Monitoring

Placement of arterial and pulmonary artery catheters is the next priority. Periodic arterial blood gas measurement will guide ventilator therapy. Intelligent use of a pulmonary artery catheter can be invaluable in choosing and titrating vasoactive drugs, as well as optimizing volume status (Fig. 4).

Blood Product Therapy

Delayed coagulopathy (disseminated intravascular coagulation) develops in 40% of patients who survive the initial insult of AFE. Concomitant uterine atony also may occur. Frequent laboratory evaluation of coagulation profiles (fibrinogen, fibrin split products, prothrombin time, partial thromboplastin time, and platelet counts) provides a basis for therapy. Treat this usually self-limited coagulopathy with factor (fresh frozen plasma) and platelet replacement. Treat uterine atony with methergonovine and avoidance of volatile anesthetics. Use prostaglandin $F_{2\alpha}$ only with extreme caution, as it may further complicate matters by inciting severe hypoxemia and hypotension (55,56).

Outcome of Survivors

Those patients fortunate enough to survive AFE without severe neurological deficit do not appear to suffer any delayed consequences of the condition. In fact, Clark (73) recently reported two patients with successful and uneventful pregnancy outcomes after recovery from AFE.

CONCLUSION

AFE syndrome remains a significant cause of maternal morbidity and mortality. Although the symptom complex involving maternal hypotension, hypoxemia, and coagulopathy clearly exists, the link to amniotic fluid remains unproven. Amniotic fluid commonly enters the maternal circulation, yet clinical AFE syndrome is rare. Amniotic fluid has a highly variable ability to activate complement and arachidonic acid pathways. Women vary tremendously in their susceptibility to complement activation and prostaglandin synthesis. Current knowledge suggests that clinical AFE syndrome results when a significant volume of amniotic fluid, high in complement-activating ability, enters the circulation of a woman predisposed to excessive complement and arachidonic acid metabolite response.

The diagnosis of AFE rests on excluding potential imitators, and therapy is essentially supportive. Early invasive monitoring helps optimize intravascular volume and use of appropriate vasoactive drugs. The finding of squamous cells and fetal debris in a pulmonary artery catheter aspirate is necessary but not sufficient for the diagnosis.

More than 40 years ago, Eastman (74) advised against making AFE syndrome "a wastebasket for all cases of unexplained death in labor." An equally sage observation is that "the diagnosis of amniotic fluid embolism has been the escape hatch through which makers of errors in judgment can gain freedom" (75). Our challenge remains to identify correctly this vexing syndrome, so that we can treat it optimally and understand it better.

REFERENCES

1. Morgan M. Amniotic fluid embolism. *Anaesthesia* 1979;34:20.
2. Ratten GJ. Amniotic fluid embolism—2 cases and a review of maternal deaths from this cause in Australia. *Aust N Z J Obstet Gynaecol* 1988;28:33.
3. Meyer JR. Embolis pulmonar-caseosa. *Brazil-Med* 1926;2:301.
4. Attwood HD. Matthew Baillie—a possible early description of amniotic fluid embolism. *Aust N Z Obstet Gynaecol* 1979;19:176.
5. Steiner PE, Lushbaugh CC. Maternal pulmonary embolism by amniotic fluid as a cause of obstetric shock and unexplained death in obstetrics. *JAMA* 1941;117:1245.
6. Liban E, Raz S. A clinicopathologic study of fourteen cases of amniotic fluid embolism. *Am J Clin Pathol* 1969;51:477.
7. Resnik R, Swartz WH, Plumer MH, et al. Amniotic fluid embolism with survival. *Obstet Gynecol* 1976;47:295.
8. Dolyniuk M, Orfei E, Vania H, et al. Rapid diagnosis of amniotic fluid embolism. *Obstet Gynecol* 1983;61:28S.
9. Agia G, Wyatt L, Re E. Pulmonary microvascular cytology: a new diagnostic application of the pulmonary artery catheter. *Chest* 1986; 90:627.
10. Clark SL, Cotton DB, Gonick B, et al. Central hemodynamic alterations in amniotic fluid embolism. *Am J Obstet Gynecol* 1988;158: 1124.
11. Clark SL, Hankins GDV, Dudley DA, et al. Amniotic fluid embolism: analysis of the national registry. *Am J Obstet Gynecol* 1995;172:1158.
12. Burrows A, Khoo SK. The amniotic fluid embolism syndrome: 10 years' experience at a major teaching hospital. *Aust N Z J Obstet Gynaecol* 1995;35:245.
13. Kaunitz AM, Hughes JM, Grimes DA, et al. Causes of maternal mortality in the United States. *Obstet Gynecol* 1985;65:605.
14. Clark SL. New concepts of amniotic fluid embolism: a review. *Obstet Gynecol Surv* 1990;45:360.
15. Shah K, Karlman R, Heller J. Ventricular tachycardia and hypotension with amniotic fluid embolism during cesarean section. *Anesth Analg* 1986;65:533.
16. Guidotti RJ, Grimes DA, Cates W. Fatal amniotic fluid embolism during legally induced abortion in the United States, 1972—1978. *Am J Obstet Gynecol* 1981;141:257.
17. Dodgson J, Martin J, Boswell J, et al. Probable amniotic fluid embolism precipitated by amniocentesis and treated by exchange transfusion. *Br Med J* 1987;294:1322.
18. Olcott CO, Robinson AJ, Maxwell TM, et al. Amniotic fluid embolism and disseminated intravascular coagulation after blunt maternal trauma. *J Trauma* 1973;13:737.
19. Masson RG, Ruggieri J, Siddiqui MM. Amniotic fluid embolism: definitive diagnosis in a survivor. *Am Rev Respir Dis* 1979;120:187.
20. Meier PR, Bowes WA. Amniotic fluid embolus-like syndrome presenting in the second trimester of pregnancy. *Obstet Gynecol* 1983;61:31S.
21. Maher JE, Wenstrom KD, Hauth JC, et al. Amniotic fluid embolism

after saline amnioinfusion: two cases and review of the literature. *Obstet Gynecol* 1994;83:851.
22. Shnider SM, Moya F. Amniotic fluid embolism. *Anesthesiology* 1961; 22:108.
23. Quance D. Amniotic fluid embolism: detection by pulse oximetry. *Anesthesiology* 1988;68:951.
24. Reeves JT, Daoud FS, Estridge M, et al. Pulmonary pressor effects of small amounts of bovine amniotic fluid. *Respir Physiol* 1974;20:231.
25. Jacques WE, Hampton JW, Bird RM, et al. Pulmonary hypertension and plasma thromboplastin antecedent deficiency in dogs. *Arch Pathol* 1960;69:248.
26. Halmajyi D, Starzecki B, Shearman RP. Experimental amniotic fluid embolism: mechanism and treatment. *Am J Obstet Gynecol* 1962;84: 251.
27. Attwood HD, Downing SE. Experimental amniotic fluid embolism. *Surg Gynecol Obstet* 1965;120:255.
28. Girard P, Mal H, Laine J-F, et al. Left heart failure in amniotic fluid embolism. *Anesthesiology* 1986;64:262.
29. Richards DS, Carter LS, Corke B, et al. The effect of human amniotic fluid on the isolated perfused rat heart. *Am J Obstet Gynecol* 1988;158: 210.
30. Phillips LL, Davidson EC. Procoagulant properties of amniotic fluid. *Am J Obstet Gynecol* 1972;113:911.
31. Lockwood CJ, Bach R, Guha A, et al. Amniotic fluid contains tissue factor, a potent initiator of coagulation. *Am J Obstet Gynecol* 1991;165: 1335.
32. Mainprize TC, Maltby JR. Amniotic fluid embolism: a report of four probable cases. *Can Anaesth Soc J* 1986;33:382.
33. Barrows JJ. A documented case of amniotic fluid embolism presenting as fetal distress. *Am J Obstet Gynecol* 1982;143:599.
34. Vartikar JV, Johnson MD, Datta S. Precordial doppler monitoring and pulse oximetry during cesarean delivery: setection of venous air embolism. *Reg Anesth* 1989;14:145.
35. Clark SL. Arachidonic acid metabolites and the patho-physiology of amniotic fluid embolism. *Semin Reprod Endocrinol* 1985;3:253.
36. Price TM, Baker VV, Cefalo RC. Amniotic fluid embolism: three case reports with a review of the literature. *Obstet Gynecol Surv* 1985;40: 462.
37. Sparr RA, Pritchard JA. Studies to detect the escape of amniotic fluid into the maternal circulation during parturition. *Surg Gynecol Obstet* 1958;107:560.
38. Talbert LM, Adcock DF, Weiss AE, et al. Studies on the pathogenesis of clotting defects during salt-induced abortions. *Am J Obstet Gynecol* 1973;115:656.
39. Roche WD, Norris HJ. Detection and significance of maternal pulmonary amniotic fluid embolism. *Obstet Gynecol* 1974;43:729.
40. Attwood HD, Park WW. Embolism to the lungs by trophoblast. *J Obstet Gynaecol Br Cmnwlth* 1961;68:611.
41. Covone AE, Johnson PM, Mutton D, et al. Trophoblastic cells in peripheral blood from pregnant women. *Lancet* 1984;1:841.
42. Lunetta P, Penttil A. Immunohistochemical identification of syncytiotrophoblastic cells and megakaryocytes in pulmonary vessels in a fatal case of amniotic fluid embolism. *Int J Legal Med* 1996;108: 210.
43. Clark SL, Pavlova Z, Greenspoon J, et al. Squamous cells in the maternal pulmonary circulation. *Am J Obstet Gynecol* 1986;154:104.
44. Kuhlman K, Hidvegi D, Tamura RK, et al. Is amniotic fluid in the central circulation of peripartum patients pathologic? *Am J Perinatol* 1985;2:295.
45. Kanayama N, Yamazaki T, Hiroo N, et al. Determining zinc coproporphyrin in maternal plasma—a new method for diagnosing amniotic fluid embolism. *Clin Chem* 1992;38:526.
46. Reis RL, Pierce WS, Behrendt DM. Hemodynamic effects of amniotic fluid embolism. *Surg Gynecol Obstet* 1965;129:45.
47. Hankins GDV, Snyder RR, Clark SL, et al. Acute hemodynamic and respiratory effects of amniotic fluid embolism in the pregnant goat model. *Am J Obstet Gynecol* 1993;168:1113.
48. Adamson K, Mueller-Heubach E, Myers R. The innocuousness of amniotic fluid infusion in the pregnant rhesus monkey. *Am J Obstet Gynecol* 1971;109:977.
49. Stolte L, Kessel HV, Seelen J, et al. Failure to produce the syndrome of amniotic fluid embolism by infusion of amniotic fluid and meconium into monkeys. *Am J Obstet Gynecol* 1967;98:694.
50. Clark SL, Motz FJ, Phelan JP. Hemodynamic alterations associated with amniotic fluid embolism: a reappraisal. *Am J Obstet Gynecol* 1985;151:617.
51. Ostergard DR. The physiology and clinical importance of amniotic fluid. *Obstet Gynecol Surv* 1970;25:297.
52. Azegami M, Mori N. Amniotic fluid embolism and leukotrienes. *Am J Obstet Gynecol* 1986;155:1119.
53. Karim SM, Delvin J. Prostaglandin content of amniotic fluid during pregnancy and labour. *J Obstet Gynaecol Br Cmnwlth* 1967;74:230.
54. Kitzmiller JL, Lucas WE. Studies on a model of amniotic fluid embolism. *Obstet Gynecol* 1972;39:626.
55. Hankins GD, Berryman GK, Scott RT, et al. Maternal arterial desaturation with 15-methyl prostaglandin F_2 alpha for uterine atony. *Obstet Gynecol* 1988;72:367.
56. Douglas MJ, Farquharson DF, Ross PLE, et al. Cardiovascular collapse following an overdose of prostaglandin F_2 alpha: a case report. *Can J Anaesth* 1989;36:466.
57. Hammerschmidt DE, Ogburn PL, Williams JE. Amniotic fluid activates complement: a role in amniotic fluid embolism syndrome? *J Lab Clin Med* 1984;104:901.
58. Horrow JC. Heparin reversal of protamine toxicity: have we come full circle? *J Cardiothorac Anesth* 1990;4:539.
59. Ogburn PL, Johnson S, Williams PP, et al. Levels of free fatty acids and arachidonic acid in pregnancy and labor. *J Lab Clin Med* 1980;95:943.
60. Keirse MJ, Hicks BR, Mitchell MD, et al. Increase in the prostaglandin precursor, arachidonic acid, in amniotic fluid during spontaneous labor. *Br J Obstet Gynaecol* 1977;84:937.
61. Lee HC, Yamaguich M, Ikenoue T, et al. Amniotic fluid embolism and leukotrienes—the role of amniotic fluid surfactant in leukotriene production. In: Baker EV: *Prostaglandins, leukotrienes and essential fatty acids.* London, United Kingdom: Longman Group Ltd, 1992:117.
62. Courtney LD. Amniotic fluid embolism. *Obstet Gynecol Surv* 1974;29: 169.
63. Dutta D, Bhargava KC, Chakravarti RN, et al. Therapeutic studies in experimental amniotic fluid embolism in rabbits. *Am J Obstet Gynecol* 1970;106:1201.
64. Peterson EP, Taylor HB. Amniotic fluid embolism: an analysis of 40 cases. *Obstet Gynecol* 1970;35:787.
65. Steingrub JS, Lopez T, Teres D, et al. Amniotic fluid embolism associated with castor oil ingestion. *Crit Care Med* 1988;16:642.
66. James FM. An evaluation of vasopressor therapy for maternal hypotension during spinal anesthesia. *Anesthesiology* 1970;33:35.
67. Forester D. Amniotic fluid embolism and emergency cardiac care. *Ann Emerg Med* 1984;13:1172.
68. Sterner S, Campbell B, Davies S. Amniotic fluid embolism. *Ann Emerg Med* 1984;13:343.
69. Oates S, Williams G, Rees GAD. Cardiopulmonary resuscitation in late pregnancy. *Br Med J* 1988;297:404.
70. DelGuercio LR, Feins NR, Cohn JD, et al. Comparison of blood flow during external and internal cardiac massage in man. *Circulation* 1982; 31:1171.
71. Albright GA. Clinical aspects of bupivacaine toxicity. Report to the Anesthetic and Life-Support Drugs Advisory Committee. Rockville: US Department of Health and Human Services, 1983.
72. Rees GAD, Willis BA. Resuscitation in late pregnancy. *Anaesthesia* 1986;43:347.
73. Clark SL. Successful pregnancy outcomes after amniotic fluid embolism. *Am J Obstet Gynecol* 1992;167:511.
74. Eastman NJ. Editorial. *Obstet Gynecol Surv* 1948;3:35.
75. Cron RS, Kilkenny GS, Wirthwein C, et al. Amniotic fluid embolism. *Am J Obstet Gynecol* 1952;64:1360.
76. Clark SL, Phelan JP, Lotton DB, eds. *Critical care obstetrics.* Cambridge, MA.: Blackwell Scientific Publications 1991.

Obstetric Anesthesia, second edition,
edited by Mark C. Norris.
Lippincott Williams & Wilkins, Philadelphia © 1999.

CHAPTER 32

Intraoperative Anesthetic Complications

Barbara L. Leighton

Obstetric anesthesia is remarkably safe, but a number of minor and major complications can and do occur. Some complications, such as hypotension, occur frequently despite our best attempts to prevent them. The incidence and consequences of such complications can be minimized by understanding the relevant pathophysiology and treatment options. Other complications, such as failed intubation, occur only rarely but can be catastrophic. In this setting, careful patient evaluation and planning are necessary preventative measures.

This chapter attempts to describe some common and uncommon obstetric anesthesia complications that are diagnosed and treated intraoperatively. Complications that present or are treated postoperatively are discussed in Chapter 39. I hope the reader will finish this chapter with the answers to the following questions:

- Why is a given event harmful to mother or fetus?
- Why is the parturient at greater risk of a given complication than her nonpregnant counterpart?
- Can the complication be prevented?
- Can the effects of the complication be minimized or eliminated even if the complication occurs?
- How can I best manage the consequences of a complication?

HYPOTENSION

Hypotension is the most common complication of obstetric regional anesthesia. The incidence of hypotension during spinal anesthesia for cesarean section can be decreased by using left uterine displacement, intravenous fluids, and intravenous venoconstrictors (1–3).

B. L. Leighton: Department of Anesthesiology, Allegheny University of the Health Sciences, City Avenue Hospital, Philadelphia, Pennsylvania 19131.

Why Are Obstetric Anesthesiologists so Worried about Hypotension?

Severe hypotension can prove fatal for both mother and fetus; "spinal shock" was once a common cause of maternal mortality (4). Infants delivered after severe hypotension lasting more than 4 minutes may be acidotic and have poor Apgar scores (5,6). Mild hypotension produces few maternal symptoms but is poorly tolerated by the fetus. Uterine blood flow falls in proportion to the decrease in maternal blood pressure (BP) (7). In one study, infants of hypotensive mothers (mean arterial pressure less than 70 mm Hg during epidural anesthesia for cesarean section) had normal Apgar scores but weak rooting and sucking reflexes for 2 days (8).

What Constitutes Treatment-requiring Hypotension in a Parturient?

Maternal and fetal conditions are unaffected if the systolic pressure remains above 100 mm Hg or it falls less than 30% (whichever is greater) (2,5,9). The fetal effects of mild to moderate maternal hypotension depend on the duration of hypotension and maternal hydration. A healthy fetus tolerates hypotension for up to 4 minutes (5,6). Generous maternal intravenous fluid administration blunts the fetal acidosis following maternal hypotension during spinal anesthesia for cesarean section. Fetal umbilical acidemia occurred less frequently if mothers received 1,000 to 1,500 mL intravenously before induction than if they received only 500 to 999 mL (10). In mothers receiving 1,500 to 2,000 mL of balanced salt solution intravenously, the incidence of fetal umbilical acidemia did not differ between the offspring of mildly to moderately hypotensive mothers (systolic BP 70 to 100 mm Hg for 0 to 15 minutes) and normotensive mothers (11).

Why Are Parturients so Susceptible to Hypotension?

Aortocaval Compression

Compression of the inferior vena cava and the aorta by the abdominal contents occurs rarely in nonpregnant patients but almost universally among parturients. The inferior vena cava is an easily collapsed blood vessel that frequently gets caught between a rock (the gravid uterus) and a hard place (the maternal vertebral bodies) (12).

The following increase the incidence and severity of aortocaval compression.

Supine Position

Obstruction of the inferior vena cava produces supine hypotension (a decrease in systolic BP of 30 mm Hg or a systolic BP of 80 mm Hg) in 6% to 11% of term parturients (Fig. 1) (13,14). Aortic compression can occur in 37% of supine term parturients (15).

Hypovolemia

The uterus compresses the vena cava in supine parturients. This compression worsens as the pressure within the vena cava falls.

Spinal or Epidural Anesthesia

Spinal and epidural blockade induce a form of distributive hypovolemia. Hypotension during spinal or epidural anesthesia occurs when the cardiac preload (not the afterload) decreases (16,17). Impedence cardiography during epidural anesthesia for cesarean section

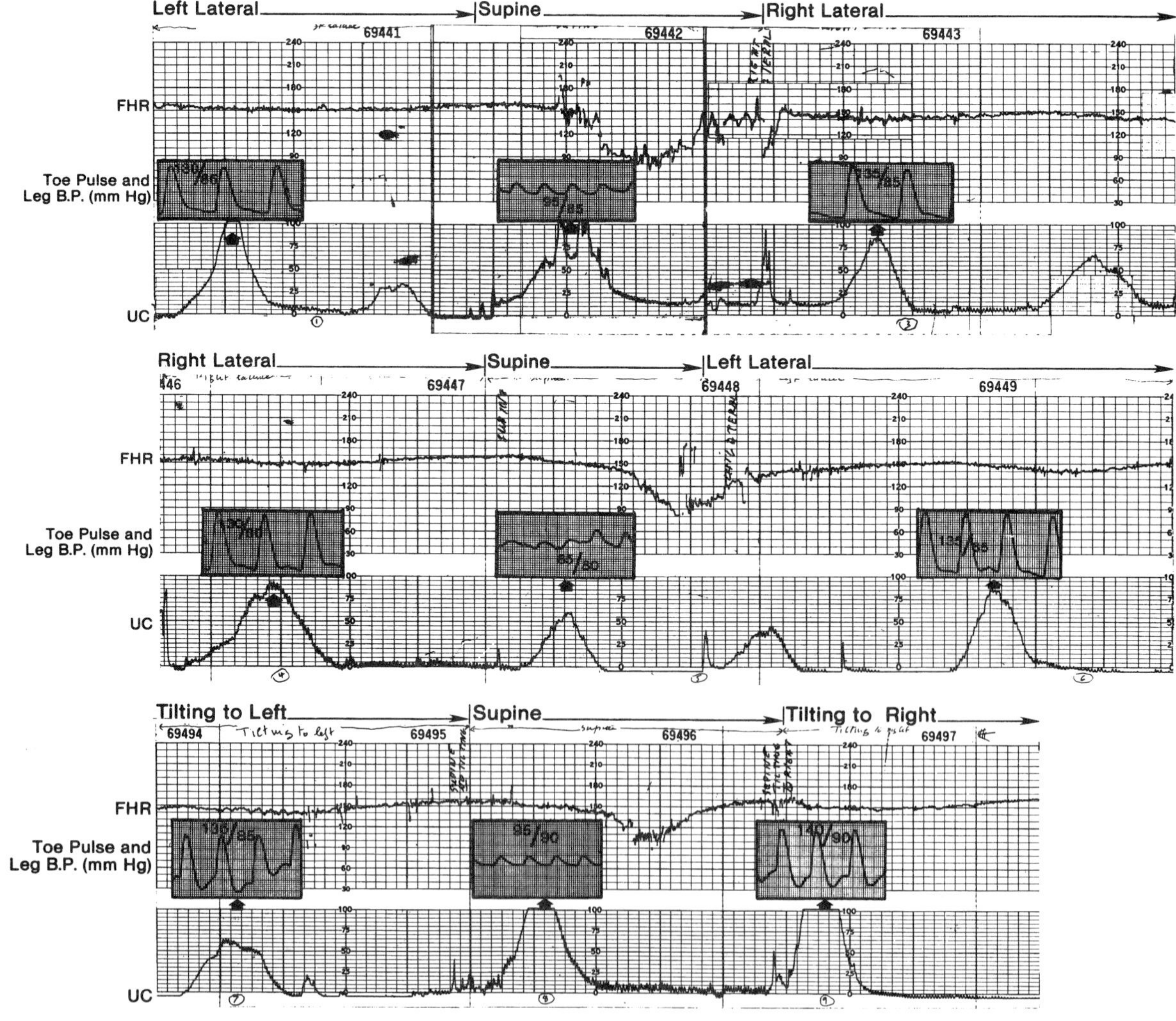

FIG. 1. An example of the effect of aortocaval compression on the fetal heart rate tracing. Several late decelerations and lower limb hypotension are seen only in the supine position. *BP*, blood pressure; *FHR*, fetal heart rate; *UC*, uterine contraction. (Reprinted from Arbitol MM. Supine position in labor and associated fetal heart rate changes. *Obstet Gynecol* 1985;65:481, with permission.)

shows that stroke volume (SV) and end-diastolic volume (EDV) diminish significantly during hypotension, while systemic vascular resistance (SVR) barely changes (Fig. 2). Ephedrine or phenylephrine treatment restores BP, SV, and EDV to baseline values while the SVR decreases further (17). Central venous pressure (CVP) falls in both normotensive and hypotensive parturients during spinal anesthesia and reaches lower values in the hypotensive patients (16).

Uterine Contractions

The uterus compresses the more posteriorly placed vena cava only between contractions (13). Maternal hypotension occurs more frequently during caval obstruction (between contractions). Aortic occlusion occurs almost exclusively during uterine contractions (12,15, 18). Regardless of maternal body position, the uterus squeezes the aorta during contractions in up to 86% of laboring women (12).

Early Labor, the Absence of Labor, or Nonengagement of the Fetal Head

Laboring women have a lower incidence of hypotension than nonlaboring parturients during epidural or spinal anesthesia for cesarean section (3,19). Aortic compression is more frequent if the cervix is dilated less than 5 cm or if the fetal head is not engaged in the pelvis (12,15,20) Occiputoposterior fetal head position also increases the risk of aortic compression (12).

Rapid Development of Sympathetic Nerve Block

Sympathetic nerve block develops more quickly in pregnant than in nonpregnant women during regional anesthesia. Intrinsic homeostatic mechanisms then are less able to compensate for this sympatholysis as it develops (21).

What Is the Best Way to Prevent or Treat Hypotension?

The Anesthesiologist Has Three Weapons in the Fight Against Hypotension:

1. Manipulation of maternal body position to prevent aortocaval compression,
2. Infusion of balanced salt or colloid solution intravenously, and,
3. Administration of a drug to constrict maternal capacitance vessels.

None of these ways is sufficient by itself; a combination must be used.

Left Uterine Displacement

Hypotension following the initiation of modified saddle block anesthesia was completely relieved by left uterine displacement in 93% of the laboring parturients (22). Left uterine displacement decreased the incidence of hypotension from 46% to 15% in hydrated laboring cesarean patients (3).

The full left or right lateral position completely relieves aortocaval compression (Fig. 1) (12). Elevating the mother's right hip 10 to 15 cm improved femoral arterial BP in all women and completely relieved aortocaval compression in 58% of term parturients (20). In some patients, tilting the uterus to the right is more effective than leftward tilt (20). Inserting a wedge under the right hip instead of using a mechanical uterine displacer better preserves femoral (and presumably uterine) arterial pressure (20,23,24).

Intravenous Hydration

Despite a 40% increase in blood volume, parturients appear hypovolemic when facing the twin assaults of a total sympathectomy and compressed abdominal blood vessels. The CVP of healthy parturients increased from 8

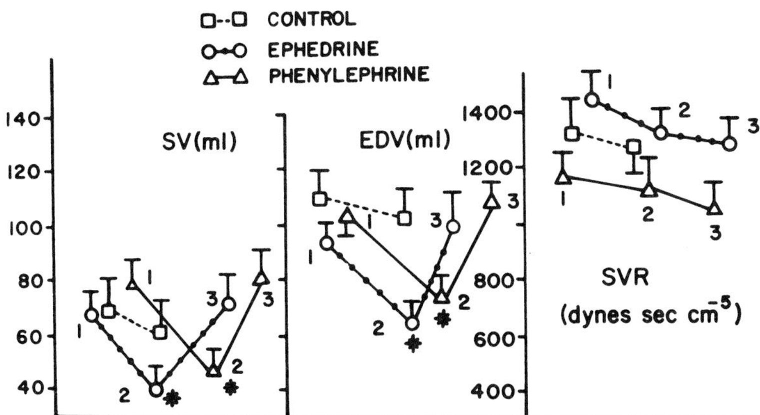

FIG. 2. Stroke volume *(SV)*, end-diastolic volume *(EDV)*, and systemic vascular resistance *(SVR)* at three time points: (1) before anesthesia, (2) during hypotension, and (3) after treatment with ephedrine or phenylephrine. *, significantly different from time points 1 and 3. Measurements in the control group were obtained before anesthesia and at the T_6 sensory level. (Reprinted from ref. 17, with permission.)

to 10 cm H_2O after rapid intravenous infusion of 1 L of D_5 Ringer's lactate with no evidence of heart failure (16). The CVP of both hydrated and nonhydrated patients fell 4 cm H_2O after induction of high spinal anesthesia. Only the nonhydrated women became hypotensive. After delivery, both groups of women had similar CVP and BP (16). One liter of the hypertonic fluid (D_5 Ringer's lactate) prevents hypotension efficiently; however, this amount of dextrose should not be infused rapidly, as it leads to neonatal hypoglycemia (3,16,25,26). One liter of balanced salt solution without dextrose before high spinal or epidural anesthesia fails to reliably prevent hypotension (19).

Rapid intravenous infusion of 2 L of balanced salt solution immediately before induction of high spinal or epidural anesthesia has been the recommended way to avoid hypotension in parturients. Early studies reported that infusion of 2 L of dextrose-free balanced salt solution produced excellent conditions in the mother (7% hypotension incidence, all CVPs less than 12 cm H_2O) and the infant (low incidence of acidosis) (11,27). Recent studies dispute that conclusion. Rout et al. (28) administered no preload or 20 mL/kg of balanced salt solution to patients presenting for elective cesarean delivery. Although the incidence of hypotension was lower in the hydrated group (55% vs 71%), hypotension was still common. The severity, timing, and duration of hypotension, ephedrine dose, and neonatal condition did not differ between the groups. Park et al. (29) found that increasing the amount of crystalloid preload from 10 to 30 mL/kg did not change maternal hemodynamics but did lower maternal colloid osmotic pressure.

Six percent hetastarch with crystalloid may be a better way to prevent hypotension than crystalloid alone. Riley et al. (30) found hypotension in 45% of patients preloaded with 500 mL of hetastarch plus 1 L of lactated Ringer's versus 85% of patients preloaded with 2 L lactated Ringer's solution (30). Similar results have been reported in postpartum tubal ligation patients (31). In pregnant normotensive sheep, hetastarch increased uterine blood flow, cardiac output, and uterine artery oxygen delivery, whereas crystalloid did not change these variables (32). Further study is needed to determine if the benefits of hetastarch sufficiently outweigh the problems (increased cost, allergic and coagulopathic risks) to justify its routine use during cesarean delivery.

So, what fluid, and how much of it, should one infuse into cesarean delivery patients before instituting spinal or epidural anesthesia? It is hard to derive a firm recommendation from the literature. The reported incidence of hypotension in patients preloaded with 2 L of balanced salt solution varies from 7% to 85% (27,30). My current practice is to infuse about 20 mL/kg (1.5 L) of balanced salt solution before inducing spinal or epidural anesthesia for cesarean delivery. Smaller amounts of intravenous fluid are needed if one is topping up an existing labor epidural.

Pressors

Pressors are double-edged swords. Administration of a small amount of a venoconstrictor to a hydrated, laterally tilted parturient can restore cardiac preload without affecting uterine blood flow (5,17). On the other hand, large doses of potent arterial constrictors decrease uterine blood flow (especially in the poorly hydrated) and further the fetal insult (5,33). The drug dose, drug venous/arterial selectivity, and patient hydration status determine whether the pressor will improve or worsen the intrauterine environment.

Ephedrine

Ephedrine remains the pressor of choice in most obstetric situations. No other agent surpasses its performance in clinical or animal studies. In hydrated parturients during cesarean section, prompt treatment of hypotension with intravenous ephedrine rapidly restores maternal BP and cardiac output. Timely therapy also ensures excellent neonatal outcome (1,3,17). Ephedrine also elevates maternal heart rate and cardiac inotropy (34). Ephedrine returned uterine blood flow to 90% of baseline during spinal anesthesia-induced hypotension in gravid ewes (5). Ephedrine did not decrease uterine blood flow in unanesthetized ewes despite producing a 50% increase in maternal BP (29). Ephedrine is the vasopressor of choice for epidural-induced hypotension in parturients receiving ritodrine (35). Ephedrine crosses the placenta, increases fetal heart rate and beat-to-beat variability, and transiently affects the neonatal electroencephalogram (36–38).

Ephedrine 5 to 10 mg intravenously, as soon as the maternal BP starts to drop, or prophylactic intravenous ephedrine infusion following spinal injection, has been reported to prevent maternal hypotension, nausea and vomiting, and neonatal acidosis, although this conclusion has been challenged recently (1,8,39). Although prophylactic intramuscular ephedrine worked well in one case series, other authors have reported a high incidence of both hypotension and excessive hypertension with this regimen (2,40,41).

Occasionally I find that ephedrine fails. Despite more than 2 L of prehydration and left lateral tilt, 50 mg or more of ephedrine increases maternal heart rate but not maternal BP. Ephedrine, a mixed α- and β-adrenergic agonist, occasionally shows predominately β-adrenergic effects. Switching to phenylephrine, an α_1 agonist, usually corrects the hypotension quickly.

Phenylephrine

In well-hydrated, laterally tilted parturients, phenylephrine 20 to 100 μg and ephedrine 5 to 10 mg are equally effective. Both restore maternal BP and cardiac preload

(Fig. 2) while ensuring good neonatal acid–base status, Apgar scores, and neurobehavioral scores (17,42,43).

Leg Wrapping

Wrapping both legs with elastic Esmarch bandages after induction of spinal anesthesia prevented hypotension in hydrated, tilted parturients at cesarean section (44). Inflatable boots and splints are ineffective (45,46).

All effective hypotension prevention and treatment regimes have the same goal: maintenance of an adequate maternal cardiac preload. Position parturients receiving regional anesthesia properly to avoid aortocaval compression. Infuse an adequate intravenous fluid preload of balanced salt solution. Give prophylactic venopressors if desired. Always be prepared to treat BP decreases with an appropriate intravenous pressor.

MALPOSITIONED EPIDURAL NEEDLES AND CATHETERS

Not all needles and catheters end up in the epidural space. Malpositioned devices should be identified and removed. In theory, an epidural anesthesia "test dose" should detect all intravenously or intrathecally located catheters. Ideally, after a negative "test dose," one could safely administer large bolus doses of epidural local anesthetic. For single-holed epidural catheters, an ideal test dose theoretically is possible but does not exist. For multiholed catheters, long used in the rest of the world and now suddenly popular in the United States, neither intrathecal nor intravenous location can be eliminated conclusively.

Mulitholed Epidural Catheters: Every Dose MUST Be a "Test Dose"!

Multiholed epidural catheters are popular because the incidence of missed segments and unilateral blocks is lower compared to single-holed catheters (47–49); however, this improved analgesia comes at a price. The epidural location of the catheter cannot be verified unless one injects contrast and radiologically determines the position of all catheter ports. The testing schemes devised for single-holed catheters will not diagnose all malpositioned multiholed catheters, for one never knows through which port(s) the "test dose" exited.

Multiholed catheters can be placed with holes in more than one compartment [i.e., the epidural space, plus either the intravenous, subarachnoid, or subdural space(s)] (50). Beck et al. (50) radiologically verified the catheter position in 113 patients who had received epidural anesthesia for lower-extremity surgery. Thirteen (12%) of the catheters were epidurovascular; of these, six patients had no signs or symptoms of intravascular catheter placement (Table 1). One of the patients with an epidurovascular catheter received, at separate times, epinephrine 10 μg via a peripheral intravenous line and the epidural catheter. The peripheral venous injection produced tachycardia and hypertension; the catheter injection did not. Three of the epidurovascular catheters provided surgical anesthesia. One of the 113 patients had an epidurosubarachnoid catheter through which cerebrospinal fluid (CSF) could not be aspirated before or after a 2-mL test dose produced T_6 sensory blockade. There are at least six additional radiologically verified two-compartment multiholed catheters reported in the literature (51–54).

TABLE 1. *Results of clinical testing of radiologically proven epidurovascular catheters*

Test	Catheter provided sufficient epidural anesthesia for surgery	Catheter did not provide sufficient anesthesia for surgery	Total
Blood aspiration	0	4	4
Toxic symptoms	1	2	3
No signs or symptoms	2	4	6
Total	3	10	13

The port through which injectate exits a multiholed catheter is determined by the fluid injection speed, the diameters of the catheter ports, the pressure outside each port, the number of ports, and catheter kinks. Slowly injected fluid exits only through the most proximal hole, whereas a rapid injection exits from all ports (55,56). For example, when 20-gauge catheters from two manufacturers were horizontally suspended in air, saline, injected at 0.06 mL/s, flowed through the proximal two holes but dribbled out the terminal hole. An injection speed of 0.2 to 0.7 mL/s produced equal jetting through all three ports. Required injection speeds are higher with air than with saline. If a catheter is positioned with the terminal port under 20 cm H_20 pressure and the two proximal ports in air, air must be injected at 4 mL/s to see bubbling via the terminal hole. Catheter manufacturing defects may add to the testing difficulties. Allegedly three-port catheters may have 0, 1, or 2 ports, and the ports may differ in diameter (56).

The clinical consequences of changing the epidural drug injection rate are illustrated in a case reported by Ward et al. (51). The initial dose and first reinjection through an aspiration-negative multiholed catheter produced appropriate levels of epidural anesthesia. A catheter kink was identified and straightened before the second reinjection, which was administered rapidly. The patient developed a total spinal block within 1 minute. The epidurosubarachnoid catheter position subsequently was identified radiologically.

Can one safely use multiport epidural catheters? Yes, but only if one never injects a bolus of local anesthetic large enough to be catastrophic if the dose is delivered intrathecally, subdurally, or intravenously. With single-holed catheters, every dose *should* be a test dose; with multiholed catheters, every dose *must* be a test dose.

UNINTENDED DURAL PUNCTURE

Diagnosis

The gold standard for clinical diagnosis of intrathecal needle or catheter position is the development of spinal anesthesia after the injection of an appropriate amount of local anesthetic. In parturients, spinal anesthesia is diagnosed by the onset of sensory anesthesia at 2 to 3 minutes and motor nerve block at 3 to 5 minutes after injection of one of the following: lidocaine 30 to 45 mg, bupivacaine 5 to 15 mg, or 2-chloroprocaine 40 to 100 mg (57–59).

Recognizing a dural puncture is simple if clear fluid flows in a continuous stream from the epidural needle or catheter. Occasionally, one can aspirate a small (0.2 to 2 mL) amount of clear fluid after injecting saline or local anesthetic. On which side of the dura did the fluid originate?

A urine dipstrip is a convenient, but not infallible, testing method (60,61). The most reliable assay is the pH (local anesthetic is pH 5, CSF is pH 7) (Table 2). CSF itself is only weakly positive for glucose. Local anesthetic tests false-positive for protein. Small amounts of fluid aspirated from epidural catheters before reinjection may have a physiologic pH and test positive for glucose despite the absence of a dural puncture (62).

Initial Management

Puncture of the dura occurs in 1% to 2.5% of attempted obstetric lumbar epidural anesthetics (63,64). Usually the dura is punctured with the needle, and CSF is visible in the needle hub. Four courses of action then are possible:

Pull the Needle Out and Insert an Epidural Catheter at Another Interspace

This choice introduces the risk of puncturing the dura a second time (65) but permits administration of a prophylactic epidural blood patch if desired (66). The incidence of unintended subdural or intrathecal cannulation is higher than if the previous dural puncture had not occurred, so epidural drug must be injected slowly and the patient tested frequently for signs of spinal anesthesia (67).

TABLE 2. *Urine test strip properties of fluids that might be aspirated from the epidural space*

Fluid	pH	Glucose	Protein
Cerebrospinal fluid	7	0–1+	Trace–1+
Saline	5	0	0
Local anesthetic	5	0	2+–4+
Epidural aspirate, no dural puncture	7	0–2+	Trace

Convert to a Single-shot Spinal Anesthetic

The tip of the epidural needle may be only partially subarachnoid. Therefore, one should insert a longer spinal needle through the epidural needle and inject through the spinal needle. Even if CSF is flowing freely, injecting bupivacaine 15 mg through the epidural needle may produce a two-dermatome epidural block (I have done it!).

Thread a Catheter and Manage as a Continuous Catheter Spinal Anesthetic

The Food and Drug Administration (FDA) has recalled spinal catheters smaller than 25 gauge, but larger catheters may be used. If one follows this course, use only isobaric drug through the spinal catheter. (Hyperbaric drug may pool and increase the risk of nerve damage.) Remember, even if CSF can be aspirated, the catheter may be subdurally or epidurally located; handle with care. In parturients, the prolonged presence of a spinal catheter does not decrease the incidence of postdural puncture headache.

Pull the Needle Back until CSF no Longer Drips and Thread a Catheter into the "Epidural Space"

Kalas and Hehre (63) attempted this maneuver in 11 patients. Eight patients had successful epidural blocks, two patients had spinal anesthetics, and no block developed in one patient.

Occasionally, the dura appears to have been punctured by the catheter: no fluid is seen in the epidural needle, but CSF is aspirated freely through the catheter. In this situation, leave the catheter in situ and initiate spinal catheter anesthesia, or remove the catheter entirely and replace it. I do not recommend withdrawing the catheter until CSF can no longer be aspirated, especially with multiport catheters.

Management of Epidural Catheters Placed after Dural Puncture

The presence of a fresh dural puncture raises the following management issues:

Should One Decrease the Epidural Dose of Local Anesthetic?

Yes, somewhat. Cases of high or total spinal anesthesia after epidural injection into an interspace adjacent to a dural puncture have been reported (68,69). Dural puncture increases drug passage across the meninges in sheep and monkeys, with the magnitude of the increased drug passage proportional to the size of the dural hole (70,71). In parturients, prior dural puncture with a 24- to 27-gauge spinal needle slightly increases the dermatomal spread of epidurally injected bupivacaine (72,73). Although the magnitude has not been determined, one would expect even greater spread of epidural local anesthetic following dural puncture with an epidural needle.

Can One Safely Administer 2-chloroprocaine?

2-Chloroprocaine has been reformulated without preservatives to minimize the problem of neurotoxicity after subarachnoid injection.[1]

Should One Administer a Prophylactic Epidural Blood Patch Through the Catheter at the End of the Anesthetic?

Early attempts at prophylactic epidural blood patch were unsuccessful, and the technique fell into disrepute. Loeser et al. (74) reported a 71% failure rate among epidural blood patches with 10-mL autologous blood performed within 24 hours of the dural puncture. The recent push to discharge all parturients from the hospital quickly has led several investigators to reexamine the practice using larger volumes of blood. Following unintended dural puncture with an 18-gauge epidural needle, 16 patients in two series received 15 to 20 mL of freshly drawn autologous blood through an epidural catheter placed at an adjacent interspace (75,76). Only one patient developed any headache, which did not require further treatment. The one randomized trial performed to date reports a definite but more realistic clinical effect. Thirty-nine patients with unintended 18-gauge dural punctures were randomized to receive an epidural injection of 15-mL autologous blood or no injection following delivery. Prophylactic epidural blood patch decreased the headache incidence from 80% to 35% ($p < 0.005$). The decrease in the need for theraputic blood patch (seven vs three patients) did not reach statistical significance.

If one decides to perform a prophylactic epidural blood patch, one should wait until the local anesthetic blockade has receded before injecting the blood. In one case, injection of 15 mL of blood through an epidural catheter when the sensory level was T_4 produced a block that was either a total subdural or a total spinal but was certainly a total clinical problem (77).

Many anesthesiologists are concerned about the possibility of causing meningitis or an epidural abscess by injecting blood through an epidural catheter that has been used intermittently for a number of hours. No such cases have been reported; however, this technique has only recently become popular.

Does a Dural Puncture Decrease the Incidence of Successful Epidural Block in a Subsequent Pregnancy?

In one review of 46 patients, dural puncture in a previous pregnancy lowered the incidence of successful epidural analgesia from 89%–92% to 59%–65% (78). Previous epidural blood patch did not affect the success rate. A second review of 47 patients found that previous dural puncture did not decrease the success of labor epidural analgesia but was associated with a greater risk of repeat dural puncture (79).

SUBDURAL ANESTHESIA

Unintended subdural, epiarachnoid anesthesia, a complication first reported by de Saram (80) and reviewed by Dawkins (64), Lubenow (81), and Reynolds and Speedy (82), is clinically recognized during 0.1% to 0.8% of attempted epidural anesthetics. The true incidence may be much higher. Mehta and Salmon (83) radiographically demonstrated partial subdural Tuohy needle position in seven of 100 attempted epidural anesthetics. Subdural injection occurs more frequently during attempted subarachnoid needle placement; subdural injection complicates 10% to 13% of attempted myelograms (84). In fact, subdural injection may be a more important cause of failed spinal anesthesia than is generally realized, for general anesthesia may be induced before the signs of subdural anesthesia appear.

The clinical picture can be confusing, for the characteristics of a subdural anesthetic are not halfway between those of spinal and epidural anesthetics. The chief clinical features of subdural anesthesia following injection of 2 to 10 mL of local anesthetic are (80):

- *Delayed anesthetic onset.*
  Most authors report a lag of 5 to 45 minutes between local anesthetic injection and the first signs of sensory block.
- *Extensive sensory block, frequently extending to cervical levels.*
  Although the sensory block is extensive, it frequently is patchy or asymmetric and may be one-sided (85,86).
- *Loss of consciousness accompanying high sensory blocks.*
  Unlike the epidural space, the subdural space does extend intracranially (87).
- *Hypotension.*
  Maternal BP requires treatment but the severity of hypotension is less than that accompanying total spinal anesthesia.

[1]Editor's note: Although preservative-free 2-chloroprocaine is available (Nesacaine-MPF), other manufacturers still sell 2-chloroprocaine containing metabisulfite for epidural use.

- *Variable motor block.*
- *Respiratory depression.*
  Respiration is usually compromised, although total apnea is uncommon.
- *Prolonged time to complete clinical recovery.*
  Most patients recover fully in 2 to 6 hours, but an 11-hour recovery has been reported (88).

Subdural anesthesia is rarely reported following injection of larger volumes of local anesthetic. Prehaps the fluid pressure from larger-volume injections ruptures the arachnoid membrane and produces a total spinal anesthetic.

Risk Factors

Factors that increase the risk of subdural anesthesia include:

- Previous back surgery (81),
- Immediately preceding dural puncture at the same or adjacent interspace (89–91), and
- Rotating the Tuohy needle 180 degrees (with gentle needle advancement) following identification of the epidural space (92).

A word must be said here in defense of the practice of rotating the epidural 90 degrees with gentle needle retraction. This technique permits one to identify the epidural space with the epidural needle bevel oriented parallel to the longitudinal dural fibers. In the event of a dural puncture, parallel needle bevel orientation decreases the headache incidence from 80% to 52% and the epidural blood patch rate from 50% to 19% (93). Following rotation, the catheter then can be threaded in the mid-line. My department has used this technique in the performance of approximately 4,000 obstetric epidural blocks with no increase in the dural puncture or subdural catheterization rates (93).

Management

The initial subdural injection usually provides a more extensive block than is desired clinically. Provide hemodynamic and respiratory support as needed. Although few authors report a second, deliberate subdural injection, the nature of a subdural block (extensive sensory analgesia with little motor or sympathetic nerve block) makes it appropriate for labor. I consider trying to continue to use the catheter. The arachnoid membrane can be punctured easily, so before any injection attempt slow, careful aspiration of the catheter with a 1- or 3-mL syringe. Then inject a small volume of dilute local anesthetic (such as 1 to 3 mL of 0.5% lidocaine) and carefully monitor the patient for at least 45 minutes. Of course, most anesthesiologists, once burned, opt to replace the subdural with an epidural catheter at a different (usually more rostral) interspace.

HIGH/TOTAL SPINAL OR SUBDURAL ANESTHESIA

Excessively extensive spinal anesthesia is seen most frequently in the following clinical circumstances:

- Unrecognized dural puncture by the epidural needle or catheter.
  Dawkins (64) reports that this event complicates 0.2% of epidural anesthetics. Treat every bolus of epidural local anesthetic as a subarachnoid test dose.
- Spinal anesthesia for cesarean section initiated immediately following institution of a patchy epidural anesthetic.
  There is at least one such case reported in the literature (94), and I am aware of several unreported cases from my institution. In this circumstance, I decrease the amount of subarachnoid bupivacaine from 15 mg to 8 to 10 mg (see Chapter 22).
- Attempted spinal or epidural anesthesia following accidental dural puncture.
  This may be either a spinal or a subdural anesthetic (see previous).
- Unexpectedly high block during a primary spinal anesthetic for cesarean section (95).
- High spinal block following administration of the initial local anesthetic "test dose."

Spinal anesthesia requiring intubation and ventilation has occurred after injection of a mere 50 mg of 2-chloroprocaine (96) and 15 mg of bupivacaine (97).

Management

If the patient develops extensive sensory and motor block, profound hypotension, apnea, and loss of consciousness, do the following (quickly!):

- Turn the patient supine with left uterine displacement.
- Ventilate with 100% oxygen via mask with cricoid pressure until intubation can be accomplished safely. Do not attempt to intubate unless appropriate supplies and a competent assistant are in the room and the patient is well oxygenated (if possible). Inject succinylcholine 1 mg/kg intravenously to optimize visualization, preceded by a small dose of thiopental if the BP permits. I advocate ventilation before intubation because the long-term consequences of hypoxia to the mother and the fetus usually are worse than the morbidity from aspiration. Once an airway is established, continue ventilation until the patient regains consciousness and can maintain a five second head lift or good hand grip.
- Administer fluids and pressors vigorously to maintain an adequate BP. The hypotension seen in this situation can be profound and difficult to treat.

Proper management of cervical (but not cerebral) levels of spinal blockade is not so obvious. At what point is a spinal too high? Most patients who appear anxious, complain vigorously of shortness of breath, and have a weaker than normal hand grip need only reassurance. I recommend induction of general anesthesia and endotracheal intubation:

- When the patient is unable to maintain oxygen saturation greater than 95% despite breathing 100% oxygen via face mask.
- When the patient can whisper but can no longer phonate. I am concerned here about the patient's ability to prevent aspiration. I recommend applying cricoid pressure, administering 1 to 3 mg/kg thiopental (based on BP), and 1.5 mg/kg succinylcholine, ventilating with 100% oxygen until the patient is well oxygenated (if necessary), intubating, and finishing the case as a general anesthetic.

UNINTENDED INTRAVENOUS PLACEMENT OF EPIDURAL NEEDLE OR CATHETER

Placing a needle or catheter into an epidural vein instead of the epidural space is all too easy to do in term-pregnant patients. During attempts to identify the epidural space, veins are cannulated in 5% to 15% of parturients versus 2.8% of nonpregnant patients (64,99,100).

Can One Lower the Incidence of Epidural Venous Cannulation?

Injecting 10 mL of saline or dilute local anesthetic before threading the epidural catheter halves the incidence of venous cannulation. Injection of 3 mL of fluid does not affect the incidence of blood vessel puncture (101).

Can One Detect All Catheters Located in Epidural Veins?

Well, no. Aspiration and careful, fractionated drug administration should always be practiced. If electing a "test dose," use one of the following. The type of epidural catheter used—single holed or multiholed—can alter the efficacy of the following "test doses." (Note the previous section on the testing of multiorifice catheters.)

Doppler Method

Precordial Doppler monitoring during injection of 1 to 2 mL of air through the epidural catheter detects most intravenously located epidural catheters (99,102,103). Because this method is independent of changes in maternal heart rate or chronotropic responsiveness, it is more appropriate than epinephrine for use in laboring women. In 313 patients with single-holed catheters, aspiration for blood or the Doppler test identified all 21 of the intravenously placed catheters, with six false-positive identifications (99). In 300 patients with multiport catheters, 11 intravenous catheters were identified: 8 by both aspiration and Doppler test, 2 only by aspiration, and 1 only by Doppler test (102).

The Doppler test is simple to perform. Insert an epidural catheter and administer a small dose of local anesthetic to test for unintended intrathecal catheter placement. Place the Doppler probe (an external fetal heart rate monitor works well) slightly to the right of the lower maternal sternum and maneuver it until clear maternal heart sounds are heard (Fig. 3). Inject air 1 to 2 mL through the epidural catheter and listen for 15 seconds for maternal heart sound changes. If the epidural catheter is in a vein, valvular maternal heart sounds ("lub-dub") become indistinct and you will hear a loud irregular swishing sound.

The Doppler test has been used at the author's institution in more than 10,000 patients with no reported complications. Intravenous entrainment of air occurs so frequently and with such rare sequelae that Doppler test safety problems are unlikely. Epidural injection of 10 mL of air during the air loss-of-resistance technique for identifying the epidural space (which has been used in millions of parturients) produces Doppler-detectable intracardiac air 43% of the time (104). Unlike the air emboli that occur in 10% to 65% of cesarean section patients, the Doppler test involves a small, known amount of air (105–107). By capitalizing on the diagnostic potential of a common clinical occurrence, the Doppler test avoids exposing the mother and fetus to the risks of intravenous local anesthetic or epinephrine.

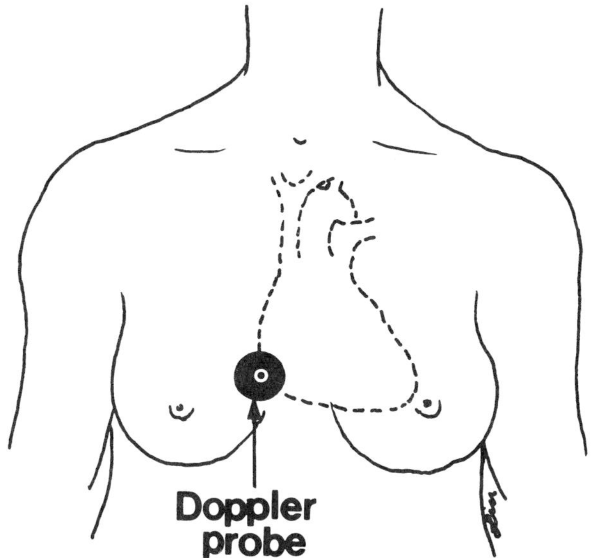

FIG. 3. Correct probe position on the maternal chest during performance of the Doppler test to detect unintended intravascular epidural catheter location.

Epinephrine 15 µg

Epinephrine 15 µg combined with local anesthetic is the most frequently used epidural anesthesia test dose. Epinephrine is not an effective way to detect intravenous cannulation in laboring parturients, for the following reasons (108):

- Healthy pregnant women are relatively insensitive to chronotropic agents. Increasing the heart rate 25 beats/min requires five times as much isoproterenol in healthy pregnant women as in nonpregnant women or mildly preeclamptic patients (109,110).
- Epinephrine, a mixed α- and β-adrenergic agonist, does not consistently produce maternal tachycardia. The mean maternal heart rate effect of epinephrine 15 µm given intravenously is tachycardia for 80 seconds followed by mild bradycardia lasting at least 3 minutes. However, some laboring women never become tachycardic (Fig. 4).
- Cyclical maternal heart rate changes occur in unanesthetized laboring women. In 12% to 45% of actively laboring women, maternal heart rate increases more than 30 beats/min with each painful uterine contraction (Fig. 5) (108,111). Maternal heart rate is more stable in nonlaboring parturients. Epinephrine seems to be a more reliable indicator in intravenous catheter location before elective cesarean section (111).

If using an epinephrine "test dose," monitor maternal pulse with a device that provides an accurate digital display of the instantaneous maternal heart rate. A finger on an artery does not suffice (109). In nonlaboring patients with a stable baseline maternal heart rate, monitor heart rate for at least 1 minute before and after injecting the epinephrine. A 25 beat/min maternal heart rate increase lasting at least 15 seconds indicates that the catheter is located in a vein. In actively laboring women, monitor maternal heart rate through at least one contraction (generally 2 to 3 minutes) to establish a baseline. A 10 beat/min increase in the peak maternal heart rate during a contraction indicates intravenous catheter location (Fig. 5). A maternal heart rate increase of 25 beats/min lasting at least 15 seconds, not occurring during a uterine contraction, also indicates an intravenous location.

Isoproterenol 5 µg

Unlike epinephrine, isoproterenol is a pure β-adrenergic agonist. In healthy term parturients, intravenous iso-

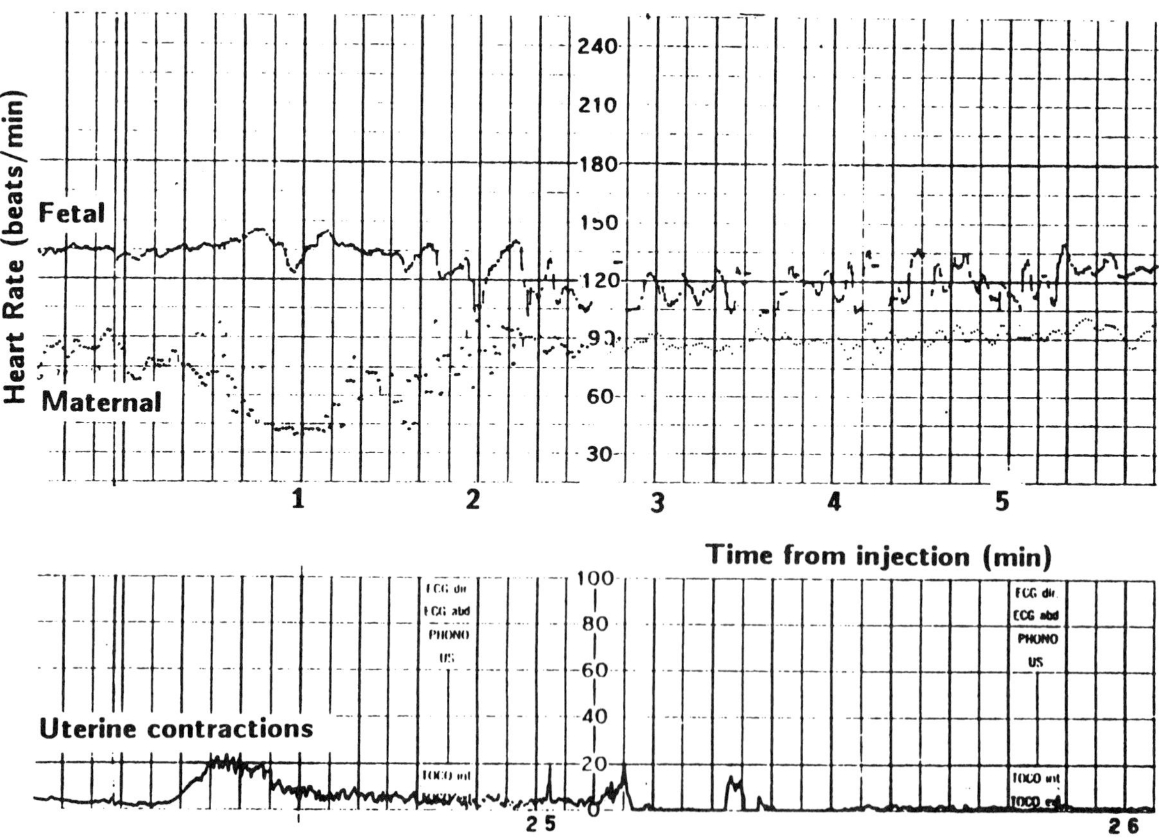

FIG. 4. Tracing of fetal heart rate **(top)**, maternal heart rate **(middle)**, and uterine contractions following maternal injection of epinephrine, 15 µg IV, at time 0. Note the maternal bradycardia at 1 minute; maternal mean arterial pressure at the time was 152 mm Hg.

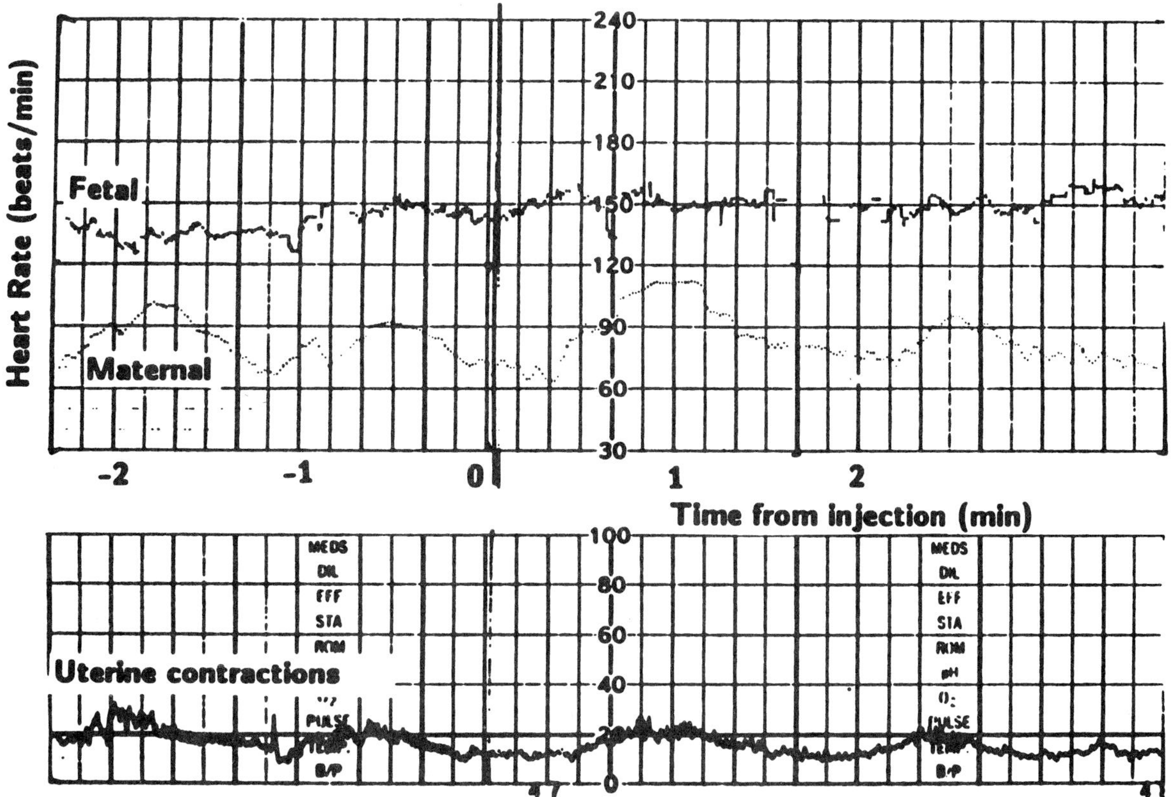

FIG. 5. Tracing of fetal heart rate **(top)**, maternal heart rate **(middle)**, and uterine contractions following matenal injection of epinephrine, 15 µm IV, at time 0. Note the marked contraction-induced variation in maternal heart rate. Maternal heart rate increases 20 to 30 beats/min with most uterine contractions and increases 40 beats/min after the epinephrine injection. (From Leighton BL. New advances in obstetric anesthesia. In: Barash PG, ed. *Refresher courses in anesthesiology,* vol 19. Philadelphia: JB Lippincott, 1991:59, with permission.)

proterenol 5 µg produces an easily detectable tachycardia without hypotension or subsequent bradycardia (109, 112). Isoproterenol also is a better indicator of intravenous injection in isoflurane-anesthetized adults and halothane-anesthetized children (113,114). Although neurotoxicity testing is not complete, two groups report no neurotoxic effects of epidural or intrathecal isoproterenol in sheep (115–117). Appropriate doses of isoproterenol have minimal hemodynamic effects in gravid ewes and guinea pigs (118,119).

When compared to epinephrine 12.5 µg, isoproterenol 5 µg hastens the onset but shortens the duration of epidural bupivacaine/sufentanil labor analgesia (120).

Which Testing Method Should Be Used?

With uniport epidural catheters, the Doppler air method by far has the best sensitivity and specificity of the three testing methods. Air must be injected quite briskly through multiport catheters (2 to 4 mL/s) to engage all holes; nonetheless, in clinical trial the Doppler method had a sensitivity of 82% and specificity of 100% (102).

Neither epinephrine nor isoproterenol "test doses" should be used in patients who are severely preeclamptic or receiving β-adrenergic tocolytic agents. Epinephrine may produce bradycardia and hypertension, whereas isoproterenol can produce marked tachycardia and hypotension.

With multiport catheters, negative test results do not rule out intrathecal, intravenous, or subdural catheter location.

I now use multiport epidural catheters routinely. To minimize the risk of catheter malposition, I inject at least 10 mL of saline or dilute local anesthetic through the epidural needle before threading the catheter. I regard all epidural catheters as potentially partially malpositioned, so I fractionate my dose and seek signs of spinal or intravenous injection with every catheter reinjection.

What Should One Do with the Catheter after Determining That it Is in a Vein?

In most cases, remove the catheter and replace it at another interspace. If you have placed a labor epidural only after great difficulty, you may attempt to rescue it by withdrawing the catheter slightly. Use it only if a repeat Doppler test is negative. Then inject lidocaine 1% (not bupivacaine) 5 to 8 mL. Watch carefully for symptoms of intravenous local anesthetic injection. The amount of local anesthetic needed for cesarean section is so large that I would abandon an intravenously located catheter and proceed to a spinal or repeat epidural anesthetic.

BUPIVACAINE: A POTENT CARDIOELECTROPHYSIOLOGIC POISON

Bupivacaine is the most popular and also the most arrhythmogenic local anesthetic currently used in parturients. Epidural injection of dilute bupivacaine provides sensory analgesia with minimal motor block, a valuable attribute during labor. Epidural bupivacaine also is used widely for cesarean section anesthesia. Initial animal studies did not suggest that bupivacaine was particularly arrhythmogenic (121,122). However, a rash of maternal deaths following unintended intravenous bupivacaine injection in cesarean section patients led the FDA to ban the epidural injection of 0.75% bupivacaine in parturients in the United States (123–125).

Pathophysiology

Bupivacaine causes arrhythmias because it dissociates from myocardial sodium channels much more slowly than it binds to them, particularly at physiologic maternal heart rates (126,127). The bupivacaine:lidocaine dose ratio for clinical effect, seizure induction, and myocardial depression is 4:1. However, bupivacaine is 16 times as potent as lidocaine in inducing cardiac arrhythmias (128). Bupivacaine blocks fast sodium channels (104), slow calcium channels (129), and potassium channels (130). Although both lidocaine and bupivacaine enter myocardial sodium channels quickly during the action potential, lidocaine is much less toxic because it dissociates ten times more quickly during diastole (time constants: 154 vs 1,557 ms) (130). Bupivacaine accumulates in myocardial sodium channels at heart rates of 60 to 150 beats/min (Fig. 6) (125). Bupivacaine impairs impulse conduction at all levels of the myocardial conduction system but does not affect sinus node automaticity. In addition to the direct effect of bupivacaine on cardiac conduction tissue, intracerebral bupivacaine produces ventricular arrhythmias and hypertension by increasing autonomic nervous system outflow from the brainstem (132,133).

Arrhythmias

There is no one pathognomonic cardiac rhythm disturbance after intravenous bupivacaine injection. The following electrocardiographic changes frequently are reported:

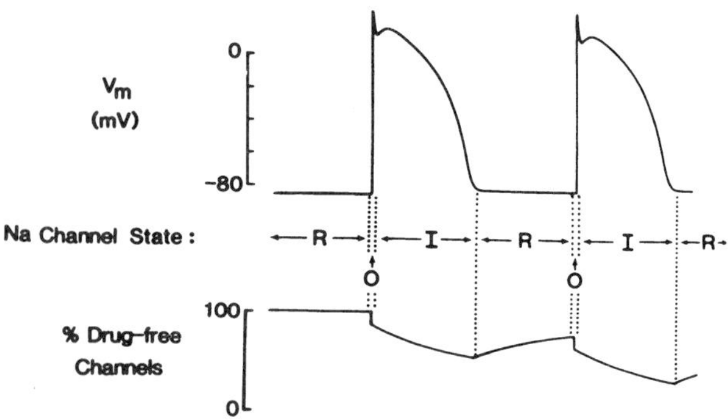

FIG. 6. Schematic diagram showing local anesthetic block of cardiac sodium (Na) channels. The drug binds to sodium channels in open (O) and inactivated (I) states (i.e., during the action potential [V_m]) but has a very low affinity for channels in the rested (R) state. Drug dissociation during diastole is time dependent and incomplete, resulting in an accumulation of drug-associated (blocked) channels with successive beats. (Reprinted from ref. 125, with permission.)

- Wide QRS complex,
- AV nodal block of varying degree,
- Polymorphic ventricular tachycardia, which can progress to torsades de pointes (Fig. 7), and
- Bradycardia with electromechanical dissociation, leading to:
- Asystole.

Confounding Factors

Factors that increase bupivacaine electrophysiologic toxicity include:

- Bupivacaine Administration by Rapid Intravenous Bolus Injection

  Bupivacaine is very lipid soluble and highly protein bound. At steady state, plasma free drug concentration is low. During rapid intravenous injection, toxic amounts of free drug can reach the heart and the brain before lipid uptake and protein binding occur. In addition, the percent of bound drug decreases with increasing serum concentrations of bupivacaine (134).
- Hypoxia and Acidosis (135,136)

  Profound hypoxia and acidosis develop within 90 seconds of the start of bupivacaine-induced convulsions in both humans and anesthetized dogs (137,138).
- Coadministration of Small Doses of Epinephrine or Phenylephrine

  In rats, bupivacaine mixed with either epinephrine or phenylephrine is more toxic than plain bupivacaine (139). This finding is surprising, because administration of massive doses of intravenous epinephrine is an integral feature of most successful animal resuscitation protocols.

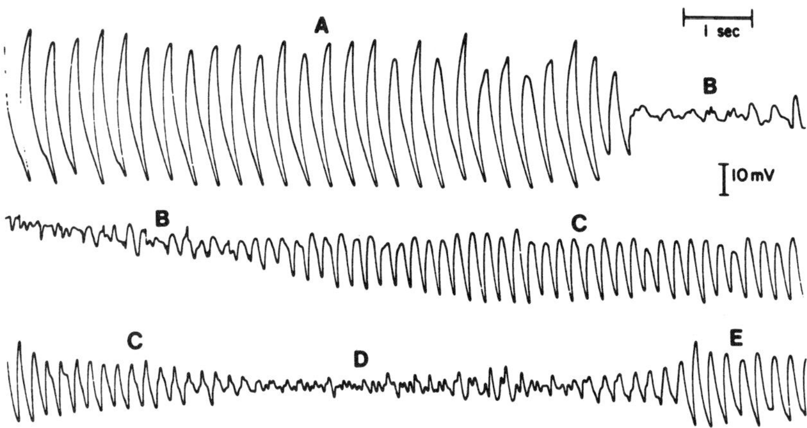

FIG. 7. Bupivacaine-induced "torsades de pointes" ventricular tachycardia in the dog. Note that periods of "typical" ventricular tachycardia **(A and C)** are followed by what appears to be ventricular fibrillation **(B and D)**, only to have "typical" ventricular tachycardia occur again **(E)**. Visual inspection revealed regular organized contractions consistent with ventricular tachycardia throughout this time. (Reprinted from ref. 143, with permission.)

- Hyperkalemia or Hyponatremia (140)
- Presence of Other Drugs That Decrease Electrical Conduction in the Heart

  This is a long list, including class I antiarrhythmics (quinidine, procainamide, lidocaine, disopyramide, etc.), calcium entry blockers (141), and b blockers (142,143).

Available Antiarrhythmics

In animals, arrhythmias have been treated successfully with the following.

Bretylium

In anesthetized dogs with constant serum bupivacaine concentrations of 7 μg/mL, bretylium 20 mg/kg proved beneficial. Bretylium corrected bupivacaine-induced alterations in cardiac output, SV, heart rate, and SVR (143). In this model, bupivacaine infusion produced no spontaneous ventricular arrhythmias but did lower the threshold for inducing sustained ventricular tachycardia. Bretylium administration returned this threshold to normal (143).

Isoproterenol

In isolated rabbit hearts, isoproterenol 1 to 2 μg/mL corrects bupivacaine-induced prolongation of electrical conduction (144). This treatment is counterintuitive, for isoproterenol induces tachycardia, which should increase sodium channel accummulation of bupivacaine. However, isoproterenol raises intracellular cyclic adenosine monophosphate concentration, thereby opening more calcium channels, which compensates for the impaired sodium flux (129). Isoproterenol is an effective antiarrhythmic in other torsades de pointes conditions.

Magnesium

Pretreating dogs with magnesium sulfate prevented widening of the QRS complex and QT interval but did not affect PR interval prolongation or the seizure dose of bupivacaine (145). Magnesium has not been used to treat bupivacaine-induced arrhythmias, although magnesium successfully treats torsades de pointes arrhythmias due to other causes.

Diazepam or Midazolam

Benzodiazepines terminate dysrhythmias caused by minute bupivacaine doses applied to the brainstem and thus may treat confounding γ-aminobutyric acid-mediated cerebral autonomic components of the arrhythmia (132,133). Benzodiazepines can treat or prevent further seizure activity.

Treatment

Treatment frequently involves a prolonged and difficult cardiac resuscitation. Because bupivacaine cardiac arrest occurs so rarely and volunteer studies have obviously not been done, the following treatment recommendations are based on animal studies, case reports, and treatments that work in related conditions.

1. *Ventilate and oxygenate immediately.*

   This is not a trivial matter in the setting of an unexpected cardiac arrest. Profound hypoxia, hypercarbia, and acidosis occur more quickly in bupivacaine cardiotoxicity than in almost any other condition (i.e., profound hypoxia develops within 90 seconds in previously well-ventilated dogs!) (138). Resuscitation is more difficult in the face of hypoxia and acidosis. Intubate the trachea quickly but do not delay ventilation pending tracheal intubation.
2. *Institute closed chest cardiac massage as needed.*
3. *Prevent any aortocaval compression.*

In anesthetized dogs, partial inferior vena cava compression lengthened the time to successful resuscitation (22 vs 2 minutes) and significantly increased the amounts of epinephrine (7 vs 1 mg) and bicarbonate (46 vs 22 mEq) required (Table 3). Because preventing aortocaval compression while maintaining effective closed chest cardiac massage may prove nearly impossible, one should strongly consider:

4. Emergency cesarean section.

In one case report, a mother could not be resuscitated until after the fetus was removed. Both the mother and the baby survived.

5. Antiarrhythmics. The following drug therapy scheme has worked successfully in dogs weighing 20 to 25 kg and in sheep weighing 40 to 50 kg (138,148):

- Ventricular tachycardia:
  Bretylium 5 mg/kg intravenously every 30 seconds to a maximum dose of 30 mg/kg.
- Ventricular fibrillation:
  Bretylium as indicated previously, plus epinephrine 1 mg intravenously, followed by direct current cardioversion.
- Bradycardia with electromechanical dissociation or asystole:
  Epinephrine 0.75 mg and atropine 0.8 mg intravenously, followed by epinephrine 0.5 mg and atropine 0.4 mg intravenously every 45 seconds until the pulse and BP are stable.

Obviously, prevention is better than cure. One of the epidural needle and catheter testing schemes described previously should be used (and used correctly!) whenever the total incremental bupivacaine dose exceeds 35 mg (124). Electrophysiologic toxicity also can occur with any other local anesthetic. However, the safety margins are larger.

FETAL HEART RATE CHANGES FOLLOWING REGIONAL ANALGESIA FOR LABOR

Fetal heart rate changes occur in about 15% of patients receiving either epidural bupivacaine or intrathecal fentanyl/sufentanil labor analgesia (149–151). After either epidural bupivacaine or intrathecal sufentanil labor analgesia, prolonged fetal bradycardia (heart rate less than 100 beats/min for more than 2 minutes) is seen in 3% to 4% of patients with previously normal fetal heart rate patterns (152,153). The fetal bradycardias generally occur about 10 to 20 minutes after the patient is pain-free. In one report, the incidence of bradycardia was much higher in patients with abnormal [21 of 33 (64%)] than with normal [9 of 267 (3.4%)] preanalgesia fetal heart rate patterns (152).

Why do these bradycardias occur? Most of them are probably secondary to tetanic uterine contractions. Uterine hypertonus accompanies the fetal bradycardia in 56% to 73% of cases (153,154). The preanalgesic frequency of uterine contractions correlates with the incidence of fetal bradycardia (153).

Why does uterine activity sometimes increase after induction of neuraxial analgesia? Maternal catecholamines (especially epinephrine) may inhibit uterine activity during painful labor (155). Physiologic plasma concentrations of catecholamines inhibit uterine activity in animals (156), and high plasma concentrations correlate with prolonged labor in humans (157). Severe labor pain increases maternal circulating epinephrine. Epinephrine, which has a serum half-life of about 3 minutes, disappears quickly after labor pain has been relieved. This decrease may disinhibit factors that promote uterine activity (i.e., oxytocin). If uterine hypertonus develops, prolonged decelerations may follow.

How should one treat these bradycardias? Turn off the oxytocin infusion. Administer oxygen by face mask. Turn the patient on her side or into knee–chest position. Palpate the abdomen for uterine contractions; recommend terbutaline or nitroglycerin if a contraction is present. Check BP; give intravenous fluids or ephedrine as needed. With intravenous fluids and tocolysis, few of these patients require emergent cesarean delivery. If an operative delivery seems indicated, recheck the fetal heart rate just before prepping the abdomen. In most cases, the fetal heart rate will have recovered during transit to the operating room.

TABLE 3. *Time and drug doses required to resuscitate dogs from bupivacaine-induced cardiovascular toxicity during partial inferior vena cava occlusion*

	Control	Partial IVC occlusion
Resuscitation time (min)	2.1 ± 0.5	22.2 ± 6.9[a]
Epinephrine dose (mg)	1.3 ± 0.4	7.1 ± 2.5[a]
$NaHCO_3$ dose (mEq)	22.4 ± 4.5	45.9 ± 10.1[a]
Survivors	6/6	5/6

Data are mean ±SD.
[a]Significantly different from control.
IVC, inferior vena cava.
Data from ref. 146.

RESPIRATORY ARREST AFTER INTRATHECAL SUFENTANIL/FENTANYL

Severe respiratory depression or respiratory arrest rarely follows intrathecal administration of fentanyl or sufentanil (158–162). Often, these patients also received parenteral opioids or more than 10 μg of sufentanil. I have participated in the resuscitation of three such patients, and each case has had the same presentation. The patient appeared sleepy but otherwise normal while she was conversing. As soon as there was no verbal stimulation, the patient lost consciousness and became apneic within seconds. The first ominous sign noted by the patient's nurse was profound fetal bradycardia. The second and third patients recovered quickly after 0.4 to 0.8 mg of intravenous naloxone was given; the first patient was intubated and ventilated instead (160).

From a respiratory standpoint, the maximum safe dose of intrathecal sufentanil or fentanyl in laboring women has yet to be determined.

MISCELLANEOUS

Broken Needles/Catheters

Needles

Open-ended needles are most prone to breakage at the junction of the hub and the shaft of the needle (163,164). Do not bury needles to the hub. Surgical exploration may be needed for needle retrieval if the hub and shaft separate (165). Needles with recessed holes (such as the Sprotte needle) may bend (and, very rarely, break) at the thinnest point of the metal after a high-velocity impact with bone. Broken needles should be removed because they can migrate and cause further tissue damage.

Epidural Catheters

The tip of an epidural catheter may shear if withdrawn through the epidural needle (166,167). Catheter shearing occurs more frequently with Teflon-coated polyvinyl chloride than with nylon or polyamide catheters (168). Such catheter tips may be left in situ if the patient is asymptomatic (64). Catheters may knot on themselves if excessive amounts are threaded into the epidural space. Most such catheters have been removed intact with gentle steady traction (169,170).

Headache of Immediate Onset

Immediate, severe headache can follow subarachnoid or subdural injection of air during attempted identification of the epidural space (87,171,172). Unlike headaches caused by low CSF pressure, subarachnoid or subdural air injection can instantly produce a headache that is not relieved, and may be exacerbated, by lying down. Patients usually recover spontaneously over 1 to 5 days.

Ulnar or Radial Nerve Injury

Automatic BP cuffs positioned over the elbow of thin parturients who are actively moving their arms may cause acute radial or ulnar nerve injury (173,174). Injury may occur after less than 1 hour of automated cuff use (173). Unlike nerve injuries under general anesthesia, which primarily are caused by ischemia of the vasa nervorum, these injuries probably are caused by mechanical intussusception of the myelin sheath (173,175).

Hypertension Secondary to Ergot Compounds and Pressors

Ergot compounds, especially when administered intravenously, can cause hypertension or coronary artery spasm in healthy parturients (41,176). Following large doses of long-acting vasopressors such as ephedrine or methoxamine, ergonovine can increase the maternal BP by up to 160 mm Hg (41). Hypertension severe enough to rupture a subarachnoid aneurysm has been reported (176).

Prevention clearly is better than cure. Use oxytocin for initial uterotonic therapy in patients who have received large doses of long-acting vasopressors. If an ergot compound is administered after pressors, give a small dose intramuscularly, not intravenously. Check the BP frequently for at least 3 hours. Ergot-induced hypertension can be treated with small doses of labetalol, trimethaphan, nitroglycerin, or nitroprusside. Chloropromazine 12.5 mg intravenously also has been used successfully (176).

Air Emboli

Air can enter the venous sinuses of the gravid uterus, especially during sexual intercourse, during manual placental extraction, during cesarean section with massive blood loss, and in patients with placenta previa (177–179). Precordial Doppler monitoring detects venous air embolism in 10% to 65% of cesarean section patients (105–107). Placing the operating table in a 5-degree reverse Trendelenburg position decreases the incidence of air emboli although flexing the head of the operating table up 5 to 10 degrees does not (180,181). Two-dimensional echocardiography verifies that the emboli detected are indeed air (182). Awake patients experiencing air emboli may complain of chest pain or dyspnea. Cyanosis, low oxygen saturation, or end-tidal carbon dioxide tension, hypotension, and cardiac dysrhythmias may occur when larger amounts of air are entrained (106). Treatment of a clinically significant air embolism consists of flooding the operative field, discontinuing nitrous oxide administration, placing the patient in steep head-down and left-tilted position, and providing cardiac resuscitation as needed (183).

Although cardiac arrest and death due to massive air embolism have been reported, morbid events occur in only a minute fraction of cesarean patients with air emboli (183,184). One should maintain a high index of suspicion for air emboli in all patients during cesarean section; however, the use of routine precordial Doppler monitoring does not seem warranted.

Electrocardiographic Changes during Cesarean Section

Electrocardiographic ST segment changes occur in 25% to 64% of cesarean section patients (185–188). The cause of this phenomenon is not known, but it is not associated with regional wall-motion abnormalities, decreased cardiac ejection fraction, abnormal postoperative 12-lead electrocardiograms, or elevated myocardial creatine kinase.

GENERAL ANESTHESIA

Failed Intubation

Failed intubation occurs roughly ten times as often during general anesthesia in parturients as in other surgical patients (189,190). Samsoon and Young (191) reported that 1 of 280 obstetric versus 1 of 2,230 other surgical patients could not be intubated. The incidence of failed intubation during general anesthesia for cesarean section ranges from 1 of 140 to 1 of 300 cases (192,193).

Intubation difficulties, with or without pulmonary aspiration, contribute heavily to maternal deaths associated with cesarean section: 33% of such deaths in Georgia from 1975 to 1976, and 26% of such deaths in England and Wales from 1982 to 1984 (Table 4) (194–196). In the United States, from 1985 to 1990, anesthetic-related death during delivery was 16.7 times more likely to occur under general than regional anesthesia. Pulmonary aspiration frequently complicates the intubation difficulties that accompany up to 5% of all obstetric general anesthetics (198). Half of the cases of pulmonary aspiration in the obstetric closed claim study occurred in association with difficult tracheal intubation, esophageal intubation, or inadequate ventilation (199).

TABLE 4. *Incidence of maternal aspiration and maternal deaths from aspiration or failed intubation*

Study	Cases/100,000 live births	
	Aspiration	Deaths
Mendelson, 1932–1945	149.92	4.54
Merrill, 1945–1949	39.06	2.36
Georgia, 1975–1976		1.88
Michigan, 1979–1986		0.82
United States, 1979–1981		0.43
United States, 1988–1990		0.17

Data from refs. 194, 197, 220, 247, 251.

Why Is Tracheal Intubation of Obstetric Patients so Difficult?

The following factors undoubtedly contribute.

1. Anatomic changes related to pregnancy
   - Edema of the larynx, nasopharynx, and tongue. Airway edema, present to some degree in all parturients, contributes to difficult intubations in some preeclamptic patients (200) and healthy patients following strenuous bearing-down efforts (201).
   - Capillary engorgement. The mucosa of the airway is friable and bleeds easily.
   - Pregnancy-induced anatomic changes can turn a difficult airway into an impossible airway. Fahy et al. (193) used x-ray laryngoscopy under local anesthesia to evaluate nonpregnant women with a history of failed intubation during pregnancy. The laryngoscopist could not view the glottis in five of the eight patients. Even when not pregnant, these women would be considered at risk for airway difficulty.
2. Mammary hyperplasia and increased anteroposterior chest diameter. These anatomic changes decrease the distance from the chin to the chest and make it more difficult to insert the laryngoscope blade in the mouth (see following for an alternative).
3. Emergency operations. The urgent or emergent clinical situation in which many obstetric general anesthetics take place leads many to proceed without sufficient airway assessment or consideration of other options.

Prevention

Decreasing the incidence of intubation failures requires careful preparation of personnel and equipment, much of which needs to occur long before the case is anticipated.

- Carefully assess the airway in all obstetric patients before inducing general anesthesia (Fig. 8). This assessment need not take much time. Honesty, not egotism, is essential in this endeavor.
- Be prepared to suggest or insist on an anesthetic plan not involving rapid sequence general anesthesia. This approach can be difficult when facing an agitated obstetrician concerned about fetal well-being; however, an excessively fetocentric view helps neither mother nor baby.
- Anticipate difficult situations and plan ahead for regional anesthesia. Spinal anesthesia for emergent cesarean section can be instituted more quickly and is accepted more readily if the anesthesiologist also uses this technique during nonemergent cesarean sections. If you anticipate airway difficulty or are seeing a preeclamptic woman with an adequate but falling platelet count, insert an epidural catheter and test its location with a small dose of local anesthetic (e.g., 5 mL of 1% lidocaine) early in the obstetric course. The epidural block does not have to be maintained if the patient is in latent labor or is feeling no pain.
- Optimize the position of the bed and the patient's head before inducing general anesthesia. In my experience, elevating the back of the operating table 5 to 15 degrees while keeping the head and the legs parallel to the floor (Fig. 9) improves laryngeal visualization in most obstetric patients. This maneuver is extremely important in obese parturients (see Chapter 25, Fig. 6). This body position permits gravity to keep the breasts and chest out of the way of the laryngoscope handle and

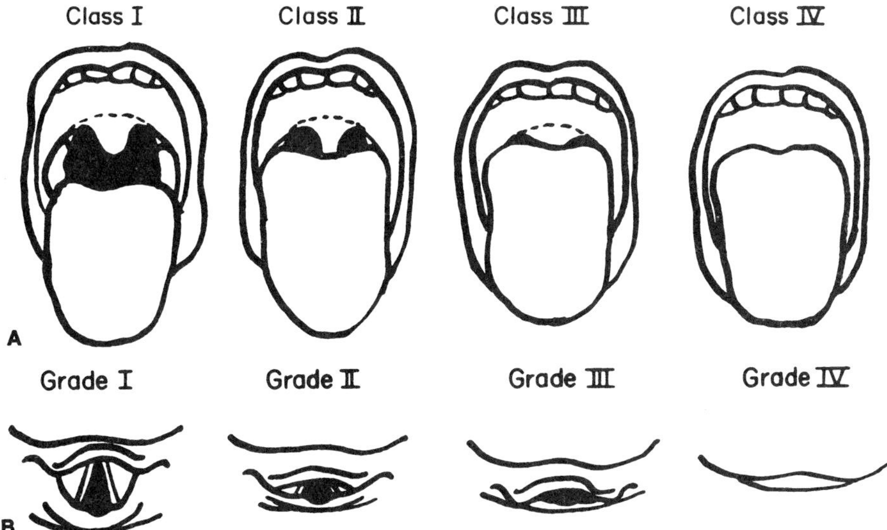

FIG. 8. A: Pictorial classification of the pharyngeal structures (modified from Mallampati). Note that in class III, the soft palate is visible, and in class IV, the soft palate is not visible. **B:** Grades of laryngoscopic views (modified from Cormack and Lehane). (Reprinted from ref. 191, with permission.)

minimizes the amount of lift necessary to expose the larynx. Although this bed position is easily accomplished on most standard operating room tables, many delivery rooms (including the one at the author's institution) have operative delivery tables in the cesarean room that do not have a separate head section. Here, use a wedge or a stack of towels and sheets for positioning.

- Never induce general anesthesia with inadequate or unchecked equipment or inadequate assistance. I feel that general anesthetic inductions proceed most smoothly with three people: one person whose only job is to hold cricoid pressure and hand the laryngoscopist the endotracheal tube, an experienced assistant who injects the drugs and assists the laryngoscopist, and the laryngoscopist. An inexperienced but reliable and well-instructed assistant can hold cricoid pressure. This assistant should adequately demonstrate cricoid-holding technique on the awake patient or the anesthetist before the induction begins.

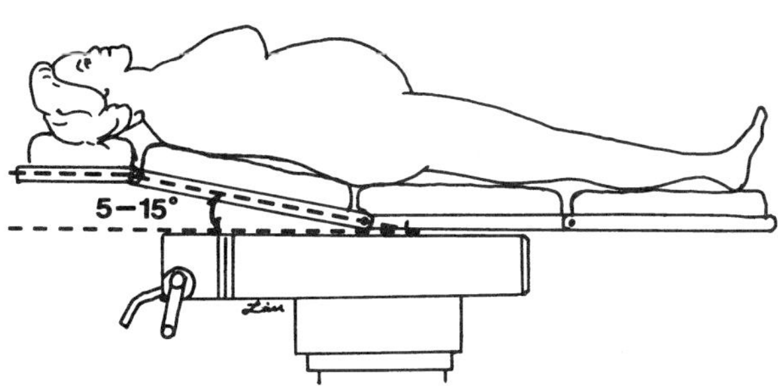

FIG. 9. Operating table position that optimizes maternal visualization in obese parturients.

- Learn and habitually use a technique for laryngoscope blade insertion that is effective in patients with increased chest anteroposterior diameter. Many anesthetists insert the laryngoscope blade in the mouth in the mid-sagittal plane and pivot in that plane to expose the larynx. Parturients often do not have enough space between the sternum and the mouth to permit this maneuver with a standard laryngoscope handle. An alternative technique (Fig. 10) is to insert the laryngoscope straight into the mouth in a plane angled 45 degrees to the right (or left) of the mid-sagittal plane, with the tip of the blade following the mid-line of the tongue, until the tip of the blade is near the uvula. Gently rotate the laryngoscope into the mid-sagittal plane and advance as usual. Be careful to keep the tip of the blade in the mid-sagittal plane to avoid getting caught in the tonsillar pillar. Learn this technique on healthy patients; do not try it for the first time during rapid sequence induction for cesarean section. The advantage of this technique is that the laryngoscope handle is never near the chest wall. Few experiences are more frustrating than an inability to get the laryngoscope in the mouth during a rapid sequence induction.
- Use smaller endotracheal tubes than one would use in nonpregnant women. I routinely use a cuffed 6.0- or 6.5-mm tube and always keep a cuffed 5.5-mm tube available.
- Develop a failed intubation protocol and review and practice it periodically. The protocol used at the author's institution is described in Fig. 11 (202).
- If the failed intubation protocol includes the use of unusual equipment, develop familiarity with that equipment during routine general anesthetics in nonpregnant patients at low risk of aspiration. Examples of

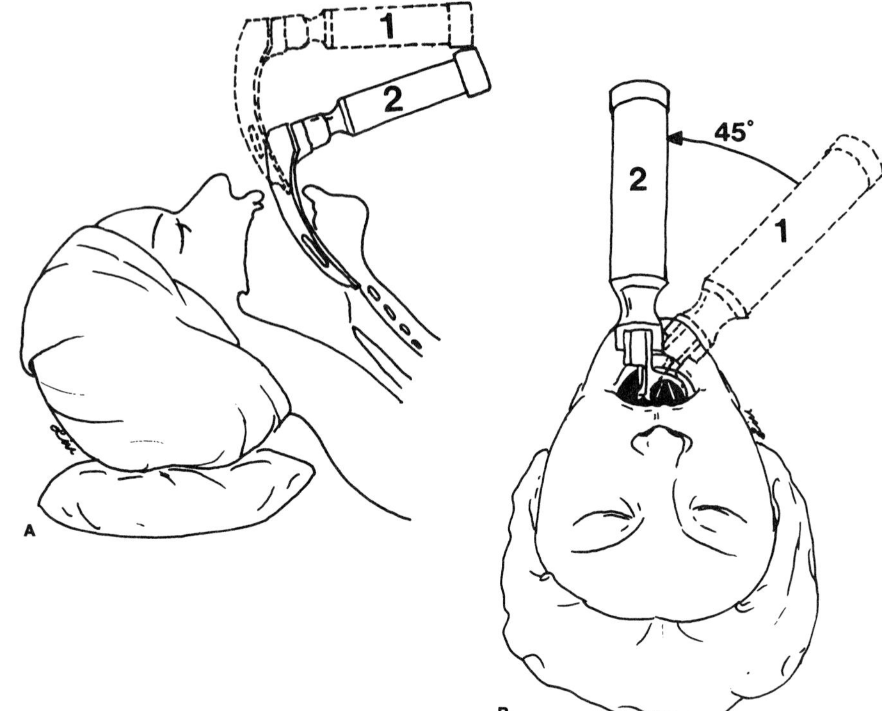

FIG. 10. Recommended technique for insertion of the laryngoscopic blade in obstetric patients. Insert the laryngoscopic blade into the mouth parallel to the floor *(A-1)* and at a 45-degree angle to the mid-sagittal plane *(B-1)*. Advance the blade tip along the mid-line of the tongue until the blade tip is at the level of the uvula. Then rotate the laryngoscopic blade into the mid-sagittal plane *(B-2)* and advance into the vellecula *(A-2)*.

such equipment include special laryngoscope blades, the light wand, the fiberoptic bronchoscope, the Bullard intubating laryngoscope, and the laryngeal mask airway (LMA) (203).

- If one cannot intubate and cannot ventilate the patient by mask, try ventilation through an LMA, which has proven to be life saving in a number of obstetric patients (204). One must remember, however, that the LMA does not protect against aspiration. Gastric reflux occurs more frequently with an LMA than with a face mask and oral airway (205,206).
- All personnel administering general anesthesia to obstetric patients must know where the relevant emergency airway/ventilation equipment is stored. Although this seems like an elementary point, it often is overlooked.

Difficult or failed intubation remains distressingly common in obstetric anesthesia. We must all work to improve our track record in this area.

Aspiration

Pulmonary aspiration has long been recognized as a clinical problem; Hippocrates described the syndrome and warned of its dangers (207). Sir James Simpson reported the first anesthetic (chloroform)-associated

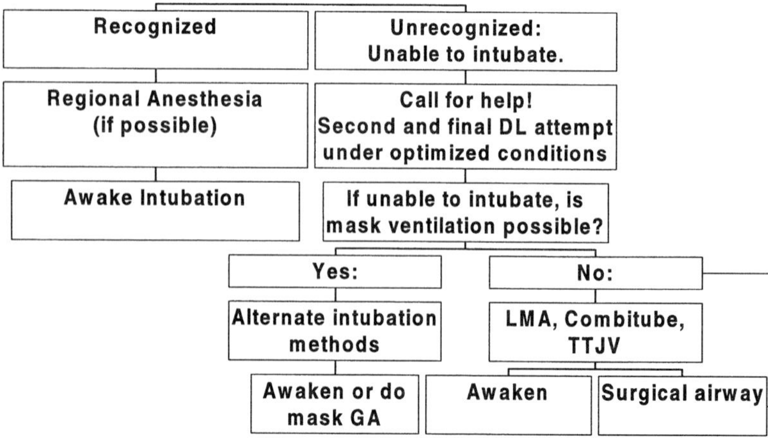

FIG. 11. Simplified version based on the ASA Difficult Airway Algorithm.

aspiration death (207). The problem remains with us to this day. In the closed claims study (cases from 1975 to 1985), 35% of the obstetric versus 2% of the nonobstetric suits involved the pulmonary aspiration of gastric contents (199).

Compared to nonpregnant women, parturients have a larger gastric volume and frequently reflux gastric contents into the esophagus. Intragastric pressure is twice as high in pregnant as in nonpregnant women (208,209). A parturient may suffer severe reflux in the absence of heartburn or a hiatal hernia (210). Pregnant women have low concentrations of plasma motilin (211) (and thus low gastric motility) and high concentrations of plasma gastrin (212) [and thus high gastric acid production (213)]. Gastric emptying, which is slowed slightly by the pain of labor and is unaffected by epidural local anesthetics, is profoundly delayed by parenteral and somewhat delayed by epidural opioids (214,215). Labor is scarcely a planned experience; patients may eat shortly before or during its early stages. Consequently, patients presenting for emergency cesarean section have much larger volumes of gastric residue than women coming for elective cesarean delivery. Laboring women may have solid food in the stomach for up to 24 hours after a meal (216).

Pathophysiology

Tracheal instillation of 1 to 4 mL/kg of any liquid produces hypoxia, hypotension, and wheezing. The further clinical course depends on the nature of the liquid aspirated (207,217–221).

- Saline: Hypoxia and hypotension are mild and completely resolve in 30 minutes with no sequelae.
- Acid: Acid produces an immediate chemical pneumonitis, the severity of which depends on the liquid's pH and volume. Instillation of liquid with a pH below a critical value (in humans, somewhere between 1.75 and 2.5) produces severe lung injury. Severe injury occurs with instillation of 0.4 mL/kg of 0.1N HCl in one lung in the monkey. However, at least 0.8 mL/kg of acid is required to produce the same injury in both lungs. Acid instillation produces moderate to severe hypoxemia and hypotension. Transudation of plasma occurs rapidly, producing intravascular hypovolemia and pulmonary edema. Adult respiratory distress syndrome then develops, with alveolar hyaline membrane formation. If the patient survives the initial event, the lungs may heal without scarring. Patients with acid aspiration uncomplicated by bacterial pneumonia recover in 4 to 5 days.
- Food: Large chunks can obstruct airways. Liquid food produces less hypoxemia, hypotension, and fluid transudation than acid but more hypercarbia and acidosis. Food aspiration heals with granuloma formation.
- Bile-contaminated gastric juice: This usually is fatal in both patients and animals.

Diagnosis

Frequently the aspiration is observed. However, one should suspect aspiration in a patient who presents with some or all of the following signs:

- Hypoxia,
- Pulmonary edema,
- Bronchospasm,
- Isolated laryngospasm (223),
- Cough,
- Apnea followed by tachypnea, tachycardia, or hypotension (207,218).

Symptoms usually present within 2 hours (218). Roentgenograms show localized or diffuse patchy alveolar infiltrates, or, in severe cases, opacification of large lung fields. Aspiration occurs most often in the right lower lobe (the straightest path from the trachea) or the most dependent lung area (frequently the right upper lobe in supine patients). The chemical pneumonitis itself can cause an initial temperature elevation; fever from bacterial overgrowth usually occurs several days later (207,218). The clinical course usually follows one of three paths:

- Rapid deterioration and death (12%),
- Rapid, sustained clinical improvement (62%), or
- Rapid improvement followed by decline due to bacterial pneumonia (26%) (218).

Superimposed bacterial pneumonia is fatal in more than 60% of the cases (218).

Therapy

Recommended therapy for symptomatic aspiration includes:

- Intubation and positive-pressure ventilation with positive end-expiratory pressure (PEEP). Use just enough oxygen to maintain oxygen saturation above 90% (207,224). Dogs receiving mechanical ventilation (tidal volume 15 mL/kg, 10 cm H_2O PEEP) for 5 hours following tracheal instillation of 2 mL/kg HCl had significantly higher oxygen saturation and improved lung histology compared to dogs not ventilated after the acid instillation (224). Because ventilation may need to be continued for several days, avoid excessively high oxygen concentrations to prevent additional damage from oxygen toxicity.
- Careful intravascular fluid replacement. Plasma volume can decrease 35% within 2 hours of a massive acid aspiration (183). Institution of mechanical ventilation with PEEP can further depress cardiac output and arterial pressure (224). Central venous or pulmonary artery pressure monitoring may be needed to guide therapy. These patients frequently have obvious pulmonary edema yet are oliguric secondary to hypovolemia (207,217). Reflex treatment of pulmonary edema with

phlebotomy and diuretics may have unnecessarily elevated mortality in early case series. One author found that patients resuscitated with colloid had less pulmonary shunt than patients resuscitated with crystalloid fluids only (219).

- Bronchoscopy ONLY if needed to clear food from the airway. Although patients certainly can die of purely mechanical airway obstruction (220) (a fate that should be prevented), bronchoscopy does not improve the course of patients who aspirate liquid gastric contents only (217).
- Rigid maintenance of asepsis during tracheal tube care. More than 60% of the patients who develop a superimposed bacterial pneumonia die (218).
- Avoidance of inhaled anesthetics. In rats with acid aspiration, inhaled anesthetics increased protein leakage, leukocyte infiltration, and mortality compared to ketamine anesthesia (225). If a general anesthetic must be continued after aspiration is diagnosed, one should consider switching to an intravenous technique.

Therapies That Are Not Recommended

Therapies that are NOT RECOMMENDED include the following:

- Lavage: Bronchial transudation neutralizes bronchial fluid pH within 30 minutes of massive acid aspiration (217). Lavage spreads the noxious aspirate to previously uninvolved lung areas and adds the negative effects (slight but appreciable) of saline aspiration (217). In dogs, 40% of lavage fluid was unrecoverable, and the dogs receiving lavage were more hypoxic than the dogs that did not (217).
- Steroids: Steroids, once enthusiastically prescribed after aspiration (226), have been shown to be clinically ineffective (207) and to impede recovery in animal models (227–229).
- Prophylactic antibiotics: Prophylactic antibiotics, also clinically ineffective, may increase late mortality by promoting the growth of resistant bacteria (207,218, 226). Obtain bronchial fluid cultures regularly and use antibiotics to treat documented bacterial infection.

Prophylaxis

Pharmacologic agents frequently are used to decrease the risk that a parturient's stomach contains dangerous amounts of acidity or gastric fluid. These agents include:

- Antacids (230): 0.3 M sodium citrate (231) (Bicitra) currently is recommended. Magnesium and aluminum-containing antacids are *not* recommended. Initial animal studies suggested that aspiration of gastric fluid was a benign clinical event as long as the pH was neutral (187,226). The first antacids widely used in laboring parturients contained magnesium or aluminum particles (232). Several parturients developed classic aspiration symptoms despite aspiration of particulate–antacid containing gastric fluid of neutral pH (233–235). Gibbs et al. (236) then demonstrated in the dog that aspiration of aluminum/magnesium hydroxide produces acute pulmonary pathology (as severe as that produced by acid instillation), which evolves into chronic granulomatous bronchopneumonitis and heals with extensive scar formation.
- Agents to raise the gastric pH: Ranitidine is now the most widely used agent from this class (237). Cimetidine or omeprazole also can be used (238).
- Metoclopramide (239): Metoclopramide increases gastric motility (240) [an effect that is blocked by opioids (241) or atropine (242)] and increases lower esophageal sphincter pressure (243).
- Anticholinergics: I do not recommend these agents. Atropine increases gastric volume (244). Atropine and glycopyrrolate either increase (245) or do not affect (246) gastric pH. Atropine decreases lower esophageal sphincter pressure (242).

Prevention

Avoiding mask general anesthesia in obstetric patients is the primary way to prevent maternal pulmonary aspiration. Most anesthesiologists preferentially perform regional anesthesia for cesarean as well as vaginal deliveries. When general anesthesia is necessary, use a rapid sequence anesthetic induction and insert a cuffed tracheal tube. Routine intubation of obstetric general anesthetic patients has decreased the incidence of maternal aspiration from 39 to 150 cases per 100,000 live births in the 1940s to nine cases per 100,000 live births in the late 1960s (220,247,248).

Although the incidence of maternal aspiration has decreased greatly in the past half century, the incidence of anesthesia-associated pulmonary deaths in obstetric patients has declined much more slowly (Table 4) (249,250) Why has the prevention of maternal aspiration had so little effect on maternal mortality?

- Now that obstetric patients receiving general anesthesia are intubated routinely, deaths from failed intubation are replacing deaths from aspiration (197,199,251).
- Many patients with anesthesia-related aspiration pneumonia aspirated while awake following a planned extubation (207,252).
- Most aspiration/failed intubation deaths occur during cesarean section, and the cesarean section rate has increased greatly in the past half century. In Georgia, from 1975 to 1976, the incidence of aspiration/failed intubation maternal deaths was 1 in 53,078 live births but 1 in 5,063 cesarean sections (194).
- Several of the agents used before 1980 for aspiration prophylaxis or treatment have been shown to be ineffective or harmful. Particulate-containing antacids,

steroids, and prophylactic antibiotics fall into this category.

- Aspiration pneumonia is a rare disease. Information on its incidence can only be gleaned from large epidemiologic studies, which usually lag 6 to 10 years behind the time studied.

No completely effective measures exist to prevent aspiration or failed intubation in parturients. A major contributing factor is that awake intubations in parturients, as currently performed, usually are so uncomfortable and time consuming that the technique is rarely seriously considered. Can new awake intubation techniques improve this situation?

SUMMARY AND CONCLUSIONS

Intraoperative complications that require prompt and effective treatment can and do occur during obstetric anesthetics. This chapter has reveiwed the diagnosis, pathophysiology, and intraoperative management of hypotension, unintended dural puncture, high/total spinal anesthesia, subdural anesthesia, unintended intravascular catheter placement, systemic bupivacaine toxicity, fetal heart rate changes associated with regional anesthesia, failed intubation, and pulmonary aspiration.

Maternal hypotension during regional anesthesia can decrease uterine perfusion and may depress neonatal Apgar and neurobehavioral scores even if the mother is asymptomatic. The gravid uterus is heavy enough to compress the inferior vena cava and the aorta, further impairing maternal BP and uterine perfusion. Generous maternal prehydration, avoidance of aortocaval compression, and judicious intravenous pressor administration can minimize the incidence and impact of maternal hypotension.

All anesthesiologists occasionally puncture the dura while identifying the epidural space. It is important to administer a "spinal size" local anesthetic dose and wait long enough for spinal anesthesia to develop before injecting larger volumes of local anesthetic through epidural needles or catheters. One must then decide whether to continue with a single shot or continuous spinal anesthetic or reidentify the epidural space.

High or total spinal anesthesia during cesarean section occurs most frequently when spinal anesthesia with an undiminished local anesthetic dose is initiated to compensate for a patchy epidural block. Extremely high spinal blocks also occur during intended spinal anesthesics and during epidural anesthesia if dural puncture is not recognized. Prompt ventilatory and hemodynamic support is critical.

Subdural anesthesia probably occurs more frequently than clinically recognized. The classic clinical presentation is a delayed anesthetic onset, extensive sensory spread with less motor and sympathetic nerve block, and delayed anesthetic regression.

Unintended intravenous placement of epidural needles and catheters occurs much more often in pregnant than in nonpregnant patients. Aspiration for blood and fractionation of the local anesthetic dose may fail to detect intravenously placed needles and catheters. Prudence dictates that every aliquot of local anesthetic injected through an epidural needle or catheter must be a "test dose."

Although bupivacaine has many desirable clinical attributes, it is extremely toxic to the conduction system of the heart. Bupivacaine binds avidly to sodium channels (and, to a lesser extent, to calcium and potassium channels) but dissociates slowly at physiologic heart rates. Hypoxia, acidosis, hyperkalemia, and the presence of other class I antiarrhythmics increase bupivacaine toxicity. Ventilation, oxygenation, external cardiac massage, if needed, and elimination of aortocaval compression (which may require cesarean section) must be instituted rapidly. Large doses of epinephrine and atropine can reverse ventricular fibrillation or bradycardia. In animal models, bretylium, isoproterenol, and magnesium successfully combat the torsades de pointes ventricular tachycardia that can occur.

Prolonged fetal bradycardia can occur in 3% to 4% of patients with previously normal fetal heart rate patterns after either epidural bupivacaine or intrathecal sufentanil labor analgesia. The fetal bradycardias generally occur about 10 to 20 minutes after the patient is pain-free. A tetanic uterine contraction frequently accompanies this bradycardia. Most of the bradycardias resolve quickly with positioning, intravenous fluids, and discontinuation of oxytocin. Tocolysis with terbutaline may be required; rarely, emergent cesarean delivery is indicated.

Failed intubation occurs ten times more often in obstetric as in surgical patients. Meticulous preparation of patient, personnel, and equipment plus honest airway assessment and the use of alternative anesthetic plans when needed are crucial to avoid this potentially lethal complication.

Pulmonary aspiration of gastric contents still occurs, albeit less frequently than in years past. Avoiding general anesthesia when possible, rapid sequence induction of general anesthesia, and minimizing maternal gastric volume and acidity before anesthetic induction may minimize the incidence and severity of aspiration.

REFERENCES

1. Kang YG, Abouleish E, Caritis S. Prophylactic intravenous ephedrine infusion during spinal anesthesia for cesarean section. *Anesth Analg* 1982;61:839.
2. Marx GF, Cosmi EV, Wollman SB. Biochemical status and clinical condition of mother and infant at cesarean section. *Anesth Analg* 1969;48:986.
3. Clark RB, Thompson DS, Thompson CH. Prevention of spinal hypotension associated with cesarean section. *Anesthesiology* 1976; 45:670.
4. Klein MD, Clahr J. Factors in the decline of maternal mortality. *JAMA* 1958;168:237.
5. Ebner H, Barcohana J, Bartoshuk AK. Influence of postspinal

hypotension on the fetal electrocardiogram. *Am J Obstet Gynecol* 1960;80:569.
6. Hon EH, Reid BL, Hehre FW. The electronic evaluation of fetal heart rate. II. Changes with maternal hypotension. *Am J Obstet Gynecol* 1960;79:209.
7. James FM, Greiss FC, Kemp RA. An evaluation of vasopressor therapy for maternal hypotension during spinal anesthesia. *Anesthesiology* 1970;33:25.
8. Hollmen AI, Joupilla R, Koivisto M, et al. Neurologic activity of infants following anesthesia for cesarean section. *Anesthesiology* 1978;48:350.
9. Datta S, Alper MH, Ostheimer GW, Weiss JB. Method of ephedrine administration and nausea and hypotension during spinal anesthesia for cesarean section. *Anesthesiology* 1982;56:68.
10. Caritis SN, Abouleish E, Edelstone DI, Mueller-Heubach E. Fetal acid–base state following spinal or epidural anesthesia for cesarean section. *Obstet Gynecol* 1980;56:610.
11. Norris MC. Hypotension during spinal anesthesia for cesarean section: does it affect neonatal outcome? *Reg Anesth* 1987;12:191.
12. Kinsella SM, Whitwam JG, Spencer JAD. Aortic compression by the uterus: identification with the Finapres digital arterial pressure instrument. *Br J Obstet Gynaecol* 1990;97:700.
13. Howard BK, Goodson JH, Mengert WF. Supine hypotensive syndrome in late pregnancy. *Obstet Gynecol* 1953;1:371.
14. Wright L. Postural hypotension in late pregnancy: the supine hypotensive syndrome. *Br Med J* 1962;1:760.
15. Goodlin RC. Importance of the lateral position during labor. *Obstet Gynecol* 1971;37:698.
16. Wollman SB, Marx GF. Acute hydration for prevention of hypotension of spinal anesthesia in parturients. *Anesthesiology* 1968;29:374.
17. Ramanathan S, Grant GJ. Vasopressor therapy for hypotension due to epidural anesthesia for caesarean section. *Acta Anaesthesiol Scand* 1988;32:559.
18. Bieniarz J, Maqueda E, Caldeyro-Barcia R. Compression of aorta by the uterus in late human pregnancy. *Am J Obstet Gynecol* 1966; 95:795.
19. Brizgys RV, Dailey PA, Shnider SM, Kotelko DM, Levinson G. The incidence and neonatal effects of maternal hypotension during epidural anesthesia for cesarean section. *Anesthesiology* 1987;67:782.
20. Eckstein KL, Marx GF. Aortocaval compression and uterine displacement. *Anesthesiology* 1974;40:92.
21. Butterworth JF, Walker FO, Lysak SZ. Pregnancy increases median nerve susceptibility to lidocaine. *Anesthesiology* 1990;72:962.
22. Kennedy RL, Friedman DL, Katchka DM, Selmantis S, Smith RN. Hypotension during obstetrical anesthesia. *Anesthesiology* 1959;20: 153.
23. Colon-Morales MA. A self-supporting device for continuous left uterine displacement during cesarean secton. *Anesth Analg* 1970;49:223.
24. Kennedy RL. An instrument to relieve inferior vena cava occlusion. *Am J Obstet Gynecol* 1970;107:331.
25. Mendiola J, Grylack LJ, Scanlon JW. Effects of intrapartum maternal glucose infusion on the normal fetus and newborn. *Anesth Analg* 1982;61:32.
26. Kenepp NB, Shelley NC, Kumar S, Gutsche BB, Gabbe S, Delivoria-Papadopoulos M. Effects on newborn of hydration with glucose in patients undergoing caesarean section with regional anaesthesia [Letter]. *Lancet* 1980;1:645.
27. Lewis M, Thomas P, Wilkes RG. Hypotension during epidural analgesia for caesarean section. *Anaesthesia* 1983;38:250.
28. Rout CC, Rocke DA, Levin J, Gouws E, Reddy D. A reevaluation of the role of crystalloid preload in the prevention of hypotension associated with spinal anesthesia for elective cesarean section. *Anesthesiology* 1993;79:262.
29. Park GE, Hauch MA, Curlin F, Datta S, Bader AM. The effects of varying volumes of crystalloid administration before cesarean delivery on maternal hemodynamics and colloid osmotic pressure. *Anesth Analg* 1996;83:299.
30. Riley ET, Cohen SE, Rubenstein AJ, Flanagan B. Prevention of hypotension after spinal anesthesia for cesarean section: six percent hetastarch versus lactated Ringer's solution. *Anesth Analg* 1995; 81:838.
31. Sharma SK, Gajraj NM, Sidawi JE. Prevention of hypotension during spinal anesthesia: a comparison of intravascular administration of hetastarch versus lactated Ringer's solution. *Anesth Analg* 1997;84:111.
32. Marcus MAE, Vertommen JD, Van Aken H. Hydroxyethyl starch versus lactated Ringer's solution in the chronic maternal-fetal sheep preparation: a pharmacodynamic and pharmacokinetic study. *Anesth Analg* 1995;80:949.
33. Ralston DH, Shnider SM, deLorimier AA. Effects of equipotent ephedrine, metaraminol, mephentermine, and methoxamine on uterine blood flow in the pregnant ewe. *Anesthesiology* 1974;40:354.
34. Zaimis E. Vasopressor drugs and catecholamines. *Anesthesiology* 1968;29:732.
35. McGrath JM, Chestnut DH, Vincent RD, et al. Ephedrine remains the vasopressor of choice for treatment of hypotension during ritodrine infusion and epidural anesthesia. *Anesthesiology* 1994;80:1073.
36. Hughes SC, Wark MG, Levinson G, et al. Placental transfer of ephedrine does not affect neonatal outcome. *Anesthesiology* 1985;63: 217.
37. Wright RG, Shnider SM, Levinson G, Rolbin SH, Parer JT. The effect of maternal administration of ephedrine on fetal heart rate and variability. *Am J Obstet Gynecol* 1981;57:734.
38. Kangas-Saarela T, Hollmen AI, Tolonen U, et al. Does ephedrine influence newborn neurobehavioural responses and spectral EEG when used to prevent maternal hypotension during caesarean section? *Acta Anaesthesiol Scand* 1990;34:8.
39. King SW, Rosen MA. Prophylactic ephedrine and hypotension associated with spinal anesthesia for cesarean delivery. *Int J Obstet Anesth* 1998;7:18.
40. Gutsche BB. Prophylactic ephedrine preceding spinal analgesia for cesarean section. *Anesthesiology* 1976;45:462.
41. Moya F, Smith B. Spinal anesthesia for cesarean section: clinical and biochemical studies of effects on maternal physiology. *JAMA* 1962;179:609.
42. Moran DH, Perillo M, Bader AM, Datta S. Phenylephrine in treating maternal hypotension secondary to spinal anesthesia. *Anesthesiology* 1989;71:A857.
43. Ramanathan S, Friedman S, Moss P, Arismendy J, Turndorf H. Phenylephrine for the treatment of maternal hypotension due to epidural anesthesia. *Anesth Analg* 1984;63:262(abst).
44. Bhagwanjee S, Rocke DA, Rout CC, Koovarjee RV, Brijball R. Prevention of hypotension following spinal anesthesia for elective caesarean section by wrapping of the legs. *Br J Anaesth* 1990;65:819.
45. James FM, Greiss FC. The use of inflatable boots to prevent hypotension during spinal anesthesia for cesarean section. *Anesth Analg* 1973; 52:246.
46. Goudie TA, Winter AW, Ferguson DJM. Lower limb compression using inflatable splints to prevent hypotension during spinal anesthesia for caesarean section. *Acta Anaesthesiol Scand* 1988;32:541.
47. D'Angelo R, Foss ML, Livesay CH. A comparison of multiport and uniport epidural catheters in laboring patients. *Anesth Analg* 1997;84: 1276.
48. Michael S, Richmond MN, Birks RJS. A comparison between open-end (single-hole) and closed-end (three lateral holes) epidural catheters: complications and quality of sensory blockade. *Anaesthesia* 1989;44:578.
49. Collier CB, Gatt SP. Epidural catheters for obstetrics: terminal hole or lateral eyes? *Reg Anesth* 1994;19:378.
50. Beck H, Brassow F, Doehn M, Bause H, Dziadzka A, Schulte am Esch J. Epidural catheters of the multi-orifice type: dangers and complications. *Acta Anaesthesiol Scand* 1986;30:549.
51. Ward CF, Osborne R, Benumof JL, Saidman LJ. A hazard of double-orifice epidural catheters. *Anesthesiology* 1978;48:362.
52. Sala-Blanch X, Martinez-Palli G, Agusti-Lasus M, Nalda-Felipe A. Misplacement of multihole epidural catheters a report of two cases. *Anaesthesia* 1996;51:386.
53. Paech MJ. Inadvertent spinal anaesthesia with 0.125% bupivacaine and fentanyl during labour. *Anaesth Intens Care* 1990;18:400.
54. Collier CB. Accidental subdural block: four more cases and a radiographic review. *Anaesth Intens Care* 1992;20:215.
55. Power I, Thorburn J. Differential flow from multihole epidural catheters. *Anaesthesia* 1988;43:876.
56. Katsiris SE, Harfa L, Leighton BL, Halpern SH, Wilson DB, Kronberg J. Testing multiorifice epidural catheters: inject briskly. *Anesthesiology Suppl* 1998:A46.
57. Abraham RA, Harris AP, Maxwell LG, Kaplow S. The efficacy of 1.5% lidocaine with 7.5% dextrose and epinephrine as an epidural test dose for obstetrics. *Anesthesiology* 1986;64:116.

58. van Zundert AA, de Wolf AM, Vaes L, Soetens M. High-volume spinal anesthesia with bupivacaine 0.125% for cesarean section. *Anesthesiology* 1988;69:998.
59. Foldes FF, McNall PG. 2-Chloroprocaine: a new local anesthetic agent. *Anesthesiology* 1952;13:287.
60. Reisner LS. Epidural test solution or spinal fluid? [Correspondence]. *Anesthesiology* 1976;44:451.
61. Rosenberg H. pH in differentiating CSF from local anesthetics in epidural anesthesia [Correspondence]. *Anesthesiology* 1976;45:579.
62. Waters J, Chuba JV, Ramanathan S, Turndorf H. Epidural catheter aspirate. *Anesthesiology* 1990;73:A959(abst).
63. Kalas DB, Hehre FW. Continuous lumbar peridural anesthesia in obstetrics. VIII. Further observations on inadvertent lumbar puncture. *Anesth Analg* 1972;51:192.
64. Dawkins CJM. An analysis of the complications of extradural and caudal block. *Anaesthesia* 1969;24:554.
65. Norris MC, Leighton BL. Continuous spinal anesthesia after unintentional dural puncture in parturients. *Reg Anesth* 1990;15:285.
66. Colonna-Romano P, Shapiro BE. Unintentional dural puncture and prophylactic epidural blood patch in obstetrics. *Anesth Analg* 1989;69:522.
67. Hodgkinson R. Total spinal block after epidural injection into an interspace adjacent to an inadvertent dural puncture. *Anesthesiology* 1981;55:593.
68. Hodgkinson R. Total spinal block after epidural injection into an interspace adjacent to an inadvertent dural perforation. *Anesthesiology* 1981;55:593.
69. Leach A, Smith GB. Subarachnoid spread of epidural local anaesthetic following dural puncture. *Anaesthesia* 1988;43:671.
70. Swenson JD, Wisniewski M, McJames S, Ashburn MA, Pace NL. The effect of prior dural puncture on cisternal cerebrospinal fluid morphine concentrations in sheep after administration of lumbar epidural morphine. *Anesth Analg* 1996;83:523.
71. Bernards CM, Kopacz DJ, Michel MZ. Effect of needle puncture on morphine and lidocaine flux through the spinal meninges of the monkey *in vitro*. *Anesthesiology* 1994;80:853.
72. Suzuki N, Koganemaru M, Onizuka S, Takasaki M. Dural puncture with a 26-gauge spinal needle affects spread of epidural anesthesia. *Anesth Analg* 1996;82:1040.
73. Leighton BL, Arkoosh VA, Huffnagle S, Huffnagle HJ, Kinsella M, Norris MC. The dermatomal spread of epidural bupivacaine with and without prior intrathecal sufentanil. *Anesth Analg* 1996;83:526.
74. Loeser EA, Hill GE, Bennett GM, Sederberg JH. Time vs. success rate for epidural blood patch. *Anesthesiology* 1978;49:147.
75. Cheek TG, Banner R, Sauter J, Gutsche BB. Prophylactic extradural blood patch is effective: a preliminary communication. *Br J Anaesth* 1988;61:340.
76. Ackerman WE, Colclough GW. Prophylactic epidural blood patch: the controversy continues. *Anesth Analg* 1987;66:913.
77. Leivers D. Total spinal anesthesia following early prophylactic epidural blood patch. *Anesthesiology* 1990;73:1287.
78. Ong BY, Graham CR, Ringaert KRA, Cohen MM, Palahniuk RJ. Impaired epidural analgesia after dural puncture with and without subsequent blood patch. *Anesth Analg* 1990;70:76.
79. Blanche R, Eisenach JC, Tuttle R, Dewan DM. Previous wet tap does not reduce success rate of labor epidural analgesia. *Anesth Analg* 1994;79:291.
80. de Saram M. Accidental total spinal analgesia: a report of three cases. *Anaesthesia* 1956;11:77-79.
81. Lubenow T, Keh-Wong E, Kristof K, Ivankovich O, Ivankovich AD. Inadvertent subdural injection: a complication of an epidural block. *Anesth Analg* 1988;67:175.
82. Reynolds F, Speedy HM. The subdural space: the third place to go astray. *Anaesthesia* 1990;45:120.
83. Mehta M, Salmon N. Extradural block. Confirmation of the injection site by X-ray monitoring. *Anaesthesia* 1985;40:1009.
84. Jones MD, Newton TH. Inadvertent extra-arachnoid injections in myelography. *Radiology* 1963;80:818.
85. Manchanda VN, Murad SHN, Shilyansky G, Mehringer M. Unusual clinical course of accidental subdural local anesthetic injection. *Anesth Analg* 1983;62:1124.
86. Smith GB, Barton FL, Watt JH. Extensive spread of local anesthetic solution following subdural insertion of an epidural catheter during labour. *Anaesthesia* 1984;39:355.
87. Katz JA, Lukin R, Bridenbaugh PO, Gunzenhauser L. Subdural intracranial air: an unusual cause of headache after epidural steroid injection. *Anesthesiology* 1991;74:615.
88. Maycock E. An epidural anaesthetic with unusual complications. *Anaesth Intens Care* 1978;6:263.
89. Stevens RA, Stanton-Hicks MD. Subdural injection of local anesthetic: a complication of epidural anesthesia. *Anesthesiology* 1985;63:323.
90. Cohen CA, Kallow T. Failure of spinal anesthesia due to subdural catheter placement. *Anesthesiology* 1972;37:352.
91. Collier C. Total spinal or massive subdural block? [Letter]. *Anaesth Intens Care* 1982;10:92.
92. Mehta M, Maher R. Injection into the extra-arachnoid subdural space; experience in the treatment of intractable cervical pain and in the conduct of extradural (epidural) analgesia. *Anaesthesia* 1977;32:760.
93. Norris MC, Leighton BL, DeSimone CA. Needle bevel direction and headache after inadvertent dural puncture. *Anesthesiology* 1989;70:729.
94. Stone PA, Thorburn J, Lamb KSR. Complications of spinal anesthesia following extradural block for caesarean section. *Br J Anaesth* 1989;62:335.
95. Russell IF. Inadvertent total spinal for caesarean section. *Anaesthesia* 1985;40:199.
96. Kim YI, Mazza NM, Marx GF. Massive spinal block with hemicranial palsy after a test dose for extradural analgesia. *Anesthesiology* 1975;43:370.
97. Stonham J, Moss P. The optimal test dose for epidural anesthesia. *Anesthesiology* 1983;58:389.
98. Kenepp NB, Gutsche BB. Inadvertent intravascular injections during lumbar epidural anesthesia. *Anesthesiology* 1981;54:172.
99. Leighton BL, Norris MC, DeSimone CA, Rosco T, Gross JB. The air test is a clinically useful indicator of intravenously placed epidural catheters. *Anesthesiology* 1990;73:610.
100. Ahn NN, Ung DA, DeFay S, Cannelli G, Rudy TE, McKenzie R. Blood vessel puncture with epidural catheters. *Anesthesiology* 1989;71:A916.
101. Rolbin SH, Halpern SH, Braude BM, Kapala D, Unger R, Radhakrisnan S. Fluid through the epidural needle does not reduce complications of epidural catheter insertion. *Can J Anaesth* 1990;37:337.
102. Topkis W, Leighton BL, Arkoosh VA, Lee SH, Huffnagle HJ, Huffnagle S. Effectiveness of the Doppler air test in diagnosing intravascular multi-orifice epidural catheters. *Anesthesiology* 1997;87:A883.
103. Leighton BL, Gross JB. Air: an effective marker of intravenously located catheters. *Anesthesiology* 1989;71:848.
104. Naulty JS, Ostheimer GW, Datta S, Knapp R, Weiss JB. Incidence of venous air embolism during epidural catheter insertion. *Anesthesiology* 1982;57:410.
105. Handler JS, Bromage PR. Venous air embolism during cesarean delivery. *Reg Anesth* 1990;15:170.
106. Malinow AM, Naulty JS, Hunt CO, Datta S, Ostheimer GW. Precordial ultrasonic monitoring during cesarean delivery. *Anesthesiology* 1987;66:816.
107. Vartikar JV, Johnson MD, Datta S. Precordial Doppler monitoring and pulse oximetry during cesarean delivery: detection of venous air embolism. *Reg Anesth* 1989;14:145.
108. Leighton BL, Norris MC, Sosis M, Epstein R, Chayen B, Larijani GE. Limitations of epinephrine as a marker of intravascular injection in laboring women. *Anesthesiology* 1987;66:688.
109. Leighton BL, DeSimone CA, Norris MC, Chayen B. Isoproterenol is an effective marker of intravenous injection in laboring women. *Anesthesiology* 1989;71:206.
110. Leighton BL, Norris MC, DeSimone CA, Darby MJ, Menduke H. Preeclamptic and healthy term pregnant patients have different chronotropic responses to isoproterenol [Correspondence]. *Anesthesiology* 1990;72:392.
111. Chestnut DH, Owen CL, Brown CK, Vandewalker GE, Weiner CP. Does labor affect the variability of maternal heart rate during induction of epidural anesthesia? *Anesthesiology* 1988;68:622.
112. Marcus MAE, Vertommen JD, Van Aken H, et al. Hemodynamic effects of intravenous isoproterenol versus saline in the parturient. *Anesth Analg* 1997;84:1113.
113. Tanaka M. Epidural test dose: isoproterenol is a reliable marker for intravascular injection in anesthetized adults. *Anesth Analg* 1996;82:1056.

114. Perillo M, Sethna NF, Berde CB. Intravenous isoproterenol as a marker for epidural test-dosing in children. *Anesth Analg* 1993;76: 178.
115. Norris MC, Arkoosh VA, Knobler R. Maternal and fetal effects of isoproterenol in the gravid ewe. *Anesth Analg* 1996;85:389.
116. Marcus MAE, Bruyninckx FL, Vertommen JD, Wouters PF, Van Aken H. Spinal somatosensory evoked potentials after epidural isoproterenol in awake sheep. *Can J Anaesth* 1997;44:85.
117. Marcus MAE, Vertommen JD, Van Aken H, Van Lommel A. Light microscopic neuropathological observations after intrathecal bolus injections of isoproterenol. *Anesthesiology* 1994;81:A1175.
118. Marcus MAE, Vertommen JD, Van Aken H, Wouters PF. Hemodynamic effects of intravenous isoproterenol versus epinephrine in the chronic maternal-fetal sheep preparation. *Anesth Analg* 1996;82:1023.
119. van de Walle AFGM, Martin CB Jr. Effect of isoproterenol on uterine blood flow and cardiac output distribution in pregnant guinea pigs. *Am J Obstet Gynecol* 1985;152:1058.
120. Marcus MAE, Vertommen JD, Van Aken H, Gogarten W, Buerkle H. The effects of the addition of isoproterenol to 0.125% bupivacaine on the quality and duration of epidural analgesia during labor in the parturient. *Anesth Analg* 1998;86:749.
121. Munson ES, Tucker WK, Ausinsch B, Malagodi MH. Etidocaine, bupivacaine, and lidocaine seizure thresholds in monkeys. *Anesthesiology* 1975;42:471.
122. Liu P, Feldman HS, Covino BM, et al. Acute cardiovascular toxicity of intravenous amide local anesthetics in anesthetized ventilated dogs. *Anesth Analg* 1982;61:317.
123. Albright GA. Cardiac arrest following regional anesthesia with etidocaine or bupivacaine [Editorial]. *Anesthesiology* 1979;51:285.
124. Albright GA. Epinephrine should be used with the theraputic dose of bupivacaine in obstetrics. *Anesthesiology* 1984;61:217.
125. Clarkson CW, Hondeghem LM. Mechanism for bupivacaine depression of cardiac conduction: fast block of sodium channels during the action potential with slow recovery from block during diastole. *Anesthesiology* 1985;62:396.
126. de Jong RH, Ronfeld RA, DeRosa RA. Cardiovascular effects of convulsant and supraconvulsant doses of amide local anesthetics. *Anesth Analg* 1982;61:3.
127. de Jong RH, Bonin JD. Deaths from local anesthetic-induced convulsions in mice. *Anesth Analg* 1980;59:401.
128. Nath S, Haggmark S, Johansson G, Reiz S. Differential depressant and electrophysiologic cardiotoxicity of local anesthetics: an experimental study with special reference to lidocaine and bupivacaine. *Anesth Analg* 1986;65:1263.
129. Coyle DE, Sperelakis N. Bupivacaine and lidocaine blockage of calcium mediated slow action potentials in guinea pig ventricular muscle. *J Pharmacol Exp Ther* 1986;242:1001.
130. Courtney KR, Kendig JJ. Bupivacaine is an effective potassium channel blocker in heart. *Biochim Biophys* 1988;939:163.
131. Lacombe P, Blaise G, Loulmet D, Hollmann C. Electrophysiologic effects of bupivacaine in the isolated rabbit heart. *Anesth Analg* 1991; 72:62.
132. Bernards CM, Carpenter RL, Rupp SM, et al. Effect of midazolam and diazepam premedication on central nervous system and cardiovascular toxicity of bupivacaine in pigs. *Anesthesiology* 1989;70:318.
133. Bernards CM, Artu AA. Hexamethonium and midazolam terminate dysrhythmias and hypertention caused by intracerebroventricular bupivacaine in rabbits. *Anesthesiology* 1991;74:89.
134. Santos AC, Pedersen H, Harmon TW, et al. Does pregnancy alter the systemic toxicity of local anesthetics? *Anesthesiology* 1989;70:991.
135. Rosen MA, Thigpen JW, Shnider SM, Foutz SE, Levinson G, Koike M. Bupivacaine-induced cardiotoxicity in hypoxic and acidotic sheep. *Anesth Analg* 1985;64:1089.
136. Sage DJ, Feldman HS, Arthur R, et al. Influence of lidocaine and bupivacaine on isolated guinea pig atria in the presence of acidosis and hypoxia. *Anesth Analg* 1984;63:1.
137. Moore DC, Crawford RD, Scurlock JE. Severe hypoxia and acidosis following local anesthetic-induced convulsions. *Anesthesiology* 1980; 53:259.
138. Kasten GW, Martin ST. Successful cardiovascular resuscitation after massive intravenous bupivacaine overdosage in anesthetized dogs. *Anesth Analg* 1985;64:491.
139. Kambam JR, Kinney WW, Matsuda F, Wright W, Holaday DA. Epinephrine and phenylephrine increase cardiorespiratory toxicity of intravenously administered bupivacaine in rats. *Anesth Analg* 1990; 70:543.
140. Timour Q, Freysz M, Mazze R, Couzon P, Bertrix L, Faucon G. Enhancement by hyponatremia and hyperkalemia of ventricular conduction and rhythm disorders caused by bupivacaine. *Anesthesiology* 1990;72:1051.
141. Edouard AR, Berdeaux A, Ahmad R, Samii K. Cardiovascular interactions of local anesthetics and calcium entry blockers in dogs. *Reg Anesth* 1991;16:95.
142. Timour Q, Freysz M, Couzon P, et al. Possible role of drug interactions in bupivacaine-induced problems related to intraventricular conduction disorders. *Reg Anesth* 1990;15:180.
143. Kasten GW, Martin ST. Bupivacaine cardiovascular toxicity: comparison of treatment with bretylium and lidocaine. *Anesth Analg* 1985; 64:911.
144. Lacombe P, Blaise G, Hollmann C, Tanguay M, Loulmet D. Isoproterenol corrects the effects of bupivacaine on the electrophysiologic properties of the isolated rabbit heart. *Anesth Analg* 1991;72:70.
145. Solomon D, Bunegin L, Albin M. The effect of magnesium sulfate administration on cerebral and cardiac toxicity of bupivacaine in dogs. *Anesthesiology* 1990;72:341.
146. Kasten GW, Martin ST. Resuscitation from bupivacaine-induced cardiovascular toxicity during partial inferior vena cava occlusion. *Anesth Analg* 1986;65:341.
147. DePace NC, Betesh JS, Koller MN. "Postmortem" cesarean section with recovery of both mother and fetus. *JAMA* 1982;248:971.
148. Kasten GW, Martin ST. Comparison of resuscitation of sheep and dogs after bupivacaine-induced cardiovascular collapse. *Anesth Analg* 1986;65:1029.
149. Cohen SE, Cherry CM, Holbrook H, El-Sayed YY, Gibson RN, Jaffe RA. Intrathecal sufentanil for labor analgesia—sensory changes, side effects, and fetal heart rate changes. *Anesth Analg* 1993;77:1155.
150. Campbell DC, Banner R, Crone LA, Gore-Hickman W, Yip RW. Addition of epinephrine to intrathecal bupivacaine and sufentanil for ambulatory labor analgesia. *Anesthesiology* 1997;86:525.
151. Nielsen PE, Erickson R, Abouleish EI, Perriatt S, Sheppard C. Fetal heart rate changes after intrathecal sufentanil or epidural bupivacaine for labor analgesia: incidence and clinical significance. *Anesth Analg* 1996;83:742.
152. Collis RE, Baxandall ML, Srikantharajah ID, Edge G, Kadim MY, Morgan BM. Combined spinal epidural (CSE) analgesia: technique, management, and outcome of 300 mothers. *Int J Obstet Anesth* 1994;3:75.
153. Eberle RL, Norris MC, Eberle AM, Naulty JS, Arkoosh VA. The effect of maternal position on fetal heart rate during epidural or intrathecal analgesia for labor. *Am J Obstet Gynecol* 179:150.
154. Clarke VT, Smiley RM, Finster M. Uterine hyperactivity after intrathecal injection of fentanyl for analgesia during labor: a cause of fetal bradycardia? [Letter] *Anesthesiology* 1994;81:1083.
155. Lederman RP, McCann DS, Work B, Huber MJ. Endogenous plasma epinephrine and norepinephrine in last-trimester pregancy and labor. *Am J Obstet Gynecol* 1977;129:5.
156. Segal S, Csavoy A, Datta S. Tocolytic effects of maternal catecholamines. *Anesthesiology* 1997;87:A915.
157. Lederman RP, Lederman E, Work B Jr, McCann DS. Anxiety and epinephrine in multiparous women in labor: relationship to duration of labor and fetal heart rate pattern. *Am J Obstet Gynecol* 1985; 153:870.
158. Hays RL, Palmer CM. Respiratory depression after intrathecal sufentanil during labor. *Anesthesiology* 1994;81:511.
159. Baker MN, Sarna MC. Respiratory arrest after second dose of intrathecal sufentanil. *Anesthesiology* 1995;83:231.
160. Ferouz F, Norris MC, Leighton BL. Risk of respiratory arrest after intrathecal sufentanil. *Anesth Analg* 1997;85:1088.
161. Palmer CM. Early respiratory depression following intrathecal fentanyl-morphine combination. *Anesthesiology* 1991;74:1153.
162. Brockway MS, Noble DW, Sharwood-Smith GH, McClure JH. Profound respiratory depression after extradural fentanyl. *Br J Anaesth* 1990;64:243.
163. Eng M, Zorotovich RA. Broken-needle complication with a disposible spinal introducer. *Anesthesiology* 1977;46:147.
164. Schlake PT, Peleman RR, Winnie AP. Separation of the hub from the shaft of a disposable epidural needle. *Anesthesiology* 1988;68:611.
165. Snow JC, Kripke BJ, Sakellarides H, et al. Broken disposable needle

during an axillary approach to block the brachial plexus. *Anesth Analg* 1974;53:89.
166. Bonica JJ. Peridural block: analysis of 3,637 cases and a review. *Anesthesiology* 1957;18:723.
167. Chun L, Karp M. Unusual complications from placement of catheters in caudal canal in obstetrical anesthesia. *Anesthesiology* 1966;27:96.
168. Hutchison GL: The severance of epidural catheters. *Anaesthesia* 1987;42:182.
169. Hehre FW, Muechler HC. Complications associated with use of extradural catheter in obstetric anesthesia. *Anesth Analg* 1965;45:245.
170. Nash TG, Openshaw DJ. Unusual complication of epidural anaesthesia. *Br Med J* 1968;2:700.
171. Wolfson B, Siker E, Gray G. Post-pneumoenceopalography headache. *Anaesthesia* 1970;25:328.
172. Heaney GAH. An interesting dural tap. *Anaesthesia* 1984;39:386.
173. Bickler PE, Schapera A, Bainton CR. Acute radial nerve injury from use of an automatic blood pressure monitor. *Anesthesiology* 1990;73:186.
174. Sy WP. Ulnar nerve palsy possibly related to use of automatically cycled blood pressure cuff. *Anesth Analg* 1981;60:687.
175. Ochoa J, Noordenbos W. Pathology and disordered sensation in local nerve lesions. In: Bonica JJ, Liebeskind JC, Albe-Fessard DG, eds. *Advances in pain research and therapy.* New York: Raven Press, 1979:68.
176. Casady GN, Moore DC, Bridenbaugh LD. Postpartum hypertension after use of vasoconstrictor and oxytocic drugs. *JAMA* 1960;172:1011.
177. Durant TM, Long J, Oppenheimer MJ. Pulmonary venous air embolism. *Am Heart J* 1947;33:269.
178. Lifschultz BD, Donoghue ER. Air embolism during intercourse in pregnancy. *J Forensic Sci* 1983;28:1021.
179. Aronson ME, Nelson PK. Fatal air embolism in pregnancy resulting from an unusual sexual act. *Obstet Gynecol* 1967;30:127.
180. Fong J, Galadalla F, Druzin M. Venous emboli occurring during caesarean section: the effect of patient position. *Can J Anaesth* 1991;38:191.
181. Karuparthy VR, Downing JW, Husain FJ, et al. Incidence of venous air embolism during cesarean section is unchanged by the use of a 5 to 10 degree head-up tilt. *Anesth Analg* 1989;69:620.
182. Fong J, Gadalla F, Pierri K, Druzin M. Are Doppler-detected venous emboli during cesarean section air emboli? *Anesth Analg* 1990;71:254.
183. Younker D, Rodriguez V, Kavanagh J. Massive air embolism during cesarean section. *Anesthesiology* 1986;65:77.
184. Waldrop GS. Fatal air embolism during term labor and the pueriperium. *Obstet Gynecol* 1953;1:450.
185. Palmer CM, Norris MC, Giudici MC, Leighton BL, DeSimone CA. Incidence of electrocardiographic changes during cesarean delivery under regional anesthesia. *Anesth Analg* 1990;70:36.
186. Zakowski MI, Ramanathan S, Baratta JB, et al. Electrocardiographic changes during cesarean section: a cause for concern? *Anesth Analg* 1993;76:162.
187. McLintic AJ, Pringle SD, Lilley S, Houston AB, Thorburn J. Electrocardiographic changes during cesarean section under regional anesthesia. *Anesth Analg* 1992;74:51.
188. Mathew JP, Fleisher LA, Rinehouse JA, et al. ST segment depression during labor and delivery. *Anesthesiology* 1992;77:635.
189. King TA, Adams AP. Failed tracheal intubation. *Br J Anaesth* 1990;65:400.
190. Cohen SE. Aspiration syndromes in pregnancy [Editorial]. *Anesthesiology* 1979;51:375.
191. Samsoon GLT, Young JRB. Difficult tracheal intubation: a retrospective study. *Anaesthesia* 1987;42:487.
192. Lyons G. Failed intubation. Six year's experience in a teaching maternity unit. *Anesthesia* 1985;40:759.
193. Fahy L, Horton WA, Charters P. Factor analysis in patients with a history of failed tracheal intubation during pregnancy. *Br J Anaesth* 1990;65:813.
194. Rubin GL, Peterson HB, Rochat RW, McCarthy BJ, Terry JS. Maternal death after cesarean section in Georgia. *Am J Obstet Gynecol* 1981;139:681.
195. Department of Health. *Report on confidential enquiries into maternal deaths in England and Wales, 1982–84.* London: Her Majesty's Stationery Office, 1989.
196. Gibb D. Confidential enquiry into maternal death [Editorial]. *Br J Obstet Gynaecol* 1990;97:97.
197. Hawkins JL, Koonin LM, Palmer SK, Gibbs CP. Anesthesia-related deaths during obstetric delivery in the United States, 1979–1990. *Anesthesiology* 1997;86:277.
198. Gibbs CP. Gastric aspiration: prevention and treatment. *Clin Anesthesiol* 1986;4:47.
199. Chadwick HS, Posner K, Caplan RA, Ward RJ, Cheney FW. A comparison of obstetric and nonobstetric anesthesia malpractice claims. *Anesthesiology* 1991;74:242.
200. Joupilla R, Joupilla P, Hollmen A. Laryngeal oedema as an obstetric anesthetic complication. *Acta Anaesthesiol Scand* 1980;24:97.
201. Mackenzie AI. Laryngeal oedema complicating obstetric anaesthesia. *Anaesthesia* 1978;33:271.
202. Malan TP, Johnson MD. The difficult airway in obstetric anesthesia: techniques for airway management and the role of regional anesthesia. *J Clin Anesth* 1988;1:104.
203. McClune S, Regan M, Moore J. Laryngeal mask airway for caesarean section. *Anaesthesia* 1990;45:227.
204. Gataure PS, Hughes JA. The laryngeal mask airway in obstetrical anaesthesia. *Can J Anaesth* 1995;42:130.
205. Barker P, Langton JA, Murphy PJ, Rowbotham DJ. Regurgitation of gastric contents during general anaesthesia using the laryngeal mask airway. *Br J Anaesth* 1992;69:314.
206. Valentine J, Stakes AF, Bellamy MC. Reflux during positive pressure ventilation through the laryngeal mask. *Br J Anaesth* 1994;73:543.
207. LeFrock JL, Clark TS, Davies B, Klainer AS. Aspiration pneumonia: a ten-year review. *Am Surg* 1979;45:305.
208. Spence AA, Moir DD, Finlay WEI. Observations on intragastric pressure. *Anaesthesia* 1967;22:249.
209. Lind JF, Smith AM, McIver DK, Coopland AT, Crispin JS. Heartburn in pregnancy-a manometric study. *Can Med Assoc J* 1968;98:571.
210. Hey VMF, Cowley DJ, Ganguli PC, Skinner LD, Ostick DG, Sharp DS. Gastro-oesophageal reflux in late pregnancy. *Anaesthesia* 1977;32:372.
211. Christofides ND, Ghatei MA, Bloom SR, Borberg C, Gillmer MDG. Decreased plasma motilin concentrations in pregnancy. *Br Med J* 1982;285:1453.
212. Attia RR, Ebeid AM, Fischer JE, Goudsouzian NG. Maternal fetal and placental gastrin concentrations. *Anaesthesia* 1982;37:18.
213. Murray FA, Erskine JP, Fielding J. Gastric secretion in pregnancy. *J Obstet Gynecol* 1957;64:373.
214. Wilson J. Gastric emptying in labour: some recent findings and their clinical significance. *J Int Med Res* 1978;6[Suppl 1]:54.
215. LaSilvia LA, Steffen EA. Delayed gastric emptying time in labor. *Am J Obstet Gynecol* 1950;59:1075.
216. Holdsworth JD. Relationship between stomach contents and analgesia in labour. *Br J Anaesth* 1978;50:1145.
217. Awe WC, Fletcher WS, Jacob SW. The pathophysiology of aspiration pneumonitis. *Surgery* 1966;60:232.
218. Bynum LJ, Pierce AK. Pulmonary aspiration of gastric contents. *Am Rev Respir Dis* 1976;114:1129.
219. Lewis RT, Burgess JH, Hampson LG. Cardiorespiratory studies in critical illness: changes in aspiration pneumonitis. *Arch Surg* 1971;103:335.
220. Mendelson CL. The aspiration of stomach contents into the lungs during obstetric anesthesia. *Am J Obstet Gynecol* 1946;52:191.
221. Teabeaut JR. Aspiration of gastric contents: an experimental study. *Am J Pathol* 1952;28:51.
222. Schwartz DJ, Wynne JW, Gibbs CP, Hood CI, Kuck EJ. The pulmonary consequences of aspiration of gastric contents at pH values greater than 2.5. *Am Rev Respir Dis* 1980;121:119.
223. Sarwar H, Sprague DH. Laryngospasm as an early indicator of aspiration. *Anesth Analg* 1978;57:119.
224. Chapman RL, Modell JH, Ruiz BC, Calderwood HW, Hood CI, Graves SA. Effect of continuous positive-pressure ventilation and steroids on aspiration of hydrochloric acid (pH 1.8) in dogs. *Anesth Analg* 1974;53:556.
225. Nader-Djalal N, Knight PR, Bacon MF, Tait AR, Kennedy TP, Johnson KJ. Alterations in the course of acid-induced lung injury in rats after general anesthesia: volatile anesthetics versus ketamine. *Anesth Analg* 1998;86:141.
226. Hamelberg W, Bosomworth PP. Aspiration pneumonitis: experimental studies and clinical observations. *Anesth Analg* 1964;43:669.
227. Wynne JW, Reynolds JC, Hood CI, Auerbach D, Ondrasick J. Steroid

therapy for pneumonitis induced in rabbits by aspiration of foodstuff. *Anesthesiology* 1979;51:11.
228. Wynne JW, DeMarco FJ, Hood CI. Physiological effects of corticosteroids in foodstuff aspiration. *Arch Surg* 1981;116:46.
229. Chapman RL, Downs JB, Modell JH, Hood CI. The ineffectiveness of steroid therapy in treating aspiration of hydrochloric acid. *Arch Surg* 1974;108:858.
230. James CF, Modell JH, Gibbs CP, Kuck EJ, Ruiz BC. Pulmonary aspiration-effects of volume and pH in the rat. *Anesth Analg* 1984; 63:665.
231. Gibbs CP, Spohr L, Schmidt D. The effectiveness of sodium citrate as an antacid. *Anesthesiology* 1982;57:44.
232. Roberts RB, Shirley MA. Reducing the risk of acid aspiration during cesarean section. *Anesth Analg* 1974;53:859.
233. Taylor G. Acid pulmonary aspiration syndrome after antacids: a case report. *Br J Anaesth* 1975;47:615.
234. Whittington RM, Robinson JS, Thompson JM. Fatal aspiration (Mendelson's) syndrome despite antacids and cricoid pressure. *Lancet* 1979;ii:228.
235. Bond VK, Stoelting RK, Gupta CD. Pulmonary aspiration syndrome after inhalation of gastric fluid containing antacids. *Anesthesiology* 1979;51:452.
236. Gibbs CP, Schwartz DJ, Wynne JW, Hood CI, Kuck EJ. Antacid pulmonary aspiration in the dog. *Anesthesiology* 1979;51:380.
237. Tordoff SG, Sweeney BP. Acid aspiration prophylaxis in 288 obstetric anaesthesia departments in the United Kingdom. *Anaesthesia* 1990; 45:776.
238. Ewart MC, Yau G, Gin T, Kotur CF, Oh TE. A comparison of the effects of omeprazole and ranitidine on gastric secretion in women undergoing elective caesarean section. *Anaesthesia* 1990;45:527.
239. Bylsma-Howell M, Riggs KW, McMorland GH, et al. Placental transport of metoclopramide: assessment of maternal and neonatal effects. *Can Anaesth Soc J* 1983;30:487.
240. Howard FA, Sharp DS. Effect of metoclopramide on gastric emptying during labor. *Br Med J* 1973;1:446.
241. Nimmo WS, Wilson J, Prescott LF. Narcotic analgesics and delayed gastric emptying during labor. *Lancet* 1975;i:890.
242. Brock-Utne JG, Rubin J, Downing JW, Dimopoulos GE, Moshal MG, Naiker M. The administration of metoclopramide with atropine. *Anaesthesia* 1976;31:1186.
243. Brock-Utne JG, Rubin J, Welman S, Dimpoulos GE, Moshal MG, Downing JW. The action of commonly used antiemetics on the lower oesophageal sphincter. *Br J Anaesth* 1978;50:295.
244. Howells TH, Khanam T, Kreel L, Seymour C, Oliver B, Davies JAH. Pharmacological emptying of the stomach with metoclopramide. *Br Med J* 1971;2:558.
245. Baraka A, Saab M, Salem M, et al. Control of gastric acidity by glycopyrrolate premedication in the parturient. *Anesth Analg* 1977;56: 642.
246. Stoelting RK. Responses to atropine, glycopyrrolate and Riopan of gastric fluid pH and volume in adult patients. *Anesthesiology* 1978;48: 367.
247. Merrill RB, Hingson RA. Study of incidence of maternal mortality from aspiration of vomitus during anesthesia occurring in major obstetric hospitals in United States. *Anesth Analg* 1951;30:121.
248. Hutchinson BR. Acid aspiration syndrome [Correspondence]. *Br J Anaesth* 1979;51:75.
249. Scott DB. Mendelson's syndrome [Editorial]. *Br J Anaesth* 1978; 50:977.
250. Cohen SE. Aspiration syndromes in pregnancy [Editorial]. *Anesthesiology* 1979;51:375.
251. Endler GC, Mariona G, Sokol RJ, Stevenson LB. Anesthesia-related maternal mortality in Michigan, 1972 to 1984. *Am J Obstet Gynecol* 1988;159:187.
252. Gibbs CP, Rolbin SH, Norman P. Cause and prevention of maternal aspiration [Correspondence]. *Anesthesiology* 1984;61:111.

Obstetric Anesthesia, second edition,
edited by Mark C. Norris.
Lippincott Williams & Wilkins, Philadelphia © 1999.

CHAPTER 33

Anesthesia and the Compromised Fetus

Kathleen A. Leavitt

Few situations in obstetric anesthesia are as anxiety provoking as sudden fetal compromise requiring emergent delivery. No anesthesiologist caring for the parturient is immune to this occurrence. Yet, more often than not, a vigorous neonate is delivered after an emergency cesarean section, mocking the frantic efforts of those trying to rescue it from a hostile in utero environment. There are several reasons for this phenomenon:

- We have limited ability to directly assess fetal status.
- There are no clearly defined criteria to determine at what point "fetal distress" will result in permanent neurological injury or death.
- Once "fetal distress" is suspected, many feel that only immediate operative delivery meets the standard of care expected of a reasonably prudent physician.

This chapter will explore these controversial issues and provide recommendations for the provision of safe, effective anesthetic care to the parturient with a potentially compromised fetus.

DEFINITION

Fetal distress is an imprecise, poorly defined term, which is applied indiscriminately to a variety of intrapartum events and fetal conditions including:

- Abnormal or "nonreassuring" fetal heart rate patterns,
- Intrauterine growth restriction,
- Oligohydramnios,
- Meconium-stained amniotic fluid, and
- Newborns born with low Apgar scores or umbilical cord blood pH.

However, none of these conditions carries much, if any, prognostic significance, because the majority of fetuses with these diagnoses are vigorous at birth and have no adverse long-term sequelae.

To better define the term *fetal distress*, we must first understand placental gas exchange. The fetus depends on placental exchange for delivery of oxygen and nutrients, and for the elimination of metabolic waste. Waste products come in two forms: volatile acids (CO_2), which readily diffuse into the maternal circulation, and organic acids (lactic acid), which slowly cross the placenta. The bidirectional exchange of oxygen and waste products takes place in the intervillous space where maternal blood bathes the fetal capillaries within the placental villi (1).

Asphyxia occurs when there is an interruption of fetal oxygen supply or respiratory gas exchange. Asphyxia leads to fetal **hypoxemia** and **hypercarbia**. Prolonged hypoxemia deprives fetal tissues of oxygen (hypoxia) and leads to anaerobic glycolysis, lactic acid production, and **metabolic acidosis** (1). However, all fetuses are born hypoxemic, with a mixed respiratory and metabolic acidosis, and are, in a sense "asphyxiated" (2). This physiologic adaptation may facilitate the prompt conversion to the adult circulatory pattern (2). Only severe, prolonged asphyxia is thought to be of consequence to the fetus.

The challenge, then, is to apply the term *fetal distress* only to those instances when the duration and extent of hypoxemia produces adverse neonatal outcome. Therefore, *fetal distress* is more accurately defined as "persistent *fetal asphyxia* that, if not corrected or circumvented, will result in permanent neurologic damage or death" (2).

PHYSIOLOGIC RESPONSE TO ASPHYXIA

The fetal response to an interruption in its blood supply has been studied in a variety of animals (3,4). One early physiologic response is decreased fetal breathing and body movement in an effort to decrease oxygen consumption (5). Then, blood flows away from splanchnic and peripheral vascular beds toward the brain, heart,

K.A. Leavitt: Department of Obstetric Anesthesia, George Washington University Hospital, Washington, DC 20037.

adrenal glands, and placenta. The wide variety of hormonal and cardiovascular mediators of this response include the sympathetic and parasympathetic nervous systems, baroreceptors, chemoreceptors, vasopressin, prostacyclin, and other prostaglandins (2).

In response to asphyxia, fetal oxygen consumption decreases by 50%, mostly from metabolic changes in underperfused vascular beds (6). Anaerobic glycolysis in these areas gradually produces a metabolic acidosis, which is completely reversible if the hypoxemia is corrected within 1 hour. With moderate degrees of hypoxemia, cardiac output is maintained. However, severe, prolonged hypoxemia impairs myocardial contractility, decreases cardiac output, and leads to intense vasoconstriction and hypoperfusion of all vascular beds (7). Both metabolic and respiratory acidosis ensue, with irreversible organ damage, hypotension, bradycardia, and eventually fetal death.

CAUSES OF FETAL DISTRESS

Although fetal distress may occur precipitously, most often fetal deterioration follows a continuum as a chronically compromised or *stressed* fetus is further deprived of nutritional blood flow and becomes hypoxemic and *distressed.* Perhaps the best analogy likens fetal stress and distress to the development of myocardial ischemia before myocardial infarction (8). As with myocardial ischemia and infarction, if fetal stress is detected, therapeutic measures may avoid irreversible ischemic damage. However, unlike myocardial ischemia, there are no clearly defined criteria, such as ST-segment depression or elevation, to determine when fetal stress or distress are present.

The exact cause of fetal distress is seldom known with certainty, but can be categorized as originating from the mother, her uterus, the placenta, the umbilical cord, or the fetus (Fig. 1). Fetal perfusion depends primarily on uterine blood flow. The uterine vessels are dilated maximally at term, and, unlike other vascular beds that undergo autoregulation, these vessels cannot dilate further in response to decreased aortic blood flow or increased fetal metabolic demand. Therefore, uteroplacental blood flow varies directly with maternal arterial perfusion pressure. Hypotension, from decreased maternal cardiac output due to aortocaval compression, sympathetic blockade, or hypovolemia, directly lowers placental perfusion. Chronic maternal vascular diseases, such as hypertension, diabetes, or systemic lupus erythematosus, produce uterine vascular insufficiency. Oxygen delivery to the fetus may be inadequate with severe maternal anemia or hypoxemia despite the preservation of adequate uterine blood flow. Although uterine blood vessels are dilated maximally at term, α-adrenergic stimulation from

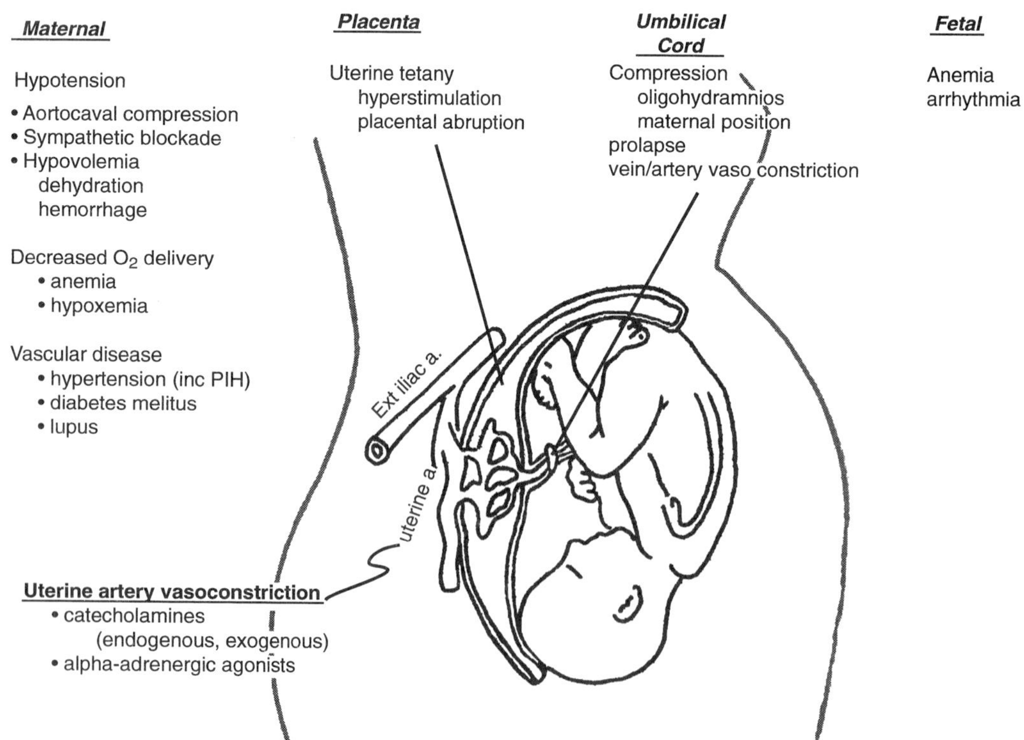

FIG. 1. Fetal distress can be categorized as originating from the mother, her uterus, the placenta, the umbilical cord, or the fetus.

endogenous or exogenous catecholamines will cause intense vasoconstriction and decrease uterine blood flow.

Because the blood supply to the placenta traverses the myometrium, uterine contractions transiently decrease intervillous blood flow in proportion to their duration, intensity, and frequency. Therefore, sustained or tetanic uterine contractions from overstimulation with oxytocin or from placental abruption significantly impair placental perfusion.

Umbilical cord occlusion can dramatically reduce blood flow to the fetus. The risk of umbilical cord compression is enhanced by the presence of oligohydramnios and also can depend on maternal position. Other conditions that predispose to sudden umbilical cord occlusion from umbilical cord prolapse include multiple gestation after the birth of the first baby and nonvertex fetal presentations with rupture of membranes.

Conditions that interfere with oxygen delivery within the fetal circulation, such as fetal anemia or arrhythmias, may result in acute fetal distress.

TABLE 1. *Diagnostic modalities used to detect fetal distress*

Antepartum
Nonstress test
Contraction stress test
Biophysical profile
Fetal breathing movement
Gross body movement
Fetal tone
Amniotic fluid volume
Fetal heart rate analysis
Doppler ultrasound
Umbilical blood flow velocity
Intrapartum
Continuous electronic fetal heart rate monitor
Intermittent auscultation of fetal heart rate
Fetal pulse oximetry
Fetal scalp capillary blood pH
Postpartum
Apgar scores
Umbilical cord blood gas analysis
Neurobehavioral testing

Diagnosis

Because the effects of moderate, transient hypoxemia are fairly reversible and of little consequence, the ultimate task of those caring for any parturient is the detection of inadequate perfusion that, if not corrected, will cause irreversible fetal damage. Detection must be followed by timely intervention to either restore fetal oxygen delivery or remove the fetus from the hostile intrauterine environment. This principle is simple, yet our inability to directly assess fetal well-being is a major obstacle to its attainment. Presently, there are no clinically useful diagnostic tests that allow us to specifically detect insufficient fetal oxygen delivery. Instead, we rely on modalities that indirectly measure fetal status (Table 1).

Antepartum

Antepartum fetal compromise can be detected by maternal assessment of fetal movement, nonstress and contraction stress testing, biophysical profile, and Doppler ultrasound measurement of umbilical blood flow velocity. The biophysical profile, which is like an in utero Apgar score, is probably the most clinically useful diagnostic modality. It evaluates the following five discrete biophysical variables:

- Fetal breathing movement,
- Gross body movement,
- Fetal tone,
- Amniotic fluid volume, and
- Fetal heart rate.

The presence of a normal parameter is awarded two points, whereas the absence of that parameter is scored as zero. The compromised fetus will attempt to conserve oxygen by suspending diaphragmatic and limb movement. Oligohydramnios may indicate poor fetal renal perfusion and is defined by an amniotic fluid index (AFI) less than or equal to 5 (9,10). AFI is calculated by dividing the uterine cavity into four quadrants and measuring the vertical diameter of the largest amniotic fluid pocket in each quadrant. These four measurements are added to obtain the AFI in centimeters. The final component of the biophysical profile consists of a nonstress test using external fetal heart rate monitoring. A low biophysical profile (less than 6) is a sensitive, specific, and highly predictive indicator of acidotic umbilical cord blood (11).

Doppler ultrasound measurement of fetal umbilical artery blood flow velocity waveforms reflects placental vascular resistance (12). Under normal conditions, vascular resistance within the placenta is extremely low and continues to decrease as the number and cross-sectional area of vascular channels increase throughout gestation. Measurement of blood flow velocity in the umbilical artery provides an estimation of the downstream vascular resistance within the placenta. When there is significant placental pathology and vascular insufficiency, increased placental vascular resistance will be detected by a decrease in diastolic blood flow through the umbilical artery. The pulsatility index (PI) is the ratio of systolic to diastolic blood flow velocity (S/D ratio). Serial measurements of PI are used to monitor suspected placental insufficiency and to assess the efficacy of therapeutic maneuvers (13,14).

Umbilical artery Doppler velocimetry may help predict poor perinatal outcome and confirm the presence of fetal compromise during labor (15). In one study of fetuses with worrisome heart rate patterns, abnormal umbilical artery blood flow velocity waveforms were highly predictive of poor perinatal outcome (i.e., small for gestational age, low Apgar score, acidosis, meconium below the neonatal vocal cords, neonatal hospital stay longer than 3 days, and neonatal intensive care unit admission) (15). Therefore, umbilical velocimetry may be a useful adjunct to intrapartum fetal heart rate analysis in detecting true fetal distress. Because only a few clinicians have mastered the use of continuous-wave Doppler velocimetry, this technique is underutilized in routine clinical practice.

Intrapartum

Fetal Heart Rate

Electronic fetal heart rate analysis remains the principal diagnostic modality used to detect fetal compromise. Observation of the baseline heart rate, variability, and periodic changes in heart rate associated with uterine contractions provides an indirect assessment of fetal status. Because these parameters are under the direct control of the central nervous system (CNS), a normal fetal heart rate tracing is thought to represent an intact axis between the CNS and cardiovascular system. Asphyxia interferes with this axis and produces characteristic changes in the fetal heart rate tracing as the fetus moves through a continuum of decompensation (Table 2).

At first, a neurologically intact fetus will develop a tachycardia in an attempt to increase cardiac output and oxygen delivery in response to asphyxia. With progressive hypoxemia and acidosis, the fetus attempts to divert blood flow to the brain, heart, and adrenal glands through intense vasoconstriction to other vascular beds. A dramatic increase in systemic vascular resistance and reflex bradycardia or deceleration of the fetal heart rate ensues.

TABLE 2. *Fetal heart rate characteristics*

	Baseline heart rate (beats/min)	Variability (beats/min)	Periodic changes
Normal	120–160	3–25	Accelerations, Early decelerations
Fetal stress	Tachycardia	>3–5	Variable decelerations, Late decelerations (moderate to severe)
Fetal distress	Bradycardia	ABSENT, unresponsive to stimuli	Variable decelerations, Late decelerations (moderate to severe)

Fetal heart rate decelerations are mediated by chemoreceptor and baroreceptor stimulation of the vagus nerve and can be categorized as early, variable, or late according to their timing in relation to the onset of a uterine contraction. Early decelerations are a benign vagal response to fetal head compression and do not indicate asphyxia.

Variable decelerations represent umbilical cord compression and often occur whenever amniotic fluid volume is decreased (i.e., oligohydramnios and premature or artificial rupture of membranes). Repetitive or prolonged umbilical cord compression can lead to progressive fetal asphyxia and acidosis, manifested by persistent fetal bradycardia. Transvaginal infusion of saline into the amniotic cavity reproduces the cushioning effect of amniotic fluid and decreases the frequency and severity of variable decelerations, end-stage bradycardia, and operative delivery for fetal distress (16,17). Amnioinfusion should be instituted prophylactically, before the development of significant fetal distress, because it may take up to 30 minutes to infuse a sufficient volume. Reported complications of amnioinfusion include umbilical cord prolapse, uterine overdistention, fetal bradycardia, dehiscence of uterine cesarean scar, and amniotic fluid embolism (18–20). Less severe umbilical cord compression often can be treated by changing maternal position.

Late decelerations are associated with more serious fetal hypoxemia from uteroplacental insufficiency. They are characterized by smooth, uniform, U-shaped decelerations that produce a delayed, but mirror, image of the uterine contraction. The latency between the onset of the contraction and the beginning of the deceleration shortens as fetal hypoxemia worsens (21).

The beat-to-beat variability of the fetal heart rate is the most important parameter in predicting fetal hypoxemia. Beat-to-beat variability represents the constant push–pull effect of the sympathetic and parasympathetic nervous systems exerted on the fetal heart and indicates an intact axis between the central nervous and cardiovascular systems. It usually ranges between 3 and 25 beats/min. Beat-to-beat variability may be diminished or absent with fetal sleep cycles, hypoglycemia, and maternally administered narcotics and sedatives. However, loss of variability caused by these conditions usually is reversed by fetal scalp or vibroacoustic stimulation. Persistent, irreversible loss of beat-to-beat variability, devoid of accelerations or decelerations in the fetal heart rate tracing, should alert the clinician to the development of true fetal distress requiring immediate delivery. Loss of baseline variability has been shown to correlate well with umbilical artery acidemia at birth (22,23).

Electronic fetal heart rate monitoring (EFM), when used correctly, can increase the chance of detecting the rare event of fetal distress. It is clear, however, that EFM has several limitations (Table 3). First, interpretation of fetal heart rate patterns is very subjective. "Experts"

TABLE 3. *Limitations of electronic fetal heart rate monitoring*

1. Interpretation is subjective
2. Uses only one physiologic variable (fetal heart rate) to assess fetal status
3. False-positive diagnosis of fetal asphyxia is high
4. False-positive tracings cause a high incidence of unnecessary operative interventions
5. Same short- or long-term neurological outcome as auscultation of fetal heart tones

differ widely in their interpretation of fetal heart rate tracings among themselves (interobserver) and by the same individual when the tracing is read on more than one occasion (intraobserver) (24). Second, EFM uses only one physiologic variable to assess fetal status. "Perhaps reminding ourselves that the EFM is nothing more than a heart rate derived from serial R-R intervals, or essentially a patient's pulse, would serve to temper our expectations. Few physicians would attempt to diagnose equally serious medical conditions in the adult by standing at the bedside and taking a pulse" (8). Third, EFM is a very sensitive, yet nonspecific, test. When applied to the general population, there will be a high incidence of false-positive diagnoses of fetal distress and many unnecessary operative interventions.

Specific fetal heart rate abnormalities do correlate with subsequent neurological damage (cerebral palsy) (25). Multiple late decelerations and decreased beat-to-beat variability are associated with an increased risk of cerebral palsy. However, in one study, those children who developed cerebral palsy represented only 0.19% of all the fetuses that displayed such fetal monitoring findings. Thus, 99.8% of fetuses who had multiple late decelerations and decreased beat-to-beat variability did not develop cerebral palsy. When these data are extrapolated to the population in the United States, approximately 10% of all electronically monitored labors will show these same fetal heart rate patterns in the absence of subsequent cerebral palsy. If operative intervention is applied to all these labors, there will be 516 unnecessary interventions performed for each child "saved" from cerebral palsy (25).

Continuous EFM was introduced into clinical practice nearly 30 years ago with the hope that it would prevent the majority of birth injuries due to hypoxemia or asphyxia. Specifically, many anticipated dramatic reductions in the incidence of cerebral palsy and long-term neurological deficits. Continuous EFM became widely used before randomized clinical studies could determine its efficacy. In the intervening years, 12 studies have been published that compare long-term neurological outcome and perinatal mortality in pregnancies monitored electronically or with intermittent auscultation. These studies found no differences in the rates of intrapartum and neonatal death, or short or long-term neurologic morbidity when continuous EFM is used instead of intermittent auscultation (26). These findings have prompted the American College of Obstetricians and Gynecologists to accept both intermittent and continuous monitoring of the fetal heart rate during labor in its standards and guidelines (27). There is an important lesson to be learned from our 30-year experience with the technology of EFM. "Continuous EFM promised much but has achieved little. Its premature acceptance highlights the need for appropriate testing of all new forms of technology before they are introduced into clinical practice" (28).

Fetal Oxygen Saturation

Currently, investigators are studying the use of fetal oxygen saturation monitoring to assess fetal well-being during labor (29,30). Oxygen saturation may prove more useful than EFM because it allows direct, noninvasive assessment of fetal oxygenation. In contrast to conventional transmission pulse oximeters, where the photodetector lies on the opposite side of the tissue bed, fetal oxygen saturation monitors use reflectance sensors with the photodetector located adjacent to the light-emitting diodes. The pulse oximeter probe is placed transvaginally between the uterine wall and the fetus and contacts the fetal presenting part, usually the fetal cheek or scalp. Application of fetal pulse oximetry has been hampered by several technical obstacles, including suboptimal sensor contact causing inadequate signal strength, artifactually lower SpO_2 values in the presence of meconium, caput formation, or thick, curly hair and a wide range of normal SpO_2 values. Before this instrument is introduced into routine clinical practice, investigators have the formidable task of correlating the duration and magnitude of "abnormal" SpO_2 values with the development of fetal acidosis, low Apgar scores, and adverse neonatal outcome.

Fetal oxygen saturation monitoring has the potential to revolutionize intrapartum obstetric management, just as the use of adult and pediatric pulse oximetry has significantly influenced all aspects of medicine. Currently, studies are attempting to determine if the combined use of fetal oxygen saturation and heart rate monitoring can reduce the frequency of cesarean section for fetal distress.

Fetal Scalp pH

The use of fetal scalp capillary blood sampling to confirm the diagnosis of fetal distress has nearly been abandoned in contemporary obstetric practice (31). It has long been realized that fetal scalp blood sampling is a technically difficult and often inaccurate test. Fetal scalp pH is affected by maternal pH, fetal scalp blood flow, and caput formation. The fetal heart rate response to scalp blood sampling is probably a more useful indicator of fetal acidemia (pH less than 7.20) (32). Significant fetal acidosis is unlikely if manual fetal scalp stimulation produces fetal heart rate acceleration or increased short-term variability.

Meconium

A discussion of intrapartum fetal monitoring would not be complete without mentioning meconium-stained amniotic fluid. Meconium has traditionally been regarded as a sign of intrapartum fetal stress. However, the significance of meconium passage is poorly understood, and some suggest that it is merely a sign of a normally functioning fetal gastrointestinal tract (33). Meconium-stained amniotic fluid occurs in up to 44% of pregnancies and has never been consistently associated with abnormal fetal heart rate tracings, acidosis, or low Apgar scores (34). Therefore, passage of meconium does not, by itself, signify fetal distress. However, its presence should prompt the obstetrician to look for other signs of fetal compromise and to take special precautions at the time of delivery to prevent the potentially devastating consequences of meconium aspiration syndrome. Intrapartum amnioinfusion of saline can wash meconium from the amniotic cavity and decrease the incidence and severity of meconium aspiration (35).

Postpartum

Apgar scores, umbilical cord blood gas analysis, and neurobehavioral testing are used in the routine evaluation of the neonate. The Apgar score, performed 1 and 5 minutes after birth, is a quick method of assessing the clinical status of the newborn and a useful index of the efficacy of resuscitative measures. Apgar scores at 1 and 5 minutes correlate poorly with subsequent neurological outcome. Persistently low Apgar scores (less than 3) at 10, 15, and 20 minutes identify infants at high risk of death or severe neurological impairment (36,37). However, it is important not to retrospectively attribute low Apgar scores to intrapartum asphyxial events. According to the most recent American College of Obstetricians and Gynecologists committee opinion, the term "asphyxia" should be reserved for clinical situations in which all of the following are present:

- Profound metabolic or mixed acidemia (pH less than 7.00) on an umbilical cord arterial blood sample,
- An Apgar score of 0 to 3 for longer than 5 minutes,
- Neonatal neurological manifestations (seizures, coma, hypotonia), and
- Multisystem organ dysfunction (cardiovascular, gastrointestinal, hematologic, pulmonary, or renal) (38).

Acidosis, identified by umbilical cord blood gas analysis, correlates poorly with neonatal status and subsequent neurological development (39). All infants are born with a mixed respiratory and metabolic acidosis, which may be a physiologic adaptation that hastens conversion to the adult circulatory and respiratory pattern (2). Most neonates with an umbilical artery pH less than 7.20 are vigorous at birth and show no adverse short- or long-term sequelae (40,41). A recent study determined the range of acid–base values in normal vigorous newborns with Apgar scores greater than 7. Mean umbilical artery pH is 7.26, but defining all values within two standard deviations of the mean as "normal" would include pH values as low as 7.10 (42). Analysis of umbilical cord blood is particularly useful to refute the presence of severe asphyxia by documenting a normal pH despite signs of intrapartum fetal distress or neonatal depression (43,44).

FETAL RESUSCITATION

Obstetric management of the stressed fetus must strike a delicate balance (Fig. 2). Surgical intervention performed too early leads to frequent cesarean section, instrumental delivery, and increases maternal morbidity. Surgery too late may produce a damaged infant. There are several noninvasive maneuvers that may improve fetal condition and avert or postpone the need for surgical intervention. Because the etiology of fetal distress often is multifactorial and seldom known with certainty, each of these measures should be implemented simultaneously with the hope that one or a combination will improve the fetal status (Table 4).

Alter Maternal Position

Changing maternal position improves fetal blood flow by relieving both aortocaval and umbilical cord compression. Aortocaval compression impairs uterine blood flow by two mechanisms. First, the gravid uterus directly compresses the aorta proximal to the origin of the uterine blood vessels, thereby decreasing uterine blood flow. Second, compression of the inferior vena cava decreases venous return to the heart, reducing right ventricular preload and maternal cardiac output. Some refer to the effects of aortocaval compression as the *supine hypotensive syndrome*. However, maternal blood pressure measured in the brachial artery may be normal when the aorta, and not the vena cava, is compressed. Aortic compression by the gravid uterus may increase maternal brachial artery blood pressure by increasing systemic vascular resistance. Blood flow to the uterus and the lower extremities will still be dramatically reduced (45). Therefore, continuous maintenance of left uterine displacement is imperative throughout labor regardless of maternal blood pressure or the presence of epidural analgesia. In some patients, the right or left lateral decubitus positions more effectively displace the gravid uterus (i.e., multiple gestation, polyhydramnios, obesity). If fetal dis-

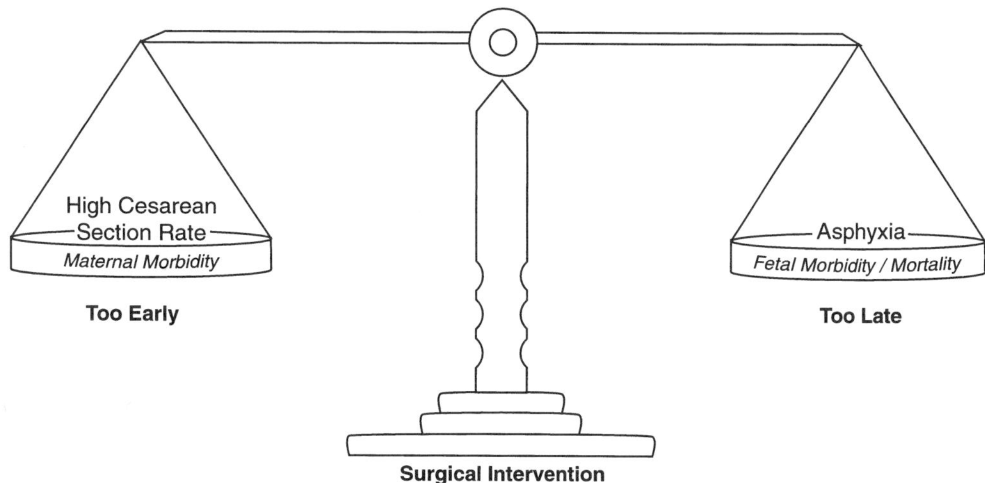

FIG. 2. Obstetric management of the stressed fetus must strike a delicate balance.

tress persists, Trendelenburg or knee–chest positions may relieve umbilical cord compression by the fetal presenting part. Vaginal examination should be performed to detect umbilical cord prolapse.

Administer Maternal Oxygen

Maternal hyperoxia can increase oxygen delivery to the fetus if uterine hypoperfusion, umbilical cord compression, or uterine hypertonus does not impede blood flow. Supplemental oxygen delivered by high-flow face mask increases maternal and fetal transcutaneous pO_2 in both normal and "high-risk" parturients in labor (46). During elective cesarean delivery with epidural anesthesia, supplemental oxygen delivered by face mask progressively increases fetal pO_2 as F_IO_2 approaches 1.0 (Table 5) (47). Although the absolute rise in umbilical venous pO_2 seems insignificant (from 28 to 47 mm Hg), it results in a dramatic increase in fetal oxygen saturation (from 65% to 87%), reflecting the steep slope of the fetal oxyhemoglobin dissociation hemoglobin curve at these pO_2 values.

TABLE 4. *Initial management of fetal distress: improve uteroplacental perfusion*

Alter maternal position
Relieve aortocaval compression
Relieve umbilical cord compression
Administer maternal oxygen
Improve maternal circulation
Give balanced salt solution, colloid, blood
Use vasopressors (ephedrine, phenylephrine)
Decrease uterine tone
Stop oxytocin
Administer tocolytics (terbutaline, nitroglycerin, $MgSO_4$)
Consider amnioinfusion
Relieve umbilical cord compression

Earlier studies reported a plateau or decline in fetal oxygen delivery when maternal p_aO_2 exceeded 300 mm Hg (48–50). These authors studied patients undergoing elective cesarean delivery with general anesthesia using nitrous oxide and volatile agent. In one such study, an increase in maternal inspired oxygen concentration from 50% to 100% did not improve fetal oxygenation (48). Marx and Mateo (49) also reported this "ceiling" effect of maternal oxygen administration at an F_IO_2 between 0.5 and 0.65. Others even reported a decline in fetal oxygen tension when maternal inspired oxygen concentrations are greater than 50% (50). However, these studies have been criticized for failing to control several important variables including:

- Anesthetic depth,
- Left uterine displacement,
- Uterine incision to delivery interval, and
- Maternal p_aCO_2.

Lack of control of anesthetic depth is the most probable explanation for the above findings. In these studies, maternal F_IO_2 was increased by decreasing the fraction of

TABLE 5. *Effect of maternal oxygen administration on maternal and fetal oxygenation*

F_IO_2	0.21	0.47	0.74	1.00
Maternal p_aO_2 (mm Hg)	96	232	312	423
UV pO_2 (mm Hg)	28	36	41	47
UV O_2 saturation (%)	65		87	
UA pO_2 (mm Hg)	15	19	21	25
UA O_2 saturation (%)	26		59	

Data from 40 healthy term parturients undergoing elective cesarean delivery with epidural anesthesia. From ref. 45.

UA, umbilical artery; UV, umbilical vein.

inspired nitrous oxide without concurrently increasing the delivered concentration of volatile agent. The resultant inadequate anesthesia allowed release of maternal catecholamines, which may have produced uterine artery vasoconstriction and compromised oxygen delivery to the fetus.

When anesthetic depth was controlled by adjusting the isoflurane concentration to reflect the use of nitrous oxide, administration of 100% oxygen and isoflurane produced a small but significant increase in umbilical venous pO_2 (51). This effect was most notable in patients undergoing emergency cesarean delivery, and fewer newborns in the 100% oxygen group needed resuscitation with supplemental oxygen. Administration of 100% oxygen to patients undergoing nonemergent cesarean delivery did not seem to offer these same advantages. No adverse maternal effects (i.e., decreased uterine contractility or increased blood loss) were observed with the use of a higher concentration of volatile agent.

Therefore, maternal oxygen administration during either general or regional anesthesia will increase umbilical venous and arterial oxygen tensions. A small rise in fetal pO_2 produces a substantial increase in fetal hemoglobin saturation and oxygen content because fetal hemoglobin resides on the steep portion of its oxyhemoglobin dissociation curve. Maternal oxygen administration may significantly improve the physiologic reserve of the compromised fetus. However, it will do little to improve fetal status if uterine, placental, or fetal perfusion is interrupted.

Improve Maternal Circulation

Maternal hypotension decreases uterine artery blood flow and intervillous perfusion. It is poorly tolerated by the compromised fetus and should be rapidly treated with nondextrose-containing crystalloid infusion and a vasopressor. The importance of nondextrose-containing fluids has been borne out by several studies showing the harmful fetal effects of maternal dextrose administration (52–54). These effects include:

- Fetal hyperglycemia leading to hypoglycemia after birth,
- Fetal lactate production causing metabolic acidosis,
- Hypoxemia, and
- Theoretically, worsened neurological outcome after global cerebral ischemia.

Recent work has questioned the ability of acute intravenous crystalloid administration to *prevent* maternal hypotension during regional anesthesia (55–57). Maternal hemodynamics and ephedrine requirements were the same in healthy parturients randomly assigned to receive 10, 20, or 30 mL/kg of crystalloid before induction of spinal anesthesia for elective cesarean section (57). A similar study found no difference in severity of hypotension, ephedrine requirement, or clinical neonatal status in parturients receiving no volume compared with those receiving 20 mL/kg (56).

Intravenous colloid administration may be more effective than crystalloids at preventing maternal hypotension before extensive regional blockade (58,59). Even with colloid administration, however, maternal hypotension frequently requires vasopressor therapy. The increased cost of colloid solutions, combined with a small increase in efficacy, precludes routine "prophylactic" administration. I reserve the use of colloid solutions for the acute replacement of intravascular volume, such as with maternal hemorrhage, when vasopressors and crystalloids alone prove ineffective.

Because fluids alone are ineffective at preventing or correcting maternal hypotension from sympathetic blockade, a vasopressor often is required. Many recommend giving a vasopressor at the first sign of falling maternal blood pressure. In obstetrics, the vasopressor of choice is ephedrine. Its β-adrenergic effects increase maternal heart rate, contractility, cardiac output, and uterine blood flow. Pure α-adrenergic agonists, such as phenylephrine, can constrict the uterine vasculature and diminish uteroplacental perfusion (60,61). However, phenylephrine reportedly lacks adverse neonatal effects when used to maintain maternal blood pressure after regional blockade for cesarean section in healthy, nonlaboring parturients (62,63). The effects of phenylephrine on the compromised fetus have not been studied. I use phenylephrine only if one of the following is present:

- Tachyphylaxis to ephedrine (more than 50 mg administered),
- Maternal heart rate greater than 100 beats/min,
- Recent β_2-agonist administration,
- Maternal cardiac disease (idiopathic hypertrophic subaortic stenosis, mitral stenosis, aortic stenosis).

Decrease Uterine Tone

Because the blood vessels that perfuse the placenta traverse the myometrium, uterine contractions decrease placental perfusion in proportion to their frequency, intensity, and duration. Even transient reductions in blood flow may cause acute decompensation in a fetus with limited placental reserve. When nonreassuring fetal signs occur, immediately stop exogenous oxytocin. Next, consider improving placental perfusion by using medications that acutely decrease uterine tone. Terbutaline 0.25 mg injected intravenously or subcutaneously significantly improves fetal heart rate tracings, fetal acid–base status, and neonatal outcome (64–68) and should be routine practice when uterine hypertonus is suspected. Terbutaline is well tolerated by most parturients but may produce mild tachycardia, hypotension from systemic vasodilation, and, in diabetics, problems with glucose homeostasis.

Other medications that can be used to treat uterine hypertonus include magnesium sulfate and nitroglycerin.

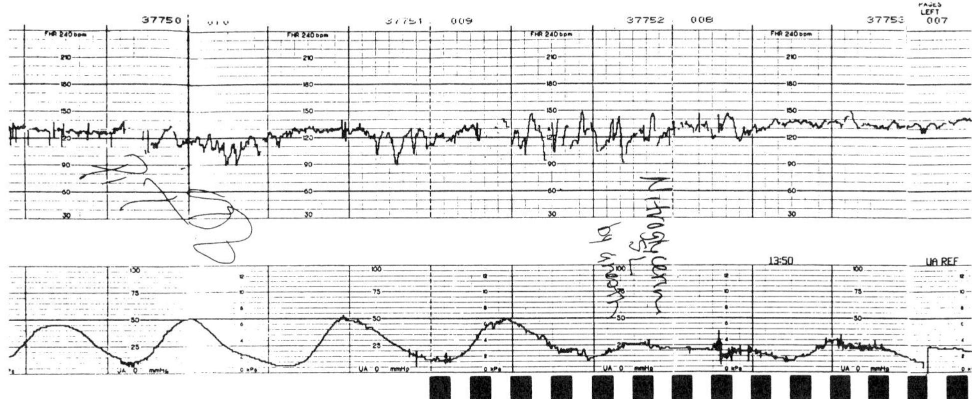

FIG. 3. Tocodynomometer strip and fetal heart rate tracing showing relaxation of a hyperstimulated uterus by sublingual nitroglycerin. (From ref. 71, with permission.)

Magnesium sulfate is probably of little benefit because of its relatively slow onset, long duration, and unwanted side effects. In addition, despite its tocolytic action, magnesium sulfate does not decrease umbilical vascular resistance (65) and adversely affects fetal lamb survival when given during maternal hemorrhage-induced hypoxemia (69).

Nitroglycerin also can provide acute uterine relaxation (70–75). It produces uterine relaxation within 30 to 90 seconds after administration, and its plasma half-life in the adult is 1 to 3 minutes (70). Bell (71) reported the use of sublingual nitroglycerin spray in a patient with recurrent late fetal heart rate decelerations from uterine hyperstimulation by intravenous oxytocin. The nitroglycerin spray was administered in a dose of 0.8 mg (72) and produced uterine relaxation (documented by a uterine pressure catheter tracing) (Fig. 3) within 1 minute. Uterine pressures gradually increased after 6 minutes, the oxytocin infusion was restarted, and the patient delivered vaginally. In sheep, nitroglycerin decreases maternal blood pressure, but does not change uterine blood flow or uterine vascular conductance (76). Because nitroglycerin has a predilection for the vascular smooth muscle within the venous circulation, clinically significant hypotension, even in patients with preexisting regional blockade or intravascular volume depletion, is uncommon (73). Although there are numerous case reports and observational studies of the ability of nitroglycerin to provide rapid, short-lived uterine relaxation, no clinical trials have compared it to other tocolytics. However, the use of nitroglycerin in the setting of uterine hyperstimulation should be considered. I make up a solution of nitroglycerin that contains 100 μg/mL and inject it in increasing bolus doses of 50, 100, 200, and 500 μg every 30 to 60 seconds until the desired effect occurs. Up to 1,000 μg has been used without significant side effects or prolonged duration (73).

Consider Amnioinfusion

Amnioinfusion has become a widely used technique for the treatment of persistent variable decelerations, which are most likely due to umbilical cord compression. Normal saline is infused transcervically through an intrauterine pressure catheter in either a set amount (250 to 500 mL) or titrated until variable decelerations resolve. The addition of this fluid to the uterine cavity seems to cushion and protect the umbilical cord from compression due to maternal position or uterine contractions. Special double-lumen intrauterine pressure catheters have been developed that allow concurrent monitoring of intrauterine pressure (77). Randomized studies comparing amnioinfusion to no therapy have shown that the technique decreases the frequency and severity of variable decelerations in labor, leads to lower instrumental and cesarean delivery rates, and improves umbilical artery and venous blood gas values (78–80). Reported complications include umbilical cord prolapse, uterine overdistention, dehiscence of a prior low-transverse cesarean section scar, fetal bradycardia, and one report of amniotic fluid embolism (77,81). In addition to treating persistent variable decelerations, amnioinfusion is used to dilute meconium and decreases the frequency and severity of meconium aspiration syndrome in the neonate (35).

ANESTHETIC MANAGEMENT: GENERAL PRINCIPLES (TABLE 6)

Anticipation

Acute fetal distress seldom arises without warning. In one study, routine preoperative evaluation predicted the need for emergency cesarean delivery for fetal distress in 87% of cases (82). Preoperative assessment allowed identification of risk factors for abdominal delivery (Table 7). Parturients with any of these risks were encouraged to have an epidural catheter placed early in labor. Early epidural analgesia allowed 70% patients to undergo operative delivery by extension of blockade. Twenty-two percent, who did not receive epidural analgesia despite preoperative risk identification, received general anesthesia for cesarean delivery. An additional 7% received general

TABLE 6. *Cornerstone principles of anesthetic management of the compromised fetus*

Anticipation
- preanesthetic evaluation of all patients presenting to the labor and delivery suite
- identify risk factors that increase the likelihood of operative delivery

Preparation
- place epidural catheter early in labor and maintain a T_{10} sensory level
- avoid combined spinal-epidural analgesia
  - potentially causes uterine hypertonicity and fetal heart rate abnormalities
  - cannot be sure that the epidural catheter is in the correct position until intrathecal analgesia subsides
- always be prepared to administer general anesthesia

Communication
- preoperative consultation should be requested by the obstetrician if risk factors for anesthetic complications are suspected
- anesthesiologist should be notified at the first sign of deterioration in fetal status

anesthesia despite the presence of an epidural catheter. Neonatal condition did not differ with the use of epidural or general anesthesia. However, maternal complications of general anesthesia that were observed included difficult intubation, bronchospasm, and awareness. These infrequent, yet serious, complications contrasted to the more frequent, but less serious, complications associated with the use of epidural anesthesia. These included discomfort during surgery requiring opiate administration (9%), hypotension treated with fluids and ephedrine (18%), nausea (20%), and vomiting (5%). These findings support the following recommendations:

- Assess all patients admitted to the labor suite.
- Identify risk factors that indicate fetal compromise and predispose to cesarean delivery.
- Inform the patient and her obstetrician about the benefits of epidural placement early in labor to help avoid the need for a rushed general anesthetic if fetal distress arises.

TABLE 7. *Characteristics of parturients who seem likely to require abdominal delivery*

Failure to progress in labor
Cephalopelvic disproportion
Nonengaged fetal head
Persistent occiput posterior head
Breech presentation
Abnormal fetal heart rate tracing
Need for fetal scalp pH analysis
Multiple gestation
Suspected intrauterine growth retardation
Vaginal birth after cesarean section
Preeclampsia

Preparation

Placing an epidural catheter early in labor should be a primary goal for the anesthesiologist caring for a parturient with suspected fetal compromise. Unfortunately, many obstetricians still believe that early induction of epidural analgesia may prolong labor (83). They may request insertion of an epidural catheter without induction of labor analgesia. An anesthetist may comply with these wishes and simply administer a "test dose" through the epidural catheter. However, a "test dose" only detects incorrect catheter location. Unless a T_{10} level of analgesia is established, one cannot be certain that the epidural catheter is positioned correctly and capable of providing anesthesia for operative delivery. Therefore, insert an epidural catheter early in labor and maintain a sensory level to the T_{10} dermatome with a continuous infusion of dilute local anesthetic and opioid. Frequently monitor the level of sensory change.

I avoid the combined spinal–epidural (CSE) technique in the presence of suspected fetal compromise. Intrathecal opioids may risk sudden fetal bradycardia (84–86). Clarke et al. (84) noted rapid onset of fetal bradycardia, unrelated to maternal hypotension, in 9 of 30 consecutive parturients receiving 50 μg of intrathecal fentanyl. Most often, tetanic uterine contractions coincided with the fetal heart rate changes and were treated with terbutaline. Nearly all of the fetal heart rate decelerations quickly resolved, but emergency cesarean section was performed in two patients when bradycardia persisted beyond 5 minutes. Herbstman et al. (85) used intrauterine pressure catheters and measured a significant increase in baseline intrauterine pressure followed by fetal heart rate deceleration in 4 of 17 laboring patients after intrathecal injection of fentanyl 25 μg. Fetal bradycardias resolved spontaneously in this series, and there were no emergency cesarean sections.

Maternal catecholamines, secreted in response to painful labor, may hinder uterine activity (87). Intrathecal opioid analgesia may allow uterine hyperstimulation by decreasing maternal catecholamine concentration.

Do fetal bradycardias occur with greater frequency after intrathecal opioid analgesia than with epidural analgesia? Fetal heart rate changes have long been observed in patients following epidural analgesia for labor. Eberle et al. (88) found that fetal bradycardias occurred with equal frequency (about 2.6%) in patients receiving a conventional epidural versus CSE for labor analgesia. No fetal heart rate change necessitated operative delivery. Nielsen et al. (89) compared the incidence of intrapartum fetal heart rate abnormalities and obstetric outcome after intrathecal sufentanil versus epidural bupivacaine. Fetal heart rate abnormalities *within the first hour* of administration were *not* more common in the group receiving intrathecal opioid. "Clinically significant" fetal heart rate abnormalities developed after

22% and 23% of patients receiving intrathecal sufentanil or epidural bupivacaine. These "clinically significant" fetal heart rate abnormalities had no effect on neonatal outcome (Apgar score and umbilical cord pH). Emergency cesarean section was performed for "fetal distress" in one patient from each group. It is unclear if the time of onset of fetal heart rate abnormalities differed between intrathecal or epidural opioid injection, because the authors only reported the occurrence of these findings within a very broad time frame (within the first hour after injection). In a letter to the editor, Kahn and Hubert (90) reported their experience with fetal bradycardia (FHR less than 90 beats/min lasting longer than 60 seconds) in women receiving CSE or epidural labor analgesia. The incidence of fetal bradycardia was 5.6% in the CSE group and 2.5% in the epidural group ($p < 0.05$). Bradycardia occurred within 5 to 15 minutes of intrathecal drug injection and within 20 to 30 minutes of epidural injection.

Albright and Forster (91) compared the incidence of emergency cesarean delivery in 1,240 patients receiving CSE analgesia for labor to 1,140 patients receiving systemic or no medication. CSE analgesia was not associated with a higher incidence of emergency cesarean delivery. Because their patient population was derived from a small community-based hospital, they caution the extrapolation of these findings to high-risk parturients found at tertiary medical centers. Nevertheless, the rapid onset of profound analgesia provided by intrathecal opioids sometimes is associated with uterine hyperstimulation and fetal heart rate deceleration. Whether these fetal heart rate abnormalities are "clinically significant" is disputable because most studies comparing CSE to epidural analgesia do not indicate differences in the rate of emergency cesarean section (92). Because the etiology and frequency of occurrence of fetal bradycardias associated with tetanic uterine contractions after CSE labor analgesia remains controversial, I avoid this technique when fetal compromise or a nonreassuring fetal heart rate tracing is present.[1]

Another drawback to the CSE technique in the presence of fetal compromise is that the exact location of the epidural catheter initially may be uncertain. Intrathecal analgesia provides rapid, effective pain relief for 60 to 120 minutes and leaves the epidural catheter "untested" for what may prove a critical period. During this time, there is no way of knowing if the epidural catheter will function adequately should surgical anesthesia be required (93).[2]

Finally, never be lulled into a false sense of security by the presence of an epidural catheter placed during labor. Properly functioning catheters can migrate intrathecally, intravascularly, or become dislodged and fail to provide adequate anesthesia for operative delivery. Medications and equipment to administer a general anesthetic must always be available and in working order. Preoperative assessment of the parturient should always include a thorough airway evaluation. Look for a history of difficult intubation or adverse reactions to anesthetic agents. In addition, consider nonparticulate oral antacids, metoclopramide, and H_2 blockers throughout labor for those patients with morbid obesity, diabetes, or potential airway difficulty.

Communication

The obstetrician should obtain antepartum consultation from an anesthesiologist when any factors are present that may increase the risks of either regional or general anesthesia. Some of these risks include:

- Intrinsic or induced coagulopathy,
- Prior back surgery with instrumentation,
- Severe scoliosis,
- Airway abnormality or history of difficult intubation, and
- Malignant hyperthermia susceptibility.

A preoperative consultation allows advance discussion about the risks and benefits of the anesthetic plan and can allay much anxiety.

Open communication among obstetric, nursing, and anesthesia personnel throughout labor is essential. At the first sign of fetal deterioration, the anesthesiologist should be notified to allow preparations for provision of anesthesia for delivery. The earlier the anesthesiologist is notified, the less likely the parturient will be subjected to a rushed general anesthetic.

ANESTHESIA FOR VAGINAL DELIVERY

When antepartum surveillance suggests that the fetus is not thriving in the intrauterine environment, prompt delivery may be indicated. Despite the possibility of fetal compromise, obstetricians often attempt to achieve either a

[1] Editor's note: A recent prospective, randomized comparison of epidural (n = 119) and CSE (n = 145) labor analgesia found no difference in the frequency of new prolonged decelerations (7.8% vs 6.9%) or late decelerations (11.6% vs 9.7%). In addition, the presence of preexisting fetal heart rate abnormalities did not increase the risk of new abnormalities after either technique. (Fogel ST, Daftary AR, Norris MC, Dalman HM, Holtmann B. The incidence of fetal heart rate abnormalities: combined spinal/epidural vs. epidural anesthesia for labor. *Abstracts of Scientific Papers.* Society for Obstetric Anesthesia and Perinatology, 1998.)

[2] Editor's note: A recent report systematically evaluated catheters placed as part of an epidural or CSE technique in laboring women. If CSF was seen in the spinal needle when using the needle-through-needle technique and the epidural catheter was not intravascular, 99% of multiorifice catheters (934 of 945) were in the epidural space and produced bilateral sensory change and analgesia. In this study, 97% of catheters (531 of 545) placed after locating only the epidural space also provided good analgesia. However, only 95% of catheters placed using either technique provided adequate anesthesia for cesarean section. (Norris MC. Are CSE catheters reliable? *Abstracts of Scientific Papers.* Society for Obstetric Anesthesia and Perinatology, 1998.)

spontaneous or instrumental vaginal delivery. Successful vaginal delivery is associated with less maternal morbidity and mortality than cesarean section (94,95). Most often, labor will be induced. Labor is stressful even to a normal fetus, and the compromised one, with marginal physiologic reserve, may decompensate. Lumbar epidural analgesia, induced early in labor, may prevent a rushed general anesthetic should fetal distress arise. Also, lumbar epidural analgesia may improve uteroplacental perfusion, probably by reducing maternal circulating catecholamines. Doppler measurement of umbilical artery flow velocity waveforms in 12 laboring parturients showed decreased placental vascular resistance after epidural analgesia with 1.5% lidocaine (96). An earlier study reported the same effect in 13 of 16 laboring women who received epidural analgesia with 3% 2-chloroprocaine (97). Both studies were performed in normal, healthy patients in spontaneous labor with no evidence of fetal stress. Jouppila et al. (98) measured intervillous blood flow using xenon clearance during labor in nine patients with severe preeclampsia. They noted dramatic improvement in intervillous blood flow after epidural analgesia with 0.25% bupivacaine. This evidence supports the beneficial effect of continuous lumbar epidural analgesia on uteroplacental perfusion, especially in the presence of a constricted placental bed. Therefore, strongly encourage parturients with evidence of fetal compromise to have epidural labor analgesia.

Should fetal compromise alter the technique of lumbar epidural analgesia for labor? The following sections consider the impact of fetal stress on the choice of local anesthetic and the use of adjuvants in labor epidural analgesia.

Choice of Local Anesthetic

In the early 1970s, Scanlon et al. (99) reported an increased incidence of "floppy but alert" newborns when lumbar epidural analgesia with lidocaine was used for labor and vaginal delivery. This result prompted numerous investigations of the neurobehavioral effects of many local anesthetics, including 2-chloroprocaine and bupivacaine (100–104). Although these studies never confirmed Scanlon's findings of neonatal hypotonia, they did detect subtle neurobehavioral effects with all local anesthetics. These effects are short-lived and correlate better with the route of delivery than the drug used. Infants delivered by cesarean section have *better* neurobehavioral scores than those delivered vaginally, despite exposure to higher concentrations of local anesthetics (104).

The phenomenon of "ion trapping" also is a consideration when fetal acidosis is possible (105). Drug accumulation may occur when the nonionized form of a weak base crosses the placenta and becomes ionized in the acidic milieu of the fetal circulation. Fetal acidosis enhances the cardiac and CNS toxicity of local anesthetics (105).

Theoretically, 2-chloroprocaine should be the local anesthetic of choice in the presence of fetal compromise. It is hydrolyzed rapidly by maternal plasma cholinesterase to an inactive metabolite. Fetal acid–base status does not affect the limited placental transfer of both the intact molecule and its major metabolite (106,107). The maternal and neonatal in vitro half-lives of 2-chloroprocaine are 21 and 43 seconds, respectively (108). However, 2-chloroprocaine possesses several undesirable characteristics that make its use for continuous lumbar epidural analgesia impractical:

- A short duration,
- Profound motor blockade, and
- Antagonism of neuraxial opioids.

In the presence of fetal compromise, I do not alter my choice of local epidural anesthetic. I use fractionated doses of dilute concentrations of bupivacaine or ropivacaine, much the same as during routine epidural labor analgesia. These long-acting local anesthetics are highly protein bound and lipid soluble. They produce minimal maternal hemodynamic effects. Fetal plasma concentration of bupivacaine remains relatively low because of binding to maternal epidural fat and serum proteins (100). Dilute concentrations of bupivacaine and ropivacaine produce minimal motor blockade and analgesia can be potentiated by epidural opioids.

For operative vaginal delivery, I use the existing epidural catheter to provide dense perineal anesthesia and pelvic relaxation. Rapid onset and minimal fetal transfer make 3% 2-chloroprocaine an ideal local anesthetic to use in this setting. I give 10 to 15 mL of pH-adjusted solution and rapidly treat any maternal hypotension that may occur. When I am concerned about maternal hemodynamic status and have time for slower onset of perineal anesthesia, I inject 10 to 15 mL of 0.5% bupivacaine. When an epidural catheter is not in place and time permits, I administer a spinal anesthetic with a small dose of either hyperbaric or isobaric lidocaine (45 to 60 mg).[3] Rarely, I rapidly induce general endotracheal anesthesia for operative vaginal delivery.

Epinephrine

I avoid epinephrine-containing solutions in parturients with suspected fetal compromise because:

- Epinephrine-containing local anesthetics can exaggerate the hypotensive response to epidural anesthesia from supplemental β_2-mediated vasodilation (109).
- Unintentional *intravascular* injection of epinephrine may produce uterine artery vasoconstriction from a direct α-agonist effect and can precipitate acute fetal distress (Fig. 4). In gravid ewes, intravenous injection

[3] Editor's note: I have abandoned the use of intrathecal lidocaine because of the risks of transient neurologic symptoms. In this setting, I often choose the CSE technique. I provide analgesia for the second stage of labor and operative vaginal delivery with sufentanil 5 to 10 μg and bupivacaine 2.5 mg (or just 5.0 to 7.5 mg bupivacaine). I also insert an epidural catheter for later use should forceps and vacuum attempts fail.

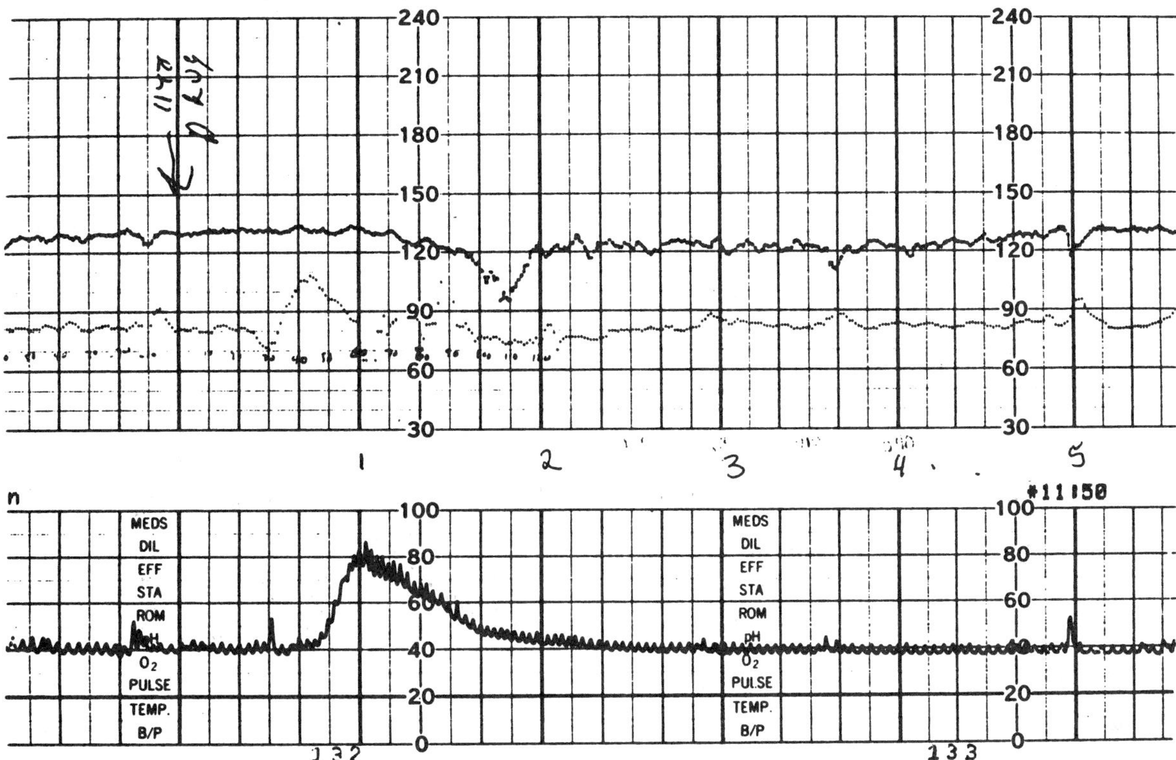

FIG. 4. Late decelerations in a previously normal fetus after maternal injection of 15-μg epinephrine. (Photograph courtesy of Barbara L. Leighton, M.D.)

of as little as 10 μg of epinephrine lowers uterine blood flow by as much as 65% (110). This decrease lasts for more than 3 minutes. Therefore, I do not use an epinephrine-containing test dose in the presence of compromised placental perfusion. Some alternatives to the epinephrine test dose are listed in Table 8.

- Epidural injection of epinephrine-containing local anesthetics in patients with underlying uteroplacental insufficiency increases placental vascular resistance. These patients seem more sensitive to the α-, rather than β-, agonist effect of epinephrine. Marx et al. (111) compared the effects of epidural injection of 8 mL of 2% lidocaine with or without epinephrine 1:200,000 on placental perfusion. In patients with normal placental vascular resistance, lidocaine plus epinephrine decreased placental vascular resistance and enhanced perfusion. However, in women with preexisting high placental vascular resistance (an indication of placental insufficiency), lidocaine plus epinephrine 1:200,000 further increased placental vascular resistance and decreased placental perfusion. Fetal distress, manifested by persistent late decelerations, developed in one patient. This study provides evidence that epinephrine-containing local anesthetics may further compromise placental perfusion when given to parturients with evidence of uteroplacental insufficiency.

TABLE 8. *Alternatives to the epinephrine "test dose" to detect and limit the consequences of unintentional intravascular injection of local anesthetics*

- Carefully aspirate through the needle or catheter using a small syringe before each injection.
- Fractionate doses of local anesthetics into 3 to 5mL aliquots.
- Frequently assess the patient for signs and symptoms of local anesthetic toxicity.
- Monitor for the onset of appropriate analgesia. Suspect intravascular injection of local anesthetic if appropriate sensory level of analgesia does not develop. Replace epidural catheter rather than administer doses of local anesthetic that could result in intravascular toxicity.
- Consider the Doppler test (see Chapter 32).

Epidural Opioids

Opioids offer several advantages when used as adjuvants to local anesthetics during labor epidural analgesia for the compromised fetus. By potentiating the effects of local anesthetics, opioids allow the use of more dilute local anesthetic solutions, thereby limiting motor blockade, hypotension, and the possibility of local anesthetic toxicity. However, epidural opioids, like systemic opioids, may affect fetal heart rate patterns and neonatal status.

TABLE 9. *Anesthetic recommendations for vaginal delivery in the presence of fetal compromise*

- Assess all parturients upon admission to the labor ward and insert an epidural catheter early in labor if risk factors for fetal distress are present.
- Provide T_{10} sensory level of analgesia with a continuous lumbar epidural infusion of dilute bupivacaine and opioid solution.
- Monitor patient hourly for signs of increasing or decreasing sensory level to detect intrathecal or intravascular migration of epidural catheter.
- Use minimum effective dose of epidural opioids.
- Avoid use of epinephrine-containing local anesthetics in the test dose, bolus dose, or by continuous infusion.

The fetal heart rate tracing is our only monitor of intrapartum fetal status. Loss of beat-to-beat or short-term variability, combined with late decelerations, raises serious concerns about fetal well-being. Maternally administered analgesics could interfere with fetal heart rate analysis by obscuring or mimicking the signs of fetal distress. Epidural injection of 50 to 75 μg of fentanyl has *no* significant impact on fetal heart rate patterns (112,113). Epidural fentanyl does not cause neonatal depression as measured by Apgar scores and respiratory rates immediately after delivery (114).

Given the benefits of epidural opioids and their apparent safety in the *absence* of fetal compromise, I believe that they also can be used in the *presence* of fetal compromise. Use the smallest effective dose to minimize fetal exposure. I add fentanyl 50 μg to my initial bolus of local anesthetic for both labor analgesia and cesarean section. If fetal heart rate variability decreases shortly after induction of epidural analgesia, a positive response to fetal scalp or vibroacoustic stimulation can rule out fetal acidosis. Table 9 summarizes my anesthetic recommendations for vaginal delivery when fetal compromise is suspected.

ANESTHESIA FOR CESAREAN SECTION

To formulate a plan to provide anesthesia for cesarean delivery of a compromised fetus:

- Determine the urgency of the situation, and
- Assess both maternal and fetal status.

In this situation, clear, unequivocal communication between obstetrician and anesthesiologist is essential. As discussed earlier, "fetal distress" is a diagnosis that is indiscriminately applied to a wide spectrum of intrapartum events and circumstances. All obstetric care providers should limit the use of this term and the arbitrary designation of "stat" to any non elective cesarean section. These terms should be applied only to emergencies that threaten the life of the mother or fetus. Optimal anesthetic care is possible only when both obstetrician and anesthesiologist have a true understanding of the urgency of the situation.

Clearly defined terminology and consensus about the time in which operative intervention should begin is required. "It should be possible, when indicated, to begin the operation within 30 minutes of the time that the decision is made to operate" (115). Many clinicians, as well as the medicolegal community, interpret this "decision to skin incision" guideline to mean they have 30 minutes to prepare the patient for surgery. Clearly, some situations (such as hemorrhage from placenta previa or abruption, umbilical cord prolapse, and uterine rupture) require a much faster response time.

Harris (116) has proposed a more useful classification of the urgency of operative delivery (Table 10). Any nonscheduled cesarean section is categorized as "emergency." These "emergencies" then are subdivided further into stable, urgent, or stat. A *stable* emergency cesarean section is one that is performed when there is evidence of chronic fetal *stress*, before acute decompensation has occurred. Delivery may take place within the next several

TABLE 10. *Classification of emergency cesarean section*

Category	Example	Preferred anesthetic
Stable	Chronic uteroplacental insufficiency Malpresentation with ruptured membranes (not in labor) Previous lower segment cesarean section (with or without labor)	Epidural, spinal
Urgent	Dystocia Active herpes with ruptured membranes Placenta previa in labor (NOT bleeding) Severe preeclampsia Chorioamnionitis Previous classic cesarean section in labor Umbilical cord prolapse WITHOUT fetal distress	Epidural (if present during labor), spinal
Stat	Agonal fetal distress	General, epidural (if T_{10} level or higher is present)
	Umbilical cord prolapse WITH fetal distress	
	Massive hemorrhage	GA Only?
	Ruptured uterus	GA Only?

After ref. 116.

hours depending on the fetal condition. Cesarean section becomes *urgent* when labor is in progress and either the fetus begins to manifest signs of *distress*, or there are maternal contraindications to vaginal delivery. Here, delivery should probably take place within the next 30 minutes. A true *stat* cesarean section is performed when either the mother or fetus faces life-threatening danger if delivery is not performed as soon as possible. Examples of these circumstances include severe maternal hemorrhage, uterine rupture, or prolonged fetal bradycardia with loss of short-term variability. These life-threatening circumstances, which fortunately are rare, require delivery within several minutes.

The anesthesiologist should be notified as soon as the surgeon even contemplates cesarean section. Once the decision to operate is made, the anesthesiologist should ask the obstetrician directly, "How much time do I have to prepare this patient for surgical incision?" This information, combined with an assessment of maternal status, should be used to formulate a mutually agreeable anesthetic plan.

Regional versus General Anesthesia

In the absence of severe maternal hemorrhage or coagulopathy, most agree that regional anesthesia is appropriate for cesarean sections categorized as *stable* or *urgent*. However, considerable controversy surrounds the choice of anesthetic for the true *stat* cesarean section. Here, the choice of anesthetic technique includes:

- An existing epidural catheter,
- A subarachnoid block, or
- A general anesthetic.

Differences among these techniques in terms of onset, as well as maternal and fetal outcome, must be considered.

Studies of anesthesia-related maternal mortality in both the United Kingdom (117) and the United States (95) clearly show that general anesthesia entails greater maternal risk than regional anesthesia. Despite an overall decline in maternal mortality between 1979 and 1990, the number of maternal deaths attributable to general anesthesia, primarily complications resulting from airway management, did not change (95). Disturbingly, during this interval:

- The use of general anesthesia in the parturient declined, and
- Pulse oximetry and end-tidal carbon dioxide monitoring came into routine clinical use.

At the same time, total regional anesthesia-related maternal mortality, primarily from local anesthetic toxicity and high neuraxial blockade, declined despite increased use of these techniques for labor and cesarean section. Why has there not been a similar reduction in general anesthesia-related maternal deaths? General anesthesia often is used in emergency situations (life-threatening maternal or fetal circumstances), and when regional anesthesia is either contraindicated (in patients with a coagulopathy due to preeclampsia or severe hemorrhage) or technically difficult (morbid obesity).

In addition, because of the increasing use of regional anesthesia, anesthesiologists are less experienced at intubating pregnant patients. Hawthorne et al. (118) conducted a prospective audit of 5,802 cesarean deliveries performed under general anesthesia between 1978 and 1994. Against a background of declining use of general anesthesia, the incidence of failed intubation increased from 1 in 300 general anesthetics in 1984 to 1 in 250 in 1994. Most failed intubations occurred outside of normal working hours, during "emergency" cesarean sections, and involved trainees. Preoperative airway examination was unremarkable in one-third of patients who were subsequently difficult to intubate. Two-thirds had previously been intubated successfully. Thus, failed intubation still represents a major cause of maternal morbidity and mortality from general anesthesia.

Few studies to date have compared neonatal outcomes between regional and general anesthesia for emergency cesarean section. A widely cited retrospective investigation by Marx et al. (119) evaluated neonatal condition after emergency cesarean section for fetal distress in 126 parturients who were allowed to "choose" their anesthetic technique. General anesthesia was used in 71, spinal anesthesia in 33, and extension of existing epidural blockade in 22 patients. The time from induction of general anesthesia to skin incision ranged from 55 to 90 seconds compared to a range of 4.5 to 6.0 minutes from induction of regional blockade to skin incision. Despite the apparent longer onset, neonates had better 1-minute Apgar scores when regional anesthesia was used. Apgar scores at 5 minutes and umbilical artery blood pH values did not differ among the groups. There were no apparent adverse maternal or fetal effects of regional anesthesia (spinal or epidural). Systolic blood pressure in the women receiving regional anesthesia did not decrease more than 15 mm Hg or drop below 100 mm Hg without the administration of a vasopressor. All patients received an 800-mL bolus of crystalloid before regional blockade. Ramanathan et al. (120) evaluated neonatal outcome in 101 emergency cesarean deliveries for fetal distress. General anesthesia was administered to 67 parturients, whereas 34 underwent extension of their epidural blockade. Apgar scores and fetal acid–base status did not differ between the two groups. Finally, Ong et al. (121) retrospectively evaluated fetal outcome in 319 cesarean deliveries performed for fetal distress under either epidural or general anesthesia. Infants whose mothers received epidural anesthesia had better Apgar scores and less need for ventilatory assistance immediately following delivery.

In the final analysis, there are probably no significant differences in neonatal status after emergency cesarean delivery using either regional or general anesthesia. At the same time, anesthesia-related maternal mortality, primarily from failed intubation and aspiration, is dramatically higher when general anesthesia is administered for cesarean section. Therefore, regional anesthesia, provided by an existing epidural catheter or subarachnoid blockade, is the safest anesthetic technique for the laboring parturient. When onset is a priority, induction of general anesthesia is faster than placement of a spinal anesthetic or extension of existing epidural blockade (119). Therefore, clear communication with the obstetrician about the urgency of the cesarean delivery and the maximum time that can elapse while preparing the patient for surgery is essential.

Preoperative Preparation

When fetal compromise is present, cesarean delivery must proceed at a more rapid pace than in the nonemergent setting. Therefore, an operating room must be available at all times, with equipment checked and in good working order. These items include, but are not limited to:

- An anesthesia machine with breathing circuit and face mask,
- Suction apparatus,
- Equipment for endotracheal intubation, including short-handled laryngoscope with an assortment of blades, cuffed styletted endotracheal tubes ranging in size from 5.5 to 7.0 mm, no. 3 and no. 4 size laryngeal mask airways, and a device for emergency cricothyrotomy and transtracheal ventilation, and
- Medications for induction and maintenance of general anesthesia.

The patient should have at least one large-bore intravenous catheter in place with an infusion of nonglucose-containing isotonic crystalloid solution. Give 30 mL of a nonparticulate antacid even if regional anesthesia is planned. Metaclopramide 10 mg can be added to increase the tone of the lower esophageal sphincter and for its antiemetic effect. However, metoclopramide does not significantly decrease gastric volume in patients undergoing emergency cesarean section (122). There is little benefit to the use of H_2-receptor antagonists. Intragastric pH does not increase for at least 30 to 40 minutes (122). Consider administering all three medications (sodium citrate, metoclopromide, and H_2-receptor antagonists) prophylactically during the intrapartum period in patients with morbid obesity, diabetes, or potential airway difficulty. Cesarean section must never proceed without adequate left uterine displacement. Administer supplemental oxygen until delivery and apply standard intraoperative monitors (electrocardiogram, pulse oximeter, and blood pressure cuff).

Finally, monitor fetal heart rate as continuously as possible until delivery (123,124). Often, the fetal heart rate abnormality will resolve or improve, and cesarean delivery can either be averted or performed in a calm and organized fashion. Stabilization of the fetal heart rate may permit the induction of epidural or spinal anesthesia. An electronic scalp electrode can be used to monitor fetal heart rate until delivery, at which time it can be disconnected under the surgical drapes or delivered through the uterine incision. Continuous assessment of fetal status can influence the speed at which surgical dissection is performed (124). It also can provide invaluable information should airway difficulties arise during induction of general anesthesia.

Epidural Anesthesia

Unless maternal hemorrhage is present, an existing epidural catheter is the technique of choice for emergency cesarean section. When a T_{10} sensory level is present, I extend the block with 15 to 20 mL of either 3% 2-chloroprocaine or 0.5% bupivacaine. I use 0.5% bupivacaine in the setting of *urgent* cesarean section, when the patient must be ready for incision within 30 minutes, for the following reasons:

- Bupivacaine provides dense sensory anesthesia without using an epinephrine-containing solution,
- Bupivacaine provides maternal hemodynamic stability because of gradual onset and lack of epinephrine, and
- Epidural opioids can be added for intraoperative anesthesia and to provide postoperative analgesia.

I reserve the use of 3% 2-chloroprocaine for *stat* cesarean section, when delivery must be accomplished as soon as possible. I begin extending the block before the patient is transported to the operating room. After a negative aspiration, I inject 20 to 25 mL of a premade 3% 2-chloroprocaine solution, which has been pH adjusted with sodium bicarbonate (1 mEq per 10 mL). I repeatedly aspirate every 5 mL and watch for overt signs of intravascular injection. Surgical anesthesia develops within 3 to 6 minutes (125). If the surgeons are ready to proceed earlier, supplemental local anesthetic can be injected in the incision or small doses (10 mg) of intravenous ketamine can be given to the parturient. Continuous reassurance that discomfort will be brief can improve patient cooperation. Because 2-chloroprocaine seems to antagonize neuraxial opioids, I place these patients on patient-controlled intravenous morphine for postoperative analgesia.

I do not use 2% lidocaine with epinephrine to extend the epidural block in the presence of fetal compromise. Epinephrine-containing solutions cause exaggerated hypotension from β_2-mediated vasodilation and can increase placental vascular resistance, especially in preeclamptic patients who have an increased sensitivity to catecholamines. Several authors, however, have reported that epidural anesthesia can be extended safely for emergency cesarean section using 1.5% or 2% lidocaine with epinephrine injected rapidly over 3 minutes (125,126,127). Price et al. (126) administered a 3-mL "test dose" of 2% lidocaine with epinephrine, monitored the maternal heart rate for 1 minute, and then injected 17 mL of drug over 3 minutes. All patients were "ready for surgery" (defined as complete loss of sensation to cold from T_6 to S_5, loss of sensation to pain to T_{10}, and Bromage grade 2 motor blockade) within 12.5 minutes. More than 90% were ready within 10 minutes. Although the rapid onset of this technique is appealing, I question the safety of injecting 2% lidocaine with epinephrine rapidly, even after a "negative test dose." Epinephrine is not a reliable indicator of intravascular placement of an epidural catheter in the obstetric population because of the wide fluctuation in maternal heart rate, especially in a tense emergency situation. Unlike lidocaine, 2-chloroprocaine is much safer to inject rapidly because local anesthetic-induced seizures from intravascular injection are short-lived owing to its rapid plasma hydrolysis. In addition, 2-chloroprocaine offers the following advantages over lidocaine:

- Onset of surgical anesthesia is faster [6 vs 12 minutes, or 3.1 vs 4.4 minutes (126)].
- Shorter maternal (21 seconds) and fetal (43 seconds) plasma half-lives. Ion trapping does not occur and toxicity from unintentional intravascular injection is short-lived.
- It produces dense sensory and motor blockade without the addition of epinephrine.

These advantages, along with the safety of rapid injection of 2-chloroprocaine, outweigh the minor disadvantages of its short duration and antagonism of neuraxial opioids.

Spinal Anesthesia

For a *stable* or *urgent* emergency cesarean section in the absence of an existing epidural catheter, I use spinal anesthesia as in the nonemergent/elective setting. After preoperative administration of a nonparticulate antacid and intravenous metoclopramide, the patient is transported to the operating room where standard intraoperative monitors are applied. I allow the intravenous fluids to infuse rapidly but do not give more than 1 L of nonglucose-containing isotonic crystalloid before induction. I have ephedrine and phenylephrine readily available. I always place the patient in the right lateral decubitus position (unless extreme obesity dictates the sitting position) to promote uniform spread of the local anesthetic once the patient is positioned supine with left uterine displacement. I inject 12 mg of hyperbaric bupivacaine with 10 μg of fentanyl and 300 μg of preservative-free morphine sulfate. A urinary catheter is inserted and surgery can begin within 5 to 10 minutes. Hyperbaric lidocaine offers little advantage over bupivacaine in terms of onset and, in my clinical practice, often fails to provide adequate duration of surgical anesthesia. I prevent high spinal blockade by elevating the head and cervical spine with pillows and by assuring that the operating room table is not in the Trendelenburg position. Treat systolic blood pressure below 100 mm Hg with ephedrine in 10-mg increments. If hypotension persists after 30 mg, or maternal heart rate is consistently more than 100 beats/min, administer phenylephrine in 40- to 50-μg boluses until maternal systolic blood pressure is greater than 100 mm Hg.

When cesarean section is categorized as *stat* and delivery must proceed as rapidly as possible, ask the obstetricians if they plan to perform a surgical scrub before the operation. If so, and there are no maternal contraindications to spinal anesthesia, I believe it is reasonable to attempt a subarachnoid block. The most experienced anesthesiologist present should make this attempt. Unless the spinal kit is prepared ahead of time with all medications drawn up into syringes, I seldom inject any local anesthetic into the skin, nor do I take time to add intrathecal opioids. I use 1.5 mL of 0.75% hyperbaric bupivacaine and add 100 μg of epinephrine to increase the density of the block.[4] Continuous monitoring of the fetal heart rate while attempting to induce spinal anesthesia can help determine how long to persist. If there is ongoing fetal distress and the block is not in place by the time the surgeons enter the operating room after washing their hands, I abandon the technique and induce general anesthesia.

General Anesthesia

In true emergency situations, when the obstetrician plans to splash betadine on the abdomen and don a surgical gown, I induce general anesthesia if I believe that the mother can be intubated successfully. When I suspect that intubation may be difficult, I have a low threshold for performing awake direct laryngoscopy and intubation. If I encounter unanticipated difficulty with intubation after induction of general anesthesia, I follow the "failed intubation" algorithm depicted in Fig. 5.

The technique of general anesthesia for cesarean delivery is described in detail elsewhere (see Chapter 20), but there are several points to consider when fetal distress is present.

Preoxygenation

When induction of general anesthesia must proceed rapidly, four maximal inspirations of 100% oxygen provide equivalent preoxygenation to that of 3 minutes of conventional oxygen administration (128).

---

[4] Editor's note: In either of these situations, I recommend 15mg hyperbaric bupivacaine ± 0.05mg morphine for spinal anesthesia.

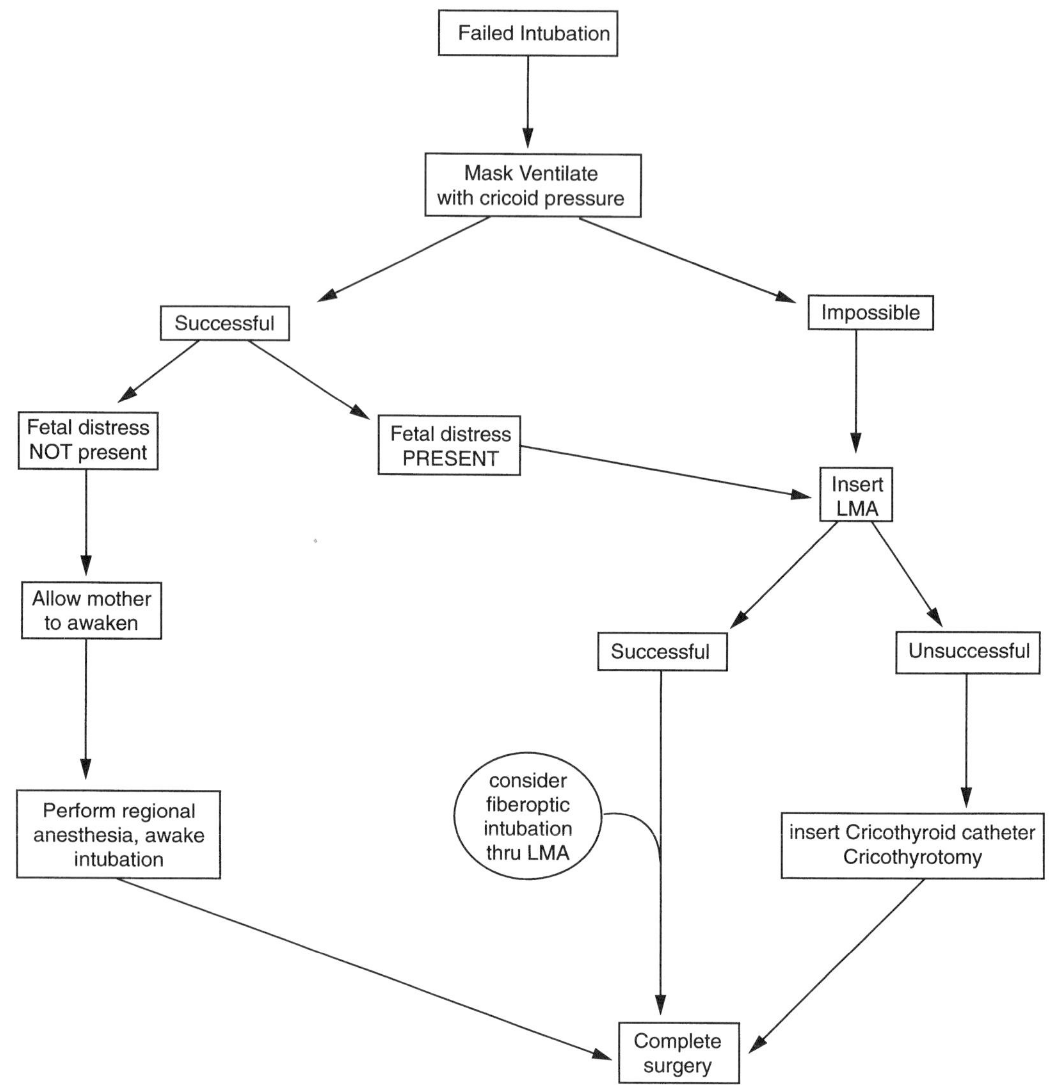

FIG. 5. Failed intubation algorithm.

Induction Agents

The ideal induction agent in the presence of fetal distress has not been determined. Thiopental is the standard against which other induction agents are compared. Peak fetal exposure after an intravenous dose of 4 mg/kg thiopental occurs in 1.5 to 3 minutes (129). Although it crosses the placenta rapidly, thiopental rarely is associated with significant neonatal depression due to at least three factors:

- Rapid redistribution in the maternal circulation,
- Dilution in the fetal inferior vena cava, and
- Uptake by the fetal liver (130,131).

There is no reason to either expedite or delay delivery after anesthetic induction to limit the depressant effects of thiopental. On the contrary, large doses of thiopental (30 mg/kg) have been administered to provide cerebral protection immediately after delivery in neonates thought to be at risk for neurological damage (132). However, significant hemodynamic instability results, with no improvement in neurological outcome. Methohexital, despite its shorter half-life, does not offer any advantage over thiopental (133).

Ketamine is a particularly well-suited induction agent when fetal distress is present. Like thiopental, ketamine 1 to 2 mg/kg rapidly crosses the placenta, and peak fetal blood concentrations develop in 1 to 2 minutes (134). Maternal mean arterial blood pressure and uterine blood flow are well preserved because of ketamine's sympathomimetic effects (135). Therefore, ketamine is an ideal induction agent for the hypotensive mother. In high doses (5 mg/kg), however, ketamine may increase both resting uterine tone and the frequency and intensity of uterine contractions (136,137). I usually limit the induction dose to 1.5 mg/kg and administer benzodiazepine after delivery to prevent dysphoria upon emergence.

Unlike other induction agents, the effects of ketamine have been studied on the asphyxiated fetus. In acidotic fetal lambs, ketamine abolishes the usual hypertensive response to umbilical cord occlusion. Nevertheless, cerebral, myocardial, and renal blood flow remain unchanged, and acid–base status does not deteriorate (138). Ketamine 2 mg/kg preserves fetal blood pressure and cerebral blood flow better than thiopental 6 mg/kg (139).

Several studies have compared neonatal outcome in humans after maternal induction with ketamine 1 mg/kg or thiopental 3-4mg/kg (140,141). Apgar scores and umbilical cord blood gas values are similar with both agents. One study, however, did report better neurobehavioral status of infants born after maternal induction with ketamine compared to thiopental for *vaginal* delivery (142). Therefore, ketamine is well suited as an induction agent in the presence of fetal compromise, especially when maternal hypotension or reactive airway disease coexist.

Etomidate 0.3 mg/kg sometimes is used as an induction agent for cesarean delivery. Compared with thiopental, etomidate produces fewer maternal hemodynamic changes and perhaps slightly better neonatal status as measured by time to sustained respiration (143,144). Propofol has been evaluated as an induction agent for elective cesarean delivery and lacks adverse effects on umbilical blood gas values or neurobehavioral scores (145). Unfortunately, these induction agents have not been studied in the asphyxiated fetus.

In summary, choice of induction agent in the presence of fetal compromise should be determined by maternal status. I use ketamine 1 to 2 mg/kg for induction of general anesthesia in the presence of maternal hemodynamic instability or reactive airway disease. Etomidate 0.3 mg/kg is another alternative when maternal hypovolemia is present. I use thiopental 3 to 5 mg/kg or propofol 1 to 2 mg/kg for induction in most other situations.

Maintenance of Anesthesia

- Maximize fetal blood flow and oxygen delivery.
- Maintain left uterine displacement.
- Give intravenous fluids and vasopressors to ensure stable maternal hemodynamics.
- Use a high inspired oxygen concentration. I give 100% oxygen before delivery of the asphyxiated fetus to maximize fetal pO_2 and oxygen saturation.
- Use enough volatile agent to provide sufficient depth of anesthesia to limit maternal catecholamine release (especially when nitrous oxide is omitted), because catecholamines can cause uterine artery vasoconstriction. I typically use 1% to 1.5% isoflurane before delivery, provided there is maternal hemodynamic stability. Brief exposure to such concentrations of volatile agent has little depressant effect on either the neonate or subsequent uterine contractility (146–148). There is no evidence to suggest that one inhalational agent is superior to another when fetal compromise is present. Brief exposure (less than 15 minutes) to moderate concentrations of inhalational agents do not significantly alter fetal compensatory responses to asphyxia (149,150).
- Maintain normocarbia. Low maternal p_aCO_2 shifts the oxyhemoglobin dissociation curve to the left, impairing oxygen delivery to the fetus (151). Aggressive positive-pressure ventilation decreases venous return, impairing maternal cardiac output and uterine perfusion (152). Profound maternal respiratory alkalosis (p_aCO_2 less than 17 mm Hg) may directly cause uterine artery vasoconstriction (153). Likewise, avoid maternal respiratory *acidosis* because it leads to fetal carbon dioxide retention and worsening acid–base status.

Local Anesthetic Infiltration

This technique is used to provide anesthesia for emergency cesarean delivery in the following rare circumstances:

- Failed or contraindicated regional anesthesia with an inaccessible airway,
- Failed intubation with ongoing fetal distress,
- Supplementation of an inadequate regional blockade, and
- Unavailability of trained personnel to administer other types of anesthesia.

The technique involves the infiltration of sequential layers in the mid-line of the lower abdominal wall with a large volume of dilute local anesthetic (typically 200 to 300 mL of 0.5% lidocaine with epinephrine) (154). Local anesthetic infiltration requires little technical skill, has a rapid onset, preserves maternal airway reflexes, and produces minimal fetal effects. However, the disadvantages of incomplete and often unsatisfactory anesthesia, combined with the potential for local anesthetic toxicity, make the use of this technique uncommon.

SUMMARY

The term “fetal distress” is applied indiscriminately to a wide variety of fetal conditions and clinical situations. The etiology of true fetal compromise often is multifactorial and seldom known with certainty. The diagnosis is hampered by our inability to directly monitor fetal status and the subjective interpretation of fetal heart rate patterns. Acute deterioration in fetal status seldom occurs without warning. Therefore, all patients presenting to the labor suite should be assessed by an anesthesiologist, and risk factors that predispose to fetal compromise and emergency cesarean delivery should be identified. High-risk patients, and their obstetric care providers, should be informed of the benefits of epidural placement early in labor to avoid the need for a rushed general anesthetic if fetal distress arises. Clear communication among obstetric, nursing, and anesthesia personnel throughout labor is critical. The anesthesiologist should be summoned at the first sign of fetal deterioration to allow formulation of an anesthetic plan without undue haste. Remember the relative safety of regional anesthesia in the presence of fetal compromise compared to the increased maternal risks of general anesthesia.

REFERENCES

1. Tucker JM, Hauth JC. Intrapartum assessment of fetal well-being. *Clin Obstet Gyn* 1990;33:515.
2. Parer JT, Livingston EG. What is fetal distress? *Am J Obstet Gynecol* 1990;162:1421.
3. Richardson BS, Carmichael L, Homan J, Johnston L, Gagnon R. Fetal cerebral, circulatory, and metabolic responses during heart rate decelerations with umbilical cord compression. *Am J Obstet Gynecol* 1996; 175:929.
4. Cohn HE, Sacks E, Heymann MA, Rudolph AM. Cardiovascular responses to hypoxemia and acidemia in fetal lambs. *Am J Obstet Gynecol* 1974;120:817.
5. Boddy K, Dawes GS, Fisher R. Foetal respiratory movements, electrocortical and cardiovascular responses to hypoxemia and hypercapnia in sheep. *J Physiol (Lond)* 1974;243:599.
6. Parer JT. The effect of acute maternal hypoxia on fetal oxygenation and the umbilical circulation in the sheep. *Eur J Obstet Gynecol Reprod Biol* 1980;10:125.
7. Yaffe H, Parer JT, Block, Llanos AJ. Cardiorespiratory responses to graded reductions in uterine blood flow in the sheep fetus. *J Dev Physiol* 1987;9:325.
8. Dellinger EH, Boehm FH. Emergency management of fetal stress and distress in the obstetric patient. *Obstet Gynecol Clin North Am* 1995; 22:2:215.
9. Phelan JP, Smith CV, Broussard P, Small M. Amniotic fluid volume assessment using the four-quadrant technique in the pregnancy between 36 and 42 weeks' gestation. *J Reprod Med* 1987;32:540.
10. Moore TR. Superiority of the four-quadrant sum over the single-deepest-pocket technique in ultrasonographic identification of abnormal amniotic fluid volumes. *Am J Obstet Gynecol* 1990;163:762.
11. Vintzileos AM, Fleming AD, Scorza WE. Relationship between fetal biophysical activities and umbilical cord blood gas values. *Am J Obstet Gynecol* 1991;165:707.
12. Trudinger BJ, Giles WB, Cook CM, Bombardieri J, Collins L. Fetal umbilical artery flow velocity waveforms and placental resistance: clinical significance. *Br J Obstet Gynaecol* 1985;92:23.
13. Brar HS, Platt LD. Antepartum improvement of abnormal umbilical artery velocimetry: does it occur? *Am J Obstet Gynecol* 1989;160:36.
14. Trudinger BJ, Giles WB. Clinical and pathological correlation of umbilical and uterine artery waveforms. *Clin Obstet Gynecol* 1989; 32:669.
15. Ogunyemi D, Stanley R, Lynch C, Edwards D, Fukushima T. Umbilical artery velocimetry in predicting perinatal outcome with intrapartum fetal distress. *Obstet Gynecol* 1992;80:377.
16. Strong TH, Hetzler G, Sarno AP, Paul RH. Prophylactic intrapartum amnioinfusion: a randomized clinical trial. *Am J Obstet Gynecol* 1990;162:1370.
17. Schrimmer DB, Macri CJ, Paul RH: Prophylactic amnioinfusion as a treatment for oligohydramnios in laboring patients: a prospective randomized trial. *Am J Obstet Gynecol* 1991;165:972.
18. Dragich DA, Ross AF, Chestnut DH, Wenstrom K. Respiratory failure associated with amnioinfusion during labor. *Anesth Analg* 1991;72: 549.
19. Miyazaki RS, Nevarez F. Saline amnioinfusion for relief of repetitive variable deceleration: a prospective randomized study. *Am J Obstet Gynecol* 1985;153:301.
20. Lameier LN, Katz VL. Amnioinfusion: a review. *Obstet Gynecol Surv* 1993;48:829.
21. Myers RE, Mueller-Heubach E, Adamsons K. Predictability of the state of fetal oxygenation from a quantitative analysis of the components of late deceleration. *Am J Obstet Gynecol* 1973;115:1083.
22. Guzman ER, Vintzileos AM, Martins M, Benito C, Houlihan C, Hanley M. The efficacy of individual computer heart rate indices in detecting acidemia at birth in growth-restricted fetuses. *Obstet Gynecol* 1996;87:969.
23. Gull I, Jaffa AJ, Oren M, Grisaru D, Peyser MR, Lessing JB. Acid accumulation during end-stage bradycardia in term fetuses: how long is too long? *Br J Obstet Gynaecol* 1996;103:1096.
24. Cibils LA. On intrapartum fetal monitoring. *Am J Obstet Gynecol* 1996;174:1382.
25. Nelson KB, Dambrosia JM, Ting TY, Grether JK. Uncertain value of electronic fetal monitoring in predicting cerebral palsy. *N Engl J Med* 1996;334:613.
26. Thacker SB, Stroup DF, Peterson HB. Efficacy and safety of intrapartum electronic fetal monitoring: an update. *Obstet Gynecol* 1995; 86:613.
27. American College of Obstetricians and Gynecologists. Intrapartum fetal heart rate monitoring. Technical Bulletin No. 132. Washington, DC: American College of Obstetricians and Gynecologists, 1989.
28. MacDonald D. Cerebral palsy and intrapartum fetal monitoring [Editorial]. *N Engl J Med* 1996;334:659.
29. Lurie S, Weissman A, Blumberg G, Hagay Z. Fetal oximetry monitoring: a new wonder or another mirage? *Obstet Gynecol Surv* 1996; 51:498.
30. Dildy GA, Clark SL, Loucks CA. Intrapartum fetal pulse oximetry: past, present, and future. *Am J Obstet Gynecol* 1996;175:1.
31. Goodwin TM, Milner-Masterson L, Paul RH. Elimination of fetal scalp blood sampling on a large clinical service. *Obstet Gynecol* 1994;83:971.
32. Clark SL, Gimovsky ML, Miller FC. Fetal heart rate response to scalp sampling. *Am J Obstet Gynecol* 1982;144:706.
33. Woods JR, Dolkart LA. Significance of amniotic fluid meconium. In: Creasy RK, Resnik R, eds. *Maternal-fetal medicine: principles and practice,* 2nd ed. Philadelphia: WB Saunders, 1989:404.
34. Meis PJ, Hobel CJ, Ureda JR. Late meconium passage in labor—a sign of fetal distress? *Obstet Gynecol* 1982;59:332.
35. Wenstrom KD, Parsons MT. The prevention of meconium aspiration in labor using amnioinfusion. *Obstet Gynecol* 1989;73:647.
36. Freeman JM, Nelson KB. Intrapartum asphyxia and cerebral palsy. *Pediatrics* 1988;82:240.
37. Nelson KB. Relationship of intrapartum and delivery room events to long-term neurologic outcome. *Clin Perinatol* 1989;16:995.
38. American College of Obstetricians and Gynecologists. ACOG committee opinion no. 174: use and abuse of the Apgar score. *Int J Gynecol Obstet* 1996;54:303.
39. Fee SC, Malee K, Deddish R, et al. Severe acidosis and subsequent neurologic status. *Am J Obstet Gynecol* 1990;162:802.
40. Tucker JM, Hauth JC. Intrapartum assessment of fetal well-being. *Clin Obstet Gynecol* 1990;33:515.
41. Josten BE, Johnson RE, Nelson JP. Umbilical cord blood pH and Apgar scores as an index of neonatal health. *Am J Obstet Gynecol* 1987;157:843.
42. Helwig JT, Parer JT, Kilpatrick SJ, Laros RK. Umbilical cord blood acid–base state: what is normal? *Am J Obstet Gynecol* 1996;174: 1807.
43. Thorp JA, Sampson JE, Parisi VM, Creasy RK. Routine umbilical cord blood gas determinations? Editors note: in either of these situations, I recommend 15 mg hyperbaric bupivacaine ± 0.05 mg morphine for spinal anesthesia. *Am J Obstet Gynecol* 1989;161:600.
44. Johnson JWC, Riley W. Cord blood gas studies: a survey. *Clin Obstet Gynecol* 1993;36:99.
45. Eckstein K, Marx GF. Aorto-caval compression and uterine displacement. *Anesthesiology* 1990;40:92.
46. Wilcourt RJ, King JC, Queenan JT. Maternal oxygen administration and fetal transcutaneous PO_2. *Am J Obstet Gynecol* 1983;146:714.
47. Ramanathan S, Gandhi S, Arismendy J, Chalon J, Turndorf H. Oxygen transfer from mother to fetus during cesarean section under epidural anesthesia. *Anesth Analg* 1982;61:576.
48. Baraka A. Correlation between maternal and foetal PO_2 and PCO_2 during cesarean section. *Br J Anaesth* 1970;42:434.
49. Marx GF, Mateo C. Effects of different oxygen concentrations during general anaesthesia for elective caesarean section. *Can Anaesth Soc J* 1971;18:587.
50. Rorke MJ, Davey DA, DuToit HJ. Foetal oxygenation during caesarean section. *Anaesthesia* 1968;23:585.
51. Piggott SE, Bogod DG, Rosen M, Rees GAD, Harmer M. Isoflurane with either 100% oxygen or 50% nitrous oxide in oxygen for caesarean section. *Br J Anaesth* 1990;65:325.

52. Philipson EH, Kalhan SC, Riha MM, Pimentel R. Effects of maternal glucose infusion on fetal acid–base status in human pregnancy. *Am J Obstet Gynecol* 1987;157:866.
53. Mendiola J, Grylack LJ, Scanlon JW. Effects of intrapartum maternal glucose infusion on the normal fetus and newborn. *Anesth Analg* 1982;61:32.
54. Blomstrand S, Hrbek A, Karlsson K. Does glucose administration affect the cerebral response to fetal asphyxia? *Acta Obstet Gynecol Scand* 1984;63:345.
55. Jackson R, Reid JA, Thorburn J. Volume preloading is not essential to prevent spinal-induced hypotension at Caesarean section. *Br J Anaesth* 1995;75:262.
56. Rout CC, Rocke DA, Levin J. A reevaluation of the role of crystalloid preload in the prevention of hypotension associated with spinal anesthesia for elective cesarean section. *Anesthesiology* 1993;79:262.
57. Park GE, Hauch MA, Curlin F, Datta S, Bader AM. The effects of varying volumes of crystalloid administration before cesarean delivery on maternal hemodynamics and colloid osmotic pressure. *Anesth Analg* 1996;83:299.
58. Vercauteren MP, Hoffmann V, Coppejans HC, Van Steenberge AL, Adriaensen HA. Hydroxyethylstarch compared with modified gelatin as volume preload before spinal anaesthesia for Caesarean section. *Br J Anaesth* 1996;76:731.
59. Riley ET, Cohen SE, Rubenstein AJ, Flanagan B. Prevention of hypotension after spinal anaesthesia for cesarean section: six percent hetastarch versus lactated Ringer's solution. *Anesth Analg* 1995; 81:838.
60. Ralston DH, Shnider SM, DeLorimier AA. Effects of equipotent ephedrine mephentermine and methoxamine on uterine blood flow in the pregnant ewe. *Anesthesiology* 1974;40:354.
61. Magness T, Rosenfeld C. Systemic and uterine responses to alpha-adrenergic stimulation in pregnant and nonpregnant ewes. *Am J Obstet Gynecol* 1986;155:897.
62. Moran DH, Perillo M, LaPorta RF, Bader AM, Datta S. Phenylephrine in the prevention of hypotension following spinal anesthesia for cesarean delivery. *J Clin Anesth* 1991;3:301.
63. Ramanathan S, Grant GJ. Vasopressor therapy for hypotension due to epidural anesthesia for cesarean section. *Acta Anaesthesiol Scand* 1988;32:559.
64. Patriarco MS, Viechnicki BM, Hutchinson TA, Klasko SK, Yeh SY. A study on intrauterine fetal resuscitation with terbutaline. *Am J Obstet Gynecol* 1987;157:384.
65. Wright JW, Patterson RM, Ridgway LE III, Berkus MD. Effect of tocolytic agents on fetal umbilical velocimetry. *Am J Obstet Gynecol* 1990;163:748.
66. Shekarloo A, Mendex-Bauer C, Cook V, Freese U. Terbutaline (intravenous bolus) for the treatment of acute intrapartum fetal distress. *Am J Obstet Gynecol* 1989;160:615.
67. Mendez-Bauer C, Shekarloo A, Cook V, Freese U. Treatment of acute intrapartum fetal distress by beta-2-sympathomimetics. *Am J Obstet Gynecol* 1987;156:638.
68. Burke MS, Porreco RP, Day D, et al. Intrauterine resuscitation with tocolysis; an alternate-month clinical trial. *J Perinatol* 1989;9:296.
69. Reynolds JD, Chestnut DH, Dexter F, McGrath J, Penning DH. Magnesium sulfate adversely affects fetal lamb survival and blocks fetal cerebral blood flow response during maternal hemorrhage. *Anesth Analg* 1996;83:493.
70. Vinatier D, Dufour P, Berard J. Utilization of intravenous nitroglycerin for obstetrical emergencies. *Int J Gynecol Obstet* 1996;55:129.
71. Bell EB. Nitroglycerin and uterine relaxation [Letter]. *Anesthesiology* 1996;85:683.
72. Redick LF, Livingston E. A new preparation of nitroglycerin for uterine relaxation. *Int J Obstet Anesth* 1995;4:14.
73. Riley ET, Flanagan B, Cohen SE, Chitkara U. Intravenous nitroglycerin: a potent uterine relaxant for emergency obstetric procedures. Review of literature and report of three cases. *Int J Obstet Anesth* 1996;5:264.
74. Wessen A, Elowsson P, Axemo P, Lindberg B. The use of intravenous nitroglycerin for emergency cervico-uterine relaxation. *Acta Anaesth Scand* 1995;39:847.
75. Desimone CA, Norris MC, Leighton BL. Intravenous nitroglycerin aids manual extraction of a retained placenta. *Anesthesiology* 1990;73:787.
76. Wheeler AS, James FM, Meis PJ, et al. Effects of nitroglycerin and nitroprusside on the uterine vasculature of gravid ewes. *Anesthesiology* 1980;52:390.
77. Lameier LN, Katz VL. Amnioinfusion: a review. *Obstet Gynecol Surv* 1993;48:829.
78. Owen J, Henson BV, Hauth JC. A prospective randomized study of saline solution amnioinfusion. *Am J Obstet Gynecol* 1990;162:1146.
79. Strong TH, Hetzler G, Sarno AP, Paul RH. Prophylactic intrapartum amnioinfusion: a randomized clinical trial. *Am J Obstet Gynecol* 1990;162:1370.
80. Schrimmer DB, Macri CJ, Paul RH. Prophylactic amnioinfusion as a treatment for oligohydramnios in laboring patients: a prospective randomized trial. *Am J Obstet Gynecol* 1991;165:972.
81. Dragich DA, Ross AF, Chestnut DH, Wenstrom K. Respiratory failure associated with amnioinfusion during labor. *Anesth Analg* 1991;72: 549.
82. Morgan BM, Magni V, Goroszenuik T. Anaesthesia for emergency caesarean section. *Br J Obstet Gynaecol* 1990;97:420.
83. Thorp JA, Hu DH, Albin RM, et al. Reply to letters to the editor regarding the effect of intrapartum epidural analgesia on nulliparous labor: a randomized prospective trial. *Am J Obstet Gynecol* 1994;171: 1396.
84. Clarke VT, Smiley RM, Finster M. Uterine hyperactivity after intrathecal injection of fentanyl for analgesia during labor: a cause of fetal bradycardia? *Anesthesiology* 1994;81:1083.
85. Herbstman CH, Zaidan JT, O'Neil L, Newman LM. Fetal bradycardia and uterine hypertonicity after intrathecal fentanyl in laboring women. Abstract, SOAP Meeting, 1997.
86. Cohen SE, Cherry CM, Holbrook H, et al. Intrathecal sufentanil for labor analgesia-sensory changes, side effects and fetal heart rate changes. *Anesth Analg* 1993;77:1155.
87. Segal S, Csavoy A, Datta S. Elevated maternal catecholamines in labor are tocolytic: an in-vitro study of the effects of physiologic concentrations of norepinephrine and epinephrine on uterine activity in the gravid rat uterus. Abstract, SOAP Meeting, 1997.
88. Eberle RL, Norris MC, Mallozzi-Eberle A, Naulty JS, Arkoosh VA. The effect of maternal position on fetal heart rate during epidural or intrathecal analgesia for labor. *Anesthesiology* 1995;83:A944.
89. Neilsen PE, Erickson R, Abouleish EI, Perriatt S, Sheppard C. Fetal heart rate changes after intrathecal sufentanil or epidural bupivacaine for labor analgesia: incidence and clinical significance. *Anesth Analg* 1996;83:742.
90. Kahn L, Hubert E. Combined spinal epidural (CSE) analgesia, fetal bradycardia, and uterine hypertonus. *Reg Anesth Pain Med* 1998;23: 111.
91. Albright GA, Forster RM. Does combined spinal-epidural analgesia with subarachnoid sufentanil increase the incidence of emergency cesarean delivery? *Reg Anesth* 1997;22:400.
92. Nageotte MP, Larson D, Rumney PJ, Sidhu M, Hollenbach K. Epidural analgesia compared with combined spinal-epidural analgesia during labor in nulliparous women. *N Engl J Med* 1997;337: 1715.
93. Mercier FJ, Bouaziz H, Benhamou D. Transition from intrathecal analgesia to epidural anesthesia for emergency cesarean section using a combined spinal epidural technique. *Anesth Analg* 1996;83:434.
94. Frigoletto FD Jr, Ryan KJ, Phillippe M. Maternal mortality rate associated with cesarean section: an appraisal. *Am J Obstet Gynecol* 1986; 136:969.
95. Hawkins JL, Koonin LM, Palmer SK, Gibbs CP. Anesthesia-related deaths during obstetric delivery in the United States, 1979–1990. *Anesthesiology* 1997;86:277.
96. Marx GF, Elstein ID, Schuss M, Anyaegbunam A, Fleischer A. Effects of epidural block with lignocaine and lignocaine-adrenaline on umbilical artery velocity wave ratios. *Br J Obstet Gynaecol* 1990;97:517.
97. Marx GF, Patel S, Berman JA, Farmakides G, Schulman H. Umbilical blood flow velocity waveforms in different maternal positions and with epidural analgesia. *Obstet Gynecol* 1986;68:61.
98. Jouppila P, Jouppila R, Hollmen A, Koivula A. Lumbar epidural analgesia to improve intervillous blood flow during labor in severe preeclampsia. *Obstet Gynecol* 1982;59:158.
99. Scanlon JW, Brown WU, Weiss JB, Alper MH. Neurobehavioral responses of newborn infants after maternal epidural anesthesia. *Anesthesiology* 1974;40:121.
100. Scanlon JW, Ostheimer GW, Lurie AO, Brown WU, Weiss JB, Alper MH. Neurobehavioral responses and drug concentrations in newborns after maternal epidural anesthesia with bupivacaine. *Anesthesiology* 1976;45:400.
101. Abboud TK, Sarkis F, Blikian A, Varakian L, Earl S, Henriksen E.

Lack of adverse neonatal neurobehavioral effects of lidocaine. *Anesth Analg* 1983;62:473.
102. Abboud TK, Kim KC, Noueihed R, et al. Epidural bupivacaine, chloroprocaine, or lidocaine for cesarean section-maternal and neonatal effects. *Anesth Analg* 1983;62:914.
103. Kileff ME, James FM, Dewan DM, Floyd HM. Neonatal neurobehavioral responses after epidural anesthesia for cesarean section using lidocaine and bupivacaine. *Anesth Analg* 1984;63:413.
104. Kuhnert BR, Harrison MJ, Linn PL, Kuhnert PM. Effects of maternal epidural anesthesia on neonatal behavior. *Anesth Analg* 1984;63:301.
105. Morishima HO, Covino BG. Toxicity and distribution of lidocaine in nonasphyxiated and asphyxiated baboon fetuses. *Anesthesiology* 1981;54:182.
106. Kuhnert BR, Kuhnert PM, Prochaska AL, Gross TL. Plasma levels of 2-chloroprocaine in obstetric patients and their neonates after epidural anesthesia. *Anesthesiology* 1980;53:21.
107. Philipson EH, Kuhnert BR, Syracuse CD. Fetal acidosis, 2-chloroprocaine, and epidural anesthesia for cesarean section. *Am J Obstet Gynecol* 1985;151:322.
108. O'Brien JE, Abbey V, Hinsvark O, et al. Metabolism and measurement of chloroprocaine, an ester-type local anesthetic. *J Pharm Sci* 1979; 68:75.
109. Grant GJ, Ramanathan S, Turndorf H. The maternal hemodynamic effects of bupivacaine-epinephrine mixture used for obstetrical anesthesia. *Acta Anaesthesiol Scand* 1990;34:543.
110. Hood DD, Dewan DM, James FM. Maternal and fetal effects of epinephrine in gravid ewes. *Anesthesiology* 1986;64:610.
111. Marx GF, Elstein ID, Schuss M, Anyaegbunam A, Fleischer A. Effects of epidural block with lignocaine and lignocaine-adrenaline on umbilical artery velocity wave ratios. *Br J Obstet Gynaecol* 1990;97:517.
112. Hoffman CT, Guzman ER, Richardson MJ, Vintzileos A, Houlihan C, Benito C. Effects of narcotic and non-narcotic continuous epidural anesthesia on intrapartum fetal heart rate tracings as measured by computer analysis. *J Matern Fetal Med* 1997;6:200.
113. Viscomi CM, Hood DD, Melone PJ, Eisenach JC. Fetal heart rate variability after epidural fentanyl during labor. *Anesth Analg* 1990;71:679.
114. Benlabed M, Dreizzen E, Ecoffey C, Escourou P, Migdal M, Gaultier C. Neonatal patterns of breathing after cesarean section with or without epidural fentanyl. *Anesthesiology* 1990;73:1110.
115. Hauth JC, Merenstein GB, eds. *Guidelines for perinatal care,* 4th ed. American Academy of Pediatrics and American College of Obstetricians and Gynecologists, 1997:112.
116. Harris AP. Emergency cesarean section. In Rogers MC, ed. *Current practice in anesthesiology.* Toronto: BC Decker, 1990:361.
117. Hibbard BM, Anderson MM, Drife JO, et al. *Report on confidential enquiries into maternal deaths in the United Kingdom 1991–1993.* London: Her Majesty's Stationery Office, 1996.
118. Hawthorne L, Wilson R, Lyons G, Dresner M. Failed intubation revisited: 17-yr experience in a teaching maternity unit. *Br J Anaesth* 1996;76:680.
119. Marx GF, Luykx WM, Cohen S. Fetal-neonatal status following caesarean section for fetal distress. *Br J Anaesth* 1984;56:1009.
120. Ramanathan J, Ricca DM, Sibai BM, Angel JJ. Epidural vs general anesthesia for fetal distress with various abnormal fetal heart rate patterns. *Anesth Analg* 1988;67:S180(abst).
121. Ong BY, Cohen MM, Palahniuk RJ. Anesthesia for cesarean section—effects on neonates. *Anesth Analg* 1989;68:270.
122. Stuart JC, Kan AF, Rowbottom SJ, Yau G, Gin T. Acid aspiration prophylaxis for emergency caesarean section. *Anaesthesia* 1996;51:415.
123. Chestnut DH. Anesthesia for fetal distress. In Chestnut DH, ed. *Obstetric anesthesia principles and practice.* St. Louis: Mosby, 1994:487.
124. Petrikovsky BM, Cohen M, Tancer ML. Usefulness of continuous fetal heart rate monitoring during cesarean section. *Am J Obstet Gynecol* 1989;161:36.
125. Gaiser RR, Cheek TG, Adams HK, Gutsche BB. Epidural lidocaine for cesarean delivery. *Int J Obstet Anesth* 1998;7:27.
126. Price ML, Reynolds F, Morgan BM. Extending epidural blockade for emergency caesarean section. *Int J Obstet Anesth* 1991;1:13.
127. Gaiser RR, Cheek TG, Gutsche BB. Epidural lidocaine versus 2-chloroprocaine for fetal distress requiring urgent cesarean section. *Int J Obstet Anesth* 1994;3:208.
128. Norris MC, Dewan DM. Preoxygenation for cesarean section: a comparison of two techniques. *Anesthesiology* 1985;62:827.
129. Kosaka Y, Takahashi T, Mark LC. Intravenous thiobarbiturate anesthesia for cesarean section. *Anesthesiology* 1969;31:489.
130. Finster M, Morishima HO, Mark LC, et al. Tissue thiopental concentration in the fetus and newborn. *Anesthesiology* 1972;36:155.
131. Woods WA, Stanski DR, Curtis J, et al. The role of the fetal liver in the distribution of thiopental from mother to fetus. *Anesthesiology* 1982; 57:A390.
132. Goldberg R, Moscoso P, Bauer C, et al. Use of barbiturate therapy in severe perinatal asphyxia: a randomized controlled trial. *J Pediatr* 1986;109:851.
133. Sliom CM, Frankel L, Holbrook RA. A comparison between methohexitone and thiopentone as induction agents for caesarean section anesthesia. *Br J Anaesth* 1962;34:316.
134. Ellingson A, Haram K, Sagen N, et al. Transplacental passage of ketamine after intravenous administration. *Acta Anaesth Scand* 1977;21:41.
135. Levinson G, Shnider SM, Gildea JE, DeLorimer AA. Maternal and foetal cardiovascular and acid–base changes during ketamine anaesthesia in pregnant ewes. *Br J Anaesth* 1973;45:1111.
136. Craft JB, Coaldrake LA, Yonekura JL, et al. Ketamine, catecholamines, and uterine tone in pregnant ewes. *Am J Obstet Gynecol* 1983; 146:429.
137. Marx GF, Hwang H, Chandra P. Postpartum uterine pressures with different doses of ketamine. *Anesthesiology* 1979;50:163.
138. Swartz J, Cumming M, Biehl D. The effect of ketamine anaesthesia on the acidotic fetal lamb. *Can J Anaesth* 1987;34:233.
139. Pickering BG, Palahniuk RJ, Cote J, et al. Cerebral vascular responses to ketamine and thiopentone during foetal acidosis. *Can Anesth Soc J* 1982;29:157.
140. Peltz B, Sinclair DM. Induction agents for caesarean section—a comparison of thiopentone and ketamine. *Anaesthesia* 1973;28:37.
141. Bernstein K, Gisselsson L, Jacobsson L, et al. Influence of two different anaesthetic agents on the newborn and the correlation between foetal oxygenation and induction-delivery time in elective caesarean section. *Acta Anesthesiol Scand* 1985;29:157.
142. Hodgkinson R, Marx GF, Kim SS, et al. Neonatal neurobehavioral test following vaginal delivery under ketamine, thiopental, and extradural anesthesia. *Anesth Analg* 1977;56:548.
143. Downing JW, Buley RJF, Brock-Utne JG, et al. Etomidate for induction of anaesthesia at caesarean section: comparison with thiopentone. *Br J Anaesth* 1979;51:135.
144. Ionescu T, Besse TC, Smalhout B. Etomidate during caesarean section, general anaesthesia in obstetrics. In: *International Congress Series,* No. 533, Seventh World Congress of Anaesthesiologists, Hamburg, West Germany. Amsterdam: Excerpta Medica, 1980:318.
145. Dailland P, Cockshott ID, Lirzin JD, et al. Intravenous propofol during cesarean section: placental transfer, concentrations in breast milk, and neonatal effects. A preliminary study. *Anesthesiology* 1989;71:827.
146. Piggott SE, Bogod DG, Rosen M, Rees GAD, Harmer M. Isoflurane with either 100% oxygen or 50% nitrous oxide in oxygen for caesarean section. *Br J Anaesth* 1990;65:325.
147. Bogod DG, Rosen M, Rees GAD. Maximum FIO_2 during caesarean section. *Br J Anaesth* 1988;61:255.
148. Tunstall ME, Sheikh A. Comparison of 1.5% enflurane with 1.25% isoflurane in oxygen for caesarean section. *Br J Anaesth* 1989;62: 138.
149. Baker BW, Hughes SC, Shnider SM, Field DR, Rosen MA. Maternal anesthesia and the stressed fetus: effects of isoflurane on the asphyxiated fetal lamb. *Anesthesiology* 1990;72:65.
150. Mokriski BK, Malinow AM. Neonatal acid–base status following general anesthesia for emergency abdominal delivery with halothane or isoflurane. *J Clin Anesth* 1992;4:97.
151. Ralston DH, Shnider SM, deLorimier AA. Uterine blood flow and fetal acid–base changes after bicarbonate administration to the pregnant ewe. *Anesthesiology* 1974;40:348.
152. Levinson G, Shnider SM, deLorimier AA, Steffenson JL. Effects of maternal hyperventilation on uterine blood flow and fetal oxygenation and acid–base status. *Anesthesiology* 1974;40:340.
153. Morishima HO, Daniel SS, Adamsons K Jr, James LS. Effects of positive pressure ventilation of the mother upon the acid–base state of the fetus. *Am J Obstet Gynecol* 1965;93:269.
154. Barth WH. Local infiltration for cesarean delivery. In: Ostheimer GW, ed. *Manual of obstetric anesthesia,* 2nd ed. New York: Churchill Livingstone, 1992:202.

Obstetric Anesthesia, second edition,
edited by Mark C. Norris.
Lippincott Williams & Wilkins, Philadelphia © 1999.

CHAPTER 34

The Premature Fetus

Holly A. Muir

Preterm birth is defined as delivery before 37 weeks completed gestation or 259 days after the first day of the last menstrual period. Low birth weight is defined as a birth weight of less than 2,500 g regardless of gestational age, and very low birth weight as less than 1,500 g at birth. In developed nations, 5% to 10% of births are preterm. Approximately 13 million preterm infants are born each year worldwide. In the United States, the incidence of preterm birth was estimated to be 10.7% in 1989 (1–3). The incidence of preterm birth was 8.9% before 1980 and 9.4% in 1981. Racial differences continue to be dramatic, with 8.8% of white and 18.9% of black births being preterm in 1989 (4–6). Approximately 45% of the preterm births follow preterm labor with intact membranes, 30% are a consequence of premature rupture of membranes (PROM), and 25% are secondary to fetal or maternal concerns. Prematurity is, by far, the leading cause of perinatal morbidity and mortality. Preterm birth accounts for between 69% and 83% of neonatal deaths.

Presently, nearly 100% of nonanomalous neonates born after at least 32 weeks' gestation survive. When birth takes place in a tertiary care center, survival rates are 90% after 29 to 30 weeks' gestation and near 50% for 26 weeks' gestation (7). Prolonging an otherwise uncomplicated pregnancy by as little as 1 week will significantly decrease neonatal morbidity. The risk of respiratory distress syndrome (RDS) declines progressively until 36 weeks. The frequency of patent ductus arteriosis and necrotizing enterocolitis fall steadily until 32 weeks. High-grade intraventricular hemorrhage (IVH) diminishes rapidly after 27 weeks and is almost absent after 32 weeks (1). The most dramatic decrease in risk occurs between weeks 25 and 26, when survival increases from 15% to 55% (2). Fewer than 15% of surviving neonates born before 26 weeks' gestation or weighing less than 800 g will have neurological handicaps (7). Therefore, efforts to salvage these infants are worthwhile and often rewarded with a normal child.

The causes of morbidity in the preterm neonate are many and formidable (Table 1). Periventricular hemorrhage and IVH have replaced RDS as the leading cause of morbidity and mortality in the preterm infant. IVH com-

TABLE 1. *Causes of morbidity and mortality in the premature neonate*

Respiratory	Respiratory distress syndrome (RDS) or hyaline membrane disease Bronchopulmonary dysplasia (BPD) Sudden infant death syndrome (SIDS) from apneic episodes Interstitial emphysema, pneumothorax
Neurologic	Periventricular and intraventricular hemorrhage (IHV) Neurological damage causing cerebral palsy, hydrocephalus, and seizure disorders Retinopathy of prematurity (ROP: benign and reversible) progressing to irreversible retrolental fibroplasis (RLF)
Circulatory	Persistent fetal circulation with patent ductus arteriosus and resultant pulmonary hypertension
Gastrointestinal	Necrotizing enterocolitis (NEC) Hyperbilirubinemia
Obstetric	Increased breech presentation (premature >25%, term <3%) Birth asphyxia Birth trauma Infection from prolonged rupture of membranes and chorioamnionitis
Miscellaneous	Increased incidence of congenital anomalies Decreased thermoregulation Decreased maternal interaction and bonding

H. A. Muir: Department of Anesthesiology, Division of Women's Anesthesia, Duke University Medical Center, Durham, NC 27701.

plicates more than 50% of preterm births with birth weights less than 1,200 g (8). Avoiding peripartum asphyxia, birth trauma, and hypothermia will minimize the incidence and morbidity of RDS, bronchopulmonary dysplasia, IVH, necrotizing enterocolitis, and retrolental fibroplasia in the preterm infant. Appropriate and skillfully administered anesthesia may limit the risks of birth trauma and perinatal asphyxia in the premature newborn (9).

OBSTETRIC CONSIDERATIONS IN PREMATURITY

Optimal anesthetic care of the woman with a preterm fetus requires familiarity with the evaluations, procedures, and medications used by the obstetrician to care for these high-risk patients (Table 2). Many of the therapeutic modalities have significant anesthetic implications.

There are a variety of conditions associated with preterm birth, including PROM with resultant premature labor (PML), infection, incompetent cervix, uterine malformations, maternal disease conditions such as preeclampsia, fetal conditions such as intrauterine fetal growth retardation, polyhydramnios, or fetal compromise and increasingly maternal substance (cocaine) abuse.

Fetal Evaluation

In utero fetal evaluation is the key to the rational therapy of PML. Two essential steps are estimating gestational age and determining fetal lung maturity. Pregnancy dates based on the last menstrual period often are in error. If performed early, diagnostic ultrasound, which is without physical risk to mother and fetus, can accurately time pregnancy within 1 week.

Fetal lung maturity usually is determined by analyzing amniotic fluid for components of lung surfactant. Historically, determining the lecithin/sphingomyelin (L/S) ratio was most common. The L/S ratio increases rapidly between 33 and 35 weeks and is usually greater than 2 at 35 weeks' gestation. In the nondiabetic parturient, an L/S ratio greater than 2 is associated with minimal risk of RDS. A value less than 1.5 predicts a significant risk of RDS. Other amniotic fluid determinations of lung maturity include both phosphatidylinositol and phosphatidylglycerol. The presence of phosphatidylglycerol in amniotic fluid virtually assures the absence of RDS.

Tocolytic Drugs

A remarkable variety of drugs have been used in attempts to stop preterm labor (Table 3). Today, β agonists and magnesium sulfate are the most widely used. Tocolytic agents act by a variety of mechanisms and have numerous side effects and anesthetic interactions, some of which can be life threatening.

β Agonists

Despite initial optimism, the advent of β-agonist tocolytic drugs has not had a significant impact on the frequency of preterm birth in Western Europe or North America (7,10). One reason for this failure may be poor patient selection. Fewer than 30% of patients presenting in PML are candidates for tocolysis (Table 4). Even though tocolytic use often is associated with a delay in delivery, it may not improve ultimate neonatal outcome. A review of 16 randomized controlled trials of β-agonist tocolytics (ritodrine, terbutaline, or isoxsuprine) published between 1966 and 1986 compared outcome in 484 treated women versus 406 controls (11). The author found "...an unequivocal effect of beta-mimetic tocolytic administration in delaying delivery and this is reflected in a reduction in the

TABLE 2. *Obstetric considerations with preterm labor*

Determine if preterm labor does indeed exist	Contractions Cervical dilatation and effacement
Treat underlying causes of preterm labor if possible	Infection Incompetent cervix: use of cerclage in early second trimester Medical conditions Surgical correction of uterine abnormalities in nonpregnant state
Fetal evaluation	Gestational age Weight Lung maturity Presence of fetal anomalies Fetal well-being: biophysical profile
Evaluation of state of pregnancy	Membranes: intact or ruptured Placental abnormalities: previa or abruptio Presentation and station of fetus
Tocolysis when indicated	
Enhancement of fetal lung maturity	Glucocorticoids
Delivery plan	Induction or trial of labor Cesarean section Attempt external version

TABLE 3. *Methods of tocolysis*

Historic and rarely used methods	Progesterone injections Ethanol: often required inebriation, associated with pulmonary acid aspiration Phosphodiesterase inhibitors (amniophylline)
Current methods	First step: bed rest Second step • β_2 agonists (ritodrine, terbutaline) • Magnesium sulphate Special use or occasional • Prostaglandin synthesis inhibitors (indomethacin) • Calcium channel blockers
New methods	Atosiban
Experimental methods	Glyceryl trinitrate Urinary trypsin inhibitor Lidocaine

frequency of preterm birth and low birthweight. However, no beneficial effect of this treatment on perinatal mortality or severe neonatal respiratory disorders could be detected." Despite these pessimistic findings, tocolysis remains a cornerstone in the treatment of PML.

β Agonists have multiple maternal physiologic effects (Table 5). Side effects, many of which have important anesthetic implications, are common (Table 6) (12).

Cardiac Effects

β-Agonist induced tachycardia, with maternal heart rates above 100 beats/min, often is associated with tremor, palpitations, and chest pain. Heart rate may exceed 140 beats/min with concurrent administration of drugs such as epinephrine, ephedrine, anticholinergics, or intravenous bolus oxytocin. Consider avoiding epinephrine-containing local anesthetics and using phenylephrine instead of ephedrine in patients with significant, symptomatic β-agonist–induced tachycardia. Arrhythmias, including premature ventricular contractions, premature nodal contractions, and atrial fibrillations have been reported with β-agonist therapy (12). Although some of these arrhythmias are benign, they often are indications for stopping β-agonist therapy. Ventricular arrhythmias may worsen with concomitant exposure to halothane.

Angina pectoris and associated electrocardiographic changes have been reported during β-agonist tocolysis (13–17). Pain usually resolves when the β agonist is stopped. Enzyme changes suggesting myocardial damage are extremely rare. Electrocardiographic changes suggestive of myocardial ischemia (including ST depression and T-wave inversion) are common and occur in over 70% of asymptomatic parturients receiving β agonists (14). These changes arise independently of patient symptoms, rate or dose of β-agonist administration, serum potassium concentration, or cardiac enzyme concentrations.

Cardiac output, elevated 40% in the third trimester of normal pregnancy, may be increased 80% above nonpregnant values with β-agonist therapy. Even the "receptor specific" β-agonist drugs have both inotropic and chronotropic effects (15).

Pulmonary Edema

The most serious complication associated with β agonists is pulmonary edema, with an reported incidence as high as 5% (18). Reported cases have involved oral, subcutaneous, and continuous intravenous infusions. The risk does not correlate with the total dose of drug or the rate of infusion. Pulmonary edema has been reported

TABLE 4. *Contraindications to tocolysis in premature labor*

Absolute	Relative
Fetal	
Mature fetus, fetal anomalies incompatible with life, severe IUFGR, chorioamnionitis	Rupture of membranes without chorioamnionitis, fetal anomaly, mild IUFGR, fetal distress
Maternal	
Severe preeclampsia or eclampsia, decompensated cardiac disease, chorioamnionitis, severe bleeding, maternal refusal or noncompliance	Controlled metabolic disease (e.g., diabetes, hyperthyroidism), cervix >4–5 cm dilated
Placental	
Significant bleeding of any cause, coagulopathy, severe abruption	Stable abruption or previa

TABLE 5. *Physiologic effects of β agonists*

β_1	β_2
Cardiac	Smooth Muscle
Increased stroke volume	Decreased uterine activity
Increased heart rate	Vasodilation
	Bronchiolar relaxation
Renal	Renal
Increased renal blood flow	Increased renin and aldosterone production
	Decreased urinary output
Metabolic	Metabolic
Lipolysis with increase in ketones	Increased insulin release
Increased intracellular K^+ with decreased in serum K^+	Increased glycogenolysis with increase in blood sugar
	Metabolic lactic acidosis

both before (during therapy) and after delivery (after cessation of therapy) (19).

The etiology of the pulmonary edema is unclear, but is likely multifactorial. Both cardiogenic and noncardiogenic mechanisms have been proposed. Possible cardiogenic causes include:

- Fluid overload,
- Catecholamine-related myocardial necrosis,
- Cardiac failure secondary to tachycardia, and
- Down regulation of cardiac β receptors due to chronic β-agonist exposure (18,20).

However, neither pulmonary artery catheterization nor echocardiography have demonstrated left ventricular failure in these women (12,21). Increased pulmonary vascular permeability and decreased colloid oncotic pressure could cause noncardiogenic pulmonary edema. The usual rapid resolution of the pulmonary edema with treatment makes this concept somewhat less plausible, as it is difficult to envisage a membrane defect that would resolve so quickly.

Whereas tocolysis stems from the β_2 actions of these drugs, pulmonary edema may be a consequence of their β_1 effects. In dogs, a selective β_1 antagonist (metoprolol) protected against pulmonary edema (22). These results suggest a role of β_1 stimulation in the genesis of this complication.

TABLE 6. *Maternal side effects of β-agonist tocolytics*

Tachycardia and palpitations
Dysrhythmias and myocardial sensitization
Vasodilation and postural hypotension
Cardiomyopathy
ECG changes of hypokalemia and ischemia
Pulmonary edema
Hypokalemia
Hyperglycemia
Lactic acidosis
Fluid retention
Apprehension
Insomnia
Tremor
Headache and exacerbation of migraine
Nausea and vomiting
Uterine atony and postpartum hemorrhage

A variety of factors may increase the risk of pulmonary edema during β-agonist tocolysis (Table 7) (22). Although once a popular theory, simultaneous administration of β agonists and glucocorticoids does not add to the incidence of pulmonary edema (12). The correlation between β-agonist and glucocorticoid therapy more likely represents an incidental association (20). The relationship between pulmonary edema and general anesthesia may represent the effect of a myocardial depressant on an already stressed cardiovascular system.

Pulmonary edema usually occurs 24 to 72 hours after initial intravenous administration of the β-agonist tocolytics, as the dose is being rapidly elevated, or when tocolysis is unsuccessful and the mother receives general anesthesia for delivery. It appears unrelated to dosage, occurs with equal frequency for all the β agonists, and only occasionally is seen once the mother is on oral maintenance. It has a significant mortality and, hence, requires rapid recognition and effective treatment, including discontinuation of the β agonist and avoidance of other tocolytic drugs, fluid restriction, the sitting position, a high inspired F_IO_2, and diuresis with furosemide. Occasionally, invasive central venous or pulmonary artery monitoring may help guide fluid and cardiac therapy. Rarely, intubation, positive pressure ventilation, and the addition of positive and expiratory pressure will be needed.

Because the etiology of pulmonary edema almost never is cardiac failure (decreased contractility), digitalis therapy rarely is indicated and may predispose to serious arrhythmias due to the coexisting hypokalemia (20).

Metabolic Effects

Metabolic changes accompanying β-agonist tocolytic therapy are hypokalemia, hyperglycemia, and lactic acidosis (23,24). Potassium concentrations of less then 3.0 mEq/L often are seen and are due to an influx of potassium into cells. This intracellular flux of potassium

TABLE 7. *Factors predisposing to the development of pulmonary edema with β-agonist tocolytic use*

Changes specific to pregnancy
Capillary wall alterations
Hypervolemia
Hypoproteinemia
Decreased colloid oncotic pressure
Fluid overload
Diseases of the heart, lungs, kidneys, and metabolism
Chorioamnionitis
Coadministration of prostaglandin antagonist
General anesthesia
Multiple gestation

results from hyperinsulinemia and direct β_2-adrenoreceptor stimulation (25). The fall in potassium occurs during initiation of intravenous therapy or within a few hours of abrupt cessation of the tocolytic (Fig. 1) (25,26). Maternal hyperventilation can exaggerate hypokalemia. As total body potassium remains normal, replacement seldom is necessary. Many of the physiologic changes associated with hypokalemia can have anesthetic implications (Table 8).

β_2-Receptor stimulation causes glycogenolysis and hyperglycemia. Metabolic lactic acidosis and a rise in maternal serum insulin concentration follow. In nondiabetic parturients, blood glucose concentrations of 140 to 160 mg/dL are common. Maternal hyperglycemia can predispose to reactive neonatal hypoglycemia. Using dextrose-free intravenous preparations before delivery may limit this risk. Using β-agonist tocolytic drugs in the diabetic parturient requires careful blood glucose monitoring and usually concomitant insulin infusion.

Maternal fluid retention is common and may decrease hemoglobin and plasma oncotic pressure (27). Other side effects of the β-agonist tocolytics include nausea, vomiting, insomnia, tremors, and headache, with an exacerbation of migraine-type headaches. Theoretically, when these drugs are used up to or near delivery, postpartum uterine atony associated with excessive maternal blood loss may occur. Uterine atony usually is treated with one or more of the following: oxytocin, ergotamine, and prostaglandin. Ergotamine has been associated with the pulmonary edema seen with β-agonist therapy (28) and should be used with caution.

The side effects of the β agonists may contraindicate their use in a variety of situations. These include:

- Cardiac lesions that contraindicate tachycardia (stenotic valvular lesions or idiopathic hypertrophic subaortic stenosis) or are associated with myocardial ischemia,
- Severe preeclampsia or eclampsia,
- Diabetes,
- Hyperthyroidism,
- Chorioamnionitis,
- Chronic hypertension,
- Hypovolemia, and
- History of cerebral vascular disorder.

Anesthetic Implications

β-Agonist tocolytics produce vasodilatation and increase cardiac output, which may alter the maternal hemodynamic response associated with epidural or spinal anesthesia. In pregnant sheep, prior administration of ritodrine did not worsen maternal hypotension, but rather helped maintain maternal cardiac output and uterine blood flow during epidural anesthesia (29). Because of the vasodilated state associated with β agonists, rapidly acting local anesthetics such as 2-chloroprocaine or lidocaine probably are safe in these patients. Overly aggressive intravenous hydration may predispose to fluid overload and decreased serum colloid oncotic pressure, which increases the risk of pulmonary edema (19,20). Incor-

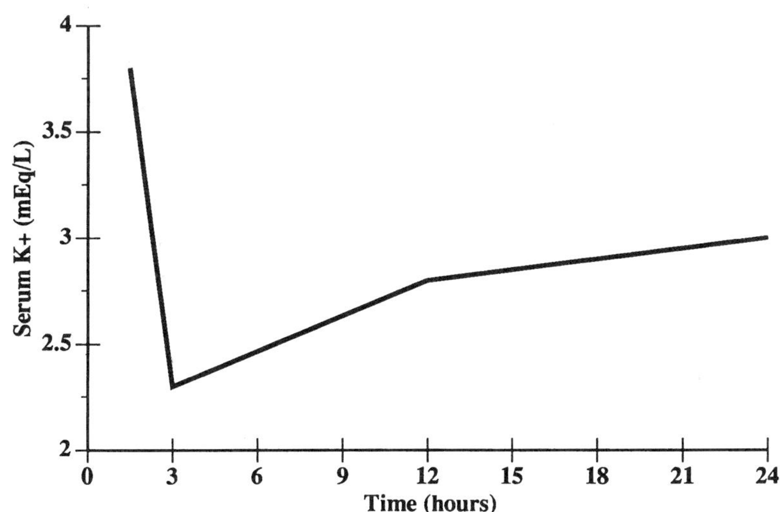

FIG. 1. Changes in serum potassium during ritodrine tocolysis. (Data from refs. 25 and 26.)

TABLE 8. *Anesthetic considerations in the presence of hypokalemia*

Autonomic neuropathy
- Orthostatic hypotension
- Decreased sympathetic reserve

Impaired myocardial contractility, aggravated by anesthetic agent with myocardial depressant properties

Electrical conduction abnormalities
- ECG changes including
  - Widened QRS
  - ST segment abnormalities
  - Decreasing T wave amplitude
  - Increasing U wave amplitude
- Arrhythmias including
  - Sinus tachycardia
  - Atrial and ventricular dysrhythmia
  - Ventricular fibrillation

Potentiation of hypokalemic state with alkalosis

Increased myocardial sensitivity to digoxin, calcium, and potassium infusion

Muscle weakness

Hypoperistalsis, delayed gastric emptying

rectly interpreting tachycardia as a sign of hypovolemia also may result in excessive intravenous fluid infusion.

Finally, the β agonists may interfere with pulmonary hypoxic vasoconstriction (30). This effect may increase the risk of maternal hypoxia, particularly under general anesthesia, and emphasizes the need for an increased F_IO_2 (31).

The magnitude of the interaction between β-agonist and anesthetic drugs depends on the time between stopping tocolytic therapy and the induction of anesthesia. Earlier studies estimated the serum half-life of ritodrine to be 50 ± 20 minutes (32). However, more recent work by Caritis et al. (33) reports a half-life of 156 minutes. The traditional teaching that general anesthesia be delayed 30 minutes, when possible, after stopping intravenous administration of a β agonist should be revised. If time allows, a delay of 2 or more hours may be more prudent.

The β-agonist tocolytics have minimal adverse effects on the fetus, although rapid intravenous infusion rates may cause a mild fetal tachycardia. If the neonate is born less than 24 hours after stopping drug infusion, neonatal hypoglycemia, hypoclacemia, and hypotension may occur. After 24 hours, there are no significant drug-related neonatal effects.

Magnesium Sulphate

Magnesium sulphate is an effective tocolytic when given intravenously in doses similar to, or slightly higher than, those used for seizure prophylaxis in women with preeclampsia/eclampsia (34). Like β agonists, magnesium sulfate frequently produces maternal side effects including vasodilation, flushing, headache, and postural hypotension. Magnesium acts at the myoneural junction to cause generalized skeletal muscle weakness and loss of deep tendon reflexes. Overdose can cause respiratory depression and arrest and even cardiac arrest. Other side effects may include drowsiness without analgesia, blurred vision, nausea, constipation, and chest pain (35,36). Of 355 patients receiving magnesium for tocolysis, 1.1% developed pulmonary edema (37). Because magnesium is excreted primarily through the kidneys, it must be used with caution in patients with compromised renal function. Deep tendon reflexes are monitored during magnesium therapy. Loss of the patellar reflex occurs with a serum magnesium concentration of about 10 mg/dL. Respiratory depression occurs at concentrations of 12 to 15 mg/dL (Table 9).

Magnesium tocolysis is preferable to β-agonist therapy in some groups of patients. Its use is not associated with hyperglycemia and metabolic lactic acidosis, rendering it more suitable for the diabetic parturient. In therapeutic doses, it does not have inotropic and chronotropic effects, making it safer for use in patients with various cardiac disorders. It is not associated with increased metabolism and, hence, is not contraindicated by hypermetabolic disorders such as hyperthyroidism. It is inexpensive and effective, but its use requires hospitalization for intravenous tocolysis, and oral use has not proven to be effective (38).

Some advocate magnesium sulphate as the drug of choice in the patient at risk of hemorrhage and in need of tocolysis. They argue that β-agonist–induced vasodilation may worsen hemorrhage and blunt the reflex vasoconstriction that occurs in response to hypovolemia (12). However, in pregnant sheep, magnesium sulphate, not ritodrine, worsened the maternal hypotensive response to hemorrhage (39). Calcium chloride, which reverses many of magnesium's side effects, did not limit magnesium's deleterious impact on the maternal response to hemorrhage (40).

Anesthetic Implications

Magnesium interacts with anesthetic drugs and techniques. In its own right, magnesium causes muscle weakness. It potentiates the nondepolarizing muscle

TABLE 9. *Effects of increasing plasma magnesium concentration*

Observed condition	mEq/L
Normal plasma concentration	1.5–2.0
Therapeutic range (may see diplopia and mild skeletal muscle weakness)	4.0–6.0
ECG changes (widened QRS and prolonged PQ interval)	5.0–10.0
Loss of deep tendon reflexes	10.0
Sinoatrial and artrioventricular block	15.0
Respiratory paralysis	15.0
Cardiac arrest	25.0

relaxants (41), including the newer drugs vecuronium (42) and rocuronium (43). Reversal of a nonpolarizing muscle relaxant with an anticholinesterase may be incomplete, as magnesium decreases the sensitivity of the motor end-plate to applied acetylocholine, reducing the efficacy of the reversal process (44).

Magnesium attenuates succinylcholine fasciculations (45). Its effect on the action of succinylcholine is variable. Magnesium does not change the onset or duration of a single dose of succinylcholine. Full intubating doses are required. Magnesium does, however, increase the duration of paralysis after repeated doses or continuous infusion of succinylcholine. Use a peripheral nerve stimulator to judge the response to, and recovery from, muscle relaxants in these patients.

Like the β agonists, magnesium produces vasodilation, but without increasing cardiac output. So, postural hypotension is more likely with magnesium than with β-agonist drugs. (Parturients receiving magnesium therapy usually are confined to bed.) Sympathetic block during regional anesthesia should be unlikely to produce hypotension. Marked preblock hydration usually is not necessary and may predispose to pulmonary edema. Magnesium also can interfere with uterine contractions following delivery, increasing the likelihood of postpartum uterine atony and excessive blood loss.

Fetal Effects

Fetal blood concentration of magnesium parallels that in maternal blood. Fetal heart rate variability may decrease. At birth, infants exposed to magnesium may exhibit decreased muscle tone, ileus, and poor feeding. However, one prospective study reported that magnesium was more likely to affect color than muscle tone (46). Neonatal weakness and respiratory or cardiac depression are unlikely in the absence of maternal toxicity. If severe neonatal depression is seen in the absence of maternal magnesium toxicity, look for other causes. If neonatal renal function is normal, the effects of magnesium dissipate within 48 hours (47–49).

Prostaglandin Synthesis Inhibitors

Indomethacin, a prostaglandin synthetase inhibitor, is an effective tocolytic (50). Maternal side effects essentially are those of aspirin: nausea, vomiting, gastritis, peptic ulcer formation, and masking of fever. Like aspirin, it can be associated with thrombocytopenia, and it interferes with platelet function. Unlike aspirin, its effects on platelets are reversible and usually dissipate within a few days of its discontinuation (51). Controversy surrounds this issue of bleeding times before regional anesthesia in patients receiving aspirin or nonsteroidal antiinflammatory agents (52,53). Bleeding time is prolonged in parturients taking indomethacin for tocolysis (54). Although this impaired hemostasis could lead to postpartum hemorrhagic complications, this has not been a clinically significant problem. The usefulness of the bleeding time now is being questioned, even by hematologists (55). The bleeding time has no predictive value in determining risk of surgical hemorrhage. We rarely use it in our practice.

Several prospective and retrospective clinical studies suggest that neuroaxial block is safe for patients receiving aspirin or other prostaglandin synthetase inhibitors. The Collaborative Low-Dose Aspirin Study in Pregnancy (CLASP) is a large, multicenter, randomized, placebo-controlled trial evaluating the effect of aspirin (60 mg/day) on the incidence of preeclampsia (56). One report from this trial reviewed the charts of 1,069 women who received epidural anesthesia, looking for evidence of hemorrhagic events (57). Aspirin therapy did not increase the risk of hemorrhagic complications. In nonpregnant patients receiving neuraxial anesthesia, there also appears to be no increased risk of hematoma or other bleeding complications associated with aspirin or other prostaglandin synthetase inhibitor use (58,59).

In animals, indomethacin, like aspirin, can induce premature closure of the ductus arteriosus, pulmonary vascular constriction, and pulmonary hypertension. These effects appear to be related to gestational age. The ductus arteriosus becomes more sensitive to prostaglandin inhibitors close to term. In clinical use, indomethacin usually is reserved for refractory PML before 34 weeks' gestation (50,60). Indomethacin also may be associated with reversible oligohydramnios (61). Contrary to previous evidence, recent studies suggest that indomethacin may reduce the risk of IVH (62).

With its lack of maternal cardiovascular and other side effects and its ease of administration, indomethacin often is used for initial tocolysis in early pregnancy. It also is a useful adjunct for the temporary control of PML in the mother being transported to a tertiary care center for delivery.

Calcium Channel Blockers

Calcium channel blockers, particularly nifedipine, are potent relaxants of uterine muscle and are effective tocolytics (63). They are potent vasodilators and often incite flushing and hypotension. Other bothersome side effects include nausea and headache. But, compared with the β agonist ritodrine, nifedipine has fewer maternal side effects. The magnitude of the cardiovascular alterations, while significant, is less than with ritodrine. Maternal heart rate increases, whereas diastolic blood pressure and mean arterial pressure decrease. Changes in glucose homeostasis accompany both nifedipine and ritodrine, although the magnitude of these changes is much less with nifedipine. Nifedipine does not significantly affect serum electrolytes, unlike the marked impact of ritodrine (63,64).

Initial studies in Rhesus monkeys and ewes suggested an increased incidence of intrauterine fetal death with calcium channel blockers. In these models, nifedipine decreased uterine blood flow and induced fetal acidosis and hypoxia (65). To date, these findings have not been substantiated in humans. Currently, use of nifedipine or ritodrine for tocolysis produces similar neonatal outcomes (63,66).

Drug Interactions

Preterm labor is a syndrome of disorders resulting from a variety of causes associated with different cellular mechanisms. Therefore, it is not unreasonable to use different tocolytic agents concurrently in the hope that their synergistic interactions may halt more resistant cases of preterm labor. However, the simultaneous use of various tocolytics increases the risk of adverse drug interaction and potentiates some side effects. For example, magnesium potentiates the hypotensive effect of nifedipine (67). In the isolated, perfused rat heart, the combination of nifedipine and magnesium depressed left ventricular systolic pressure and left ventricular contractility more than either drug alone (68). Also, nifedipine potentiates the effects of magnesium on neuromuscular function (69). This interaction may further exaggerate the response of patients on magnesium sulphate to nondepolarizing muscle relaxants.

Anesthetic Effects

Calcium channel blockers interact with various anesthetics. Both inhalation and local anesthetics exhibit some calcium channel blocking properties. Animal models have looked at the hemodynamic interactions between calcium channel blockers and inhalational anesthetics. Both have similar impact on the cardiovascular system, namely, vasodilation and myocardial depression. In the dog, during light halothane anesthesia (1%), nifedipine induced transient hypotension with a compensatory increase in cardiac output and heart rate. More significant hypotension arose under deep halothane anesthesia (2%), presumably because of attenuation of the compensatory increase in heart rate (70). Isoflurane or enflurane, when given in conjunction with other calcium channel blocking agents, yield similar results (71). Although deep volatile anesthesia generally is contraindicated in the obstetric population, there are circumstances where uterine relaxation may be indicated in which this drug interaction could have significant consequence.

The interactions between lidocaine or bupivacaine and verapamil or diltiazem have been examined in conscious dogs in an attempt to reproduce the clinical situation of epidural anesthesia (72). When animals receiving an intravenous infusion that produces serum bupivacaine concentrations seen with epidural anesthesia are given calcium channel blockers, both mean arterial pressure and myocardial contractile force decrease significantly. The combination of either lidocaine or bupivacaine and a calcium channel blocker prolongs the PR interval. Calcium channel blockers plus bupivacaine also can induce high-degree atrioventricular nodal block. In mice, calcium channel blockers (verapamil, diltiazem, or bepridil) increase the risk of bupivacaine-induced mortality (73). To date, this interaction has not been seen in humans.

Atosiban

Atosiban (1-deamino 2D-tyr-(OE+)-4-thr-8-orn-vasotocin/oxytocin Mpa, D-Tyr(E+)^2,Thr^4,Orn^8-oxytocin) is a competitive inhibitor of oxytocin. Preliminary studies in animals and humans (74–79) report a reduction in preterm uterine activity versus placebo. When compared to β agonists and magnesium, atosiban has relatively few side effects. In animals, atosiban lacks effect on maternal or fetal cardiovascular parameters (80). Atosiban is expected to be available for widespread clinical use in the near future. To date, there are no published reports of interactions between atosiban and anesthetics.

Experimental Tocolytics

Glyceryl Trinitrate

Glyceryl trinitrate is a nitric oxide donor. Uterine nitric oxide production is associated with the maintenance of a quiescent uterine state. Promising results have been reported in one small study of PML treated with glyceryl trinitrate patches (81). Further work is needed to investigate its value as a tocolytic agent and to evaluate maternal and fetal safety.

Urinary Trypsin inhibitor

Urinary trypsin inhibitor is present in amniotic fluid and has both antiinflammatory and anticytokine effects. It may have a role in maintaining normal pregnancy and preventing preterm delivery. Preliminary studies have shown that urinary trypsin inhibitor can suppress myometrial contractions (82,83).

Lidocaine

Lidocaine, a well-known local anesthetic, recently has received some attention as a potential tocolytic agent. In animals, lidocaine selectively blocks myometrial Na^+ channels, reducing muscle exitability (84). Lidocaine, when used as a local anesthetic for epidural anesthesia, has been implicated in neonatal neurobehavioral abnormalities (85) and has been shown to accumulate in the acidotic preterm sheep fetus (86). Little information is available on the fetal or neonatal effects of maternal intravenous infusion of lidocaine. Fetal serum concentration is lower than the maternal concentration. Lidocaine appears to accumulate in the amniotic fluid (87). One case report details the use of lidocaine as a tocolytic for preterm twins. The infants were delivered at 27 weeks' gestation with Apgar scores of 1 and 1. Central nervous and cardiovascular toxicity of lidocaine may have contributed to the poor condition at delivery. If lidocaine finds a role in the treatment of preterm labor, it will present some unique anesthetic challenges.

ANESTHETIC MANAGEMENT OF THE PRETERM DELIVERY

The obstetric anesthesiologist has several goals when caring for a mother and her preterm infant. Try to ensure the most atraumatic delivery possible. A sudden, uncontrolled delivery, will markedly increase the likelihood of intracerebral hemorrhage, the leading cause of morbidity and mortality in preterm birth. For vaginal delivery, the obstetrician will strive for an atraumatic delivery over a wide episiotomy. Take all possible measures to prevent fetal asphyxia and hypothermia. The premature infant tolerates asphyxia poorly. The asphyxiated preterm infant has an increased incidence of RDS, IVH, and necrotizing enterocolitis. Before vaginal or cesarean delivery, position the mother carefully to prevent aortocaval compression. Give supplemental oxygen (88). Avoid or aggressively treat maternal hypotension. Continuous electronic fetal monitoring may detect early signs of fetal asphyxia.

Preterm birth risks both maternal and fetal morbidity. Maternal hemorrhage from placenta previa, placenta abruption, or uterine atony from attempted tocolysis can complicate preterm birth. The incidence of breech in the preterm birth is 25% compared to 3% at term. Maternal, fetal, and neonatal infection are more frequent in preterm birth, often resulting from prolonged rupture of membranes. Fetal heart rate changes and prolapsed cord are more common in PML than at term. Expeditious cesarean section is indicated if the fetus shows any evidence of compromise.

Delivery in a tertiary care center, instead of transfer after birth, lowers neonatal mortality (89,90). The preterm fetus and newborn, with its less developed lungs, liver, and kidneys, may have difficulty metabolizing and excreting depressant analgesic and anesthetic drugs. Despite this possibility, most experts recommend the use of appropriate analgesics when needed (91).

Finally, the anesthetist involved in a preterm birth must be acquainted with the side effects of the various tocolytics and their interactions with anesthetic techniques and drugs (see previous).

Vaginal Delivery

When the mother delivering a preterm infant is to have a trial of labor, lumbar epidural analgesia, initiated early and maintained throughout labor and delivery, is the most desirable option (Table 10). When using epidural analgesia/anesthesia in the management of the preterm delivery, keep the following principles in mind:

- The preterm infant may require urgent or emergent cesarean delivery. Make certain that the epidural catheter is functioning properly. Local anesthetics should produce bilateral sensory change that ascends with additional drug.
- Minimize the effects of epidural block on the duration of labor. Try not to hinder maternal expulsive efforts during the second stage of labor.
- Avoid precipitous delivery. Most obstetricians like to control delivery of the fetal head by gradually stretching the perineum, cutting a generous episiotomy, or using forceps. These maneuvers require good perineal anesthesia.
- Avoid drugs that can cause fetal compromise.

Many of these principles conflict. How does one assure the ability to move rapidly to operative delivery while preserving maternal motor function? How does one avoid the use of drugs that can cause fetal compromise (e.g., opioids) without hindering maternal expulsive efforts? Or, how can one preserve maternal motor function and still provide adequate perineal analgesia? Previously, experts advocated generous doses of concentrated local anaesthetics without additional opioids (92). Although this approach met some of the noted principles, it often prolonged the second stage of labor and necessitated operative delivery.

Patient Positioning

If the fetal head is low in the vagina or labor is progressing rapidly, identify the epidural or subarachnoid space with the mother on her side to prevent fetal head compression. To reduce the risk of cord prolapse, apply this same precaution if the membranes have ruptured but

TABLE 10. *Advantages of epidural analgesia for vaginal delivery of the preterm infant*

Alert, cooperative, pain-free mother
Ideal conditions for a vaginal delivery
Mother can control pushing on command
Allows operative delivery (forceps or vacuum extraction)
Allows wide episiotomy and repair
Decreases likelihood of precipitous delivery
Minimizes the risk of pulmonary edema associated with β agonists, magnesium, and general anesthesia
Not associated with newborn drug depression
Stable maternal cardiovascular system
Protects mother and fetus from the stress of painful labor with associated metabolic acidosis and increased maternal catecholamines
Can be rapidly extended for an emergency cesarean section

the fetal head remains out of the pelvis or the fetal breech is presenting.

Anesthetic Technique

A balanced anesthetic approach can successfully meet the goals discussed. After inserting an epidural catheter and giving an appropriate preload (depending on previous tocoytic therapy and hydration), induce analgesia with the mother in the left lateral decubitus position. Inject drug in small increments via the epidural catheter. (Although drug injection through the epidural needle may provide good initial analgesia, a poorly functioning epidural catheter will be useless for subsequent cesarean section.) I use 15 to 20 mg of bupivacaine (i.e., 15 to 20 mL of 0.1%, 10 to 15 mL of 0.125%, or 10 mL of 0.187%). To minimize the risk of drug-induced fetal depression, I avoid epidural opioids. Freshly added epinephrine (5 µg/mL) and bicarbonate (0.1 mL of 8.4% solution to 20 mL of bupivacaine) will hasten the onset and prolong the duration of blockade. Look for sensory change 15 to 20 minutes after drug injection. The goal is complete perineal analgesia and a sensory level to at least T_8.

Use an infusion of bupivacaine (0.1% to 0.125%) with fentanyl 2 µg/mL at 6 to 12 mL/h to maintain the block. Althoug the advantages of a continuous infusion are well documented, remember to monitor the block closely to ensure adequate perineal analgesia without excessive maternal motor blockade. The use of fentanyl in the continuous infusion may appear to compromise the fourth principle; however, the actual dose delivered is very small (12 to 24 µg/h) and appears to be well tolerated by the fetus. The addition of opioid allows a reduction in the concentration of local anaesthetic, allowing preservation of some motor power. Give the mother supplemental oxygen throughout labor.

Combined Spinal–Epidural Analgesia

Combined spinal–epidural (CSE) analgesia has gained popularity in recent years. Intrathecal injection of an opioid and a small dose of local anesthetic (i.e., sufentanil 5 to 10 µg and bupivacaine 2.5 mg) will rapidly provide excellent labor analgesia (and perineal anesthesia) with minimal motor blockade. Despite its popularity, the CSE technique has some limitations (93,94). Foremost is the questionable location of the epidural catheter. Initiation of labor analgesia using the CSE technique does not allow testing of the epidural catheter to ensure appropriate functioning should urgent cesarean delivery be required within a couple hours of induction. The use of intrathecal opioids in labor may be associated with profound fetal bradycardia. The etiology of this event is unclear. Some postulate uterine hypertonus (95,96). Although usually of a relatively brief duration, bradycardia may not be well tolerated by preterm fetuses.

A rare potential complication of CSE is bacterial contamination of the cerebrospinal fluid (CSF) on puncture of the dura. Meningitis has been reported as a complication of CSE in healthy laboring patients. One etiology of preterm labor is either subclinical or overt (i.e., chorioamnionitis) infection. In untreated bacteremic rats, bacterial seeding of the CSF follows dural puncture (97). This risk essentially disappears in animals receiving appropriate antibiotic treatment. Central nervous system infection was not seen in two retrospective reviews of laboring women with chorioamnionitis who received spinal or epidural anesthesia (98,99).

With the risk of fetal bradycardia, introducing a CSF contaminant and the uncertainty of placement and function of the epidural catheter, I find it difficult to justify the routine use of the CSE technique for labor analgesia with a preterm fetus.

A modification of the classic CSE technique can be used in the rapidly progressing labor, using a higher dose of local anesthetic and little or no opioid. It is useful to keep a supply of long spinal needles on hand for that epidural for labor analgesia that suddenly becomes an anesthetic for delivery in the middle of block placement. Five milligrams of bupivacaine (2 mL of 0.25% or 4 mL 0.125%) provides excellent analgesia for the second stage of labor and delivery.

Local Anesthetic

The choice of local anesthetic for epidural labor analgesia has generated controversy over the years. In the mid 1970s, Scanlon et al. (100) described the alert but floppy baby after delivery with epidural block using lidocaine or mepivacaine. Others reported that acidosis increased the fetal uptake of lidocaine (101). These findings led to a marked decrease in the use of lidocaine for epidural anesthesia. This trend was especially marked when neonatal adaptation was critical and the risk of fetal asphyxia was high, as with the preterm fetus. 2-Chloroprocaine became favored. It has a very short half-life (43 seconds in cord blood) and seemed to have no adverse neonatal effects.

Many experts disputed Scanlon's findings. Subsequent studies found no clinically significant neonatal effects attributable to epidural lidocaine (102–107). Further studies also failed to confirm the superiority of 2-chloroprocaine. Indeed, one report suggested that term infants delivered after bupivacaine epidural anesthesia did better on neurobehavioral tests than those delivered after 2-chloroprocaine anesthesia (108). However, lidocaine may have some adverse effects in premature infants. In asphyxiated preterm fetal lambs, lidocaine significantly decreases in fetal pH compared with controls receiving saline (86). Similarly, clinically relevant concentrations of bupivacaine adversely affect the cardiovascular adaptations to asphyxia in fetal lambs (109). Clinically, 1.5% to 2% lidocaine continues to be a reliable agent for rapidly providing epidural anesthesia for cesarean delivery. Its speed of onset and the quality of blockade are comparable to 3% 2-chloroprocaine.

Ropivacaine may be an attractive local anesthetic for the management of the preterm vaginal delivery. Even without supplemental opioids, it provides good analgesia for labor with a reduced incidence of motor block (110–112). However, ropivacaine's pharmacokinetics may be problematic in the preterm fetus. Compared to bupivacaine, ropivacaine is less lipid soluble, less completely protein bound, and has a longer free plasma clearance time (113,114). At cesarean delivery, these factors produce a higher free ropivacaine concentration in fetal umbilical blood versus bupivacaine (115,116). However, in term infants, neonatal adaptive capacity scores and Apgar scores are similar after either bupivacaine or ropivacaine. Ropivacaine does have a shorter terminal elimination half-life than bupivacaine. As yet, there are no studies evaluating ropivacaine and the preterm fetus. Thus, at the present time, it is difficult to advocate the use of ropivacaine as the drug of choice for preterm delivery.

Alternatives to Neuraxial Analgesia

If epidural or subarachnoid block is contraindicated by lack of time, maternal refusal, hypovolemia, abnormal coagulation, etc., analgesia for delivery can be provided by inhalation of 50% nitrous oxide in oxygen. Intravenous ketamine 0.25 mg/kg (15 to 25 mg) can provide additional analgesia and often will allow the use of forceps or vaccuum. Should prolonged analgesia be required, additional 0.125 to 0.25 mg/kg doses may be used. Avoid loss of consciousness and limit the total dose of ketamine to 1.0 mg/kg before delivery. Pudendal block or at least local infiltration of the perineum help decrease the need for systemic analgesics for episiotomy and application of forceps or vaccuum. Although this technique has its uses, it is not as effective as epidural or subarachnoid block. It does not abolish the reflex urge to bear down. It does not assure a controlled delivery. It does not assure a cooperative mother.

General anesthesia rarely is required for vaginal delivery. Should it be, take precautions to prevent pulmonary aspiration. Avoid inducting anesthesia in the lithotomy position. Use a rapid sequence induction with cricoid pressure.

Cesarean Section

Cesarean section often is indicated for the viable preterm neonate and accounts for a large proportion of these deliveries. Although it offers little or no long-term benefit, the use of cesarean section for very low birth weight infants (500 to 1,499 g) has been rising steadily over the past 15 years (117).

Choice of Anesthetic

Although the choice of anesthetic can influence neonatal condition at birth, there is little evidence of any long-lasting effects. A retrospective analysis of 509 preterm infants delivered over 5 years in Toronto revealed significantly higher 1- and 5-minute Apgar scores in infants delivered using epidural anesthesia compared with those delivered using general anesthesia (118). Regression analysis suggested variables significantly related to low 1-minute Apgar scores were anesthetic technique, malpresentation, primiparity, low gestational age, and the presence of RDS and IVH. In term infants, 1-minute Apgar scores and umbilical venous pH values are significantly higher in the infants delivered with spinal anesthesia versus general anesthesia (119).

Regional Anesthesia

Still, for both maternal and fetal reasons, lumbar epidural or spinal block is our method of choice anesthesia for cesarean section. Several points need to be reemphasized. In a breech or nonvertex presentation, doing the block in the sitting position may predispose to prolapse of the umbilical cord. A mother who has just received a β-agonist tocolytic should have cautious and minimal intravenous prehydration. An F_IO_2 of 0.5 from the time of block until delivery may significantly improve neonatal oxygenation at birth.[1]

Uterine Relaxation

Some anesthesiologists traditionally have avoided regional anesthesia for cesarean delivery of the preterm infant because general anesthesia provides uterine relaxation if needed for delivery of the head. Intravenous nitroglycerin 50 to 200 μg also is a potent uterine relaxant and is useful in obstetric emergencies such as cesarean delivery of the breech fetus (120). A prudent approach for the delivery of the preterm fetus is to administer nitroglycerin 100 μg to induce acute uterine relaxation (approximately 30-second onset) to assist in the delivery of the fetal head. Although a potential risk, maternal hypotension following nitroglycerin administration usually is transient.

[1] Editor's note: James et al. examined the spread of hyperbaric bupivacaine 11.25 mg in 25 term parturients and 25 women presenting for cesarean section at 28 to 35 weeks' gestation. This dose of bupivacaine produced sensory change to at least T_4 in all term parturients but in only 16% of the preterm women. Onset of blockade also was slower in the preterm group. While others have not reported diminished spread of spinal anesthesia in preterm women, this observation is intriguing and potentially significant. (James KS, McGrady E, Patrick A. Combined spinal-extradural anaesthesia for preterm and term caesarean section: is there a difference in local anaesthetic requirements? *Br J Anaesth* 1997;78:498.)

General Anesthesia

Occasionally, general anesthesia may be indicated for various conditions, including severe fetal distress in a mother without a functioning epidural catheter, maternal refusal of an epidural or a subarachnoid block, and conditions contraindicating major conduction block.

Do not reduce the dose of the induction agents for general anesthesia. With proper technique, fetal drug exposure is minimal and not associated with perinatal asphyxia. As with all general anesthetics given to the parturient, use appropriate maneuvers to prevent aspiration. Maintain left uterine displacement until delivery. Use a high F_IO_2 (0.5 to 1.0) until delivery. Maintain anesthesia and help assure maternal amnesia with 0.75 minimum alveolar concentration of a potent inhaled agent. Nitrous oxide can be used if desired. Monitor end-tidal CO_2 and avoid maternal hyperventilation. Remember the potential for interactions between tocolytics (particularly the β agonists, magnesium, and the calcium channel blockers), anesthetics, and muscle relaxants.

MANAGEMENT OF THE COCAINE-ADDICTED OR INTOXICATED PATIENT IN PRETERM LABOR

Cocaine use during pregnancy is associated with an increased incidence of preterm labor. An estimated 30 million Americans have used cocaine at least once, and more than 5 million are using it regularly. Fifteen percent of these regular users are women of reproductive age. The reported prevalence of cocaine use in pregnancy is as high as 10% to 15% (121,122).

In addition to causing preterm labor, cocaine use in pregnancy is associated with an increased incidence of intrauterine growth retardation, abruptio placenta, and pregnancy-induced hypertension. Pregnant women who use cocaine on a regular basis also are at risk for sudden death, myocardial and vascular toxicity (infarction, dysrhythmia, aortic rupture, and myocarditis), cerebrovascular accidents, subarachnoid hemorrhage, hypertension, seizures, hyperpyrexia, intestinal ischemia, and pulmonary edema (123). Any of these conditions can complicate the anesthetic management of delivery, but their existence in an acutely intoxicated patient can create problems of nightmarish proportions.

Cocaine acts mainly by blocking presynaptic reuptake of norepinephrine and dopamine, increasing the availability of these neurotransmitters at the postsynaptic receptor. The resultant sympathetic nervous system stimulation produces vasoconstriction, tachycardia, hypertension, and cardiac dysrhythmias. Cocaine is detoxified by plasma and liver cholinesterases, and its water-soluble metabolites are excreted in the urine. Plasma cholinesterase concentration decreases during pregnancy, potentially prolonging cocaine's duration. Cocaine produces greater increases in heart rate, blood pressure, systemic vascular resistance, and myocardial oxygen consumption and more significant decreases in cardiac output in pregnant, compared with nonpregnant, animals (124–128).

Anesthetic Considerations

Anesthetic considerations for the cocaine-abusing parturient delivering a preterm fetus must include both maternal and fetal drug effects as well as interaction between the cocaine and anesthetic agents or techniques. Long-term intravenous users can present problems of venous access. Peripheral veins may be thrombosed. Some addicts even self-inject via their internal jugular veins. The subclavian veins may be the only option. These patients also are at high risk for infection with human immunodeficiency virus and hepatitis.

Acute cocaine intoxication can precipitate a placental abruption and, at the same time, produce sympathetic stimulation that masks the degree of blood loss and volume depletion. As the drug effect wanes, catecholamine concentrations decrease and blood pressure may fall. Vasopressors may be needed to restore maternal blood pressure and placental perfusion. However, ephedrine (the drug of choice in pregnancy) acts indirectly by inducing release of endogenous catecholamines. Ephedrine may prove ineffective in cocaine users with depleted catecholamine reserves. Phenylephrine, a direct acting agent, is a good alternative.

Consider the cardiovascular effects of cocaine when choosing anesthetics. Use caution with agents with arrythmogenic potential in the face of elevated catecholamines (halothane), those that may further stimulate the cardiovascular system (ketamine), or myocardial depressants (high-dose thiopental or volatile agents).

In addition to the usual problems of prematurity, these neonates may be at a higher risk for periventricular hemorrhage, IVH, and necrotizing enterocolitis (122). The fetus acutely intoxicated with cocaine has arterial hypoxemia and increases in blood pressure, heart rate, and cerebral blood flow (124). The neonates of cocaine-addicted mothers have a higher incidence of genitourinary tract and central nervous system defects (129).

CARE OF THE PREMATURE NEWBORN

Ideally, care of the premature newborn begins well before delivery. When time permits, mother and fetus should be transferred intact to a center that can appropriately care for preterm infants.

Maternal antenatal corticosteroids can hasten fetal lung maturity and decrease the incidence of RDS. Initially, the benefits of maternal steroid therapy appeared limited to infants with a gestational age of 30 to 34 weeks and whose mothers had received at least 24 hours of treatment before delivery. There also appeared to be little benefit in white male infants or in multiple gestation (130,131).

More recent data suggest that maternal steroid therapy can benefit most preterm infants. A multicenter study examined outcome of 11,718 low birth weight infants (500 to 1,500 g) born between 1988 and 1992 (132). Maternal antenatal steroid therapy was associated with significant reductions in the risk of RDS, IVH, and death before 28 days of life. These benefits were seen in all infants, regardless of gestational age, sex, race, multiple gestation, surfactant administration, and time between maternal therapy and delivery. Other studies have confirmed these results (133,134).

The most significant risk of antenatal corticosteroids appears to be a slight increase in the incidence of neonatal sepsis. This risk is greatest in infants receiving only a partial course of steroids (less than 24 hours), but was not increased by the presence of ruptured membranes (132,134). Although once thought to represent a contraindication for administration, the use of corticosteroids in the presence of PROM appears to be increasing (135).

Antenatal steroid therapy incurs some maternal risk. Demargination of neutrophils increases the white blood cell count, which can make it difficult to accurately detect maternal infection. Corticosteroids interfere with glucose homeostasis and increase blood glucose concentration. Immunosuppression may increase the risk of maternal infection.

The value of prophylactic maternal antibiotics is unclear. Antibiotics benefit the mother by reducing the incidence of chorioamnionitis and postpartum infection. Prophylactic maternal antibiotics offer little neonatal benefit in PML with intact membranes (136), but may offer some benefit in the presence of PROM (137).

Other therapies that appear to improve neonatal outcome include surfactant for the prevention and treatment of RDS (138–142) and inhaled nitric oxide in the treatment of persistent pulmonary hypertension of the newborn, congenital diaphragmatic hernia, and some forms of congenital heart disease (143). These improvements in management of the preterm neonate reiterate the importance of delivery in a center with a tertiary care level neonatal unit.

Before the birth, qualified pediatricians or neonatologists should be notified and be prepared to care for the newborn. Initial care focuses primarily on the prevention or treatment of asphyxia and maintenance of body temperature. Although hyperoxia is a concern because of the fear of retrolental fibroplasia and pulmonary oxygen toxicity, one should not hesitate to give a high F_IO_2 (greater than 0.9) if there are signs of hypoxemia (144). A pale or markedly cyanotic premature neonate requires oxygen to avoid the devastating consequences of hypoxia. If intubation is required, either continuous positive airway pressure or positive end-expiratory pressure will be necessary to maintain alveolar expansion. The premature infant has a large surface area for a small mass and rapidly loses heat, for which the infant cannot compensate. Hypothermia can lead to acidosis and increased oxygen consumption. It should be prevented by immediately drying the neonate at birth and placing the child under radiant heat in an area protected from drafts.

Premature infants are prone to develop hypoglycemia and hypocalcemia, particularly those whose mothers recently received β agonists for tocolysis. And, finally, because these neonates, especially those weighing less than 2,000 g, require much monitoring and intensive care, mother and fetus, as a unit, should be promptly transported to a tertiary center where this care is available.

SUMMARY

Premature birth still accounts for about 75% of perinatal mortality. Although great strides in the care of the premature infant over the past two decades have markedly decreased mortality, the incidence of premature birth unfortunately has not changed greatly. The use of tocolysis, particularly β agonists and magnesium sulfate, may delay birth and allow maturation. However, these drugs have many side effects that, if not recognized, can cause serious maternal morbidity and even mortality. These drugs, and other less widely used tocolytics, have important anesthetic implications. To assure optimal outcomes, preterm infants should be delivered in a tertiary center that is ready to attend to their needs.

Major conduction analgesia, particularly continuous lumbar epidural blockade, is an ideal form of maternal pain relief for the delivery of most premature neonates. Properly administered, this technique maintains maternal physiology, does not produce newborn drug depression, provides for a controlled atraumatic vaginal delivery, and has little interaction with tocolytics and may protect against some of their potential side effects.

Epidural block is ideal for a trial of labor and, if initiated early, will allow for emergency cesarean delivery. Continuous lumbar epidural and subarachnoid block are superb for the elective or urgent cesarean section. However, when their use is contraindicated, inhalation analgesia for vaginal delivery or general anesthesia for cesarean section can be administered safely without compromise of either mother or child. *Expertly administered anesthesia is not a luxury but an indispensable requirement for an optimal outcome in a premature delivery.*

REFERENCES

1. Greasy RK. Preterm birth prevention: where are we? *Am J Obstet Gynecol* 1993;168:1223.
2. Keirse MJNC. New perspectives for the effective treatment of preterm labor. *Am J Obstet Gynecol* 1995;173:618.
3. Lockwood CJ. Recent advances in elucidating the pathogenesis of preterm delivery, the detection of patients at risk and preventative therapies. *Curr Opin Obstet Gynecol* 1994;6:7.
4. US Department of Health and Human Services, Public Health Service,

National Center for Health Statistics. Vital Statistics of the United States 1980. Hyattsville, MD: US Department of Health and Human Services, 1984:1.
5. Fuchs F. Prevention of prematurity. *Am J Obstet Gynecol* 1986;126: 809.
6. Rush RW, Keirse MJNC, Howat P, Baum JD, Anderson ABM, Turnbull AC. Contribution of preterm delivery to perinatal mortality. *Br Med J* 1976;2:965.
7. Main DM, Main EK. Management of preterm labor and delivery. In: Gabbe SG, Neigyl JR, Simpson JL, eds. *Obstetrics: normal and problem pregnancies.* New York: Churchill Livingston, 1986:689.
8. Horbar JD, Pasnick M, McAuliffe TL, Lucey JF. Obstetric events and risks of periventricular hemorrhage in premature infants. *Am J Dis Child* 1983;137:678.
9. Mayhew JF, Bourke DL, Guinee WS. Evaluation of the premature infant at risk for postoperative complications. *Can J Anaesth* 1987; 34:627.
10. Eggleston MK. Management of preterm labor and delivery. *Clin Obstet Gynecol* 1986;29:230.
11. King JF, Grant A, Kierse MHNC, Chalmers I. Beta-mimetics in preterm labor: an overview of the randomized controlled trials. *Br J Obstet Gynaecol* 1988;95:211.
12. Benedetti T. Maternal complications of parenteral beta-sympathomimetic therapy for PML. *Am J Obstet Gynecol* 1983;154:1.
13. Hosenpud JD, Morton MJ, O'Grady JP. Cardiac stimulation during ritodrine hydrochloride tocolytic therapy. *Obstet Gynecol* 1983;62:52.
14. Ying YK, Tejani NA. Angina pectoris as a complication of ritodrine hydrochloride therapy in premature labor. *Obstet Gynecol* 1982;60:385.
15. Tye KH, Desset KB, Benchimol A. Angina pectoris associated with terbutaline treatment for preterm labor. *JAMA* 1980;244:692.
16. Michalak D, Klein V, Marquette G. Myocardial ischemia: a complication of ritodrine tocolysis. *Am J Obstet Gynecol* 1983;146:861.
17. Hendricks SK, Keroes J, Katz M. Electrocardiographic changes associated with ritodrine-induced maternal tachycardia and hypokolemia. *Am J Obstet Gynecol* 1986;154:921.
18. Hawker F. Pulmonary edema associated with β2-sympathomimetic treatment of premature labor. *Anesth Intens Care* 1984;12:143.
19. Jacobs MM, Knight AB, Arias F. Maternal pulmonary edema resulting from beta-mimetic and glucocorticoid therapy. *Obstet Gynecol* 1980;56:56.
20. Pisani J, Rosenow EC. Pulmonary edema associated with tocolytic therapy. *Ann Intern Med* 1989;110:714.
21. Philipsen T, Eriksen PS, Lynggard F. Pulmonary edema following ritodrine-saline infusion in premature labor. *Obstet Gynecol* 1981;58:304.
22. Strigl R, Pfeiffer U, Aschenbrenner G. Influence of the beta-1 elective blocker, metoprolol on the development of pulmonary edema in tocolytic therapy. *Obstet Gynecol* 1986;67:537.
23. Gross TL, Sokol RJ. Maternal metabolic complications following ritodrine or terbutaline therapy. *Birth Defects* 1982;18:191.
24. Cotton DB, Strassner HT, Lipson LG, Goldstein DA. The effect of terbutaline on acid base, serum electrolytes and glucose homeostasis during the management of preterm labor. *Am J Obstet Gynecol* 1981; 141:617.
25. Cano A, Tobar I, Parilla JJ. Metabolic disturbances during intravenous use of ritodrine: increased insulin levels and hypokalemia. *Obstet Gynecol* 1985;65:359.
26. Young DC, Toofanian A, Leveno KJ. Potassium and glucose concentration without treatment during ritodrine tocolysis. *Am J Obstet Gynecol* 1983;145:105.
27. Armson BA, Samuels P, Miller F, Verbalis J, Main EK. Evaluation of maternal fluid dynamics during tocolytic therapy with ritodrine hydrochloride and magnesium sulfate. *Am J Obstet Gynecol* 1992;167:758.
28. Adverse reactions from treating premature labor with beta-agonist. *FDA Drug Bulletin* 1981;11:13.
29. Chestnut DH, Pollack KL, Thompson CS. Does ritodrine worsen maternal hypotension during epidural anesthesia in gravid ewes? *Anesthesiology* 1990;72:315.
30. Conover WB, Benumof JL, Key TL. Ritodrine inhibition of hypoxic pulmonary vasoconstriction. *Am J Obstet Gynecol* 1983;146:652.
31. Marx GF, Mateo CV. Effects of different oxygen concentrations during general anesthesia for elective cesarean section. *Can Anesth Soc J* 1971;18:587.
32. Holleboom CAG, Merkus JMWM, van Elferen LWN. Loading dose infusion scheme for intravenous tocolysis with ritodrine: a pilot study. *Eur J Obstet Gynaecol Reprod Biol* 1987;26:119.
33. Caritis SN, Venkataramanan R, Darby MJ, et al. Pharmacokinetics of ritodrine administered intravenously: recommendations for changes in the current regime. *Am J Obstet Gynecol* 1990;162:429.
34. Hollander DI, Nagey DA, Pupkin MJ. Magnesium sulfate and ritodrine hydrochloride: a randomized comparison. *Am J Obstet Gynecol* 1987;156:631.
35. Skaredoff MN, Roaf ER, Datta S. Hypermagnesemia and anesthetic management. *Can J Anesth* 1982;29:35.
36. Gambling DR, Birmingham CL, Jenkins C. Magnesium and the anesthetist. *Can J Anesth* 1988;35:644.
37. Elliott J. Magnesium sulfate as a tocolytic agent. *Am J Obstet Gynecol* 1983;147:277.
38. Rust OA, Bofill JA, Arriola RM, Andrew ME, Morrison JC. The clinical efficacy of oral tocolytic therapy. *Am J Obstet Gynecol* 1996; 175:838.
39. Chestnut DH, Thompson CS, McLaughlin GL. Does the infusion of ritodrine or magnesium sulphate alter the hemodynamic response to haemorrhage in gravid ewes? *Am J Obstet Gynecol* 1988;159:1467.
40. Vincent RD, Chestnut DH, Sipes SL, et al. Calcium chloride administration during hemorrhage hypotension does not increase maternal pressure or uterine blood flow in hypermagnesiemic gravid ewes. Abstract, SOAP Meeting, 1991.
41. Giesecke AG, Morris RE, Dalton MD, Stephen CR. On magnesium, muscle relaxants, toxemic patients and cats. *Anesth Analg* 1980;47:689.
42. Sinatra RS, Phillip BK, Naulty JS, Ostheimer GW. Prolonged neuromuscular blockade with vecuronium in a patient treated with magnesium sulfate. *Anesth Analg* 1985;64:1220.
43. Gaiser RR, Seem EH. Use of rocuronium in a pregnant patient with an open eye injury, receiving magnesium medication, for preterm labor. *Br J Anaesth* 1996;77:669.
44. James MFM, Cork RC, Dennett JE. Succinylchloline pretreatment with magnesium sulphate. *Anesth Analg* 1986;65:373.
45. DeVore JS, Astrani R. Magnesium sulfate prevents succinylchloine-induced fasciculations in toxemic parturients. *Anesthesiology* 1980;52:76.
46. Pruett KM, Kirshon B, Cotton D, Adam K. Doody K. The effects of magnesium sulphate on Apgar scores. *Am J Obstet Gynecol* 1988; 159:1047.
47. Lipsitz PJ. The clinical and biochemical effects of excess magnesium in the newborn. *Pediatrics* 1981;47:3.
48. Peaceman AM, Meyer BA, Thorp JA. The effect of magnesium sulphate tocolysis on the fetal biophysical profile. *Am J Obstet Gynecol* 1989;161:771.
49. Green KW, Key TO, Coen R. The effects of maternally administered magnesium sulphate on the neonate. *Am J Obstet Gynecol* 1983;146:29.
50. Dudley DKL, Hardie MJ. Fetal and neonatal effects of indomethacin used as a tocolytic agent. *Am J Obstet Gynecol* 1985;151:181.
51. Kocsis JJ, Hernandovich J, Silver JJ, et al. Duration of inhibition of platelet prostaglandin formation and aggregation by ingested aspirin or indomethacin. *Prostaglandins* 1973;3:141.
52. MacDonald R. Aspirin and extradural blocks. *Br J Anaesth* 1991;66:1.
53. Hindman BJ, Koka BV. Usefulness of post-aspirin bleeding time. *Anesthesiology* 1986;64:368.
54. Lunt CC, Satin AJ, Bath WH, Hankins GD. The effect of indomethacin tocolysis on maternal coagulation status. *Obstet Gynecol* 1994; 84:820.
55. Channing Rodgers RP, Levin J. A critical reappraisal of the bleeding time. *Semin Thromb Hemost* 1990;16:1.
56. CLASP Collaborative Group. CLASP: a randomized trial of low dose aspirin for the prevention and treatment of preeclampsia among 9,364 pregnant women. *Lancet* 1994;343:619.
57. DeSwiet M, Redman CWG. Aspirin, extradural anaesthesia and the MRC collaborative low-dose aspirin study in pregnancy (CLASP) [Letter]. *Br J Anaesth* 1992;69:109.
58. Horlocker TT, Wedel DJ, Offord KP. Does preoperative anti-platelet therapy increase the risk of hemmorhagic complications associated with regional anesthesia? *Anesth Analg* 1990;70:631.
59. Horlocker TT, Wedel DJ, Schroeder DR, et al. Preoperative anti-platelet therapy does not increase the risk of spinal hematoma associated with regional anesthesia. *Anesth Analg* 1995;80:303.
60. Moise KH, Huhta JC, Sharif DS. Indomethacin in the treatment of premature labor: effects on the fetal ductus arteriosus. *N Engl J Med* 1988;319:327.

61. Hickok DE, Hollenback KA, Reilly SF. The association between decreased amniotic fluid volume and treatment with non-steroidal anti-inflammatory for preterm labor. *Am J Obstet Gynecol* 1989;160:1525.
62. Ment LR, Oh W, Ehrenkranz RA, et al. Low dose indomethacin and prevention of intraventricular hemorrhage: a multicenter randomized trial. *Pediatrics* 1994;93:543.
63. Read MD, Wellby DE. The use of a calcium antagonist (nifedipine) to suppress preterm labor. *Br J Obstet Gynaecol* 1986;93:933.
64. Ferguson JE, Dyson DC, Holbrook RH, Schultz T, Stevenson DK. Cardiovascular and metabolic effects associated with nifidipine and ritodrine tocolysis. *Am J Obstet Gynecol* 1989;161:788.
65. Harake B, Gilbert RD, Ashwal S, Power GG. Nifedipine: effects on fetal and maternal hemodynamics in pregnant sheep. *Am J Obstet Gynecol* 1987;157:1003.
66. Ferguson JE, Dyson DC, Schultz T, Stevenson DK. A comparison of tocolysis with nifedipine or ritodrine analysis of efficacy and maternal fetal and neonatal outcome. *Am J Obstet Gynecol* 1990;163:105.
67. Waisman GD, Mayorga LM, Camera MI. Magnesium plus nifedipine: potentiation of the hypotensive effect in preeclampsia. *Am J Obstet Gynecol* 1988;159:308.
68. Thorp JM, Spielman FJ, Valea FA, et al. Nifedipine enhances the cardiac toxicity of magnesium sulphate in the isolated perfused Sprague-Dawley rat heart. *Am J Obstet Gynaecol* 1990;163:655.
69. Snyder S, Cardwell MS. Neuromuscular blockade with magnesium sulfate and nifidipine. *Am J Obstet Gynecol* 1989;161:35.
70. Tosone S, Reves J, Kissin I, Smith I, Fournier S. Hemodynamic responses to nifedipine in dogs anesthetized with halothane. *Anesth Analg* 1983;62:903.
71. Merin R, Calcium channel blocking drugs and anaesthetics: is the drug interaction beneficial or detrimental? *Anesthesiology* 1987;66:111.
72. Eduard A. Bordeaux A, Ahmand R, Samii K. Cardiovascular interactions of local anesthetics and calcium entry blockers in conscious dogs. *Reg Anesth* 1991;16:95.
73. Bruguerolle B. Effects of calcium channel blockers on bupivacaine-induced toxicity. *Life Sci* 1993;53:349.
74. Hahn DW, Demarest KT, Ericson E, et al. Evaluation of 1-deamino-[d-try(O-ethyl)2, Thr4, Orn8] vasotocin, an oxytocin antagonist, in animal models of uterine contractility and preterm labor: a new tocolytic agent. *Am J Obstet Gynecol* 1987;157:977.
75. Goodwin TM, Millar L, North L, Abrams LS, Weglein RC, Hollans ML. The pharmacokinetics of the oxytocin antagonist atosiban in pregnant women with preterm uterine contractions. *Am J Obstet Gynecol* 1995;173:913.
76. Akerlund M, Stromberg P, Hauksson A, et al. Inhibition of uterine contractions of premature labor with an oxytocin analog. Results from a pilot study. *Br J Obstet Gynaecol* 1984;94:1040.
77. Goodwin TM, Paul R, Silver H, et al. The effect of the oxytocin antagonist atosiban on preterm uterine activity in the human. *Am J Obstet Gynecol* 1994;170:474.
78. Andersen LF, Lyndrup J, Akerlund M, Melin P. Oxytocin receptor blockade: a new principle in the treatment of preterm labor? *Am J Perinatol* 1989;6:196.
79. Goodwin TM, Valenzuela GJ, Silver H, Creasy G, and the Atosiban Study Group. Dose ranging study of the oxytocin antagonist atosiban in the treatment of preterm labor. *Obstet Gynecol* 1996;88:331.
80. Greig PC, Massman GA, Demarest KT, Weglein RC, Holland ML, Figuerora JP. Maternal and fetal cardiovascular effects and placental transfer of the oxytocin antagonist atosiban in late gestation pregnant sheep. *Am J Obstet Gynecol* 1993;169:897.
81. Lee SC, Campbell S, Jauniaux E, et al. Arrest of preterm labour and prolongation of gestation with glyceryl trinitrate, a nitric oxide donor. *Lancet* 1994;343:1325.
82. Kaga N, Katsuki Y, Futamara Y, Obata M, Shibutani Y. Role of urinary trypsin inhibitor in the maintenance of pregnancy in mice. *Obstet Gynecol* 1996;88:872.
83. El-Maradny E, Kanayama N, Halim A, Maehara K, Kobayashi T, Tera OT. Effects of urinary trypsin inhibitor or myometrial contraction in term and preterm deliveries. *Gynecol Obstet Invest* 1996;41:96.
84. Kao CY, Wang S. Effect of lidocaine on rat myometrial sodium channels and implications for the management of preterm labor. *Am J Obstet Gynecol* 1994;171:446.
85. Scanlon JW, Brown WU, Weiss JB, Alper MH. Neurobehavioural responses of newborn infants after maternal epidural anaesthesia. *Anesthesiology* 1974;40:121.
86. Morishima HO, Pedersen H, Santos AC, et al. Adverse effects of maternally administered lidocaine on the asphyxiated preterm fetal lamb. *Anesthesiology* 1989;71:110.
87. Banzai M, Sato S, Tezuka N. Komiya H, Chimura T, Hiroi M. Placental transfer of lidocaine hydrochloride after prolonged continuous maternal intravenous administration. *Can J Anaesth* 1995;42:338.
88. Bassell GM, Marx GF. Optimization of fetal oxygenation. *Int J Obstet Anesth* 1995;4:238.
89. Crenshaw C, Payne P, Blackmon L, et al. Prematurity and the obstetrician. *Am J Obstet Gynecol* 1983;147:125.
90. Kitchen W, Ford G, Orgill A, et al. Outcome in infants with a bright weight 500 to 999 gm: a regional study of 1979 and 1980 births. *J Pediatr* 1984;104:921.
91. Myers RE, Myers SE. Use of sedative, analgesic, and anesthetic drugs during labor and delivery. Bane or boon? *Am J Obstet Gynecol* 1979;133:83.
92. Gutsche BB, Samuels P. Anesthetic consideration in premature birth. *Int Anesthesiol Clin* 1990;28:33.
93. Norris M, Arkoosh V. Spinal opioid analgesia for labor. *Int Anesthesiol Clin* 1994;32:69.
94. Gamlin FMC, Lyons G. Spinal analgesia in labor. *Int J Obstet Anesth* 1997;6:161.
95. Clark VT, Smiley RM, Finster M. Uterine hyperactivity after intrathecal injection of fentanyl for analgesia during labor: a cause of fetal bradycardia? *Anesthesiology* 1994;4:1083.
96. Friedlander JD, Fox HE, Cain CF, Dominiguez CL, Smiley RM. Fetal bradycardia and uterine hyperactivity following subarachnoid administration of fentanyl during labor. *Reg Anesth* 1997;22:378.
97. Carp H, Bailey S. The association between meningitis and dural puncture in bacteremic rats. *Anesthesiology* 1992;76:739.
98. Ramanathan J, Vaddadi A, Mercer BM, Sibai B, Angel JJ. Epidural anesthesia in women with chorioamnionitis. *Anesth Rev* 1992;19:35.
99. Goodman E, DeHorta E, Taguiam J. Safety of spinal and epidural anesthesia in parturients with chorioamnionitis. *Reg Anesth* 1996; 21:436.
100. Scanlon JW, Brown WI, Weiss JB, et al. Neurobehavioral responses of newborn infants after maternal epidural anesthesia. *Anesthesiology* 1974;40:121.
101. Biehl D. Placental transfer of lidocaine: effects of fetal acidosis. *Anesthesiology* 1978;48:409.
102. Abboud TK, Williams V, Miller F, et al. Comparative fetal, maternal, and neonatal responses following epidural analgesia with bupivacaine, chloroprocaine and lidocaine. *Anesthesiology* 1981;55:A315.
103. Abboud TK, Khoo SS, Miller F, et al. Maternal, fetal, and neonatal responses after epidural anesthesia with bupivacaine, 2-chloroprocaine or lidocaine. *Anesth Analg* 1982;61:638.
104. Datta S, Corke BC, Alper MH, et al. Epidural anesthesia for cesarean section: a comparison of bupivacaine, chloroprocaine and etidocaine. *Anesthesiology* 1980;52:48.
105. Kileff M, James FM, Dewan E, et al. Neonatal neurobehavioral responses after epidural anesthesia for cesarean section with lidocaine and bupivacaine. *Anesthesiology* 1982;57:A403.
106. Merkow AJ, McGuinness GA, Erenberg A, et al. The neonatal neurobehavioral effects of bupivacaine, mepivacaine, and 2-chloroprocaine used for pudendal block. *Anesthesiology* 1980;52:309.
107. Kuhnert BR, Harrison MJ, Linn PL, Kuhnert PM. Effects of maternal epidural anesthesia on neonatal behavior. *Anesth Analg* 1984;63:301.
108. Kuhnert BR, Kennard MJ, Linn PL. Neonatal neurobehavior after epidural anesthesia for cesarean section. *Anesth Analg* 1988;67:64.
109. Santos AC, Yun EM, Bobby PD, Noble G, Arthur GR, Finster M. The effects of bupivacaine, L-Nitro-L-Arginine-Methyl Ester, and phenylephrine on cardiovascular adaptations to asphyxia in the preterm fetal lamb. *Anesth Analg* 1997;85:1299.
110. Muir HA, Writer WDR, Weeks S, Douglas JD. A double-blind comparision between epidural ropivacaine 0.25% and bupivacaine 0.25% for the relief of childbirth pain: report of a Canadian multicentre study. *Can J Anaesth* 1997;44:599.
111. Eddelston JM, Holland JJ, Griffin RP, et al. A double-blind comparison of 0.25% ropivacaine and 0.25% bupivacaine for extradural analgesia in labour. *Br J Anaesth* 1996;76:66.
112. Benhamou D, Hamza J, Eledjam J, et al. Continuous extradural infusion of ropivacaine 2 mgml-1 for pain relief during labour. *Br J Anaesth* 1997;78:748.
113. Arthur GR, Feldman HS, Covino BG. Comparative pharmacokinetics

of bupivacaine and ropivacaine, a new amide local anesthetic. *Anesth Analg* 1988;67:1053.
114. Katz JA, Bridenbaugh PO, Knarr DC, et al. Pharmacodynamics and pharmacokinetics of epidural ropivacaine in humans. *Anesth Analg* 1990;70:16.
115. Datta S, Camann W, Bader A, et al. Clinical effects and maternal and fetal plasma concentrations of epidural ropivacaine versus bupivacaine for cesarean section. *Anesthesiology* 1995;82:1346.
116. Ala-kokko TI, Alahahta S, Jouppila P, Korpi K. Westerling P, Vahakangas K. Fetal-maternal distribution of ropivacaine and bupivacaine after epidural administration for cesarean section. *Int J Obstet Anesth* 1997;6:147.
117. Malloy M, Rhoads G, Schramm W, Land G. Increasing cesarean section rates in very low-birth weight infants. Effect on outcome. *JAMA* 1989;262:1475.
118. Rolbin S, Cohen M, Levinter D, Kelly E, Farne D. The premature infant: anesthesia for cesarean delivery. *Anesth Analg* 1994;78:912.
119. Hodgson CA, Wauchob TD. A comparison of spinal and general anesthesia for elective caesarean section: effect on neonatal condition at birth. *Int J Obstet Anaesth* 1994;3:25.
120. Riley ET, Flanagan B, Cohen SE, Chitkara U. Intravenous nitroglycerine: a potent uterine relaxant for emergency obstetric procedures. Review of literature and report of three cases. *Int J Obstet Anaesth* 1996;5:264.
121. Rozenak D, Diamant YZ, Yoffe H, et al. Cocaine: maternal use during pregnancy and its effects on the mother, the fetus and the infant. *Obstet Gynecol Surv* 1990;45:348.
122. Slutster L. Risks associated with cocaine use during pregnancy. *Obstet Gynecol* 1992;79:778.
123. Cregler L, Marx H. Medical complications of cocaine abuse. *N Engl J Med* 1986;315:1495.
124. Chao C. Cardiovascular effects of cocaine during pregnancy. *Semin Perinatol* 1996;20:107.
125. Morishima HO, Cooper TB, Hara T, et al. Pregnancy alters the hemodynamic responses to cocaine in the rat. *Dev Pharmacol Ther* 1992;19:69.
126. Woods JR, Plessinger MA. Pregnancy increases cardiovascular toxicity to cocaine. *Am J Obstet Gynecol* 1990;162:529.
127. Plessinger MA, Woods JR. Progesterone increases cardiovascular toxicity to cocaine in nonpregnant ewes. *Am J Obstet Gynecol* 1990;75:725.
128. Woods JR, Scott KL, Plessinger MA, et al. Pregnancy enhances cocaine's actions on the heart and within the peripheral circulation. *Am J Obstet Gynecol* 1994;170:1027.
129. Scafidi FA, Fuld TF, Wheeden A, et al. Cocaine exposed preterm neonates show behavioral and hormonal differences. *Pediatrics* 1996; 97:851.
130. Collaborative Group on Antenatal Steroid Therapy. Effect of antenatal dexamethasone administration on the prevention of respiratory distress syndrome. *Am J Obstet Gynecol* 1981;141:276.
131. Morales WJ. Preparing the fetus for preterm birth. *Ballieres Clin Obstet Gynaecol* 1993;7:601.
132. Wright L, Verter J, Younes N, et al. Antenatal corticosteriod administration and neonatal outcome in very low birthweight infants: the NICHD Neonatal Research Network. *Am J Obstet Gynecol* 1995;173: 269.
133. Crowley P. Antenatal corticosteriod therapy: a meta-analysis of the randomized trials, 1972 to 1994. *Am J Obstet Gynecol* 1995;73:322.
134. Andrews EB, Marcucci G, White A, Long W. Association between use of antenatal corticosteriods and neonatal outcomes within the exosurf. Neonatal Treatment Investigational New Drug Program. *Am J Obstet Gynecol* 1995;173:290.
135. Doyle M, Hamilton R, Johanson R, O'Brien S. The use of corticosteroids for maturation of fetal lungs in patients with preterm prelabour rupture of the membranes. *Br J Obstet Gynaecol* 1994;101:1078.
136. Egarter C, Leifich H, Husslein P, Kaider A, Schemper M. Adjunctive antibiotic treatment in preterm labor and neonatal morbidity: a meta-analysis. *Obstet Gynecol* 1996;88:303.
137. Mercer B, Arheart K. Antimicrobial therapy in expectant management of preterm premature rupture of membranes. *Lancet* 1995;346:1271.
138. Long WA, Corbet AJ, Cotton R, et al. A controlled trial of synthetic surfactant in infants weighing 1250 g or more with respiratory distress syndrome. *N Engl J Med* 1991;325:1696.
139. Corbet AJ, Long WA, Murphy DJ, et al. Reduced mortality in small premature infants treated at birth with a single dose of synthetic surfactant. *J Paediatr Child Health* 1991;27:245.
140. Canadian EXOSURF Pediatric Study Group. Effects of two rescue doses of EXOSURF Pediatric in 342 750–1249 gram infants. *Pediatr Res* 1990;27:200A.
141. Smyth J, Allen A, Sankaran K, et al. Effects of two rescue doses of EXOSURF Neonatal in 221 500–749 gram infants. *Pediatr Res* 1991;29:330A.
142. Stevenson D, Walther F, Long W, et al. Controlled trial of a single dose of synthetic surfactant at birth in premature infants weighing 500 to 699 grams. *J Pediatr* 1992;120:S3.
143. Davidson D. Nitric oxide from bench to bedside: a perinatal perspective—Part I and Part II. *Int J Obstet Anesth* 1996;5:181,244.
144. Merritt JC, Kraybill EN. Retrolental fibroplasia: a five-year experience in a tertiary perinatal center. *Ann Ophthalmol* 1988;65:67.

Obstetric Anesthesia, second edition,
edited by Mark C. Norris.
Lippincott Williams & Wilkins, Philadelphia © 1999.

CHAPTER 35

Fetal Malpresentation and Multiple Birth

Yaakov Beilin and Howard H. Bernstein

Birth trauma, neonatal hypoxemia, prematurity and maternal hemorrhage are just some of the possible complications when malpresentation of the fetus or multiple gestation occurs. Appropriate anesthetic management of these patients can play a critical role in ensuring successful outcomes for both mother and baby. In this chapter, we review the obstetric and anesthetic considerations associated with malpresentation and multiple gestation. Understanding these issues will help formulate an appropriate anesthetic plan.

FETAL MALPRESENTATION

Definitions

The lie of the fetus is the relative position of the long axis of the fetus to that of the uterus. Fetal lie can be longitudinal, transverse, or oblique. Vertex and breech presentations are longitudinal lies. A spontaneous vaginal delivery can be achieved only from a longitudinal lie. The presentation of the fetus is defined by the body part that overlies the pelvic inlet. The most common presentations are cephalic (vertex), breech, or shoulder. The presenting, most dependent, part of the fetus will be palpated first during vaginal examination. The attitude of the fetal head is either flexion, with the chin approaching the chest, or extension, with the occiput approaching the back. The lie, presentation, presenting part, and attitude of the fetus are important factors in determining the likelihood and safety of a vaginal delivery.

Vertex presentation with flexion is associated with the greatest chance of a safe vaginal delivery, because the fetal skull enters the pelvis first with the smallest presenting diameter. Any variation in presentation or attitude is referred to as a malpresentation, and the prognosis for a safe vaginal delivery is decreased. Malpresentations include breech, occiput posterior, face, brow, and military presentations.

Y. Beilin and H.H. Bernstein: Departments of Anesthesiology, and Obstetrics, Gynecology, and Reproductive Sciences, Mount Sinai School of Medicine, New York, New York 10029.

Breech Presentation

In breech presentation, the fetal lie is longitudinal with the sacrum presenting over the pelvic inlet. The prevalence of breech presentation decreases with increasing gestational age. The incidence of breech presentation is about 25% at the end of the second trimester, 17% at 30 weeks, and 3.5% at term (1,2). There are four types of breech presentation, defined by the presenting part and whether the hips and knees are flexed or extended (Fig. 1).

1. Complete breech: The buttocks present with both hips and knees flexed.
2. Frank breech: The buttocks present with the hips flexed and the knees extended. This is the most common breech presentation.
3. Footling breech: One or both feet present, and both hip(s) and knee(s) are in extension.
4. Kneeling: One or both knees present. The hips are extended and the knees flexed.

The biologic mechanisms leading to breech presentation are unknown (Table 1). Associated maternal factors are uterine anomalies, primiparity, high parity, established maternal diabetes, older maternal age, and smoking during pregnancy. Fetal factors include multiple gestation, low birth weight, prematurity, hydrocephalus, and congenital abnormalities (2,3). The incidence of congenital abnormalities in the fetus with a breech presentation is about 3 times that of the vertex fetus (4).

Fetal Risks

The hazards of breech presentation were described by Edmund Piper at the 1928 annual meeting of the American Medical Association (5). He attributed the increased

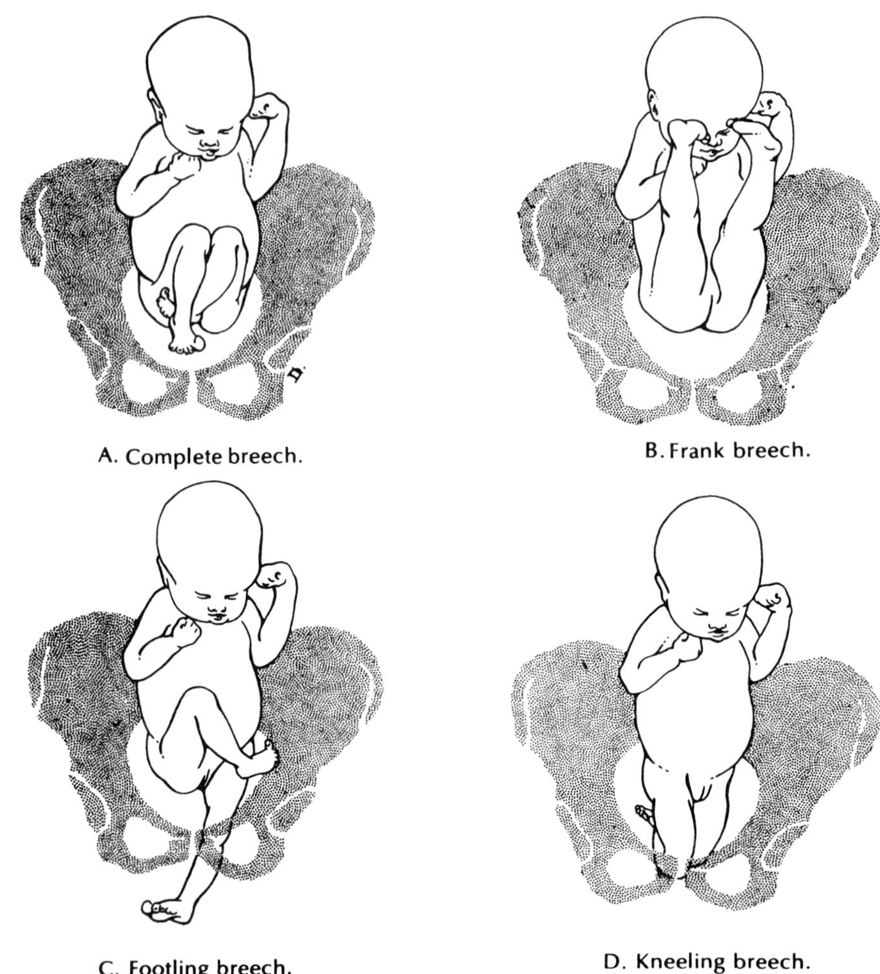

FIG. 1. Attitudes of breech presentation. (From ref. 2, with permission.)

risk of perinatal morbidity and mortality with breech presentation to umbilical cord accidents including cord compression and prolapse, the occurrence of a nuchal arm, and difficulty with the aftercoming head. These problems can cause either fetal mechanical injury, such as skull fracture or brachial plexus damage, or anoxic brain injury and death. Neonatal mortality with breech presentation is about 5 times greater than that of term cephalic presentations (6,7).

The incidence of umbilical cord prolapse is about 5% in complete breech presentation and 10% in footling breech presentation. In a frank breech presentation, the presenting part, the buttocks, fills the maternal pelvic inlet, and the risk of cord prolapse, 0.5%, is the same as with a vertex presentation (8).

TABLE 1. *Known factors associated with breech presentation and possible reasons for failure to assume the vertex presentation*

Factors	Possible reasons
Uterine and placental	
Bicornuate to double uterus	Aberrant shape of pregnant uterine cavity
Placenta previa or placenta in cornua of uterus	Aberrant shape of pregnant uterine cavity
Fetal	
Twins	Aberrant crowding
Prematurity	Less uterine constraint to fetal positioning
Low birth weight	Less uterine constraint to fetal positioning
Polyhydramnios	Less uterine constraint to fetal positioning
Oligohydramnios	Undue uterine constraint to fetal movement
Abnormalities in form or function of the fetus	Limitation in the capacity of the fetus to assume the vertex position

Maternal Risks

The mother delivering a baby in the breech presentation also is at increased risk. Much of this increased morbidity is related to the use of cesarean section for delivery. One prospective study of breech deliveries reported maternal morbidity of 49.3% in cesarean sections versus 6.7% in vaginal deliveries (9). However, vaginal breech delivery also increases maternal risk compared with vertex delivery. Intrauterine manipulation, common during a vaginal breech delivery, increases the risk of infection, and the need for uterine relaxation to aid in the breech delivery increases the risk of uterine atony and hemorrhage.

External Cephalic Version

External cephalic version is the procedure in which a fetus is turned from a breech to a cephalic presentation by using manipulations through the abdominal wall. Successful version will reduce the cesarean section rate for breech presentation (10–12). Most versions are performed after week 36 of gestation because the spontaneous version rate after this time is low, and only about 2% will revert to the breech position (1). Using a tocolytic agent may improve the success rate of version, especially in nulliparous mothers (13,14).

Potential complications of version, although rare, include placental abruptio, fetal–maternal hemorrhage, isoimmunization, preterm labor, uterine rupture, fetal distress and death, and maternal mortality (15). Contraindications to external cephalic version include uterine anomalies, placenta previa, abruptio placenta, and nonreassuring signs of fetal well-being (1).

Anesthetic Considerations

The role of neuraxial anesthesia in external version is controversial. Both epidural analgesia and intrathecal opioids improve maternal comfort. Maternal analgesia also may improve chances of successful version. One nonrandomized study reported a higher success rate of external cephalic version at term in women who received an epidural anesthetic versus those who did not (59% vs 24%) (16). Epidural block was not associated with any increased fetal or maternal morbidity, but some obstetricians use maternal discomfort to gauge the pressure they apply during a version attempt. A recent prospective randomized trial also reported more successful versions in women receiving epidural anesthesia (2% lidocaine with 1:200,000 epinephrine) compared with women who received no analgesia (69% vs 32%) (17).

Obstetric Management

There are three methods of vaginal breech delivery; spontaneous, partial extraction, or total extraction. In a spontaneous breech delivery, the infant delivers without any obstetric manipulations. With partial breech extraction, the baby delivers without assistance up to the umbilicus at which point the obstetrician assists with the delivery of the thorax and aftercoming head. With total breech extraction, the obstetrician assists in the delivery of the entire fetus, usually by applying traction to the legs or ankles. Except for the delivery of a second twin, total breech extraction is almost never performed.

The choice between cesarean and vaginal delivery for a baby presenting as a breech is controversial. Before 1945, maternal mortality after cesarean section was as high as 16% (1). Although the fetal risks of vaginal breech delivery were understood, the maternal risks of cesarean section were unacceptably high, and the vaginal route was preferred. As the risks of cesarean section decreased, its use for breech presentation increased. By 1955, about 11% of viable breech presentations were delivered abdominally. In 1959, Wright (18) argued that advance prediction of successful vaginal delivery was impossible, and recommended cesarean section for all viable breech fetuses. Two recent meta-analyses of the available obstetric literature on breech deliveries reported a fourfold to tenfold increase in the risk of fetal trauma with a vaginal breech delivery compared with abdominal delivery (19,20). Now the cesarean section rate for breech presentations is 80% to 100% (1) and accounts for 15% of cesarean sections, costing society about $1.4 billion per year (21).

Over the last decade, the debate about the benefit of universal cesarean delivery for breech presentation has continued. Although neonatal outcomes may be better after cesarean delivery for breech presentation, maternal morbidity is several times higher (22,23).

Term Breech Deliveries

The advantage of routine cesarean section for the term breech fetus has been questioned. Danielian et al. (24) performed a population-based study comparing the outcome until school age of term breech infants delivered by elective cesarean section versus those delivered vaginally. They did not find any difference between the groups in terms of severe handicap, developmental delays, neurologic deficit, or psychiatric referral. Schiff et al. (25) performed a retrospective chart review of 846 breech deliveries to look at the effect of route of delivery on morbidity and mortality. There were no statistically significant differences between the groups in the frequency of low Apgar scores, need for endotracheal intubation, or neonatal intensive care unit admissions. There was a trend toward more birth trauma in infants delivered vaginally. Others reported similar findings (26–28).

Preterm Breech Deliveries

Even greater controversy surrounds the route of delivery for preterm infants in breech presentation. Kaplan et al. (29) reviewed the charts of 185 breech infants weighing between 1,000 and 2,500 grams. Vaginal delivery had no statistically significant impact on perinatal mortality or morbidity compared with cesarean section. Cibils et al. (30) performed an observational study of 262 consecutive breech deliveries of infants weighing between 500 and 1,500 grams. Here, prematurity was the most frequent cause of neonatal death, and there was no correlation with the mode of delivery. These same authors (31), in another study, also found no influence of route of delivery on neonatal outcome in infants weighing more than 1,500 grams.

In a nationwide collaborative study in The Netherlands, perinatal data were collected on 899 live-born, singleton, non-malformed, preterm, breech infants who presented at younger than 32 weeks' gestation or less than 1,500 grams (32). They found that preterm breech infants born by cesarean section had a lower morbidity rate than those delivered vaginally. However, 5 years after delivery, the incidence of minor and major handicaps was the same in both groups. Weissman et al. (33) compared the fetal mortality and morbidity in vaginal versus cesarean delivery in breech infants weighing 1,000 to 2,000 grams. Contrary to the results of these studies (28–31), these authors found greater neonatal morbidly and mortality associated with vaginal delivery. Infants weighing less than 1,500 grams were at greatest risk.

Cesarean delivery also may not benefit breech infants weighing less than 1,000 grams. In a retrospective analysis of 83 viable singleton preterm breech infants, route of delivery did not affect survival in the infants who weighed less than 1,000 grams (34).

Two attempts were made at randomizing women with breech babies to either cesarean section or vaginal delivery (35,36). Unfortunately too few patients were recruited in either study to reach any conclusions. In one study, 25% of infants in the vaginal trial group required cesarean section for fetal indications.

In 1994 the International Federation of Gynecology and Obstetrics (FIGO) Committee on Perinatal Health, based on a review of the available literature, published guidelines for choosing a trial of labor for a singleton breech fetus (Table 2) (23).

TABLE 2. *FIGO criteria for a trial of labor for a singleton breech delivery*

- Term infant weighing <4,000 g
- Gestational age >34 weeks: cesarean section recommended for fetus between 28 and 34 weeks' gestational age
- Adequate pelvimetry: radiography or magnetic resonance imaging pelvimetry
- Rule out hyperextension of head
- Rule out hydrocephalus
- Rule out severe fetal malformations
- Frank or complete breech presentation only
- Electronic fetal monitoring and fetal blood gas analysis should be available
- An experienced obstetrician should be present at the delivery

FIGO, International Federation of Gynecology and Obstetrics.

From ref. 23, with permission.

Anesthetic Considerations

Vaginal Delivery

Epidural Analgesia

In the past, breech presentation was a relative contraindication to epidural analgesia because of concerns about prolonged labor and impaired maternal expulsive efforts (37). More recently, however, epidural block has become the preferred method of labor analgesia in breech presentation (Table 3). As early as 1960, less neonatal morbidity was noted in breech births managed with caudal anesthesia (38). This benefit was attributed to the avoidance of general anesthetics and improved obstetric management. In 1974, Crawford (39) reported a series of 247 singleton breech deliveries of which 56 received epidural analgesia with bupivacaine, 0.375%. Despite a slightly prolonged second stage (44 minutes in the epidural group vs 34 minutes in the nonepidural group), neonatal condition was better, and there was no increased incidence of fetal extractions in the epidural group.

In the 1970s, three other retrospective reviews assessed the use of epidural analgesia for attempted vaginal delivery of breech presentations (40–42). In these studies, epidural analgesia did not influence Apgar scores or umbilical cord acid–base values. Epidural analgesia was associated with a longer second-stage labor but not with the frequency of breech extraction or emergency cesarean section. Breeson et al. (43), in a prospective study, found no increase in the duration of labor, a decreased need for breech extraction, and improved neonatal condition with epidural analgesia. The authors strongly recommended the use of epidural analgesia in the management of all breech deliveries.

In contrast, Confino et al. (44) retrospectively compared 94 vaginal breech deliveries with, and 277 deliveries without, epidural analgesia. In the epidural group, mean duration of the second stage of labor was increased, and 1-minute Apgar scores were lower in fetuses weighing more than 2,500 grams. However, 5-minute Apgar scores, perinatal morbidity, and maternal complications were the same in both groups.

Whereas epidural analgesia may prolong the second stage of labor, the importance of this association is unclear. In nulliparous women who delivered term breech babies under epidural analgesia, the length of the second stage of labor did not correlate with the risk of fetal trauma or low Apgar scores (45).

TABLE 3. *Epidural analgesia for vaginal breech deliveries*

Authors	Study design	Effects on labor and delivery	Effects on neonatal outcome	Method(s) of neonatal evaluation
Crawford (39) (1974)	Retrospective: epidural vs no epidural	Prolonged second stage; no increase in breech extractions	Decreased neonatal depression	Apgar scores, "postnatal course"
Bowen-Simpkins and Fergusson (40) (1974)	Retrospective: epidural vs "other forms of analgesia"	Prolonged second stage; no increase in manipulative delivery	No adverse effects	Apgar scores
Donnai and Nicholas (41) (1975)	Retrospective: no control	Low incidence of breech extraction	87% 1-min Apgar scores <6	Umbilical vein pH, Apgar scores
Darby and Hunter (42) (1976)	Retrospective: epidural vs parenteral	Prolonged first and second stage; no increase in breech extractions or emergency cesarean section	Higher 5-min Apgar scores	Apgar scores
Breeson et al. (43) (1978)	Prospective: epidural vs historic control group	No increase in duration of labor; decrease in breech extraction	Improved fetal condition	Fetal blood sampling, Apgar scores
Confino et al. (44) (1985)	Retrospective: epidural vs no epidural	Prolonged second stage if birth weight >2,500 g	Lower 1-min Apgar scores but similar 5-min Apgar scores; no change in perinatal morbidity	Apgar scores epidural vs no epidural
Van Zundert et al. (46) (1991)	Retrospective: vaginal breech vs vaginal vertex and cesarean breech, all with epidural	Mean duration second stage 31 min; 9 min mean "expulsion time"; 6% instrumental deliveries	Lower 1-min Apgar scores vs. vertex or cesarean section; similar 5-min Apgar scores	Apgar scores
Chadha et al. (47) (1992)	Retrospective: epidural vs no epidural	Longer first and second stage labor; greater use of pitocin; higher cesarean section rate in the second stage of labor	No difference in Apgar scores or need for neonatal intensive care	Apgar scores
Perl et al. (45) (1996)	Retrospective: all patients had an epidural; compared length of second stage with risk of neonatal injury	N/A	No correlation between length of second stage and risk of fetal trauma or low Apgar scores	Apgar scores, neonatal examination

Van Zundert et al. (46) reported their 10-year experience with epidural analgesia for vaginal breech delivery. All patients with a breech presentation for a trial of labor received epidural analgesia with bupivacaine, 0.125%, and epinephrine, 1:800,000. They recorded the duration of the second stage of labor, time from diagnosis of full dilatation to delivery, and the expulsion time. Expulsion time was defined as time from the first expulsive effort (push) until delivery. They found a mean expulsion time of 8.7 minutes (range, 1 to 40 minutes). Only four women pushed for more than 20 minutes. Although the 1-minute Apgar scores were lower in breech infants than after singleton vertex deliveries, there were no differences in 5-minute Apgar scores. These authors concluded that epidural analgesia is indicated for all vaginal breech deliveries.

In contrast, Chadha et al. (47) performed a retrospective study to determine the effect of epidural analgesia on the outcome of spontaneous labor in women with a term singleton breech baby. Women who had an epidural anesthetic had a significantly longer first and second stage of labor and greater need for oxytocin augmentation than women who did not have an epidural anesthetic. The cesarean section rate during the first stage of labor was the same in both groups. However, the cesarean-section rate in the second stage of labor was significantly greater in women who received an epidural anesthetic. Perinatal outcome, as determined by Apgar scores and the need for neonatal intensive care was the same in both groups. They concluded that epidural analgesia was associated with longer first and second stages of labor, greater need for oxytocin augmentation, and a greater cesarean-section rate in the second stage of labor.

Although conflicting data exist, epidural analgesia for vaginal delivery of the breech fetus has become the anesthetic of choice. As with vertex presentation, there are several advantages of epidural analgesia:

- Excellent pain relief for labor and vaginal examination,
- Diminution of bearing-down reflex before full cervical dilatation,
- Ability to extend level of analgesia rapidly to allow breech extraction or cesarean section,
- Avoidance of general anesthesia,
- Pelvic floor relaxation, allowing a controlled delivery of the aftercoming head, and
- Safe delivery of the fetus without increased perinatal morbidity.

We use bupivacaine, 0.125% to 0.25%, to initiate labor analgesia, and then begin a continuous infusion of 0.0625% bupivacaine with fentanyl, 2 μg/mL, at 10 to 15 mL per hour. If this concentration of local anesthetic is inadequate to prevent premature maternal pushing, give additional bupivacaine, 0.25%, with or without an opioid. If breech extraction becomes necessary, lidocaine, 2%, with epinephrine, 1:200,000, or 2-chloroprocaine, 3%, may be administered to attain rapidly an appropriate level of anesthesia. When rapid analgesia is desired, as in a patient in advanced labor, consider subarachnoid fentanyl, 25 μg, or sufentanil, 5 to 10 μg, ± bupivacaine, 2.5 mg, as part of a combined spinal–epidural technique (48).

Uterine Relaxation

During vaginal delivery, immediate uterine relaxation may become necessary to assist in delivery of the aftercoming head. General endotracheal anesthesia with a potent inhalation agent will provide uterine relaxation. Either halothane, enflurane, or isoflurane will provide uterine relaxation in equipotent doses (49). Intravenous nitroglycerin, 50 to 100 μg (50), or sublingual aerosol spray of nitroglycerin, 0.8 mg (51), also will reliably produce uterine relaxation and may preclude the need for general anesthesia. We currently use nitroglycerin as our first modality to achieve uterine relaxation, and then general anesthesia, if necessary.

Cesarean Section

Anesthetic considerations for cesarean section of a breech baby are similar to those with vertex presentations. We use regional anesthesia whenever possible to lower the risk of maternal morbidity and mortality (52). As with babies who present as a vertex, it is unclear whether regional anesthesia offers any neonatal benefit over general anesthesia (53,54).

Emergency cesarean section for cord prolapse or severe fetal distress will be performed under either general anesthesia or spinal anesthesia, depending on the clinical scenario. If a functioning epidural catheter is already in place, a rapid level of anesthesia may be attained with 2-chloroprocaine, 3%, or lidocaine, 2%, with epinephrine, 1:200,000. Darby and Hunter (55) noted no difference in neonatal outcome after spinal or general anesthesia for emergency cesarean section.

Entrapment of the aftercoming head may occur during cesarean section because of uterine muscle contraction. Relaxation of the uterus can be accomplished with an inhalational agent or nitroglycerin, as described for vaginal deliveries (56).

Malpresentation of the Vertex

During labor, the smallest anteroposterior (AP) diameter of the fetal skull normally presents into the pelvis (Fig. 2). Before labor, the fetal head is partially flexed, with the occipitofrontal diameter presenting (11.5 cm). As contractions intensify, and the fetus begins to descend into the pelvis, resistance to descent normally forces flexion of the fetal head, and the chin approaches the chest. Thus the presenting diameter changes to the smaller suboccipitobregmatic diameter (9.5 cm), and allows easier descent of the fetal head. Malpresentation of the vertex (Fig. 3) occurs when the fetal head is not flexed [i.e., military attitude (no flexion or extension), or brow (partial extension), or face (complete extension) present]. In these situations, a larger AP diameter of the fetal head presents to the maternal pelvis than in the flexed attitude (Table 4).

The most common factor associated with malpresentation of the vertex is cephalopelvic disproportion, due to large fetal size or a contracted maternal pelvis. Cephalopelvic disproportion may inhibit flexion and rotation of the fetal head. Other associated risk factors include multiparity, neoplasms, uterine anomalies, abnormal placental size and location (57), and polyhydramnios.

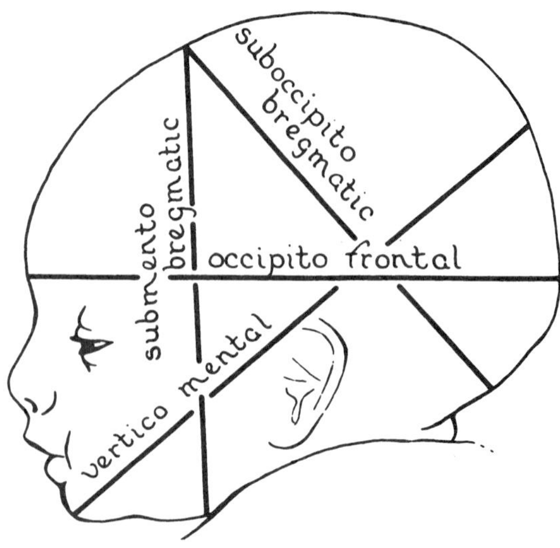

FIG. 2. Landmarks and diameters of fetal skull. (From ref. 2, with permission.)

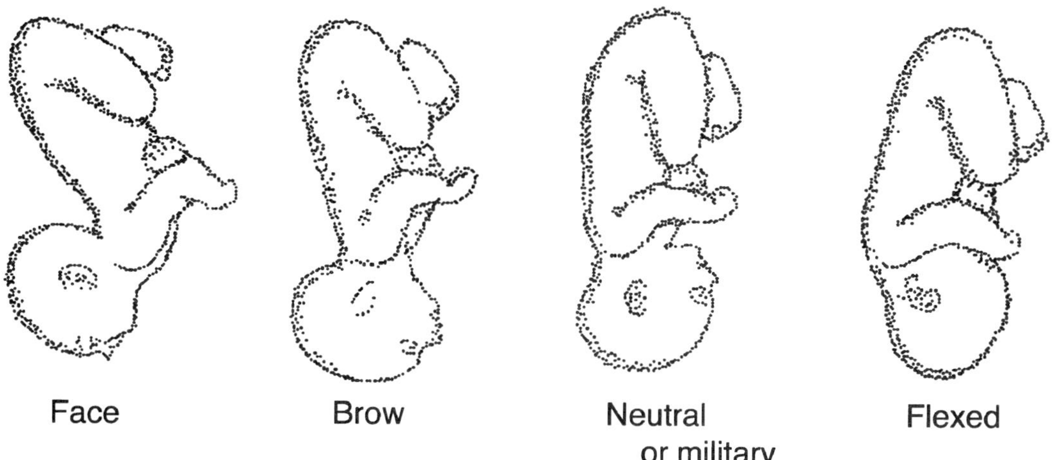

FIG. 3. Attitudes of the vertex.

The prognosis for vaginal delivery of a face presentation depends on the direction of the mentum (chin). Seventy percent to 80% may deliver vaginally in a mentum anterior (chin-up) position (58). In the mentum posterior position, the prognosis for vaginal delivery is poor, unless the fetus is very small. In the mentum posterior position, the fetal brow is compressed against the maternal symphysis, preventing flexion of the fetal head (59).

In contrast to face presentation, the prognosis for vaginal delivery in brow presentation is very poor. Here, the largest fetal AP diameter presents into the pelvis. Only with a small, preterm infant will vaginal delivery possibly occur. Fortunately, most brow presentations spontaneously convert to either a face or occiput presentation (60).

Persistent occiput posterior presentation (OPP) is not uncommon, occurring in about 5% of births. Because a larger cephalic diameter presents into the pelvis, the frequency of cephalopelvic disproportion is greater, the length of the first and second stages of labor is longer, and the frequency of operative deliveries higher with OPP than with an occiput anterior presentation (61,62). Pearl et al. (63) reported a significantly greater risk of maternal morbidity and neonatal Erb's and facial palsies with OPP. Both maternal and neonatal hospital stays were prolonged with OPP. Of importance, babies who present as OPP have an increased incidence of abnormal fetal heart-rate tracings, leading to a higher incidence of cesarean section for fetal indications than babies who present in the occiput anterior position (61,64).

Anesthetic considerations for the management of labor with babies who present with malpresentation of the vertex are not different from those who present with an occiput anterior presentation. Epidural anesthesia is commonly used, with low concentrations of local anesthetics. Of interest is the possible association of epidural analgesia use during labor and malpresentation. A retrospective cohort study found a significant increase in the risk of occiput malposition when epidural analgesia was placed before engagement of the fetal vertex (65). In contrast, Floberg et al. (66), found a correlation between decreased pelvic capacity and occiput posterior position, but not between epidural anesthesia and malpresentation.

Shoulder Presentation

Shoulder presentation is uncommon, about one in 350 pregnancies (58), and requires cesarean section for safe delivery of the fetus. Etiologic factors include placenta

TABLE 4. *Malpresentation of the vertex*

Attitude	Presenting part	Presenting diameter (cm)	Incidence at delivery	Prognosis for vaginal delivery
Flexion	Vertex (posterior)	Suboccipitobregmatic (9.5)	60%–70%	Good
Military	Vertex (median)	Occipitofrontal (11.5)		Good
Partial extension	Brow	Verticomental (13.5)	1/3,000	Poor
Complete extension	Face	Submentobregmatic (9.5)	1/250	Good
Occiput posterior (flexion)	Vertex (anterior)	Suboccipitofrontal (10.5)	15%–30%	Good
Occiput posterior (incomplete flexion)	Vertex (median)	Occipitofrontal (11.5)		Poor

From ref. 2, with permission.

previa, prematurity, multiparity, and cephalopelvic disproportion. As the presenting part cannot engage, the risk of cord prolapse is increased. During cesarean section, difficulty with delivery of the fetus may occur, leading to prolonged uterine incision-to-delivery time. As with breech presentation, uterine contraction may interfere with delivery, and uterine relaxation may be needed.

Compozund Presentation

Compound presentation occurs when both an extremity and the vertex or breech enter the pelvis and complicates about one in 1,000 deliveries (67). A compound presentation is usually a vertex/arm presentation, but may be vertex/arm/foot, vertex/foot, or breech/arm. Compound presentation is most commonly associated with prematurity but also may occur at term. Women with a baby who has a compound presentation may be allowed to labor, as the presenting extremity will usually withdraw as labor progresses (68).

MULTIPLE B IRTH

Incidence

Twin gestation occurs in approximately one in 90 pregnancies, triplets in one in 9,800 pregnancies, and quadruplets in one in 70,000 pregnancies. Twin gestation may either be monozygotic (MZ), occurring from a single ovum, or dizygotic (DZ), occurring from two ova. MZ twins are almost always genetically identical and occur from fertilization of a single ovum that subsequently divides. The frequency of MZ twins is fairly constant throughout the world at approximately four per 1,000 deliveries. DZ twins account for approximately two thirds of all twins and are as genetically distinct as any other siblings born to the same parents. The rate of DZ twinning is affected by nationality and maternal factors (Table 5). The highest rate of twins is in Nigeria (rate, 50 per 1,000 deliveries), and the lowest rate is in Japan (rate, four per 1,000) (69). Older women, those of higher parity (70), and taller women (71) have a higher incidence of multiple births. The use of ovulation-induction drugs for the treatment of infertility and a greater proportion of older pregnant women has increased the incidence of multiple births.

TABLE 5. *Twinning per 1,000 deliveries by zygosity in different countries*

	Monozygotic	Dizygotic	Total
Nigeria	5	49	54
United States			
Black	4.7	11.1	15.8
White	4.2	7.1	11.3
England and Wales	3.5	8.8	12.3
India (Calcutta)	3.3	8.1	11.4
Japan	3.0	1.3	4.3

From ref. 69, with permission.

Placentation

All DZ twins develop a dichorionic diamniotic placenta. The timing of cell division in MZ twins affects the subsequent placental-membrane relation (Fig. 4) and has a significant impact on morbidity and mortality (Table 6). Vascular anastomoses leading to twin-to-twin transfusions occurs in approximately 1% of monochorionic gestations. Twin-to-twin transfusion syndrome occurs when blood is shunted from one twin, the donor, who has anemia, growth retardation, and oligohydramnios, to the second twin, the recipient, who develops polyhydramnios and becomes plethoric, macrosomic, and hydropic. High perinatal mortality rates (60% to 85%) have been reported. Outcome of twin-to-twin transfusion syndrome is particularly poor when:

- It occurs in the second versus the third trimester,
- Hydrops is present in one or both of the twins, or
- The mother develops severe hydramnios.

Treatment modalities include elective termination, selective feticide, therapeutic amniocenteses, laser ablation of vascular anastomoses, and medical therapy. The most promising strategy appears to be aggressive therapeutic amniocenteses. Elliott et al. (72) reported 17 cases of twin-to-twin transfusion syndrome diagnosed at 16 to 28 weeks of gestation and managed with aggressive therapeutic amniocenteses. They prophylactically removed enough amniotic fluid to maintain "normal" volume in each sac. The procedure was repeated as often as needed. They had a 79% survival rate in contrast to the 100% mortality rate reported by Weir et al. (73) without this treatment.

Monoamniotic placentation occurs in fewer than 2% of all twin pregnancies but also carries a high perinatal mortality rate because of the potential for cord entanglement. Before sonography, the type of placentation was diagnosed only at delivery. High-resolution sonography now allows earlier diagnosis. This development has produced management dilemmas in the presence of monoamniotic placentation. To avoid fetal loss, some experts recommend intensive fetal surveillance after 25 weeks' gestation and early cesarean delivery after documentation of lung maturity (74,75). Early cesarean delivery was questioned by Tessen and Zlatnick (76), who found no fetal deaths beyond 32 weeks' gestation. More than half the patients in their series delivered vaginally without adverse sequelae. They hypothesized that the absence of cord-related deaths beyond 32 weeks was related to crowding that prevented further cord entanglement.

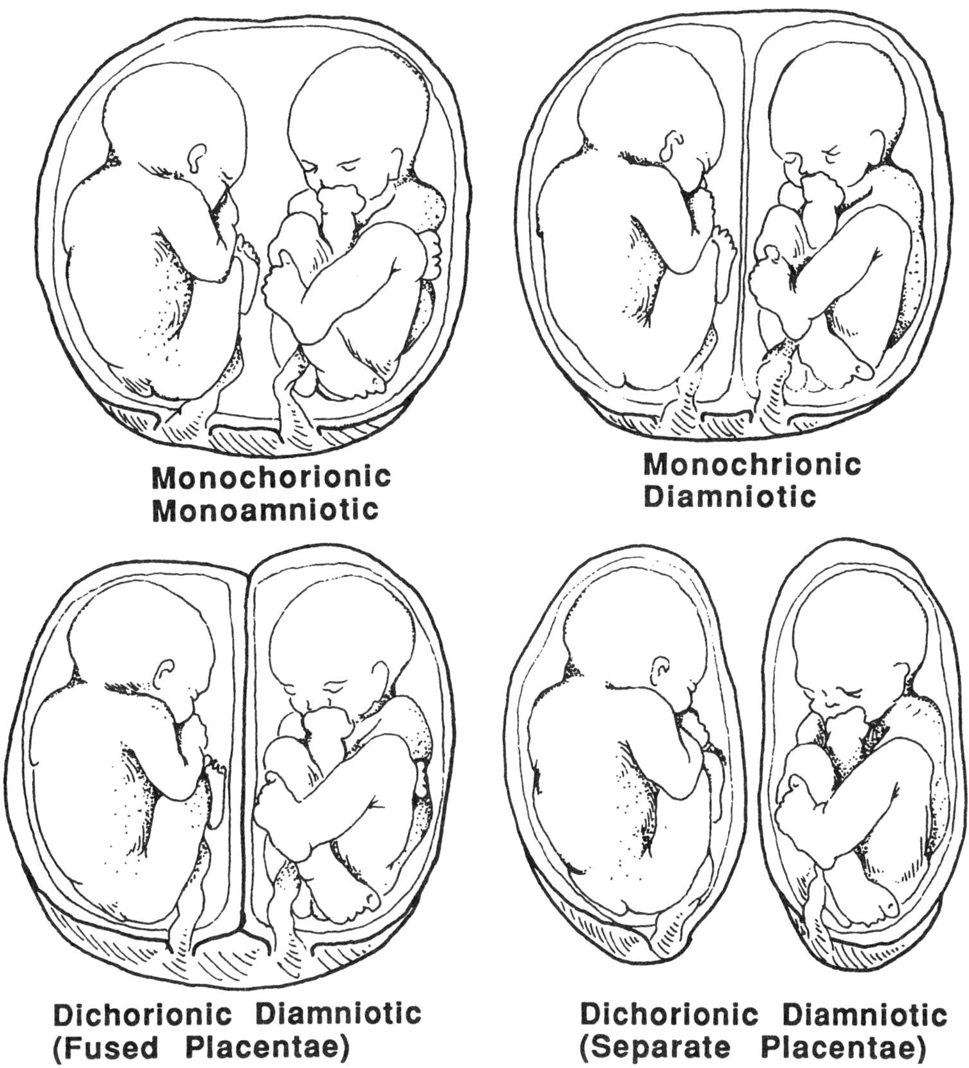

FIG. 4. Placentation in twin pregnancies. (Reprinted from Gabbe SG, Niebyl JR, Simpson JL, eds. *Obstetrics: normal and problem pregnancies.* 2nd ed. New York: Churchill Livingstone, 1991, with permission.)

Fetal Risks

Twin delivery increases perinatal mortality 6 to 8 times above that with singleton deliveries (Table 7). The risk of morbidity and mortality in multifetal pregnancy is primarily related to prematurity. In one prospective study of twin pregnancies, 28 of 29 neonatal deaths were due to prematurity (77). Twins deliver prematurely because the uterus does not remain quiescent until term (78) or because of insufficient uterine blood flow (79). Even when a twin pregnancy reaches term, the infants are still at increased risk. One study examined 1,253 twin pregnancies and a randomly selected control group of 5,119 singleton pregnancies delivering between 1982 and 1987.

TABLE 6. *Monozygotic twins*

Chorion	Amnion	Time to division (days)	Rate (%)	Perinatal mortality (%)	Comments
Dichorionic	Diamniotic	0–3	30	9	Two single placentas or one distinct placenta
Monochorionic	Diamniotic	4–8	68	25	Cord anomalies, placental vascular anomalies
Monochorionic	Monoamniotic	>8	5	>50	High mortality from cord intertwining

TABLE 7. *Fetal Risks*

Placental problems	Developmental problems	Obstetric problems
Cord entanglement	Prematurity	Interlocking twins
Cord prolapse	Intrauterine growth retardation	Malpresentation
Velamentous cord insertion	Perinatal asphyxia	Malposition
Vasa previa	Polyhydramnios	
	Acardia	
	Conjoined twins	
	Congenital abnormalities	
	Hypocalcemia	
	Hyperbilirubinemia	
	Decreased intelligence quotient	

The perinatal mortality rate for twin A was 48.8 per 1,000, and for twin B, 64.1 per 1,000. In contrast, the mortality rate of a single gestation was only 10.4 per 1,000 (80). When segregating mortality by birthweight, twins weighing more than 2,500 grams were at greater risk of death than the singleton controls. The twin mortality rate was lower than the singleton rate in babies weighing less than 2,500 grams. These data suggest that infants of multiple gestation are more mature at the same weight than are low-birth-weight singletons (76). Advances in both maternal–fetal medicine and neonatal care have decreased the perinatal mortality rate over the last 20 years. Between 1952 and 1962, at the University of North Carolina Hospital, the perinatal death rate for both twins was 16%. At these same hospitals, between 1983 and 1993, these rates had decreased to 10% for twin A and 11% for twin B (81). Triplet gestation also has a higher perinatal mortality rate than that for singletons but not greater than that of twins (82).

The second twin may be at greater risk of morbidity and mortality than the first. After delivery of the first twin, partial separation of the placenta, reduced uterine size, and clamping of the first umbilical cord can reduce intervillous blood flow and oxygenation to the second twin. Several groups reported an increased perinatal mortality rate in the second twin compared with the first (76,83,84). However, more recent studies (85,86) reported similar outcome for both twins, even if delivery of the second twin is delayed beyond 15 minutes. This improved outcome probably stems from the use of continuous fetal heart-rate monitoring and improved neonatal resuscitation. However, some studies still reported small differences in Apgar scores and umbilical acid–base values between the first and second twin. Young et al. (87) found statistically significant differences in 1-minute Apgar score, umbilical venous pH, pO_2, and pCO_2, and umbilical arterial pO_2, which favored twin A. In contrast, Antoine et al. (88) reported no statistically significant differences in biochemical tests or Apgar scores between the third baby in a triplet gestation and the first two.

Malpresentation is more likely to occur in multiple gestations because of growth retardation and polyhydramnios. The risk of umbilical cord prolapse also increases with the greater incidence of malpresentations, malpositions, and premature rupture of membranes. Interlocking of twins occurs when the vertex of a breech-presenting first twin interlocks with the chin of a vertex-presenting second twin. If not recognized before labor, the traction normally applied during delivery of the breech can result in fetal death. The incidence of interlocking twins is about one in 1,000 twin deliveries and carries a high mortality rate. Successful disimpaction of interlocked twins has been reported with the aid of epidural anesthesia (89).

Compared with singletons, the fetal growth of twins, triplets, or quadruplets is retarded beyond 32, 30, and 28 weeks' gestation, respectively. Intrauterine growth retardation is more common in MZ twins because they usually share the same placenta. The intrauterine death of one fetus is uncommon, occurring in about 4% of all twin gestations, but can lead to disseminated intravascular coagulation in the mother (90,91).

The incidence of conjoined twins is approximately one in 50,000 deliveries. Seventy percent of conjoined twins are thoracopagi, and up to 95% are female (92). The etiology of conjoined twins is unknown but probably occurs because of incomplete division of an MZ embryo at approximately 13 to 15 days after ovulation.

Maternal Risks

The mother carrying a multiple gestation faces both physiologic and obstetric risks (Table 8).

Physiologic Risks

The physiologic changes that occur during a singleton gestation are exaggerated in mothers with multiple gestations. In single gestation, cardiac output (as measured by echocardiography) increases to an average of 7.6 L/min by 20 weeks. It remains at this level for the remainder of the pregnancy (89). Twining is associated with an additional 15% increase in cardiac output (93,94). This difference may be related to a greater increment in heart rate

TABLE 8. *Maternal Risks*

Physiologic risks	Obstetric risks
Increased cardiac stress	Pregnancy-induced hypertension
Supine hypotensive syndrome	Preeclampsia
Anemia	Antepartum hemorrhage
Hypoxemia	Postpartum hemorrhage
Pulmonary edema	Placenta previa
	Abruptio placentae
Aspiration	Premature labor
Polyhydramnios	Increased use of tocolytic agents
	Premature rupture of membranes
	Cord prolapse
	Cesarean section
	Uterine atony
	Infection
	Increased hospitalization

but not stroke volume (89) or to increases in both heart rate and stroke volume (90).

The greatly enlarged uterus that occurs in a multiple gestation increases the incidence of supine hypotensive syndrome (95). A 32-week uterus of a twin gestation is as big as a term uterus containing a single fetus and gets progressively larger.

Anemia occurs 2.4 times more often in the woman with a twin gestation than in one with a singleton gestation. In twin gestation, intravascular volume increased by 59%, plasma volume by 67%, and red cell mass by 40% (96). In comparison, these values increase by 42%, 49%, and 31%, respectively, in single pregnancies. These changes are further exaggerated in the triplet gestation (92).

Hypoxemia, especially in the supine position, also is more likely to occur in the woman with a twin gestation. This risk is related to:

- A decrease in the functional residual capacity from displacement of the diaphragm by the enlarged uterus,
- An increase in the closing volume, and
- An increase in oxygen consumption (97).

The woman with a multiple gestation also is at greater risk for aspiration of stomach contents. The enlarged uterus displaces the pylorus more cephalad than during a singleton gestation. Displacement of the pylorus changes the angle between the stomach and the esophagus, making the lower esophageal sphincter incompetent. Furthermore, progesterone, which decreases gastric emptying, and gastrin, which increases the production of hydrogen ions, are produced in greater amounts than during a singleton gestation (98).

Obstetric Risks

The mother with a multiple gestation faces a higher risk of obstetric complications than one carrying a single fetus (Tables 8, 9, and 10). Pregnancy-induced hypertension and preeclampsia are 5 times more common during a twin gestation than a singleton pregnancy (99). Uterine atony, because of the overdistended uterus in multiple gestations, increases the risk of postpartum hemorrhage by two- to threefold (100). There also is an increased incidence of antepartum hemorrhage from abruptio placentae and placenta previa (80). Premature rupture of membranes occurs more frequently in multiple gestations, leading to preterm labor (101). Tocolytic agents, especially the β-adrenergic agonists and magnesium sulfate (102), are associated with maternal pulmonary edema. Premature rupture of membranes coupled with fetal malpresentation and malposition leads to an increased incidence of umbilical cord prolapse. Malpresentation also leads to a greater frequency of cesarean section and postoperative infection (103). Polyhydramnios occurs in approximately 12% of all multiple gestations and may herald congenital abnormalities (gastrointestinal and central nervous system) (104).

Obstetric Management

Antepartum management of multiple gestation is geared toward preventing complications, especially preterm delivery. Early diagnosis reduces perinatal morbidity and mortality (105). Diagnosis can be made on historical or clinical grounds but should be confirmed with ultrasound (106). The patient should be counseled as to the high-risk nature of the pregnancy and taught to recognize early signs of labor. Prophylactic bed rest, cervical cerclage, prophylactic tocolysis, and early elective hospitalization have been suggested to prevent premature labor and its sequelae. It is difficult, however, to

TABLE 9. *Maternal antepartum complications in twin versus singleton pregnancies*

Complications	Twins (n = 1,253)	Singletons (n = 5,119)	Odds ratio	95% CI
Hypertension	12.9%	5.6%	2:5	2.1–3.2
Abruptio placentae	2.2%	0.8%	3:0	1.9–4.7
Anemia	9.4%	4.1%	2:4	1.9–3.0
Urinary tract infection	8.7%	6.7%	1:4	1.1–1.7
Pyelonephritis	0.7%	0.3%	2:1	0.9–4.5
Postdates	1.2%	3.1%	2:6	1.6–4.4

CI, confidence interval.
From ref. 80, with permission.

TABLE 10. *Prenatal and neonatal complications of triplet versus twin pregnancies*

Complication	Triplet (n = 15)	Twin (n = 15)	*p* Value	Relative risk
Anemia	2 (13.3%)	1 (6.7%)	—	0.5
Preterm labor	12 (80.0%)	6 (40.0%)	0.03	2.0
PPROM	4 (26.7%)	1 (6.7%)	—	4.0
Pregnancy-induced hypertension	1 (6.7%)	2 (13.3%)	—	0.5
Gestational diabetes	0	1 (6.7%)	—	—
Intrauterine fetal death	1 (6.7%)	1 (6.7%)	—	1.0
Gestational age of infants (wk)	33 ± 5.1	36.6 ± 3.4	0.03	—
Mean average birth weight (g)	1,720 ± 700	2,475 ± 628	0.16	—
Mean lowest birth weight (g)	1,438 ± 599	2,285 ± 628	0.006	—
Mean average hospital (days)	29 ± 46.2	8.5 ± 11.5	0.05	5.0

PPROM, premature premature rupture of membranes.
From ref. 82, with permission.

document any benefit from these measures. A study of elective hospitalization could find no benefit in admitted women (n = 285) versus nonadmitted controls (n = 237) (107). Prophylactic cervical cerclage also does not prolong twin gestation and may be detrimental because it risks preterm labor, chorioamnionitis, bleeding, and premature rupture of membranes (108). Prophylactic cerclage does benefit triplet and quadruplet pregnancies (109). In randomized, blinded studies, prophylactic tocolysis failed to prolong twin gestation (110). A protocol of reduced physical activity, with 2 hours of rest during the day, and obstetric management by a specialized care team has been shown to prolong twin gestations (111,112).

Intrapartum Management

Obstetricians often elect to deliver twins by cesarean section. However, outside of a few widely accepted indications (Table 11), few data support this choice. Laros et al. (113) reviewed 206 twin deliveries over a 10-year period and found no difference in outcome between twins delivered by elective cesarean section and twins who had attempted vaginal deliveries. Women with a previous cesarean section also can have successful twin vaginal delivery (114).

The intrapartum management of a twin gestation is determined by the intrauterine position of the twins. The possibilities include:

- Twin A vertex, twin B vertex (42.5%);
- Twin A vertex, twin B nonvertex (38.4%); and
- Twin A nonvertex (19.1%; Fig. 5).

When twin A and twin B are in the vertex position, most experts agree that vaginal delivery should be attempted (85,115).

When twin A presents as a vertex and twin B is in a nonvertex position, management is controversial. Whereas some recommend cesarean delivery (110), others argue for a trial of labor (116–118). After delivery of the first baby, a decision must be made as how to deliver the second baby. Options include external cephalic version, internal podalic version and total breech extraction, or cesarean section. Chervenak et al. (119) documented the safety and successful outcome of external cephalic version in 25 women and also noted that epidural analgesia made the version easier. If version fails, the baby can either be delivered vaginally as a breech or by cesarean section. As is the case when a singleton fetus presents as a breech, vaginal delivery of the breech should be attempted only if the estimated fetal weight is greater than 1,500 grams (120). Internal podalic version and breech delivery yields the same neonatal outcome as vertex delivery (121). The time between delivery of the first and second twin is not critical as long as fetal heart-rate tracing of twin B remains reactive (85,86). Cesarean delivery is usually chosen when twin A is in a nonvertex presentation.

Although triplets can be safely delivered vaginally (122), most authorities recommend cesarean section for all women with three or more fetuses (123,124).

Anesthetic Management

Labor and Delivery

All women with multiple gestations should have a large-bore i.v. placed on admission to the labor floor and early consultation with an anesthesiologist. A delivery plan should be discussed early in labor with the obstet-

TABLE 11. *Factors favoring cesarean delivery with multiple gestation*

Malpresentation of twin A
Discordancy, with twin B larger than twin A
Intrauterine death of one fetus
Twin–twin transfusion
Congenital deformities
Decreased uteroplacental reserve (positive oxytocin challenge test or nonreactive nonstress test)
Fetal cardiac decelerations of either twin
Prematurity
Three or more fetuses

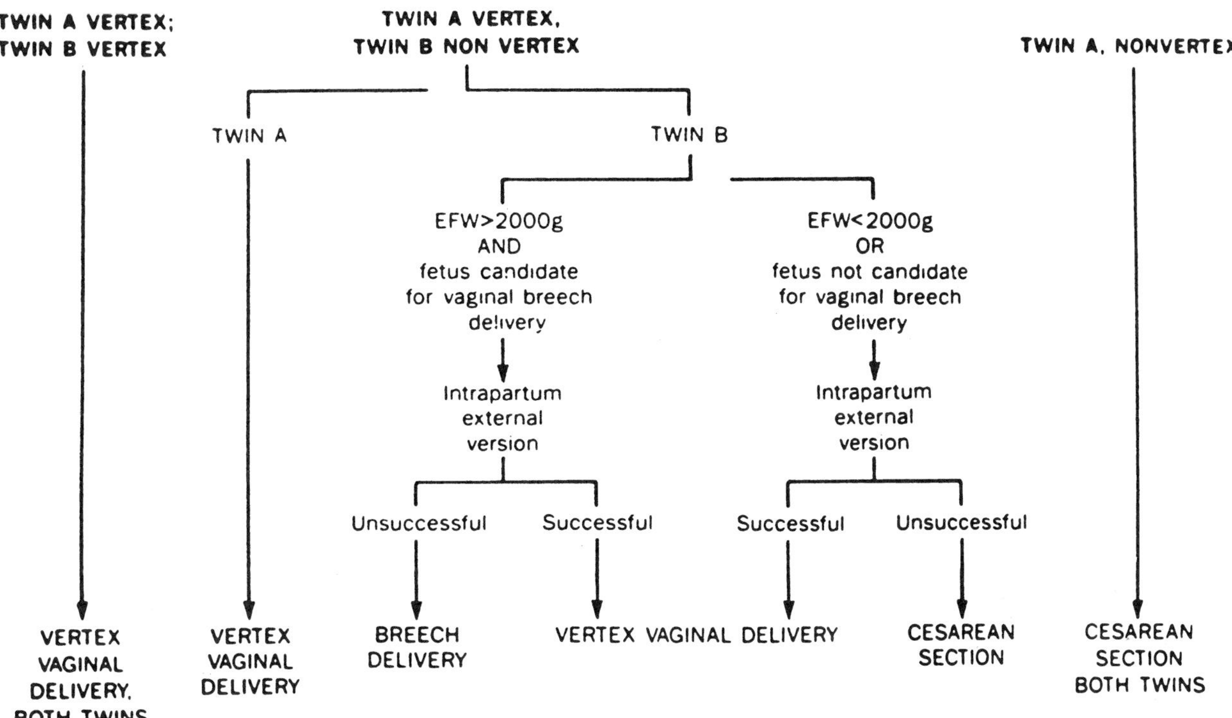

FIG. 5. Outline of proposed intrapartum management of twin gestation. (From ref. 85, with permission.)

ricians. Because of the increased risk of emergency cesarean section, we encourage the early placement of an epidural catheter. The advantages of an epidural anesthetic include:

- Elimination of the need for parenteral narcotics,
- Provision of good perineal analgesia, which prevents reflex bearing down by the mother and permits a more controlled delivery over a relaxed perineum,
- Provision of optimal conditions for instrumental delivery,
- Limitation of the need for general anesthesia for emergency cesarean section,
- Provision of maternal analgesia for external cephalic version or internal podalic version, and
- Decrease of maternal catecholamine levels through pain relief and possible improvement of uterine blood flow.

Until the mid 1970s, when a number of investigators documented the safety of regional anesthesia, the effects of epidural analgesia on the outcome of twin deliveries was controversial. In 1958, Little and Friedman (83) reported a higher mortality rate in twin B associated with maternal caudal anesthesia. In the same year, Guttmacher and Kohl (84) reported a higher perinatal death rate in either twin when caudal anesthesia was used. At the same time, however, Aaron and Halperin (125) reported a lower mortality rate in twins whose mothers had a caudal anesthetic (5.4% vs 14%). The higher mortality rate associated with the use of caudal anesthesia may have been related to a failure to provide left uterine displacement, the inability to monitor the fetal heart rate continuously, the large amounts of local anesthetic usually injected, or the preferential use of caudal anesthesia in complicated or high-risk cases.

In 1975, Crawford (126) retrospectively reviewed the outcome of 102 multiple pregnancies. He included women carrying twins (n = 99) or triplets (n = 3) who underwent a vaginal delivery with (n = 55) or without (n = 47) epidural anesthesia. Apgar scores for twin A did not differ between the epidural and nonepidural groups. Epidural anesthesia was associated with a longer time from full cervical dilation and delivery of the first twin and with lower 1-minute Apgar scores in twin B. However, the time between delivery of the first and second twin was shorter in the epidural group. Of the seven infant deaths, five were in the nonepidural group. He concluded that, overall, neonates of a twin gestation derived significant benefit from maternal epidural anesthesia.

In a follow-up study, James et al. (127) compared Apgar scores and maternal arterial and umbilical vessel blood gas values in twins deliveries (n = 14) with those of singleton deliveries (n = 10). All mothers had epidural anesthetics during labor. They found that all outcomes were similar in twin A and in infants born of single gestations. The second twins had lower 1-minute Apgar scores, umbilical artery pH, and venous pO_2 values than the single babies. These differences were exaggerated when twin B was nonvertex. Again, the authors concluded that epidural analgesia did not adversely alter the outcome of twin pregnancy.

Three other studies, published in 1977, reported no adverse effects of the use of epidural analgesia in twin gestations. Weekes et al. (128) examined labor course and outcome in twin gestations managed with epidural analgesia (n = 50) or parenteral narcotics (n = 92). They found no differences in morbidity (including the duration of the first and second stages of labor, Apgar scores, incidence of assisted deliveries with twins in vertex position or breech extractions) or mortality. Jaschevatzky et al. (129) reviewed their experience with epidural analgesia for twin delivery (n = 58) and compared their results with those of women who did not receive an epidural anesthetic for a twin delivery (n = 44). For term infants, they too found similar outcomes between the groups and noted that all obstetric maneuvers were easily accomplished with the use of epidural analgesia. They did, however, find a higher perinatal mortality rate in the premature infants of mothers who had an epidural anesthetic. Because of the small numbers involved and the potential for selection bias, no definitive conclusion about the effect of epidural analgesia on the premature infant can be drawn from this study. In the only prospective, randomized study of epidural analgesia (n = 28) versus no epidural analgesia (n = 24) for twin deliveries, Gullestad and Sagen (130) found no difference in the Apgar scores or neonatal course between the two groups. They did, however, find that 11 of the women who did not have an epidural anesthetic required general anesthesia for intrauterine manipulation of the second baby versus none in the epidural group.

In the most recent and largest study to date, Crawford (131) prospectively studied the neonatal outcome of 200 consecutive twin deliveries. He grouped patients by epidural anesthetic and mode of delivery. In babies delivered vaginally, twin A in the epidural group had slightly better Apgar scores and acid–base balance than did twin A in the nonepidural group. Although there were no differences in outcome between twin A and twin B in the epidural group, twin B did worse than twin A in the nonepidural group. Women who had an epidural had fewer cesarean sections for twin B than those who did not have an epidural. Within the epidural group, eliminating reflex maternal expulsive efforts also was associated with better condition of twin B. All of these advantages existed despite a longer second stage and greater incidence of instrumental deliveries in the epidural group. For infants of women who had an elective cesarean section under epidural versus general anesthesia, there were no differences in Apgar score or umbilical artery analyses of either twin A or twin B.

Suggested Technique

During the early stages of labor, use a local anesthetic that offers good analgesia while minimizing motor block. Bupivacaine, 0.25% boluses, followed by an infusion of 0.125% bupivacaine or 0.0625% bupivacaine with fentanyl, 2 μg/mL, have proven effective. Throughout labor, and especially after induction of epidural analgesia, the parturient should be positioned with adequate left uterine displacement. Twins should be delivered in an operating room prepared for a cesarean section. On transfer to the delivery room, the mother should receive a nonparticulate antacid. In the delivery room, place appropriate monitors and give supplemental oxygen. Two pediatric teams should be present for resuscitation of the neonates. Immediately before delivery of twin A, inject a more concentrated local anesthetic (i.e., lidocaine, 2%) to achieve a dermatomal level of about T_{10}. This step provides perineal anesthesia, analgesia for any intrauterine manipulations of twin B, and decreases the time necessary to extend the block should cesarean section be required. If uterine relaxation is needed for intrauterine manipulation of twin B, use either nitroglycerin, 50 to 100 μg i.v. (132), or general anesthesia with a high concentration of a volatile anesthetic agent. After delivery, be prepared for uterine atony and postpartum hemorrhage. Uterine atony may require the use of oxytocin, methylergonovine, or 15-methyl prostaglandin $F_{2\alpha}$.

Cesarean Section

There are no prospective randomized trials regarding epidural versus general anesthesia for cesarean section of twins or triplets. Crawford (131) reported no differences in outcome, as measured by umbilical artery blood gas values or Apgar scores, in twins delivered by epidural anesthesia (n = 9) versus those delivered by general anesthesia (n = 7) (131). Because regional anesthesia seems to decrease maternal morbidity and mortality (52), we prefer it for women with multiple gestations undergoing cesarean section. Monitoring is similar to that described for vaginal delivery, with careful attention to left uterine displacement to prevent aortocaval compression.

For elective cesarean section, we prefer spinal anesthesia with 12.5 mg of hyperbaric bupivacaine. Twin gestation does not appear to increase the risk of hypotension or the spread of sensory block associated with spinal anesthesia (133). If an epidural catheter was placed for labor and a cesarean section is necessary, we use it and extend the level of anesthesia with lidocaine, 2%, with epinephrine, 1:200,000. With either spinal or epidural anesthesia, we use preservative-free morphine sulfate for postoperative analgesia.

For urgent or emergency cesarean section, if the woman does not have an epidural catheter in place, we use either a spinal or a general anesthetic depending on the clinical situation. General anesthesia is preceded by preoxygenation, cricoid pressure, and rapid-sequence induction with thiopental, 4 to 5 mg/kg, and succinylcholine, 100 mg, to facilitate endotracheal intubation. Before delivery, give N_2O, 50% in oxygen, and isoflurane, 0.2% to 0.4%, for amnesia. After delivery of the babies, the volatile agent may need to be discontinued because of uterine atony.

The anesthetic management of triplet and higher-order pregnancies is similar to the previously described except that all the concerns are magnified. The woman is at greater risk for gastric acid aspiration, difficult endotracheal intubation, and aortocaval compression. Keeping these concerns in mind, we use spinal anesthesia for cesarean section. Yarnell et al. (134) compared the maternal and neonatal outcomes of triplets delivered under spinal, epidural, or general anesthesia. Although there was a greater initial decrease of blood pressure under spinal anesthesia, all mothers were easily resuscitated with fluid and ephedrine, and there were no differences noted in neonatal outcome.

REFERENCES

1. Scorza WE. Intrapartum management of breech presentation. *Clin Perinatol* 1996;23:31.
2. Oxorn H. *Oxorn-Foote: Human labor and birth.* 5th ed. Norwalk, CT: Appleton & Lange, 1986:221.
3. Rayl J, Gibson PJ, Hickok DE. A population-based case-control study of risk factors for breech presentation. *Am J Obstet Gynecol* 1996;174:28.
4. Brenner WE, Bruce RD, Hendricks CH. The characteristics and perils of breech presentation. *Am J Obstet Gynecol* 1974;118:700.
5. Piper EB, Bachman C. The prevention of fetal injuries in breech delivery. *JAMA* 1929;92:217.
6. Hall JE, Kohl S. Breech presentation: a study of 1,456 cases. *Am J Obstet Gynecol* 1956;72:977.
7. Morgan HS, Kane SH. An analysis of 16,327 breech births. *JAMA* 1964;187:262.
8. Morley GW. Breech presentation: a 15-year review. *Obstet Gynecol* 1967;30:745.
9. Collea JV, Chein C, Quilligan EJ. The randomized management of term frank breech presentation: a study of 208 cases. *Am J Obstet Gynecol* 1980;137:235.
10. Foote AJ. External cephalic version from 34 weeks under tocolysis: factors influencing success. *J Obstet Gynaecol* 1995;21:127.
11. Kornman MT, Kimball KT, Reeves KO. Preterm external cephalic version in an outpatient environment. *Am J Obstet Gynecol* 1995;172:1734.
12. Megory E, Ohel G, Fisher O, Ruach M. Mode of delivery following external cephalic version and induction of labor at term. *Am J Perinatol* 1995;12:404.
13. Marquette GP, Boucher M, Theriault D, Rinfkret D. Does the use of a tocolytic agent affect the success rate of external cephalic version? *Am J Obstet Gynecol* 1996;175:859.
14. Chung T, Neale E, Lau TK, Rogers M. A randomized, double blind, controlled trial of tocolysis to assist external cephalic version in late pregnancy. *Acta Obstet Gynecol Scand* 1996;75:720.
15. Cunningham FG, MacDonald PC, Grant NF, et al. *Williams Obstetrics.* 20th ed. Stamford, CT: Appleton & Lange, 1997:495.
16. Carlan SJ, Marshall JD, Huckaby T, Whittington EC, Shaefer D. The effect of epidural anesthesia on safety and success of external cephalic version at term. *Anesth Analg* 1994;79:525.
17. Schorr SJ, Speights SE, Ross EL, et al. A randomized trial of epidural anesthesia to improve external cephalic version success. *Am J Obstet Gynecol* 1997;177:1133.
18. Wright RC. Reduction of perinatal mortality and morbidity in breech delivery through use of cesarean section. *Obstet Gynecol* 1959;14:758.
19. Cheng M, Hannah M. Breech delivery at term: a critical review of the literature. *Obstet Gynecol* 1993;82:605.
20. Gifford DS, Morton SC, Fiske M, Kahn K. A meta-analysis of infant outcomes after breech delivery. *Obstet Gynecol* 1995;85:1047.
21. Eller DP, VanDorsten JP. Breech presentation. *Curr Opin Obstet Gynecol* 1993;5:664.
22. Petitti DB. Maternal mortality and morbidity in cesarean section. *Clin Obstet Gynecol* 1985;28:763.
23. Kunzel W. Recommendations of the FIGO committee on perinatal health on guidelines for the management of breech delivery. *Int J Gynecol Obstet* 1994;44:297.
24. Danielian PJ, Wang J, Hall MH. Long-term outcome by method of delivery of fetuses in breech presentation at term: population based follow up. *BMJ* 1996;312:1451.
25. Schiff E, Friedman SA, Mashiach S, et al. Maternal and neonatal outcome of 846 term singleton breech deliveries: seven-year experience at a single center. *Am J Obstet Gynecol* 1996;175:18.
26. Christian SS, Brady K, Read JA, Kopelman JN. Vaginal breech delivery: a five-year prospective evaluation of a protocol using computed tomographic pelvimetry. *Am J Obstet Gynecol* 1990;163:848.
27. Croughan-Minihane MS, Petitti DB, Gordis L, Golditch I. Morbidity among breech infants according to method of delivery. *Obstet Gynecol* 1990;75:821.
28. Roumen FJ, Luyben AG. Safety of term vaginal breech delivery. *Eur J Obstet Gynecol Reprod Biol* 1991;40:171.
29. Kaplan B, Rabinerson D, Hirsch M, et al. Intrapartum management of the low-birth-weight breech fetus. *Clin Exp Obstet Gynecol* 1995;22:307.
30. Cibils LA, Karrison T, Brown L. Factors influencing neonatal outcomes in the very-low-birth-weight fetus (<1500 grams) with a breech presentation. *Am J Obstet Gynecol* 1994;171:35.
31. Brown L, Karrison T, Cibils LA. Mode of delivery and perinatal results in breech presentation. *Am J Obstet Gynecol* 1994;171:28.
32. Gravenhorst JB, Schreuder AM, Veen S, et al. Breech delivery in very preterm and very low birthweight infants in the Netherlands. *Br J Obstet Gynaecol* 1993;100:411.
33. Weissman A, Blazer S, Zimmer EZ, Jakobi P, Paldi E. Low birthweight breech infant: short-term and long-term outcome by method of delivery. *Am J Perinatol* 1988;5:289.
34. Gilady Y, Battino S, Reich D, Gilad G, Shalev E. Delivery of the very low birthweight breech: what is the best way for the baby? *Isr J Med Sci* 1996;32:116.
35. Zlatnik FJ. The Iowa premature breech trial. *Am J Perinatol* 1993;10:60.
36. Penn ZJ, Steer PJ, Grand A. A multicentre randomised controlled trial comparing elective and selective caesarean section for the delivery of the preterm breech infant. *Br J Obstet Gynaecol* 1996;103:684.
37. Bonica JJ, McDonald JS. *Principles and practice of obstetric analgesia and anesthesia.* 2nd ed. Philadelphia: Williams & Wilkins, 1995:941.
38. Boyson WA, Simpson JW. Breech management with caudal anesthesia. *Am J Obstet Gynecol* 1960;79:1121.
39. Crawford JS. An appraisal of lumbar epidural blockade in patients with a singleton fetus presenting by the breech. *J Obstet Gynaecol Br Commonw* 1974;81:867.
40. Bowen-Simpkins P, Fergusson IL. Lumbar epidural block and the breech presentation. *Br J Anaesth* 1974;46:420.
41. Donnai P, Nicholas AD. Epidural analgesia, fetal monitoring and the condition of the baby at birth with breech presentation. *Br J Obstet Gynaecol* 1975;82:360.
42. Darby S, Hunter DJ. Extradural analgesia in labour when the breech presents. *Br J Obstet Gynaecol* 1976;83:35.
43. Breeson AJ, Kovacs GT, Pickles BG, Hill JG. Extradural analgesia: the preferred method of analgesia for vaginal breech delivery. *Br J Anaesth* 1978;50:1227.
44. Confino E, Ismajovich B, Rudick V, David MP. Extradural analgesia in the management of singleton breech delivery. *Br J Anaesth* 1985;57:892.
45. Perl FM, Friederichs Vieten W, Klock FK. Progress of labor and neonatal morbidity in primiparity with breech presentation. *Z Geburtshilfe Neonatol* 1996;200:56.
46. Van Zundert A, Vaes L, Soetens M, et al. Are breech deliveries an indication for lumbar epidural analgesia? *Anesth Analg* 1991;72:399.
47. Chadha YC, Mahmood TA, Dick MJ, et al. Breech delivery and epidural analgesia. *Br J Obstet Gynaecol* 1992;99:96.
48. Campbell DC, Camann W, Datta S. The addition of bupivacaine to intrathecal sufentanil for labor analgesia. *Anesth Analg* 1995;81:305.
49. Munson ES, Embro WJ. Enflurane, isoflurane and halothane and isolated human uterine muscle. *Anesthesiology* 1977;46:11.

50. Effer SB, McMorland GH. Breech presentation, malpresentation, multiple gestation. In: Datta S, ed. *Anesthetic and obstetric management for high-risk pregnancy.* 1st ed. Chicago: Mosby-Year Book, 1991:74.
51. Redick LF, Livingston E. A new preparation of nitroglycerin for uterine relaxation. *Int J Obstet Anesth* 1995;4:14.
52. Hawkins JL, Koonin LM, Palmer SK, Gibbs CP. Anesthesia-related deaths during obstetric delivery in the United States, 1979-1990. *Anesthesiology* 1997;86:277.
53. James FM III, Crawford JS, Hopkinson R, Davies P, Naiem H. A comparison of general anesthesia and lumbar epidural analgesia for elective cesarean section. *Anesth Analg* 1977;56:228.
54. Crawford JS, Davies P. Status of neonates delivered by elective caesarean section. *Br J Anaesth* 1982;54:1015.
55. Darby S, Hunter DJ. Extradural analgesia in labour when the breech presents. *Br J Obstet Gynaecol* 1996;83:35.
56. Mayer DC, Weeks SK. Antepartum uterine relaxation with nitroglycerin at caesarean delivery. *Can J Anaesth* 1992;39:166.
57. Gardberg M, Tuppurainen M. Anterior placental location predisposes for occiput posterior presentation near term. *Acta Obstet Gynecol Scand* 1994;73:151.
58. Cruikshank DP, White CA. Obstetric malpresentations: twenty years' experience. *Am J Obstet Gynecol* 1973;116:1097.
59. Duff P. Diagnosis and management of face presentation. *Obstet Gynecol* 1981;57:105.
60. Cruikshank DP, White CA. Obstetric malpresentations: twenty years' experience. *Am J Obstet Gynecol* 1973;116:1097.
61. Gardberg M, Tuppurainen M. Persistent occiput posterior presentation: a clinical problem. *Acta Obstet Gynecol Scand* 1994;73:45.
62. Macara LM, Murphy KW. The contribution of dystocia to the cesarean section rate. *Am J Obstet Gynecol* 1994;171:71.
63. Pearl ML, Roberts JM, Laros RK, Hurd WW. Vaginal delivery from the persistent occiput posterior position: influence on maternal and neonatal morbidity. *J Reprod Med* 1993;38:955.
64. Ingemarsson E, Ingemarsson I, Solum T, Westgren M. Influence of occiput posterior position on the fetal heart rate pattern. *Obstet Gynecol* 1980;55:301.
65. Robinson CA, Macones GA, Roth NW, Morgan MA. Does station of the fetal head at epidural placement affect the position of the fetal vertex at delivery? *Am J Obstet Gynecol* 1996;175:991.
66. Floberg J, Belfrage P, Ohlsen H. Influence of the pelvic outlet capacity on fetal head presentation at delivery. *Acta Obstet Gynecol Scand* 1987;66:127.
67. Cunningham FG, MacDonald PC, Gant NF. *Williams' obstetrics.* 20th ed. Norwalk, CT: Appleton & Lange, 1997:448.
68. Goplerus J, Eastman NJ. Compound presentation: a survey of 65 cases. *Obstet Gynecol* 1953;1:59.
69. MacGillivray I. Epidemiology of twin pregnancy. *Semin Perinatol* 1986;10:4.
70. Bulmer MG. The effect of parental age, parity and duration of marriage on the twinning rate. *Ann Hum Genet* 1959;23:454.
71. Anderson WRJ. Stillbirth and neonatal mortality in twin pregnancy. *J Obstet Gynaecol Br Emp* 1956;63:205.
72. Elliott JP, Urig MA, Clewell WH. Aggressive therapeutic amniocentesis for treatment of twin-twin transfusion syndrome. *Obstet Gynecol* 1991;77:537.
73. Weir PE, Ratten GJ, Beischer NA. Acute polyhydramnios: a complication of monozygous twin pregnancy. *Br J Obstet Gynaecol* 1979;86: 849.
74. Rodis JF, Vintzileos AM, Campbell WA, et al. Antenatal diagnosis and management of monoamniotic twins. *Am J Obstet Gynecol* 1987;157: 1255.
75. Aisenbrey GA, Catanzarite VA, Hurley TJ, et al. Monoamniotic and pseudoamniotic twins: sonographic diagnosis, detection of cord entanglement, and obstetric management. *Obstet Gynecol* 1995;86: 218.
76. Tessen JA, Zlatnik FJ. Monoamniotic twins: a retrospective controlled study. *Obstet Gynecol* 1991;77:832.
77. Sehgal NN. Perinatal mortality in twin pregnancies: implication for clinical management. *Postgrad Med* 1980;68:231.
78. McKeown T, Record RG. Observations on foetal growth in multiple pregnancy in man. *J Endocrinol* 1952;8:386.
79. Morris N, Osborn SB, Wright HP. Effective circulation of the uterine wall in late pregnancy measured with ^{24}NaCl. *Lancet* 1955;1:323.
80. Spellacy WN, Handler A, Ferre CD. A case-control study of 1253 twin pregnancies from a 1982-1987 perinatal data base. *Obstet Gynecol* 1990;75:168.
81. Saacks CB, Thorp JM, Hendricks CH. Cohort study of twinning in an academic health center: changes in management and outcome over 40 years. *Am J Obstet Gynecol* 1995;173:432.
82. Sassoon DA, Castro LC, Davis JL, Hobel CJ. Perinatal outcome in triplet versus twin gestations. *Obstet Gynecol* 1990;75:817.
83. Little WA, Friedman EA. Anesthesia for the twin delivery. *Anesthesiology* 1958;19:515.
84. Guttmacher AF, Kohl SG. The fetus of multiple gestations. *Obstet Gynecol* 1958;12:528.
85. Chervenak FA, Johnson RE, Youcha S, Hobbins JC, Berkowitz RL. Intrapartum management of twin gestation. *Obstet Gynecol* 1985;65: 119.
86. Rayburn WF, Lavin JP, Miodovnik M, Varner MW. Multiple gestation: time interval between delivery of the first and second twins. *Obstet Gynecol* 1984;63:502.
87. Young BK, Suidan J, Antoine C, et al. Differences in twins: the importance of birth order. *Am J Obstet Gynecol* 1985;151:915.
88. Antoine C, Kirshenbaum NW, Young BK. Biochemical differences related to birth order in triplets. *J Reprod Med* 1986;31:330.
89. Kenney A, Koh LS, Pole YL. A case of locked twins managed under lumbar epidural analgesia. *Anaesthesia* 1978;33:32.
90. Gaucherand P, Rudigoz RC, Piacenza JM. Monofetal death in multiple pregnancies: risks for the co-twin, risk factors and obstetrical management. *Eur J Obstet Gynecol Reprod Biol* 1994;55:111.
91. Landy HJ, Weingold AB. Management of multiple gestation complicated by an antepartum fetal demise. *Obstet Gynecol Surv* 1989;44:171.
92. Harper RG, Kenigsberg K, Sia CG, et al. Xiphopagus conjoined twins: a 300-year review of the obstetric, morphopathologic, neonatal and surgical parameters. *Am J Obstet Gynecol* 1980;137:617.
93. Robson SC, Hunter S, Boys RJ, Dunlop W. Hemodynamic changes during twin pregnancy. A Doppler and M-mode echocardiographic study. *Am J Obstet Gynecol* 1989;161:1273.
94. Veille JC, Morton MJ, Burry KJ. Maternal cardiovascular adaptations to twin pregnancy. *Am J Obstet Gynecol* 1985;153:261.
95. Kim Y, Chandra P, Marx GF. Successful management of severe aortocaval compression in twin pregnancy. *Obstet Gynecol* 1975;46:362.
96. Rovinsky JJ, Jaffin H. Cardiovascular hemodynamics in pregnancy. I. Blood and plasma volume in multiple pregnancy. *Am J Obstet Gynecol* 1965;93:1.
97. Redick LF. Anesthesia for twin delivery. *Clin Perinatol* 1988;15:107.
98. Craft JB, Levinson G, Shnider SM. Anaesthetic considerations in caesarean section for quadruplets. *Can Anaesth Soc J* 1978;25:236.
99. Kauppila A, Jouppila P, Koivisto M, Moilanen I, Ylikorkala O. Twin pregnancy. A clinical study of 335 cases. *Acta Obstet Gynecol Scand* 1975;44:5.
100. Little WA, Friedman EA. The twin delivery factors influencing second twin mortality. *Obstet Gynecol Surv* 1958;13:611.
101. Rayburn W, Piehl E, Schork MA. Intravenous ritodrine therapy: a comparison between twin and singleton gestations. *Obstet Gynecol* 1986;67:243.
102. Elliott JP. Magnesium sulfate as a tocolytic agent. *Am J Obstet Gynecol* 1983;147:277.
103. Thompson SA, Lyons TL, Makowski EL. Outcome of twin gestations at the University of Colorado Health Sciences Center. *J Reprod Med* 1987;32:328.
104. Cetrulo CL, Ingardia CJ, Sbarra AJ. Management of multiple gestation. *Clin Obstet Gynecol* 1980;23:533.
105. Persson PH, Grennert L, Gennser G, Kullandor S. On improved outcome of twin pregnancies. *Acta Obstet Gynaecol Scand* 1979;58:3.
106. Hays PM, Smeltzer JS. Multiple gestation. *Clin Obstet Gynecol* 1986; 29:264.
107. Andrews WW, Leveno KJ, Sherman ML, et al. Elective hospitalization in the management of twin pregnancies. *Obstet Gynecol* 1991;77:826.
108. Weekes AR, Menzies DN, De Boer CH. The relative efficacy of bed rest, cervical suture, and no treatment in the management of twin pregnancy. *Br J Obstet Gynaecol* 1977;84:161.
109. Goldman GA, Dicker D, Peleg D, Goldman JA. Is elective cerclage justified in the management of triplet and quadruplet pregnancy? *Aust NZ J Obstet Gynaecol* 1989;29:9.
110. O'Connor MC, Murphy H, Dalrymple IJ. Double blind trial of ritodrine and placebo in twin pregnancy. *Br J Obstet Gynaecol* 1979;86:706.

111. Newman RB, Ellings JM. Antepartum management of the multiple gestation: the case for specialized care. *Semin Perinatol* 1995;19: 387.
112. Vergani P, Ghidini A, Bozzo G, Sirtori M. Prenatal management of twin gestation: experience with a new protocol. *J Reprod Med* 1991;36:667.
113. Laros RK Jr, Dattel BJ. Management of twin pregnancy: the vaginal route is still safe. *Am J Obstet Gynecol* 1988;158:1330.
114. Gilbert L, Saunders N, Sharp F. The management of multiple pregnancy in women with a lower-segment caesarean scar: is a repeat caesarean section really the "safe" option? *Br J Obstet Gynaecol* 1988;95:1312.
115. Cetrulo CL. The controversy of mode of delivery in twins: the intrapartum management of twin gestation (Part 1). *Semin Perinatol* 1986; 10:39.
116. Gocke SE, Nageotte MP, Garite T, Towers CV, Dorcester W. Management of the nonvertex twin: primary cesarean section, external version, or primary breech extraction. *Am J Obstet Gynecol* 1989;161:111.
117. Rabinovici J, Barkai G, Reichman B, Serr DM, Mashiach S. Randomized management of the second nonvertex twin: vaginal delivery or cesarean section. *Am J Obstet Gynecol* 1987;156:52.
118. Mazor M, Leiberman JR, Dreval D, et al. Management and outcome of vertex-breech and vertex-vertex presentation in twin gestation: a comparative study. *Eur J Obstet Gynecol Reprod Biol* 1986;22:69.
119. Chervenak FA, Johnson RE, Berkowitz RL, Hobbins JC. Intrapartum external version of the second twin. *Obstet Gynecol* 1983;62:160.
120. Goldenberg RL, Nelson KG. The premature breech. *Am J Obstet Gynecol* 1977;127:240.
121. Blickstein I, Schwartz-Shoham Z, Lancet M, Borenstein R. Vaginal delivery of the second twin in breech presentation. *Obstet Gynecol* 1987;69:774.
122. Dommergues M, Mahieu-Caputo D, Mandelbrot L, et al. Delivery of uncomplicated triplet pregnancies: is the vaginal route safer? *Am J Obstet Gynecol* 1995;172:513.
123. Udom-Rice I, Skupski DW, Chervenak FA. Intrapartum management of multiple gestation. *Semin Perinatol* 1995;19:424.
124. Cunningham FG, MacDonald PC, Grant NF, et al. *Williams obstetrics.* 20th ed. Stamford, CT: Appleton & Lange, 1997:889.
125. Aaron JB, Halperin J. Fetal survival in 376 twin deliveries. *Am J Obstet Gynecol* 1955;69:794.
126. Crawford JS. An appraisal of lumbar epidural blockade in labour in patients with multiple pregnancy. *Br J Obstet Gynaecol* 1975;82:929.
127. James FM III, Crawford JS, Davies P, Naiem H. Lumbar epidural analgesia for labor and delivery of twins. *Am J Obstet Gynecol* 1977; 127:176.
128. Weekes AR, Cheridjian VE, Mwanje DK. Lumbar epidural analgesia in labour in twin pregnancy. *Br Med J* 1977;2:730.
129. Jaschevatzky OE, Shalit A, Levy Y, Grunstein S. Epidural analgesia during labour in twin pregnancy. *Br J Obstet Gynaecol* 1977;84:327.
130. Gullestad S, Sagen N. Epidural block in twin labour and delivery. *Acta Anaesth Scand* 1977;21:504.
131. Crawford JS. A prospective study of 200 consecutive twin deliveries. *Anaesthesia* 1987;42:33.
132. Abouleish AE, Corn SB. Intravenous nitroglycerin for intrapartum external version of the second twin. *Anesth Analg* 1994;78:808.
133. Jawan B, Lee JH, Chong ZK, Chang CS. Spread of spinal anaesthesia for caesarean section in singleton and twin pregnancies. *Br J Anaesth* 1993;70:639.
134. Yarnell RW, Steinbok VS, Goudas LC, et al. Maternal and fetal outcomes following anesthesia for triplet birth: a review of 55 consecutive cases [Abstract]. *Society for Obstetric Anesthesia and Perinatology* 1997:113.

Obstetric Anesthesia, second edition,
edited by Mark C. Norris.
Lippincott Williams & Wilkins, Philadelphia © 1999.

CHAPTER 36

Neonatal Resuscitation

Valerie A. Arkoosh

At birth, numerous physiological changes must occur as a fetus makes the transition to a neonate. Despite the complexity of this process, only 6% of newborns require life support in the delivery room (1). This percentage increases quickly among newborns who weigh less than 1,500 grams. Delivery room personnel must understand the neonatal adaptations to extrauterine life, make provision for resuscitation, understand the predictors of need for resuscitation, and respond appropriately. Additionally, hospital policies designating who answers calls for neonatal resuscitation may have important medicolegal consequences for the anesthesiologist.

NEONATAL ADAPTATIONS TO EXTRAUTERINE LIFE

The fetus depends on placental blood flow for gas exchange. Pulmonary vascular resistance (PVR) is high, with 90% of right ventricular output shunting across the ductus arteriosus. Systemic vascular resistance (SVR) is low: 40% of cardiac output flows to the low-resistance placenta. During vaginal delivery, compression of the infant thorax expels fluid from the mouth and upper airways. With crying, the lungs fill with air, surfactant is released, and oxygenation increased. These changes greatly decrease PVR. Simultaneously, clamping of the umbilical cord removes the low-resistance placental bed from the circulation, increasing SVR. Within minutes, the right-to-left shunt across the foramen ovale and ductus arteriosus is substantially reduced (2,3).

Transient hypoxemia or acidosis is well tolerated by a normal newborn, and prompt intervention usually prevents any permanent sequelae. Prolonged hypoxemia or acidosis impedes the transition from fetal to neonatal physiology. The fetus/neonate initially responds to hypoxemia by redistributing blood flow to the heart, brain, and adrenal glands. Tissue oxygen extraction increases. Eventually, myocardial contractility and cardiac output decrease. Hypoxemia and acidosis promote patency of the ductus arteriosus, counteracting the normal neonatal increase in pulmonary artery blood flow. Ventilatory drive is reduced by both indirect central nervous system and direct diaphragmatic depression. The net result of these physiological responses is a neonate with persistent pulmonary hypertension and little or no ventilatory drive. These babies require prompt intervention.

V.A. Arkoosh: Department of of Anesthesiology, Allegheny University of the Health Sciences, Allegheny University Hospital for Women, Philadelphia, Pennsylvania 19131.

PREPARATION

Preparation for neonatal resuscitation encompasses a number of activities including acquisition and maintenance of the proper equipment, identification, education and training of responding personnel, and development of contingency plans for additional personnel, if needed. Equipment and medications should be conveniently located, checked frequently for proper functioning and expiration date, and replenished immediately after use (Table 1) (1).

At least one person skilled in newborn resuscitation should attend every delivery (i.e., certified to provide neonatal advanced life support; NALS). Additional personnel should be available if a high-risk delivery is anticipated. An obstetric anesthesia work-force survey, conducted in 1992, found that anesthesiologists performed neonatal resuscitation in fewer than 10% of cesarean deliveries (4). This percentage has decreased from 23% in 1981. The remainder of resuscitations were performed by either pediatricians, obstetricians, nurse specialists, family practitioners, respiratory therapists, or CRNAs not medically directed by an anesthesiologist. In a 1991 survey of midwestern community hospitals, routine involvement of anesthesia personnel in neonatal resuscitation was noted by 31% of respondents (5). Looking forward,

TABLE 1. *Equipment and medications for neonatal resuscitation*

Suction equipment	Bag and mask equipment
Bulb syringe	Neonatal resuscitation bag with pressure-relief valve
Mechanical suction	
Suction catheters, 5F–10F	Face masks: newborn and premature sizes
Meconium aspirator	Oral airways
	Oxygen with flowmeter and tubing
Intubation equipment	**Medications**
Laryngoscope	Epinephrine, 1:10,000
Straight blades, 0 and 1	Naloxone hydrochloride, 0.4 mg/mL or 1.0 mg/mL
Extra bulbs and batteries	Volume expander
Endotracheal tubes, 2.5–4.0 mm	Sodium bicarbonate, 4.2% (5 mEq/10 mL)
Stylet	Dextrose, 10%
Scissors and gloves	Sterile water and normal saline
Miscellaneous	
Radiant warmer	Umbilical artery catheterization tray
Stethoscope	Umbilical tape
ECG	Umbilical catheters, 3.5F, 5F
Adhesive tape	Three-way stopcocks
Syringes and needles	Feeding tube, 5F
Alcohol sponges	

the need for anesthesia personal to participate in neonatal resuscitation may increase as pediatric residents spend more time in primary-care training and less in neonatology.

In determining need for personnel trained in neonatal resuscitation, remember Guideline VII of the American Society of Anesthesiology, *Guidelines for Regional Anesthesia in Obstetrics,* which states:

> Qualified personnel, other than the anesthesiologist attending the mother, should be immediately available to assume responsibility for resuscitation of the newborn. The primary responsibility of the anesthesiologist is to provide care to the mother. If the anesthesiologist is also requested to provide brief assistance in the care of the newborn, the benefit to the child must be compared to the risk to the mother.

ASSESSMENT OF RISK

With careful ante- and intrapartum fetal assessment, the need for neonatal resuscitation can be predicted in about 80% of cases. Antepartum assessment includes evaluation for major fetal anomalies and identification of maternal factors that may influence fetal well-being (Table 2) (1,2). Intrapartum events often predict the need for neonatal resuscitation (Table 3) (1,2). Assessment must continue throughout labor, as the clinical situation can change rapidly. Intrapartum evaluation includes fetal heart-rate monitoring with, when indicated, fetal scalp or vibroacoustic stimulation, or fetal scalp-blood sampling for pH determination.

TABLE 2. *Maternal and fetal factors associated with need for resuscitation*

Maternal diabetes	Postterm gestation
Pregnancy-induced hypertension	Preterm gestation
Chronic hypertension	Multiple gestation
Previous Rh sensitization	Size–dates discrepancy
Previous stillbirth	Polyhydramnios
Bleeding in the second or third trimester	Oligohydramnios
Maternal infection	Maternal drug therapy
Lack of prenatal care	Reserpine, lithium carbonate
Maternal substance abuse	Magnesium, adrenergic-blocking drugs
Known fetal anomalies	

Intrapartum fetal heart rate (FHR) monitoring is the first line of fetal assessment (6). FHR monitoring is most reliable in confirming fetal well-being. A reassuring tracing is more than 90% accurate in predicting a 5-minute Apgar score greater than 7 (7,8). In predicting fetal compromise, however, FHR monitoring has a false-positive rate of 35% to 50% (8,9). A recent study compared FHR tracings of singleton infants with birth weights at least 2,500 grams and moderate to severe cerebral palsy with FHR strips from control children (10). The 21 children with cerebral palsy who had multiple late decelerations or decreased HR variability represented 0.19% of the infants who had these FHR findings. Thus the false-positive rate in this patient population was 99.8%. Nonetheless, practitioners have little else with which to judge fetal well-being, and clinical decisions regarding delivery are often based on a careful evaluation of the FHR tracing.

Evaluation of the FHR tracing includes evaluation of the baseline HR, baseline HR variability, and identification of HR decelerations. The normal FHR ranges between 120 and 160 beats/min. Parasympathetic nervous activity increases near term, resulting in a lower

TABLE 3. *Intrapartum events associated with need for resuscitation*

Cesarean delivery	General anesthesia
Abnormal fetal presentation	Uterine tetany
Premature labor	Meconium-stained amniotic fluid
Rupture of membranes >24 h	Prolapsed cord
Chorioamnionitis	Abruptio placentae
Precipitate labor	Uterine rupture
Prolonged labor >24 h	Difficult instrumental delivery
Prolonged second state >3–4 h	Maternal systemic narcotics within 4 h of delivery
Nonreassuring fetal heart-rate patterns	

baseline HR in a term fetus compared with a preterm fetus. Bradycardia, mediated by increased vagal activity, is the first response to acute hypoxemia. If hypoxemia is prolonged, catecholamine release may produce fetal tachycardia. Maternal fever, intrauterine infection, or exogenous drugs also can cause fetal tachycardia. Finally, the fetus may have a tachy- or bradyarrhythmia from an intrinsic anatomic or functional aberration.

FHR variability includes both short-term and long-term variability. Fetal scalp-electrode monitoring provides the most reliable means of evaluation, as external monitors may overestimate variability. Normal short-term (beat-to-beat) variability is a two-to-three beat/min difference between adjacent heart beats. Normal long-term variability consists of a sine wave–like pattern that occurs 3 to 6 times per minute and varies by at least 6 beats/min. The presence of normal FHR variability predicts early neonatal health (8).

FHR decelerations are classified by their temporal relation to the uterine contraction. Early decelerations mirror the uterine contraction and have an amplitude of ten to 20 beats/min. Reflex vagal activity resulting from mild hypoxemia or fetal head compression is the likely cause of early decelerations. If good variability is present, this FHR change is not ominous. Late decelerations begin after the contraction has begun and end after the contraction has ended. They are often smooth and repetitive and may signal fetal hypoxemia. Combined with decreased or absent FHR variability, repetitive late decelerations are a sign of fetal stress. Variable decelerations have an abrupt start and finish and an amplitude of more than 30 beats/min. They may vary in shape and duration. Umbilical cord compression produces this type of pattern. Unless severe (FHR below 60 to 80 beats/min), the healthy fetus can usually tolerate these HR changes.

In the presence of a nonreassuring FHR trace, the practitioner may wish confirmatory studies of fetal well-being or lack thereof. Digital stimulation of the fetal scalp or vibroacoustic stimulation through the maternal abdomen will result in FHR accelerations in a healthy, nonacidotic fetus. Fetal scalp pH determination can confirm or exclude fetal acidosis. A pH of less than 7.2 is considered abnormal and, if confirmed by a second measurement, may indicate the need for delivery.

RESPONSE

Intrapartum

Intrapartum resuscitation is attempted once fetal compromise is identified. Identify and correct maternal factors that may impair oxygen delivery to the fetus. These problems may include maternal hypotension or decreased cardiac output resulting from aortocaval compression, sympathectomy, hemorrhage, or cardiac disease. Consider and, if appropriate, treat disease states that may interfere with maternal oxygenation, such as asthma, pneumonia, or pulmonary edema.

Remember, uterine hyperstimulation, tetany, abruption, or rupture may interfere with blood flow to the fetus. If needed, stop oxytocin infusion or give a tocolytic agent to reduce uterine tone. Emergency delivery will be required if abruption or rupture is severe.

Consider umbilical cord prolapse if FHR changes are sudden, severe, and prolonged. Oligohydramnios is a risk factor for umbilical cord compression and variable decelerations. Saline amnioinfusion may help alleviate cord compression (11). Amnioinfusion also is being tried in cases of thick meconium in an attempt to dilute the meconium and (we hope) to decrease the severity of meconium aspiration syndrome (12).

At Birth

The first step in neonatal resuscitation is to minimize heat loss (Fig. 1) (13,14). Depressed, asphyxiated infants often have an unstable thermal regulatory system. In addition, cold stress leads to hypoxemia, hypercarbia, and metabolic acidosis, which will promote persistence of the fetal circulation and hinder resuscitation. Within the first 20 seconds of life, the newborn should be dried, placed under a radiant warmer, and undergo suctioning of mouth and nose (tracheal suctioning if meconium is present).

The second step (within 30 seconds of birth) is assessment of neonatal respiration. If the infant is gasping or apneic, begin positive-pressure ventilation (PPV) at a rate of 40 to 60 breaths per minute with 100% oxygen (14). Peak inspiratory pressures of 30 to 40 cm H_2O or higher are necessary for initial lung expansion (13). The majority of infants requiring any resuscitation will respond to these first two steps. Indications for endotracheal intubation include ineffective bag-and-mask ventilation, anticipated need for prolonged mechanical ventilation, or as a route for administration of medicine. With prolonged bag-and-mask ventilation, a nasal or orogastric tube should be inserted to decompress the stomach.

The third step is assessment of neonatal heart rate. Chest compressions are required in only 0.03% of deliveries (13). Neonatal cardiac arrest is generally the result of respiratory failure, producing hypoxemia and tissue acidosis. The result of these metabolic changes is bradycardia, decreased cardiac contractility, and eventually cardiac arrest. Chest compressions should be instituted at a rate of 120 per minute when, after 15 to 30 seconds of PPV, the heart rate is below 60 or between 60 and 80 and not increasing (14). Chest compressions should be stopped when heart rate is greater than 80. Chest compressions can be performed by using either the thumb method or the two-finger method (Fig. 2). In most neonates with adequate ventilation, cardiac function normalizes quickly.

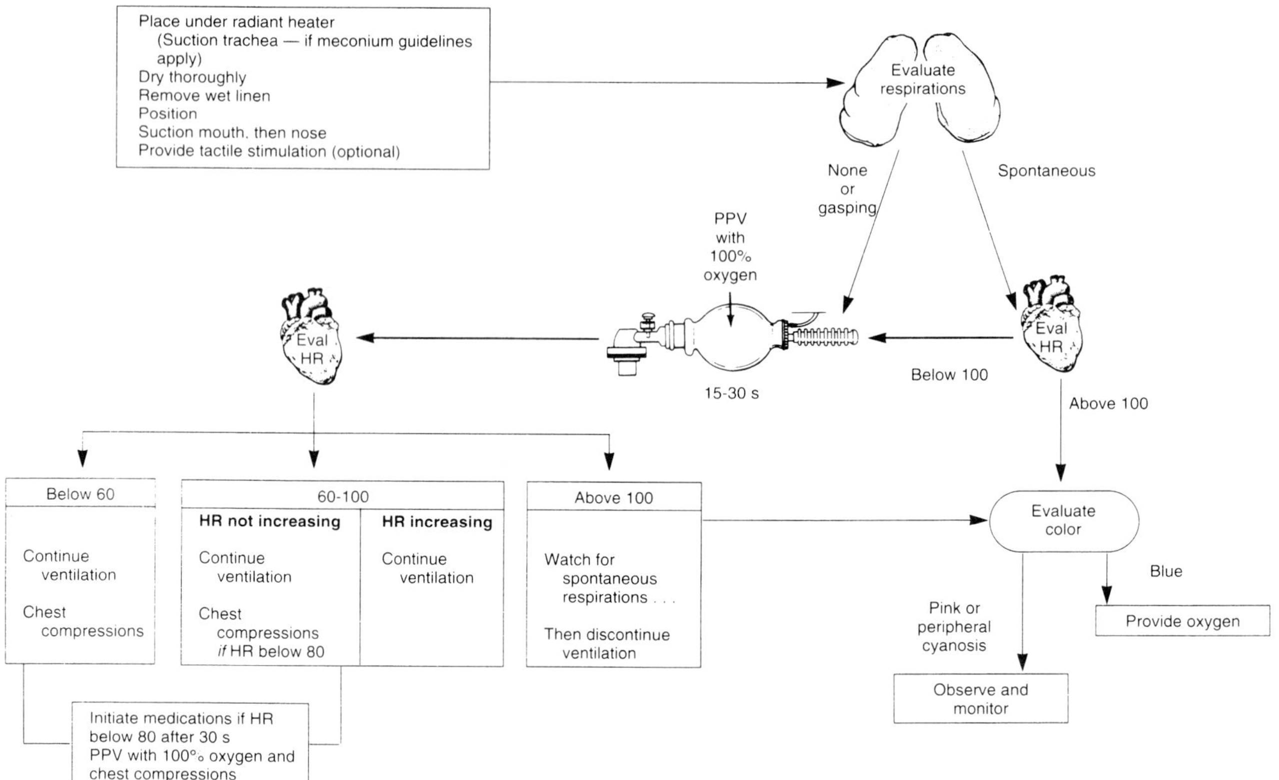

FIG. 1. Overview of resuscitation in the delivery room. (Reprinted from ref. 14, with permission.)

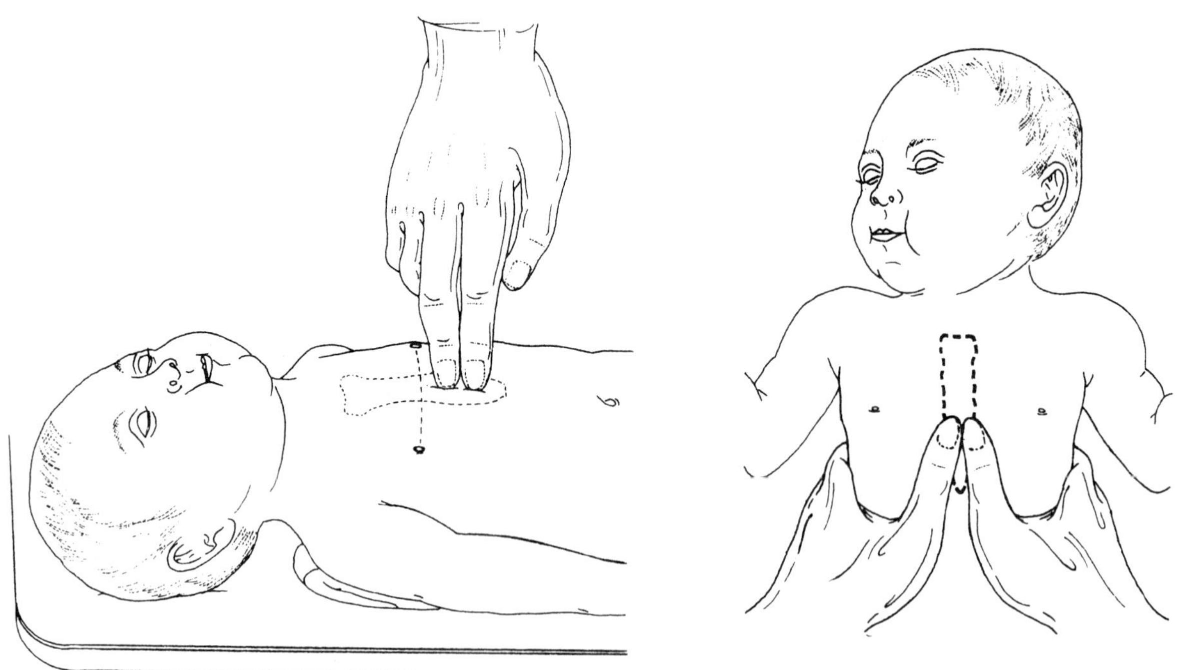

FIG. 2. Positions for performing chest compressions. Two-finger method: The tips of the middle and index or ring fingers should be used for compression. Thumb method: The balls of the thumbs should be used for compression. (Reprinted from ref. 14, with permission.)

TABLE 4. *APGAR scoring system*

Sign	0	1	2
Heart rate	Absent	<100	>100
Respiratory effort	Absent	Slow, irregular	Crying
Muscle tone	Flaccid	Some flexion of extremities	Active motion
Reflex irritability	No response	Grimace	Vigorous cry
Color	Blue, pale	Blue extremities	Completely pink

These three steps should occur within the first minute of life. Although 1- and 5-minute Apgar scores (Table 4) are recorded as one way of assessing neonatal response to resuscitation, the practitioner *should not* wait for the 1-minute score to begin resuscitation. If the 5-minute score is less than 7, additional scores should be obtained every 5 minutes until 20 minutes have passed or until two successive scores are greater than or equal to 7 (15). In a study of stillborn infants, 66.6% were resuscitated and left the delivery room alive (16). Of these, 39% survived beyond the neonatal period. Survival is unlikely if the Apgar score is 0 at 10 minutes of age (16).

Medications are indicated if, after adequate ventilation with 100% oxygen and chest compressions for 30 seconds, HR remains below 80 beats/min. Medications, doses, and routes of administration are given in Table 5.

TABLE 5.

Medication	Concentration to administer	Preparation	Dosage/route	Total dose/infant: Weight	Total dose	Total mL	Rate/precautions
Epinephrine	1:10,000	1 mL	0.1–0.3 mL/kg	1 kg		0.1–0.3 mL	Give rapidly
				2 kg		0.2–0.6 mL	May dilute with normal saline to 1–2 mL if giving ET
				3 kg		0.3–0.9 mL	
			IV or ET	4 kg		0.4–1.2 mL	
Volume expanders	Whole blood 5% Albumin-saline Normal saline Ringer's lactate	40 mL	10 mL/kg IV	1 kg		10 mL	Give over 5–10 min
				2 kg		20 mL	
				3 kg		30 mL	
				4 kg		40 mL	
Sodium bicarbonate	0.5 mEq/mL (4.2% solution)	20 mL or two 10-mL prefilled syringes	2 mEq/kg IV	1 kg	2 mEq	4 mL	Give *slowly,* over at least 2 min
				2 kg	4 mEq	8 mL	
				3 kg	6 mEq	12 mL	
				4 kg	8 mEq	16 mL	Give only if infant is being effectively ventilated
Naloxone hydrochloride	0.4 mg/mL	1 mL	0.1 mg/kg (0.25 mL/kg) IV, ET IM, SQ	1 kg	0.1 mg	0.25 mL	Give rapidly IV, ET preferred IM, SQ acceptable
				2 kg	0.2 mg	0.50 mL	
				3 kg	0.3 mg	0.75 mL	
				4 kg	0.4 mg	1.00 mL	
	1.0 mg/mL	1 mL	0.1 mL/kg (0.1 mL/kg) IV, ET IM, SQ	1 kg	0.1 mg	0.1 mL	
				2 kg	0.2 mg	0.2 mL	
				3 kg	0.3 mg	0.3 mL	
				4 kg	0.4 mg	0.4 mL	
Dopamine	$\frac{6 \times \text{Weight (kg)} \times \text{Desired dose } (\mu g/kg/min)}{\text{Desired fluid (mL/h)}}$ = mg of dopamine per 100 mL of solution		Begin at 5 µg/kg/min (may increase to 20 µg/kg/min if necessary) IV	1 kg	Total µg/min: 5–20 µ/min		Give as a continuous infusion using an infusion pump Monitor heart rate and blood pressure closely Seek consultation
				2 kg	10–40 µg/min		
				3 kg	15–60 µg/min		
				4 kg	20–80 µg/min		

IM, intramuscular; ET, endotracheal; IV, intravenous; SQ, subcutaneous.
From ref. 14, with permission.

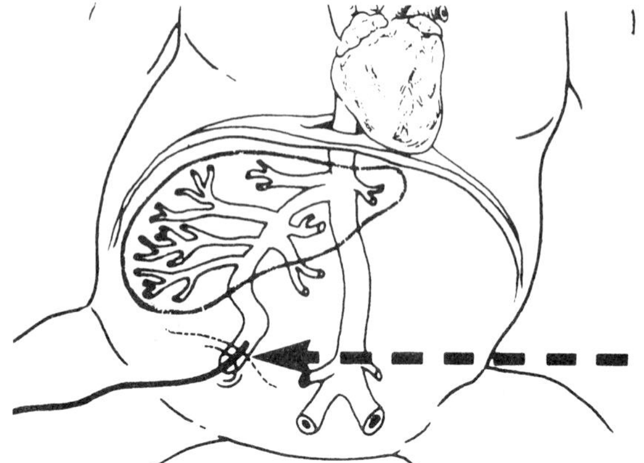

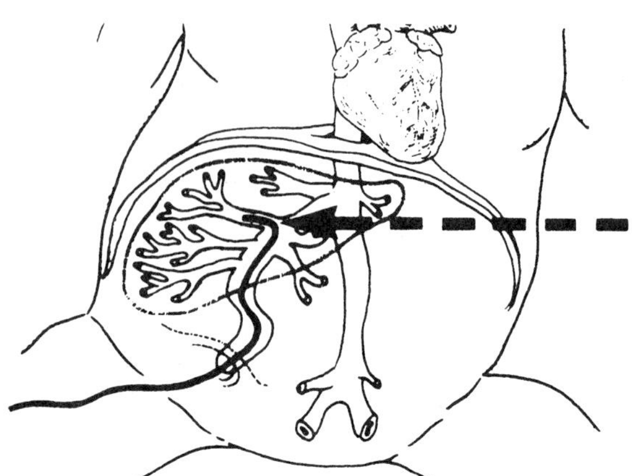

FIG. 3. Umbilical vein catheter placement. (Reprinted from ref. 14, with permission.)

Naloxone hydrochloride is indicated specifically for neonatal respiratory depression due to maternal opioid administration. It should not be given to a neonate exposed to long-term maternal opiates as it can precipitate acute withdrawal. Sodium bicarbonate should be used only when ventilation is adequate (or respiratory acidosis will replace metabolic acidosis) *and* metabolic acidosis is documented or presumed, or all other measures have been unsuccessful (13,17). Atropine is not indicated in neonatal resuscitation because vagal stimulation is rarely the cause of bradycardia in a newborn requiring resuscitation (13). Direct laryngoscopy, however, may cause a transient decrease in HR.

Once the need for medications is established, there are three possible routes of administration: umbilical vein, peripheral veins, or endotracheal instillation. The umbilical vein is cannulated by using a 3.5F or 5.0F radiopaque catheter with a single end hole. The catheter should be inserted into the vein of the umbilical stump until the tip is just below the skin level (Fig. 3). Free flow of blood should be present. If inserted too far, the catheter may enter the liver, which can be damaged by direct infusion of vasoactive drugs. Catheter location should be confirmed radiographically as soon as possible after insertion. Peripheral veins are adequate for resuscitation but may be difficult to cannulate in an emergency. While establishing intravenous access, both epinephrine and naloxone can be instilled into the trachea.

ANCILLARY ISSUES

Neonatal Hypoglycemia

Approximately 10% of healthy term neonates have transient hypoglycemia (18). Other neonates at risk include those born of diabetic mothers or mothers who received a large amount of intravenous dextrose during labor. Macrosomic, pre- or postmature neonates also are prone to hypoglycemia. A dextrose strip is easily obtained on any infant at risk and also should be obtained from neonates who appear lethargic at birth without obvious cause. If the glucose concentration is fewer than 40 to 45 mg/dL, the neonate should be treated either with oral feedings (2 to 3 mL/kg D_{10} in water) or by intravenous infusion (8 mg/kg/min).

Laryngeal-Mask Airway

Recently, the size 1 laryngeal-mask airway (LMA) has been used successfully to resuscitate newborns requiring PPV at birth (19–21). In a descriptive study by Paterson et al. (19), eligible newborns weighed at least 2.5 kg and were at least 35 weeks estimated gestational age. Twenty of 21 neonates were successfully resuscitated with the LMA. One neonate underwent tracheal intubation to facilitate administration of epinephrine. Time for LMA insertion averaged 8.6 seconds; circuit pressure at audible leak averaged 22 cm H_2O, and peak circuit pressure obtained averaged 37 cm H_2O. Gastric distention was not observed during the resuscitation procedure. The successful use of the LMA also was described in neonates with Pierre Robin syndrome in whom both bag-and-mask ventilation and endotracheal intubation had failed (22,23). Further studies are needed to assess the reliability of this technique of airway management in the neonate requiring resuscitation.

Pulse Oximeter Placement

The right-to-left shunt at the ductus arteriosus persists for some time after birth and may affect oxygen saturation readings obtained by pulse oximetry. Measurements of arterial oxygen saturation taken at birth simultaneously from the right hand and the right foot are consistently higher in the right hand (24). An oxygen saturation measurement obtained from the right hand is a better index of neonatal cerebral oxygenation than that obtained from the lower extremities.

MEDICOLEGAL ASPECTS FOR THE OBSTETRIC ANESTHESIOLOGIST

In establishing hospital policy for neonatal resuscitation, it is critically important to define who is responsible for the actual resuscitation and what procedures will be followed if additional personnel are needed. These policies should not conflict with Guideline VII of the American Society of Anesthesiology, *Guidelines for Regional Anesthesia in Obstetrics* (see the preceding).

It is clear that an anesthesiologist caring for a woman during her labor has a duty to care for that patient. There is, however, no reason to assume that a patient–physician relationship exists between the newborn infant and the anesthesiologist. In the absence of a pediatrician at delivery, frequently the anesthesiologist is assumed to have responsibility for the resuscitation of the baby. Good Samaritan statutes prevent a person from being liable for negligent acts or omissions committed while voluntarily providing emergency care. An appellate court was asked to determine whether a Good Samaritan statute provided immunity to an anesthesiologist asked to resuscitate an infant. The court found no immunity for the anesthesiologist where he has an employment duty to resuscitate the infant. However, if a duty to the infant does not exist before delivery, then it is not suddenly created because the anesthesiologist is present and has a relationship with the mother (25).

In a recent review of obstetric anesthesia closed malpractice claims, 13% (5) of the claims were due to problems with neonatal resuscitation (26). Three were for lack of or delay in tracheal intubation and one for lack of recognition of esophageal intubation. Adverse outcomes in two of the cases were judged by the closed-claim reviewers to be related to the management by anesthesia personnel.

A compilation of obstetric anesthesia malpractice suits since 1985 found the 12 of 69 (17.4%) included neonatal resuscitation claims against anesthesia personnel (27). There was a payout to the plaintiff in ten of the 12 cases.

Risk management dictates that an anesthesiologist who is expected to perform neonatal resuscitation maintain a high level of skill in that area and that a different anesthesiologist should have primary responsibility for the mother. Any obstetric anesthesiologist, even if he or she is not a designated resuscitator, should be capable of basic neonatal-resuscitation steps that could be initiated in an unanticipated emergency while awaiting designated personnel. Finally, written hospital policies delineating who is responsible for neonatal resuscitation are the best protection for the anesthesiologist who becomes involved with neonatal resuscitation only under unusual circumstances. In this scenario, Good Samaritan statutes may apply.

ETHICAL ASPECTS FOR THE OBSTETRIC ANESTHESIOLOGIST

When faced with the need to resuscitate a very low birth weight infant (fewer than 750 grams), a stillborn infant, or an infant with severe congenital anomalies that may preclude long-term survival, the obstetric health care team may have conflicting feelings about how to proceed (28). A survey of neonatologists in Alberta, Canada, revealed that factors extremely important or important to the decision-making process included gestational age, birth weight, multiple anomalies, and parental requests (29). Factors classified as not important included financial costs to parents, hospital, or society; medicolegal factors; physician's own moral or religious beliefs; and potential adoption of the infant. There was disagreement concerning the importance of apnea and asystole at birth. Likelihood of neonatal death or severe handicap also was considered important, but only when these outcomes were greater than 75% certain to occur. Ideally, discussions are held between the parents, neonatology and obstetric staff, and hospital ethics committee (when necessary) before delivery. In the complete absence of such discussions, my opinion is that it is best to attempt resuscitation.

SUMMARY

Successful neonatal resuscitation requires an understanding of neonatal physiology and adequate preparation of personnel and supplies. Good ante- and intrapartum assessment will identify the majority of infants who will require resuscitation. Those who frequent the delivery room, even when not designated as primary responders to neonatal resuscitations, should understand how to initiate neonatal resuscitation.

REFERENCES

1. American Heart Association. Standards and guidelines for cardiopulmonary resuscitation and emergency care. *JAMA* 1992;268:2276.
2. Wimmer JE. Neonatal resuscitation. *Pediatr Rev* 1994;15:255.
3. Ostheimer GW. Anaesthetists' role in neonatal resuscitation and care of the newborn. *Can J Anaesth* 1993;40:R50.
4. Hawkins JL, Gibbs CP, Orleans M, Schmid K. Obstetric anesthesia workforce survey: 1992 versus 1981. *Anesthesiology* 1994;81:A1128.
5. Heyman HJ, Joseph NJ, Salem MR, Heyman K. Anesthesia personnel, neonatal resuscitation, and the courts. *Anesthesiology* 1991;75:A1074.
6. Guay J. Fetal monitoring and neonatal resuscitation: what the anaesthetist should know. *Can J Anaesth* 1991;38:R83.
7. Krebs HB, Petres RE, Dunn LJ, Jordan HVF, Segreti A. Intrapartum fetal heart rate monitoring I. Classification and prognosis of fetal heart rate patterns. *Am J Obstet Gynecol* 1979;133:762.
8. Schifrin BS, Dame L. Fetal heart rate patterns: prediction of Apgar score. *JAMA* 1972;219:1322.
9. Tejani N, Mann LI, Bhakthavathsalan A. Correlation of fetal heart rate patterns and fetal pH with neonatal outcome. *Obstet Gynecol* 1976;48: 460.

10. Nelson KB, Dambrosia JM, Ting TY, Grether JK. Uncertain value of electronic fetal monitoring in predicting cerebral palsy. *N Engl J Med* 1996;334:613.
11. Sivan E, Seidman DS, Barkai G, Atlas M, Dulitzky M, Mashiach S. The role of amnioinfusion in current obstetric care. *Obstet Gynecol Surv* 1992;47:80.
12. Macri CJ, Schrimmer DB, Leung A, Greenspoon JS, Paul RH. Prophylactic amnioinfusion improves outcome of pregnancy complicated by thick meconium and oligohydramnios. *Am J Obstet Gynecol* 1992;167: 117.
13. Leuthner SR, Jansen RD, Hageman JR. Cardiopulmonary resuscitation of the newborn. *Pediatr Clin North Am* 1994;41:893.
14. American Heart Association and American Academy of Pediatrics. *Textbook of neonatal resuscitation.* Dallas: American Heart Association, 1994.
15. Jain L, Vidyasagar D. Controversies in neonatal resuscitation. *Pediatr Ann* 1995;24:540.
16. Jain L, Ferre C, Vidyasagar D, Nath S, Sheftel D. Cardiopulmonary resuscitation of apparently stillborn infants: survival and long-term outcome. *J Pediatr* 1991;118:778.
17. Hein HA. The use of sodium bicarbonate in neonatal resuscitation: help or harm? [Letter]. *Pediatrics* 1993;91:496.
18. Fanaroff AA, Martin RJ, eds. *Neonatal-perinatal medicine: diseases of the fetus and infant.* 5th ed. St. Louis: Mosby Year Book, 1992.
19. Paterson SJ, Byrne PJ, Molesky MG, Seal RF, Finucane BT. Neonatal resuscitation using the laryngeal mask airway. *Anesthesiology* 1994; 80:1248.
20. Brimacombe J. The laryngeal mask airway for neonatal resuscitation [Letter]. *Pediatrics* 1994;93:874.
21. Lavies NG. Use of the laryngeal mask airway in neonatal resuscitation [Letter]. *Anaesthesia* 1993;48:352.
22. Denny NM, Desilva KD, Webber PA. Laryngeal mask airway for emergency tracheostomy in a neonate. *Anaesthesia* 1990;45:895.
23. Baraka A. Laryngeal mask airway for resuscitation of a newborn with Pierre Robin syndrome [Letter]. *Anesthesiology* 1995;83:645.
24. Dimich I, Singh PP, Adell A, Hendler M, Sonnenklar N, Jhaveri M. Evaluation of oxygen saturation monitoring by pulse oximetry in neonates in the delivery system. *Can J Anaesth* 1991;38:985.
25. Knapp RM. Medicolegal aspects of obstetric anesthesia. In: Ostheimer GW, ed. *Manual of obstetric anesthesia.* New York: Churchill-Livingstone, 1992:412.
26. Chadwick HS, Posner K, Caplan RA, Ward RJ, Cheney FW. A comparison of obstetric and nonobstetric anesthesia malpractice claims. *Anesthesiology* 1991;74:242.
27. Heyman HJ. Neonatal resuscitation and anesthesiologist liability [Letter]. *Anesthesiology* 1994;81:783.
28. Landwirth J. Ethical issues in pediatric and neonatal resuscitation. *Ann Emerg Med* 1993;22:502.
29. Byrne PJ, Tyebkhan JM, Laing LM. Ethical decision-making and neonatal resuscitation. *Semin Perinatol* 1994;18:36.

PART III

After Delivery

Obstetric Anesthesia, second edition,
edited by Mark C. Norris.
Lippincott Williams & Wilkins, Philadelphia © 1999.

CHAPTER 37

Anesthesia for Postpartum Sterilization

Sung-Hee Rhim Lee and Barbara L. Leighton

Patients requesting postpartum tubal ligation (PPTL) present special anesthetic concerns. Postpartum physiology resembles that of the term parturient. Yet postpartum patients cannot be treated as though they are "a little bit pregnant," for important differences exist. For example:

- Postpartum patients have variable blood volumes,
- Cardiac output is greater immediately after delivery, and
- The duration of succinylcholine and vecuronium is prolonged in these women.

There are no fetal issues, but the condition of the neonate must be considered before permanent sterilization. Health care costs of postpartum sterilization are lower than interval sterilization at 6 to 8 weeks after delivery. For most patients, postpartum tubal sterilization is at least as safe as interval sterilization. In this chapter, we discuss unique features of postpartum physiology and suggest ways to increase the safety of anesthesia for PPTL.

OBSTETRIC AND GYNECOLOGIC ISSUES

Advantages

Postpartum tubal ligation offers several surgical, anesthetic, and logistic advantages. After delivery, the fallopian tubes are easily accessible by minilaparotomy. Interval tubal sterilization requires laparoscopy, which has a higher risk of bowel and vascular injury (1). If the PPTL is performed within 4 to 12 hours of delivery, additional hospitalization can be avoided (2), and the epidural catheter placed for labor analgesia may be reused (3,4). For most women with an uncomplicated peripartum course, postpartum tubal ligation is an uneventful and convenient option.

S.-H. Rhim Lee: Department of Anesthesiology, New York Presbyterian Hospital-Cornell Medical Center, New York, New York 10021.
B. L. Leighton: Department of Anesthesiology, Allegheny University of the Health Sciences Hospital–City Avenue Hospital, Philadelphia, Pennsylvania 19131.

Certain conditions, however, are incompatible with postpartum tubal sterilization. The American College of Obstetricians and Gynecologists (ACOG) recommends that tubal ligation be deferred in patients who have had medical or obstetric complications, and that we reaffirm the desire for sterilization after the neonate has been assessed (5). Obstetricians may defer operating on patients with risk factors for subsequent regret, such as young age, low parity, low socioeconomic status, or the decision to undergo sterilization made by someone other than the patient (6). Postpartum tubal ligations that are performed in the labor and delivery ward may be cancelled if staffing is insufficient (5).

Morbidity and Mortality

Tubal ligations have a good safety record. Numerous investigators, including those from developing countries, report a low incidence of complications with tubal ligations performed under general, local, epidural, or spinal anesthesia immediately after delivery (7–11). The Committee on Obstetrics of the American College of Obstetricians and Gynecologists supports the practice of postpartum tubal ligation, barring any maternal or neonatal contraindication (12). The World Federation of Health Agencies for the Advancement of Voluntary Surgical Contraception endorses tubal ligations performed within 48 hours of delivery (13).

The reported mortality rate for all tubal sterilizations, interval and postpartum, has been reported as four (0.004%) of 100,000 (14). Mask general anesthesia has been a causative factor in many perioperative tubal-ligation deaths. In New York City, from 1980 to 1984, one death resulted from anesthesia during tubal ligation (postpartum vs interval not specified) (15). The Centers for Disease Control (CDC) surveyed deaths associated with tubal ligation, both postpartum and interval, from 1977 to 1981. Five of the eight deaths concurrent with pregnancy termination (seven vaginal deliveries and one hysterotomy abortion) were attributed to complications of general anesthesia: hypoventilation (two cases) and unexplained cardiorespiratory arrest (three cases). All but one of these deaths occurred during mask general anesthesia (16). A survey of maternal mortality in Michigan, 1972 to 1984, attributed one death during tubal ligation to cardiac arrest after mask general anesthesia. This death, however, was most likely caused by the chronic myocarditis diagnosed at autopsy, rather than by anesthetic mishap (17). Regional block has replaced mask general anesthesia as the most popular anesthetic technique for postpartum surgery. It remains to be seen how this trend will affect anesthetic-related mortality.

POSTPARTUM PHYSIOLOGY

Relevant physiologic alterations include changes in the cardiovascular, respiratory (pulmonary function and airway anatomy), hematologic, hormonal, and gastrointestinal systems. By 6 weeks, patients have almost entirely returned to nonpregnant physiology.

Cardiovascular

Cardiac output increases to 150% of nonpregnant values at 32 weeks' gestation to support the needs of the mother and the rapidly growing fetus (18). Blood volume increases during pregnancy to 145% of nonpregnant values (19). Cardiac output reaches its peak level immediately after delivery, increasing to up to 240% to 270% of nonpregnant values in patients with normal intrapartum blood loss (20). The return of blood to the circulation from the involuting uterus causes this increased cardiac output, which may be poorly tolerated by patients with cardiac disease (19). However, excessive blood loss from lacerations, uterine atony, placenta accreta, or coagulopathy can lead to hypovolemia and decreased cardiac output in the postpartum patient. Cardiac output gradually returns to nonpregnant values, with most of the decrease occurring within the first 2 weeks after delivery (21).

Respiratory

Minute ventilation at term increases to 150% of nonpregnant values (obtained 4 to 9 months postpartum) in subjects followed serially during pregnancy (22). One to 2 weeks after delivery, minute ventilation is still 28% higher than nonpregnant values. This increase is primarily caused by a higher tidal volume, rather than increased respiratory rate (22). The functional residual capacity, decreased during pregnancy, expands to within 5% of the nonpregnant value by 1 to 2 weeks after delivery (22,23).

The anatomic abnormalities associated with difficult intubation in term pregnant patients (obesity, short neck, receding mandible, protruding maxillary incisors, and Mallampati classification of 3 or 4) persist postpartum (24,25). In addition, postpartum patients, especially those with preeclampsia, may have developed laryngeal edema during intense, prolonged second-stage Valsalva maneuvers (26,27). Successful regional anesthesia allows us to avoid manipulating these potentially difficult airways.

Central Nervous System

The increased sensitivity of the parturient to spinal or epidural local anesthetics decreases soon after delivery. Studying the same subjects at term and 36 to 48 hours after delivery, Assali and Prystowsky (28) found a three- to fourfold increase after delivery in the dose of procaine required to achieve the same level of spinal anesthesia. Both hormonal and mechanical postpartum changes may contribute to this effect. Datta et al. (29) compared plasma and cerebrospinal fluid (CSF) progesterone in pregnant women at term and 12 to 18 hours after delivery. They found that progesterone decreases rapidly after delivery, with the spread of intrathecal lidocaine decreasing as CSF progesterone decreased ($r = -0.6$; $p = 0.03$). Barclay et al. (30) demonstrated the mechanical effects of pregnancy on spinal anesthesia by comparing the dermatomal spread of spinal anesthesia in nonpregnant subjects, term pregnant patients, and nonpregnant patients fitted with abdominal binders pressurized to simulate the mechanical effects of the gravid uterus. The dermatomal anesthetic level was significantly higher in the subjects given abdominal compression compared with the nonpregnant controls, but similar to the response in pregnant patients.

Risk of Aspiration

Some of the gastrointestinal changes associated with pregnancy persist after delivery. Decreased esophageal sphincter pressure, delayed gastric emptying, and increased gastric volume increase the risk of aspiration of gastric contents. Anesthesiologists caring for postpartum patients must consider whether, and if so, how long and to what extent, these patients remain at increased risk for aspiration of gastric contents.

Reflux

Esophageal reflux is common during pregnancy. Pregnant women with symptoms of reflux have lower esophageal pressures than either pregnant women without heartburn or nonpregnant control subjects (31). The incidence of esophageal reflux decreases after delivery. Vanner (32) studied 25 women both at term and 36 hours after delivery, by using an esophageal pH probe to detect reflux. At term, 17 (68%) of the women had a total of 29 episodes of reflux, whereas after delivery, five (20%) of the women had one reflux episode each (Fig. 1).

Gastric Emptying

Gastric emptying of liquids is not delayed during pregnancy, in laboring women who do not receive opioids, or

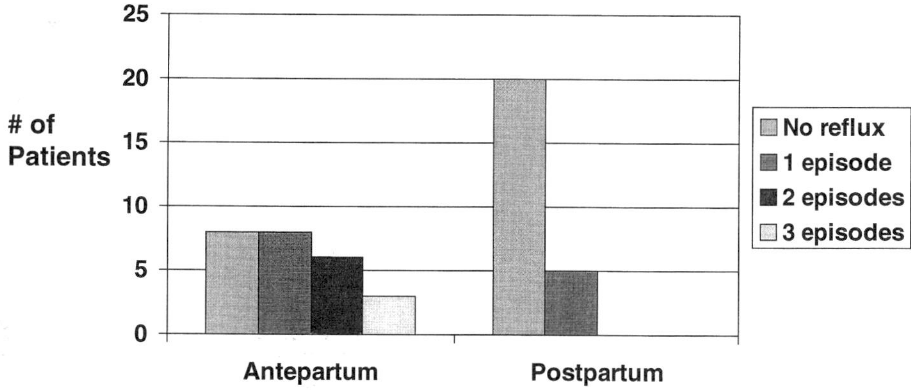

FIG. 1. The incidence of esophageal reflux at term and after delivery. (Data from ref. 32, with permission.)

in the postpartum period. Gin (33) found no difference in acetaminophen absorption times among postpartum patients 12 to 36 hours, 60 to 84 hours, and 6 weeks after delivery. Whitehead (34) found no difference in gastrointestinal acetaminophen absorption between nonpregnant women and women 1 to 5 days after delivery. (Acetaminophen is absorbed only in the small intestine, so the drug must leave the stomach before it can appear in serum.) Women 2 hours after delivery had delayed gastric emptying, reflected by delayed appearance of serum acetaminophen; however, 24% of the subjects had received opioid labor analgesia. Sandhar et al. (35), by using applied potential tomography, found rapid gastric emptying (11 to 15 minutes) in women during the third trimester, at 2 to 3 days before delivery, and at 6 weeks after delivery.

Gastric emptying of solid food is delayed after delivery. Jayaram et al. (36) used ultrasonography to compare the stomach contents of postpartum patients 9.0 ± 6.3 hours after delivery with nonpregnant volunteers. Four hours after ingestion of a standardized meal, four (19%) of 21 volunteers had detectable food in the stomach, whereas 19 of 20 of the postpartum patients had gastric food particles. The authors indicated that six of the postpartum patients had received opioid medication 14.5 ± 6.9 hours before eating. Of the patients presenting for postpartum tubal ligation, 11 of 28 had food particles detectable by ultrasonography, compared with none of 24 gynecologic patients. Narcotic medication, labor epidural analgesia, duration of fasting, or interval since delivery lacked impact on the presence of gastric food.

Opioids are the most important cause of delayed gastric emptying in parturients. Nimmo et al. (40) performed acetaminophen absorption studies on postpartum patients, unmedicated laboring women, and laboring women who received intramuscular opioids with or without metoclopramide (Fig. 2). Gastric emptying was rapid in all unmedicated patients but delayed by 4 hours in those who

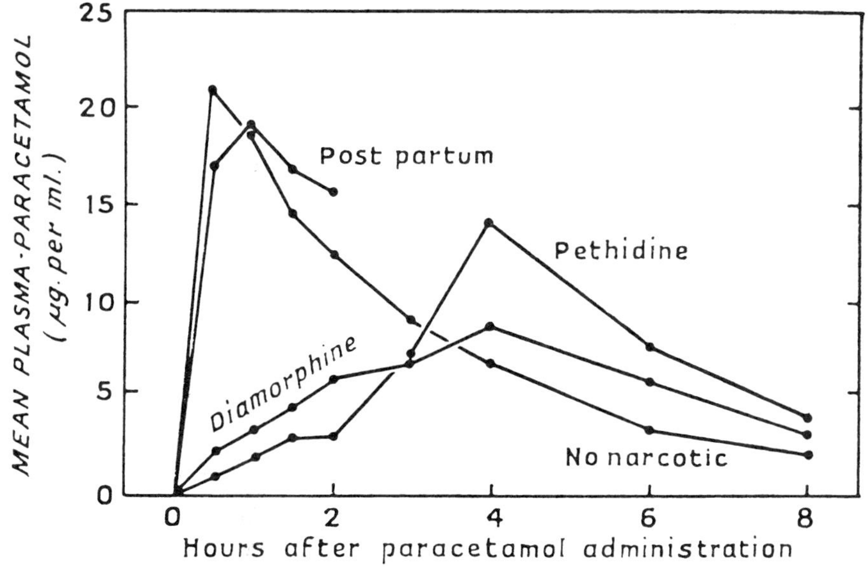

FIG. 2. Effect of meperidine and diamorphine on paracetamol absorption in laboring women. (Reprinted from ref. 40, with permission.)

TABLE 1. *Gastric volumes and pH of postpartum and nonpregnant women*

	Mean gastric volume (mL) (range)	Subjects with gastric volume >25 mL (%)	Mean pH (range)	Subjects with pH <2.5 (%)
1–8 h postpartum	39.1 (7–73)	73	1.53 (1.27–2.24)	100
9–23 h postpartum	24.0[a] (6–56)	40	1.48 (1.14–2.07)	100
24–45 h postpartum	40.9 (8–73)	73	1.40 (0.98–2.80)	80
Nonpregnant	38.1 (10–82)	67	1.56 (1.08–6.47)	80

[a]Significantly differs from other postpartum groups, $p < 0.05$.
Data from ref. 46, with permission.

had received opioids. By using an epigastric impedance technique, O'Sullivan et al. (37) found the same results. Naloxone reverses the delay in gastric emptying in laboring women given meperidine (38). Methylnaltrexone, an opioid antagonist that does not cross the blood–brain barrier, prevents delays in gastric motility when given concomitant with morphine (39). Metoclopramide does not reverse this opioid effect (40). Cisapride, on the other hand, speeds opioid-delayed gastric emptying in nonpregnant subjects (41).

How much opioid can we give a laboring patient before gastric emptying is delayed? Zimmerman et al. (42) reported that epidural fentanyl, 50 μg, followed by an infusion of fentanyl, 20 μg/h, did not delay acetaminophen absorption. However, Ewah et al. (43) and Wright et al. (44) found that bolus administration of epidural fentanyl, 50 or 100 μg, or epidural diamorphine, 5 mg, delayed acetaminophen absorption. Parenteral meperidine, 150 mg, diamorphine, 10 mg, or pentazocine, 60 mg, markedly delay gastric emptying; the effects of smaller doses of opioids have not been studied.

Gastric Volume and pH

Gastric volume and pH do not differ between nonpregnant and postpartum patients. Blouw (45) compared 21 patients 9 to 42 hours after delivery with nonpregnant control subjects undergoing interval tubal ligation by using a turbidimetric method. Wide ranges of gastric volumes and pH were found, with no intergroup differences. Many but not all of these patients received atropine and a narcotic before surgery. By using the same turbidimetric technique, James et al. (46) measured gastric volumes in nonpregnant subjects and patients 1 to 8, 9 to 23, and 24 to 45 hours after delivery (Table 1). The authors did not report whether patients had received opioid labor analgesia, but stated that all patients had fasted for at least 15 hours. Mean gastric volume was the same in patients 1 to 8 and 24 to 45 hours after delivery and in nonpregnant subjects, but was lower in patients 9 to 23 hours after delivery. Of note, 62% of postpartum patients and 67% of nonpregnant control patients had gastric volumes greater than 25 mL. All postpartum patients had a gastric pH of 2.8 or less (46). Lam et al. (47) looked at gastric pH and volume in patients up to 5 days after delivery undergoing tubal ligation with general anesthesia. All patients fasted at least 8 hours, and then half of the postpartum patients were given 150 mL of water to drink 2 to 3 hours before surgery. There were no differences in gastric volume or pH between nonpregnant and postpartum patients. Drinking 150 mL of water 2 to 3 hours before surgery did not increase gastric volume in postpartum patients compared with the NPO postpartum patients or the nonpregnant patients (47).

Summary

In postpartum patients who have not received opiates, gastric emptying of liquids is rapid, and the incidence of esophageal reflux is lower than that in pregnant patients. Solid food empties from the stomach more slowly in postpartum than in nonpregnant patients. Administration of opiates during labor increases gastric volume and slows gastric emptying. Epidural labor analgesia with minimal or no opiates may minimize aspiration risk.

ANESTHESIA

Spinal, epidural, local, or general anesthesia may be used for PPTL. Because minilaparotomy does not require pneumoperitoneum, which greatly increases the patient's work of breathing during laparoscopic surgery, regional and local anesthesia are feasible. Because intubation is riskier in postpartum than in nonpregnant patients, many anesthetists favor local and regional techniques. When general anesthesia is used, differences in physiology and pharmacokinetics in the postpartum patient may alter the sensitivities to various drugs.

Regional Anesthesia

Regional anesthesia offers the advantages of excellent surgical anesthesia, avoidance of airway manipulation, and, when labor epidural catheters are successfully reused, avoidance of an additional anesthetic procedure.

Patient refusal is a contraindication to regional anesthesia. Gajraj et al. (48) surveyed 100 patients who had refused regional anesthesia for obstetric procedures, including postpartum tubal ligation. The most common reasons cited were fear of backache (33%), fear of the needle (28%), fear of seeing or hearing during the procedure (10%), and fear of paralysis (8%). On further discussion, 21 of these patients consented to regional anesthesia. A reassuring preoperative interview may increase patient acceptance of regional anesthesia.

Spinal Anesthesia

Spinal anesthesia provides reliable surgical anesthesia with rapid onset. Lidocaine, meperidine, and bupivacaine are the most frequently used spinal anesthetic agents.

Lidocaine

The quick onset and short duration of lidocaine give it an excellent pharmacodynamic profile for tubal ligation. Lidocaine has a long history of safe use in spinal anesthesia (49). Recent reports of transient neurologic symptoms (TNS), which consist of radicular back and lower extremity pain after isobaric 2% or hyperbaric 5% lidocaine, have led some anesthesiologists to avoid using lidocaine for spinal anesthesia (50–52).

Meperidine

Meperidine is an opioid that produces local anesthetic effects after intrathecal injection. Norris et al. (53) compared meperidine, 60 mg, with lidocaine, 70 mg, in 20 postpartum patients (Fig. 3). Patients receiving meperidine had similar levels of sensory and motor block but longer times to first request for analgesia (448 ± 184 min vs 83 ± 33 min) than patients receiving lidocaine (Fig. 4). Curran (54) compared intrathecal meperidine, 50 to 80 mg, with lidocaine, 60 to 90 mg (dose adjusted for patient height). Patients receiving meperidine also had a shorter duration of motor block, a longer time to first request for postoperative analgesia, and a decreased postoperative requirement for intravenous patient-controlled anesthesia (PCA) morphine. Both studies reported more pruritus but no increase in nausea among the meperidine-group patients (Fig. 5) (53,54).

Respiratory depression was reported with intrathecal meperidine in patients also receiving benzodiazepines. Curran (54) administered up to 2 mg i.v. midazolam to patients receiving intrathecal meperidine or lidocaine and found a nonsignificant increase in the incidence of oxygen desaturation in the meperidine group. The oxygen desaturation resolved with naloxone, 0.1 mg (54). A postpartum patient receiving intrathecal meperidine, 50 mg, and midazolam, 2 mg i.v., experienced oxygen desaturation that was successfully treated with supplemental oxygen and verbal encouragement. Respiratory depression has not been seen beyond the first hour after intrathecal meperidine injection (55).

Bupivacaine

Bupivacaine may be used to provide spinal anesthesia for postpartum tubal ligations despite its long duration. Abouleish (56) gave intrathecal bupivacaine, with doses height-adjusted by formula, to patients 8 to 24 hours after delivery and to term pregnant patients. All patients were in the right lateral decubitus position during spinal injection. Although postpartum patients received larger doses of bupivacaine (11.3 mg vs 9.1 mg), the upper level of sensory anesthesia was higher in term pregnant patients (T_3 vs T_4). The time to complete recovery was 146 minutes (motor) and 162 minutes (sensory) in postpartum patients (56).

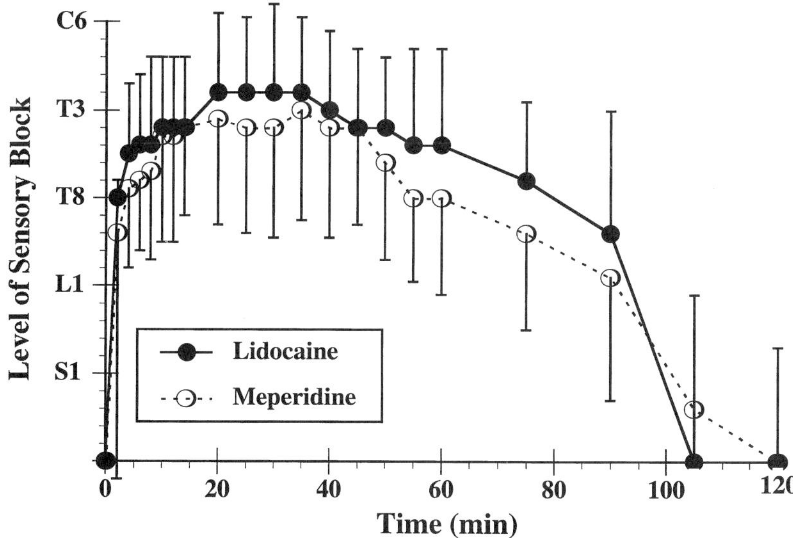

FIG. 3. Onset of analgesia after subarachnoid meperidine or lidocaine for postpartum tubal ligation. (Reprinted from ref. 53, with permission.)

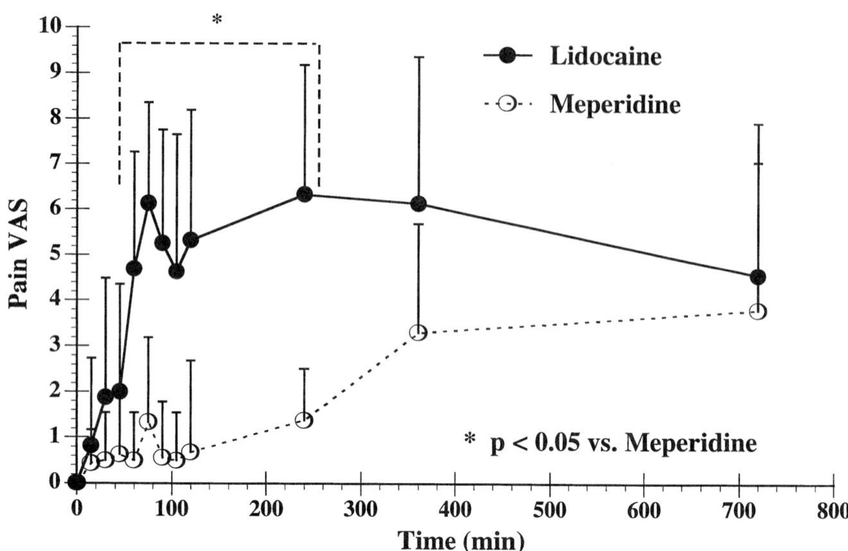

FIG. 4. Visual analog pain scores after subarachnoid meperidine or lidocaine for postpartum tubal ligation. Meperidine provided postoperative analgesia for a longer time. (Reprinted from ref. 53, with permission.)

Huffnagle et al. (57) found that 7.5 mg hyperbaric bupivacaine, administered with the patient in the lateral position, provided good anesthesia for postpartum tubal ligation in 10 of 11 patients, with an average duration of motor block of 74.4 minutes. Average time spent in the postanesthetic care unit (PACU) was 37.7 minutes. Patients receiving larger doses of hyperbaric bupivacaine had significantly longer recovery room stays. Bupivacaine, 5 mg, did not provide adequate sensory block for tubal ligation.

Although many anesthesiologists choose a local anesthetic dose based on the patient's height or weight, this adjustment is not needed for postpartum patients of normal height and weight. In patients receiving intrathecal hyperbaric lidocaine, 75 mg, in the lateral position for PPTL within 48 hours of delivery, height had only a small influence on the dermatomal level to pinprick and cold. Body mass index and vertebral column length did not affect the extent of sensory anesthesia (58).

It is our strong clinical impression that patient position during spinal administration has a large influence on the final block height in postpartum patients. If hyperbaric local anesthetic is injected while the patient is in the lateral position, a higher sensory block is obtained. Consequently, adequate spinal anesthesia can be achieved with a lower dose of hyperbaric local anesthetic when the drug is injected into laterally positioned patients. For example, hyperbaric bupivacaine, 7.5 mg, provides adequate anesthesia for tubal ligation in laterally positioned patients, yet in my experience, a minimum of 10 mg seems to be necessary in sitting patients. Unfortunately, no clinical trials have addressed this issue.

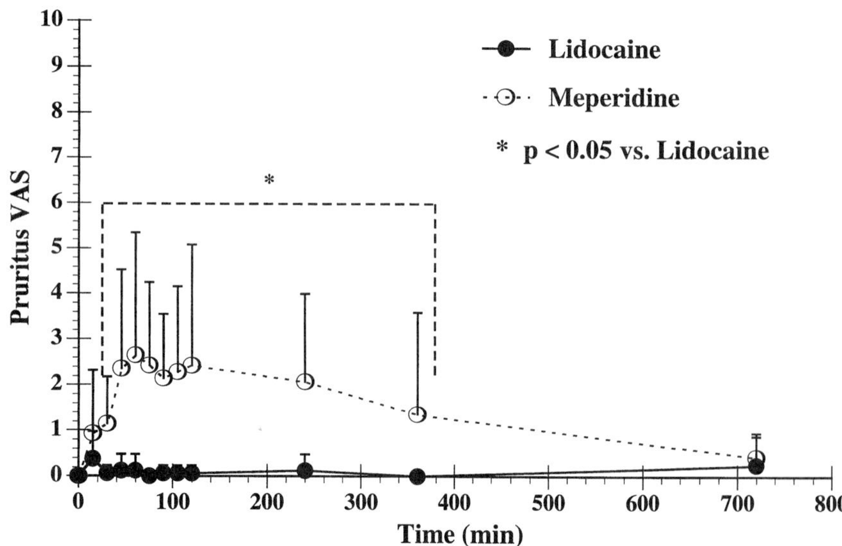

FIG. 5. Pruritus after subarachnoid meperidine or lidocaine for postpartum tubal ligation. (Reprinted from ref. 53, with permission.)

Epidural Anesthesia

An epidural catheter placed for labor analgesia may be used for postpartum tubal ligation. If reactivation of the catheter is unsuccessful, however, valuable operating room time is lost. Viscomi et al. (59) retrospectively compared labor epidural catheter reactivation (n = 45) with spinal anesthesia (n = 75; 20 patients with and 55 patients without prior epidural analgesia). Ten (26%) of the epidural catheters failed, which increased anesthesia-provider time and added an average of $176 to patient costs and 12 minutes to operating room time compared with patients receiving spinal anesthesia. There was a trend toward improved reactivation rates among patients undergoing postpartum tubal ligation within 4 hours of delivery (59).

Three retrospective studies reported that a short delivery-to-surgery time improves the success of labor epidural reactivation. The only prospective study of this question found no such association. Vincent et al. (3) found that a delivery-to-surgery time of less than 4 hours was associated with a higher rate of successful epidural catheter reactivation (95% vs 67%; $p = 0.029$; Fig. 6), whereas length of catheter insertion and patient demographics were not. Kopacz (4) reported a 63% success rate in reactivating epidural catheters (43 of 68 patients). Epidural catheters placed specifically for PPTL had a success rate of 81% (25 of 31 patients). Spinal anesthesia had a success rate of 93% (102 of 110 patients). All 13 catheters reinjected within 8 hours of delivery were successfully reactivated, whereas catheters reinjected later than 8 hours had a 55% success rate. Patteson et al. (60) reported that successfully reactivated catheters had a mean delivery-to-operation time of 9.2 hours, as compared with 13.6 hours in unsuccessful reactivation attempts. However, Norman et al. (61) prospectively examined epidural catheter reactivation in 50 consecutive patients. Seventy-eight percent of the catheters were successfully reactivated, and there was no association with delivery-to-surgery interval.

How can these studies be reconciled? Several of the retrospective studies date back to a time when catheters were routinely inserted no more than 3 cm into the epidural space. If an epidural catheter is inserted shallowly and the delivery-to-surgery time is long enough for the patient to ambulate, the catheter may be pulled out of the epidural space by patient motion. If, however, the catheter is inserted 5 to 8 cm into the epidural space, there may be a smaller chance that patient motion will dislodge the catheter.

Controversy exists on whether the choice of local anesthetic affects epidural reactivation success rates. Patteson et al. (60) found no reactivation failures by using 2-chlorprocaine, 3%, in 13 patients, compared with a 33% (12 of 36 patients) failure rate with lidocaine, 2%. Another study found no influence of the choice of local anesthetics on the success rate; however, patients with lidocaine had a shorter delivery-to-operation time (9.2 vs 13.6 hours) (61).

Buffering 2-chloroprocaine does not hasten its onset. Glosten et al. (62) compared 2-chloroprocaine buffered to a pH of 7.08 with unbuffered 2-chloroprocaine (pH 3.74). The time to attain a T_4 level did not differ between the groups. A pH of 7.08 may not have been high enough to affect onset time, however, for the high pKa of 2-chloroprocaine (8.7) still leaves much of the drug in the ionized form at that pH.

Prolonged duration of 2-chloroprocaine anesthesia has been reported in a postpartum patient with pseudocholinesterase deficiency. A patient was excessively somnolent and had an unusually prolonged anesthetic duration (3 hours) after epidural 2-chloroprocaine administration. Serum drawn 15 minutes and 5 hours after drug injection revealed unusually high concentrations of 2-chloroprocaine. Dibucaine numbers and pseudocholinesterase activity immediately and 6 weeks postpartum were abnormally low (63).

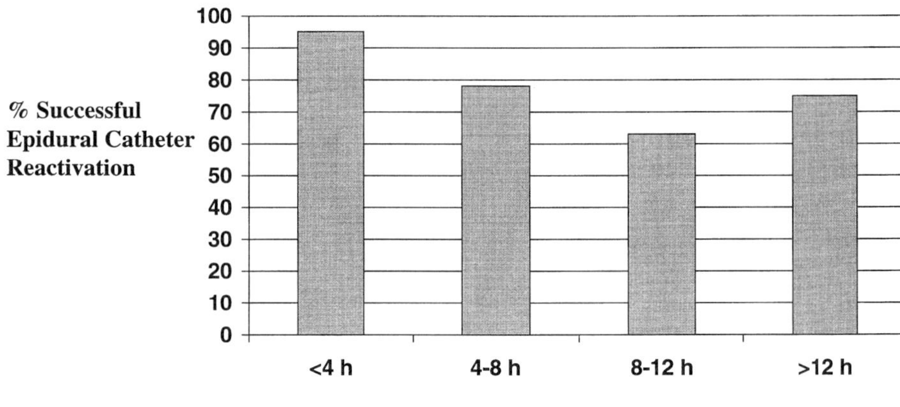

FIG. 6. Success rate of reactivation of labor epidural catheters for postpartum tubal ligation. (Data from ref. 3, with permission.)

Local Anesthesia

Patients can undergo postpartum tubal ligations comfortably with only local anesthesia. This option is frequently used in developing nations (11), especially in thin patients and in areas underserved by anesthesia providers (2). Two similar-local anesthetic techniques have been described. The senior author (B.L.L.) successfully used Cruikshank's method (see later), substituting fentanyl and midazolam for alphaprodine and diazepam. Remember, do not sedate the patient so heavily that she risks unconsciousness and loss of her protective airway reflexes.

Cruikshank et al. (64) injected 20 mL lidocaine, 0.5%, subcutaneously to allow skin incision and entry into the intraperitoneal space and then instilled 80 mL intraperitoneal lidocaine, 0.5%. All patients were premedicated with alphaprodine, 15 mg, and diazepam, 15 mg, intravenously. Nineteen of 26 patients had excellent anesthesia. The remainder experienced some discomfort with skin incision, which resolved by waiting longer for the subcutaneous lidocaine to take effect. No patients required general anesthesia or exhibited signs or symptoms of lidocaine toxicity (64). Dey et al. (65) premedicated patients with meperidine, 100 mg i.m., and diazepam, 10 mg i.v., and then injected 20 mL prilocaine, 1%, subcutaneously. Two hundred five of 208 patients tolerated the procedure, although some patients required additional diazepam. Three patients received general anesthesia for "uncooperativeness" or because intraabdominal adhesions increased the complexity of the surgery.

General Anesthesia

Maternal physiologic changes after delivery affect the response of postpartum patients to some commonly used general anesthetic drugs.

Succinylcholine

Succinylcholine, which is degraded by plasma cholinesterase, is the muscle relaxant of choice to facilitate tracheal intubation in peripartum patients. In pregnancy and after delivery, however, plasma cholinesterase activity decreases. This decrease in enzyme activity starts by 4 to 8 weeks of gestation and continues throughout pregnancy. Plasma cholinesterase activity is even lower during the first 7 days after delivery (66).

This diminished activity of plasma cholinesterase prolongs the duration of succinylcholine after delivery but not during gestation. Ganga et al. (67) compared the response to succinylcholine in women 1 to 2 days after delivery and in nonpregnant women. Postpartum subjects require a lower dose to attain 80% twitch depression. The time to 95% twitch recovery after succinylcholine, 20 mg, is longer in postpartum than in nonpregnant patients (627 vs 434 seconds). Leighton et al. (68) compared the plasma cholinesterase activities and the time to return to 25% twitch height in term pregnant patients, patients approximately 33 hours after delivery, and nonpregnant patients (Table 2). Whereas plasma cholinesterase activity was significantly decreased in both term pregnant and postpartum patients, the time to 25% twitch-height recovery after succinylcholine, 1 mg/kg, was significantly prolonged only in the postpartum group (postpartum, 685 seconds vs pregnant, 470 seconds vs nonpregnant, 501 seconds).

Metoclopramide is often used as a premedication to speed gastric emptying. Metoclopramide, however, may prolong the duration of succinylcholine. Kao et al. (69) found that adding metoclopramide to an in vitro preparation of succinylcholine and plasma decreased the production of choline, a succinylcholine degradation product. In nonpregnant women, intravenous metoclopramide, 10 mg, increases the time to 25% twitch-height recovery after succinylcholine, 20 mg (366 vs 276 seconds). Metoclopramide may directly inhibit acetylcholinesterases, thus leading to cholinergic effects, while also inhibiting the degradation of succinylcholine.

Nondepolarizing Muscle Relaxants

The postpartum decrease in plasma cholinesterase activity also prolongs the duration of mivacurium, a nondepolarizing muscle relaxant that is metabolized by plasma cholinesterase. Gin et al. (70) compared the duration of mivacurium in women 30 to 39 hours after delivery with that in nonpregnant control subjects and found

TABLE 2. *Recovery from succinylcholine, 1 mg/kg, in pregnant and nonpregnant women*

	Time to 25% recovery (s)	Time from 25% to 75% recovery (s)	Cholinesterase activity (U/mL)	Dibucaine number
Nonpregnant (n = 14)	501 ± 21	102 ± 6	5.01 ± 0.33	82.5 ± 0.4
Oral contraceptive (n = 7)	499 ± 29	104 ± 8	4.81 ± 0.63	80.7 ± 0.8
Term pregnant (n = 5)	470 ± 56	83 ± 6	3.66 ± 0.39[b]	82.4 ± 1.0
Postpartum (n = 8)	685 ± 22[a]	95 ± 11	2.84 ± 0.35[c]	82.7 ± 0.9

[a] $p < 0.001$ vs all other groups.
[b] $p < 0.05$ vs nonpregnant group.
[c] $p < 0.05$ vs nonpregnant and oral-contraceptive groups.
Data from ref. 68, with permission.

that the time to recovery of 25% twitch height was 3.1 minutes longer in the postpartum group. This increase in mivacurium duration correlated with decreased plasma cholinesterase activity.

The duration of vecuronium, but not atracurium, is prolonged in postpartum patients. Camp et al. (71) studied the onset and duration of vecuronium in patients undergoing tubal ligation 24 to 48 hours after delivery and in nonpregnant women. The onset did not differ among the groups; however, vecuronium blockade lasted significantly longer in postpartum patients (63 vs 35 minutes). Khuenl-Brady et al. (72) also found a significant increase in vecuronium duration in postpartum patients (49 minutes) compared with nonpregnant patients (32 minutes). However, the duration of 0.5 mg/kg atracurium did not differ between postpartum and nonpregnant subjects (72).

Volatile Anesthetics

The minimal alveolar concentration (MAC) of volatile anesthetic agents is reduced in pregnant women. The MAC of isoflurane also is decreased for a short period immediately after delivery. Zhou et al. (73) recorded the response to a standardized electrical stimulation under isoflurane anesthesia in patients presenting for postpartum tubal ligations within 12 hours after delivery, 12 to 24 hours after delivery, and 6 weeks after delivery. Less than 12 hours after delivery, isoflurane MAC was 0.75%, 28% less than MAC at 6 weeks postpartum. However, isoflurane MAC did not differ between women studied 12 to 24 hours after delivery (0.95%) and at 6 weeks (1.04%).

High concentrations of volatile anesthetic agents may interfere with both spontaneous contraction of the uterus and the contractile response to oxytocin in postpartum patients. Marx et al. (74) measured intrauterine pressures during general anesthesia with nitrous oxide in oxygen and varying concentrations of either halothane or enflurane. Both spontaneous contraction and the response to oxytocin were not inhibited with up to 0.5% of either halothane or enflurane. At higher inhaled concentrations, halothane, 2%, or enflurane, 1.5%, uterine contraction was depressed, an effect that reversed quickly when the volatile anesthetic was discontinued.

ADMINISTERING ANESTHESIA FOR POSTPARTUM TUBAL LIGATIONS

- **Identify the patient early in her labor; obtain early anesthetic consultation.** Determine the time of last solid food consumption and predelivery hematocrit. Carefully examine the airway. Evaluate any medical and obstetric conditions that might interfere with the planned surgery. Urge the patient and obstetrician to use epidural rather than systemic opiate analgesia.
- **Minimize gastric pH and volume.** Clear liquids are rapidly cleared from the stomach; consumption of modest amounts of liquid up to 1 to 2 hours before surgery should not increase gastric volume. Solid food empties from the stomach more slowly in postpartum than nonpregnant women; ideally, the patient should not have eaten solid food for at least 8 hours. Ranitidine, 1.5 mg/kg p.o. or i.v., will decrease gastric volume and pH. Ranitidine has been used extensively before cesarean delivery with few reported problems. Sodium citrate, 0.3 *M,* 30 mL, will increase gastric pH and may be used in addition to or in place of the H_2 blocker.
- **Maximize gastric emptying, especially if solid food was eaten shortly before admission.** Avoid i.m., i.v., and epidural opioids; if possible, provide analgesia with epidural local anesthetic. Epidural fentanyl should be kept to less than 100 μg. We consider this a reasonable goal because most postpartum tubal patients are multiparous with rapidly progressing labors.*
- **Postpone or cancel surgery in patients with medical or obstetric conditions that would interact negatively with the anesthesia or surgery.** Immediate postpartum tubal ligation (particularly with a general anesthetic with volatile agent) is not appropriate in patients in whom there is difficulty maintaining uterine tone. Patients with moderate to severe preeclampsia should wait until the preeclampsia has resolved and magnesium therapy is stopped. Patients with valvular heart disease may not tolerate the stress of a general anesthetic on top of postpartum increase in cardiac output.
- **Assess the blood loss and intravascular volume status before initiating anesthesia.** In patients who did not receive conduction anesthesia for labor, perform a tilt test immediately before initiating regional anesthesia. Patients with an ongoing epidural anesthetic should not be hypotensive or tachycardic before the block is extended for tubal ligation. Every now and then, we discover profound hypotension (and hypovolemia) by performing a postpartum tilt test. In patients with adequate predelivery hemoglobins and minimal blood loss, little information is gained by an immediate postpartum hemoglobin test.
- **Perform regional anesthesia if possible.** Consider spinal anesthesia rather than attempting to reactivate an epidural catheter if the delivery-to-tubal interval is more than 8 hours. Reactivate an epidural catheter with 15 to 20 mL 2% lidocaine with 1:200,000 epinephrine, or 3% 2-chloroprocaine, which should raise the sensory level to at least the sixth thoracic dermatome. In patients without an epidural block, spinal anesthesia may be induced by using hyperbaric lidocaine, 60 mg, bupivacaine, 7.5 to 10 mg, or meperidine, 50 mg, with the

*Editor's note: I do not alter my labor analgesic technique for patients requesting PPTL.

patient in the lateral position. If the patient sits during spinal drug injection, use slightly higher drug doses.

- **Provide general anesthesia if safe and needed.** Avoid rapid-sequence induction of general anesthesia in patients with identified difficult airways. General anesthesia can be safely performed after delivery. Look carefully for predictors of difficult intubation (poor mouth opening, short neck, protruding incisors, and receding chin, etc.). Replacing the standard supine position with a back-elevated position eases intubation in obese parturients (see Fig. 6, Chapter 25). Remember, the duration of succinylcholine is moderately prolonged in the postpartum patient. When a nondepolarizing muscle relaxant is needed, consider atracurium (or cisatracurium) instead of vecuronium, as the duration of vecuronium is prolonged after delivery. If volatile anesthetics are given to patients within hours of delivery, MAC is decreased by approximately 30%. High concentrations of these agents may interfere with the effects of oxytocin and cause excessive uterine relaxation.
- **Consider performing selected tubal ligations under local rather than general anesthesia.** Patients who refuse regional anesthesia may be candidates for intraperitoneal lidocaine anesthesia.

CONCLUSION

Postpartum tubal ligation is an elective procedure that may be safely performed shortly after delivery. Without taking precedence over safety concerns, social and financial issues may favor the performance of tubal ligations soon after delivery. Before administering anesthesia for these patients, consider the immediate postpartum changes in maternal physiology and pharmacology, and carefully evaluate the relative risk of morbidity for each individual. Assess obstetric issues, anesthetic risk, and neonatal concerns. If the patient is a good candidate for tubal ligation, a variety of anesthetic options exist.

REFERENCES

1. Rozier JR. Immediate postpartum tubal ligation. *Am J Obstet Gynecol* 1973;117:226.
2. Chi I, Gates D, Thapa S. Performing tubal sterilizations during women's postpartum hospitalization: a review of the United States and international experiences. *Obstet Gynecol Surv* 1992;47:71.
3. Vincent RD Jr, Reid RW. Epidural anesthesia for postpartum tubal ligation using epidural catheters placed during labor. *J Clin Anesth* 1993; 5:289.
4. Kopacz DJ. Postpartum tubal ligation: timing and choice of regional anesthetic technique [Abstract]. *Reg Anesth* 1990;15:753.
5. American College of Obstetrics and Gynecology Committee Opinion. Committee on obstetrics: maternal and fetal sterilization: postpartum tubal sterilization. *Int J Gynecol Obstet* 1992;39:244.
6. Chi I, Gates D, Thapa S. Performing tubal sterilizations during women's postpartum hospitalization: a review of the United States and international experiences. *Obstet Gynecol Surv* 1992;47:71.
7. Rozier JR. Immediate postpartum tubal ligation. *Am J Obstet Gynecol* 1993;117:226.
8. Lu T, Chun D. A long-term follow-up study of 1055 cases of postpartum tubal ligation. *J Obstet Gynaecol Br Emp* 1967;74:875.
9. Whitacre FE, Loeb WM, Loeb L. The timing for postpartum tubal sterilization. *Am J Obstet Gynecol* 1946;52:1041.
10. Esposito JM, Mastellone AT, Rubino G. Minilaparotomy: an approach to postpartum tubal sterilization. *N Y State J Med* 1987;87:622.
11. World Health Organization. Mini-incision for postpartum sterilization of women: a multicenter, multinational prospective study. *Contraception* 1982;26:495.
12. American College of Obstetrics and Gynecology Committee Opinion. Committee on Obstetrics: maternal and fetal Sterilization: postpartum tubal sterilization. *Int J Gynecol Obstet* 1992;39:244.
13. World Federation of Health Agencies for the Advancement of Voluntary Surgical Contraception. *Safety and voluntary surgical contraception: guidelines for service programs.* 1988.
14. Peterson HB, Destefano F, Greenspan JR, Ory HW. Mortality risk associated with tubal sterilization in United States hospitals. *Am J Obstet Gynecol* 1982;143:125.
15. Syverson C, Chavkin W, Atrash HK, Rochat RW, Sharp ES, King GE. Pregnancy-related mortality in New York City, 1980 to 1984: causes of death and associated factors. *Am J Obstet Gynecol* 1991;164:603.
16. Peterson HB, Destefano F, Rubin GL, Greenspan JR, Lee NC, Ory HW. Deaths attributable to tubal sterilization in the United States, 1977 to 1981. *Am J Obstet Gynecol* 1983;146:131.
17. Endler GC, Mariona FG, Sokol RJ, Stevenson LB. Anesthesia-related maternal mortality in Michigan, 1972 to 1984. *Am J Obstet Gynecol* 1988;159:187.
18. Robson SC, Hunter S, Boys RJ, Dunlop W. Serial study of factors influencing changes in cardiac output during human pregnancy. *Am J Physiol* 1989;256:H1060.
19. Ueland K. Maternal cardiovascular hemodynamics. VII. Intrapartum blood changes. *Am J Obstet Gynecol* 1976;126:671.
20. Ueland K, Hansen JM. Maternal cardiovascular dynamics. *Am J Obstet Gynecol* 1969;103:8.
21. Robson SC, Hunter S, Moore M, Dunlop W. Haemodynamic changes during the puerperium: a Doppler and M-mode echocardiographic study. *Br J Obstet Gynaecol* 1987;94:1028.
22. Cugell DW, Frank NR, Gaensler EA, Badger TL. Pulmonary function in pregnancy: i. serial observations in normal women. *Am Rev Tubercul* 1953;67:568.
23. Gee JBL, Packer BS, Millen JE, Robin ED. Pulmonary mechanics during pregnancy. *J Clin Invest* 1967;46:945.
24. Rocke DA, Murray WB, Rout CC, Gouws E. Relative risk analysis of factors associated with difficult intubation in obstetric anesthesia. *Anesthesiology* 1992;77:67.
25. Samsoon GLT, Young JRB. Difficult tracheal intubation: a retrospective survey. *Anaesthesia* 1987;42:487.
26. Jouppila R, Jouppila P, Hollmen A. Laryngeal oedema as an obstetric anaesthesia complication. *Acta Anaesth Scand* 1980;24:97.
27. Mackenzie AI. Laryngeal oedema complicating obstetric anaesthesia: three cases. *Anaesthesia* 1987;33:271.
28. Assali NS, Prystowsky H. Studies on autonomic blockade: I. comparison between the effects of tetraethylammonium chloride (TEAC) and high selective spinal anesthesia on blood pressure of normal and toxemic pregnancy. *J Clin Invest* 1950;29:1354.
29. Datta S, Hurley RJ, Naulty JS, et al. Plasma and cerebrospinal fluid progesterone concentrations in pregnant and nonpregnant women. *Anesth Analg* 1986;65:950.
30. Barclay DL, Renegar OJ, Nelson EW Jr. The influence of inferior vena cava compression on the level of spinal anesthesia. *Am J Obstet Gynecol* 1969;101:792.
31. Hey VMF, Cowley DJ, Ganguli PC, Skinner LD, Ostick DG, Sharp DS. Gastro-oesophageal reflux in late pregnancy. *Anaesthesia* 1977;32:372.
32. Vanner RG, Goodman NW. Gastro-oesophageal reflux in pregnancy at term and after delivery. *Anaesthesia* 1989;44:808.
33. Gin T, Cho AMW, Lew JKL, et al. Gastric emptying in the postpartum period. *Anaesth Intens Care* 1991;19:521.
34. Whitehead EM, Smith M, Dean Y, O'Sullivan G. An evaluation of gastric emptying times in pregnancy and the puerperium. *Anaesthesia* 1993;48:53.
35. Sandhar BK, Elliott RH, Windram I, Rowbotham DJ. Peripartum changes in gastric emptying. *Anaesthesia* 1992;47:196.
36. Jayaram A, Bowen MP, Deshpande S, Carp HM. Ultrasound examina-

tion of the stomach contents of women in the postpartum period. *Anesth Analg* 1997;84:522.
37. O'Sullivan GM, Sutton JA, Thompson SA, Carrie LE, Bullingham RE. Noninvasive measurement of gastric emptying in obstetric patients. *Anesth Analg* 1987;66:505.
38. Frame WT, Allison RH, Moir DD, Nimmo WS. Effect of naloxone on gastric emptying during labor. *Br J Anaesth* 1984;56:263.
39. Murphy DB, Sutton JA, Prescott LF, Murphy MB. Opioid-induced delay in gastric emptying. *Anesthesiology* 1997;87:765.
40. Nimmo WS, Wilson J, Prescott LF. Narcotic analgesics and delayed gastric emptying during labor. *Lancet* 1975;1:890.
41. Rowbotham DJ, Bamber PA, Nimmo WS. Comparison of the effect of cisapride and metoclopramide on morphine-induced delay in gastric emptying. *Br J Clin Pharmacol* 1988;26:741.
42. Zimmerman DL, Breen TW, Fick G. The effect of epidural fentanyl on gastric emptying in laboring patients. *Anesth Analg* 1995;82:612.
43. Ewah B, Yau K, King M, et al. Effect of epidural opioids on gastric emptying in labour. *Int J Obstet Anesth* 1993;2:125.
44. Wright PMC, Allen RW, Moore J, Donnelly JP. Gastric emptying during lumbar extradural analgesia in labour: effect of fentanyl supplementation. *Br J Anaesth* 1992;68:248.
45. Blouw R, Scatliff J, Craig DB, Palahniuk RJ. Gastric volume and pH in postpartum patients. *Anesthesiology* 1976;45:456.
46. James CF, Gibbs CP, Banner T. Postpartum perioperative risk of aspiration pneumonia. *Anesthesiology* 1984;61:756.
47. Lam KK, So HY, Gin T. Gastric pH and volume after oral fluids in the postpartum patient. *Can J Anaesth* 1993;40:218.
48. Gajraj NM, Sharma SK, Souter AJ, Pole Y, Sidawi JE. A survey of obstetric patients who refuse regional anesthesia. *Anaesthesia* 1995; 50:740.
49. Phillips OC, Ebner H, Nelson AT, Black MH. Neurologic complications following spinal anesthesia with lidocaine. *Anesthesiology* 1969; 30:284.
50. Pollock JE, Neal JM, Stephenson CA, Wiley CE. Prospective study of the incidence of transient radicular irritation in patients undergoing spinal anesthesia. *Anesthesiology* 1996;84:1361.
51. Hampl KF, Schneider MC, Bont A, Pargger H. Transient radicular irritation after single subarachnoid injection of isobaric 2% lignocaine for spinal anesthesia. *Anaesthesia* 1996;51:178.
52. Albrecht A, Hogg M, Robinson S. Transient radicular irritation as a complication of spinal anaesthesia with hyperbaric 5% lignocaine. *Anaesth Intens Care* 1996;24:508.
53. Norris MC, Honet JE, Leighton BL, Arkoosh VA. A comparison of meperidine and lidocaine for spinal anesthesia for postpartum tubal ligation. *Reg Anesth* 1996;21:84.
54. Curran C, Dickerson SE, Bailey SL. Efficacy of intrathecal meperidine as the sole anesthetic for postpartum tubal ligation [Abstract]. *Anesthesiology* 1992;77:A1004.
55. Ong B, Segstro R. Respiratory depression associated with meperidine spinal anaesthesia. *Can J Anaesth* 1994;41:725.
56. Abouleish EI. Postpartum tubal ligation requires more bupivacaine for spinal anesthesia than does cesarean section. *Anesth Analg* 1986; 65:897.
57. Huffnagle SL. The optimal dose of bupivacaine for spinal anesthesia for postpartum tubal ligation. *Soc Obstet Anesth Perinatol,* 1998.
58. Huffnagle SL, Norris MC, Leighton BL, Arkoosh VA, Huffnagle HJ. Intrathecal hyperbaric bupivacaine dose resonse in postpartum tubal ligation patients. *Anesthesiology* 1998;89:A1071.
59. Viscomi CM, Rathmell JP. Labor epidural catheter reactivation or spinal anesthesia for delayed postpartum tubal ligation: a cost comparison. *J Clin Anesth* 1995;7:380.
60. Patteson SK, Baird MA, Chesney JT. Efficacy of labor epidurals for postpartum tubal ligation: effect of elapsed time from placement and choice of local anesthetic [Abstract]. *Anesthesiology* 1992;77:A1033.
61. Norman PF, Werhan CF, Robertson KM. Reactivation of labor epidural catheters for delayed postpartum tubal ligation: a prospective trial [Abstract]. *Anesth Analg* 1994;78:S318.
62. Glosten B, Dailey PA, Preston PG, et al. pH-Adjusted 2-chloroprocaine for epidural anesthesia in patients undergoing postpartum tubal ligation. *Anesthesiology* 1988;68:948.
63. Kuhnert BR, Philipson EH, Pimental R, Kuhnert PM. A prolonged chloroprocaine epidural block in a postpartum patient with abnormal pseudocholinesterase. *Anesthesiology* 1982;56:477.
64. Cruikshank DP, Laube DW, De Backer LJ. Intraperitoneal lidocaine anesthesia for postpartum tubal ligation. *Obstet Gynecol* 1973;42:127.
65. Dey A, Mackay G. Postpartum tubal ligation and local anaesthesia. *Br Med J* 1974;252.
66. Evans RT, Wroe JM. Plasma cholinesterase changes during pregnancy. *Anaesthesia* 1980;35:651.
67. Ganga CC, Heyduk JV, Marx GF, Sklar GS. A comparison of the response to suxamethonium in post-partum and gynaecological patients. *Anaesthesia* 1982;37:903.
68. Leighton BL, Cheek TG, Gross JB, et al. Succinylcholine pharmacodynamics in peripartum patients. *Anesthesiology* 1986;64:202.
69. Kao YJ, Turner DR. Prolongation of succinylcholine block by metoclopramide. *Anesthesiology* 1989;70:905.
70. Gin T, Derrick JL, Chan MTV, Chui PT, Mak TWL. Postpartum patients have slightly prolonged neuromuscular block after mivacurium. *Anesth Analg* 1998;86:82.
71. Camp C, Tessem J, Adenwala J, Joyce TH III. Vecuronium and prolonged neuromuscular blockade in postpartum patients. *Anesthesiology* 1997;67:1006.
72. Khuenl-Brady KS, Koller J, Mair P, Puhringer F, Mitterschiffthaler G. Comparison of vecuronium and atracurium-induced neuromuscular blockade in postpartum and nonpregnant patients. *Anesth Analg* 1991; 72:110.
73. Zhou HH, Norman P, DeLima LGR, Mehta M, Bass D. The minimum alveolar concentration of isoflurane in patients undergoing bilateral tubal ligation in the postpartum period. *Anesthesiology* 1995;82:1364.
74. Marx GF, Kim YI, Lin C, Halevy S, Schulman H. Postpartum uterine pressures under halothane or enflurane anesthesia. *Obstet Gynecol* 1978;51:695.

Obstetric Anesthesia, second edition,
edited by Mark C. Norris.
Lippincott Williams & Wilkins, Philadelphia © 1999.

CHAPTER 38

Postoperative Analgesia

Craig M. Palmer

Cesarean delivery is probably the most frequently performed in-patient operation in the United States, with more than 860,000 done in 1993 [American College of Obstetricians and Gynecologists (ACOG)]. Such a large number of procedures in a relatively homogeneous population provides a ready opportunity to evaluate and compare many analgesic options. Although differences in study design often complicate comparison, in few other areas of medicine have such a variety of techniques and drugs been investigated. This chapter discusses clinical experience with postoperative analgesia in parturients.

Intramuscular and intravenous narcotics have long been the mainstay of pain therapy after cesarean delivery. In some hospitals, they are still the most widely practiced analgesic technique. The last two decades, however, have seen a major shift in the methods used for postoperative analgesia in obstetric patients. The discovery, beginning in the 1970s, of widely distributed receptor systems (both opioid and non-opioid) within the central nervous system, combined with the escalating use of regional anesthesia (1), produced a radically different approach to postoperative pain control.

EPIDURAL ANALGESIA

Morphine

In 1979, Behar et al. (2) reported that epidurally injected morphine effectively relieved pain in nonobstetric patients. Subsequently, multiple studies appeared analyzing the analgesic efficacy of epidural morphine.

Youngstrom et al. (3) reported a prospective, double-blind study of 35 patients who randomly received either epidural morphine, 4 mg, or intramuscular morphine, 4 mg, after epidural anesthesia for cesarean. A single dose of epidural morphine provided more profound and prolonged analgesia than did the same dose of intramuscular morphine (Table 1).

Writer et a1. (4) studied a larger series (207) of both obstetric and nonobstetric patients. Subjects randomly received either epidural morphine, 5 mg, or epidural placebo. Both the obstetric and nonobstetric patients who received epidural morphine had longer postoperative analgesia with lower supplemental narcotic requirements than did placebo patients. Parturients had longer pain relief after the same dose of morphine than did nonobstetric patients (18.3 ± 1.3 hours vs 9.2 ± 1.2 hours). In a similar study, 83% of parturients receiving 5 mg of epidural morphine reported good to excellent postoperative analgesia. Fifty-two percent needed no other analgesics for more than 24 hours (Fig. 1) (5).

An early dose–response study of epidural morphine involved 40 patients who received lumbar epidural anesthesia for cesarean delivery. They were prospectively randomized to one of four groups for postoperative analgesia: morphine, 7.5 mg intramuscularly, or morphine, 2.0, 5.0, or 7.5 mg epidurally. Women in the intramuscular-morphine group had pain relief for 1 to 3 hours after injection. Most patients receiving more than 2 mg epidural morphine had significant analgesia for more than 12 hours (Fig. 2) (6).

Palmer et al. (7) further defined the dose–response relation of epidural morphine for postcesarean analgesia in a prospective, randomized study of 60 parturients. Patients were randomly assigned to one of five groups and received between 0 and 5 mg epidural morphine at cesarean section; they then were given a patient-controlled analgesia (PCA) pump. Analysis of postoperative PCA use allowed quantification of the degree of analgesia provided by the epidural morphine. Supplemental PCA morphine use decreased significantly as dose of epidural morphine increased, up to an epidural dose of 3.75 mg. PCA use did not differ between the 3.75- and 5.0-mg epidural dose groups (Fig. 3). Using PCA to

C.M. Palmer: Department of Anesthesiology, University Medical Center, Tucson, Arizona 85724.

TABLE 1. *Median of hourly and total 6-hour visual-analog pain scores after epidural or intramuscular morphine*

Group	n	MS dose (mg)	Hour 1	2	3	4	5	6	Total
A	5	4 i.m.	4	3	3	4	4	3	19
BC	19	4 epidural	2	1	1[a]	1[a]	1[b]	1[b]	7[b]

Group A received morphine, 4 mg i.m., and epidural placebo. Groups B and C received epidural morphine, 4 mg, in 10 mL normal saline and i.m. placebo. In group C, 1:200,000 epinephrine was added to the epidural morphine solution.
[a] $p < 0.05$.
[b] $p < 0.01$, Wilcoxon rank-sum test. Data from ref. 3, with permission.

quantify postoperative analgesia allowed the authors to show a modest (PCA) morphine-sparing effect at low doses of epidural morphine (7).

Volume of diluent does not appear to be factor in the production of analgesia with epidural morphine. A randomized study of 60 parturients examining a 10-fold range of volume (2 to 20 mL) for dilution of 4 mg morphine found no difference among groups in the resulting quality of analgesia (7).

Today morphine remains the most widely used epidural opioid for analgesia after cesarean section. A number of reports confirmed the efficacy of epidural morphine (9–12). Although currently 5 mg is probably the most commonly used dose, it likely represents a modest overdose (7). Patients usually have good analgesia with lower doses. Four milligrams provides comparable analgesia for most patients and may decrease the incidence of side effects (10). A higher failure rate (i.e., diminished analgesia) becomes apparent if the dose is reduced further.

Side Effects of Epidural Morphine

Some of the initial enthusiasm for epidural morphine was dampened by the high incidence of accompanying side effects. As epidural morphine has become the "gold standard" against which other methods of postcesarean analgesia are inevitably compared, the following section characterizes its side effects in more detail before reviewing the use of other opioids for epidural analgesia.

Pruritus

Nearly all investigators studying epidural morphine have reported itching as a side effect; reports differ only in its frequency and severity (Table 2) (6,12–14). The pruritus associated with epidural morphine is characteristically mild. It occurs most commonly on the face or trunk, although it also may be generalized. In the clinically used range, itching is not significantly related to dose (Fig. 4) (7).

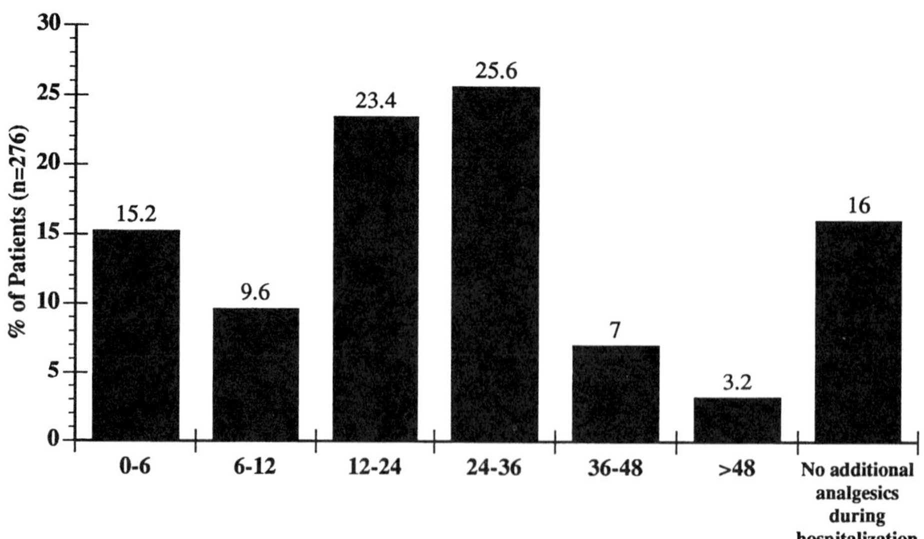

FIG. 1. Time to first request for additional analgesia after epidural morphine, 5 mg, after cesarean delivery. (Redrawn from ref. 5, with permission.)

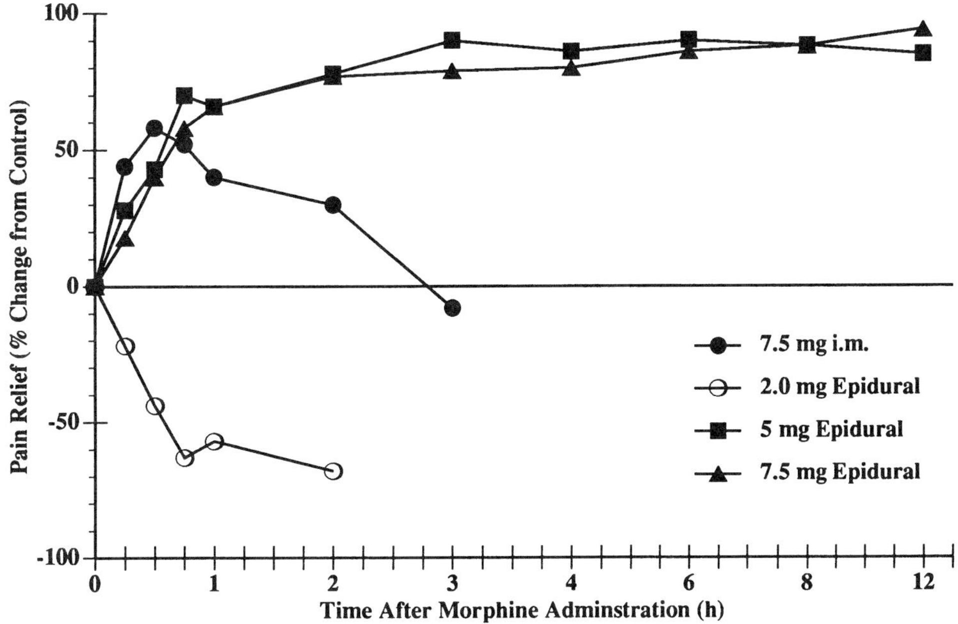

FIG. 2. Percentage changes in pain relief (from control) in parturients after cesarean section with either epidural or intramuscular morphine. Data represent average values with 10 women in each group. (Redrawn from ref. 6, with permission.)

The exact mechanism by which epidural morphine causes pruritus is unknown. Although pruritus resulting from epidural opioids is often dismissed as a simple μ receptor–related phenomenon, a careful review of the available data indicates this to be a much more complex issue, a full discussion of which is beyond the scope of this chapter (15,16). The role of opioid receptors in pruritus may be primarily by facilitation of other excitatory neuronal pathways and protective reflexes. A full understanding of this phenomenon awaits further investigation.

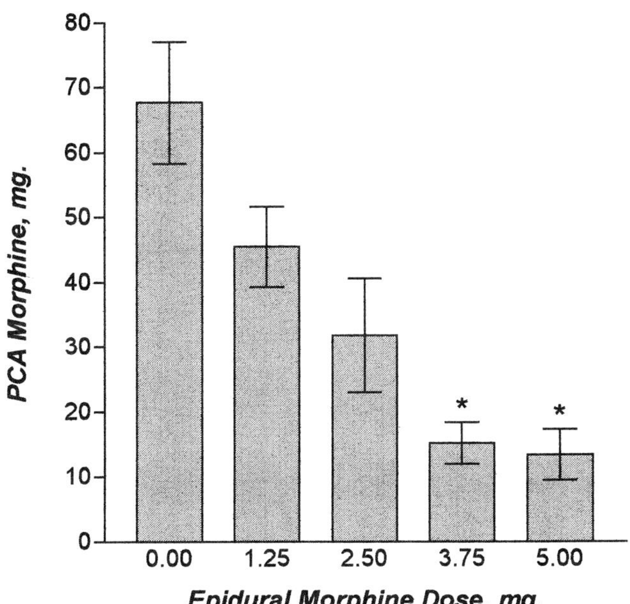

FIG. 3. Patient-controlled analgesia (PCA) morphine consumption over a 24-hour period versus dose of epidural morphine after cesarean delivery. PCA morphine use decreased significantly as dose of epidural morphine increased, up to 3.75 mg. (Data from ref. 7, with permission.)

Nausea and Vomiting

Nausea or vomiting occur less frequently after epidural morphine than does pruritus. Without differentiating nausea from vomiting, Leicht et al. (12) reported an incidence of 20% in a survey of 1,000 parturients. Kotelko et al. (5) reported nausea in 18% and vomiting in 11% of parturients who received 5 mg of epidural morphine. Fuller et al. (17) reported a 30% incidence of nausea and vomiting after unspecified doses of epidural morphine in their retrospective review of 4,880 parturients. Not all nausea and vomiting after cesarean delivery is due to epidural opioid. We found no difference in the incidence of nausea and vomiting between epidural morphine and placebo (7).

Epidural morphine can cause nausea and vomiting by stimulating the chemoreceptor trigger zone located in the base of the fourth ventricle of the brain. Morphine, a highly hydrophilic compound, remains free in the cerebrospinal fluid (CSF) for a long time. Morphine concentration in the cervical CSF increases slowly. It is undetectable for the first hour after lumbar epidural injection. Morphine concentration in cervical CSF peaks 3 to 4 hours after injection (Fig. 5) (18). In nonpregnant volunteers, Bromage et al. (19,20) found progressive rostral

TABLE 2. *Pruritus after epidural morphine*

Study	Dose epidural morphine (mg)	Pruritus (%)	Severe (or requiring treatment)
Ackerman et al. (13)	5	60	—
Gieraerts et al. (14)	5	80	—
Kotelko et al. (5)	5	68	28%
Leicht et al. (12)	5	27	4%

spread of cutaneous hyperalgesia after the injection of 10 mg epidural morphine, which was accompanied by nausea about 4 hours after injection in more than half the subjects. Radiographic studies of other water-soluble compounds confirmed that cephalad migration in the CSF does occur (21).

Respiratory Depression

Respiratory depression was recognized as a serious complication of epidural morphine shortly after its introduction to clinical use (22,23). The incidence of this potentially disastrous complication, and whether it is lower in the obstetric population, has been the subject of some debate. The risk is low enough that it can only be characterized by a large series of patients. A retrospective review of 4,880 parturients receiving an unspecified dose of epidural morphine after cesarean delivery found a respiratory rate less than 10 in only 12 patients, or 0.25% (17). A prospective study of 1,000 parturients who received morphine, 5 mg epidurally, reported four patients with a respiratory rate of less than 10 (12). Two of these women were observed and received no treatment. One, with a respiratory rate of nine breaths per minute and a normal arterial blood gas, received naloxone. The last had a respiratory rate of four to six breaths per minute, a p_aCO_2 of 76 mm Hg, and recovered without sequelae after intravenous naloxone. These reports suggest that the incidence of clinically significant respiratory depression after epidural morphine at doses of 5 mg or less in the obstetric population is at most 0.2% to 0.3%.

Respiratory depression after epidural morphine is often described as "late," with an onset between 6 and 12 hours after administration. Such late depression usually manifests as a decline in respiratory rate that, if untreated, will lead to progressive respiratory acidosis. The cause, as with nausea and vomiting, is the cephalad migration of morphine within the CSF, which leads to direct central depression of respiration. Based on case reports, the risk of respiratory depression probably increases as dose increases, at least beyond 5 mg.

Early respiratory depression after epidural morphine also is possible. This event probably arises from rapid systematic uptake or intravascular injection of the drug.

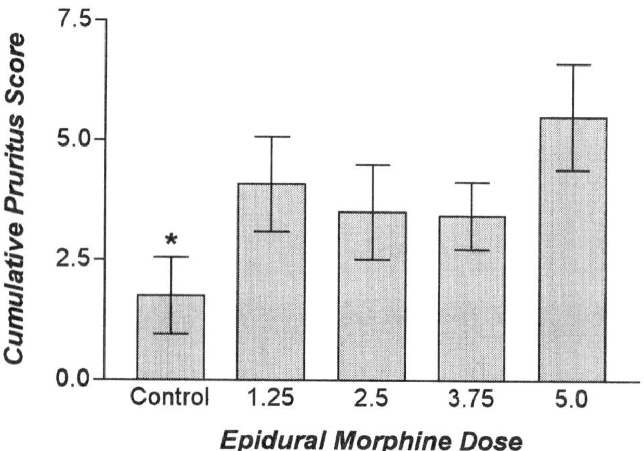

FIG. 4. Pruritus after epidural morphine in parturients after cesarean delivery. The severity of pruritus did not correlate with the dose of epidural morphine. (From C.M. Palmer, unpublished data, with permission.)

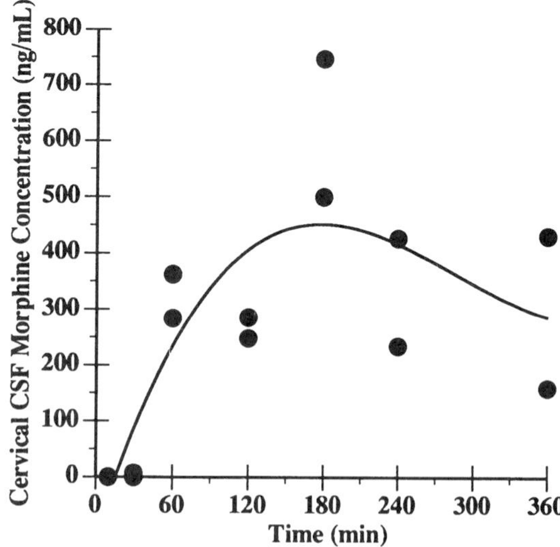

FIG. 5. Cervical cerebrospinal fluid (CSF) morphine concentrations at various times after lumbar epidural administration of 10 mg morphine. The patients were randomly allocated to have the CSF collection at the recorded times. Each point represents data from a single patient. Each patient had one CSF sample collected from the C_7 to T_1 interspace. (Data from ref. 18, with permission.)

In the absence of cephalad migration causing central depression of respiration, epidural morphine does not appear to have any characteristic effect on respiratory patterns. Slow respiratory rates and brief apneic periods occur both in patients who receive epidural morphine and those who receive intramuscular morphine. Brose and Cohen (24) monitored oxygen saturation in parturients receiving either epidural, intramuscular, or intravenous opioids after cesarean delivery. Some patients in all groups had periods of arterial desaturation (S_aO_2 less than 95%). Patients receiving epidural morphine or intramuscular meperidine were at greatest risk of transient periods of severe desaturation (S_aO_2 less than 85%). Similarly, Pan and James (25) found parturients receiving epidural morphine were more likely to experience mild desaturation (S_aO_2 90% to 95%) and to have lower respiratory rates 8 to 14 hours after surgery than parturients receiving parenteral morphine.

Herpes Simplex Labialis

In 1987, Gieraerts et al. (14) reported a prospective, nonrandomized study of 44 parturients after cesarean delivery. Twenty-six of these women received epidural morphine, 5 mg intraoperatively, and 3 to 5 mg up to twice daily thereafter. Another 18 women received intramuscular morphine, 10 mg, every 6 hours as needed for pain. Recurrent herpes simplex labialis (HSL) lesions appeared in nine of the 26 patients in the epidural group, but in none of the patients in the intramuscular group. The authors speculated that scratching to relieve epidural morphine-induced pruritus led to reactivation of the virus. Crone et al. (26) corroborated this report a year later, reporting HSL lesions recurred in 9.7% of patients who received epidural morphine after cesarean delivery, but in only 0.6% of those who did not. Boyle (27), reporting a series of more than 800 parturients, found that those who received epidural morphine were 11.5 times more likely to develop HSL lesions than were those who received parenteral morphine.

Other investigators have been unable to verify this association. Norris et al. (28) prospectively followed 203 parturients after cesarean delivery: 24 patients received epidural morphine, 3 to 5 mg; 81 patients received intrathecal morphine, 0.15 mg; and 98 patients received systemic opioids. They found that HSL developed in six of 105 patients receiving neuraxial morphine and in four of 98 patients receiving systemic opioids. Further, they noted no differences in the risk of HSV recurrence between general and regional anesthesia, or spinal and epidural anesthesia (Fig. 6).

Boyle (29) speculated that morphine reaching the trigeminal nucleus somehow decreases cell-mediated immunity, leading to recrudescence of latent herpes simplex virus-1 (HSV-1) lesions. The disparity in the findings of these different series may represent differences in the study populations that have not yet been characterized, or other recognized factors.

James (30) reported a case of herpes simplex blepharitis in a parturient after receiving 6.5 mg epidural morphine over a period of 2 days after cesarean delivery. As complications of such an infection are potentially more serious than oral herpes simplex, James thought a history of herpes infection in less common areas may be a relative contraindication to the use epidural morphine. It is difficult to make such a recommendation from a single case report. As clarification of any association between epidural morphine and the recurrence of oral herpes awaits further study (and a better understanding of the possible mechanism), most clinicians do not consider a history of oral herpes infection as a contraindication to epidural morphine.

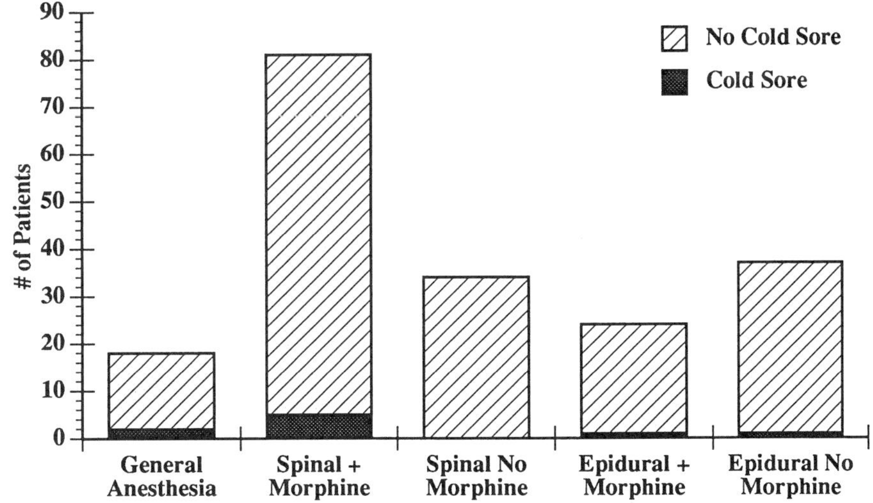

FIG. 6. Incidence of cold sore versus type of anesthesia, ± neuraxial morphine (n = 203). Neither type of anesthetic nor the use of neuraxial morphine correlated with the development of oral lesions. (Data from ref. 28, with permission.)

Treatment of Side Effects

Most cases of pruritus are mild and do not require treatment. Diphenhydramine, 25 to 50 mg, usually provides adequate symptomatic relief. The sedation associated with diphenhydramine may be as instrumental in providing relief as its antihistaminergic effect. Naloxone, 0.04 to 0.2 mg intravenously, also can relieve the itching, but must be titrated carefully to eliminate pruritus without reversing analgesia. Because of its short duration, a continuous infusion of naloxone may be needed to prevent recurrent itching. Start at 0.4 to 0.6 mg/h and titrate as needed.

In a case report, intravenous nalbuphine successfully stopped both pruritus and nausea associated with epidural opioid administration (31). A randomized, double-blind comparison of intravenous naloxone, 0.2 to 0.6 mg, and nalbuphine, 5 to 15 mg, found nalbuphine better at relieving the side effects of epidural morphine (32). Wang et al. (33) reported that a continuous infusion of nalbuphine reduced side effects from epidural morphine without affecting analgesia in nonobstetric patients. Kendrick et al. (34) compared naloxone and nalbuphine infusions for prophylaxis of epidural morphine-induced pruritus. Both infusions decreased the severity of pruritus, but higher doses also tended to decrease analgesia.

Propofol has been advocated as a treatment for epidural morphine-induced pruritus. One series compared propofol, 10 mg i.v., with naloxone, 2 μg/kg i.v., for treatment of severe pruritus (35). Both treatments had the same efficacy, but the level of discomfort (pain) increased in significantly more patients given naloxone. However, Warwick et al. (36) found this same dose of propofol ineffective. Although propofol may be an effective antipruritic, its current packaging (in 20-mL ampules) probably does not make it a cost-effective treatment.

Horta and Horta (37) found that large doses (2.5 mg!) of droperidol were effective in decreasing the incidence and severity of pruritus after epidural morphine but, not surprisingly, increased the incidence of somnolence. Finally, a recent report noted ondansetron to be an effective, but expensive, treatment for pruritus (38). This wide array of reported treatments by widely differing classes of agents underscores our lack of knowledge about opioid-related pruritus.

I have had good success treating morphine-induced pruritus with nalbuphine, 10 to 20 mg, i.v.* This treatment also may augment analgesia from the epidural opioid (31). Routinely using prophylactic or continuous infusions of nalbuphine or naloxone seems a cumbersome and expensive method of treating this side effect. Nalbuphine lasts longer than naloxone, so a continuous infusion should rarely be necessary. Further, nalbuphine reportedly reverses epidural opioid-induced respiratory depression (39,40).

Treatment options for nausea and vomiting include antiemetics and opioid antagonists. As noted, nausea and vomiting in this setting are often not due to the epidural morphine (4,7) and conventional antiemetics will be more effective. Droperidol, 2 mg intramuscularly, suffices (5). In my experience, intravenous ondansetron, 4 mg, and droperidol, 0.625 mg, are faster, more effective treatments. Intravenous nalbuphine, 5 to 10 mg, can relieve opioid-induced nausea and vomiting (31). Likewise, intravenous naloxone, 0.1 to 0.2 mg, also should work if the nausea is due to a morphine effect.

Early or late, the treatment of choice for respiratory depression is intravenous naloxone. Institute artificial or mechanical support of ventilation immediately if the patient is obtunded while waiting for naloxone to have effect.

Prevention of Side Effects

Several investigators have attempted to prevent the side effects of epidural morphine. Naloxone will reverse pruritus, nausea, and respiratory depression but also can reverse analgesia. Naloxone infusion can prevent side effects as well. Because naloxone must be carefully titrated and it can only be given intravenously, it has not found wide use as prophylactic therapy. Intravenous nalbuphine, although an effective treatment, does not prevent side effects after epidural morphine (30).

Naltrexone is a long-acting, orally administered opioid antagonist that may effectively limit the side effects of epidural morphine. In one study of patients after cesarean delivery, naltrexone, 5 mg orally, 1 hour after epidural morphine, 5 mg, decreased the incidence of pruritus, nausea, and vomiting compared with placebo (41). Neither pain scores nor the need for supplemental analgesics differed between the two groups. Abboud et al. (42) studied the effects of two different doses of naltrexone on analgesia and side effects. Women received 4 mg of epidural morphine after cesarean section. Those receiving naltrexone reported significantly less pruritus compared with placebo. The incidence of inadequate analgesia increased as the dose of naltrexone rose from 6 to 9 mg. The duration of analgesia (as determined by time to first remedication) decreased as the dose of naltrexone increased. Other studies involving the use of oral naltrexone after intrathecal morphine found that naltrexone decreased the incidence of side effects after intrathecal morphine but also tended to reverse the analgesia (43,44).

Some investigators attempted to reduce side effects by adding other drugs to epidural morphine. Lawhorn et al. (45) reported that the addition of 3 mg epidural butorphanol to 4 mg epidural morphine eliminated pruritus and nausea without hindering analgesia. Gambling et al.

*Editor's note: I routinely order nalbuphine, 5 mg i.v., q 4 to 6 h, as needed for itching.

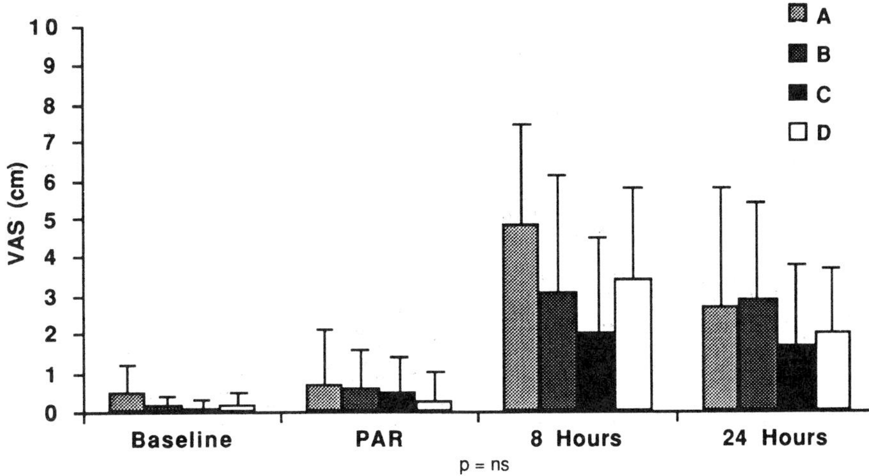

FIG. 7. Visual-analog scores for pruritus at preoperative baseline and 2, 8, and 24 hours after delivery in patients receiving epidural morphine with or without butorphanol. There were no significant differences among the groups. PAR, postanesthesia recovery, 2 hours after delivery. Groups (all medications injected via epidural catheter): A, 3 mg morphine + 1 mg butorphanol; B, 3 mg morphine + 2 mg butorphanol; C, 3 mg morphine + 3 mg butorphanol; D, 3 mg morphine alone. (Reprinted from ref. 46, with permission.)

(46) compared three doses of epidural butorphanol (1, 2, and 3 mg) or placebo as additives to 3 mg epidural morphine. They did not find any differences among the groups in pain, nausea, pruritus, or satisfaction, but did note significantly higher somnolence scores in the butorphanol groups (Fig. 7). Finally, Wittels et al. (47) examined epidural butorphanol, 3 mg, epidural nalbuphine, 10 mg, oral naltrexone, 6 mg, or placebo and epidural morphine, 4 mg. Pain scores were significantly higher in patients who received nalbuphine or naltrexone in the early postoperative period but were not different among the morphine (control) and butorphanol groups. Patients who received placebo were most likely to require treatment for pruritus. In all, these studies suggest that epidural butorphanol may modestly reduce, but not eliminate, epidural morphine side effects, but may cause side effects (somnolence) of its own.

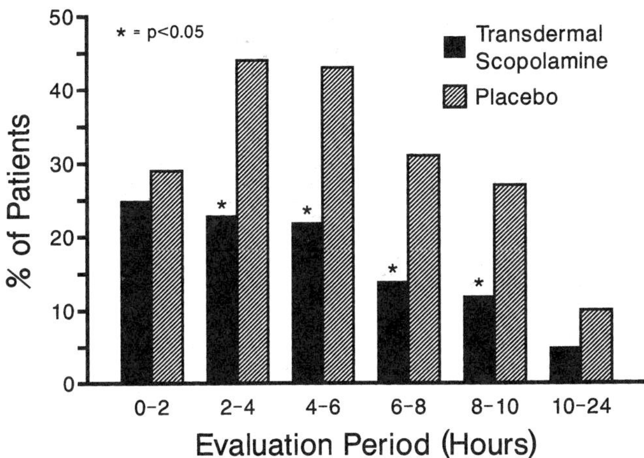

FIG. 8. Nausea and transdermal scopolamine. All women received 4 mg epidural morphine for analgesia after cesarean section. Patients receiving transdermal scopolamine experienced significantly less nausea during the first 12 hours after surgery. (Reproduced from ref. 48, with permission.)

Finally, prophylactic transdermal scopolamine decreases the incidence of nausea and vomiting during the first 24 hours after cesarean delivery (Fig. 8) (48). The scopolamine patch must be applied several hours in advance. Some patients then complain of dry mouth.

Other Epidural Opioids

Fentanyl

Morphine, although an excellent epidural analgesic, has limitations. The occurrence of side effects and a prolonged latency and duration complicate its use. These restraints have led investigators to try other compounds in a quest for a more "perfect" epidural analgesic. An early alternative explored was fentanyl, a phenylpiperidine derivative. Unlike morphine, fentanyl is highly lipid soluble. This characteristic accounts for much of the difference between the two compounds. Fentanyl is much more rapidly acting, has a shorter duration, and has greater potency.

In a dose–response study, 30 patients undergoing cesarean delivery with epidural bupivacaine randomly received one of six doses of epidural fentanyl. The investigators injected epidural fentanyl, 0 to 100 μg, after delivery (no intravenous fentanyl control group was included) (49). The onset of analgesia was rapid, and its duration was dose dependent. At 50 μg, all patients reported pain scores of 0 (Fig. 9). Twenty-five micrograms provided partial analgesia. Duration of pain relief increased as dose approached 50 μg. The duration of complete analgesia at this dose was about 4.5 hours (Fig. 10). Whereas these authors found that epidural fentanyl, 50 to 100 μg, reduced 24-hour morphine consumption, another group found that 100 μg of epidural fentanyl had no effect on 24-hour i.v. PCA morphine consumption (50). A similar

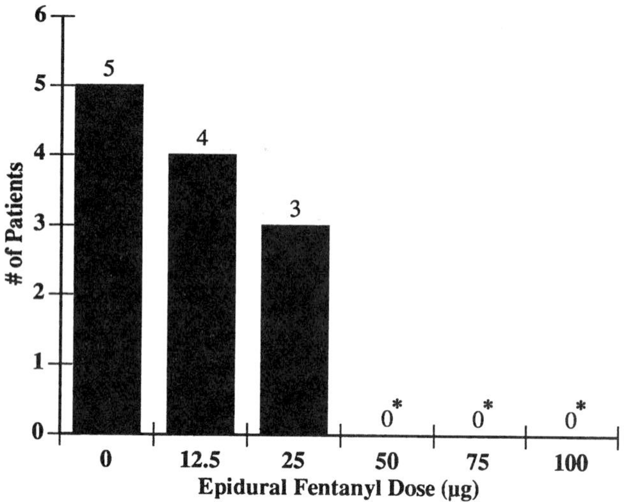

FIG. 9. Number of patients feeling pain during cesarean section after varying doses of epidural fentanyl. Six patients were in each group. All patients received 0.75% bupivacaine for epidural blockade for cesarean delivery. *$p < 0.1$ vs 0 μg. (Redrawn from ref. 49, with permission.)

study found better and longer-lasting perioperative analgesia with 75 μg or more epidural fentanyl (51).

The analgesic properties of fentanyl differ significantly from those of morphine. Epidural fentanyl, 75 μg, provides faster pain relief than epidural morphine, 2 mg. Epidural morphine has a markedly longer duration (52).

Adding epidural fentanyl to epidural morphine offers some advantages. Kotelko et al. (53) retrospectively reviewed 219 patients who received either no epidural opioids or epidural morphine, 3.5 mg, with either 100, 50, or 0 μg fentanyl. Only 4% of the patients who received epidural fentanyl required further intraoperative analgesics, compared with 37% who received epidural morphine alone and 71% of those who received no epidural opioids. The time to first analgesic request tended to be longer with the highest dose of fentanyl (100 μg).

Epidural fentanyl may have a direct spinal action, or it may produce analgesia only indirectly via systemic absorption. A randomized study of 40 parturients addressed this issue by comparing patient-controlled consumption of epidural and i.v. fentanyl (54). Patients in the epidural group reported lower pain scores and used less fentanyl compared with the intravenous group. The failure rate in the intravenous group (i.e., the number of parturients who requested discontinuation because of inadequate analgesia) was 45% compared with 0 in the epidural group. These data support the hypothesis that epidural fentanyl works primarily via a direct spinal action, or at least that this route of administration is more effective at delivering fentanyl to its primary site of action.

Opioid-related side effects also are common with epidural fentanyl. Forty percent of patients who received 25 μg of epidural fentanyl complained of itching (49). James et al. (55) reported pruritus in 75% of patients with a bolus technique and 100% of patients receiving a continuous epidural infusion. The itching required treatment in 12.5% to 20% of patients. Helbo-Hansen et al. (51) noted that pruritus increased with the dose of fentanyl up to 100 μg but characterized it as mild to moderate in almost all patients. Nausea and vomiting occurred less frequently, between 4% with a bolus technique (49) and 30% in patients receiving an epidural infusion (55). In some studies, epidural fentanyl protected against nausea and vomiting compared with control groups (51). Some patients also complained of drowsiness (49).

Respiratory depression was reported in one woman who received epidural fentanyl, 100 μg, at cesarean delivery. The depression responded rapidly to i.v. naloxone (56). Unlike epidural morphine, epidural fentanyl produces early-onset respiratory depression. This property in

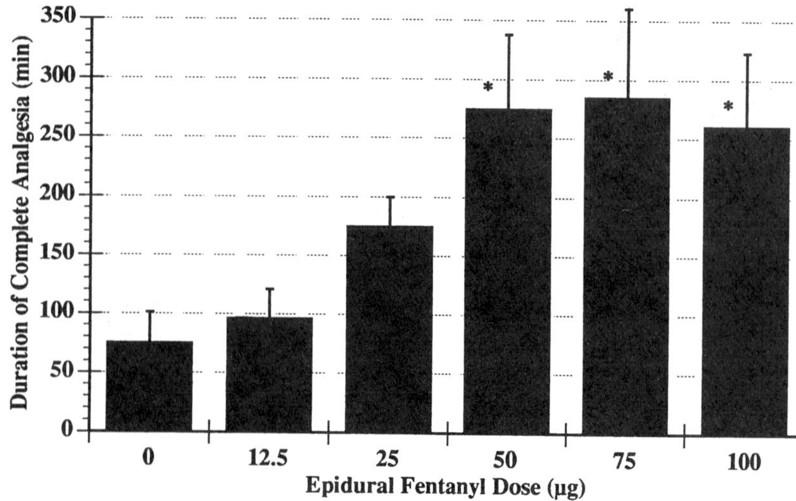

FIG. 10. Duration of complete analgesia (pain score, 0) after varying doses of epidural fentanyl. Values represent the mean ± SEM of six patients in each group. All patients received 0.75% bupivacaine for epidural blockade for cesarean delivery. *$p < 0.1$ vs 0 μg. (Redrawn from ref. 49, with permission.)

some ways lessens the risks of epidural fentanyl, as respiratory depression is likely to occur when the patient is still under the anesthesiologist's direct care and supervision, rather than hours later.

Gourlay et a1. (57) studied the pharmacokinetics of lumbar epidural fentanyl, 1 μg/kg, in patients with chronic pain. Fentanyl rapidly crossed the dura and underwent cephalad migration. Cervical CSF fentanyl concentrations were approximately 10% of lumbar CSF concentrations. Peak cervical CSF concentration varied considerably. The mean time to peak concentration was 22 minutes (Fig. 11.)

In summary, epidural fentanyl, 50 to 100 μg, rapidly provides profound analgesia for up to 4 hours. Increasing the dose further neither improves nor prolongs pain relief. The short duration limits fentanyl's utility as a postoperative analgesic. Like epidural morphine, epidural fentanyl can cause both bothersome and serious side effects.

Sufentanil

Sufentanil, like fentanyl, is a phenylpiperidine derivative. Intravenously, sufentanil is approximately 10 times as potent as fentanyl. Sufentanil is even more lipid soluble than is fentanyl and possesses a high affinity for the μ receptor. In 1987, Madej and Strunin (58) compared the analgesia provided by a single 100-μg bolus of epidural fentanyl with four different doses of epidural sufentanil in a randomized, blinded study of 50 parturients. The

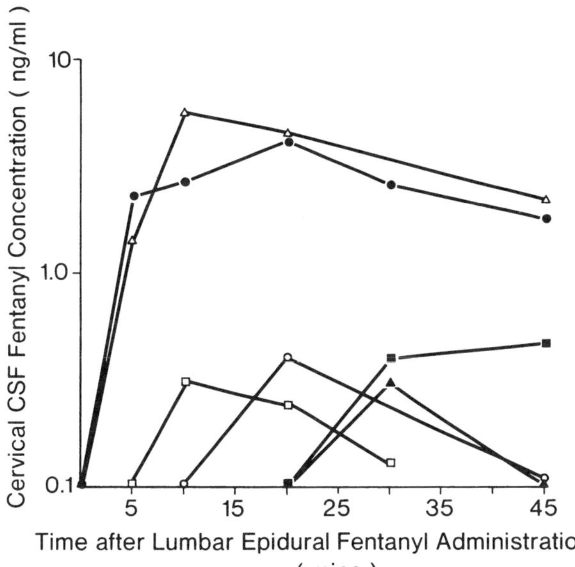

FIG. 11. Cerebrospinal fluid (CSF) fentanyl concentrations as a function of time after lumber epidural administration of 1 μg/kg body weight of fentanyl to patients with chronic pain. Each line represents values from a single patient. (Reprinted from ref. 57, with permission.)

duration of pain relief was related to dose, but was similar, after either drug (Fig. 12). Drowsiness and sedation appeared to increase with larger doses of sufentanil. Nausea and vomiting increased with 30 μg of sufentanil. Pruritus was common in all groups.

Others have compared intravenous and epidural sufentanil (59) and epidural morphine with epidural sufentanil (60). Epidural sufentanil, 50 μg, produced more prolonged pain relief than did intravenous sufentanil, 30 μg. Epidural sufentanil, 30 to 60 μg, delivered prompt, short-lasting analgesia. In contrast, epidural morphine, 5 mg, had a long latency and a long duration. Side effects were common in both studies. Itching occurred regardless of sufentanil dose or route of administration. Nausea and vomiting occurred in 20% of patients after either epidural morphine and sufentanil, 60 μg. Both studies concluded that 30 μg of epidural sufentanil was an effective dose for postoperative analgesia.

Like fentanyl, the major advantage of epidural sufentanil over epidural morphine is its rapid onset. The incidence of side effects is comparable to, or higher than, equianalgesic doses of epidural morphine. Larger doses slightly prolong epidural sufentanil analgesia. Nonetheless, morphine provides much longer-lasting pain relief. None of the currently available studies is large enough to evaluate the risk of respiratory depression. When given intravenously at these doses, sufentanil can produce profound respiratory depression.

Meperidine

Meperidine, also known as pethidine, is another phenylpiperidine derivative. In a study that combined patients with cesarean section with those with lower abdominal surgery, Brownridge and Frewin (61) compared epidural meperidine, 50 mg, with epidural bupivacaine, 25 mg, or intramuscular meperidine, 100 mg. Epidural meperidine produced a lower pain score than did intramuscular meperidine or epidural bupivacaine. The duration of all three treatments ranged between 150 and 200 minutes. Patients preferred epidural meperidine to the other two analgesics. Perriss et a1. (62) compared epidural meperidine, 50 mg, with intramuscular meperidine, 100 mg, in patients after cesarean section. Epidural meperidine had a faster onset than intramuscular meperidine, but the same duration. Epidural meperidine provided significantly better analgesia in all patients. The incidence of sedation, nausea, and vomiting was low in both groups, and pruritus was not reported. Ngan Kee et al. (63) looked at the dose–response relation of epidural meperidine. Speed of onset and duration increased as the dose increased from 12.5 to 25 mg, but increasing the dose to 100 mg provided no additional benefit (Table 3). All doses more than 25 mg provided effective pain relief for about 165 minutes. Side effects were infrequent except at the very highest dose (100 mg). Although epidural meperi-

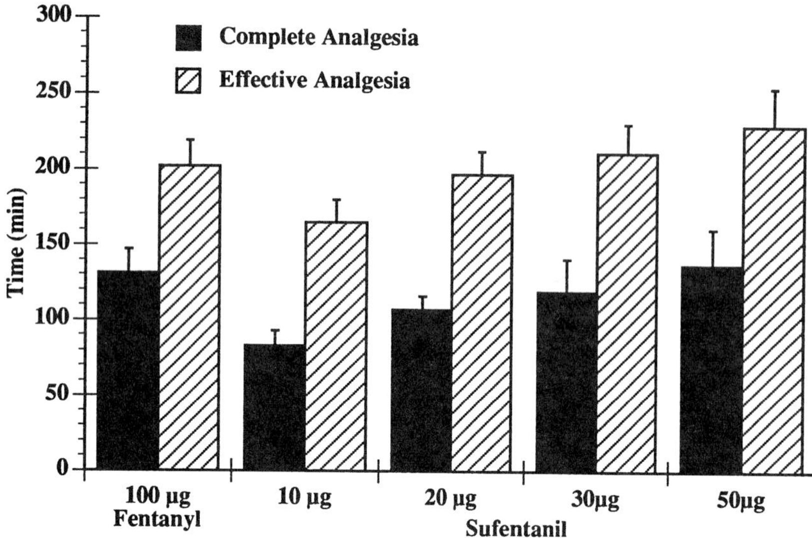

FIG. 12. Duration of complete analgesia (pain score, 0) and effective analgesia (time to first request for additional analgesia) after 100 µg of epidural fentanyl or varying doses of epidural sufentanil. All patients received 2% lidocaine with 1:200,000 epinephrine for epidural anesthesia for cesarean delivery. Values represent the mean ± SEM. The duration of pain relief was related to dose but similar after either drug. (Data from ref. 58, with permission.)

dine would appear to be an effective postoperative analgesic, its clinical utility is limited by its short duration.

Hydromorphone

Hydromorphone, commonly known as Dilaudid, is a semisynthetic derivative of morphine that is available in a preservative-free solution. Its analgesic potency, administered systemically, is roughly twice that of morphine. Henderson et a1. (64) compared epidural hydromorphone, 1.0 mg, with intramuscular hydromorphone, 2 mg, in 30 parturients after cesarean delivery. The mean time to first request for additional analgesia was 19.3 hours in the epidural group versus 5.0 hours in the intramuscular group. Visual-analog pain scores were significantly lower in the epidural group between 4 and 12 hours after injection. Halpern et al. (65) compared epidural morphine, 3 mg, with epidural hydromorphone, 0.6 mg, and found no differences in duration of analgesia or the incidence of side effects. In a randomized, blinded study of 40 parturients, epidural injection of both hydromorphone, 1.0 mg, and morphine, 5.0 mg, provided good pain relief, but morphine provided significantly longer analgesia (21.1 vs 12.0 hours for hydromorphone) (66).

Side effects after epidural hydromorphone are at least as common as those after epidural morphine. Chestnut et al. (67) reported a 42% incidence of nausea and vomiting and a 58% incidence of pruritus after epidural hydromorphone, 1.0 mg. Others reported no significant differences in side effects between epidural morphine and hydromorphone (65,68). None of these series reported respiratory depression, although the numbers of patients were too small to gauge the risk of this complication accurately.

Other Opioids

Epidural methadone provides more rapid onset of analgesia than does epidural morphine. In one study, the mean duration of analgesia after epidural methadone, 4 mg, was 4.8 hours (69), whereas another reported a median duration of 6.5 hours after 5 mg (70).

Diamorphine (heroin) has been used as an epidural analgesic. Roulson et al. (71) found the duration of analgesia to be 15 to 17 hours after 2.5 mg, whereas Haynes et al. (70) reported the median duration after 5 mg to be

TABLE 3. *Time to first patient-controlled epidural analgesia (PCEA) demand and total 24-hour meperidine consumption by PCEA*

	Dose epidural meperidine (mg)				
	12.5	25	50	75	100
First PCEA demand (min)	83 (44–116)	165 (127–213)	175 (117–232)	188 (127–254)	170 (122–246)
24 hour meperidine consumption (mg)	260 (160–500)	200 (140–340)	240 (160–425)	300 (160–415)	220 (140–360)

Values expressed as median (interquartile range). Duration of analgesia was longer after 25 mg vs 12.5 mg ($p = 0.0005$), but there were no differences between 25 mg and any of the larger doses.
Data from ref. 63, with permission.

14 hours, and still others reported only 5.7 hours (72). Diamorphine is not readily available in the United States.

Agonist/Antagonists

Butorphanol

Butorphanol is a mixed opioid agonist/antagonist. It has both agonist and antagonist actions at the μ receptor. It is a pure agonist at the δ and κ receptors. Hoping to avoid the side effects of epidural morphine, specifically nausea, pruritus, and respiratory depression, several investigators studied the epidural use of butorphanol in obstetric patients.

Naulty et al. (73) reported that 2 mg of epidural butorphanol prolonged postoperative analgesia after cesarean delivery under epidural anesthesia. Increasing the dose of butorphanol increased the duration of analgesia and led to a dose-related decrease in supplemental narcotic use. No patient complained of nausea or pruritus. The only side effect reported was somnolence, occurring in 13 of 14 patients who received 2 mg or more of epidural butorphanol. The somnolence lasted approximately 6 hours, although patients were reportedly "easily arousable." Epidural butorphanol has a faster onset but a shorter duration than epidural morphine (Fig. 13) (74). Epidural injection of both morphine and butorphanol slightly decreased central sensitivity to carbon dioxide (74).

The low incidence of pruritus after epidural butorphanol is its major advantage. The short duration and high incidence of somnolence are significant shortcomings. Combining morphine and butorphanol for postcesarean epidural analgesia may modestly decrease pruritus compared with morphine alone (45–47). It may not be appropriate, however, to give a new mother a treatment with a high likelihood of causing drowsiness during an important time in her and her new baby's lives.

Nalbuphine

Nalbuphine is another mixed opioid agonist/antagonist. It has antagonist effects at the μ receptor, agonist effects at the σ receptor, and partial agonist effects at the κ receptor. Its antagonist properties may limit the potential for respiratory depression and other side effects after epidural administration but also may limit its analgesic potency.

Camann et al. (75) studied the dose–response relation of epidural nalbuphine for post–cesarean section analgesia. Epidural nalbuphine, 10 mg, afforded just over an hour of analgesia, whereas doses of 20 to 30 mg increased the duration to more than 3 hours. The only significant side effect was somnolence, which was seen in up to 50% of patients after 30 mg. They concluded that nalbuphine was "disappointing" as an analgesic after cesarean section.

α_2 Agonists

Clonidine

Clonidine is an α-adrenergic type 2–receptor agonist. After oral administration, it has significant antihypertensive actions. After epidural or spinal injection, it produces significant analgesia. Only a few of the data on the analgesic effects of neuraxial clonidine come from parturients.

In 1989, a report appeared describing the use of epidural clonidine in six women after cesarean delivery (76). These women received epidural clonidine, 800 to

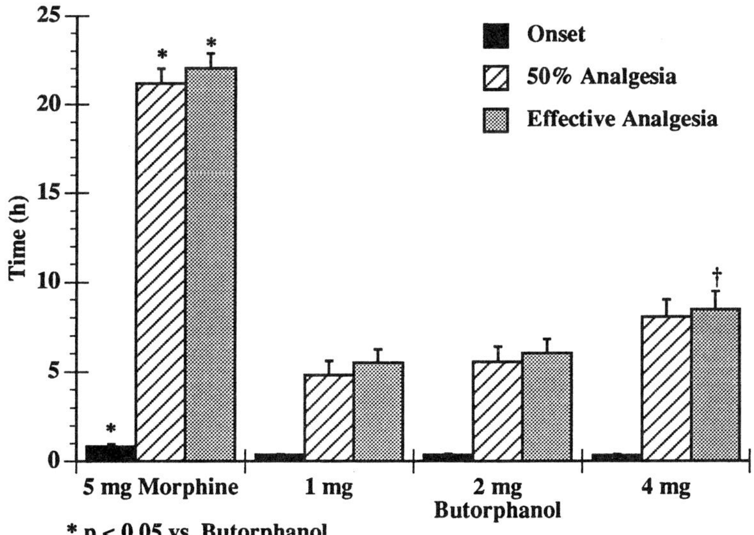

FIG. 13. Onset and duration of 50% analgesia [pain relief 50% by visual analog score (VAS)] and effective analgesia with epidural morphine or various doses of epidural butorphanol. Values represent the mean ± SEM. All patients received 2% lidocaine with 1:200,000 epinephrine for epidural anesthesia for cesarean delivery. (Redrawn from ref. 74, with permission.)

900 μg, on the first complaint of pain. They self-administered intravenous morphine for additional pain relief. No patient required morphine within 4 hours after clonidine injection. Twenty-four-hour morphine use (23 mg) was less than a historical control group (62 mg). Sedation was the only side effect reported and was described as "prominent" in the first hour after injection.

These investigators then studied the analgesic effects of continuous infusions of epidural clonidine (77). One group received clonidine, 400 μg epidurally, followed by an infusion at 10 μg/h; a second group received clonidine, 800 μg epidurally and a 20-μg/h infusion; and a control group received a saline bolus and infusion. Further analgesia was provided by intravenous morphine through a PCA pump. Both clonidine groups reported better analgesia for 6 hours after injection than did the saline control group. Only the higher infusion rate decreased 24-hour opioid use (Fig. 14). Decreased heart rate and blood pressure occurred in both clonidine groups. The decreased opioid use may have reflected the prolonged sensory blockade produced by epidural clonidine. In a separate study (78), a bolus of 400 μg clonidine followed by a 40-μg/h clonidine infusion provided analgesia equivalent to an 800-μg bolus followed by a similar infusion; interestingly, 2-chloroprocaine inhibited much of the clonidine-induced analgesia (see later).

Capogna et al. (79) studied the addition of either 75 or 150 μg clonidine to an epidural bolus dose of morphine, 2 mg, with 0.125% bupivacaine and epinephrine. They found a dose-dependent increase in the duration of analgesia and a reduction in the total dose of morphine administered. They found no difference in hemodynamic or respiratory parameters between the clonidine groups and a control group.

Eisenach et al. (80) used an isobolographic method to determine whether the interaction between epidural clonidine and epidural opioids, in this case, fentanyl, is additive or synergistic. In a study of 90 postcesarean parturients, they found that the median effective dose (ED_{50}) of the combination of clonidine and fentanyl was only 52% of that predicted by an additive interaction, though there was wide variability of response (Fig. 15).

These studies revealed several consistent side effects associated with epidural clonidine. In human volunteers, epidural clonidine produces sedation, decreases blood pressure and heart rate, and appears to increase peripheral blood flow (81). These effects largely parallel those seen in animals (82). Sympathectomy and decreased cardiac filling pressures are the probable mechanism of hypotension. An infusion of crystalloid restores all variables. Epidural clonidine appears to have no negative inotropic effects. Oral clonidine appears to share many of the analgesic properties of epidural clonidine (83).

These studies suggest that as a postoperative analgesic, the usefulness of clonidine will be limited. Epidural clonidine is largely without the usual side effects associated with epidural opioids (pruritus, nausea, vomiting, respiratory depression), but appears to have its own set of side effects (sedation, decreased blood pressure) that could prove equally bothersome. Finally, the short duration of epidural clonidine means an infusion is necessary beyond the immediate postoperative period. It may prove useful as an adjunct to other agents when a continuous-infusion technique is used for postoperative analgesia.

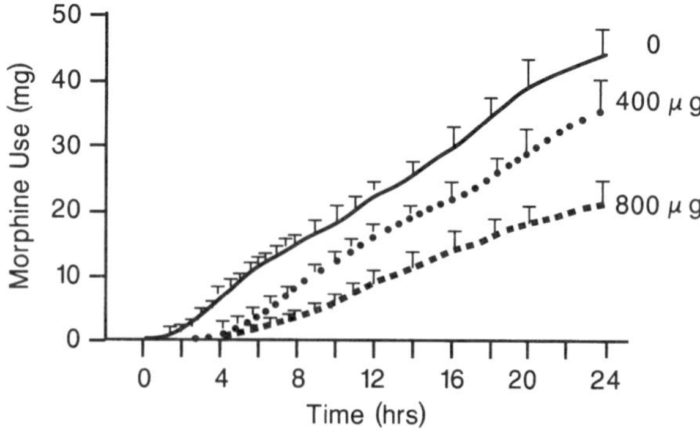

FIG. 14. Cumulative mean patient-controlled anesthesia (PCA) morphine use by patients receiving either 800 μg, 400 μg, or no epidural clonidine as a bolus after cesarean delivery under epidural anesthesia. (Reprinted from ref. 77, with permission.)

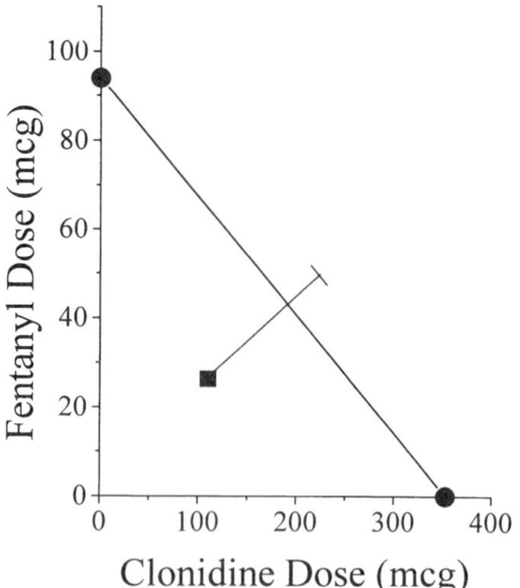

FIG. 15. Isobologram of epidural clonidine and fentanyl. The points on each axis represent the median effective duration (ED_{50}) of each drug alone. The interconnecting line is the line of additivity. The point in the center of the graph represents the combination of clonidine and fentanyl. The confidence intervals for this point include the line of additivity, indicating that the effect produced by a combination of these two drugs does not differ from an additive one. (Reprinted from ref. 80, with permission.)

Epinephrine

Epinephrine, a naturally occurring catecholamine with both α- and β-adrenergic agonist actions, has been used with a variety of epidural analgesics. The primary aim of this combination is to prolong analgesia, and secondary goals are to decrease the incidence of side effects and decrease systemic uptake. A point often overlooked is epinephrine's α_2-adrenergic agonist property. α_2 Agonism is presumed to be the basis for clonidine-mediated analgesia, and this mechanism may give epinephrine some of its intrinsic analgesic properties (84,85).

Most investigators have focused on using epinephrine to enhance the duration of the shorter-acting epidural opioids. One randomized, blinded study compared analgesia after cesarean delivery with epidural fentanyl alone with epidural fentanyl with epinephrine, 1:400,000 (86). Each patient received two injections of her assigned study solution. No difference was found between groups in speed of onset or duration of analgesia after the first injection. Duration of analgesia after the second injection was longer in the epinephrine group. More women (44%) in the epinephrine group complained of itching than in the control group (17%).

Leicht et al. (87) found that epinephrine, 300 μg, significantly prolonged the duration of analgesia provided by epidural sufentanil, 50 μg (348 vs 266 min). Side effects occurred with equal frequency in both groups, but with greater severity in the epinephrine group. Another series found no prolongation of analgesia from sufentanil, 30 μg, by epinephrine, 1:200,000 (50 μg, a much smaller epinephrine dose than earlier) (88).

Dougherty et al. (89) added epinephrine, 1:200,000 (total dose of epinephrine, 50 μg), to epidural hydromorphone, 1.5 mg, for analgesia after cesarean delivery. Compared with patients who received the same amount of epidural hydromorphone alone, the epinephrine group had a slightly faster onset and slightly better analgesia over the initial 12 hours after injection. The duration of effective analgesia was somewhat longer in the epinephrine group: 24.3 hours versus 18.2 hours. The epinephrine patients requested fewer additional analgesics. Pruritus was common in both groups (more than 70%). All patients received prophylactic intravenous nalbuphine and droperidol, however, making comparison with other series difficult. Smith et al. (72) reported a modest increase in the duration of analgesia of epidural diamorphine, 5 mg, with the addition of epinephrine.

In parturients, epinephrine may prolong the analgesic effects of shorter-acting opioids. This prolongation often comes at the expense of an increased incidence or severity of side effects. Except for hydromorphone, the duration of analgesia still is well short of that obtained with epidural morphine alone. If used as a component of a continuous epidural infusion, epinephrine may reduce the infusion rate and total amount of opioid.

Controversies

Youngstrom (3) reported marked and prolonged analgesia in parturients who received epidural morphine after 2-chloroprocaine anesthesia. Later, Kotelko et al. (90) reported that the use of 2-chloroprocaine for epidural anesthesia impaired the analgesic efficacy of epidural morphine. They speculated that the low pH of the chloroprocaine solution interfered with the action of epidural morphine, possibly by causing the morphine to remain highly ionized in the epidural space (91). 2-Chloroprocaine remains a popular local anesthetic in obstetrics, and this observation ignited a lingering controversy.

A randomized, prospective comparison of epidural morphine after either 2-chloroprocaine or lidocaine anesthesia for cesarean section also found poorer analgesia in the 2-chloroprocaine group (92). Using even small (7 mL) doses of 2-chloroprocaine to "test" epidural catheters significantly impairs subsequent epidural morphine analgesia (93). Other investigators reported no differences in the duration of epidural morphine analgesia after different local anesthetics (94).

The inhibitory effect of 2-chloroprocaine is not limited to epidural morphine. Epidural fentanyl, 50 μg, provides significantly shorter analgesia after lidocaine or 2-chloroprocaine than after bupivacaine or lidocaine with epinephrine (95). Grice et al. (96) also found a shorter duration of epidural fentanyl in laboring women after 2-chloroprocaine compared with lidocaine.

The mechanism of 2-chloroprocaine's inhibitory effect has been elusive. At first, relatively low pH of the then available formulation was blamed (91). Other possibilities included a "window" effect, due to the rapid regression of 2-chloroprocaine sensory blockade (91,97). Others suggested that a metabolite of 2-chloroprocaine is a μ-receptor antagonist (98). Finally, a μ-receptor action of the local anesthetic itself has been considered. 2-Chloroprocaine adversely affects fentanyl analgesia (μ-receptor mediated), but not butorphanol analgesia (κ-receptor mediated) (99).

The most thorough investigation of this phenomenon was reported by Coda et al. (100), who used an in vitro preparation to study the affinity of 2-chloroprocaine, its metabolites, and various μ- and κ-receptor agonists for these receptors. While 2-chloroprocaine does have some affinity for μ (and κ) receptors, the concentrations at which this affinity becomes significant make it an unlikely cause of 2-chloroprocaine's observed in vivo opioid antagonism.

The preponderance of recent evidence indicates that 2-chloroprocaine can significantly decrease the analgesia resulting from epidural morphine and fentanyl, although the exact mechanism remains elusive. Epidural administration of opioids has become widespread in obstetrics. When using 2-chloroprocaine, be aware that epidural opioid analgesia may not be ideal, and be prepared to offer an alternative form of pain relief.

Summary

There are a variety of ways to provide epidural opioid analgesia after cesarean delivery. The following recommendations reflect the current practice at the University of Arizona. Most commonly, we rely on fentanyl and morphine for postoperative analgesia after a bupivacaine or lidocaine epidural anesthetic. We avoid using 2-chloroprocaine except in the most urgent situations owing to its negative interaction with epidural opioids. Fentanyl, 50 to 100 μg, mixed with the local anesthetic, enhances intraoperative comfort and provides early postoperative analgesia. Morphine is still the longest-lasting epidural opioid available and is the mainstay of postoperative analgesia in our practice. Immediately after delivery, we give morphine, 4 mg, in a volume of 8 mL.

We have had good success treating pruritus, and to a lesser extent, nausea and vomiting with intravenous nalbuphine. Not all patients will respond predictably, however, and other medications may be required.

These recommendations, and those presented in the studies cited, are applicable to most parturients. While it is convenient to think of this patient population in terms of means and averages, individual responses are distributed along a bell-shaped curve. It is impossible to predict how any individual will respond. Despite the fact that most patients will have sufficient analgesia with this regimen, others will require significant additional medications. If a parturient requires significant amounts of additional analgesics in the early postoperative period, we do not hesitate to give them a PCA device for additional analgesia (see later).

Because of the theoretical risk of respiratory depression and the occurrence of side effects, we find standard postoperative orders very useful (Table 4). Nurses check and record respiratory rates hourly for 24 hours after epidural morphine. If respiratory rate decreases below eight breaths per minute, the nurse should immediately inject naloxone and notify the anesthesiologist. In the absence of other sedatives or narcotics, respiratory depression of this degree is extremely uncommon. A review of our experience over the last 8 years encompassing more than 4,500 cesarean births (the vast majority of whom received neuraxial morphine) revealed no incidents of respiratory depression requiring naloxone reversal.

TABLE 4. *Postoperative neuraxial opioid orders*

1. Epidural/intrathecal__________,_____mg, administered at _____ hours on _____ (date).
2. No sedatives or narcotics administered except by order of anesthesiologist.
3. One ampule naloxone at bedside at all times.
4. Maintain i.v. access or heparin-lock at all times.
5. Measure and record respiratory rate q 1 h; for respiratory rate $<$8/min, give naloxone, 0.2 mg i.v., slowly over 2 min; notify anesthesiologist.
6. Supplemental analgesics: nalbuphine, 10–20 mg i.v. q 4 h p.r.n. pain.
7. For pruritus: nalbuphine, 10–20 mg i.v. q 4 h p.r.n. itching.
8. For nausea/vomiting: nalbuphine, 10–20 mg i.v. q 4 h p.r.n. nausea and vomiting.
9. For pain, pruritus, or nausea/vomiting unresponsive to above, page anesthesiologist on call.
10. This protocol covers 24 h after each dose of neuraxial narcotic.

SUBARACHNOID ANALGESIA

The past decades have seen the resurgence of spinal anesthesia for cesarean delivery. As the use of spinal anesthesia has increased, so has the use of intrathecal opioids for postoperative analgesia.

Morphine

In 1979, Wang et al. (101) reported that small doses of intrathecal morphine provided prolonged analgesia in patients with chronic pain. In parturients, subarachnoid morphine produces excellent pain relief after cesarean section. The duration of analgesia ranges from 18.6 hours after 0.1 mg to 27.7 hours after 0.25 mg (102). Women not receiving subarachnoid morphine typically request analgesics 3.4 hours after cesarean delivery with intrathecal bupivacaine (Fig. 16). In a retrospective review, 0.3 to 0.5 mg of intrathecal morphine provided pain relief for more than 20 hours in 78% of women (103). A tendency toward longer-lasting analgesia was noted with higher doses. Zakowski et al. (104) prospectively compared the duration of analgesia after 0.2, 0.4, or 0.6 mg of intrathecal morphine administered with 12 mg of bupivacaine for spinal anesthesia. After 0.6 mg, analgesia lasted 44 hours.

Palmer et al. (105 and unpublished data) studied the dose–response relation of intrathecal morphine in more detail. Parturients were randomized to one of nine groups, receiving between 0 and 0.5 mg intrathecal morphine at cesarean delivery, and then given i.v.-PCA morphine after surgery. Surprisingly, intrathecal morphine provided effective analgesia at very small doses; whereas self-administered PCA morphine use was predictably highest in the 0 and 0.025-mg intrathecal morphine groups, there was no difference in PCA morphine use over the wide range of 0.1 to 0.5 mg intrathecal morphine. The incidence of pruritus and the need for treatment interventions increased significantly as the dose of intrathecal morphine increased, although the incidence of nausea and vomiting did not (Fig. 17). These data indicate that the steep portion of the intrathecal morphine analgesia dose–response curve lies below 0.1 mg (Fig. 18). They concluded the optimal dose of intrathecal morphine for postcesarean analgesia was between 0.1 mg and 0.2 mg. Similar conclusions were reached in

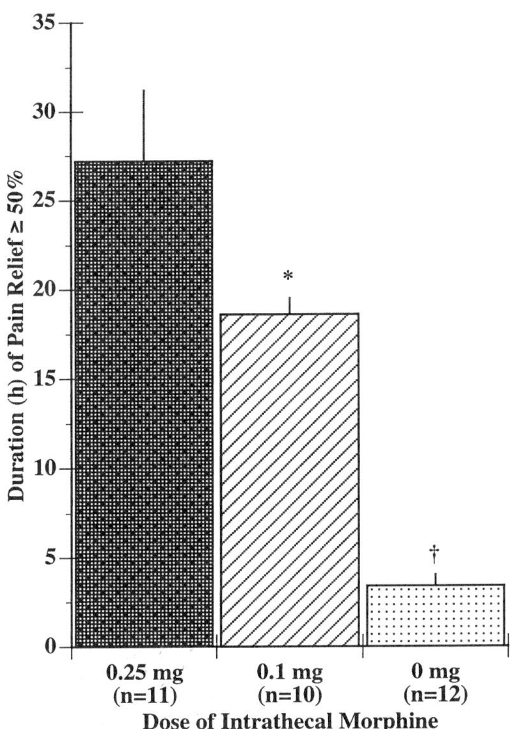

FIG. 16. Duration of subjective pain relief as assessed by visual-analog score in parturients receiving intrathecal morphine or placebo after cesarean section. $^{*}p < 0.05$ vs 0 mg morphine, $^{\dagger}p < 0.05$ vs 0.1 and 0.25 mg morphine. (Data from ref. 102, with permission.)

subsequent series studying doses of intrathecal morphine of 0.2 mg or less (106,107).

Patients continued to self-medicate with PCA morphine at a constant rate despite a 5-fold to 10-fold increase in the dose of intrathecal morphine. Increasing the dose of spinal morphine did not improve analgesia, but concurrently administering parenteral morphine did. These results suggest that optimal analgesia requires occupation of opiate receptors at two distinct sites; intrathecal morphine occupies spinal receptors, and parenteral (PCA) morphine acts at supraspinal receptors. Support for this spinal–supraspinal receptor synergy can be found in animal models (108) and also has been hypothesized to be important for the effects of spinally administered sufentanil (109).

Side effects reported after intrathecal morphine are comparable to those seen after epidural morphine. Pruritus occurs in 40% to 80% of patients and appears to be dose dependent (102,103, C.M. Palmer, unpublished data). Huffnagle et al. (106) found no difference between control and treatment groups in the degree of pruritus, but the pruritus in the control group may have been due to systemic (PCA) morphine, which also can cause pruritus. Vomiting occurs rarely after low doses (0.1 mg) of morphine, but in up to one third of patients receiving larger doses (0.25 mg) (102,103), Palmer et al. (unpublished data) could find no relation between the dose of intrathecal morphine and nausea or vomiting. Clinically significant respiratory depression is rare (103) but has been reported (110–113). Abboud et al. (102) reported no depression of respiratory response to carbon dioxide challenge in patients receiving 0.1 to 0.25 mg subarachnoid morphine (Fig. 19). Subarachnoid morphine, 0.2 mg, rarely produced clinically significant respiratory depression in a series of more than 1,600 parturients (114). Eight markedly obese patients had episodes of respiratory depression (S_aO_2 less than 85% or respiratory rate less than 10 per minute).

The optimal dose of subarachnoid morphine is between 0.1 and 0.2 mg, which should provide more than 20 hours of good analgesia while avoiding an excessive

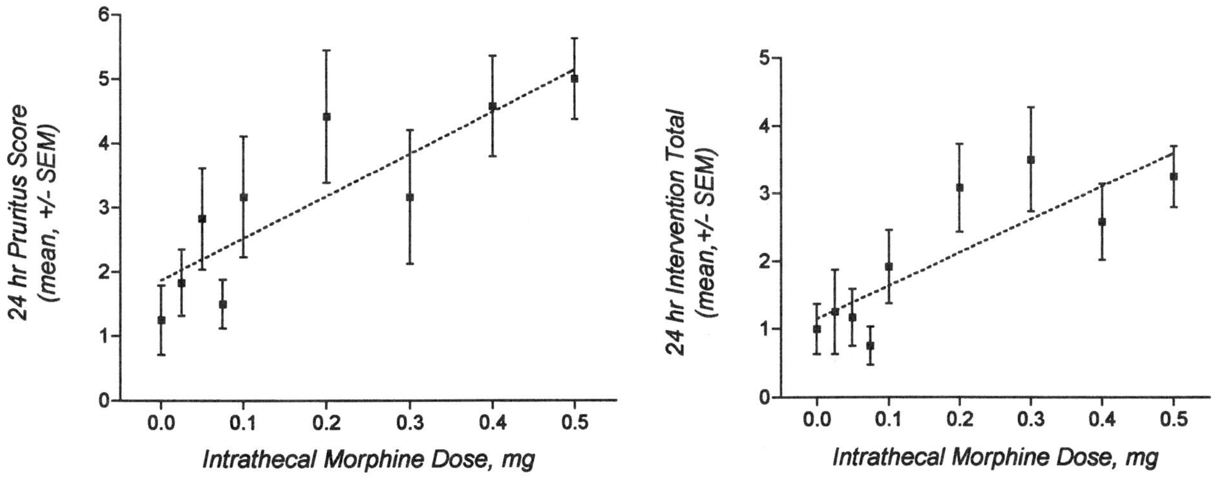

FIG. 17. Twenty-four-hour pruritus score **(A)** and the need for treatment intervenous **(B)** as an intrathecal morphine dose increases from 0 to 0.5 mg in parturients at cesarean delivery. The trends (dotted lines) are highly significant (linear regression, $p = 0.003$ and $p = 0.0002$, **A** and **B**, respectively). (Unpublished data from C.M. Palmer, Tucson, Arizona, with permission.)

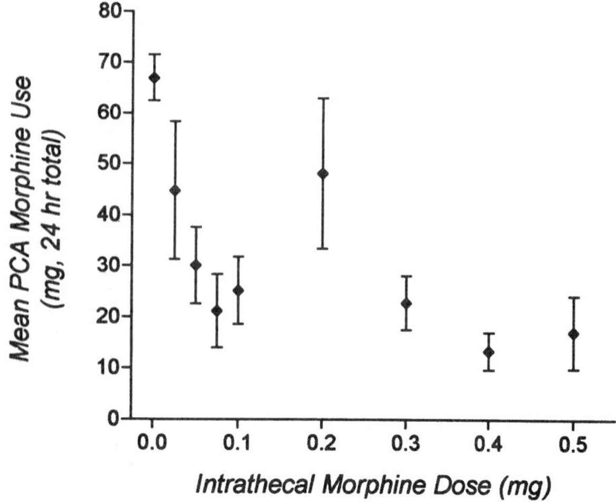

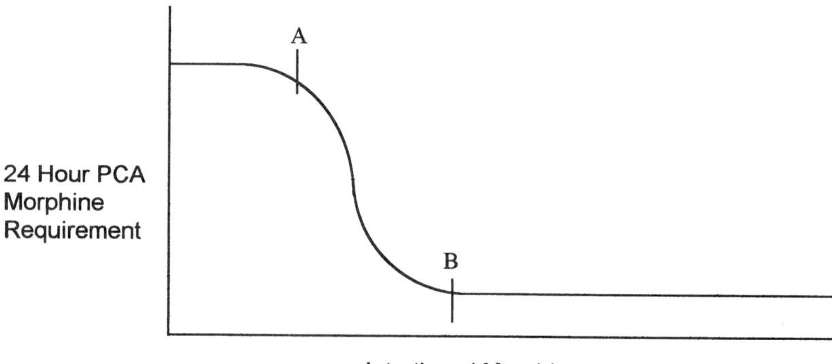

FIG. 18. A: Mean 24-hour patient-controlled anesthesia (PCA) morphine use in nine groups of parturients after cesarean delivery (n = 108). Parturients were randomized to receive between 0 and 0.5 mg intrathecal morphine and then allowed free access to PCA morphine. **B:** Hypothetical shape of the dose–response curve for intrathecal morphine for postcesarean analgesia based on data in A. The inflection points of the curve, A and B, lie at or about 0.025 mg and 0.075 mg, respectively. (Unpublished data from C.M. Palmer, Tucson, Arizona, with permission.)

incidence of side effects. Intrathecal morphine cannot completely eliminate the need for supplemental analgesics however (105,106), and the best way to ensure excellent analgesia may be through a combination of intrathecal morphine and PCA supplementation.

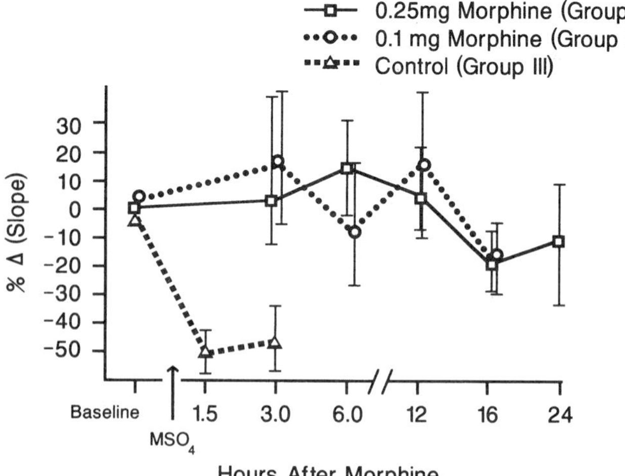

FIG. 19. Percentage change in slope of CO_2 response curve after administration of either 0.1 mg or 0.25 mg intrathecal morphine at cesarean delivery in healthy parturients. (Redrawn from ref. 102, with permission.)

Fentanyl

Fentanyl also has been used at cesarean delivery. Hunt et al. (115) published a prospective, randomized dose–response study of subarachnoid fentanyl in combination with bupivacaine in parturients. The amount of fentanyl administered ranged from 0 to 50 μg, and the bupivacaine dose varied with patient height. Fentanyl did not shorten the latency of anesthesia, but higher doses did transiently slow regression of blockade. The duration of complete analgesia increased with the dose of fentanyl and plateaued at 6.25 μg. Likewise, the duration of effective analgesia increased from 71.8 minutes without fentanyl to 192 minutes with 6.25 μg of fentanyl (Fig. 20). Twenty-four-hour narcotic use did not vary among the groups. Pruritus occurred frequently in all the fentanyl groups, and nausea occurred less often. Palmer et al. (116) studied fentanyl as an adjunct to lidocaine spinal anesthesia for cesarean delivery. Again, fentanyl, 15 μg, prolonged the duration of effective analgesia from 71 to 101 minutes, but did not significantly alter 4- or 24-hour PCA morphine use.

The short duration of effective analgesia even at the higher doses limits the value of subarachnoid fentanyl as a postoperative analgesic. Respiratory depression was reported in association with intrathecal fentanyl at cesarean delivery (117).

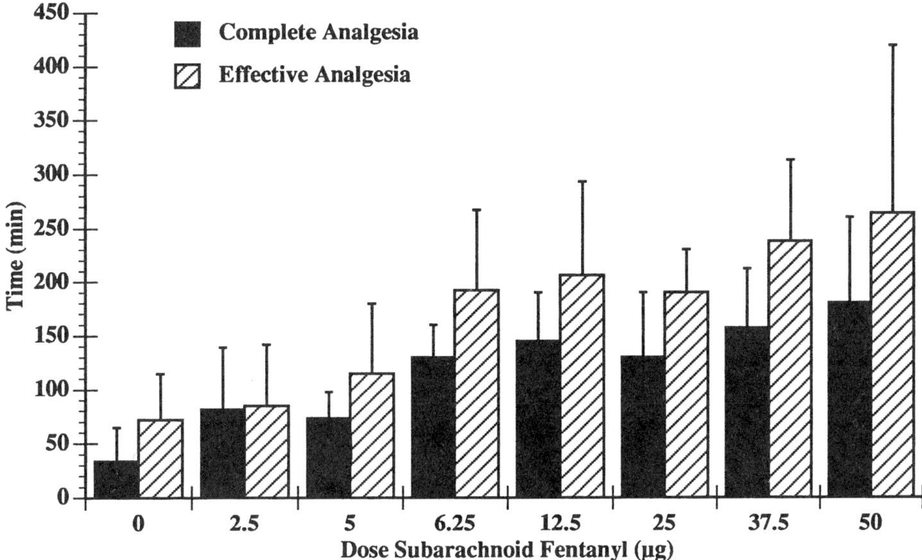

FIG. 20. Mean duration of complete analgesia (pain score, 0) and effective analgesia (time to first request for additional analgesia) after varying doses of intrathecal fentanyl and hyperbaric bupivacaine for cesarean section. *$p < 0.05$ vs 0μg fentanyl. (Redrawn from ref. 115, with permission.)

Other Opioids

Subarachnoid sufentanil, 10 μg, provided 5.4 hours of analgesia after cesarean delivery (118). Patients who did not receive sufentanil needed pain medication 2.8 hours after induction. Sufentanil patients used fewer narcotics in the first 4 postoperative hours, but by 8 hours, both groups required similar amounts of additional analgesics. Pruritus, usually of short duration, occurred in more than half of the patients with sufentanil. As with fentanyl, a short duration limits the usefulness of sufentanil as a postoperative analgesic.

Subarachnoid buprenorphine, 0.045 mg, prolonged the pain-free interval after bupivacaine spinal anesthesia for cesarean delivery from 109 minutes in controls to 420 minutes (119). Nausea and vomiting developed slightly more often in the buprenorphine group. The incidence of pruritus after buprenorphine was 13.3%.

Other subarachnoid opioids that have been used in nonpregnant populations include methadone and oxymorphone. Methadone produces analgesia of shorter duration and less consistent quality than morphine, even at doses as high as 20 mg (120,121). Oxymorphone provides approximately 16 hours of analgesia when administered intrathecally, with predictable side effects of pruritus, nausea, and vomiting (122). Optimal dose ranges and advantages and disadvantages await further study.

Nalbuphine has been administered intrathecally as an adjunct to intrathecal morphine in an attempt to decrease the side effects of the morphine. Hays et al. (123) administered three doses of nalbuphine (0.05 to 0.15 mg) in conjunction with 0.15 mg intrathecal morphine. There were no differences among treatment and control groups in the incidence or severity of pruritus, or in supplemental postoperative analgesic use, but a trend toward more nausea was found with increasing nalbuphine dose.

Nonopioids

As with epidural techniques, epinephrine is often added to intrathecal injections to prolong the duration of anesthesia. However, epinephrine does not appear to augment intrathecal morphine postoperative analgesia. Abouleish et al. (124) studied the addition of epinephrine to intrathecal morphine, 0.2 mg. Whereas the quality of intraoperative analgesia was somewhat improved, there was no increase in the duration of postoperative analgesia or decrease in supplemental analgesic requirements after cesarean delivery. A study in nonpregnant patients undergoing gynecologic surgery reported similar findings (125).

Epinephrine added to a lidocaine–fentanyl mixture, but not to a lidocaine anesthetic alone, prolonged analgesia after postpartum tubal ligation (126). Epinephrine may delay absorption of fentanyl or act synergistically to prolong analgesia. It may be useful in prolonging the short duration of analgesia of subarachnoid fentanyl.

Although most interest has been focused on clonidine as an epidural analgesic, it also has been studied as an intrathecal agent. Filos et al. (127) compared intrathecal clonidine, 150 μg, with placebo in parturients who had received general anesthesia for cesarean delivery. The duration of analgesia after clonidine was significantly longer (more than 6 hours) than after placebo. Clonidine significantly decreased systolic, diastolic, and mean arterial pressures, and also significantly increased sedation.

These systemic effects parallel those seen after epidural clonidine.

Recent studies have elucidated some of the spinally mediated neurochemical responses to pain. Specifically, painful stimuli release norepinephrine (NE) from descending inhibitory pathways. NE stimulates α_2-adrenoreceptors, which activate spinal cholinergic neurons. Painful stimuli increase NE and acetylcholine (ACh) concentrations in CSF (128), and spinal neostigmine prevents the breakdown of synaptically released ACh, enhancing analgesia (129,130).

In parturients, a single injection of intrathecal neostigmine produces a dose-related decrease in morphine consumption after cesarean section for about 10 hours (131). Unfortunately, neostigmine also incites dose-related postoperative nausea and vomiting.

Intrathecal neostigmine and an epidural clonidine infusion, when used in combination, have an additive effect in enhancement of analgesia. The combination did not increase side effects and tended to reduce clonidine-induced hypotension (132). In a nonpregnant population undergoing abdominal surgery under spinal anesthesia, fentanyl plus neostigmine also provided dose-related postoperative analgesia (133). Nausea and vomiting did not increase with fentanyl, 25 μg, and neostigmine, 25 μg.

These studies indicate that both clonidine and neostigmine have significant analgesic potential when administered intrathecally and are free of some of the side effects common to the opioids. They both have significant side effects of their own, however, which may ultimately limit their clinical utility. Further investigation is necessary before either agent can be recommended for routine clinical practice.

Summary

Morphine remains the best choice for postoperative subarachnoid analgesia. Our current practice is to combine 0.15 mg of morphine and 15 μg of fentanyl with either lidocaine or bupivacaine for spinal anesthesia for cesarean delivery. The morphine provides up to 24 hours of good to excellent postoperative analgesia for most parturients, but if a patient is having significant discomfort, we do not hesitate to provide supplemental analgesia, usually PCA morphine. Many parturients advance directly to oral pain medications on the first postoperative day, completely eliminating the need for parenteral analgesics. Fentanyl may enhance intraoperative comfort and provide some early postoperative analgesia. Because of the very small volumes of opioids used with this technique, we measure these drugs in tuberculin syringes to minimize the risk of accidental overdose. Although the addition of opioid to hyperbaric local anesthetic solution will predictably lower its baricity, these solutions remain hyperbaric, and we have not found the dermatomal level of anesthesia to be appreciably different. As with epidural opioid analgesia, close postoperative monitoring of patients is essential. Postoperative orders are identical to those used after epidural opioids (Table 4).

PATIENT-CONTROLLED ANALGESIA

In recent years, PCA has become a popular and effective method of providing postoperative analgesia after a wide range of surgical procedures. Several studies examined the use of PCA in the obstetric population. One prospective, randomized study compared intramuscular narcotics on an as-needed schedule; morphine, 5 mg epidurally, and PCA morphine for analgesia in 60 patients after cesarean delivery (134). After a loading dose of morphine in the recovery room, patients in the PCA group received a morphine bolus with a 15-minute lockout interval. The intramuscular group received either meperidine or morphine intramuscularly as ordered by their obstetrician. Patients rated their pain on a 5-point scale every 2 hours, while awake, for 24 hours. Twenty-four-hour narcotic use was lowest in the epidural group. Analgesia, as determined by patient ratings, did not differ significantly between the intramuscular and PCA groups. Analgesia was significantly better in the epidural group than in the intramuscular group. Patient satisfaction was higher in both the PCA and epidural groups when compared with the intramuscular group, with patient satisfaction being highest in the PCA group (Table 5).

Harrison et al. (135) and Cade and Ashley (136) confirmed these results in similar studies. Harrison et al. found that patients receiving epidural morphine had significantly lower pain scores in the first 16 hours after surgery than did women receiving either intramuscular or PCA morphine. Again, no difference in analgesia was found between intramuscular and PCA groups. The incidence of pruritus was highest in the epidural morphine group. Patient satisfaction with PCA was comparable to that with epidural morphine, despite poorer pain control in the PCA group. Cade and Ashley found that whereas pain scores were significantly lower in parturients who had received epidural morphine, patient satisfaction was greatest in parturients who had received intravenous meperidine PCA.

Sinatra et a1. (137) compared postcesarean analgesia using PCA with morphine, meperidine, and oxymorphone. Equipotent solutions of each opioid were used (1 mL contained either 1.5 mg of morphine, 15 mg of meperidine, or 0.25 mg of oxymorphone). On first complaint of pain, patients received 1-mL increments of one of the opioids until comfortable and then could self-administer 1.2-mL boluses with a lockout interval of 8 minutes. Patient-satisfaction scores were very high with all three opioids, and no differences in analgesia at rest were found. A few very slight differences were reported. The meperidine group more frequently reported severe pain with movement. Nausea was highest in the oxymor-

TABLE 5. *Patient responses to questions about analgesia and satisfaction with three alternate methods of postoperative analgesia*

Parameter	i.m. Therapy (%)	Patient-controlled analgesia (%)	Epidural morphine (%)
Analgesia (overall quality)			
Comfortable	25	40	65[a]
Mildly uncomfortable	55	60	30[a]
Very uncomfortable	10	0	0
In pain	10	0	5
Satisfaction (vs previous cesarean section)			
Much prefer current therapy	25	90[b]	65[a]
Prefer current therapy	30	10	30
Don't care	30	0[a]	0[a]
Prefer PRN i.m. therapy	15	0	5

[a] $p < 0.05$ vs i.m. group.
[b] $p < 0.001$ vs i.m. group.
Data from ref. 133, with permission.

phone group. Sedation was highest in the morphine group. Howell et al. (138) compared morphine and fentanyl for postcesarean PCA analgesia and found only that patients receiving fentanyl were more likely to require supplemental doses.

The effect of using a basal infusion plus intermittent bolus PCA also was studied by Sinatra's group (139). Thirty-two patients received either morphine or oxymorphone PCA, with or without a basal infusion of the same opioid, after cesarean delivery. Basal infusion did not change 24-hour opioid use, but it did significantly decrease pain scores with movement. The incidence of nausea was higher in the groups receiving the basal infusion. This finding is in agreement with studies in nonobstetric populations that have shown that a background infusion adds nothing to on-demand PCA (140,141). If PCA therapy is used as a supplement to neuraxial opioids, a background infusion may increase the risk of respiratory depression.

Russell et al. (142) added droperidol to i.v. PCA morphine in an attempt to decrease postoperative nausea and vomiting. While this strategy effectively decreased the incidence of these two side effects, it increased the incidence of drowsiness and decreased overall patient satisfaction.

A number of other studies also investigated the use of PCA in this population, but this sampling illustrates most of the relevant points. Although intravenous PCA may not provide the same degree of analgesia as do neuraxial opioids, the ability to control analgesia directly provides a significant level of patient satisfaction. The choice of opioid does not appear markedly to affect analgesia or satisfaction. Morphine, however, may have fewer neonatal effects. Breast-feeding neonates of mothers using morphine PCA scored consistently higher in "alertness" and "human orientation" measures on the Brazelton Neonatal Assessment Scale than did neonates whose mothers used meperidine PCA (143). Also, PCA is an excellent adjunct to neuraxial techniques for postcesarean analgesia, and it is an effective way to titrate postoperative analgesia to individual needs.

Patient-Controlled Epidural Analgesia

Epidural PCA (PCEA) allows the use of both local anesthetics and opioids and nonopioid adjuncts for postoperative analgesia. As might be imagined, this approach allows a large and sometimes bewildering array of options.

Yu and Gambling (144) compared the efficacy of a single dose of epidural morphine with that of fentanyl-based PCEA. Parturients in the morphine group received 3 mg epidural morphine, whereas those in the PCEA group received a loading dose of 100 μg fentanyl intraoperatively, and then up to two self-administered doses of 50 μg doses each hour. Mean 24-hour fentanyl use in the PCEA group was 680 μg. There were no differences between groups in analgesia, satisfaction, or use of supplemental analgesics. Nausea was equally common in both groups, although pruritus scores were lower in the fentanyl group.

Opioid use of this magnitude raises the question of whether PCEA is really better than PCA, as systemic concentration of drug may be similar. In addressing this question, it must be remembered that observations related to one opioid may not necessarily apply to a different opioid. Paech et al. (145) considered this question in a blinded, cross-over study comparing PCEA with PCA meperidine. They found comparable onset but significantly lower pain scores in the PCEA group. Although there was no difference in nausea between groups, sedation scores were higher in the PCA group. Meperidine use was approximately 50% less when administered epidurally (Fig. 21).

Fentanyl and sufentanil are the opioids most often used for PCEA administration because of their rapid onset and efficacy. As with patients who receive intravenous PCA, a basal infusion does not significantly improve the quality of pain relief with PCEA (146). Background infusion does increase sedation.

Local anesthetics, particularly bupivacaine, are often used for postsurgical epidural analgesia and can be added to PCEA for analgesia after cesarean section. The concentration of local anesthetic must be carefully chosen to enhance analgesia without producing sensory or motor blockade, as many of these patients are ambulatory within hours of surgery. PCEA with fentanyl or buprenorphine plus 0.03% bupivacaine produces effective analgesia but interferes with ambulation (147). Patients receiving PCEA with fentanyl or sufentanil plus 0.01% bupivacaine "could ambulate easily" (148). However, the dose of fentanyl consumed was comparable to that reported with fentanyl PCEA alone (54,144). Thus it is unclear what benefit, if any, is provided by including dilute bupivacaine in a PCEA solution. Adding local anesthetic to PCEA also may increase the risk of significant complications, such as pressure sores (147,149).

The nonopioid agents epinephrine and clonidine also have been used as adjuncts to opioid PCEA. In a randomized study, of 60 parturients receiving sufentanil PCEA with either no additives, epinephrine, or clonidine (150), both epinephrine and clonidine significantly reduced epidural sufentanil use. Epinephrine tended to increase pruritus. Parker et al. (151) studied the addition of nalbuphine to PCEA hydromorphone to attempt to decrease opioid-related side effects. This study illustrates the difficulty of finding a dose of nalbuphine to decrease side effects without also limiting analgesia. Epidural nalbuphine did produce some dose-dependent decreases in the incidence of epidural opioid-induced urinary retention, pruritus, and nausea. As the dose increased, however, a partial reversal of analgesia and an increase in drowsiness and pruritus was noted.

Clearly PCEA is an effective technique for analgesia after cesarean section. Whether it offers distinct advantages over epidural or intrathecal morphine is a matter of dispute. PCEA requires maintaining a functioning epidural catheter in the postoperative period, not always a simple task. Further, in many practices, cesarean delivery is more likely to be accomplished with spinal than with epidural anesthesia, which precludes use of the technique or subjects the parturient to a second procedure. Still PCEA may be a useful technique for selected patients and populations.

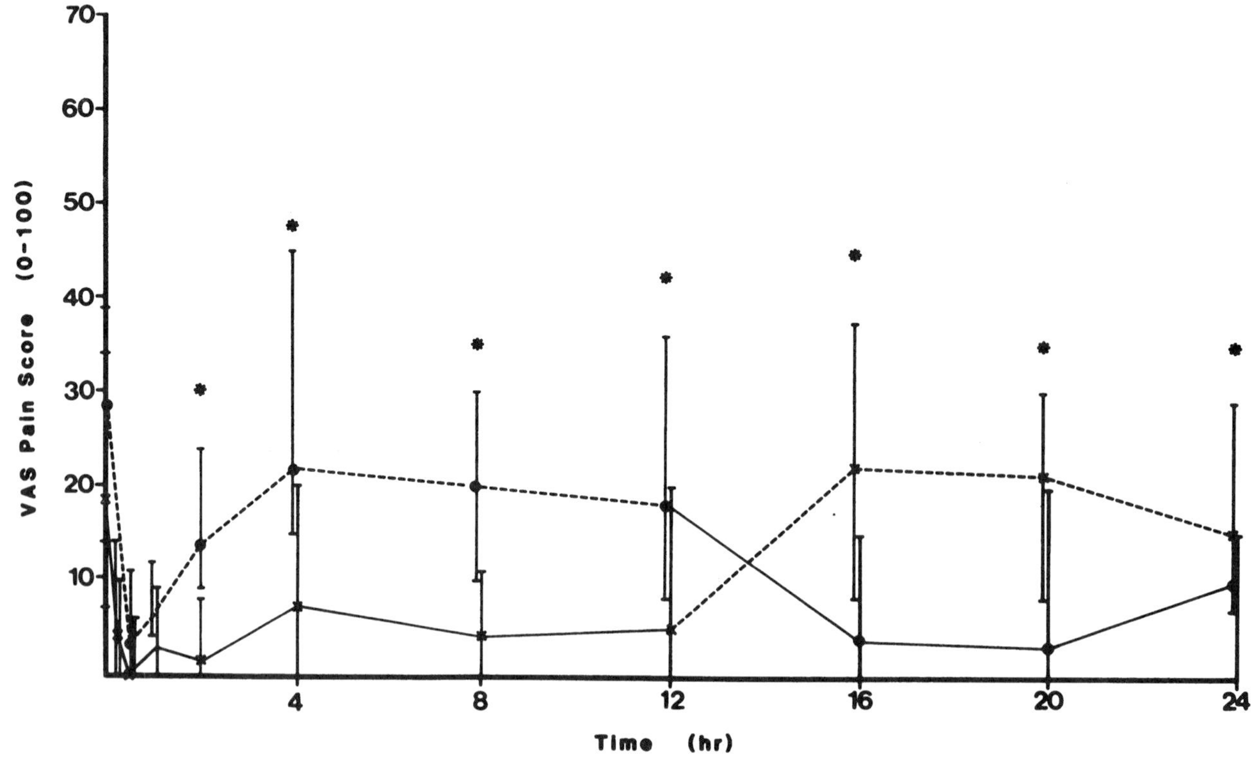

FIG. 21. Visual-analog pain score at rest (median and quartile range for 24 hours after cesarean delivery). *Solid line,* period of patient-controlled epidural anesthesia (PCEA); *dotted line,* period of i.v.-PCA. *$p < 0.05$, Wilcoxon's rank-sum test. (Reprinted from ref. 144, with permission.)

ALTERNATIVE APPROACHES

Ilioinguinal Nerve Block

Bunting and McConachie (152) in 1988 reported the use of ilioinguinal nerve block to provide postoperative analgesia after cesarean delivery (via Pfannenstiel incision). In a prospective study, patients receiving general anesthesia for cesarean delivery randomly received either bilateral ilioinguinal nerve blocks or conventional intramuscular papaveretum injections for postoperative analgesia. The block was performed by using bupivacaine, 0.5%, 10 mL bilaterally (Fig. 22). Patients in both groups had equal access to intramuscular analgesics. Patients in the nerve-block group had significantly lower visual-analog pain scores at four of the five intervals recorded between 0 and 24 hours after surgery. The mean 24-hour dose of papaveretum administered was significantly lower in the block group. Ganta et al. (153) reported similar findings in parturients undergoing general anesthesia and also found wound infiltration with bupivacaine, 0.5%, to be comparable to the nerve block.

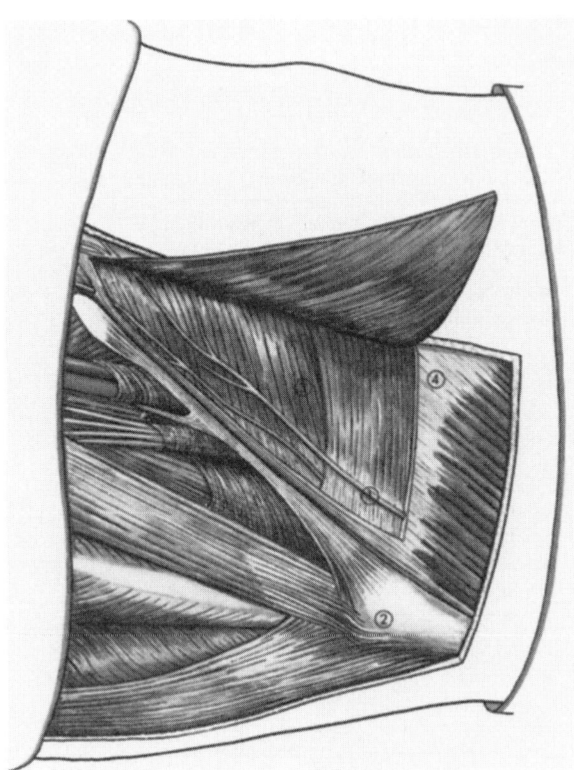

FIG. 22. Course of the ilioinguinal nerve (1), as it proceeds between the internal oblique muscle (3) and the external oblique muscle (4), just medial to the anterior superior iliac spine (2). Block the nerve at a point 2.5 cm medial to the anterior superior iliac spine on a line between this landmark and the umbilicus. (Reproduced from Nolte W. Ilioinguinal nerve block. In: Hoerster W, Kreuscher H, Niesel HC, Zenz M, eds. *Regional anesthesia,* 2nd ed. St. Louis: Mosby Year Book, 1990:278, with permission.)

Huffnagle et al. (154) studied both the use and timing of ilioinguinal nerve block in parturients undergoing spinal anesthesia for cesarean delivery. Patients had the block performed either before or after surgery and were compared with a control group receiving no block. They found no difference in postoperative analgesic use or patient satisfaction among any of the groups and concluded that the block was of no value as an adjunct to spinal anesthesia. Spinal anesthesia, in and of itself, may decrease postoperative analgesic requirements.

Witkowski et al. (155) studied ilioinguinal nerve block as an alternative or supplement to intrathecal morphine in patients receiving spinal anesthesia for cesarean delivery, again via Pfannenstiel incision. Patients received either morphine, 0.15 mg, intrathecally, bilateral ilioinguinal nerve block with bupivacaine 0.5%, 10 mL, or both. Postoperative narcotic orders were standardized. The three groups did not differ in pain scores or supplemental narcotic use. The women getting intrathecal morphine had a higher incidence of pruritus. These authors concluded that bilateral ilioinguinal nerve block could be used as a substitute for, or supplement to, intrathecal morphine, although they stopped short of actually recommending their use.

Transnasal

Transnasal administration of medications has recently proven effective in pediatric patients. In parturients after cesarean section, one randomized, prospective study compared transnasal and intravenous butorphanol (156). All patients had effective pain relief. Intravenous butorphanol worked faster. Butorphanol, 2 mg transnasally, either as a single dose or in two equal portions, provided longer analgesia than did butorphanol, 2 mg intravenously (4.5 vs 3.0 hours). Somnolence was a frequent side effect (more than 70%) in both groups.

Nonsteroidal Antiinflammatory Drugs

In recent years, several parenteral nonsteroidal antiinflammatory agents (NSAIDs) have been developed. Gin et al. (157) compared analgesia after a single intramuscular dose of ketorolac, 30 mg, or meperidine, 75 mg, and found them to be equally efficacious, but not surprisingly, the ketorolac was somewhat inconsistent and of short duration. Parker et al. (158) found some modest advantages to the addition of ketorolac to PCA opioids after abdominal hysterectomy. Rosarius et al. (159) compared continuous intravenous infusions of either diclofenac or ketoprofen to placebo for analgesia after cesarean and found that both NSAIDs decreased postoperative analgesic requirements by about 40% when compared with placebo. Belzarena (160) reported a similar reduction in postoperative analgesic requirements from a single intravenous dose of tenoxicam before delivery.

TABLE 6. *Intrathecal morphine and systemic NSAIDs: Visual-analog pain scores (0–10) and patients requiring supplemental analgesics*

	24-h VAS pain	Supplementary analgesics
Morphine, 0.1 mg + diclofenac q 8 h	$0.22 \pm 0.40^{a,b}$	0/20
Morphine, 0.1 mg	0.26 ± 0.29^{a}	$9/20^{b}$
Morphine, 0.05 mg + diclofenac q 8 h	0.35 ± 0.29^{b}	0/20
Morphine, 0.05 mg	0.54 ± 0.40	$12/20^{b}$
Morphine, 0.025 mg + diclofenac q 8 h	0.23 ± 0.30^{b}	0/20
Morphine, 0.025 mg	0.66 ± 0.62	$15/20^{b}$

NSAIDs, nonsteroidal antiinflammatory drugs; VAS, visual-analog scale.
$^{a}p < 0.05$, morphine, 0.1 mg < morphine, 0.05 mg = morphine, 0.025 mg.
$^{b}p < 0.05$ morphine + diclofenac vs morphine only.
Data from ref. 163, with permission.

Cohen et al. (161) compared analgesia among parturients given intrathecal morphine, 0.2 mg, intravenous ketorolac, 30 mg, intravenously each every 6 hours, or both, at cesarean delivery. Supplemental analgesic use was comparable among all groups in the postoperative period, and the major difference between groups was the lower incidence of pruritus in the ketorolac group. They concluded that ketorolac provided similar analgesia to intrathecal morphine and that the addition of ketorolac to intrathecal morphine was of no advantage. In contrast, Sun et al. (162) found that a single dose of intramuscular diclofenac as a supplement to intrathecal morphine at cesarean section reduced uterine contraction pain. In nonobstetric patients, Wittels and Toledano (163) found that the addition of intravenous ketorolac to intrathecal morphine significantly enhanced analgesia and reduced the need for supplemental analgesics; the dose of intrathecal morphine (0.55 to 0.8 mg) they used was significantly greater than that injected in Cohen's study, however.

Recently Cardoso et al. (164) reported that diclofenac significantly enhanced the analgesia provided by intrathecal morphine. Parturients received 0.025, 0.05, or 0.1 mg intrathecal morphine and either diclofenac, 75 mg i.m. every 8 hours, or only on request. Patients receiving diclofenac every 8 hours reported lower pain scores and were less likely to need supplementary analgesics (Table 6). Severe pruritus was most common among women who received 0.1 mg intrathecal morphine.

The conflicting results reported in these studies indicates that further work is necessary to elucidate the advantages of combination neuraxial opioid and parenteral NSAID therapy. Although it appears that at least in some situations, NSAIDs can decrease postoperative opioid use, one limiting factor may be the significantly higher cost associated with these newer agents.

CONCLUSION

The past two decades have seen remarkable advances in our understanding of pain pathways and the pharmacology of opioid and nonopioid receptors. We also have the technology to make use of this knowledge. These developments have provided anesthesiologists with myriad options for providing analgesia after cesarean delivery. Neuraxial opioids, PCA, and PCEA are no longer interesting research topics, they are therapeutic modalities that can and should be options in every clinical practice. The use of PRN intramuscular analgesics for analgesia after cesarean section should continue to become increasingly uncommon.

REFERENCES

1. Hawkins JL, Koonin LM, Palmer SSK, Gibbs CP. Anesthesia-related deaths during obstetric delivery in the United States, 1979-1990. *Anesthesiology* 1997;86:277.
2. Behar M, Magora F, Olshwang D, et al. Epidural morphine in treatment of pain. *Lancet* 1979;1:527.
3. Youngstrom PC, Cowan RI, Sutheimer C, et al. Pain relief and plasma concentrations from epidural and intramuscular morphine in post-cesarean patients. *Anesthesiology* 1982;57:404.
4. Writer WDR, Hurtig JB, Edelist G, et al. Epidural morphine prophylaxis of postoperative pain: report of a double-blind multicentre study. *Can Anaesth Soc J* 1985;32:330.
5. Kotelko DM, Dailey PA, Shnider SM, et al. Epidural morphine analgesia after cesarean delivery. *Obstet Gynecol* 1984;63:409.
6. Rosen MA, Hughes SC, Shnider SM, et al. Epidural morphine for the relief of postoperative pain after cesarean delivery. *Anesth Analg* 1983;62:666.
7. Palmer CM, Petty JV, Nogarmi WM, Marquez RC, Van Maren G, Alves DM. What is the optimal dose of epidural morphine for post-cesarean analgesia? A dose response study. *Anesthesiology* 1996;85:A909.
8. Asantila R, Eklund P, Rosenberg PH. Epidural analgesia with 4 mg of morphine following caesarean section: effect of injected volume. *Acta Anaesthesiol Scand* 1993;37:764.
9. Chambers WA, Mowbray A, Wilson J. Extradural morphine for the relief of pain following caesarean section. *Anaesthesia* 1983;55:1201.
10. Kanto J, Erkkola R, Aaltonen L, et al. Epidural morphine as postoperative analgesic following cesarean section under epidural analgesia. *Int J Clin Pharm Ther Toxicol* 1985;23:43.
11. Webster NR, Lyons G, Macdonald R. Forum: sleep and comfort after caesarean section. *Anaesthesia* 1986;41:1143.
12. Leicht CH, Hughes SC, Dailey PA, et al. Epidural morphine sulfate for analgesia after cesarean section: a prospective report of 1000 patients. *Anesthesiology* 1986;65:A366.
13. Ackerman WE, Juneja MM, Kaczoramski DM, Colclough GW. A comparison of the incidence of pruritus following epidural opioid administration in the parturient. *Can J Anaesth* 1989;36:388.
14. Gieraerts R, Navalgund A, Vaes L, et al. Increased incidence of itch-

ing and herpes simplex in patients given epidural morphine after cesarean section. *Anesth Analg* 1987;66:1321.
15. Ballantyne JC, Loach AB, Carr DB. Itching after epidural and spinal opiates. *Pain* 1988;33:149.
16. Kam PC, Tan KH. Pruritus-itching for a cause and relief? *Anaesthesia* 1996;51:1133.
17. Fuller JG, McMorland GH, Douglas J, et al. Epidural morphine for postoperative pain after caesarean section: a report of 4880 patients. *Can J Anaesth* 1990;37:636.
18. Gourlay GK, Cherry DA, Cousins MJ. Cephalad migration of morphine in CSF following lumbar epidural administration in patients with cancer pain. *Pain* 1985;23:317.
19. Bromage PR, Camporesi EM, Curant PAC, Nielsen CH. Nonrespiratory side effect of epidural morphine. *Anesth Analg* 1982;61:490.
20. Bromage PR, Camporesi EM, Durant PAC, Nielsen CH. Rostral spread of epidural morphine. *Anesthesiology* 1982;56:431.
21. Drayer BP, Rosenbaum AE. Studies of the third circulation, amipaque CT cisternography and ventriculography. *J Neurosurg* 1978; 48:946.
22. Christensen V. Respiratory depression after extradural morphine. *Br J Anaesth* 1980;52:841.
23. Glynn CJ, Mather LE, Cousins MJ, Wilson PR, Graham JR. Spinal narcotics and respiratory depression. *Lancet* 1979;2:356.
24. Brose WG, Cohen SE. Oxyhemoglobin saturation following cesarean section in patients receiving epidural morphine, PCA, or IM meperidine analgesia. *Anesthesiology* 1989;70:948.
25. Pan PH, James CF. Anesthetic-postoperative morphine regimens for cesarean section and postoperative oxygen saturation monitored by a telemetric pulse oximetry network for 24 continuous hours. *J Clin Anesth* 1994;6:124.
26. Crone LA, Conly JM, Clark KM, et al. Recurrent herpes simplex virus labialis and the use of epidural morphine in obstetric patients. *Anesth Analg* 1988;37:318.
27. Boyle RK. Herpes simplex labialis after epidural or parenteral morphine: a randomized prospective trial in Australian obstetric population. *Anaesth Intens Care* 1995;23:433.
28. Norris MC, Weiss JH, Carney MD, Leighton BL, Torjman M. Incidence of recurrent herpes simplex virus labialis after cesarean section. *Int J Obstet Anesth* 1994;3:127.
29. Boyle RK. A review of anatomical and immunological links between epidural morphine and herpes simplex labialis in obstetric patients. *Anaesth Intens Care* 1995;23:425.
30. James CF. Recurrence of herpes simplex virus blepharitis after cesarean section and epidural morphine. *Anesth Analg* 1996;82:1094.
31. Henderson SK, Cohen H. Nalbuphine augmentation of analgesia and side effects following epidural hydromorphone. *Anesthesiology* 1986; 65:216.
32. Cohen SE, Ratner EF, Kreitzman TR, Archer JH, Mignano LR. Nalbuphine is better than naloxone for treatment of side effects after epidural morphine. *Anesth Analg* 1992;75:747.
33. Wang JJ, Ho ST, Hu OY. Comparison of intravenous nalbuphine infusion versus saline as an adjuvant for epidural morphine. *Reg Anesth* 1996;21:214.
34. Kendrick WD, Woods AM, Daly MY, et al. Naloxone versus nalbuphine infusion for prophylaxis of epidural morphine-induced pruritus. *Anesth Analg* 1996;82:641.
35. Salah M, Borgeat A, Wilder-Smith OHG, Rifat K, Suter PM. Epidural morphine-induced pruritus: propofol versus naloxone. *Anesth Analg* 1994;78:1110.
36. Warwick JP, Kearns CF, Scott WE. The effect of subhypnotic doses of propofol on the incidence of pruritus after intrathecal morphine for caesarean section. *Anaesthesia* 1997;52:270.
37. Horta ML, Horta BL. Inhibition of epidural morphine-induced pruritus by intravenous droperidol. *Reg Anesth* 1993;18:118.
38. Larijani GE, Goldberg ME, Rogers KH. Treatment of opioid-induced pruritus with ondansetron: report of four patients. *Pharmacotherapy* 1996;16:958.
39. Latasch L, Probst S, Dudziak R. Reversal by nalbuphine of respiratory depression caused by fentanyl. *Anesth Analg* 1984;63:814.
40. Penning JP, Samson B, Baxter A. Nalbuphine reverses epidural morphine induced respiratory depression. *Anesth Analg* 1986;65:S119.
41. Cullen M, Altstatt AH, Kwon NJ, Benzuly S, Naulty JS. Naltrexone reversal of the side effects of epidural morphine. *Anesthesiology* 1988;69:A336.
42. Abboud TK, Afrasiabi A, Davidson J, et al. Prophylactic oral naltrexone with epidural morphine: effect on adverse reactions and ventilatory responses to carbon dioxide. *Anesthesiology* 1990;72:233.
43. Norris MC, Leighton BL, DeSimone CA. Naltrexone and subarachnoid morphine following cesarean section. *Anesthesiology* 1989; 71:A873.
44. Abboud TK, Lee K, Zhu J, et al. Prophylactic oral naltrexone with intrathecal morphine for cesarean section: effects on adverse reactions and analgesia. *Anesth Analg* 1990;71:367.
45. Lawhorn CD, McNitt J, Fibuch EE, Leadle RJ. Epidural morphine with butorphanol for postoperative analgesia following cesarean delivery. *Anesth Analg* 1991;72:53.
46. Gambling DR, Howell P, Huber C, Kozak S. Epidural butorphanol does not reduce side effects from epidural morphine after cesarean birth. *Anesth Analg* 1994;78:1099.
47. Wittels B, Glosten B, Faure EAM, et al. Opioid antagonist adjuncts to epidural morphine for postcesarean analgesia: maternal outcomes. *Anesth Analg* 1993;77:925.
48. Kotelko DM, Rottman RL, Wright WC, Stone JJ, Yamashiro AY, Rosenblatt RM. Transdermal scopolamine decreases nausea and vomiting following cesarean section in patients receiving epidural morphine. *Anesthesiology* 1989;71:675.
49. Naulty JS, Datta S, Ostheimer GW, et al. Epidural fentanyl for postcesarean delivery pain management. *Anesthesiology* 1985;63:694.
50. Sevarino FB, McFarlane C, Sinatra RS. Epidural fentanyl does not influence intravenous PCA requirements in the post-caesarean patient. *Can J Anaesth* 1991;38:450.
51. Helbo-Hansen HS, Bang U, Lindholm P, Klitgaard NA. Maternal effects of adding epidural fentanyl to 0.5% bupivacaine for caesarean section. *Int J Obstet Anesth* 1993;2:21.
52. Blanco J, Blanco E, Carceller JM, et al. Epidural analgesia for post-caesarean pain relief: a comparison between morphine and fentanyl. *Eur J Anaesth* 1987;4:395.
53. Kotelko DM, Rottman RL, Wright WC, et al. Improved surgical and post-cesarean analgesia with epidural fentanyl/morphine combination. *Anesthesiology* 1987;67:A622.
54. Cooper DW, Ryall DM, Desira WR. Extradural fentanyl for postoperative analgesia: predominant spinal or systemic action? *Br J Anaesth* 1995;74:184.
55. James CF, Banner CE, Hanna PG, et al. Comparison of epidural fentanyl via bolus with or without continuous infusion after cesarean section. *Anesthesiology* 1988;69:A682.
56. Brockway MS, Noble DW, Sharwood-Smith GH, McClure JH. Profound respiratory depression after extradural fentanyl. *Br J Anaesth* 1990;14:243.
57. Gourlay GK, Murphy TM, Plummer JL, Kowalksi SR, Cherry DA, Cousins MJ. Pharmacokinetics of fentanyl in lumbar and cervical CSF following lumbar epidural and intravenous administration. *Pain* 1989; 38:253.
58. Madej TH, Strunin L. Comparison of epidural fentanyl with sufentanil. *Anaesthesia* 1987;42:1156.
59. Cohen SE, Tan S, White PF. Sufentanil analgesia following cesarean section: epidural versus intravenous administration. *Anesthesiology* 1988;68:129.
60. Rosen MA, Daily PA, Hughes SC, et al. Epidural sufentanil for postoperative analgesia after cesarean section. *Anaesthesiology* 1988;68:448.
61. Brownridge P, Frewin DB. A comparative study of techniques of postoperative analgesia following caesarean section and lower abdominal surgery. *Anaesth Intens Care* 1985;13:123.
62. Perriss BW, Latham BV, Wilson IH. Analgesia following extradural and i.m. pethidine in post-caesarean section patients. *Br J Anaesth* 1990;64:355.
63. Ngan Kee WD, Lam KK, Chen PP, Gin T. Epidural meperidine after cesarean section. *Anaesthesiology* 1996;85:289.
64. Henderson SK, Matthew EB, Cohen H, Avram MJ. Epidural hydromorphone: a double-blind comparison with intramuscular hydromorphone for postcesarean section analgesia. *Anesthesiology* 1987;66: 825.
65. Halpern SH, Arellano R, Preston R, O'Leary G, Sandler A. Epidural morphine vs hydromorphone in post-caesarean section patients. *Can J Anaesth* 1996;43:595.
66. Matthew EB, Henderson SK, Avram MJ, et al. Epidural hydromorphone versus epidural morphine for post-cesarean section analgesia. *Anesth Analg* 1987;66:S112.

67. Chestnut DH, Choi WW, Isbell TJ. Epidural hydromorphone for postcesarean analgesia. *Obstet Gynecol* 1986;68:65.
68. Albright G. Epidural morphine, hydromorphone, and meperidine for post C-section pain relief utilizing a respiratory apnea monitor. *Anesthesiology* 1983;59:A416.
69. Beeby D, MacIntosh KC, Bailey M, Welch DB. Postoperative analgesia for caesarean section using epidural methadone. *Anaesthesia* 1984;39:61.
70. Haynes SR, Davidson I, Allsop JR, Dutton DA. Comparison of epidural methadone with epidural diamorphine for analgesia following caesarean section. *Acta Anaesthesiol Scand* 1993;37:375.
71. Roulson BJ, Bennett J, Shaw M, Carli F. Effect of extradural diamorphine on analgesia after caesarean section under subarachnoid block. *Br J Anaesth* 1993;71:810.
72. Smith ID, Klubein KE, Wood ML, Macral DJ, Carli F. Diamorphine analgesia after caesarean section: comparison of intramuscular and epidural administration of four dose regimens. *Anaesthesia* 1991;46:970.
73. Naulty JS, Weintraub S, McMahon J, et al. Epidural butorphanol for post-cesarean delivery pain management. *Anesthesiology* 1984;61:A415.
74. Abboud TK, Moore M, Zhu J, et al. Epidural butorphanol or morphine for the relief of section pain: ventilatory responses to carbon dioxide. *Anesth Analg* 1987;66:887.
75. Camann WR, Hurley RH, Gilbertson LI, Long ML, Datta S. Epidural nalbuphine for analgesia following caesarean delivery: dose-response and effect of local anaesthetic choice. *Can J Anaesth* 1991;38:728.
76. Viscomi CM, Eisenach JC. Epidural clonidine for post cesarean section analgesia. *Anesthesiology* 1989;71:640.
77. Mendez RM, Eisenach JC, Kashtan K. Epidural clonidine infusion following cesarean section. *Anaesthesiology* 1990;73:848.
78. Huntoon M, Eisenach JC, Boese P. Epidural clonidine after cesarean section, appropriate dose and effect of prior local anesthetic. *Anesthesiology* 1992;6:187.
79. Capogna G, Celleno D, Zangrillo A, Constantino P, Foresta S. Addition of clonidine to epidural morphine enhances postoperative analgesia after cesarean delivery. *Reg Anesth* 1995;20:57.
80. Eisenach JC, D'Angelo R, Taylor C, Hood DD. An isobolographic study of epidural clonidine and fentanyl after cesarean section. *Anesth Analg* 1994;79:285.
81. Eisenach J, Detweiler D, Hood D. Hemodynamic and analgesic actions of epidurally administered clonidine. *Anaesthesiology* 1993;78:277.
82. Weiler RL, Wardell GC. Hemodynamic study of epidural clonidine in awake sheep. *Anaesth Analg* 1988;67:S252.
83. Park J, Forrest J, Kolesar R, et al. Oral clonidine reduces postoperative PCA morphine requirements. *Can J Anaesth* 1996;43:900.
94. Collins JG, Kitahata LM, Matsumoto M, Homma E, Suzukawa M. Spinally administered epinephrine suppresses noxiously evoked activity of WDR neurons in the dorsal horn of the spinal cord. *Anaesthesiology* 1984;6:269.
85. Reddy SVR, Maderdrut JL, Yakash TL. Spinal cord pharmacology of adrenergic agonist-mediated antinociception. *J Pharmacol Exp Ther* 1980;213:525.
86. Robertson K, Douglas MJ, McMorland GH. Epidural fentanyl, with and without epinephrine for post-caesarean section analgesia. *Can Anaesth Soc J* 1985;32:502.
87. Leicht CH, Kelleher AJ, Robinson DE, Dickerson SE. Prolongation of postoperative epidural sufentanil analgesia with epinephrine. *Anaesth Analg* 1990;70:323.
88. McMorland GH, Douglas MJ, Kim JH, et al. Epidural sufentanil for post-caesarean section analgesia: lack of benefit of epinephrine. *Can J Anaesth* 1990;37:432.
89. Dougherty TB, Baysinger CL, Henenberger JC, Gooding DJ. Epidural hydromorphone with and without epinephrine for postoperative analgesia after cesarean delivery. *Anaesth Analg* 1989;68:318.
90. Kotelko DM, Thigpen JW, Shnider SM, et al. Postoperative epidural morphine analgesia after various local anesthetics. *Anaesthesiology* 1983;59:A413.
91. Hughes SC, Wright RG, Murphy D, et al. The effect of pH adjusting 3% 2-chloroprocaine on the quality of postcesarean section analgesia with epidural morphine. *Anaesthesiology* 1988;69:A689.
92. Phan CQ, Azar I, Osborn IP, et al. The quality of epidural morphine analgesia following epidural anesthesia with lidocaine or chloroprocaine for cesarean delivery. *Anaesth Analg* 1988;67:S172.
93. Eisenach JC, Schlairet TJ, Dobson CE, Hood DH. Effect of prior anesthetic solution on epidural morphine analgesia. *Anaesth Analg* 1991;73:119.
94. Durkan WJ, Baker LT, Leicht CH. Postoperative epidural morphine analgesia after 3% 2-chloroprocaine (Nesacaine-MPF) or lidocaine epidural anesthesia. *Anaesthesiology* 1989;71:A834.
95. Naulty JS, Hertwig L, Hunt CO, et al. Duration of analgesia of epidural fentanyl following cesarean delivery-effects of local anesthetic drug selection. *Anaesthesiology* 1986;65:A180.
96. Grice SC, Eisenach JC, Dewan DM. Labor analgesia with epidural bupivacaine plus fentanyl: enhancement with epinephrine and inhibition with 2 chloroprocaine. *Anesthesiology* 1990;72:623.
97. Malinow AM, Mokriski BLD, Wakefield ML, et al. Anesthetic choice affects postcesarean epidural fentanyl analgesia. *Anesth Analg* 1988;67:S138.
98. Naughton NN, Pelligrino DA, Albrecht RF. A principal metabolite of 2-chloroprocaine does not act as a μ-opiate receptor antagonist in the dog [Abstract]. *Anesthesiology* 1988;69:S137.
99. Camann WR, Hartigan PM, Gilbertson LI, Johnson MD, Datta S. Chloroprocaine antagonism of epidural opioid analgesia: a receptor-specific phenomenon? *Anesthesiology* 1990;73:860.
100. Coda B, Bausch S, Haas M, Chavkin C. The hypothesis that antagonism of fentanyl analgesia by 2-chloroprocaine is mediated by direct action on opioid receptors. *Reg Anesth* 1997;22:43.
101. Wang JK, Nauss LA, Thomas JE. Pain relief by intrathecally applied morphine in man. *Anesthesiology* 1979;50:149.
102. Abboud TK, Dror A, Mosaad P, et al. Mini-dose intrathecal morphine for the relief of post-cesarean section pain: safety, efficacy, and ventilatory responses to carbon dioxide. *Anesth Analg* 1988;67:137.
103. Chadwick HS, Ready LB. Intrathecal and epidural morphine sulfate for postcesarean analgesia: a clinical comparison. *Anesthesiology* 1988;68:925.
104. Zakowski M, Ramanathan S, Turndorf H. Intrathecal morphine for postcesarean section analgesia. *Anesthesiology* 1989;71:A870.
105. Palmer CM, Voulgaropoulos D, Van Maren G, Emerson SS, Alves D. What is the optimal dose of subarachnoid morphine for post-cesarean analgesia? A dose response study. *Anesthesiology* 1994;81:A1151.
106. Palmer CM, Tucson, Arizona. Unpublished data.
107. Huffnagle HJ, Norris MC, Leighton BL, Arkoosh VA, Huffnagle SL. A dose-response study of intrathecal morphine for post cesarean section analgesia. Annual Meeting of the Society for Obstetric Anesthesia and Perinatology. Tucson, 1996:199.
108. Milner AR, Bogod DG, Harwood RJ. Intrathecal administration of morphine for elective caesarean section: a comparison between 0.1 mg and 0.2 mg. *Anaesthesia* 1996;51:871.
109. Yeung JC, Rudy TA. Multiplicative interaction between narcotic agonisms expressed at spinal and supraspinal sites of antinociceptive action as revealed by concurrent intrathecal and intracerebroventricular injections of morphine. *J Pharmacol Exp Ther* 1980;215:633.
110. Ferouz F, Norris MC, Arkoosh VA, et al. Baricity, needle direction, and intrathecal sufentanil labor analgesia. *Anesthesiology* 1997;86:592.
111. Cousins MJ, Mather LE. Intrathecal and epidural administration of opioids. *Anesthesiology* 1984;61:271.
112. Gloss PSA. Respiratory depression following only 0.4 mg of intrathecal morphine [Letter]. *Anesthesiology* 1984;60:256.
113. Odoom JA, Sih IL. Respiratory depression after intrathecal morphine [Letter]. *Anesth Analg* 1982;61:70.
114. Abouleish E, Rawal N, Rashad MN. The addition of 0.2 mg subarachnoid morphine to hyperbaric bupivacaine for cesarean delivery: a prospective study of 856 cases. *Reg Anesth* 1991;16:137.
115. Hunt CO, Naulty JS, Bader AM, et al. Perioperative analgesia with subarachnoid fentanyl-bupivacaine for cesarean delivery. *Anesthesiology* 1989;71:535.
116. Palmer CM, Voulgaropoulos D, Alves D. Subarachnoid fentanyl augments lidocaine spinal anesthesia for cesarean delivery. *Reg Anesth* 1995;20:389.
117. Palmer CM. Case report: early respiratory depression following intrathecal fentanyl-morphine combination. *Anesthesiology* 1991;74:1153.
118. De Sousa H, De la Vega S. Spinal sufentanil. *Reg Anesth* 1988;13:23.
119. Cellano D, Capogna G. Spinal buprenorphine for postoperative analgesia after caesarean section. *Acta Anaesthesiol Scand* 1989;33:236.
120. Jacobson L, Chabal C, Brody MC, et al. Intrathecal methadone and morphine for postoperative analgesia: a comparison of the efficacy, duration and side effects. *Anesthesiology* 1988;69:A352.
121. Jacobson L, Chabal C, Brody MC, et al. Intrathecal methadone: a

dose-response study and comparison with intrathecal morphine. *Anesthesiology* 1989;71:A695.

122. De Sousa H, Klein E. Intrathecal and epidural oxymorphone. *Anesthesiology* 1989;71:A699.
123. Hays RL, Palmer CM, Van Maren GA, Alves DM. Does intrathecal nalbuphine decrease side effects of intrathecal morphine analgesia post-cesarean delivery? *Anesthesiology* 1995;83:A982.
124. Abouleish E, Rawal N, Tobon-Randall B, et al. A clinical and laboratory study to compare the addition of 0.2 mg of morphine, 0.2 mg of epinephrine, or their combination to hyperbaric bupivacaine for spinal anesthesia in cesarean section. *Anesth Analg* 1993;77:457.
125. Paech MJ. The influence of adrenaline on postoperative analgesia after subarachnoid morphine. *Anaesth Intens Care* 1993;21:79.
126. Malinow AM, Mokriski BLK, Nomura MK, et al. Effect of epinephrine on intrathecal fentanyl analgesia. *Anesthesiology* 1990;73:381.
127. Filos KS, Goudas LC, Patroni O, Polyzon V. Intrathecal clonidine as a sole analgesic for pain relief after cesarean section. *Anesthesiology* 1992;77:267.
128. Eisenach JC, Detweiler DJ, Tong C, et al. Cerebrospinal fluid norepinephrine and acetylcholine concentrations during acute pain. *Anesth Analg* 1996;82:621.
129. Eisenach JC. Three novel spinal analgesics: clonidine, neostigmine, amitriptyline. *Reg Anesth* 1996;21:81.
130. Bouaziz H, Tong C, Eisenach JC. Postoperative analgesia from intrathecal neostigmine in sheep. *Anesth Analg* 1995;80:1140.
131. Krukowski JA, Hood DD, Eisenach JC, Mallak KA. Intrathecal neostigmine for post-cesarean section analgesia: dose response. *Anesthesiology* 1996;85:A903.
132. Hood DD, Mallak KA, Eisenach JC, Tong C. Interaction between intrathecal neostigmine and epidural clonidine in human volunteers. *Anesthesiology* 1996;85:315.
133. Lauretti GR, Lima ICPR, Reis MP, Mattos AL. Dose related analgesic effect of intrathecal fentanyl associated with intrathecal neostigmine. *Anesthesiology* 1996;85:A724.
134. Eisenach JC, Grice SC, Dewan DM. Patient-controlled analgesia following cesarean section: a comparison with epidural and intramuscular narcotics. *Anesthesiology* 1988;68:444.
135. Harrison DM, Sinatra R, Morgese L, Chung JH. Epidural narcotic and patient-controlled analgesia for post-cesarean section pain relief. *Anesthesiology* 1988;68:454.
136. Cade L, Ashley J. Towards optimal analgesia after caesarean section: comparison of epidural and intravenous patient-controlled opioid analgesia. *Anaesth Intens Care* 1993;21:416.
137. Sinatra RS, Lodge K, Sibert K, et al. A comparison of morphine, meperidine, and oxymorphone as utilized in patient-controlled analgesia following cesarean delivery. *Anesthesiology* 1989;70:585.
138. Howell PR, Gambling DR, Pavy T, McMorland G, Douglas MJ. Patient-controlled analgesia following caesarean section under general anaesthesia: a comparison of fentanyl with morphine. *Can J Anaesth* 1995;42:41.
139. Sinatra R, Chung KS, Silverman DG, et al. An evaluation of morphine and oxymorphone administered via patient-controlled analgesia (PCA) or PCA plus basal infusion in postcesarean delivery patient. *Anesthesiology* 1989;71:502.
140. Parker RK, Holtmann B, White PF. Patient-controlled analgesia. Does a concurrent opioid infusion improve pain management after surgery? *JAMA* 1991;266:1947.
141. Parker RK, Holtmann B, White PF. Effects of a nighttime opioid infusion with PCA therapy on patient comfort and analgesic requirements after abdominal hysterectomy. *Anesthesiology* 1992;76:362.
142. Russell D, Duncan LA, Frame WT, Higgins SPJ, Asbury AJ, Millar K. Patient controlled analgesia with morphine and droperidol following caesarean section under spinal anaesthesia. *Acta Anaesthesiol Scand* 1996;40:600.
143. Wittels B, Scott DT, Sinatra RS. Exogenous opioids in human breast milk and acute neonatal behavior: a preliminary study. *Anesthesiology* 1990;73:864.
144. Yu PYH, Gambling DR. A comparative study of patient-controlled epidural fentanyl and single dose epidural morphine for post-caesarean analgesia. *Can J Anaesth* 1993;40:416.
145. Paech MJ, Moore JS, Evans SF. Meperidine for patient-controlled analgesia after cesarean section. *Anesthesiology* 1994;80:1268.
146. Vercauteren MP, Coppejans HC, Broecke PWT, Steenberge AL, Adriaensen HA. Epidural sufentanil for postoperative patient-controlled analgesia (PCA) with or without background infusion: a double-blind comparison. *Anesth Analg* 1995;80:76.
147. Cohen S, Amar D, Pantuck CB, Pantuck EJ, Weissman AB. Adverse effects of epidural 0.03% bupivacaine during analgesia after cesarean section. *Anesth Analg* 1992;75:753.
148. Cohen S, Amar D, Pantuck CB, et al. Postcesarean delivery epidural patient-controlled analgesia. *Anesthesiology* 1993;78:486.
149. Smet IGG, Vercauteren MP, De Jongh RF, Vundelinckx GJM, Heylen RJ. Pressure sores as a complication of patient-controlled epidural analgesia after cesarean delivery. *Reg Anesth* 1996;21:338.
150. Vercauteren MP, Vandeput DM, Meert TF, Adriaensen HA. Patient-controlled epidural analgesia with sufentanil following caesarean section: the effect of adrenaline and clonidine admixture. *Anaesthesia* 1994;49:767.
151. Parker RK, Holtmann B, White PF. Patient-controlled epidural analgesia: interactions between nalbuphine and hydromorphone. *Anesth Analg* 1997;84:757.
152. Bunting P, McConachie I. Ilioinguinal nerve blockade for analgesia after cesarean section. *Br J Anaesth* 1988;61:773.
153. Ganta R, Samra SK, Maddineni VR, Furness G. Comparison of the effectiveness of bilateral ilioinguinal nerve block and wound infiltration for postoperative analgesia after caesarean section. *Br J Anaesth* 1994;72:229.
154. Huffnagle HJ, Norris MC, Leighton BL, Arkoosh VA. Ilioinguinal iliohypogastric nerve blocks: before or after cesarean delivery under spinal anesthesia? *Anesth Analg* 1996;82:8.
155. Witkowski TA, Leighton BL, Norris MC. Ilioinguinal nerve blocks: an alternative or supplement to intrathecal morphine. *Anesthesiology* 1990;73:A962.
156. Abboud TK, Zhu J, Gangolly J, et al. Transnasal butorphanol: a new method for pain relief in post-cesarean section pain. *Acta Anaesthesiol Scand* 1991;35:14.
157. Gin T, Kan AF, Lam KK, O'Meara ME. Analgesia after caesarean section with intramuscular ketorolac or pethidine. *Anaesth Intens Care* 1993;21:420.
158. Parker RK, Holtmann B, Smith I, White PF. Use of ketorolac after lower abdominal surgery: effect on analgesic requirement and surgical outcome. *Anesthesiology* 1994;80:6.
159. Rorarius MGF, Suominen P, Baer GA, Romppanen O, Tuimala R. Diclofenac and ketoprofen for pain treatment after elective caesarean section. *Br J Anaesth* 1993;70:293.
160. Belzarena SD. Evaluation of intravenous tenoxicam for postoperative cesarean delivery pain relief. *Reg Anesth* 1994;19:408.
161. Cohen SE, Desai JB, Ratner EF, Riley ET, Halpern J. Ketorolac and spinal morphine for postcesarean analgesia. *Int J Obstet Anesth* 1996;5:14.
162. Sun HL, Wu CC, Lin MS, Chang CF. Effects of epidural morphine and intramuscular diclofenac combination in postcesarean analgesia: a dose-range study. *Anesth Analg* 1993;76:284.
163. Wittels B, Toledano A. Intravenous ketorolac and subarachnoid opioid analgesia in the management of acute postoperative pain. *Reg Anesth* 1995;20:395.
164. Cardoso MMSC, Carvalhlo JCS, Amaro AR, Prado AA, Cappelli EL. Small doses of intrathecal morphine combined with systemic diclofenac for postoperative pain control after cesarean delivery. *Anesth Analg* 1998;86:538.

Obstetric Anesthesia, second edition,
edited by Mark C. Norris.
Lippincott Williams & Wilkins, Philadelphia © 1999.

CHAPTER 39

Postoperative Complications Associated with Regional Anesthesia in the Parturient

Mark I. Zakowski

Obstetric anesthesia is generally a positive experience for the parturient and her family. A woman may be worried about the pain of labor and have fears of regional anesthesia and its potential effects on her and the baby. These women and all patients need reassurance and an explanation of regional anesthesia and its potential complications. If a problem does occur, it must be dealt with promptly and with expertise. This chapter discusses the signs, symptoms, diagnostic clues, laboratory tests, and management of complications related to regional anesthesia and delivery. Topics include headache, backache, infections, neurological deficits, and how to conduct a neurological examination.

HEADACHE

Headache is very common postpartum. Many causes of headache are unrelated to the recent administration of anesthesia. However, post–dural puncture headache (PDPH) is the most common postoperative complication of regional anesthesia in obstetric patients. Health care professionals should be familiar with the various causes, presentations, and treatments of headache. A careful history, including symptoms past and present, physical examination, and laboratory tests, if indicated, are essential in guiding proper diagnosis and management.

The differential diagnosis of headache includes nonspecific headache, migraine, preeclampsia, incipient eclampsia, and PDPH (Table 1). Almost 40% of women experience headaches in the first week after delivery (1). Although delivery is generally a happy time, many adjustments are required and stress is common. Stress headaches are typically pounding, temporal, or circumferential. Risk factors for nonspecific headache include history of migraine, depression, stress, or caffeine withdrawal.

TABLE 1. *Differential diagnosis: headache*

Nonspecific headache: stress
Migraine headache
Post–dural puncture headache (PDPH)
Hypertension/preeclampsia/incipient eclampsia
Caffeine withdrawal
Lactation headache
Sinusitis
Subdural hematoma
Hypoglycemia
Meningitis
Cortical vein thrombosis
Subarachnoid hemorrhage
Tumor
Drugs (e.g., $MgSO_4$)

Tension Headache

Tension headaches last 30 minutes to 7 days and have at least two of the following: pressing/tightening (nonpulsating) character, mild or moderate intensity, bilateral location, and are not aggravated by physical activity. Nausea and photophobia are absent (2). Treatment is with simple analgesics: acetaminophen or nonsteroidal antiinflammatory drugs (NSAIDs).

Migraine Headache

Migraine headaches occur more often in women, with a prevalence of 15% to 20% (3). Uncommonly, migraines may first occur during pregnancy, particularly in the first trimester. The hormonal changes of pregnancy result in an improvement of migraine symptoms for more than 66% of women. Headaches frequently recur postpartum (3). Migraine headaches typically last 4 to 72 hours, and

M. I. Zakowski: Department of Obstetric Anesthesia, Department of Anesthesiology, Cedars–Sinai Medical Center, Los Angeles, California 90048.

have two of the following: unilateral location, pulsating quality, moderate or severe intensity, and are aggravated with physical activity. Nausea, vomiting, or photophobia also are present. Prodromes may occur in 15% of patients, with visual changes being the most common. Ergotamine tartarate, 2 mg, is one of the classic treatments for migraine headaches. However, higher dose aspirin, acetaminophen, or NSAIDs also may work. Sumatriptan, a 5-hydroxytryptamine (5-HT_1)-receptor agonist, administered as 6 mg s.c. or 25 to 100 mg p.o., is very effective (2).

Hypertension/Preeclampsia/Eclampsia

Severe hypertension may cause headaches. Ergot preparations like methergine may produce or exacerbate hypertension (4). Preeclampsia is associated with headache, possible visual changes, nausea, and vomiting. Postpartum preeclampsia or eclampsia may first manifest as a complaint of headache (5).

Brain Tumor

Headache associated with brain tumor is typically generalized, or has a dull, deep, aching quality. It is usually intermittent and relieved by simple analgesics. Symptoms may overlap with migraine and tension-type headache. In pain clinics specializing in headaches, the incidence of brain tumors is less than 1% (2).

Cortical Vein Thrombosis

Pregnancy is a hypercoaguable state that may rarely lead to cortical vein thrombosis (CVT), with an incidence of one in 6,000 (6). In the United Kingdom, the incidence of CVT is one in 3,000 with a 25% maternal mortality rate (1988–1990 Report on Confidential Enquiries). The superior longitudinal sinus or the cortical veins may thrombose, impeding venous drainage. The increased venous pressure reduces cerebrospinal fluid (CSF) absorption from the arachnoid villi and increases intracranial pressure (ICP) (6). Venous stasis may produce arterial stasis and focal cerebral infarction.

Symptoms may occur before delivery or within 48 hours after delivery and include severe headache, nausea, focal neurological signs, seizures, and altered mental status (7). Diagnosis is made by contrast computed tomography (CT) scan, magnetic resonance imaging (MRI), or cerebral angiogram. Once the diagnosis is confirmed, treatment aims at seizure prophylaxis, and reducing ICP and cerebral edema by mechanical ventilation and steroids. Anticoagulation is controversial in the treatment of CVT because it may risk intracerebral hemorrhage (7,8).

Subdural Hematoma

Dural puncture can rarely result in a subdural hematoma (9). Take particular care with patients receiving any form of anticoagulation or thromboprophylaxis (10,11). The CSF leaks through the dural puncture, reducing ICP and allowing the cerebral vessel to dilate. When the patient is upright, downward movement of the brain may disrupt cerebral vessels, causing subdural hematoma. Headache should be nonpositional and persistent. In addition to headache, there may be symptoms of nausea/vomiting, confusion, or altered mental status. Focal neurological signs may be present. A noncontrast CT scan or MRI will reveal the hematoma. Surgical drainage is usually required.

Subarachnoid Hemorrhage

Symptoms of subarachnoid hemorrhage include severe headache, nausea and vomiting, neck stiffness, and decreased mental status. Focal neurological deficits may be present. A noncontrast CT scan or MRI will reveal the hematoma. Surgery may be required. Nimodipine, a selective cerebrovascular calcium channel blocker, may help prevent cerebral vasospasm.

Meningitis: Septic/Aseptic

Infectious meningitis is rare after regional anesthesia (12). Bacterial meningitis resulting from endocarditis occurs in one of 8,000 deliveries (12). Symptoms of meningitis typically include severe headache, fever, stiff neck, Kernig and Brudzinski signs (pain when extending the knee with the hip flexed and flexion of the lower extremities with neck flexion). Decreased mental status, vomiting, and seizures also may occur. Aseptic meningitis appears like bacterial meningitis, but no organisms are found in the CSF. Chemical irritation is thought to be the cause (13). Symptoms occur 6 to 24 hours after spinal anesthesia and are similar to those of bacterial meningitis (see later, Infections).

Pneumocephalus

Air may be introduced into the subarachnoid space during either spinal or epidural placement (14,15). Intracranial air may cause sudden severe headache, possibly with neck or back pain. In one series of more than 3,700 epidural injections, the use of air during loss-of-resistance technique resulted in significantly more headaches (PDPH) compared with saline (32 vs 5, respectively) in spite of an equal number of accidental dural punctures (48 vs 51). Intrathecal air bubbles were seen on CT scan in the deep brain structures (ventricles, sylvian fissures, and cisterns) as well as the superficial subarachnoid space in the air group only (16). Reabsorption of air over a period of several hours to days will eliminate the cause of the headache. Breathing 100% oxygen may hasten air reabsorption by denitrogenation.

Caffeine Withdrawal

Caffeine is almost ubiquitous in beverages today. Patients with a moderate daily dose of caffeine (235 mg;

2.5 cups coffee) may develop caffeine-withdrawal headaches. The average daily caffeine consumption should be checked as a cause of postoperative headache. Even people who consume low or moderate amounts of caffeine may have withdrawal syndrome: 52% develop moderate to severe headache, 10% depression/anxiety, and even decreased fine-motor performance (17). Caffeine sodium benzoate may be administered intravenously for replacement therapy while the patient has nothing by mouth (NPO). Incidentally, caffeine, 500 mg i.v., also has been used to treat PDPH (see later).

Lactation Headache

The hormonal changes of lactation have been reported to cause headaches (18).

Iatrogenic/Medications

Certain medications also may cause headache. Patients receiving $MgSO_4$ may develop flushing, nausea, and headaches. The headache may be due to the underlying preeclampsia or to cerebral vasodilatation. Allergies to food or flowers also may cause nasal stuffiness, sinusitis, and headaches. Hypoglycemia may cause headache and tachycardia. Electrolyte disturbances also may cause headaches. A patient with hypomagnesemia received an epidural blood patch (EBP) as a misdirected treatment for her headache (19).

Psychogenic

Patients should be told of the risk of headache with any regional anesthetic. There is no evidence for widespread psychogenic headaches. The incidence of headache after spinal anesthesia was the same whether the patients knew about it ahead of time or received it unknowingly (and probably without consent) during general anesthesia (20).

Post–Dural-Puncture Headache

Headache may follow intentional or unintentional puncture of the dura mater (PDPH). Previously called "spinal headache," this syndrome has been known for almost a century. CSF loss after dural puncture produces a low-intracranial-pressure headache. In the supine position, there are few or no symptoms. Changing to the sitting or standing position results in traction on the intracerebral venous sinuses, dural structures, cranial nerves, or tentorium (Fig. 1) (21). Symptoms include a rapid onset of a severe headache, neck pain, and cranial nerve symptoms (vision or hearing changes). Pain originating above the tentorium is transmitted via the trigeminal nerve to the frontal region, whereas pain from below the tentorium is transmitted via the vagus and upper cervical nerves to the occipital region and neck (22). This *positional* headache may be frontal, or circumferential. A headache that does not change in severity with position is not a PDPH. Nausea and, less frequently, vomiting may occur, but are not typical. Tinnitus, deafness, photophobia, and diplopia also are rarely possible. The sixth cranial nerve has a tortuous intracranial course and is more susceptible to traction and clinical symptoms. Abducens nerve paresis occurs in one in 5,000 to 8,000 PDPHs (23,24).

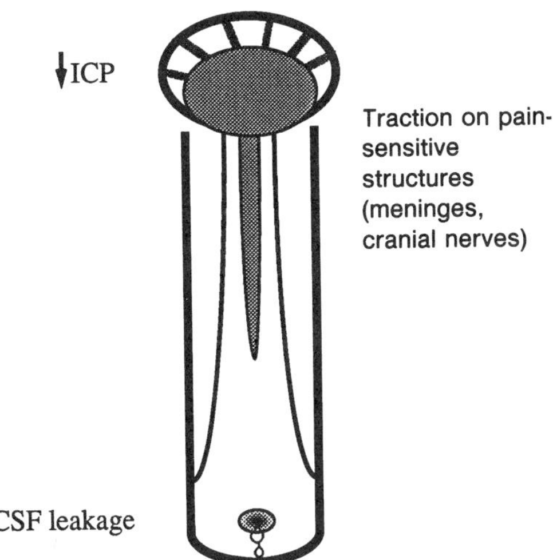

FIG. 1. Mechanical pathophysiology of post–dural puncture headache (PDPH). Cerebrospinal fluid (CSF) loss reduces lumbar and CSF intracranial pressure (ICP). When the patient assumes the upright position, this loss of CSF causes a shift in the brain relative to the dura and creates traction on pain-sensitive tentorial and meningeal structures and pain-sensitive cerebral vessels. Headache follows. (Drawing courtesy of M. Norris, M.D., with permission.)

Incidence

The overall risk of dural puncture during epidural catheter placement is 1.2% to 2.6% in residency training programs (25–29) and as low as 0.6% in one series (28). Risk factors for PDPH include age younger than 40, female, pregnant, increasing needle size, cutting beveled needle, orientation of needle, and history of PDPH (Table 2) (30). PDPH is infrequent after age 60 years,

TABLE 2. *Multivariate relation between PDPH and other factors after spinal anesthesia in the general surgical patient population*

Factor	*p*
Age	0.0001
Previous PDPH	0.0018
Direction of needle bevel	0.022
Gender	0.118
Needle size	0.105
Multiple attempts	0.091
Duration of postoperative recumbency (>4 or <4 h)	0.65

Modified from ref. 30, with permission.
PDPH, post–dural puncture headache.

possibly due to stiffening or calcification of dural and cerebral vessels. Women had twice the incidence of PDPH compared with men (20). Pregnancy may further increase the risk of PDPH in women. Bearing down during delivery did not affect the incidence of PDPH after accidental dural puncture with a large-gauge needle (31). The rate of CSF leak and the incidence of PDPH are related to the size of the dural hole (27,32,33). Dural puncture with a 17-gauge epidural needle may cause headache in 50% to 86% of parturients (26,29).

The newer blunt or pencil-point spinal needles only carry a 1% to 2% incidence of headache (Table 3). If a cutting-edged needle is used, orienting the needle bevel parallel to the longitudinal axis of the back (caudad–cephalad) decreases the size of the dural hole and the incidence of headache compared with perpendicular orientation (Fig. 2) (25,30). In one in vitro study, orienting the bevel perpendicular to the dura resulted in an increased rate of transdural fluid leak (32). Another author found no effect of bevel orientation on fluid leak (33).

The paramedian approach also has been advocated to decrease the incidence of headache by creating a flap valve that would close and decrease CSF leakage. Although one in vitro study supported this hypothesis (32), others have not achieved the success of Hatfalvi (34), who reported no headaches in 600 paramedian, 20-gauge spinal anesthetics. Another series showed no difference in the incidence of PDPH after midline or paramedian approach (35). History of a PDPH increases the likelihood of another PDPH after spinal anesthesia (30).

Continuous spinal anesthesia (CSA) via an indwelling catheter has been suggested as a means of reducing PDPH after accidental dural puncture. Fibrin deposits along the catheter may plug the dural hole on removal. In parturients, CSA after accidental dural puncture did not reduce the incidence of PDPH (Fig. 3) (36). Other, uncontrolled studies reported a smaller-than-expected incidence (1% to 16%) of PDPH associated with CSA (37–40). Use of microcatheter CSA for postoperative analgesia was associated with only a 1% chance of PDPH (41).

Pathophysiology

The normal adult has 150 mL of CSF and produces about 450 mL per day. In the horizontal position, lumbar CSF pressure is around 10 cm H_2O and increases to 50 cm H_2O in the upright position. The loss of CSF may cause some sagging of intracranial contents in the upright position, putting traction on pain-sensitive structures like the meninges, cranial nerves, bridging veins, and tentorium (Fig. 1). The acute loss of as little as 20 mL CSF caused symptoms of PDPH (42). Intrathecal injection of up to 20 mL glucose or saline immediately improved PDPH in 100% of patients (43). In this report, recumbent lumbar CSF pressure was 0 to 9 cm H_2O and 0 to 20 cm H_2O when sitting. After injection, the lumbar CSF pressure increased by about 10 to 15 cm H_2O (43). Leakage of CSF will continue until the dural hole seals, in 7 to 14 days, although headache usually resolves within 1 week (44).

Cerebral vasodilatation resulting from low ICP may produce PDPH (Fig. 4). The symptomatic relief offered by some cerebral vasoconstrictors (e.g., caffeine) supports this theory. Transcranial Doppler studies show significant changes in cerebral blood flow that correlate with symptoms of PDPH. Patients who develped PDPH after diagnostic lumbar puncture had asymmetric distribution of cerebral blood flow and lower blood flow velocity (suggesting vasodilation) in the middle cerebral artery compared with patients who did not develop a headache (45). In contrast, patients who had PDPH and developed seizures had cerebral vasoconstriction and decreased blood flow (46).

Reduction in intracranial CSF volume after lumbar puncture has been demonstrated on MRI (47). There was a trend toward a correlation between the reduction in CSF volume and the incidence of PDPH. The sagging of the

TABLE 3. *Post–dural puncture headache in obstetrics: effects of needle gauge and tip design*

	Needle type and gauge									
	Epidural		Quincke			Gertie Marx	Sprotte		Whitacre	Atraucan
Author	17	22	25	26	29	24	22	24	25	26
Stride (26)	86%									
Costigan (29)	50%									
Lambert (27)				5.2%					1.2%	
Flaatten (244)				6.7%	0%					
Dahl (245)					1%					
Wang (53)		25%								
Schultz (246)										2.7%
Sharma (247)									4.3%	4%
Douglas (248)									2.5%	
Lynch (249)					2%					
Jackson (250)						1%				
Sears (251)							1.6%	1.6%		

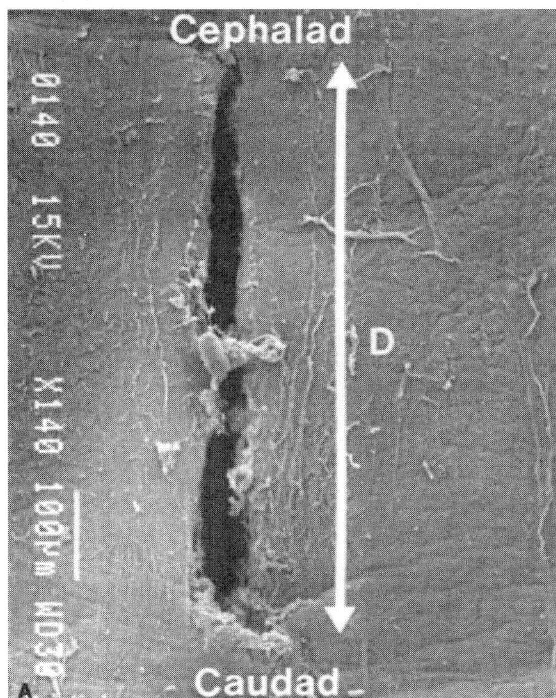

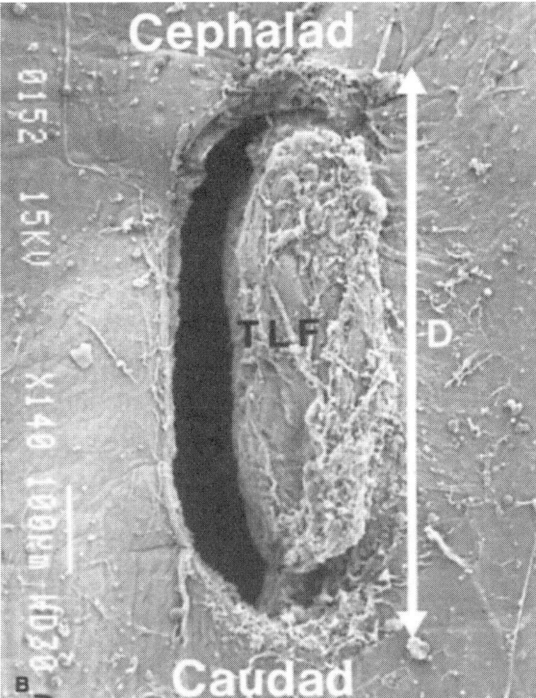

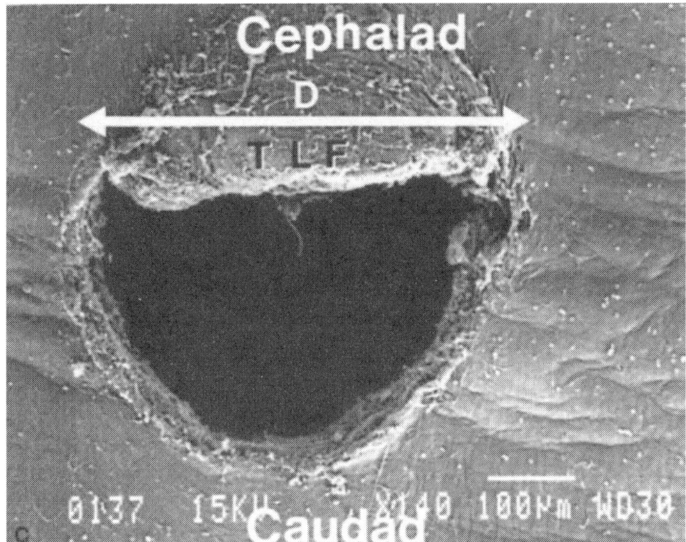

FIG. 2. Micrographs of dural defects produced by 22-gauge needles. **A:** Whitacre type (pen-point). **B:** Quincke, with the bevel oriented parallel to the longitudinal dural axis. **C:** Quincke, with the bevel oriented perpendicular to the longitudinal dural axis. Magnification 140×. D, diameter of the defect; TLF, "Tin-lid" flap. (Photograph courtesy of K. Sami, M.D., Naperville, Illinois, with permission.)

intracranial contents in the erect position may cause tears in the bridging veins, producing a subdural hematoma. Rarely, there also may be sufficient tugging on cranial nerves to produce symptoms like visual changes or buzzing in the ears (23,48). There was also a report of uncal herniation against the tentorium cerebelli due to sagging of the brain (49).

Hearing Loss

Auditory side effects of dural puncture may include a transient decrease in low-frequency hearing (50). A decreased CSF pressure may cause a similar decrease in the perilymphatic pressure of the inner ear via a patent cochlear aqueduct (51). Hearing loss may be unilateral and is related to size of dural puncture (52,53). Hearing loss resolved after epidural blood patch (54,55).

Course/Treatment

Although the onset of PDPH can be immediate or delayed, headache begins within 2 days of dural puncture in 66% of obstetric patients (Fig. 5) (26). PDPH usually resolves in 1 week, but prolonged headache for months or even years has rarely been reported. In a large series from the 1950s with 16- to 24-gauge cutting-edge needles,

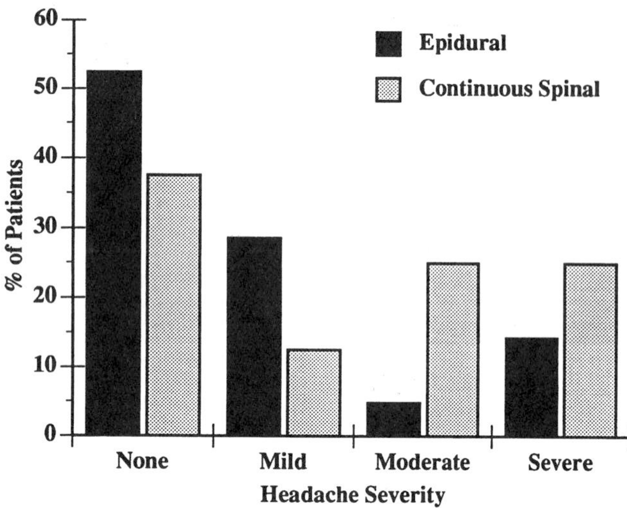

FIG. 3. Headache severity in parturients after dural puncture with a 17- or 18-gauge Hustead needle. Women in the epidural group received conventional lumbar epidural analgesia for labor and delivery. Women in the continuous spinal group had a 20-gauge polyamide catheter inserted into their subarachnoid space for labor pain relief. (Redrawn from ref. 36, with permission.)

75% of headaches lasted less than 1 week; 8%, less than 2 weeks; 5%, 3 to 6 weeks; 2%, 3 to 6 months; and 9%, 7 to 12 months (Fig. 6) (20). Needle size affects the duration of PDPH with headache after 20-, 22-, and 23-gauge (cutting) needles lasting 5.4, 4.9, and 2.7 days, respectively (56). Most headaches resolved within 8 days after

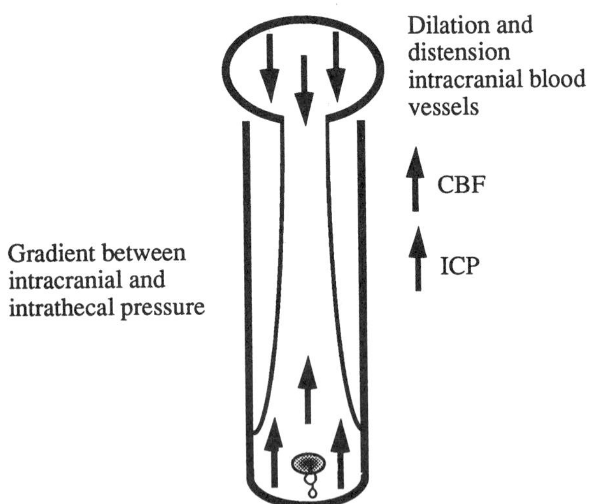

FIG. 4. Vascular mechanism of post–dural puncture headache (PDPH). Short-term loss of cerebrospinal fluid (CSF) produces a gradient between lumbar and CSF intracranial pressure (ICP). A reflex increase in cerebral blood flow (CBF) follows. This augmented CBF increases ICP and produces dilation and distention of intracranial blood vessels. Both of these effects can incite headache. (Drawing courtesy of M. Norris, M.D., with permission.)

accidental dural puncture with a 16-gauge Touhy needle (29). A delayed (more than 2 days) onset is associated with a shorter duration of headache (26). Treatment of PDPH is usually symptomatic. Any medication that ameliorates the pain, allows time for the dural puncture to heal and the headache to spontaneously resolve. Although an EBP is considered the definitive treatment for PDPH, it is usually elective in nature. If a patient shows signs of cranial nerve traction (diplopia, tinnitus), then EBP becomes an urgent necessity.

In the past, preventive bedrest had been suggested to avoid PDPH. Although patients do not have a headache while supine, the incidence of PDPH is not affected by bedrest (57,58).

Oral or intravenous hydration used to be recommended for treatment of PDPH (59). The incidence of PDPH after saddle block was reduced from 16% to 6.7% with the administration of 1 L of D_5NS after delivery (59). Whereas CSF resorption depends on CSF pressure, the rate of production does not (60). Hydration does not increase CSF production. Prophylactic oral hydration of 3 L did not reduce the incidence of PDPH (60).

Abdominal binders also are an old treatment of PDPH (61). The binder increases intraabdominal pressure, increasing epidural and vertebral venous pressure, resulting in increased intracranial pressure. The use of abdominal binders after spinal anesthesia for saddle block reduced the incidence of headache from 18% to 4% (61). However, abdominal binders are not commonly used today.

Cerebral Vasoconstrictors

Caffeine has been used to treat PDPH for more than 50 years (62). By producing cerebral vasoconstriction, caffeine may treat PDPH by counteracting the cerebral vasodilatation caused by low ICP. Caffeine sodium ben-

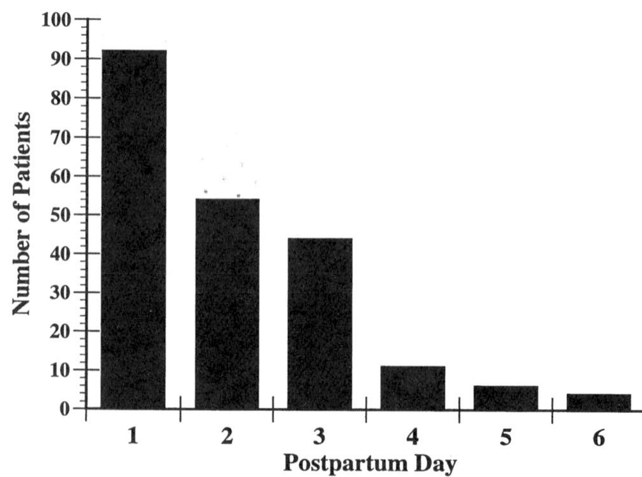

FIG. 5. Onset of post–dural puncture headache (PDPH) among 209 parturients with accidental dural puncture with a 16-gauge needle. (Redrawn from ref. 26, with permission.)

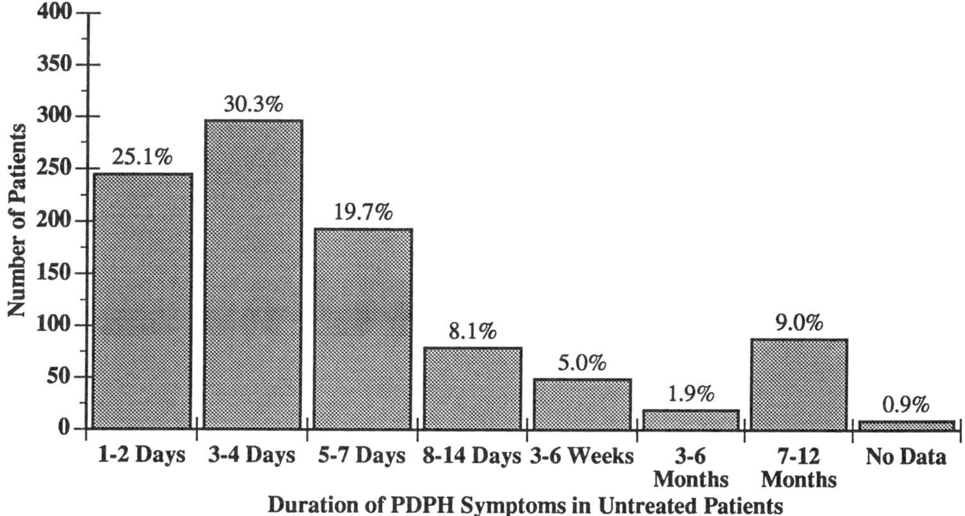

FIG. 6. Duration of symptoms after dural puncture in 1,011 patients. Spinal anesthesia was performed with 24- to 16-gauge needles in patients ranging between ages 10 and 89 years. (Redrawn from ref. 20, with permission.)

zoate, 500 mg i.v., relieved PDPH in 75% of patients after one dose and in 85% of patients after a second dose (63,64). Only 30% of patients whose headache improved had a return of the headache (65). Oral caffeine, 300 mg, reduced the visual-analog pain score (VAS, rated 100 to 0) from 66 to 33, whereas placebo reduced the VAS from 60 to 49 (Fig. 7) (66). Side effects of i.v. caffeine include dizziness and flushing. It has even been reported to cause seizures (67,68). Caffeine toxicity occurs in doses of more than 15mg/kg, when serum caffeine concentrations are greater than 30 mg/mL, and may result in seizures (69). The half-life of caffeine is increased nearly twofold in pregnancy to 8 to 12 hours (70).

Theophylline, another methylxanthine, also has been useful to reduce headache after dural puncture. Oral theophylline was better than placebo for the treatment of PDPH (71,72).

Sumatriptan, a serotonin (5-HT_1) agonist, has been reported to be effective in the treatment of PDPH, but not in all cases (73,74). Sumatriptan, 6 mg s.c., relieved PDPH in all patients (n = 6) (73). This effect is further evidence of a vascular role in the development of PDPH (75,76).

Nonsteroidal Antiinflammatory Drugs

Nonsteroidal antiinflammatory drugs help relieve PDPH. Indomethacin, 100 mg orally, decreased the incidence of PDPH from 18% to 10% after spinal anesthesia (77). Ibuprofen, 400 to 600 mg p.o., also has been helpful in my clinical practice.

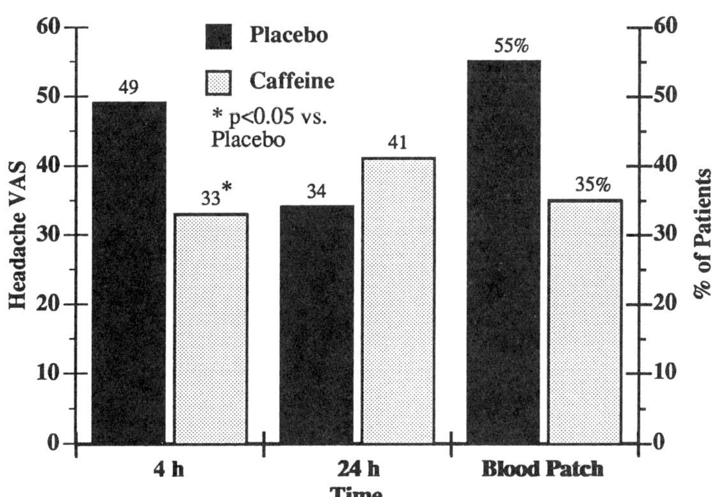

FIG. 7. Oral caffeine provides transient relief of post–dural puncture headache (PDPH). Forty parturients who complained of PDPH received either placebo or a single 300-mg dose of oral caffeine. Women in the caffeine group had less pain 4 hours later. Both groups had the same degree of pain by 24 hours. The need for therapeutic epidural blood patch did not differ between the groups. (Redrawn from ref. 66, with permission.)

Epidural Morphine

Epidural morphine may help alleviate symptoms of PDPH. All six patients with PDPH (five after 25-gauge needle, one after 19-gauge needle) reported relief of headache after 3.5 to 4.5 mg lumbar epidural morphine. Only the 28-year-old woman with the 19-gauge dural puncture needed a second dose of epidural morphine to obtain permanent relief (78).

Epidural Saline

Epidural saline has been used to treat PDPH for nearly 50 years (79). Lumbar epidural saline (10 to 20 mL) increased lumbar epidural and CSF pressure for up to 10 minutes (80). Rapid injection produced higher pressure than did slow injection, with an increase in dizziness, nausea, and lumbar back pain (80). Epidural injection of up to 60 mL or infusion of 1,000 mL saline was reported to relieve the headache, at least for the short term. Two prophylactic injections of 60 mL saline via the epidural catheter decreased the incidence of PDPH from 76% to 13% (81). In parturients, prophylactic epidural infusion of 1 to 1.5 L Hartman's solution per 24 hours decreased the incidence and severity of PDPH to 31%, with mild headaches only, compared with 77% among a historical control group (82). Epidural saline boluses of 20 to 30 mL were repeated until resolution of headache (average, 82 mL) in patients with PDPH. Patients had no return of headache (45%) or return of only a mild headache (55%) (81). Another study had an 80% cure rate with epidural saline injection (80). However, others found no improvement with epidural saline (28,83). Excessive epidural volume may produce side effects of back, neck, and orbital pain (82). Retinal hemorrhages were reported after an epidural bolus of 120 mL saline while under general anesthesia (84).

Epidural Blood Patch

Epidural blood patch (EBP) is considered the definitive treatment for PDPH and has been used for more than 35 years (85). The original report of EBP only used 2 to 3 mL of autologous blood. With 10 mL autologous blood, a 91% cure rate for PDPH was reported (86). Further increasing the injected volume to 20 mL resulted in a 98% cure rate (87). Currently successful treatment rates for EBP are commonly described as greater than 95% (87,88). These high reported success rates may reflect the short duration of follow-up in some studies. With longer follow-up, headache may return in 30% of patients (89).

Epidural blood spreads more in the cephalad direction than in the caudad direction (88). In one study, patients receiving EBP for PDPH had technetium-99m added to their autologous blood. Spread was determined with a gamma counter. Blood was injected into the epidural space until the patient complained of pain. The average

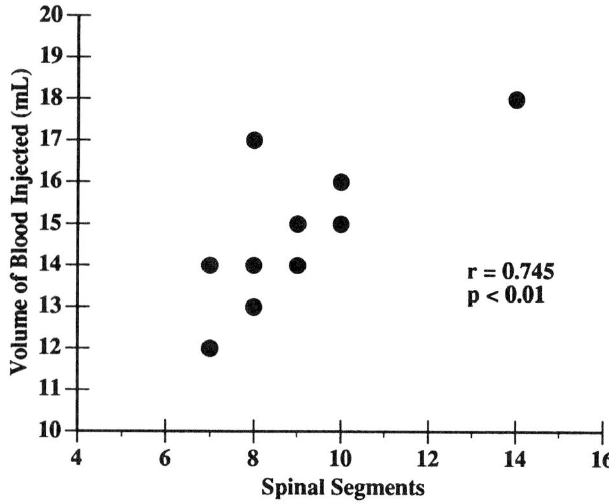

FIG. 8. Correlation between the amount of radiolabeled blood injected into the epidural space and the spread of gamma radiation. (Redrawn from ref. 90, with permission.)

volume injected was 15 mL, which spread nine spinal segments (1.6 mL/segment; Fig. 8). In another study, compression of the thecal sac from L_2 to T_{11}, predominantly cephalad spread, and a small amount of intrathecal blood were noted 30 minutes after EBP on MRI (90). Most of the blood extended over three to five spinal segments with a mass effect present until 3 hours. Clot resolution occurred by 7 hours. The nerve roots were temporarily displaced, perhaps causing the radicular pain that may occur with EBP. A small amount of blood was noticed in the CSF, forming a clot on the dural surface within the thecal sac. Spread of blood back into the subcutaneous tissues may account for the occurrence of low back pain after EBP (22,90). Vakharia et al. (91) used MRI to locate the site of dural puncture and to show the tamponade effect of injected blood on the thecal sac. EBP had mean spread of 4.6 intervertebral spaces and altered CSF flow.

Side Effects

Transient side effects, including back pain, neck ache, paresthesia, radiculitis, and cranial nerve dysfunction, are seen with up to 35% of EBPs (22,92). A few patients with PDPH treated with EBP had some backache for an average of 28 days (92). Although cranial nerve paresis can occur after one in 5,000 lumbar punctures, one case reports sixth cranial nerve weakness after EBP (23). Rarely mental status may change after an EBP. In two case reports, patients had other intracranial pathology (93,94). These exceedingly rare cases reinforce the need for a proper history and physical examination before performing EBP.

Histopathology

Animal studies examined the histopathologic effects of EBP. Epidural injection of 2 mL of blood produced a clot but no harmful tissue reaction in goats (95). Epidural blood resulted in fibroblastic activity and collagen formation. Dural puncture alone resulted in fibroblastic activity on the dura, which, after 3 weeks to 6 months, was similar to that of the EBP group (95).

In vitro studies examined the effects of blood on occluding holes in cadaver dura. Control puncture sites leaked at 1.5 cm H_2O, whereas blood-treated dura did not leak up to 40 to 50 cm H_2O pressure, which is the lumbar thecal pressure achieved in the erect position (96).

Jehovah's Witnesses

Jehovah's Witnesses may allow EBP if a continuous circuit for the blood is made from the vein into the epidural space. Variations of this technique have been described (97,98). The details of the technique must be discussed and permission obtained. Also, dextran 40 or powdered gelatin may be used as an alternate epidural injectate (see later).

Prophylactic Epidural Blood Patch

Early studies showed prophylactic EBP did not prevent PDPH (99,100). Seventy percent of patients developed a headache if they had EBP performed within 24 hours of dural puncture, compared with only 4% if EBP was done after 24 hours (99). These early studies used smaller volumes of blood (10 mL). More recent studies suggested better efficacy of prophylactic EBP (101–105) (Table 4). After placing the epidural catheter in a different interspace from the dural puncture and administering medication for labor analgesia or cesarean section, Colonna-Romano and Shapiro randomly assigned patients to receive 15 mL EBP or conservative therapy. Only 21% in the EBP group reported PDPH compared with 80% in the control group (101). In another study, only 10% of parturients who received a prophylactic EBP developed headache (104). After spinal anesthesia with a 25-gauge Quincke needle, prophylactic epidural saline was associated with a 45% incidence of headache compared with an 8% incidence in those receiving prophylactic EBP (105). EBP immediately after epidural anesthesia may fail because of residual local anesthetic impairing coagulation of blood (106).

Should all patients with an accidental dural puncture with an epidural needle receive a prophylactic EBP? Routine EBP would subject the 10% to 45% of patients who do not develop a PDPH to an unnecessary treatment. How soon is soon enough? There is a case report of total spinal anesthesia after an immediate prophylactic EBP (107). Others, however, performed immediate EBP without complications (108). One option is to leave the epidural catheter in place for 24 hours and then use it for EBP if a PDPH occurs. However, contamination of the epidural catheter is a theoretic risk. Leaving the epidural catheter might be helpful if it was very difficult to insert the first time. It is usually easy to identify the epidural space during EBP. I prefer to wait 24 hours and perform a new epidural needle insertion for EBP and not be concerned about catheter-tip location (midline vs lateral) or migration. The patient must give informed consent before any EBP is performed.

Dextran 40

Epidural administration of low-molecular-weight dextran (Dextran 40) also has been used successfully to treat PDPH (109). Patients for whom conservative therapy failed, as well as EBP, received 20 to 30 mL of Dextran 40 with a 100% cure of PDPH (n = 56). Side effects were dysesthesia (7%) and burning sensation (3.5%) at time of injection with no long-term sequelae. Another series of 13 patients for whom EBP failed were cured with a bolus of 20 mL epidural Dextran 40 followed by an infusion at 3 mL/h until 12 hours after headache disappeared. All patients had relief of symptoms within 20 hours (mean, 9.5 hours) (110,111). The prophylactic use of 20 mL of Dextran 40 after accidental dural puncture with an epidural needle successfully prevented any patient from getting a PDPH (n = 17; three parturients) (112). In sheep, epidural dextran was not neurotoxic and produced no pathologic changes in the epidural, subdural, or subarachnoid tissues (113). Dextran 40 may be effective because it is slowly absorbed from the epidural space, allowing more time for the dural puncture to heal.

Gelatin

Epidural gelatin also has been described in the treatment of PDPH. Gelatin powder (Gelfoam; Upjohn Co, Kalamazoo, MI), 600 to 700 mg, was dissolved in 10 mL of autologous plasma and injected epidurally in two patients for the treatment of PDPH. The solution was viscous, requiring increased pressure for injection via a plas-

TABLE 4. *The incidence of PDPH (%) with or without prophylactic epidural blood patch*

Number PDPH (%)		Volume	
+ PEBP (n)	− PEBP (n)	PEBP (mL)	Author
4/19 (23)	16/20 (80)	15	Colonna-Romano (101)
1/10 (10)		17–20	Cheek (104)
11/29 (38)	7/15 (47)	10–20	Mandell (103)
6/11 (55)	44/75 (57)	5–10	Palahniuk (100)

PEBP, prophylactic epidural blood patch; PDPH, post–dural puncture headache.

tic syringe. Gelfoam adheres to the area and causes a tissue reaction similar to a blood clot (114).

Technique for Epidural Blood Patch

The technique of performing an EBP is similar to that for labor analgesia. With strict aseptic technique, the epidural space is approached at or close to the site of dural puncture. The lower space may be preferred to a higher interspace because epidural blood spreads more cephalad than caudad. I prefer to perform EBP in the sitting position; it is somewhat easier to perform, and immediate relief of the headache confirms the epidural placement of the blood. Although transient (12 seconds) relative bradycardia (from 89 to 51 beats/min) was reported within 2 minutes after the performance of EBP, blood pressure, pulse oximetry, and EEG were unchanged (115). Thus intermittent monitoring of blood pressure and pulse is probably sufficient. The loss-of-resistance technique may be used with either air or normal saline. Local anesthetic should not be injected into the epidural space, as lidocaine in large proportion to blood serves as an anticoagulant (106). A few drops of CSF originating from the epidural space may be seen. Do not inject blood intrathecally! It may cause severe aseptic meningitis. Inject blood slowly, to a total volume of 15 mL. Commonly the patient complains of some pressure or pain in her back during injection. When this occurs, stop injecting, wait 1 minute, and then inject slowly until symptoms appear again. The needle may then be withdrawn. Patients should be left supine for 1 to 2 hours to maximize the efficacy of blood patch (Fig. 9) (116). Patients may then be discharged with instructions to return to the hospital if the headache returns, gets worse, or if visual or hearing disturbances develop.

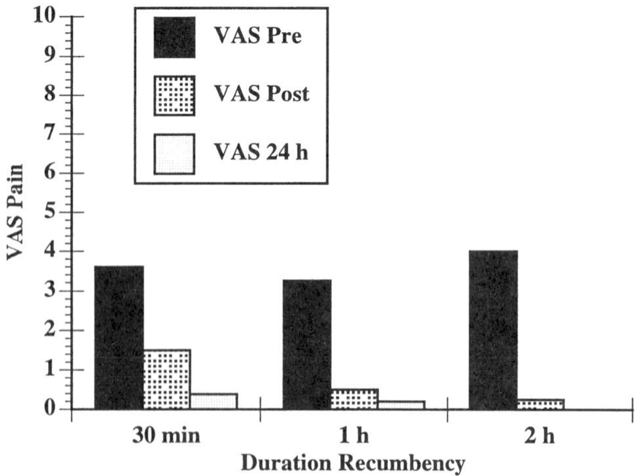

FIG. 9. Duration of recumbency and efficacy of epidural blood patch. Parturients were randomly assigned to remain flat for 30, 60, or 120 minutes after epidural blood patch. Patients lying flat for only 30 minutes had more pain when they first stood up and 24 hours later. (Redrawn from ref. 116, with permission.)

Subsequent Epidural Analgesia

Some patients will return for epidural analgesia in the years after accidental dural puncture and EBP. The rate of subsequent dural puncture is higher in those with a history of dural puncture (30). Although some reported restricted spread of epidural analgesia in patients with a history of EBP (117,118), other authors reported normal analgesia (119,120). In a retrospective study of 29 women with prior EBP, only 59% had good epidural analgesia. Of 17 parturients who had dural puncture but no EBP, only 65% achieved good analgesia compared with a historic control of 90% (118). However, a case–control study of 47 women with a previous dural puncture found no decrease in the efficacy of a subsequent labor epidural catheter (93% previous dural puncture vs 89% matched control subjects) (120).

Recurrent Headache

Symptoms of PDPH may improve after an EBP for only a short while. When symptoms return, a repeated EBP may be needed. These patients usually will do well. If the original EBP never worked, the technique or diagnosis should be questioned. If symptoms are still present after a second EBP, radiologic imaging may be warranted. A CT scan of the head may reveal other causes of headache (see earlier). I usually do not perform more than two EBPs, and never more than three. One patient had signs of spinal subdural hematoma after six EBPs (121).

Human Immunodeficiency Virus and Epidural Blood Patch

EBP may be performed in patients who are HIV seropositive. In a study monitoring six patients for up to 2 years after EBP, no neurocognitive or other adverse neurological or infectious complications could be found (122). Regional anesthesia in HIV-seropositive parturients had no neurological or immunologic sequellae (123). During EBP, blood can leak into the CSF (90), theoretically introducing infection and causing concern about EBP in HIV (124). However, HIV is neurotropic and present in the central nervous system (CNS), so dural puncture or EBP is unlikely to alter the course of the disease (125). However, EBP in HIV-seropositive individuals may be most prudently performed after failure of conservative measures (124).

BACKACHE

Another problem commonly encountered after delivery is backache.

Background

Low back pain is a nearly ubiquitous problem in the general population. Indeed, the lifetime prevalence of back pain is 70%, with a 1-year prevalence of 25% to 45%. Chronic back pain is present in 3% to 7% of the adult population (126). Sciatica accompanies back pain in up to 25% of cases. Herniated lumbar disc has a prevalence of 13% in both those with back pain and the general population. More than 90% of surgeries for removal of herniated disc are performed at the L_4 to L_5 level, yet only 10% to 15% of people with low back pain have an organic cause. Pain may originate from a herniated intervertebral disc, a nerve root that is compressed or stretched, lumbar facet joints, paraspinous muscle, posterior longitudinal ligament, or from the local blood vessels and nerves (126). Clearly the high prevalence and multiple causes of low back pain in the general population must be kept in mind when treating backache during or after delivery.

Pregnancy

Low back pain continues to be a common problem for parturients. The physiological changes of pregnancy predispose to back pain during pregnancy, with an incidence approaching 50% (127). The body releases a polypeptide named relaxin that loosens ligaments. The increasing size of the gestation exaggerates the lumbar lordosis. These changes may permit excessive range of motion, causing back pain. In one series, low back pain occurred in 40% of pregnant women and sacroiliac pain in 50% (128). Pain also may be caused by compression of the lumbosacral nerves. Weinreb et al. (129) found that 53% of pregnant women and 54% of nonpregnant women showed evidence of disc abnormalities on MRI. Radicular symptoms may often accompany low back pain. However, true sciatica with a dermatomal distribution is uncommon (1%) (127). In another study, a herniated nucleus pulposus occurred in only one in 10,000 pregnancies (130,131). After delivery, back pain is very common, occurring in about 40% of new mothers (132).

Regional Anesthesia

Several studies have examined the effects of regional anesthesia on the incidence of low back pain in parturients after delivery. Although three retrospective studies reported an increased risk of back pain after epidural analgesia (133–135), other prospective studies found no increased risk (132,136,137).

A retrospective study from England found a significantly greater incidence of low back pain in women receiving epidural labor analgesia compared with those who did not (18.9% vs 10.5%; $p < 0.05$) (137). Women who had an elective cesarean section with epidural anesthesia did not have an increased incidence of back pain. This retrospective study was conducted by postal survey and included deliveries over the previous 8 years. Reporting bias probably played a role in these results. It also is possible that the relatively high concentrations of local anesthetic (0.375% to 0.5% bupivacaine) used for labor analgesia during the survey period produced greater relaxation of the lumbar musculature and allowed the patient to remain in positions that might otherwise have been too painful. With the same database, MacArthur et al. (138) found that the only predictor of long-term backache was backache immediately after birth. Women who delivered spontaneously and without anesthesia had significantly more back pain compared with those whose deliveries were assisted with forceps or vacuum (40% vs 25%) (139). Thus the duration of second stage of labor may influence the incidence of backache.

Several prospective studies also examined the affect of regional anesthesia on low back pain. In one study of 1,036 parturients, the incidence of back pain was 32%. Risk factors associated with back pain were history of back pain, multiparity, and epidural analgesia (140). In a small study, there was a significantly greater incidence of long-term backache after epidural anesthesia compared with general anesthesia for manual removal of placenta (6.25% vs 33%) (141). In a prospective postal survey of 262 patients who received epidural analgesia, backache was associated with a shorter length of labor compared with those with no backache (9.75 hours vs 11.75 hours; $p = 0.01$). This finding suggests that more intense, painful labors may produce backache. No association was found between backache and age, height, weight, parity, or mode of delivery (142). Risk factors for long-term backache included nulliparity, Asian race, young maternal age, prolonged second stage, and lower social class (133).

In another prospective study, women who received epidural labor analgesia had a higher incidence of low back pain on the first postpartum day, (53% vs 43%), but the incidence of low back pain was similar at 1 and 6 weeks after delivery (136). In an institution where residents insert most epidural catheters, the incidence of back pain after childbirth was 44% in those receiving epidural analgesia and 45% in those who did not (132). The type of delivery [normal spontaneous vaginal delivery (NSVD) or cesarean] did not affect back pain. The best predictor of low back pain after delivery was back pain during pregnancy. Even new-onset back pain was not associated with epidural analgesia. However, increased maternal weight was associated with an increased chance of back pain (132). The epidural analgesia solution used in this study was bupivacaine, 0.04% to 0.125%, with fentanyl ± epinephrine. These relatively low doses of local anesthetic may preserve muscle function and prevent stretching of the spinous ligaments, muscles, and nerves. However, in another study, the duration of epidural analgesia and degree of sensory and motor block were not related to the long-term back pain (138).

In a prospective cohort study, there was no difference in the prevalence of back pain 1 year after delivery between women who received epidural analgesia and those who did not (10% vs 14%) (137). In this study, women received bupivacaine, 0.25%, for both the initial and repeated doses of epidural analgesia. Lidocaine, 2%, or 2-chloroprocaine, 3%, were used for anesthesia at time of delivery. This study also suggested that the concentration of local anesthetic lacks impact on the incidence of low back pain.

In discussing epidural analgesia with patients who are concerned about back pain, I try to mention the following points:

- Back pain is common with or without regional anesthesia,
- Back pain is a chronic disease: a history of back pain predicts future pain,
- Epidural analgesia does not affect the incidence of back pain after delivery in prospective studies, and
- Epidural injections are used in the treatment of acute back pain.

Discussing these points with a parturient anxious about the effects of epidural analgesia on postpartum back pain usually allays the fears.

2-Chloroprocaine

The use of 2-chloroprocaine-MPF has been associated with severe back pain lasting up to 36 hours. The original formulation of 2-chloroprocaine used metabisulfite as a preservative. However, after reports of accidental intrathecal injection causing cauda equina syndrome, the bisulfite concentration was reduced and then eliminated. Sodium EDTA (ethylenediaminetetraacetic acid) became the preservative used in the MPF formulation from Astra Pharmaceuticals. However, reports of back pain after the use of 2-chloroprocaine with EDTA soon proliferated. Back pain occurred in 40% of patients receiving epidural injection of 25 to 29 mL of drug (143,144). Although gross muscle spasm was not noted, this pain was possibly due to paraspinous muscle spasm caused by localized EDTA-related hypocalcemia (145). EDTA injected into the epidural space caused tetanic muscle contractions in the rat (146). Indeed, intravenous calcium chloride has been used to treat the back pain (147). 2-Chloroprocaine–induced back pain may be moderate or even severe in intensity but resolves by the following day. The most recent preparation of 2-chloroprocaine (Nesicaine-MPF) lacks both bisulfite and EDTA.

Prevention

In a letter to the editor, Peng et al. (148) reported that the use of a field block to anesthetize the segmental recurrent spinal nerves before epidural anesthesia significantly reduced the incidence of back pain and eliminated long-term back pain. Administration of less than 25 mL of 2-chloroprocaine will help prevent backache (see earlier). Proper positioning during labor, delivery, or cesarean section also may help.

Treatment

Treatment of back pain is symptomatic with analgesics. Heat and physical therapy may help. Exercise and proper posture are important in the long-term prevention of backache.

INFECTIONS

Serious infections related to neuraxial anesthesia are very rare. Epidural or subarachnoid infections can produce permanent disability or death. Rapid diagnosis and treatment are essential. Issues of localized or generalized infection (e.g., herpes, severe acne) may complicate regional anesthesia. Erythema at the site of epidural insertion is not uncommon because of irritation of the catheter or a minor localized infection. Infections of the skin and subcutaneous tissues are readily treated with antibiotic therapy, if needed.

Prevention

Infection can start by introduction of bacteria during a procedure, or when bacteremia causes "seeding" of an indwelling foreign body (e.g., epidural catheter). Strict aseptic technique is essential, not only during insertion of the epidural catheter, but during subsequent injections as well. The hub and cap of the epidural catheter must be kept sterile. Only sterile solutions should be injected. Some anesthesiologists use a micropore filter during epidural injection. However, filters with a pore size of 1 μm will only filter microscopic particles of glass produced by opening ampoules. A pore size of 0.2 μm is needed to filter bacteria. Such a filter lacked benefit in healthy obstetric patients (149). Because microscopic glass particles may enter the solution, clean the neck of ampoules with alcohol before opening.

Epidural Abscess

Epidural abscess is fortunately rare but can be devastating if not promptly recognized and treated. The estimated incidence is 0.2 to 1.2 per 10,000 tertiary hospital admissions (150). Epidural abscess usually occurs as a complication of infection elsewhere in the body, with bacteria seeding the epidural space (151). In one review of 39 cases of epidural abscess, only one was associated with an epidural catheter (152). Another review also found no spinal infections related to epidural anesthesia among 35 cases (153). Epidural abscess usually becomes symptomatic a few days to a few weeks after delivery.

One epidural abscess was reported in a bacteremic patient 16 days after delivery in a series of more than

26,000 epidural anesthetics in parturients. In a series of more than 500,000 obstetric epidural blocks, only one patient had an epidural abscess (154). She had diabetes and developed an epidural abscess 11 months after delivery. A recent survey of more than 13,000 blocks reported one abscess after prolonged epidural labor analgesia (88 hours) (155). At my institution, only one case of epidural abscess has occurred in more than 50,000 regional anesthetics in parturients. This patient had predisposing risk factors for infection (e.g., obesity, intravenous drug abuse).

Epidural abscess usually becomes symptomatic a few days to weeks after delivery (151). Typical symptoms include fever, malaise, headache, and back pain at the level of the infection. On physical examination, there is tenderness to deep palpation over the site of infection and pain with movement (flexion greater than extension). On routine laboratory examination, the white blood cell count will be increased with a polymorphonuclear leukocytosis, and blood cultures may be positive for bacteria. Nerve-root pain develops 1 to 3 days after onset. Neurological deficits will develop as the abscess progresses and impinges on the spinal cord and its blood supply. Lower-extremity pain, weakness, bowel and bladder dysfunction, and paraplegia may occur (Table 5) (151,156).

Diagnostic tests include prompt imaging of the spinal canal. The preferred imaging technique for spinal infections is MRI with gadolinium enhancement (157). If MRI is unavailable, a CT scan also may be used. A myelogram is less informative and more invasive. Especially if neurological symptoms are present, spinal decompression by laminectomy must be performed immediately. Treatment with antibiotics but not surgical drainage is not sufficient. Neurological compromise is usually reversible if the spinal cord is decompressed within 6 to 12 hours of symptoms (158).

Some controversy exists concerning regional anesthesia in patients who are presumed or documented to be bacteremic. An invasive procedure and introduction of a foreign body (e.g., epidural catheter) may provide a nidus for infection. A small amount of blood may be introduced into the spinal canal during regional anesthesia by puncture of the epidural veins, serving as a culture medium for bacteria. Debate often centers on the use of epidural catheters in parturients with chorioamnionitis, a potential source of bacteremia. Several retrospective studies suggested that continuous epidural analgesia is safe in women who may have chorioamnionitis (see Chapter 29) (159–161).

Meningitis

Bacterial meningitis is very rare after epidural or spinal anesthesia. Proper sterile technique allows the use of continuous spinal anesthesia or epidural catheter use after accidental dural puncture. Although there are a couple of case reports of meningitis in parturients (162,163), they are assumed to be related to a breach in sterile technique. Interestingly, 30% of rats injected with *Escherichia coli* developed meningitis if the dura was punctured compared with none if the dura remained intact (164). Meningitis also was reported after the combined spinal–epidural technique (165). Bacterial meningitis usually is seen 24 to 48 hours after regional anesthesia, with fever, headache, and stiff neck (150). The CSF will show increased white blood cells (polymorphonuclear), decreased glucose, increased protein, and organisms seen on Gram stain.

Aseptic meningitis appears like bacterial meningitis except that no organisms are found in the CSF. This syndrome was more common when reusable equipment was improperly cleaned and sterilized (166–168). In one large series, only two cases of aseptic meningitis occurred in 780,000 regional anesthetics (169). Aseptic meningitis is probably due to chemical irritation of the spinal cord and meninges. Detergent residue on a reusable glass syringe was reported to produce aseptic meningitis (13). Symptoms usually occur 6 to 24 hours after spinal anesthesia, are similar to those of bacterial meningitis, and include

TABLE 5. *Differential diagnosis of epidural abscess, epidural hematoma, and anterior spinal artery syndrome*

	Epidural abscess	Epidural hematoma	Anterior spinal artery syndrome
Age	Any age	Older > younger	Elderly
History	Diabetes, infection(?)	Anticoagulants: heparin, coumadin	Vascular disease, hypotension (?)
Onset	Delayed	Sudden	Sudden
Symptoms	Fever, back pain, tenderness Progressive motor deficits (hours-days)	Sharp back and radicular pain Progressive motor deficits (hours)	None Acute motor deficit
Sensory	None or paresthesias	Variable, late	Minor
Motor	Flaccid paralysis, later spastic	Flaccid paralysis	Flaccid paralysis
Reflexes	Decreased	Decreased	Decreased
MRI/CT scan	Extradural compression	Extradural compression	Normal
Cerebrospinal fluid	↑WBC	Normal	Normal
Labs	↑WBC	Possible ↑PT/PTT, ↓fibrinogen	Normal

WBC, white blood cell count; PT, prothrombin time; PTT, partial thromboplastin time.
Modified from ref. 150, with permission.

headache, fever, stiff neck (nuchal rigidity), and photophobia (13). CSF analysis shows increased white blood cells (usually lymphocytosis), normal glucose, increased protein, and no bacteria on Gram stain (165).

Herpes Simplex Virus

Active herpes simplex virus (HSV) type 2 infection in the genital area is an indication to perform a cesarean section in women who are in labor or who have ruptured amniotic membranes. The neonate may acquire HSV infection during passage through the birth canal, causing serious CNS infection with potential permanent sequelae (170). Although antiviral therapy decreases the severity of neonatal infection, cesarean section is still indicated.

Pregnant women are more prone to serious neurological sequelae from HSV (171). During primary HSV infection, viremia occurs and may cause CNS symptoms. Regional anesthesia during primary HSV infection is controversial. In theory, regional anesthesia may introduce the virus into the CNS. However, HSV normally resides in dorsal root ganglia and is inherently a neurotropic virus. The presence of an epidural catheter or a dural puncture is unlikely to alter the eventual presence of virus within the CNS.

During episodes of recurrent genital herpes, regional anesthesia was reported to be safe by many authors (172–174). One patient with a primary HSV infection had weakness of one leg for 1 week after delivery. It cannot be ascertained whether the spinal anesthetic altered the course of the disease.

There have been a few reports of epidural morphine increasing the risk of recurrence of oral herpes simplex lesions after cesarean section (175–177). In a randomized prospective study, 15% of patients had facial pruritis and reactivation of herpes labialis after epidural morphine compared with none in an i.m. opioid group (175). However, in a prospective study of 357 parturients, the incidence of herpes simplex labialis after cesarean delivery was similar in the groups receiving neuraxial and i.m. morphine (3.5% vs 2.6%, respectively) (178). Whether herpes labialis reactivation could be due to a direct drug effect or due to the facial pruritus and scratching cannot be determined (176). Current evidence points to morphine affecting trigeminal nerve opioid activity, resulting in facial itching. This influence may be through the tract of Lissauer in the dorsal horn, which is continuous with the spinal (caudal) nucleus of the trigeminal nerve. However, the itching is thought to be a marker, not a direct trigger for HSV reactivation (170).

NEUROLOGICAL DEFICITS

The most feared complication of regional anesthesia is a neurological deficit. Fortunately, such problems are very rare in obstetric patients. After delivery, most neurological injuries have obstetrical, not anesthetic, causes. A complete history, physical examination, and diagnostic testing are important for proper diagnosis and treatment of these events.

Neurological Examination and Testing

Symptoms of back or extremity pain, weakness, paresthesia, or numbness must be evaluated promptly. Although most of these complaints are minor in origin (e.g., nonspecific low back discomfort or tenderness at the epidural insertion site), some are potentially catastrophic (i.e., epidural hematoma) (Table 6). The best approach to possible postpartum neurological deficits is to:

- Take a good history,
- Perform a full neurologic examination,
- Request additional diagnostic testing, if needed, and then
- Decide on management and the need for consultations.

History

A proper history of the current complaint is essential. Elicit the precise onset, location, and radiation of symp-

TABLE 6. *Differential diagnosis of prolonged neural blockade*

Drug effect
Prolonged duration of local anesthetic
Slow regression of block
More common after multiple doses (e.g., bupivacaine)
Neurotoxicity
Rare effect of usual drug (e.g., lidocaine, 5%)
Wrong drug administered (e.g., potassium chloride)
Trauma
Peripheral nerve
Compression from positioning
Known peripheral nerve pattern
Central nervous system
Impingement during needle insertion
Paresthesias, pain with insertion
External compression of root or spinal cord
Herniated intervertebral disc
Epidural hematoma (early)
Epidural abscess (late)
Spinal stenosis
Vascular
Hemorrhage: spinal AVM
Decreased blood supply: no signs of recovery/ permanent injury
Anterior spinal artery syndrome
Compression of the arterial blood supply by fetal head
Severe hypotension
After cardiac arrest
Emboli: air, thrombotic, amniotic fluid
Neurological disease: preexisting and new
Multiple sclerosis
HIV
Guillain-Barré

AVM, arteriovenous malformation; HIV, human immunodeficiency virus.

toms. Did they start during needle insertion or drug injection? Is the anesthetic block prolonged, or was there a period of full recovery? Is the pain/deficit in a dermatomal pattern, part of a peripheral nerve distribution, or perhaps nonanatomic? Note any history of back pain, numbness, or weakness. Investigate positioning and management of second stage of labor. Use of forceps and excessive or prolonged hyperflexion of the hips may result in injury to the muscles or nerves.

Physical Examination

Perform and document a detailed neurological examination. Fully test cranial nerves, upper and lower extremities, sensory and motor function, reflexes, and Babinski signs. Have the patient perform a straight-leg raise. Careful mapping of symptoms may reveal a pattern consistent with a peripheral nerve injury or a single root lesion (Fig. 10). Detailed documentation in the chart is very important to good patient care and may serve in your future defense.

Areas to check on physical examination include sensory as well as motor tone of the paraspinous muscles (soft vs knotted, innervated by the posterior rami of the nerve root), tenderness to deep palpation of the processes (transmits pressure to epidural space, pain elicited with an intraspinal mass), localized area of erythema or purulence, and sacroiliac joint tenderness. Pay particular attention to distribution of symptoms along a peripheral nerve or an individual nerve root.

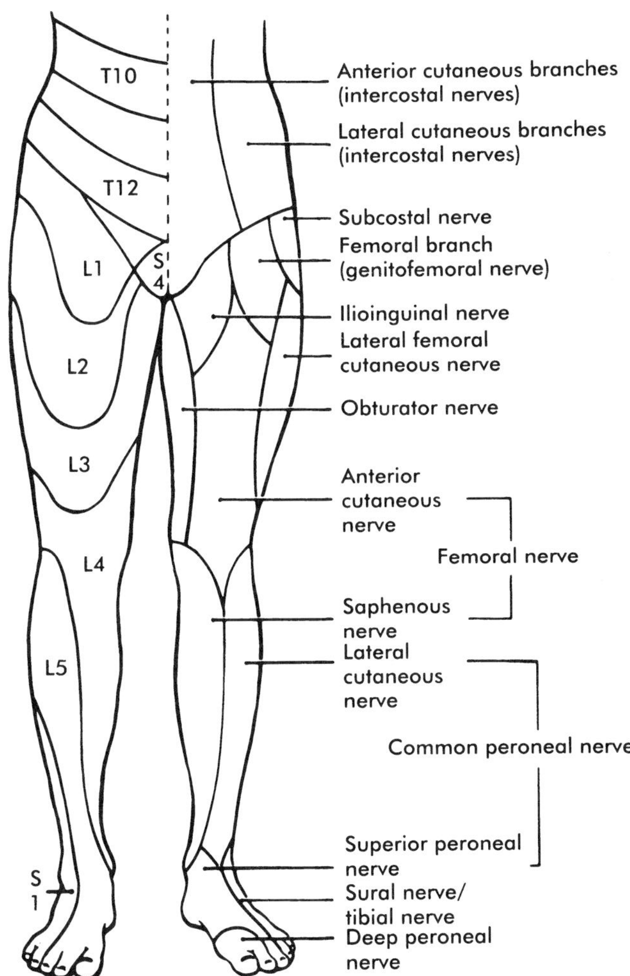

FIG. 10. Anterior diagram of segmental (left side) and peripheral (right side) sensory nerve distributions useful in distinguishing central from peripheral nerve injury. (Reprinted from ref. 179, with permission.)

Diagnosis

The common peroneal nerve is frequently injured where it lies above the fibula, just below the knee. This nerve may be compressed when the legs are in stirrups. Common peroneal nerve injury produces lateral calf paresthesia with foot drop and inversion. The lateral femoral cutaneous nerve provides sensation along the lateral aspect of the thigh. Pressure on the nerve may produce numbness there. Recovery usually occurs within 6 weeks. During flexion of the hip, the inguinal ligament may compress the femoral nerve. Symptoms include quadriceps weakness and hypalgesia in thigh and calf. The lumbosacral trunk may be injured within the pelvis by the fetal head (especially forceps, occiput posterolateral). Symptoms may be unilateral or bilateral and may affect the quadriceps, hip adduction, and foot drop (Table 7).

Routine Tests

If the problem is a peripheral nerve injury (e.g., common peroneal nerve), further testing may not be needed. If fever accompanies back pain or headache, a white blood cell count and differential should be performed. An examination of the CSF may rarely be indicated to rule out septic or aseptic meningitis.

Advanced Testing

The diagnosis of certain neurological deficits will be aided by sophisticated imaging, neurophysiologic, or electrodiagnostic tests. If a patient has symptoms isolated to a particular nerve root, then obtain CT or MRI of the affected area. History of a recent regional anesthetic does not prove causation. An occult herniated disc may become symptomatic after the stress of labor and delivery. Neurophysiologic testing can help document the location and severity of an injury. Electrodiagnostic testing will localize a problem to the CNS or to the periphery at the individual nerve, root, or plexus. Electodiagnostic testing also may help differentiate a neurapraxia, which will resolve in 1 to 5 months, from an axonotmesis with axonal interruption, which may last longer (180).

TABLE 7. *Peripheral nerve injuries in obstetric patients*

Nerve	Root value	Mechanism of injury	Clinical picture
Lumbosacral trunk	$L_{4,5}$, S_1	Forceps Fetal head	Foot drop Quadriceps and hip adductors affected
Femoral nerve	L_2, L_3, L_4	Fetal head Retractor	Quadriceps weakness Weak hip flexion Absent patellar reflex Hypalgesia in thigh and calf
Lateral cutaneous nerve	L_2, L_3	Stirrups	Hypalgesia in the front thigh
Common peroneal nerve	L_4–S_2	Stirrups	Foot drop Hypesthesia in the lateral calf
Obturator nerve	L_2–L_4	Fetal head	Weakness of thigh adduction Hypesthesia in the medial aspect of thigh

Nerve may be compressed by the fetal head or by the stirrups because of improper positioning.
From Ramanathan S. *Obstetric anesthesia.* Philadelphia: Lea & Ferbiger, 1988: 102, with permission.

CT scanning is faster and less expensive than MRI. CT is superior to MRI in detecting intracranial blood, especially subarachnoid hemorrhage, and in defining cortical bone structure of the skull and spine. MRI is contraindicated if the patient has implanted metallic objects (e.g., pacemaker). MRI is superior for intracranial and intraspinal soft-tissue lesions, permitting better three-dimensional information, and also can show blood or CSF flow. Gadolinium-enhanced MRI increases the sensitivity for neoplastic and inflammatory lesions, like epidural abscess (181). However, MRI takes longer, is more expensive, and some patients are unable to complete the study because of claustrophobia.

Electromyography (EMG) will help to document the time and location of injury. A recording needle is placed directly into the muscle. After denervation, the muscle fibers begin to discharge spontaneously, but muscle-fibrillation potentials do not change for 2 to 3 weeks after nerve injury. Thus an EMG with abnormalities within the first week after delivery will document preexisting disease (i.e., before regional anesthesia). If an interval change occurs 4 to 6 weeks after delivery, then the injury occurred around the time of delivery. If the nerve root is injured, both the anterior and posterior rami should be involved. Thus the paraspinous area should be affected. If not, then the level of nerve injury is distal to the nerve root and not caused as a direct result of central regional anesthesia.

Unlike EMG, conduction-velocity studies can provide immediate information about both motor and sensory nerves. The efferent pathway is stimulated at the level of either the nerve root or the descending pathways of the brain or spinal cord. The response is measured at the muscle or along a distal portion of the nerve. A supramaximal stimulus is applied to ensure that all nerve fibers are activated, the latency is measured, and the conduction velocity is calculated. The conduction velocity represents the fastest-conducting fibers, and surface recordings may miss disease in small-diameter nerve fibers. Lesions proximal to the dorsal root ganglia do not affect the sensory potential and thus help to distinguish radicular from peripheral nerve disease (180).

Proximal nerve segments can be indirectly evaluated by using the late-response studies (F responses, H reflex). The F response is a measure of proximal nerve conduction from the point of peripheral nerve stimulus to the anterior horn cells and back along the nerve. The H reflex is found in the tibial nerve/soleus system, occurs during submaximal stimulation, and is thought to be a monosynaptic reflex with an afferent and efferent limb. A prolonged H reflex with a normal F response in the same nerve identifies dorsal root pathology (180,182).

Somatosensory evoked potentials (SSEPs) will monitor the dorsal columns of the spinal cord. An electrical stimulus is applied over the posterior tibial or median nerve, and electrical activity is measured in the brain. The afferent sensory pathways conduct from the periphery through the gray matter of the lumbar spinal cord, brainstem, and primary somatosensory cortex. SSEPs are sensitive to spinal cord damage produced by compression, mechanical distraction, and ischemia (182).

Motor evoked potentials (MEPs) measure the integrity of the descending motor pathways in the anterior part of the spinal cord. A magnetic field is used to stimulate the motor cortex, and compound muscle actions potentials are then recorded over the distal muscles. This technique may not be widely available, even in major hospital centers (182).

Management

Management of a neurological deficit is specific to the particular injury. A neurologist should be consulted if a deficit is identified. Discuss the patient's symptoms and your differential diagnosis with the neurologist or other specialist to facilitate obtaining the diagnostic tests that you think are indicated. Steroids are frequently used to reduced swelling and inflammation. Physical therapy may be appropriate for intermediate and long-term neurological deficits.

OBSTETRIC INJURIES

Injuries to the nervous system occur during NSVDs in patients who do not receive regional or general anesthesia. Parturients may experience compression nerve injury, or rarely, an ischemic spinal cord injury. The incidence of neurological deficits up to the early 1960s was as high as to one in 2,100 (183–185). Obstetric practice during this time allowed protracted labor and the frequent use of forceps. A more recent survey of almost 24,000 deliveries from 1975 to 1983 found transient neurological deficits in one of 4,167 deliveries without anesthesia (186). All of the neurological deficits in this study were transient, lasting fewer than 3 days (Table 8). Patients receiving anesthesia during labor and delivery have a higher risk of transient neurological deficits (one in 280) that is independent of technique (general vs regional) (186). Of note, in one study, only 20% of these mild, transient neurological deficits were noted in the patient's chart.

The fetal head may compress and injure the lumbosacral plexus as it crosses the ala of the sacrum or the posterior brim of the pelvis (Fig. 11). This injury is more common in nulliparae with platypelloid pelves, large babies, cephalopelvic disproportion, vertex presentation, and forceps delivery (187,188). This injury can be unilateral (75%) or bilateral (25%). Compressive nerve injuries of this type may involve multiple root levels and appear as injuries to the femoral nerve or obturator nerve with sensory impairment in the fourth and fifth lumbar ($L_{4\text{-}5}$) dermatomes (Fig. 10). The superior gluteal nerve also may be affected.

Femoral nerve injury decreases sensation over the anterior thigh and medial calf and impairs quadriceps strength, hip flexion, and patellar reflex (Table 7). Proximal lesions at the level of the lumbosacral plexus also may impair hip flexion because of iliopsoas weakness. Mild weakness of knee extension (quadriceps) is well compensated in walking by intact hip extensors that bring the knee into extension. This adaptation permits walking on flat surfaces, but not on stairs or uneven ground.

The obturator nerve can be compressed against the lateral pelvic wall or in the obturator canal, resulting in decreased sensation over the medial thigh and weakness in hip adduction and internal rotation (180,188). Electrophysiologic evaluation will differentiate obturator nerve injury from $L_{3\text{-}4}$ radiculopathy and lumbar plexopathy.

Compression injuries are more common at sites peripheral to the sacrum. Most peripheral nerve injuries are due to positioning problems, with the common peroneal nerve being among the most frequently affected. The common peroneal nerve exits the popliteal fossa by winding around the fibular head before dividing into the deep and superficial branches. The nerve may be compressed at the level of the neck of the fibula during lithotomy position in stirrups or with the legs leaning against the bed rail. Common peroneal nerve compression results in paresthesia over the lateral calf and dorsum of the foot, with foot drop and inversion (i.e., difficulty with dorsiflexion and eversion of the foot) and sensory loss on the dorsal surface of the foot just proximal to the first and second toes. Electrophysiologic testing will show focal slowing of motor conduction across the fibular head. A false-negative test result may occur because the motor response is measured in the extensor digitorum brevis, which may receive an anomalous motor branch in up to 22% of patients (180).

The femoral nerve also may be compressed at the level of the inguinal ligament during flexion of the hip during the second stage of labor. Extreme flexion of the hips during pushing should be avoided, and the legs rested between contractions/pushing (179,189). The use of a squatting bar to keep the hips hyperflexed during second stage of labor has resulted in femoral nerve injury.

The lateral femoral cutaneous nerve of the thigh arises from the lumbar plexus ($L_{2\text{-}3}$) and provides sensation to the anterolateral thigh. The nerve enters the thigh by passing under the lateral inguinal ligament, where it may become compressed. Injury produces paresthesia in the anterolateral thigh, also called meralgia paresthetic. No treatment is necessary, and sensation usually returns within 6 weeks. In obese patients, weight reduction may help (180).

Ischemic injury also may produce neurological deficits. The spinal cord may become ischemic during periods of severe hypotension or by compression of its blood supply. The lower spinal cord receives blood from the artery of Adamkiewicz (arteria magna) and the internal iliac arteries. About 85% of people have the majority of arterial blood supplied by the artery of Adamkiewicz, which arises from the lower thoracic or upper lumbar segment of the aorta (T_9 to L_2) (190,191). The other 15% of people have spinal cord blood supplied by a branch of the

TABLE 8. *Maternal neurological deficit associated with parturition*

Author	Year	Number of cases	Transient incidence/10,000	Permanent incidence/10,000
Holdcroft (207)	1995	48,066	—	4
Ong (186)	1987	12,725	2.4	0
Hill (184)	1962	13,093	—	3.8
Cole (187)	1946	45,000	—	1.6
Tillman (183)	1935	18,800	—	4.8

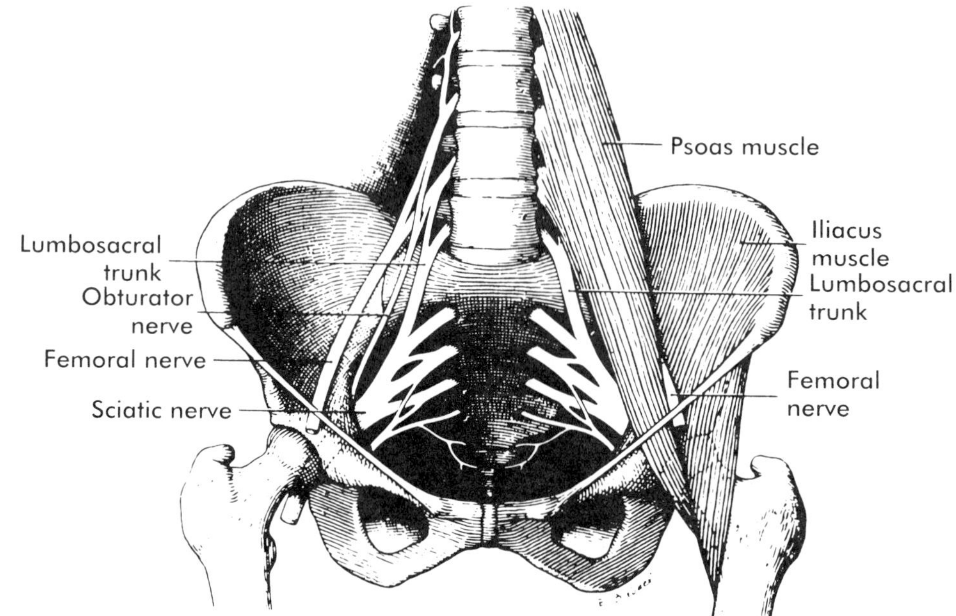

FIG. 11. The lumbosacral trunk and obturator and femoral nerves lying on the ala of the sacrum and exposed to pressure in cases of cephalopelvic disproportion, especially in patients with platypelloid pelves. (Reprinted from ref. 185, with permission.)

iliac arteries when the artery of Adamkiewicz originates high off the aorta (T_5). These feeder vessels from the iliac artery may be compressed as they cross the lumbosacral trunk. This mechanism of injury is suggested by a series from Nigeria. Here, 15% of postpartum neurological deficits, occurring in women who had not received anesthesia, produced permanent paraparesis (192).

Neurological deficit also may occur because of anterior spinal artery syndrome. The artery of Adamkiewicz supplies the anterior two thirds of the spinal cord, and injury (compression or extreme hypotension) may result in ischemic injury. Loss of the anterior two thirds of the spinal cord results in loss of motor function, pain, and temperature below the level of the lesion. The dorsal column is supplied by vertebral arteries and carries vibration and joint sensation, which are spared. Rarely, vasoconstriction of the anterior spinal artery may result in neurological injury. Although epinephrine has been coexistent in several case reports, a causal relation remains in question. Intrathecal epinephrine does not decrease spinal cord blood flow (193,194). Epinephrine may cause vasoconstriction of blood vessels within the epidural space, perhaps affecting the artery of Adamkiewicz or the feeding arteries derived from the iliac artery (169,195). In one series of 17,733 regional anesthetics, there was one case of anterior spinal artery syndrome (196).

Arteriovenous malformation (AVM) within the spinal cord can cause paraplegia. The spinal venous pressure may be increased, predisposing the spinal cord to decreased flow and stasis during periods of moderate hypotension or compression. AVMs may be intradural or on the external surface of the dura. Spinal AVM occurs at the same dermatome level in 20% of patients with a cutaneous arteriovenous abnormality (197–199). Dural AVMs most commonly are seen as pain (of the back, root, or remote) in 39%, leg weakness in 29%, or sensory symptoms in 24%. Progression of symptoms is usually slow, and spontaneous hemorrhage is less common than in spinal cord AVMs (197).

ANESTHESIA-RELATED NEUROLOGICAL DEFICITS

Serious neurological complications related to regional anesthesia are fortunately very rare (200,201). Neurological complications can be due to direct nerve trauma, severe hypotension, cardiac arrest, equipment problems, adverse drug effect, administration of the wrong drug, and wrong site of drug administration.

Nerve Trauma

Neurological deficits related to nerve trauma during regional anesthesia are very uncommon. The old adage "the customer is always right" serves us well here. If the patient reports localized pain with insertion of an epidural or spinal needle or catheter, stop immediately! Then differentiate benign pressure from a true paresthesia. Transient paresthesia with threading an epidural catheter is common and probably related to the catheter-tip design and stiffness (202). The combined spinal–epidural needle-through-needle technique also is associated with frequent transient paresthesae (203). Stop advancing and withdraw immediately in the face of severe radicular pain with involuntary leg movement. Direct trauma to nervous tissue may occur at the level of the spinal cord, nerve root, or peripheral nerve. Epidural needle insertion is most likely to stimulate a nerve root. Spinal needles may touch nerve roots inside or outside of the thecal sac or directly injure the spinal cord. The spinal cord usually ends at the first intervertebral disc, but may extend lower to the L_{2-3} intervertebral disc (Fig. 12) (204). Although the superior iliac crest denotes the L_4 spinous process or L_{4-5} interspace in 79% of patients, Tuffier's line is as high as the L_{3-4} interspace in 4% and as low as the L_5-S_1 interspace in another 4% (205). Use caution at any level of insertion. Two thirds of neurological complications are associated with either paresthesia (nerve trauma) or pain during injection (intraneuronal injection) (200).

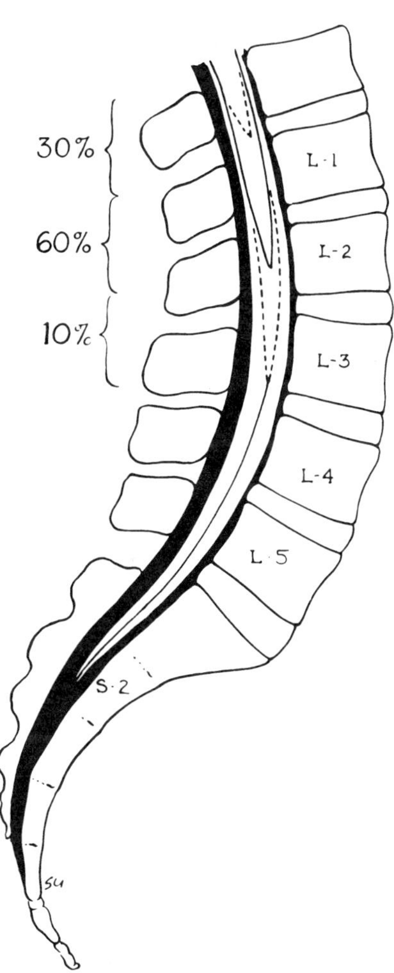

FIG. 12. Variations of the level of termination of the spinal cord. The figures (left) indicate the approximate percentage of each level that was found among 129 specimens. Extradural space is shown in black and subarachnoid space in white. (Reprinted from Bonica JJ. *Principles and practice of obstetric anesthesia,* vol 1. Philadelphia: Davis, 1969:552, with permission.)

Auroy et al. prospectively monitored neurological complications associated with more than 103,000 regional anesthetics performed in France (200). All deficits were present within 48 hours after anesthesia. Twenty-nine of 34 neurological complications were transient with recovery occurring between 48 hours and 3 months (200). Spinal anesthesia was significantly more likely to result in both neurological injury (5.9 vs 2 per 10,000) and radiculopathy (4.7 vs 1.7 per 10,000) compared with epidural anesthesia (200). All patients with radicular deficits after paresthesia resolved except one (spinal anesthesia with bupivacaine). Of the patients who had neurological deficits without paresthesia, 12 of 13 followed spinal anesthesia, with nine of 12 receiving 5% lidocaine. Although patients commonly fear paralysis, this complication is extremely rare. In this series, only one patient (of 103,730) became paraplegic due to spinal cord ischemia: an elderly man who had a prolonged period of hypotension (Table 9).

Other authors have investigated neurological complications associated with regional anesthesia (Table 9). One series included 17,733 regional anesthetics for general surgery. Here, neurological problems complicated 2.4 per 10,000 spinal and 3.2 per 10,000 epidural anesthetics (196). Surgery, concurrent disease (i.e., diabetes mellitus) and degeneration probably accounted for some of the observed deficits. In addition, anticoagulation contributed to the three epidural-related complications: epidural hematoma.

In a series of 2,580,000 obstetric deliveries with 505,000 epidural blocks, there were 38 single-root neuropathies (0.75 per 10,000). All deficits resolved between 2 weeks and 3 months, except for one (0.02 per 10,000) (154). In a similar study 5 years later involving 123,000 obstetric regional anesthetics, 46 cases of single nerve root neuropathy were reported (3.7 per 10,000). Complete recovery was reported in all patients between 1 and 12 weeks (206). In another series of more than 13,000 obstetric epidural blocks, one woman had a prolonged paresthesia along a nerve root. Similarly, Paech et al. reported only one mononeuropathy in 11,000 obstetric epidural anesthetics (Table 9) (208).

Cardiac Arrest

In France, cardiac arrest occurred significantly more frequently after spinal anesthesia compared with epidural anesthesia for all types of surgeries (6.4 vs 1 per 10,000) (200). Fatal cardiac arrest occurred more in the elderly, with a longer time from spinal anesthesia to arrest. Five of six were undergoing total hip arthroplasty. Hypoxic brain damage may ensue if blood pressure and oxygenation are not promptly restored. Fortunately, no neurological sequelae were observed in 25 patients who recovered from cardiac arrest (200). In obstetric patients, there were three cases of cardiac arrest in 505,000 epidural anesthet-

TABLE 9. *Anesthesia-related neurological deficit*

Author	Year	Number of cases	Transient incidence/10,000	Prolonged/Permanent incidence/10,000
Paech (213)	1998	10,995	0.9	0
Auroy (206)	1997	103,730	3.3	0.1
Dahlgren (196)	1995	17,733	—	2.8 (1.2)[a]
Holdcroft (212)	1995	13,007	—	0.77
Scott (211)	1995	122,989	5.6	0.08
Scott (155)	1990	505,000	0.97	0.1
Ong (184)	1987	23,827	18.9	0
Usubiaga (170)	1975	780,000	—	0.91

[a]Higher rate due to three cases of epidural hematoma related to anticoagulation. The lower rate of 1.2/10,000 is without those cases.

ics (0.06 of 10,000). Two patients recovered, and one had brain damage after severe hypotension after a "top-up" (154). In the follow-up study, two patients had a cardiac arrest (0.16 of 10,000); one patient died because of amniotic fluid embolism, and one recovered from a total spinal block (206).

Equipment Problems

Epidural catheters usually slide out easily when pulled. If resistance is encountered on withdrawal, reposition the patient into the exact position used during insertion. If the catheter starts to stretch, be very cautious. Most catheters are fairly strong and will not break, even when mildly stretched (209,210). However, it may be advisable to leave the catheter in place and wait a few hours. Spontaneous movement of the patient may loosen the catheter. If pain is encountered during epidural catheter withdrawal, stop immediately! The catheter may entrap a nerve root. An imaging procedure may be necessary (MRI or CT after injecting a little contrast media into the epidural catheter). If a knot in the catheter is found or if it is encircling a root, a radiologist may be able to untangle it under fluoroscopy.

If a catheter breaks or becomes sheared off (usually during placement), the patient must be informed. Epidural catheters meet the ANSI Z-29 implantation standards and are nonirritating. Attempting surgical removal of a catheter fragment will cause more trauma than leaving it in place. However, if neurological symptoms are attributable to the catheter fragment (e.g., radicular pain), then surgical removal may become necessary (211). A microspinal catheter that was withdrawn from commercial availability (TFX Medical, Deluth, GA) had a ferro-metallic component. Patients with metallic particles/objects should not have MRI, as the strong magnetic field may move the fragment and cause tissue damage. The Sprotte spinal needle has been reported to bend at the tip (212). Again, unless neurological irritation occurs, the risk/benefit analysis is not in favor of surgical retrieval.

Adverse Drug Effect

After reports of cauda equina syndrome, the Food and Drug Administration removed microspinal catheters (28 and 30 gauge) from commercial use in 1992. The small-diameter/high-resistance catheters required slow injection allowing pooling of local anesthetic in the sacral area. When doses of 5% lidocaine exceeded 100 mg, localized high concentrations of lidocaine resulted in neurotoxicity and cauda equina syndrome (213). A spinal canal model showed that pooling of drug could occur in the sacral area with the use of microspinal catheters (214,215). Lidocaine neurotoxicity has become a controversial topic. Although it has been used for many years, recent data show that lidocaine can be neurotoxic (216,217). Indeed, transient neurological symptoms (TNS) associated with intrathecal lidocaine now seem relatively commonplace.

Transient Neurological Symptoms

The term "transient neurological symptoms" (TNS; also known as transient radicular irritation) is used to describe a syndrome of pain and dysesthesia in the buttocks, thighs, or calves that can follow spinal anesthesia and resolves within 72 hours. Most reports of TNS are associated with the use of 5% hyperbaric lidocaine. Although 5% lidocaine in dextrose has been used since 1948, TNS has only recently been recognized. More thorough follow-up or the introduction of small-bore atraumatic spinal needles in the late 1980s may explain this phenomenon. Factors associated with TNS include atraumatic small-bore needles with side hole directed caudad, lithotomy position, and high dose and concentration of lidocaine (218,219). Hyperbaricity is not a causative factor (216,220). One study reported that the incidence of TNS was related to the concentration of intrathecal lidocaine (16% incidence of TNS with 5% lidocaine, 5% incidence with 2% lidocaine, and none with bupivacaine) (221). Transient neurological symptoms were found in 37% of patients receiving 5% lidocaine and only 0.7% after 0.5% bupivacaine (222). Even 2% lidocaine was reported to cause transient radicular pain (223). Spinal anesthesia with bupivacaine provides a similar duration as lidocaine with epinephrine, so bupivacaine may be preferred for spinal anesthesia for cesarean section, although tetracaine also may be used.

Chemical Contamination

The epidural space is remarkably tolerant to chemical contamination. However, subarachnoid injection of chemical contaminants may produce neurotoxicity. Several factors may help protect against nerve injury from chemical contaminants injected into the epidural space. The epidural space is vascular and has a high degree of systemic absorption (224). The dura also serves as a protective barrier to the spinal cord unless there has been a dural puncture. Drugs accidentally injected into the epidural space include thiopental, methohexital (158), magnesium sulfate, and potassium chloride. Thiopental and methohexital caused no neurological sequelae (225,226). Magnesium infusion into the epidural space resulted in a burning sensation with no neurological sequelae (227). Epidural administration of potassium chloride produced profound motor and sensory block. Two patients recovered within 9 hours, but the patient who received the largest dose (15 mL of 11.25% KCl) remained paraplegic (228–230). Amazingly, not even hyperosmolar solutions (e.g., total parenteral nutrition) produced neurological sequelae after epidural injection (231).

Accidental Intrathecal or Intravascular Injection

A drug administered by the wrong route may produce neurotoxicity. Unrecognized intrathecal injection of most local anesthetics may produce excessive sensory and motor block, but prompt diagnosis and treatment should prevent adverse outcomes (see Chapter 32). Some reports of neurological deficit after accidental intrathecal injection of 2-chloroprocaine were reported (see later). Intravenous injection of local anesthetics can produce convulsions and possibly cardiac arrest. Cardiac arrest caused by intravenous bupivacaine requires prolonged resuscitation and possibly cardiopulmonary bypass to allow the bupivacaine to dissociate from the Na^+ channel (232). Suggested treatment of bupivacaine-induced cardiac arrest includes the use of bretylium (see Chapter 32).

The local anesthetic 2-chloroprocaine may produce neurotoxicity. The original formulation of epidural 2-chloroprocaine contained sodium bisulfite as an antioxidant. There were several reported cases of cauda equina syndrome when large doses of this formulation were injected into the subarachnoid space (233–235). The manufacturer (Astra Pharmaceuticals) reformulated the drug, decreasing the concentration of bisulfite, and eventually adding EDTA as a preservative. In rabbits, intrathecal EDTA also was neurotoxic (146). In addition, back pain may follow the epidural injection of large volumes (more than 25 mL) of 2-chloroprocaine containing sodium EDTA (143,144). Formulations of 2-chloroprocaine without any preservative are now available (Nescaine–MPF).

Human Immunodeficiency Virus

Testing for HIV is now mandatory for pregnant women in many states. The HIV virus is neurotropic and may produce neurological symptoms. The use of regional anesthesia in parturients with HIV did not adversely affect the course of their disease (123). EBP also has been used in HIV-infected patients without neurological complications (122). HIV may produce gross neurological symptoms as the disease progresses (e.g., demyelinating neuropathy, dementia) (125). When women with HIV were followed up for 2 years after delivery, neither regional nor general anesthesia had any detectable effect on the maternal immune system (236). In these women, the choice of anesthetic technique should be based on the usual obstetric and clinical considerations.

EPIDURAL HEMATOMA

Epidural hematoma is a rare complication of central regional anesthesia, with an estimated frequency of one in 150,000 to one in 250,000 in the healthy patient (237). A damaged blood vessel requires vessel contraction, formation of a platelet plug, and activation of the clotting cascade for bleeding to stop (238). Patients at risk for thromboembolism are given aspirin, coumadin, heparin, or dextran. Most epidural hematomas associated with regional anesthesia occur in patients with a hemostatic abnormality (239). Epidural hematomas have been noted after both insertion and removal of the catheter in anticoagulated patients. Thus epidural catheters should be inserted and removed only when the coagulation status is normal. Most of our information is from the orthopedic surgical population, in whom some form of anticoagulation is used to prevent deep vein thrombosis and pulmonary embolism. In a few studies, no complications of regional anesthesia were found in patients who had received aspirin or anticoagulants before, during, or after surgery (237,240,241). After reports of epidural and spinal hematomas after regional anesthesia in patients receiving low-molecular-weight heparin (10), the Food and Drug Administration released a public health advisory warning of this risk (11).

Signs/Symptoms

Epidural hematoma is characterized by bilateral leg weakness, urinary incontinence, absent rectal sphincter tone, and decreased lower-extremity reflexes (242). These severe neurological deficits may be preceded by sharp pain in the back and legs, with progression of symptoms over a few hours. If a hematoma occurs during surgical anesthesia, the sensory level of anesthesia may decrease slightly or not at all. Continued motor paralysis without regression of the block should raise suspicions. Check for any hemostatic alterations that would increase the risk of epidural hematoma. If suspected, immediate CT or MRI is indicated. Surgical decompression should occur within 6 hours for best chance of full neurological recovery (Table 5) (158).

REFERENCES

1. Stein G, Morton J, Marsh A, et al. Headaches after childbirth. *Acta Neurol Scand* 1984;69:74.
2. Schoenen J, Maertens de Noordhout A. Headache. In: Wall PD, Melzack R. eds. *Textbook of pain*. London: Churchill Livingstone, 1994:495.
3. Uknis A, Silberstein SD. Review article: migraine and pregnancy [Review]. *Headache* 1991;31:372.
4. Shah JL. Severe headache following an epidural "top-up." *Int J Obstet Anesth* 1991;1:29.
5. Ariola SE, Russo TO, Marx GF. Postdural puncture headache or incipient eclampsia? *Int J Obstet Anesth* 1991;1:33.
6. Younker D, Jones MM, Adenwala J, Citrin A, Joyce TH. Maternal cortical vein thrombosis and the obstetric anesthesiologist. *Anesth Analg* 1986;65:1007.
7. Ravindran RS, Zandstra GC, Viegas OJ. Postpartum headache following regional analgesia: a symptom of cerebral venous thrombosis. *Can J Anaesth* 1989;36:705.
8. Mallaiah S, Tailby CH. Unusual early presentation of cerebral venous thrombosis. *Int J Obstet Anesth* 1994;3:228.
9. Rudehill A, Gordon E, Rahn T. Subdural haematoma: a rare but life-threatening complication after spinal anaesthesia. *Acta Anaesthesiol Scand* 1983;27:376.
10. Sternlo JE, Hybbinette CH. Spinal subdural bleeding after attempted epidural and subsequent spinal anaesthesia in a patient on thromboprophylaxis with low molecular weight heparin. *Acta Anaesthesiol Scand* 1995;39:557.
11. Lumpkin MM. Reports of epidural or spinal hematomas with the concurrent use of low molecular weight heparin and spinal/epidural anesthesia or spinal puncture. *FDA Public Health Advisory* 12. U.S. Department of Health and Human Resources.
12. Ready LB, Helfer D. Bacterial meningitis in parturients after epidural anesthesia. *Anesthesiology* 1989;71:988.
13. Bert AA, Laasberg LH. Aseptic meningitis following spinal anesthesia: a complication of the past? *Anesthesiology* 1985;62:674.
14. Ash KM, Cannon JE, Biehl DR. Pneumocephalus following attempted epidural anaesthesia. *Can J Anaesth* 1991;38:772.
15. Roderick L, Moore DC, Artru AA. Pneumocephalus with headache during spinal anesthesia. *Anesthesiology* 1985;62:690.
16. Aida S, Taga K, Yamakura T, Endoh H, Shimoji K. Headache after attempted epidural block: the role of intrathecal air. *Anesthesiology* 1998;88:76.
17. Silverman K, Evans SM, Strain EC, Griffiths RR. Withdrawal syndrome after the double-blind cessation of caffeine consumption. *N Engl J Med* 1992;327:1109.
18. Askmark H, Lundberg PO. Lactation headache: a new form of headache? *Cephalalgia* 1989;9:119.
19. Ravindran RS, Carrelli A. Neurologic dysfunction in postpartum patients caused by hypomagnesemia. *Anesthesiology* 1987;66:391.
20. Vandam LD, Dripps RD. Long-term follow-up of patients who received 10,098 spinal anesthetics. *JAMA* 1956;161:586.
21. Brownridge P. The management of headache following accidental dural puncture in obstetric patients. *Anaesth Intens Care* 1983;11:4.
22. Carrie LE. Postdural puncture headache and extradural blood patch [Editorial]. *Br J Anaesth* 1993;71:179.
23. Heyman HJ, Salem MR, Klimov I. Persistent sixth cranial nerve paresis following blood patch for postdural puncture headache. *Anesth Analg* 1982;61:948.
24. Greene NM. Neurologic sequelae of spinal anesthesia. *Anesthesiology* 1961;22:682.
25. Norris MC, Leighton BL, DeSimone CA. Needle bevel direction and headache after inadvertent dural puncture. *Anesthesiology* 1989;70:729.
26. Stride PC, Cooper GM. Dural taps revisited: a 20-year survey from Birmingham maternity hospital. *Anaesthesia* 1993;48:247.
27. Lambert DH, Hurley RJ, Hertwig L, Datta S. Role of needle gauge and tip configuration in the production of lumbar puncture headache. *Reg Anesth* 1997;22:66.
28. Okell RW, Sprigge JS. Unintentional dural puncture: a survey of recognition and management. *Anaesthesia* 1987;42:1110.
29. Costigan SN, Sprigge JS. Dural puncture: the patients' perspective: a patient survey of cases at a DGH maternity unit 1983-1993. *Acta Anaesthesiol Scand* 1996;40:710.
30. Lybecker H, Moller JT, May O, Nielsen HK. Incidence and prediction of postdural puncture headache: a prospective study of 1021 spinal anesthesias. *Anesth Analg* 1990;70:389.
31. Ravindran RS, Viegas OJ, Tasch MD, Cline PJ, Deaton RL, Brown TR. Bearing down at the time of delivery and the incidence of spinal headache in parturients. *Anesth Analg* 1981;60:524.
32. Ready LB, Cuplin S, Haschke RH, Nessly M. Spinal needle determinants of rate of transdural fluid leak. *Anesth Analg* 1989;69:457.
33. Cruickshank RH, Hopkinson JM. Fluid flow through dural puncture sites: an in vitro comparison of needle point types. *Anaesthesia* 1989;44:415.
34. Hatfalvi BI. The dynamics of post-spinal headache. *Headache* 1977;17:64.
35. Stasiuk RB, Jenkins LC. Post spinal headache: a comparison of midline and laminar approaches. *Can J Anaesth* 1990;37:S58.
36. Norris MC, Leighton BL. Continuous spinal anesthesia after unintentional dural puncture in parturients. *Reg Anesth* 1990;15:285.
37. Cohen S, Amar D, Pantuck EJ, Singer N, Divon M. Decreased incidence of headache after accidental dural puncture in caesarean delivery patients receiving continuous postoperative intrathecal analgesia. *Acta Anaesthesiol Scand* 1994;38:716.
38. Denny N, Masters R, Pearson D, Read J, Sihota M, Selander D. Postdural puncture headache after continuous spinal anesthesia. *Anesth Analg* 1987;66:791.
39. Giuffrida JG, Bizzarri DV, Masi R, Bondoc R. Continuous procaine spinal anesthesia for cesarean section. *Anesth Analg* 1972;51:117.
40. Benedetti C, Chadwick HS, Mancuso JJ, Ross BK, Tiengo M. Incidence of postspinal headache after continuous subarachnoid analgesia for labor using a 32 ga microcatheter [Abstract]. *Anesthesiology* 1990;73:A922.
41. Standl T, Eckert S, Schulte AE. Microcatheter continuous spinal anaesthesia in the post-operative period: a prospective study of its effectiveness and complications. *Eur J Anesth* 1995;12:273.
42. Kunkle EC, Ray BS, Wolff HG. Experimental studies on headache: analysis of the headache associated with changes in intracranial pressure. *Arch Neurol Psychiatry* 1943;49:323.
43. Ahearn RE. Management of severe postlumbar puncture headache. *N Y State J Med* 1948;48:1495.
44. Ostman PL. Complications associated with regional anesthesia in the obstetric patient. In: Norris MC, ed. *Obstetric anesthesia.* Philadelphia: JB Lippincott, 1993:763.
45. Gobel H, Klostermann H, Lindner V, Schenkl S. Changes in cerebral haemodynamics in cases of post-lumbar puncture headache: a prospective transcranial Doppler ultrasound study. *Cephalalgia* 1990;10:117.
46. Shearer VE, Jhaveri HS, Cunningham FG. Puerperal seizures after post-dural puncture headache. *Obstet Gynecol* 1995;85:255.
47. Grant R, Condon B, Hart I, Teasdale GM. Changes in intracranial CSF volume after lumbar puncture and their relationship to post-LP headache. *J Neurol Neurosurg Psychiatry* 1991;54:440.
48. Lee JJ, Roberts RB. Paresis of the fifth cranial nerve following spinal anesthesia. *Anesthesiology* 1978;49:217.
49. Eerola M, Kaukinen L, Kaukinen S. Fatal brain lesion following spinal anaesthesia: report of a case. *Acta Anaesthesiol Scand* 1981;25:115.
50. Wang LP, Fog J, Bove M. Transient hearing loss following spinal anaesthesia. *Anaesthesia* 1987;42:1258.

51. Wang LP, Schmidt JF. Central nervous side effects after lumbar puncture: a review of the possible pathogenesis of the syndrome of postdural puncture headache and associated symptoms [Review]. *Dan Med Bull* 1997;44:79.
52. Lee CM, Peachman FA. Unilateral hearing loss after spinal anesthesia treated with epidural blood patch. *Anesth Analg* 1986;65:312.
53. Fog J, Wang LP, Sundberg A, Mucchiano C. Hearing loss after spinal anesthesia is related to needle size. *Anesth Analg* 1990;70:517.
54. Lybecker H, Andersen T. Repetitive hearing loss following dural puncture treated with autologous epidural blood patch. *Acta Anaesthesiol Scand* 1995;39:987.
55. Lybecker H, Andersen T, Helbo-Hansen HS. The effect of epidural blood patch on hearing loss in patients with severe postdural puncture headache. *J Clin Anesth* 1995;7:457.
56. Kovanen J, Sulkava R. Duration of postural headache after lumbar puncture: effect of needle size. *Headache* 1986;26:224.
57. Carbaat PA, van Crevel H. Lumbar puncture headache: controlled study on the preventive effect of 24 hours' bed rest. *Lancet* 1981;2: 1133.
58. Hilton-Jones D, Harrad RA, Gill MW, Warlow CP. Failure of postural maneuvers to prevent lumbar puncture headache. *J Neurol Neurosurg Psychiatry* 1982;45:743.
59. Jacobs MW. Prevention of the postpartum spinal headache. *Am J Obstet Gynecol* 1962;83:320.
60. Dieterich M, Brandt T. Incidence of post-lumbar puncture headache is independent of daily fluid intake. *Eur Arch Psychiatr Neurol Sci* 1988;237:194.
61. Beck WW Jr. Prevention of the postpartum spinal headache. *Am J Obstet Gynecol* 1973;115:354.
62. Holder HG. Reactions after spinal anesthesia. *JAMA* 1944;124:56.
63. Sechzer PH, Abel L. Post-spinal anesthesia headache treated with caffeine: evaluation with demand method. Part I. *Curr Ther Res* 1978; 24:307.
64. Jarvis AP, Greenawalt JW, Fagraeus L. Intravenous caffeine for postdural puncture headache [Letter]. *Anesth Analg* 1986;65:316.
65. Sechzer PH. Post-spinal anesthesia headache treated with caffeine. Part II: intracranial vascular distention: a key factor. *Curr Ther Res* 1979;26:440.
66. Camann WR, Murray RS, Mushlin PS, Lambert DH. Effects of oral caffeine on postdural puncture headache: a double-blind, placebo-controlled trial. *Anesth Analg* 1990;70:181.
67. Cohen SM, Laurito CE, Curran MJ. Grand mal seizure in a postpartum patient following intravenous infusion of caffeine sodium benzoate to treat persistent headache. *J Clin Anesth* 1992;4:48.
68. Bolton VE, Leicht CH, Scanlon TS. Postpartum seizure after epidural blood patch and intravenous caffeine sodium benzoate [Comments]. *Anesthesiology* 1989;70:146.
69. Paech M. Unexpected postpartum seizures associated with post-dural puncture headache treated with caffeine. *Int J Obstet Anesth* 1996; 5:43.
70. Aldridge A, Bailey J, Neims AH. The disposition of caffeine during and after pregnancy. *Semin Perinatol* 1981;5:310.
71. Feuerstein TJ, Zeides A. Theophylline relieves headache following lumbar puncture: placebo-controlled, double-blind pilot study. *Klin Wochenschr* 1986;64:216.
72. Schwalbe SS, Schiffmiller MW, Marx GF. Theophylline for post-dural puncture headache [Abstract]. *Anesthesiology* 1991;75:A1082.
73. Carp H, Singh PJ, Vadhera R, Jayaram A. Effects of the serotonin-receptor agonist sumatriptan on postdural puncture headache: report of six cases. *Anesth Analg* 1994;79:180.
74. Lhuissier C, Mercier FJ, Dounas M, Benhamou D. Sumatriptan: an alternative to epidural blood patch? [Letter]. *Anaestheisa* 1996;51: 1078.
75. Rohmer C, Le Bourlot G. Headache after spinal anesthesia treated with sumatriptan [Letter]. [French]. *Ann Fr Anesth Reanim* 1995;14: 237.
76. Stallard N, Barry P. Another complication of the combined extradural-subarachnoid technique [Letter]. *Br J Anaesth* 1995;75:370.
77. Kaukinen S, Kaukinen L, Kannisto K, Kataja M: The prevention of headache following spinal anaesthesia. *Ann Chir Gynaecol* 1981;70: 107.
78. Eldor J, Guedj P, Cotev S. Epidural morphine injections for the treatment of postspinal headache [Letter]. *Can J Anaesth* 1990;37:710.
79. Rice GG, Dabbs CH. The use of peridural and subarachnoid injections of saline solution in the treatment of severe postspinal headache. *Anesthesiology* 1950;11:17.
80. Usubiaga JE, Usubiaga LE, Brea LM, Goyena R. Effect of saline injections on epidural and subarachnoid space pressures and relation to postspinal anesthesia headache. *Anesth Analg* 1967;46:293.
81. Craft JB, Epstein BS, Coakley CS. Prophylaxis of dural-puncture headache with epidural saline. *Anesth Analg* 1973;52:228.
82. Crawford JS. The prevention of headache consequent upon dural puncture. *Br J Anaesth* 1972;44:598.
83. Bart AJ, Wheeler AS. Comparison of epidural saline placement and epidural blood placement in the treatment of post-lumbar-puncture headache. *Anesthesiology* 1978;48:221.
84. Clark CJ, Whitwell J. Intraocular haemorrhage after epidural injection. *BMJ* 1961;1612.
85. Gormley JB. Treatment of postspinal headache. *Anesthesiology* 1960; 21:565.
86. DiGiovanni AJ, Dunbar BS. Epidural injections of autologous blood for postlumbar-puncture headache. *Anesth Analg* 1970;49:268.
87. Crawford JS. Experiences with epidural blood patch. *Anaesthesia* 1980;35:513.
88. Szeinfeld M, Ihmeidan IH, Moser MM, Machado R, Klose KJ, Serafini AN. Epidural blood patch: evaluation of the volume and spread of blood injected into the epidural space. *Anesthesiology* 1986;64:820.
89. Taivainen T, Pitkanen M, Tuominen M, Rosenberg PH. Efficacy of epidural blood patch for postdural puncture headache. *Acta Anaesthesiol Scand* 1993;37:702.
90. Griffiths AG, Beards SC, Jackson A, Horsman EL. Visualization of extradural blood patch for post lumbar puncture headache by magnetic resonance imaging. *Br J Anaesth* 1993;70:223.
91. Vakharia SB, Thomas PS, Rosenbaum AE, Wasenko JJ, Fellows DG. Magnetic resonance imaging of cerebrospinal fluid leak and tamponade effect of blood patch in postdural puncture headache. *Anesth Analg* 1997;84:585.
92. Abouleish E, Vega S, Blendinger I, Tio TO. Long-term follow-up of epidural blood patch. *Anesth Analg* 1975;54:459.
93. Beers RA, Cambareri JJ, Rodziewicz GS. Acute deterioration of mental status following epidural blood patch. *Anesth Analg* 1993;76:1147.
94. Sperry RJ, Gartrell A, Johnson JO. Epidural blood patch can cause acute neurologic deterioration [published erratum appears in *Anesthesiology* 1994;82:1310] [Comments]. *Anesthesiology* 1995;82:303.
95. DiGiovanni AJ, Galbert MW, Wahle WM. Epidural injection of autologous blood for postlumbar-puncture headache: II. Additional clinical experiences and laboratory investigation. *Anesth Analg* 1972;51: 226.
96. Rosenberg PH, Heavner JE. In vitro study of the effect of epidural blood patch on leakage through a dural puncture. *Anesth Analg* 1985; 64:501.
97. Kanumilli V, Kaza R, Johnson C, Nowacki C. Epidural blood patch for Jehovah's Witness patient [Letter]. *Anesth Analg* 1993;77:872.
98. Brimacombe J, Clarke G, Craig L. Epidural blood patch in the Jehovah's Witness [Letter]. *Anaesth Intens Care* 1994;22:319.
99. Loeser EA, Hill GE, Bennett GM, Sederberg JH. Time vs. success rate for epidural blood patch. *Anesthesiology* 1978;49:147.
100. Palahniuk RJ, Cumming M. Prophylactic blood patch does not prevent post lumbar puncture headache. *Can Anaesth Soc J* 1979;26:132.
101. Colonna-Romano P, Shapiro BE. Unintentional dural puncture and prophylactic epidural blood patch in obstetrics. *Anesth Analg* 1989; 69:522.
102. Ackerman WE, Juneja MM, Kaczorowski DM. The attenuation of postdural puncture headache with a prophylactic blood patch in labor patients. *Anesth Analg* 1989;68:S1.
103. Mandell G, Ramanathan S. Effectiveness of prophylactic blood patches in laboring parturients: A prospective study. *Anesth Analg* 1996;82:S291.
104. Cheek TG, Banner R, Sauter J, Gutsche BB. Prophylactic extradural blood patch is effective: a preliminary communication. *Br J Anaesth* 1988;61:340.
105. Sengupta P, Bagley G, Lim M. Prevention of postdural puncture headache after spinal anaesthesia for extracorporeal shockwave lithotripsy: an assessment of prophylactic epidural blood patching. *Anaesthesia* 1989;44:54.
106. Tobias MD, Pilla MA, Rogers C, Jobes DR. Lidocaine inhibits blood coagulation: implications for epidural blood patch. *Anesth Analg* 1996;82:766.

107. Leivers D. Total spinal anesthesia following early prophylactic epidural blood patch. *Anesthesiology* 1990;73:1287.
108. Quaynor H, Corbey M. Extradural blood patch—why delay? *Br J Anaesth* 1985;57:538.
109. Barrios-Alarcon J, Aldrete JA, Paragas-Tapia D. Relief of post-lumbar puncture headache with epidural Dextran 40: a preliminary report. *Reg Anesth* 1989;14:78.
110. Aldrete JA. Persistent post-dural-puncture headache treated with epidural infusion of dextran. *Headache* 1994;34:265.
111. Reynvoet ME, Cosaert PA, Desmet MF, Plasschaert SM. Epidural Dextran 40 patch for postdural puncture headache. *Anaesthesia* 1997; 52:886.
112. Salvador L, Carrero E, Castillo J, Villalonga A, Nalda MA. Prevention of post dural puncture headache with epidural-administered Dextran 40 [Letter] [published erratum appears in *Reg Anesth* 1993;18:202]. *Reg Anesth* 1992;17:357.
113. Lander CJ, Korbon GA. Histopathologic consequences of epidural blood patch and epidurally administered Dextran 40 [Abstract]. *Anesthesiology* 1988;69:A410.
114. Ambesh SP, Kumar A, Bajaj A. Epidural gelatin (Gelfoam) patch treatment for post dural puncture headache. *Anaesth Intens Care* 1991;19:444.
115. Andrews PJ, Ackerman WE, Juneja M, Cases-Cristobal V, Rigor BM. Transient bradycardia associated with extradural blood patch after inadvertent dural puncture in parturients. *Br J Anaesth* 1992;69:401.
116. Martin R, Jourdain S, Clairoux M, Tetrault JP. Duration of decubitus position after epidural blood patch. *Can J Anaesth* 1994;41:23.
117. Crawford JS. Epidural blood patch [Letter]. *Anaesth Intens Care* 1983;11:384.
118. Ong BY, Graham CR, Ringaert KR, Cohen MM, Palahniuk RJ. Impaired epidural analgesia after dural puncture with and without subsequent blood patch. *Anesth Analg* 1990;70:76.
119. Abouleish E, Wadhwa RK, de la Vega S, Tan RNJ, Lim UN. Regional analgesia following epidural blood patch. *Anesth Analg* 1975;54:634.
120. Blanche R, Eisenach JC, Tuttle R, Dewan DM. Previous wet tap does not reduce success rate of labor epidural analgesia. *Anesth Analg* 1994;79:291.
121. Tekkok IH, Carter DA, Brinker R. Spinal subdural haematoma as a complication of immediate epidural blood patch. *Can J Anaesth* 1996;43:306.
122. Tom DJ, Gulevich SJ, Shapiro HM, Heaton RK, Grant I. Epidural blood patch in the HIV-positive patient: review of clinical experience San Diego HIV Neurobehavior Research Center. *Anesthesiology* 1992;76:943.
123. Hughes SC, Dailey PA, Landers D, Dattel BJ, Crombleholme WR, Johnson JL. Parturients infected with human immunodeficiency virus and regional anesthesia: clinical and immunologic response. *Anesthesiology* 1995;82:32.
124. Newman P, Carrington D, Clarke J, Shapiro HM. Debate: epidural blood patch is contraindicated in HIV-positive patients. *Int J Obstet Anesth* 1994;3:167.
125. Price RW, Worth RJ. Management of neurologic complications of HIV-1 infection and AIDS. In: Sande MA, von Rosen F, eds. *The medical management of AIDS.* Philadelphia: WB Saunders, 1995:261.
126. Cavanaugh JM, Weinstein JN. Low back pain: epidemiology, anatomy and neurophysiology, In: Wall PD, Melzack R, eds. *Textbook of pain.* New York: Churchill Livingstone, 1994:441.
127. Berg G, Hammar M, Moller-Nielsen J, Linden U, Thorblad J. Low back pain during pregnancy. *Obstet Gynecol* 1988;71:71.
128. Ostgaard HC, Anderson GB, Karlsson K. Prevalence of back pain in pregnancy. *Spine* 1991;16:549.
129. Weinreb JC, Wolbarsht LB, Cohen JM, Brown CE, Maravilla KR. Prevalence of lumbosacral intervertebral disk abnormalities on MR images in pregnant and asymptomatic nonpregnant women. *Radiology* 1989;170:125.
130. LaBan MM, Perrin JC, Latimer FR. Pregnancy and the herniated lumbar disc. *Arch Phys Med Rehabil* 1983;64:319.
131. Rathmell JP, Viscomi CM, Ashburn MA. Management of nonobstetric pain during pregnancy and lactation [Review]. *Anesth Analg* 1997; 85:1074.
132. Breen TW, Ransil BJ, Groves PA, Oriol NE. Factors associated with back pain after childbirth. *Anesthesiology* 1994;81:29.
133. MacArthur C, Lewis M, Knox EG, Crawford JS. Epidural anaesthesia and long term backache after childbirth. *BMJ* 1990;301:9.
134. Russell R, Groves P, Taub N, O'Dowd J, Reynolds F. Assessing long term backache after childbirth. *BMJ* 1993;306:1299.
135. MacLeod J, Macintyre C, McClure JH, Whitwell J. Backache and epidural analgesia. *Int J Obstet Anesth* 1995;4:21.
136. Macarthur A, MacArthur C, Weeks S. Epidural anaesthesia and low back pain after delivery: a prospective cohort study. *BMJ* 1995;311: 1336.
137. Macarthur AJ, MacArthur C, Weeks SK. Is epidural anesthesia in labor associated with chronic low back pain? A prospective cohort study. *Anesth Analg* 1997;85:1066.
138. MacArthur C, Lewis M. Anaesthetic characteristics and long-term backache after obstetric epidural anaesthesia. *Int J Obstet Anesth* 1996;5:8.
139. Grove LH. Backache, headache and bladder dysfunction after delivery. *Br J Anaesth* 1973;45:1147.
140. Lecoq G, Hamza J, Narchi P, Jullien P, Attane D. Risk factors associated with postpartum backache in obstetric patients [Abstract]. *Anesthesiology* 1990;73:A966.
141. Vickers RJ, May AE. Long-term backache after extradural or general anaesthesia for manual removal of placenta: preliminary report. *Br J Anaesth* 1993;70:214.
142. Clark VA, McQueen MA. Factors influencing backache following epidural analgesia in labour. *Int J Obstet Anesth* 1993;2:193.
143. Fibuch EE, Opper SE. Back pain following epidurally administered Nesacaine-MPF. *Anesth Analg* 1989;69:113.
144. Stevens RA, Chester WL, Artuso JD, Bray JG, Nellestein JA. Back pain after epidural anesthesia with chloroprocaine in volunteers: preliminary report. *Reg Anesth* 1991;16:199.
145. Hynson JM, Sessler DI, Glosten B. Back pain in volunteers after epidural anesthesia with chloroprocaine. *Anesth Analg* 1991;72:253.
146. Wang BC, Li D, Hiller JM, Simon EJ, Budzilovich G, Turndorf H. Epidural EDTA induces tetanic contractions in rats [Abstract]. *Anesth Analg* 1991;72:S312.
147. Dirkes WE Jr. Treatment of nesacaine-MPF-induced back pain with calcium chloride [Letter; comment]. *Anesth Analg* 1990;70:461.
148. Peng AT, Behar S, Blancato LS. Reduction of postlumbar puncture backache by the use of field block anesthesia prior to lumbar puncture [Letter]. *Anesthesiology* 1985;63:227.
149. Abouleish E, Amortegui AJ, Taylor FH. Are bacterial filters needed in continuous epidural analgesia for obstetrics? *Anesthesiology* 1977;46: 351.
150. Wedel DJ, Horlocker TT. Risks of regional anesthesia—infectious, septic [Review]. *Reg Anesth* 1996;21:57.
151. Hulme A, Dott NM. Spinal epidural abscess. *BMJ* 1954;1:64.
152. Baker AS, Ojemann RG, Swartz MN, Richardson EP Jr. Spinal epidural abscess. *N Engl J Med* 1975;293:463.
153. Danner RL, Hartman BJ. Update on spinal epidural abscess: 35 cases and review of the literature. *Rev Infect Dis* 1987;9:265.
154. Scott DB, Hibbard BM. Serious non-fatal complications associated with extradural block in obstetric practice. *Br J Anaesth* 1990;64:537.
155. Kindler C, Seeberger M, Siegemund M, Schneider M. Extradural abscess complicating lumbar extradural anaesthesia and analgesia in an obstetric patient. *Acta Anaesthesiol Scand* 1996;40:858.
156. Crawford JS. Pathology in the extradural space. *Br J Anaesth* 1975;47: 412.
157. Teman AJ. Spinal epidural abscess: early detection with gadolinium magnetic resonance imaging. *Arch Neurol* 1992;49:743.
158. Bromage PR. Neurologic complications of labor, delivery, and regional anesthesia. In: Chestnut DH, ed. *Obstetric anesthesia: principles and practice.* St. Louis: Mosby-Year Book, 1994:621.
159. Bader AM, Gilbertson L, Kirz L, Datta S. Regional anesthesia in women with chorioamnionitis. *Reg Anesth* 1992;17:84.
160. Vaddadi ARJ, Angel JJ, Sibai B. Epidural anesthesia in women with chorioamnionitis [Abstract]. *Anesthesiology* 1990;70:A863.
161. Goodman EJ, DeHorta E, Taguiam JM. Safety of spinal and epidural anesthesia in parturients with chorioamnionitis. *Reg Anesth* 1996;21: 436.
162. Berga S, Trierweiler MW. Bacterial meningitis following epidural anesthesia for vaginal delivery: a case report. *Obstet Gynecol* 1989; 74:437.
163. Roberts SP, Petts HV. Meningitis after obstetric spinal anaesthesia. *Anaesthesia* 1990;45:376.
164. Carp H, Bailey S. The association between meningitis and dural puncture in bacteremic rats. *Anesthesiology* 1992;76:739.

165. Harding SA, Collis RE, Morgan BM. Meningitis after combined spinal-extradural anaesthesia in obstetrics. *Br J Anaesth* 1994;73:545.
166. Goldman WM, Sanford JP. An "epidemic" of chemical meningitis. *Am J Med* 1960;29:94.
167. Denson JS, Joseph SI, Koons RA, Murry WE, Bissonette HW. Effects of detergents intrathecally. *Anesthesiology* 1957;18:143.
168. Gibbons RB. Chemical meningitis following spinal anesthesia. *JAMA* 1969;210:900.
169. Usubiaga JE. Neurological complications following epidural anesthesia. *Int Anesth Clin* 1975;13:1.
170. Boyle RK. A review of anatomical and immunological links between epidural morphine and herpes simplex labialis in obstetric patients [Review]. *Anaesth Intens Care* 1995;23:425.
171. Martins. Infections. In: Gilstrap LC, Faro S, eds. *Infections in pregnancy.* New York: Wiley-Liss, 1990:277.
172. Crosby ET, Halpern SH, Rolbin SH. Epidural anaesthesia for caesarean section in patients with active recurrent genital herpes simplex infections: a retrospective review. *Can J Anaesth* 1989;36:701.
173. Ramanathan S, Sheth R, Turndorf H. Anesthesia for cesarean section in patients with genital herpes infections: a retrospective study. *Anesthesiology* 1986;64:807.
174. Bader AM, Camann WR, Datta S. Anesthesia for cesarean delivery in patients with herpes simplex virus type-2 infections. *Reg Anesth* 1990;15:261.
175. Crone LA, Conly JM, Storgard C, et al. Herpes labialis in parturients receiving epidural morphine following cesarean section. *Anesthesiology* 1990;73:208.
176. Gieraerts R, Navalgund A, Vaes L, Soetens M, Chang JL, Jahr J. Increased incidence of itching and herpes simplex in patients given epidural morphine after cesarean section. *Anesth Analg* 1987;66:1321.
177. Crone LA, Conly JM, Clark KM, et al. Recurrent herpes simplex virus labialis and the use of epidural morphine in obstetric patients. *Anesth Analg* 1988;67:318.
178. Norris MC, Weiss J, Carney M, Leighton BL. The incidence of herpes simplex virus labialis after cesarean delivery. *Int J Obstet Anesth* 1994;3:127.
179. Schaumburg HH, Berger AR, Thomas PK. *Disorders of peripheral nerves.* Philadelphia: FA Davis, 1992:240.
180. Redick LF. Maternal perinatal nerve palsies. *Postgrad Obstet Gynecol* 1992;12:1.
181. Chan S, Khandji AG, Hilal SK. CT and MRI. In: Rowland LP, ed. *Merritt's textbook of neurology.* Baltimore: Williams & Wilkins, 1995:59.
182. Lange DJ, Trojaborg W. Electromyography and nerve conduction studies in neuromuscular disease. In: Rowland LP, ed. *Merritt's textbook of neurology.* Baltimore: Williams & Wilkins, 1995:77.
183. Tillman AJB. Traumatic neuritis in the puerperium. *Am J Obstet Gynecol* 1935;29:660.
184. Hill EC. Maternal obstetric paralysis. *Am J Obstet Gynecol* 1962;83:1452.
185. Murray RR. Maternal obstetrical paralysis. *Am J Obstet Gynecol* 1964;88:399.
186. Ong BY, Cohen MM, Esmail A, Cumming M, Kozody R, Palahniuk RJ. Paresthesias and motor dysfunction after labor and delivery. *Anesth Analg* 1987;66:18.
187. Cole JT. Maternal obstetric paralysis. *Am J Obstet Gynecol* 1946;52:372.
188. Graham JG. Neurological complications of pregnancy and anaesthesia. *Clin Obstet Gynaecol* 1982;9:333.
189. Vargo MM, Robinson LR, Nicholas JJ, Rulin MC. Postpartum femoral neuropathy: relic of an earlier era? *Arch Phys Med Rehabil* 1990;71:591.
190. Lazorthes G, Poulhes J, Bastide G, Gouaze A. La vascularization de la moelle epiniere (etude anatomique et physiologique). *Rev Neurol* 1962;106:535.
191. Lazorthes G, Gouaze A, Bastide G, Poulhes J. La vascularization arterielle du renflement lumbaire: etudes des variations et des suppleances. *Rev Neurol* 1966;114:109.
192. Bademosi O, Osuntokun BO, Van de Werd HJ, Bademosi AK, Ojo OA. Obstetric neuropraxia in the Nigerian African. *Int J Gynaecol Obstet* 1980;17:611.
193. Kozody R, Palahniuk RJ, Wade JG, Cumming MO, Pucci WR. The effect of subarachnoid epinephrine and phenylephrine on spinal cord blood flow. *Can Anaesthet Soc J* 1984;31:503.
194. Dohi S, Takeshima R, Naito H. Spinal cord blood flow during spinal anesthesia in dogs: the effects of tetracaine, epinephrine, acute blood loss, and hypercapnia. *Anesth Analg* 1987;66:599.
195. Ackerman WE, Juneja MM, Knapp RK. Maternal paraparesis after epidural anesthesia and cesarean section [Review]. *South Med J* 1990;83:695.
196. Dahlgren N, Tornebrandt K. Neurological complications after anaesthesia: a follow-up of 18,000 spinal and epidural anaesthetics performed over three years. *Acta Anaesthesiol Scand* 1995;39:872.
197. Symon L, Kuyama H, Kendall B. Dural arteriovenous malformations of the spine: clinical features and surgical results in 55 cases. *J Neurosurg* 1984;60:238.
198. Doppman JL, Wirth FPJ, Di Chiro G, Ommaya AK. Value of cutaneous angiomas in the arteriographic localization of spinal-cord arteriovenous malformations. *N Engl J Med* 1969;281:1440.
199. Hirsch NP, Child CS, Wijetilleka SA. Paraplegia caused by spinal angioma—possible association with epidural analgesia. *Anesth Analg* 1985;64:937.
200. Auroy Y, Narchi P, Messiah A, Litt L, Rouvier B, Samii K. Serious complications related to regional anesthesia: results of a prospective survey in France. *Anesthesiology* 1997;87:479.
201. Eisenach JC. Regional anesthesia: vintage Bordeaux (and Napa Valley) [Editorial]. *Anesthesiology* 1997;87:467.
202. Yoshii WY, Rottman RL, Rosenblatt RM, et al. Epidural catheter-induced traumatic radiculopathy in obstetrics. *Reg Anesth* 1994;19:132.
203. Herbstman CH, Jaffee JB, Tuman KJ, Newman LM. An in vivo evaluation of four spinal needles used for the combined spinal-epidural technique. *Anesth Analg* 1998;86:520.
204. Bromage PR. Neurologic complications of regional anesthesia for obstetrics. In: Shnider SM, Levinson G, eds. *Anesthesia for obstetrics.* Baltimore: Williams & Wilkins, 1993:433.
205. Render CA. The reproducibility of the iliac crest as a marker of lumbar spine level. *Anaesthesia* 1996;51:1070.
206. Scott DB, Tunstall ME. Serious complications associated with epidural/spinal blockade in obstetrics: a two-year prospective study. *Int J Obstet Anesth* 1995;4:133.
207. Holdcroft A, Gibberd FB, Hargrove RL, Hawkins DF, Dellaportas CI. Neurological complications associated with pregnancy. *Br J Anaesth* 1995;75:522.
208. Paech MJ, Godkin R, Webster S. Complications of obstetric epidural analgesia and anaesthesia: a prospective analysis of 10,995 cases. *Int J Obstet Anesth* 1998;7:5.
209. Ley SJ, Jones BR. Strength of continuous spinal catheters. *Anesth Analg* 1991;73:394.
210. Davies R, Vaughan RS, Richards J. Epidural catheters: breaking and extraction forces. *Anaesthesia* 1993;48:900.
211. Blanchard N, Clabeau JJ, Ossart M, Dekens J, Legars D, Tchaoussoff J. Radicular pain due to a retained fragment of epidural catheter. *Anesthesiology* 1997;87:1567.
212. Lipov EG, Sosis MB, McCarthy RJ, Ivankovich AD. Does the design of the Sprotte spinal needle reduce the force needed to deform the tip? *J Clin Anesth* 1994;6:411.
213. Rigler ML, Drasner K, Krejcie TC, et al. Cauda equina syndrome after continuous spinal anesthesia. *Anesth Analg* 1991;72:275.
214. Ross BK, Coda B, Heath CH. Local anesthetic distribution in a spinal model: a possible mechanism of neurologic injury after continuous spinal anesthesia. *Reg Anesth* 1992;17:69.
215. Rigler ML, Drasner K. Distribution of catheter-injected local anesthetic in a model of the subarachnoid space. *Anesthesiology* 1991;75:684.
216. Lambert LA, Lambert DH, Strichartz GR. Irreversible conduction block in isolated nerve by high concentrations of local anesthetics. *Anesthesiology* 1994;80:1082.
217. Denny NM. Continuous spinal anaesthesia and cauda equina syndrome [Letter]. *Anaesthesia* 1995;50:474.
218. Beardsley D, Holman S, Gantt R, et al. Transient neurologic deficit after spinal anesthesia: local anesthetic maldistribution with pencil point needles? *Anesth Analg* 1995;81:314.
219. Tong D. Transient radicular irritation: is there an appropriate alternative to 5% hyperbaric lidocaine? *Educ Synop Anesth Crit Care Med* 1997;4:2.

220. Hampl KF, Schneider MC, Thorin D, Ummenhofer W, Drewe J. Hyperosmolarity does not contribute to transient radicular irritation after spinal anesthesia with hyperbaric 5% lidocaine. *Reg Anesth* 1995;20:363.
221. Pollock JE, Neal JM, Stephenson CA, Wiley CE. Prospective study of the incidence of transient radicular irritation in patients undergoing spinal anesthesia. *Anesthesiology* 1996;84:1361.
222. Hampl KF, Schneider MC, Ummenhofer W, Drewe J. Transient neurologic symptoms after spinal anesthesia. *Anesth Analg* 1995;81: 1148.
223. Fenerty J, Sonner J, Sakura S, Drasner K. Transient radicular pain following spinal anesthesia: review of the literature and report of a case involving 2% lidocaine. *Int J Obstet Anesth* 1996;5:32.
224. Zakowski MI, Ramanathan S, Sutin K, Grant GJ, Turndorf H. Pharmacokinetic profile of morphine in parturients following intravenous or epidural administration. *Reg Anesth* 1994;19:119.
225. Forestner JE. Inadvertent epidural injection of thiopental: a case report. *Anesth Analg* 1975;54:406.
226. Wells D, Davies G, Wagner D. Accidental injection of epidural methohexital. *Anesthesiology* 1987;67:846.
227. Dror A, Henriksen E. Accidental epidural magnesium sulfate injection. *Anesth Analg* 1987;66:1020.
228. Shanker KB, Palkar NV, Nishkala R. Paraplegia following epidural potassium chloride. *Anaesthesia* 1985;40:45.
229. Tessler MJ, White I, Naugler-Colville M, Biehl DR. Inadvertent epidural administration of potassium chloride: a case report. *Can J Anaesth* 1988;35:631.
230. Lin D, Becker K, Shapiro HM. Neurologic changes following epidural injection of potassium chloride and diazepam: a case report with laboratory correlations. *Anesthesiology* 1986;65:210.
231. Patel PC, Sharif AM, Farnando PU. Accidental infusion of total parenteral nutrition solution through an epidural catheter [Letter]. *Anaesthesia* 1984;39:383.
232. Hogan Q. Local anesthetic toxicity: an update [Review]. *Reg Anesth* 1996;21:43.
233. Ravindran RS, Bond VK, Tasch MD, Gupta CD, Luerssen TG. Prolonged neural blockade following regional analgesia with 2-chloroprocaine. *Anesth Analg* 1980;59:447.
234. Reisner LS, Hochman BN, Plumer MH. Persistent neurologic deficit and adhesive arachnoiditis following intrathecal 2-chloroprocaine injection. *Anesth Analg* 1980;59:452.
235. Moore DC, Spierdijk J, vanKleef JD, Coleman RL, Love GF. Chloroprocaine neurotoxicity: four additional cases. *Anesth Analg* 1982;61: 155.
236. Gershon RY, Manning-Williams D. Anesthesia and the HIV-infected parturient: a retrospective study. *Int J Obstet Anesth* 1997;6:76.
237. Horlocker TT. Regional anesthesia and analgesia in the patient receiving thromboprophylaxis [Editorial]. *Reg Anesth* 1996;21:503.
238. Macdonald R. Aspirin and extradural blocks [Editorial]. *Br J Anaesth* 1991;66:1.
239. Vandermeulen EP, Van Aken H, Vermylen J. Anticoagulants and spinal-epidural anesthesia [Review]. *Anesth Analg* 1994;79:1165.
240. Wu CL, Perkins FM. Oral anticoagulant prophylaxis and epidural catheter removal [Comments]. *Reg Anesth* 1996;21:517.
241. Horlocker TT, Wedel DJ, Schlichting JL. Postoperative epidural analgesia and oral anticoagulant therapy. *Anesth Analg* 1994;79:89.
242. Lao TT, Halpern SH, MacDonald D, Huh C. Spinal subdural haematoma in a parturient after attempted epidural anaesthesia. *Can J Anaesth* 1993;40:340.
243. Flaatten H, Rodt S, Rosland J, Vamnes J. Postoperative headache in young patients after spinal anaesthesia. *Anaesthesia* 1987;42:202.
244. Dahl JB, Schultz P, Anker-Moller E, Christensen EF, Staunstrup HG, Carlsson P. Spinal anaesthesia in young patients using a 29-gauge needle: technical considerations and an evaluation of postoperative complaints compared with general anaesthesia. *Br J Anaesth* 1990; 64:178.
245. Schultz AM, Ulbing S, Kaider A, Lehofer F. Postdural puncture headache and back pain after spinal anesthesia with 27-gauge Quincke and 26-gauge Atraucan needles. *Reg Anesth* 1996;21:461.
246. Sharma SK, Gambling DR, Joshi GP, Sidawi JE, Herrera ER. Comparison of 26-gauge Atraucan and 25-gauge Whitacre needles: insertion characteristics and complications. *Can J Anaesth* 1995;42: 706.
247. Douglas MJ, Ward ME, Campbell DC, Bright SB, Merrick PM. Factors involved in the incidence of post-dural puncture headache with the 25 gauge Whitacre needle for obstetric anesthesia. *Int J Obstet Anesth* 1997;6:220.
248. Lynch J, Arhelger S, Krings-Ernst I. Post-dural puncture headache in young orthopaedic in-patients: comparison of a 0.33 mm (29-gauge) Quincke-type with a 0.7 mm (22-gauge) Whitacre spinal needle in 200 patients. *Acta Anaesthesiol Scand* 1992;36:58.
249. Jackson JL, Ravindran RS. The use of Gertie Marx spinal needle for tubal ligation in postpartum patients. Presented at the Midwest Anesthesiology Residents Conference, 1997 [Abstract]. Indianapolis, IN.
250. Sears DH, Leeman MI, Jassy LJ, O'Donnell LA, Allen SG, Reisner LS. The frequency of postdural puncture headache in obstetric patients: a prospective study comparing the 24-gauge versus the 22-gauge Sprotte needle. *J Clin Anesth* 1994;6:42.

PART IV

Organizing an Obstetric Anesthesia Service

Obstetric Anesthesia, second edition,
edited by Mark C. Norris.
Lippincott Williams & Wilkins, Philadelphia © 1999.

CHAPTER 40

Toward the Next Millennium: A Guide to Managing a State-of-the-Art Obstetric Analgesia/Anesthesia Service

John W. Downing, Ramiah Ramasubramanian, Beth H. Minzter, and Walter U. Brown

The combined life expectancy of a woman and her child is 110 to 130 years. The delivery of a healthy baby to a happy mother and father represents a significant investment in our future. Obstetric anesthesiologists therefore bear a singular responsibility for the health and welfare of their community. Obstetrics and obstetric anesthesia are high-risk medical and medicolegal environments. Obstetric anesthesiologists are unique in that they care for more than one patient at a time. Furthermore, the legal statutory limit for the fetus is 21 years. Injuries that occur during an obstetric anesthetic can alter the lives of two people and haunt both obstetrician and anesthesiologist for years. The largest punitive award after an obstetric anesthetic misadventure that the authors are aware of is $13 million.[1] Reports of $10 million and $8 million jury verdicts were published in 1997[2] and 1998.[3] These misadventures involved human error during regional anesthetic administration. Against these gargantuan sums, the funding required to provide dedicated anesthesia coverage staffed by trained obstetric anesthesiologists, and thus to insure the safety of mothers and their babies, pales into insignificance.

These statements remain as true today as they were in 1991 when they appeared in the first edition of this book. However, managerial and, in particular, fiscal issues have changed radically in the ensuing years. Emphasis has shifted from the everyday clinical problems of providing first-class medical care for mothers and their babies to a more cost-oriented approach toward the same laudable goal. Recent publications show that obstetric anesthesia is not alone in having to face the fact that managing money is now the key to both survival and success (1–6). Obstetric anesthesiologists must of necessity learn to "think thrifty and smart." Why so? Because the shifting economics of anesthesia in particular and of medicine in general now demand a more frugal approach to spending the health care dollar. In addition, the growing competition among patient care centers for ever-decreasing funds has created a contest that seldom favors our future citizens or their parents. Consequently, the move toward value-based obstetric anesthesia care gains momentum by the day. These facts must be confronted and understood. To quote: "Why must the practice of. . . [obstetric] . . . anesthesiology change? It's economics, Doctor!"(2).

The goals of this chapter are therefore:

- To justify the creation of a dedicated, physician-directed, obstetric anesthesia service;
- To present guidelines for how this end may best be achieved today;
- To define the short- and long-term implications, both social and fiscal, of this type of community service;
- To consider the potential impact of for-profit managed care and capitation on the present and future conduct of an obstetric analgesia/anesthesia service; and
- To suggest innovations for the efficient and economic delivery of obstetric anesthesia services in an increasingly competitive environment.

J. W. Downing, R. Ramasubramanian, B. H. Minzter, and W. U. Brown: Department of Anesthesiology and Obstetrics, Vanderbilt Clinic, Vanderbilt University School of Medicine, Nashville, Tennessee 37232.

[1]Medical Malpractice: Verdicts, Settlements & Experts. 4, 1, 1988.
[2]Anesthesia Malpractice Prevention: 2, 93, 1997.
[3]Anesthesia Malpractice Prevention: 3, 22, 1998.

BACKGROUND

In 1942, Bert Hershenson was appointed Chief of Anesthesiology at the Boston Hospital for Women, making him the first Director of Obstetric Anesthesia in the United States (7). Meanwhile, in New York, Gertie Marx argued that obstetric anesthesia should meet the special needs of the parturient, and championed the cause of obstetric anesthesia resident education. Earlier, "anesthesiology residents received meager instruction in obstetric anesthesia, which was still thought to be a superfluous subspecialty" (8). In October 1952, Daniel Moore and his colleagues at the Virginia Mason Clinic in Seattle inaugurated a full-time obstetric anesthesia service and were the first to share their experiences in print (9–11).

The early 1970s saw recognition of a need to consolidate obstetric services and to provide dedicated 24-hour obstetric anesthesia care (12,13). In 1974, Sheldon wrote:

> Even though it is estimated that 60 to 90 per cent of obstetric patients deliver their babies without complications, obstetrics must be considered an emergency service. Various support equipment, material, and personnel must be available quickly to support life in situations of hemorrhage, cardiorespiratory collapse, and metabolic disturbances. . . . It is logical to assume that anesthesiology support is an integral part of modern obstetrics, not only to provide pain relief with conduction and inhalation anesthesia but also to maintain vital functions during both normal and surgical deliveries (13).

By 1988, the American College of Obstetricians and Gynecologists (ACOG) recognized the important role of anesthetic services in the care of the laboring parturient and issued the following declaration: "Ideally, hospitals in which obstetric care is provided should have anesthesia services available on a 24-hour basis. These units require the availability of sophisticated monitoring equipment and specially trained professional nursing personnel." (ACOG. Technical Bulletin 112, January 1988.)

A similar proclamation was issued more recently in the United Kingdom (U.K.):

> The standards expected for anaesthesia care of the obstetric patient should be equal to those described by the Association of Anaesthetists as necessary for surgical patients. No unit should undertake the responsibility of providing anaesthesia for the obstetric patient unless it is able to offer the level of care considered routine for other surgical patients. Standards in the obstetric operating room and recovery area should be the same as in other theatre suites. (Obstetric Anaesthesia Association: Recommended Minimum Standards for Obstetric Anesthesia Services. January, 1995.)

Both statements clearly emphasize that investments in both manpower and capital equipment are a priority to assure the safety of the parturient and her offspring.

As alluded to earlier, recent changes in the economics of medicine will have a significant impact on the provision of obstetric anesthesia services. No longer can a mother, unless she is self-funded, choose the hospital in which she wishes to have her baby. Instead, her choice of Health Management Organization (HMO) or Preferred Provider Organization (PPO) largely dictates where her child will be born. Contracts between insurers and hospitals are often based on cost, not quality. Even more disturbing, some health care insurers are currently attempting to discourage women from requesting epidural labor analgesia. Others are refusing payment for epidural labor analgesia absent a "medical indication." "Overall, about 25 percent of anesthesiologists report they have been denied reimbursement for labor epidurals." (Joy Hawkins, ASA Newsletter, 1995;59:11.)

In an attempt to combat some of these trends, the ACOG and the American Society of Anesthesiologists (ASA) have proclaimed that "Labor results in severe pain for many women. There is no other circumstance where it is considered acceptable for a person to experience severe pain, amenable to safe intervention, while under a physician's care. . . . Maternal request is a sufficient justification for pain relief during labor. Third party payers . . . should not deny reimbursement for epidural anesthesia because of an absence of other 'medical indications'" (ACOG Committee Opinion # 118-January 1993 approved by the ASA House of Delegates on October 21, 1992).

Obstetric services delivering 2,000 to 2,500 babies annually have the best morbidity and mortality statistics (13). The safety and success of an obstetrics program depend largely on the ready availability of an obstetric anesthesia service fully staffed by knowledgeable, competent, and caring obstetric anesthesiologists. In our opinion, a cost-effective obstetric service should perform no fewer than 2,000 and no more than 5,000 deliveries a year. A delivery rate of less than 2,000 per annum may provide too little work to justify a dedicated obstetric anesthesia service. Exceptions to this rule are those tertiary referral units with fewer than 2,000 annual deliveries but that frequently care for parturients considered "at risk" of serious pregnancy-related complications and medical problems. A workload exceeding 5,000 deliveries in a year can easily overburden obstetric, anesthesia, and nursing staff, as well as available hospital facilities. We consider ideal a delivery rate of 3,000 (±500) a year.

STANDARDS, GUIDELINES, AND PROTOCOLS (CLINICAL PATHWAYS)

In 1958, Sappenfield, as president of the ASA, established a Committee on Maternal Welfare to address the special problems related to the administration of obstetric anesthesia. A link was forged between the ASA Committee on Maternal Welfare and the ACOG Committee on Maternal Welfare in 1963. These committees formulated standards for obstetric analgesia/anesthesia that were published in the ACOG Manual of Standards one year later. In 1966, John Bonica, then president of the ASA, engineered a change in name from Committee on Maternal Welfare to Committee on Obstetrical Anesthesia, to emphasize that obstetric anesthesiologists were concerned with both fetal/neonatal and maternal well-being (8,14).

In 1988, the ASA published the Standards for Conduction Anesthesia in Obstetrics, a document generated collectively over several years by the ASA Committees on Obstetrical Anesthesia and Standards of Care. ACOG reviewed and approved its contents, but its adoption provoked considerable concern and argument. As a result, in 1990, the two ASA committees that coauthored the original standards recommended that they be withdrawn and replaced with a new set of guidelines. The 1990 ASA House of Delegates voted to leave the standards in place but renamed them Guidelines for Conduction Anesthesia in Obstetrics. Meanwhile, the two ASA committees set about generating new guidelines based on the previous standards. The resultant Guidelines for Regional Anesthesia in Obstetrics were accepted by the ASA House of Delegates on October 30, 1991, and remain in effect today (Appendix A).

ASA and ACOG in concert periodically update their recommendations concerning the safe practice of obstetric anesthesia. Their latest joint proclamations focus on several issues:

- Personnel on the labor and delivery floor should be trained in resuscitation and life-support techniques;
- Qualified anesthetic care for the parturient should be available within 30 minutes or less; and
- The quality of equipment, facilities, and support personnel should at least equal or perhaps exceed that provided in the surgical operating suite (Obstetric Analgesia and Anesthesia. ACOG Technical Bulletin no. 225, July, 1996).

In current use, the terms "standards" and "guidelines" have specific, different meanings. "Experts in setting practice guidelines have defined *standards* as hard and fast rules that should always be followed. . . . *Guidelines* are intended to be more flexible. They should be followed under most circumstances, but depending on the patient, the circumstances, and other factors, they can and should be tailored to fit individual needs." (Sheila E. Cohen: "Obstetrical Anesthesia: An Overview of Growth and Change." ASA Newsletter, 1991;55:17–20.) "Guidelines should be used to inform medical decision making, not to enforce medical decisions. . . . physicians must be free to diverge from official guidelines and to tailor diagnostic strategies and therapies when the patient's clinical state demands it. Properly developed, guidelines could be a valuable benchmark against which practices could be assessed" (15).

Meanwhile, at the 1998 meeting of the Society for Obstetric Anesthesia and Perinatology (SOAP), a draft of a proposal entitled "Practice Guidelines for Obstetrical Anesthesia" was unveiled for comment and suggestions. ASA commissioned the Task Force on Obstetrical Anesthesia to develop practice guidelines that ". . . provide recommendations that are supported by analysis of the current literature and by a synthesis of expert opinion, open forum commentary, and clinical feasibility data." Unfortunately, because of the dearth of appropriate literature concerning the practice of obstetric anesthesia, these guidelines are based less on evidence than on opinion or consensus. Although these guidelines are still being developed, if approved by ASA, they will have a significant impact on the practice of obstetric anesthesia in the United States.

[The Task Forces' frequent need to draw on expert and consensus opinion rather than literature-based evidence to reach their conclusions presents a ringing challenge to obstetric anesthesiologists. The practice of obstetric anesthesia, like that of the rest of medicine, can be greatly improved by the results of well-conducted clinical outcome studies (16).]

In the context of standards and guidelines, it is appropriate to raise the relatively new issue of "clinical pathways" (17,18). These are patient-management protocols or strategies that address familiar clinical scenarios. In theory, a systematic approach to common clinical conditions will improve both the quality and the efficiency of medical care. Clinical pathways should be formulated with great care, if at all. Ideally, anesthesia-related clinical pathways should be crafted in such a way as to describe broadly the care to be provided without defining clinical management so narrowly and precisely that they could be interpreted by attorneys at law as standards and thus create unnecessary medicolegal hazards.

A related issue is the creation of a departmental handbook describing policies and protocols (19). Such publications provide concise guidelines outlining acceptable alternative approaches to common clinical events. The handbook can be a useful reference for all members of the perinatal care team.

Although standards and practice guidelines are growing in popularity, there is little information to show that they improve clinical outcome (20). In the U.K., the Obstetric Anaesthetists Association (OAA) issued standards for obstetric anesthesia in 1987 and updated them in 1995. The effect of these standards on the quality of practice is unclear.

> Whilst a great deal of attention has been paid to defining and measuring quality and to setting standards, there is still a need to evaluate methods for producing change and improvement in service quality. . . . Whilst standard setting has been promoted as an important component of clinical audit, in itself it may be insufficient to ensure changes in facilities and practice. . . .Comparison of practice standards may improve quality, but further incentives may be needed to promote change. Features of the NHS reforms, including the purchaser-provider interaction, and the inclusion and monitoring of quality clauses within contracts, may offer a further means of stimulating change, although their capacity to do so has been brought into question (20).

Obstetric anesthesiologists should familiarize themselves with these and future standards, guidelines and clinical pathways and adopt them, as appropriate, into their practices.

Relatives & Friends

Father of Infant

MOTHER AND INFANT NUMERO UNO!

Neonatologists/ Pediatricians Obstetric Nurses

Anesthesiologists/ Anesthetists Technical Staff

Obstetricians/ Midwives Ancillary/Service Staff

* Consultant Services
* Administrative Services
* Domestic Services
* Laboratory Services
* Diagnostic Services
* Supportive Services (e.g., ICU)

[Ancillary services include: Prenatal/parenting class tutors, diagnostic facilities (laboratory, radiology, etc.), consultant services (cardiology, pulmonary, nephrology, surgery, internal medicine, etc.) housekeeping (cleaners, janitors, hazardous waste disposal experts, laundry, linen supplies, etc.), catering service (dietetic, food preparation, cooking), transport (in house, ambulance, hospital vehicles), and any other service or facility contributing to care and welfare of mother and child.]

FIG. 1. The perinatal team.

THE "PERINATAL TEAM"

Adoption of the perinatal team concept (Fig. 1), is essential for proper care of the mother and her infant(s). Anesthesiologists can make a major contribution to the perinatal team. To create and preserve a spirit of camaraderie and cooperation, team members should meet regularly for clinical rounds on patients and medical seminars. Informal communication in a communal recreational setting over coffee and doughnuts is equally important to team morale. We highly recommend acceptance of the "Big Cs" (Table 1) by the perinatal team as guiding principles for interpersonal relationships. Kindness and humanity to patients and co-workers alike are the keys to the perinatal team's success. The growing popularity of patient-care centers, developed largely in response to the need to rationalize expenses, conserve staff, and redistribute resources, now demands that the cooperative process be expedited and facilitated by all available means.

TABLE 1. *The "Cardinal Cs"*

Compassion
Cooperation
Concern
Courtesy
Communication
Consideration
Coordination
Confidence

From Bonica JJ. *Principles and practice of obstetric analgesia and anesthesia.* Philadelphia: FA Davis, 1967 with permission.

MANAGING AN OBSTETRIC ANESTHESIA SERVICE

"Obstetric anesthesia is immediate, not emergent" (attributed to the late Robert Hodgkinson, M.D.).

Obstetric anesthesia services fall broadly into two categories, teaching and nonteaching. Teaching usually occurs in a "public" institution, university hospital, or university-affiliated medical center. University hospitals and their affiliates can be funded privately, by the state, or both. These hospitals provide teaching, clinical care, and research. A nonteaching unit, more often located in a busy private institution or smaller state hospital, devotes itself almost entirely to patient care.

Managing an Obstetric Anesthesia Teaching Program

"The transformation of the health care system to a market-driven, price-competitive structure poses a significant threat to the ability of medical schools and teaching hospitals to maintain an environment for research and innovation. There is a growing sense that changes in the health care marketplace are endangering this base of support" (Diana Beattie, Ph.D., Chair-elect, AAMC's Council of Academic Societies).

Staffing Requirements

An academic obstetric anesthesia program begins with a structured staff cohort, headed by a Director of Obstetric Anesthesia and affiliated with the faculty of a recognized anesthetic teaching department (12,21). In theory, the Director should provide a balanced academic program based on the academic tripod of excellent patient care, resident teaching (practical and didactic), and clinical and laboratory research (Fig. 2A). Each leg of the tripod is of equal importance and thus deserves the same amount of attention, dedication, and support. Regrettably, current economic realities have shifted the emphasis in a manner best represented by the four-legged structure depicted in Fig. 2B. Many academic centers now place heavy emphasis on clinical activities as a means to economic survival. With government and private insurers no longer willing indirectly to subsidize teaching and research through generous reimbursement for clinical care, only institutions with significant internal or external resources [i.e., National Institutes of Health (NIH) or pharmaceutical industry funding] can afford active clinical and laboratory research programs. Most academic obstetric anesthesiologists are becoming more committed by the day to clinical activities. Nonclinical academic time is now a rare luxury.

An additional priority for the service director or leader is personnel management. A happy work force produces the best team effort. The leader should offer constructive criticism and, when necessary, issue reprimands. The service leader should give praise and place trust where they are due. Recognition of a job well done boosts self-worth, reinforces morale, and inspires loyalty. Keep in mind that success at home and at work are interdependent. An employee with problems at home, whether due to financial difficulties, personal or family illness, or relationship problems, will be unlikely to give of her or his best at work. "Success on the job depends upon success at home" (Tobias, CEO Eli-Lilly).

A good leader can delegate duties and responsibilities to capable associates. Empowering others challenges them to succeed and enhances their importance to the organization. Success adds to an individual's sense of achievement and encourages further effort. Recognition may include citations, gifts, financial rewards, and material incentives. Appropriate delegation can reward leadership as well by freeing limited nonclinical time for reading, writing, and research activities.

As an aside, most chairmen, directors, and chiefs of clinical academic departments and divisions in the fairly recent past have been to a large degree appointed on the basis of their clinical skills and academic prowess. Few boast a background or training in management methods. But with the drastic changes currently rocking academic and private medicine, business acumen and personnel skills are becoming important prerequisites for departmental and institutional leaders. In response, some physicians are addressing this deficiency in their training by attaining an advanced business degree. Others appoint suitably qualified laypersons to head the business and personnel aspects of their division, department, or institution. In addition, we suggest hiring a private billing and collection service. These organizations are obviously motivated to maximize departmental income because they are paid a percentage of their collections. Although they are sometimes foreign to academic medical institutions, financial incentives can be a potent motivator of employee performance, whether faculty, administrative, or support personnel.

An adequate number of clinically capable but academically oriented faculty is essential. This number will vary with the size of the obstetric service and the availability of support for nonclinical time. In most settings, a cohort of four to five anesthesiologists will be needed to consistently cover the weekday work on labor and delivery. Because of the heavy burden of poorly reimbursed or totally uncompensated care born by most academic obstetric services, these anesthesiologists will usually

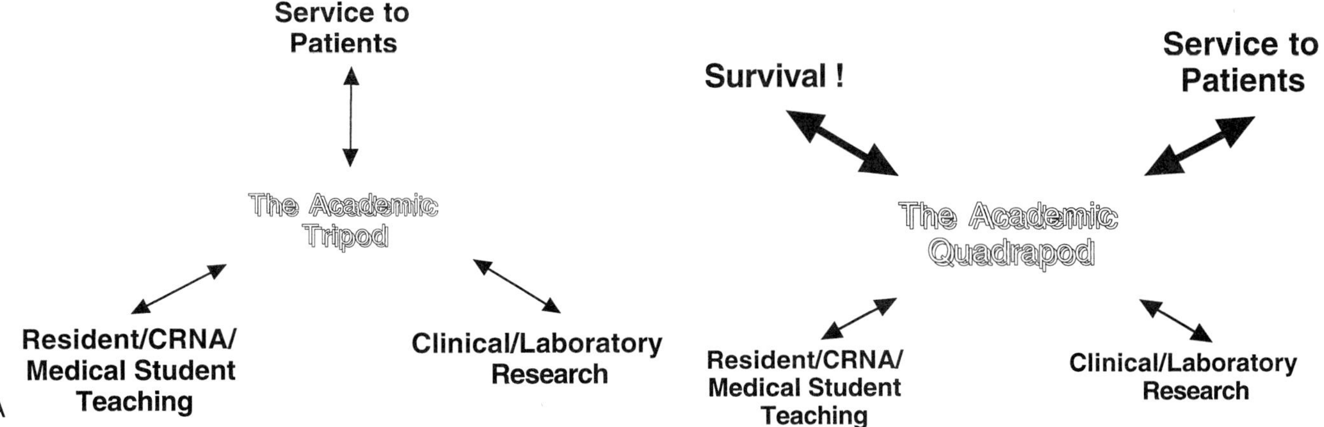

FIG. 2. A: The academic tripod. **B:** The academic "quadrapod."

have to perform other clinical duties to generate enough income to cover their salaries. Alternatively, the institution may be persuaded to subsidize obstetric anesthesia services.

General anesthesia faculty without specific obstetric anesthesia training but with an interest in the field can participate. They may be recruited to help teach residents and provide staff coverage for nights, weekends, and holidays. Often the entire anesthesia department attending staff can provide coverage for both the surgical operating rooms and obstetric suite at night and over weekends and holidays. Larger services may justify 24-hour coverage by a dedicated obstetric anesthesiologist, as may smaller units caring for a high proportion of "at risk" mothers and babies. Obstetric anesthesia faculty should contribute to the surgical/obstetric anesthesiologist call roster. In addition, an obstetric anesthesiologist must constantly be available for consultation or assistance. To help communication, besides a beeper, the latter should carry a cellular telephone.

Academic obstetric anesthesia services will rarely generate enough income to cover their salaries and expenses. At Vanderbilt University Hospital, approximately 45% of obstetric patients are now insured by Tenncare or Medicaid. Reimbursement for labor epidural analgesia and anesthesia for cesarean section for these patients averages $208 and $246, respectively. As a result, like our own, most academic obstetric anesthesia services are subsidized by other clinical revenues or institutional support. However, the benefits that can accrue to a hospital from reliable, around-the-clock, obstetric anesthesia coverage may well be worth the modest investment needed to provide this level of care.[4]

Obstetric anesthesia faculty also should provide operating room anesthesia services. Skills seldom used but vital to obstetric anesthetic practice can thus be retained.

The Trainees

Preparation

Residents should administer analgesia for vaginal delivery, as well as regional and general anesthesia for cesarean section. But obstetric patients may present special difficulties in placing epidural catheters and face greater danger from general anesthesia. Therefore in the best of circumstances, trainees should have successfully performed a reasonable number of epidural and subarachnoid blocks before entering the obstetric anesthesia teaching program. Recommendations as to a "reasonable number" range from 20 to 100, depending upon the authority consulted. We believe that 50 epidural and 25 subarachnoid blocks will provide the necessary preemptive experience. [Editor's note: In some programs, residents will be in their final year of training before they do 50 epidural blocks outside of obstetrics. Closely supervised residents can safely learn the techniques of epidural and spinal anesthesia on labor and delivery after only 4 to 6 months of training to ensure their ability to manage complications. The authors of this chapter have recently had to adopt this policy. They, however, still believe that this pragmatic approach remains far from the ideal in terms of both resident competence and hence confidence on the obstetric floor. The ability of close supervision to reduce iatrogenic (resident)-induced anesthetic complications should not be underestimated.][5]

Before arriving on the obstetric anesthesia service, residents should be able to perform a rapid-sequence induction of general endotracheal anesthesia. Although decreasing in frequency, general anesthesia will still be needed for occasional obstetric emergencies. Skill in airway management, including the potentially lethal difficult-to-impossible intubation/ventilation scenario, is essential. Residents should be readily able to manage local anesthetic or eclampsia-induced seizures. Trainees also should be adept at cardiopulmonary resuscitation (CPR). They should understand that the immediate relief of aortocaval occlusion that follows expedient abdominal delivery much improves the mother's chances of intact survival.

As a minimum, residents should have 6 to 12 months' experience (500 cases) before beginning their obstetric anesthesia training. A higher incidence of anesthetic complications such as accidental dural puncture (due to maternal lumbar lordosis, softening of the ligaments of the back during pregnancy, etc.) and failed intubation (but, we hope, not failed ventilation) can be expected in a teaching environment. Constant faculty supervision and assistance for obstetric anesthesia trainees is desirable, if not essential.[5] Protocols dealing with immediate obstetric anesthesia complications should be conscientiously taught and prominently displayed.

The Rotation

Obstetric anesthesia guidelines must be issued to residents at the start of their rotation. We strongly recommend the creation of an introductory obstetric anesthesia guideline booklet for use by all obstetric anesthesia care providers. These notes should not be so detailed as to distract from the literature. Relevant books and journals should be readily available so residents can study when the service is quiet.

An obstetric anesthesia resident rotation should last 2 to 3 months. Senior residents with a special interest in the field can take an optional 3- to 6-month training. Those

[4]"Birth Room with a View, and a Jacuzzi. Public Hospitals Add Amenities to Lure Back Maternity Patients." Article in the New York *Times*, Sunday, February 8, 1998.

[5]Hoyt MR. Epidural complication rates in a training program which utilizes close attending supervision and reusable Touhy needles. Abstracts of Scientific Papers, 29th Annual Meeting of the Society for Obstetric Anesthesia and Perinatology, 1997:71.

planning an academic career dedicated to obstetric anesthesia may opt for a more rigorous 1- to 2-year fellowship that allows time for clinical and laboratory research.

With the population of anesthesia trainees changing every 2 to 3 months, familiarity with the unit layout, anesthesia equipment, and functional aspects of the service can be deficient. This difficulty can be somewhat offset by staggering rotations such that trainees overlap month by month with the aim of providing better continuity. This worthy intent is further served by the constant presence of competent anesthesia faculty. If inadequate staffing makes these approaches impractical, a continuous Certified Registered Nurse Anesthetist (CRNA) commitment to obstetric anesthesia offers a sensible alternative. In some settings, a trained anesthesia technician is a cheaper, workable option. The technician's familiarity with facilities and equipment provides excellent backup for obstetric anesthesia residents and faculty.

A Recommended System

For an "ideal" obstetric service performing 3,000 deliveries/year,[6] with a 70% use of epidural analgesia (Fig. 3) and a cesarean section rate of 20%, we recommend the following staffing:

- Academic Director of Obstetric Anesthesia: 1,
- Obstetric anesthesia faculty anesthesiologists: 3,
- CRNAs providing 24-hour coverage: 5,

or:

- Senior residents (CA3) working 1 in 3 × 24 hours: 3,[7]
- Residents (CA2-3): 3 to 4,[7] and
- Anesthetic technicians, daytime hours only: 2.[8]

A service of 3,000 deliveries/year with a 70% use of epidural analgesia would provide about 175 procedures per month. Each resident/trainee would perform on average 60 epidural blocks for labor and delivery in a 2-month rotation (Fig. 4). A 3-month rotation would yield approximately 90 procedures. Each resident/trainee would anesthetize on average 17 patients for cesarean section in a 2-month rotation and 25 in a 3-month rotation (Fig. 5). However, 95% of these cases will likely receive regional anesthesia, and only 5%, general anesthesia. Therefore resident experience in the performance of rapid-sequence induction of general anesthesia will be limited (22,23). This deficiency should be corrected by exposing residents to emergency surgical and trauma anesthesia before their obstetric anesthesia rotation.

$$\frac{\text{Epidural Blocks} \times 100}{\text{Total Deliveries} - \text{Cesarean Deliveries}} = \%\ \text{Epidural Analgesia}$$

FIG. 3. Calculation of the percentage of patients receiving epidural labor analgesia.

Certified Registered Nurse Anesthetists

In our opinion, CRNAs assigned to obstetrics should be allowed to perform conduction analgesia/anesthesia. Qualified CRNAs doing epidural blocks should not seriously dilute trainee experience. A CRNA presence on the obstetric floor also is a source of educated assistance and resident backup. This view is controversial in the light of the ASA Statement on Regional Anesthesia (Appendix A). This promulgation recommends that only physicians do regional blocks.

Qualified anesthesiologists interested in obstetric analgesia/anesthesia are at a premium (24–34). At least 60% to 70% of primigravid women experience severe to excruciating pain during labor and delivery (35). Epidural block can control the pain of childbirth in 85% of these women and reduce suffering in a further 12% to 13%. Also, once a mother has experienced a successful epidural block for childbirth, she is likely to choose to do so again. Institutions with skilled obstetric anesthesia personnel therefore can expect a 60% to 90% epidural rate.

In 1992, 51% of women delivering in hospitals performing more than 1,500 deliveries/year received epidural blockade (vs 22% in 1983) (31,34). Anesthesiologists or medically directed residents or CRNAs placed 95% of these blocks (vs 79% in 1983). In smaller hospitals (500 to 1,500 deliveries per year), 33% of women received epidural labor analgesia (vs 13% in 1983), 79% (vs 61% in 1983) being provided by either an anesthesiologist or a medically directed resident or CRNA.

In 1991, the original authors of this chapter (J.W.D. and W.U.B.) canvassed 802 members of SOAP about the role of CRNAs in obstetric anesthetic practice and opinions about the 1983 ASA "Statement on Regional Anesthesia." Of the 802 questionnaires mailed, 60 were returned undelivered. Of the remaining 742 questionnaires, 216 replies were received, a response rate of 29.3%. After review, we considered 210 of 216 eligible for inclusion.

$$\frac{3{,}000\ \text{Deliveries/Year} \times 70\%\ \text{Epidural Analgesia}}{6\ \text{Trainees/Month} \times 12\ \text{Months/Year}} \times 100 = 29\ \text{Procedures/Trainee/Month}$$

FIG. 4. Average number of epidural blocks per trainee per month.

[6]Others consider an annual delivery rate of 2,000 to 2,500 optimal. We believe this number too low, with tertiary care obstetric and neonatal referral units excepted.

[7]After call day off. Maximum of ten 24-hour calls with one long week end (Friday through Sunday) off per month. Clinical assignment [e.g., GYN, MOR anesthesia, or Acute Pain Service (APS)] on day 3, limited to 4 to 5 (10- to 12-hour days) per month. Each resident thus works an average of 68 to 70 hours per week for the 3 months of rotation. If CRNAs are involved in the service, only three or four trainees are reasonably able to rotate at any one time.

[8]As noted, an alternative to CRNAs, 24-hour technical coverage with five technicians, may be entertained.

$$\frac{3{,}000 \text{ Deliveries/Year} \times 20\% \text{ Cesarean Sections}}{6 \text{ Trainees/Month} \times 12 \text{ Months/Year}} \times 100 = \text{8.3 Cesarean Sections/Trainee/Month}$$

FIG. 5. Average number of anesthetics for cesarean section per trainee per month.

Of these 210 respondents, 108 (51.4%) worked with CRNAs. Of these, 46 (42.6%) of 108 reported that CRNAs administered conduction anesthesia for obstetrics. Of the remaining 62 who admitted functioning with CRNA help, 16 (25.8%) of 62 did not permit CRNAs to do conduction anesthesia because of the 1983 ASA Statement on Regional Anesthesia; 18 (29.0%) of 62 gave other reasons; and 28 (45.2%) of 62 chose not to answer the question.

Thus despite the stance taken by the ASA, CRNAs perform a significant number of regional anesthetics in the United States. Given the more than twofold increase in the use of labor epidural analgesia noted previously, there is reason to believe that CRNAs are even more frequently involved in the administration of obstetric analgesia today.

Therefore we (some of us reluctantly) must concur with Frederick Hehre, who in 1975 stated,

> I firmly believe that an elite group of nurse anesthetists should be developed into obstetrical anesthesia specialists, and, after training and certification, be allowed to administer conduction anesthesia. Pragmatically, the nurse anesthetist presently makes certain medical decisions and administers drugs and treatment; for example, treatment of hypotension with vasopressors, administration of blood, choice of anesthetic agent, etc. (An important analogy seems to exist here between the obstetric nurse anesthetist and the intensive care nurse.) It is more sensible to allow qualified individuals to make the decision to administer conduction anesthesia to an obstetrical patient with a known full stomach than to risk aspiration of vomitus with inhalation anesthesia, which is the leading anesthetic cause of maternal death (36).

We hasten to add that, in our unanimous opinion, these specially trained CRNAs should practice their art whenever possible under the direction of a qualified obstetric anesthesiologist.

A joint statement issued by ACOG/ASA appears to recognize that CRNAs do, in practice, administer conduction anesthesia for obstetrics:

> Qualifications for administering anesthesia. A qualified anesthesiologist responsible for all anesthetics administered should be appointed. In many obstetric units, obstetricians or obstetrician-supervised nurse anesthetists administer the anesthetics. The administration of general or regional anesthesia requires numerous medical judgments and technical skills. Nurse anesthetists are not trained as physicians and cannot be expected to make medical decisions. Obstetricians seldom have sufficient training or experience in administering anesthesia to allow them to properly supervise nurse anesthetists [ACOG and ASA recommended obstetric anesthesia goals. *ACOG Newsletter* 1988;32(September):9,10].

This statement stressed the need for direct CRNA supervision by a qualified anesthesiologist rather than by an obstetrician. Training in obstetrics cannot guarantee the prerequisite anesthetic skills and knowledge needed for adequate CRNA surveillance.

In its own proclamations, the ASA recommends that only properly trained physicians perform regional anesthesia (see Appendix E). We prefer the more pragmatic approach taken in the joint ACOG/ASA statement. It provides sensible latitude for those institutions that allow the administration of obstetric regional anesthesia by appropriately supervised CRNAs. In rural areas, small towns, and some large cities, anesthesiologists interested in the practice of obstetric anesthesia are in short supply. Here, CRNAs provide most of the direct obstetric anesthesia care, including epidural analgesia. The actual number of obstetric regional blocks performed by CRNAs annually in North America is unknown but is undoubtedly significant. We emphasize again, ideally obstetric CRNAs should practice under the direct supervision of qualified obstetric anesthesiologists.

Caring for the Obstetric Patient at High Risk

Clinical management of obstetric patients who are hypertensive, bleeding, or who have a critical medical or surgical condition is detailed elsewhere. However, this chapter would be incomplete if it failed to address the issues of facilities and staffing for the care of these women (37–39). Ideally, a Critical Care Obstetrics or CCOB facility should be located close to the obstetric delivery suite, as are dedicated obstetric operating rooms in most institutions that deliver babies. The CCOB unit should include sophisticated electronic monitors for the direct measurement and display of arterial, central venous, pulmonary artery, and pulmonary capillary occlusion pressures. Evaluation of cardiac output and peripheral and mixed venous oxygen saturation should be possible. Monitors must be situated permanently in the obstetric suite and placed in an area designated for the care of the critically ill. A versatile lung ventilator that can compensate for decreased lung compliance and increased airway resistance should be at hand. A nearby automated biochemical laboratory performing arterial and mixed venous blood gas/acid–base analyses provides data for calculation of tissue O_2 consumption, O_2 delivery, and $\dot{V}O_2/\dot{D}O_2$ ratios. Other biochemical parameters essential to patient management can be measured as well.

The CCOB unit should have a director or two codirectors who are responsible for addressing all administrative and clinical policy issues. The CCOB unit should, like other subspecialty critical care units, use a multidisciplinary approach to all critically ill patients to deliver high-quality critical care. A major component in the successful treatment of the critically ill parturient is the constant presence of an ICU-trained obstetric nurse. Vanderbilt University Medical Center maintains an elite cadre of intensive care–trained nurses. The obstetric anesthesia service provides the technical expertise for the insertion of arterial and central lines. The obstetric anesthesiologists help with interpretation of monitored data and advise on patient management.

Obstetricians, anesthesiologists, and obstetric nurses commissioned to develop an obstetric intensive care program should meet in advance to review and agree on management strategies and define treatment protocols. This goal particularly applies to severe preeclampsia, where singular controversy exists. Obstetric anesthesiologists largely agree about the anesthetic management and intravenous fluid therapy for this complex syndrome. Consensus among obstetricians working together is far less frequent. More conservative obstetric ideas may even hamper anesthesia care of the severe preeclamptic. As an example, patients are kept "dry" without the benefit of central venous or pulmonary artery pressure monitoring to avoid "iatrogenic pulmonary edema." This strategy may be considered safer obstetrically in a poorly equipped and understaffed peripheral hospital. But profound volume depletion makes perilous the induction of anesthesia, regional or general. Swift transport by air or road argues for transfer of critically ill parturients to tertiary obstetric care centers with intensive care facilities.

Established management guidelines should be reviewed on a monthly or quarterly basis and amended when necessary. A chain of command must be fashioned by designating a single physician (the duty obstetric chief/senior resident) to prescribe all patient therapy in writing. This precaution ensures that orders given to the ICU obstetric nurses do not conflict.

Seriously ill parturients may need to be delivered hurriedly, frequently by cesarean section. Sophisticated anesthesia equipment, ventilators, and electronic monitors held in standby mode should be ready for instant action in the obstetric operating rooms. A modular system of monitors reduces the need for costly duplication. Expensive cardiac-output and mixed venous oxygen saturation modules can be moved between the operating room and intensive care area as required.

In short, we agree with the statement made by Palmer and Gibbs: "No matter what obstetric anesthesia protocols are adopted, one overriding rule applies: that obstetric patients receive the same standard of care, including quality of anesthetic equipment and monitors, that patients in the general operating room receive" (39).

Obstetric Anesthesia Teaching and Research

A balanced academic program ensures good resident education (12,41). A series of didactic presentations on obstetric anesthesia must be included in the departmental lecture program. Try to set aside time during the working day for faculty and residents to meet informally. Another anesthesiologist or a qualified CRNA can cover clinical duties during these sessions to avoid interruptions. Tutorials and literature discussions may be scheduled two to three times a week. The goal should be to inculcate in residents the life-long habit of reading current literature as a means of keeping up to date and enabling them to practice evidence-based medicine whenever possible.

Obstetric anesthesia clinical and laboratory research depends on the motivation of the director and faculty. Funding is essential, particularly for laboratory research. Faculty need reasonable (50%) nonclinical time to draft protocols, write grant proposals, and do research studies. For the foreseeable future, this amount of nonclinical time will be available only to faculty with significant external grant funding. Still, successful academic anesthesia departments must devise a way to allocate available nonclinical time to potentially productive younger faculty. A substantial portion of this nonclinical time needs to be allotted to reading current literature, preparing and delivering lectures and tutorials, and writing abstracts, papers, and book chapters. Sharing laboratory space, facilities, and staff within the Department of Anesthesiology cuts costs and may allow more productive use of scarce nonclinical time. Obstetric anesthesia research fellowships of 1 to 2 years' duration should be created to attract young, inquisitive people. After completing their training, fellows may remain or move to bolster the cause of obstetric anesthesia elsewhere. Either way, the reputation of a department's obstetric anesthesia fellowship and resident programs will be enhanced.

Fellows should aim to complete one or two worthwhile projects. Here, the experience and guidance of the director (or other mentor) are critical. A poorly designed, irrelevant study consumes as much energy, time, and money as does a worthwhile, carefully constructed project. The director must channel the fellow's energy and enthusiasm in productive directions. Only with this guidance can the fellow acquire the necessary intellectual skills to turn an interesting research idea into an acclaimed publication in a peer-reviewed journal.

Managing a Nonteaching Obstetric Anesthesia Service

The basic management tenets outlined stand also in the organization of a nonteaching obstetric anesthesia service. However, important differences exist regarding staffing. Two distinct staffing patterns prevail in larger (more than 1,500 deliveries per annum) nonteaching obstetric anesthesia units. Structural differences are dictated mainly by local anesthesiologists' attitudes to CRNAs in obstetrics.

Many nonteaching institutions, including some with large obstetric services (4,000 to 5,000 deliveries per year) provide obstetric analgesia/anesthesia services with a cohort of CRNAs. A suitably qualified physician directs the Obstetric Anesthesia Service. The director and other members of the anesthesiology practice supervise these CRNAs. The anesthesiologist should be free to help if immediate problems or complications arise.

The contrasting situation can be found in physician-based obstetric anesthesia services. Although this arrangement is exemplary, it works well only if sufficient numbers of well-trained obstetric anesthesiologists are available continuously to meet the clinical workload. Practical problems may arise in hospitals with large obstetric services and a high use of epidural analgesia. The scenario then changes to one of clinical overload, leading inevitably to compromise in the quality of clinical care and poor documentation. Considerations such as cost structure, price competition, and a large clinical workload may lead some anesthesiology departments to implement the anesthesia-care team approach, as outlined earlier, to meet the needs of their laboring patients.

Staffing with a cohort of CRNAs offers a better way to cope with this situation. A CRNA inserts the epidural catheter under the supervision of the duty anesthesiologist. The CRNA then remains at the bedside and monitors vital signs for the next 20 minutes or until the patient is comfortable and hemodynamically stable. The CRNA is trained to respond appropriately to maternal hypotension, seizures, high subarachnoid or insidious subdural block, and so on. Other CRNAs are available to help should an obstetric emergency arise demanding immediate assisted vaginal or abdominal delivery. The need for an epidural "top-up," or infusion syringe or pump refill, or treatment of an anesthetic complication draws a quick and appropriate reaction. Such dedicated patient coverage by physicians is expensive, and in areas where anesthesiologists are hard to find, impossible.

MISCELLANEOUS MATTERS

Patient Evaluation and Anesthetic Documentation

A thorough preanesthetic assessment is vital. Complete obstetric, medical, surgical, anesthetic, drug, allergic, and family histories are prerequisite to patient safety and optimal anesthesia care. They alert the anesthesiologist to potential problems. The ASA "Basic Standards for Preanesthesia Care" (approved by the House of Delegates on October 14, 1987; Appendix F) and the more recent Guideline III as promulgated in the ASA Guidelines for Regional Anesthesia in Obstetrics (approved by the House of Delegates on October 12, 1988, and last amended on October 30, 1991; Appendix A) provide direction here.

A further ASA statement, which appears in "Documentation of Anesthesia Care" (approved by the House of Delegates on October 12, 1988; Appendix J), emphasizes the importance of documenting the preanesthetic patient evaluation and maintaining a detailed time-based record of perianesthesia events. "Documentation is a factor in the provision of quality care, and is the responsibility of an anesthesiologist." We recommend using a preprinted, preanesthetic form, which will become part of the patient's anesthesia record. Thus important questions that the patient should answer will not be overlooked. A permanent record of the preanesthesia interview also will be available in the patient's chart.

In the ideal world, the parturient should be interviewed by an anesthesiologist well in advance (at 34 to 36 weeks' gestation) of delivery. To attain this ideal requires a considerable degree of cooperation and coordination between the obstetrician and anesthesiologist. And even if such a utopian policy exists, it cannot predict the sudden onset of preterm labor or antepartum bleeding. In practice, most women who have experienced an uncomplicated pregnancy are likely to meet their anesthesiologist on admission to the labor suite. The preanesthetic interview should be conducted as soon as possible after the patient's admission to allow adequate time to discuss the patient's anesthetic options.

An obstetric anesthesia record differs from that used in the main operating rooms, but the two should originate from the same root and bear a close resemblance. This similarity will simplify the task of keeping good anesthetic records, especially for those working in both the operating rooms and the obstetric suite. Recovery and the postpartum anesthetic visit also should be documented.

All anesthesia documentation should be of the highest caliber. A meticulous anesthesia record is considered evidence of good care, an important consideration in the highly charged legal climate of obstetrics. Automated anesthesia records (AARs) can offer more accurate documentation and contribute to patient care.[9] But problems, such as artifact rejection and cost remain unresolved. A computerized anesthesia data-management system is presently in an advanced stage of development at the Vanderbilt University Department of Anesthesiology. The preanesthetic portion, generated during the patient's visit to the Vanderbilt Preoperative Evaluation Clinic (VPEC) is already in operation. Although this system suits the economic demands of modern day anesthesia and surgery, it has its limitations. An individual anesthesiologist's ability to establish rapport with the patient is limited. Occasionally, serious omissions in both the history and physical examination arise. Anesthesiologists using these computerized systems are well advised to spend some time talking to and getting to know their patients while confirming the recorded findings.

[9]Merritt TW. Can anesthesiologists adapt and benefit from use of automated record keeping devices? Anesthesiology News, The McMahon Group, New York: July, 1991.

Higgins MS. (1998) Preoperative data management. Systems for recording and management of preoperative data. Chapter in preparation.

Analgesia and Anesthesia Techniques

Indications for obstetric epidural blockade vary from one institution to the next. Obstetric anesthesiologists can play an important role in educating their obstetric colleagues about the risks and benefits of appropriate labor analgesia. Differences of opinion also can confound the anesthetic management of complicated obstetric cases. For example, should parturients with pregnancy-induced hypertension, breech presentation, multiple gestation, preterm labor, or diabetes receive epidural blockade? Regular meetings and literature reviews with obstetric colleagues can help coordinate the care of these women at high risk. The collegial relations that these regular interactions foster will help create a healthy, low-stress working environment.

Acute Pain Consultants

The role of acute pain service (APS) or as we prefer, acute pain consultants (APCs) in obstetrics deserves attention. Good recovery from surgery and patient satisfaction with anesthesia depends on effective postoperative analgesia. Postoperative patient mobility is a key factor in avoiding deep vein thrombosis and pulmonary venous embolism. Satisfactory analgesia greatly facilitates maternal ambulation. The parturient can then begin to interact with and care for her baby. The patient can cough and breathe deeply, too, making postoperative bronchopneumonia less likely. Both epidural morphine and patient-controlled epidural analgesia can effectively meet these ends.

The juxtaposition of obstetric anesthesia and the APC makes good sense. Both are concerned with acute pain management. In some institutions, anesthesiologists share duties in these two mutually compatible areas. Involvement in the APC benefits patients, expands the interests of obstetric anesthesiologists, and adds stature to the specialty. Income from an APC may help to subsidize the costs of continuous obstetric anesthesia coverage.

Management of the Patient Requiring Abortion

Controversy may surround the use of conduction analgesia for mid-trimester abortion. Staff opposed to abortion on religious or conscientious grounds may refuse to become involved. Some anesthesiologists believe the risks of epidural blockade outweigh the benefits in this setting. Because the baby's welfare is not at issue, they argue for liberal use of potent intravenous analgesic, anxiolytic, and amnestic agents.

An induced abortion can be painful, and conduction analgesia may be indicated. Regardless of indication, the patient's suffering is real. No patient requesting help in this situation should be denied regional analgesia on other than medical grounds. The feelings of the patient's husband, significant other, or immediate family concerning relief of her anxiety and pain should not be overlooked and need to be addressed, but their opinions do not supersede the patient's wishes and needs. Institutional policies can help avoid embarrassment or unpleasantness for all concerned.

Medicolegal Issues: Informed Consent

Others have succinctly confronted the medicolegal implications of obstetric anesthesia (42), and excellent guidelines are available for risk management in this setting (39). Informed consent plays an important role in minimizing the medicolegal risks of obstetric anesthesia (43,44). To avoid litigation, most important, adopt an open and honest approach to the patient, her partner, and close relatives. Without being patronizing, take the time to explain frankly the proposed anesthetic procedure, with its benefits, risks, and potential complications.

The patient should appreciate that in a training institution, some complications may be more common. Provide a fair estimate of the degree of extra risk involved, based on your practice and the current literature. For example, accidental dural puncture may occur in 1% to 3% of patients managed by residents. The incidence in more experienced hands may be less than 0.5%. The risks of more serious complications, such as epidural abscess or blood clot, permanent nerve damage, or local anesthetic–induced seizures or cardiac arrest, should be minimal in any setting.

Providing the patient with appropriate information during the consent process demands a delicate and individual approach (44). Too detailed a description of anesthesia-related complications can frighten even the most balanced individual. Emphasize that effective methods exist (i.e., blood patch) to deal with anesthetic complications (i.e., postdural puncture headache). Admit the possibility of an imperfect or failed block. Outline the potential remedies, including replacement of the epidural catheter, repeated spinal blockade, or on rare occasions, general anesthesia.

Should a serious complication occur, take an honest and forthright approach to all concerned. Accurately inform the patient and her support persons. Keep them apprised of developments, whether good or bad. Most important, convey that the perinatal team has the patient's best interests at heart and that its members are doing all they can to make her better. Once the crisis passes, again take time to explain matters to ensure reasonable understanding. A further visit or telephone call about a month after the patient leaves the hospital will impress on her that she has been and continues to be well cared for. As her anesthesiologist, you in turn will be reassured that no misconceptions exist about the recent critical events. Misinformation and misunderstanding cause confusion, anger, and frustration. All members of the perinatal care team should provide consistent, nonjudgmental information to patient and family.

Financial Implications of an Obstetric Anesthesia Service

> Health care reform in the United States is on a collision course with economic reality. . . . In industry after industry, the underlying dynamic is the same: competition compels companies to deliver increasing value to customers. The fundamental driver of this continuous quality improvement and cost reduction is in innovation. Without incentives to sustain innovation in health care, short-term cost savings will soon be overwhelmed by the desire to widen access, the growing health needs of an aging population, and the unwillingness of Americans to settle for anything less than the best treatments available. Inevitably, the failure to promote innovation will lead to lower quality or more rationing of care: two equally undesirable results (45).

American medicine is based on free-market principles. Despite the disadvantages of this practice, its benefits clearly predominate (45). Rivalry among community hospitals for patients is, and will continue to become, increasingly competitive. With the growth of managed care, hospitals must compete for extended contracts, often covering hundreds of thousands of lives. To attract individual patients and these managed care contracts, many hospitals have adopted the idea of a Women's Pavilion or Patient Care Center. This approach offers convenient, cost-effective specialized obstetric and gynecologic patient care all under one roof.

A significant factor contributing to patient satisfaction is the presence of an efficient, available, obstetric analgesia/anesthesia service. Many private institutions have established such services, and 60% to 90% of their clients now request epidural labor analgesia. An obstetric anesthesia service can be profitable despite the major commitment to staff and equipment involved, even when anesthesiologists, not CRNAs, provide care. If the hospital fails to make a direct profit from obstetric anesthesia, it can still benefit from an increase in patient referrals.

State and university-based hospitals face somewhat different issues. They often serve an uninsured or underinsured patient population. Obstetric care, usually delivered by residents, is more complicated and less efficient than that in nonacademic institutions. Consequently, obstetric anesthesia care will cost more but be reimbursed less than in private hospitals. Continuous clinical coverage plus resident education and research demands manpower and funding. It is the rare academic obstetric anesthesia service that will cover these expenses solely from clinical revenues. The running expenses of an obstetric anesthesia division must therefore be shared. Augmented patient referrals offset financial losses incurred by the hospital. Furthermore, a good obstetric anesthesia service enhances a hospital's reputation and prestige within the community it serves. These facts are worth emphasizing when negotiating with hospital administrators.

Confounding these issues, insurers are limiting their costs by negotiating for discounted and capitated fees. Some are even attempting to limit the use of epidural labor analgesia to "medical indications." Our patients may become our allies in combating these trends. "As. . .the search continues to find means of decreasing medical expenses, consumerism may play an even greater role in the survival of our specialty. For example, the response of American women to the information that labor analgesia will no longer be covered by their insurance policies may force insurers to reconsider." Anesthesiologists should "take a proactive role in educating our prospective patients and our obstetric colleagues regarding the safety, benefits, and affordability of analgesia for childbirth" (Birnbach DJ. The economics of obstetric anesthesia: what's in our future? *SOAP Newsletter* 1995, Winter). Birnbach enumerates a number of useful suggestions for minimizing expenses and maximizing reimbursement associated with obstetric anesthesia services (Editor's note: I do not endorse the wholesale implementation of the thought-provoking ideas that follow):

- Enforce cost-conscious behavior by the perinatal team, patients included;
- Take advantage of the savings offered by bulk buying (of epidural and spinal kits, for example);
- Negotiate with insurers (see later);
- Make public a list of insurers who refuse to cover the costs of epidural analgesia for labor (see ASA and ACOG joint statement-Committee Opinion 118, 1993);
- Increase the number of personally administered anesthetics;
- Agree on reasonable capitation payments with insurers or hospital administration;
- Have an anesthesiologist on committees that negotiate HMO contracts;
- Establish prepayment plans whereby patients wanting epidural labor analgesia are required to register and prepay for the anticipated anesthetic service;
- Offer and charge for advance anesthetic consultations for parturients at increased risk for complications;
- Participate in postoperative pain management (see our earlier comments on the role of the APC);
- Increase the demand for epidural labor analgesia through public relations and education;
- Maximize collections through more efficient and creative billing practices, such as acceptance of credit cards; and
- Establish rapport with the patient and her family to help them understand the importance and value of the services provided by the obstetric anesthesiologist.

Current consensus is lacking about the basis for billing and reimbursement of obstetric anesthesia services. Some of the commonly used approaches include:

- Base units + time (at 4 units/hour);
- Base units + time (at 1 unit/hour);
- Base units + time spent in direct patient care;

- Flat fee;
- Scaled fee (i.e., rate A for continuous labor analgesia at 4 hours, or rate B for duration greater than 4 hours); or
- Capitation.

None of these choices is ideal. Whereas time-based methods ensure some correlation between the anesthesiologist's work and charges, without a "cap," the bill can assume unconscionable size. Although a flat fee offers simplicity, some question the fairness of charging the same for 30 minutes of care as for 24 hours of care.

Marketing and Communication

In the light of the suggestions summarized, it may be said there are few anesthetic subspecialties for which marketing and communication are more important than obstetric anesthesia. Prospective parents should have access to both verbal and printed information about obstetric analgesia and anesthesia. Participation by an obstetric anesthesiologist in institutional parenting classes can provide a firm foundation for establishing good patient/physician rapport. A brief, but professionally produced and narrated, videotape can be a useful alternative to a live presentation. An informational pamphlet about obstetric anesthesia, comprehensible and devoid of medical jargon, will allow the patient and her partner to read about conduction analgesia and general anesthesia at their leisure. The patient can then make informed decisions about her pain control well in advance of labor.

Childbirth classes can provide valuable skills that help the parturient cope with the rigors of childbirth (46). Classes also teach "natural childbirth" methods featuring regulated breathing patterns and muscle relaxation that may help some women accommodate the pain of labor (35,46). But when these techniques fail, women often then request epidural blockade. Patients should not view this situation as a personal failure. Childbirth is itself quite "natural." Relieving pain and suffering does not eliminate that natural element; it simply makes the experience safer and less unpleasant. Because women whose expectations of labor are violated by actual experience report more severe pain (35), patients should have realistic expectations about the efficacy of relaxation and breathing methods and recognize that conduction blockade is a safe and effective option for pain control.

CONCLUSION

A pregnant woman and her anesthesiologist can expect a smooth course and joyous outcome to childbirth. Obstetric anesthesia also can provide some of the greatest challenges to an anesthesiologist's technical skills. The obvious case is the parturient with an unsuspected difficult airway. The knowledge and expertise of the obstetric anesthesiologist also can be tested when managing less urgent, but equally menacing situations. For example, severe preeclampsia is a syndrome so diverse in its presentation that it sometimes confuses even the most erudite clinician.

A well-staffed and efficiently organized obstetric anesthesia division, equipped with appropriate anesthesia and monitoring equipment, promotes patient well-being and safety. It also can provide a happy and challenging work environment. Communication between patient, obstetrician, and anesthesiologist is essential. An open and honest approach to the patient and her supporters will help in making all anesthetic-related decisions. Potential complications associated with conduction analgesia and general anesthesia should be discussed clearly beforehand. Untoward events, should they occur, must be dealt with efficiently and candidly. This approach should largely offset any concurrent medicolegal threat. Full participation by the anesthesiologist in the perinatal team is a prerequisite to patient satisfaction and safety. Despite the risks and frustrations they confront, obstetric anesthesiologists generally can lead a demanding but exciting and satisfying existence.

REFERENCES

1. Fisher DM, Macario A. Editorial views: special section economics: economics of anesthesia care. *Anesthesiology* 1997;86:1018.
2. Shapiro BA. Why must the practice of anesthesiology change? It's economics, Doctor! *Anesthesiology* 1997;86:1020.
3. Lubarsky DA, Glass PSA, Ginsberg B, et al. The successful implementation of pharmaceutical practice guidelines. *Anesthesiology* 1997;86:1145.
4. Lubarsky DA, Sanderson IC, Gilbert WC, et al. Using an anesthesia information management system as a cost containment tool. *Anesthesiology* 1997;86:1161.
5. Sperry RJ. Principles of economic analysis. *Anesthesiology* 1997;86:1197.
6. Watcha MF, White PF. Economics of anesthetic practice. *Anesthesiology* 1997;86:1170.
7. Marx GF. Foreword. In: Datta S, ed. *Anesthetic and obstetric management of high risk pregnancy.* St. Louis: Mosby Year Book, 1991:xi.
8. Marx G. Personal reflections on 50 years of obstetric anesthesia. *Reg Anesth* 1990;15:232.
9. Moore DC, Bridenbaugh LD. Is it practical for medical anesthetists to supply a twenty-four hour obstetrical service? *West J Surg Obstet & Gynecol* 1955;63:382.
10. Moore DC. Twenty-four hour coverage of obstetrical deliveries by physician anesthetists. *Acta Anaesthesiol Scand Suppl* 1966;25:350.
11. Moore DC, Bridenbaugh LD, Bridenbaugh PO. Twenty-four hour coverage of obstetric deliveries by anesthesiologists. *Anesth Analg* 1969;48:401.
12. Kalas DB, Hehre FW. Departmental evolution of obstetric anesthesia: a 12 year survey. *Obstet Gynecol* 1970;36:156.
13. Sheldon RS. Consolidation of hospital obstetric services. *Med Clin North Am* 1974;58:885.
14. Marx GF. Obstetric anesthesia organizations in the United States [Letter]. *Anesthesiology* 1974;41:308.
15. Kassirer JP. The quality of care and the quality of measuring it [Editorial]. *N Engl J Med* 1993;329:1263.
16. Goodman NW. Anaesthesia and evidence-based medicine. *Anesthesia* 1998;53:353.
17. Horne M. Involving physicians in clinical pathways: an example for perioperative knee arthroplasty. *J Qual Improv* 1996;22:115.
18. Servis KW, Ferarra EP. Practice guidelines: the New York State Task Force on Clinical Guidelines and Medical Technology Assessment. *J Qual Improv* 1996;22:134.

19. McDonagh J, Clarke F, Veale D. How to do it: write a departmental handbook for junior staff. *Br Med J* 1993;307:553.
20. Thomson RG, Bryson M, Donaldson LJ. Obstetric anesthesia: an approach to improving the standards of service. *Int J Obstet Anesth* 1997;6:250.
21. Marx GF. Obstetric anesthesia in New York City [Letter]. *Am J Obstet Gynecol* 1976;124:440.
22. Hawkins JL, Gibbs CP. General anesthesia for cesarean section: are we really prepared? *Int J Obstet Anesth* 1998;7:145.
23. Tsen LC, Pitner R, Camann WR. General anesthesia for cesarean section at a tertiary care hospital 1990–1995: indications and implications. *Int J Obstet Anesth* 1998;7:147.
24. Phillips OC, Frazier TM. Obstetric anesthesia care in the United States. *Obstet Gynecol* 1962;19:796.
25. Shnider SM. Obstetric anesthesia coverage: problems and solutions. *Obstet Gynecol* 1969;34:615.
26. Taylor G. Obstetric anaesthesia services in the United Kingdom. *Br Med J* 1971;1:101.
27. Rasmussen J, George T, Reisman A, Cull WA, Gravenstein JS. Obstetric anesthesiology practices and attitudes in hospitals in Cuyahoga County, Ohio: a survey. *Ohio State Med J* 1977;73:139.
28. Palahniuk RJ. Survey of obstetric anaesthesia practice in British Columbia [Editorial]. *Can Anaesth Soc J* 1986;33:123.
29. McMorland GH, Jenkins LC, Douglas MJ. A survey of obstetric anaesthesia practice in British Columbia. *Can Anaesth Soc J* 1986;33:185.
30. Levinson G, Shnider SM. Obstetric anesthesia coverage: a continuing problem [Editorial]. *Anesthesiology* 1986;65:245.
31. Gibbs CP, Krischer J, Peckham BM, Sharp H, Kirschbaum TH. Obstetric anesthesia: a national survey. *Anesthesiology* 1986;65:298.
32. Reynolds F. Obstetric anaesthetic services [Editorial]. *Br Med J* 1986; 293:403.
33. MacDonald R, Webster DCS. Obstetric anaesthetic services in the Yorkshire region. *Br Med J* 1986;293:431.
34. Hawkins JL, Gibbs CP, Orleans M, et al. Obstetric anesthesia work force survey, 1981 versus 1992. *Anesthesiology* 1997;87:135.
35. Melzack R. The myth of painless childbirth (The John J. Bonica Lecture). *Pain* 1984;19:321.
36. Hehre FW. Observations, philosophy and opinions on obstetric anesthesia coverage. In: Safer P, ed. *Clinical anesthesia: public health aspects of critical care medicine and anesthesiology.* Philadelphia: FA Davis, 1976:10.
37. Graham SG, Luxton MC. The requirement for intensive care support for the pregnant population. *Anaesthesia* 1989;44:581.
38. Mabie WC, Sibai BM. Treatment in an obstetric intensive care unit. *Am J Obstet Gynecol* 1990;162:1.
39. Palmer SK, Gibbs CP. Risk management in obstetric anesthesia. *Int Anesth Clin* 1989;27:188.
40. Umo-Etuk J, Lumley J, Holdcroft A. Critically ill parturient women and admission to intensive care: a 5-year review. *Int J Obstet Anesth* 1996; 5:79.
41. Shnider SM. Training in obstetric anesthesia in the United States. *Am J Obstet Gynecol* 1965;93:243.
42. Karp D, Craddick M. Obstetric anesthesia and lawsuits. In: Shnider SM, Levinson G, ed. *Obstetric anesthesia.* 2nd ed. Baltimore: Williams & Wilkins, 1987:334.
43. Gild WM. Informed consent: a review. *Anesth Analg* 1989;68:649.
44. Stenchever MA. Too much informed consent? [Editorial]. *Am J Obstet Gynecol* 1991;77:631.
45. Tiesberg EO, Porter ME, Brown GB. Making competition in health care work. *Harvard Bus Rev* 1994;July-August:131.
46. Hetherington SE. A controlled study of the effect of prepared childbirth classes on obstetric outcomes. *Birth* 1990;17:86.

Obstetric Anesthesia, second edition,
edited by Mark C. Norris.
Lippincott Williams & Wilkins, Philadelphia © 1999.

CHAPTER 41

Legal and Ethical Issues in Obstetric Anesthesia

L Michael Newman

LEGAL ISSUES

"Pain during childbirth leads to $2.4-million lawsuit" said an article about a suit brought by a woman against a hospital and three physicians (1). The patient alleged that she did not receive adequate analgesia for the birth of her twin boys. A seemingly unsupervised "resident in anesthesiology that had little experience" attempted to place an epidural shortly after the patient arrived at the hospital. The patient, whose husband is a physician, stated that she brought the suit so others would not have to suffer as she did. The patient maintained she was offered no other forms of analgesia such as nitrous oxide, a pudendal block, or intravenous medications, all of which she knows have been administered to other women in labor. This event took place in a tertiary care center in Canada, and the patient opined: "You can bet that this would not have happened in a private hospital in the U.S." Perhaps not, but let us examine the problem of medical negligence in the United States.

Scope of the Problem

Lawsuits alleging medical malpractice have increased steadily over the last decade in Cook County, Illinois (Fig. 1) (2,3). This situation is not unique to the midwestern United States, but is representative of trends throughout the country. Statistics from the National Practitioner Data Bank show an increase in both payments and number of suits filed between 1993 and 1994 (Table 1).

In Illinois, medical malpractice is an industry with a healthy 3.6% annual growth rate (Fig. 1). The rate of guilty verdicts has remained stable at around 33% (Table 2). A look at the award pattern shows an average yearly total of $34.4 million (actual dollars, not adjusted for inflation). Of the tort cases that settled for more than $1 million between 1 July 1995 and 30 June 1996, 34 (42%) of 81 were medical malpractice actions and about one third of these were related to birth injuries for failure to monitor labor or perform a cesarean section for fetal distress. In the calendar year 1995, the Cook County Jury Verdict Reporter listed seven cases categorized as birth injury to child (2). Of these seven, two were plaintiff verdicts (guilty), two settled, and the defendant prevailed in the remaining three. There were two cases of Erb's palsy, one of which resulted in a not guilty verdict, and the other was settled for $500,000. Because there is no information on how often any given outcome occurs (e.g., Erb's palsy), there is no way of knowing whether these data suggest that the tort system works or not (4).

There is no paucity of information about medical malpractice readily available to the public. The Internet has in excess of 750,000 listings under the term Medical Malpractice. Attorneys and instructions about whether you may have a suit are available. Consumer's Union, in a press release in 1994, claimed that the "Harvard Study" proves that doctors kill 80,000 patients a year. The Harvard Study refers to a collection of reports that present the results of an examination of a weighted sample of 31,429 of 2,671,863 case records from nonpsychiatric patients discharged from nonfederal acute care hospitals in New York (5–9). The details of this study are beyond the scope of this chapter, but we are saddled with its principal conclusions:

- Medical malpractice is frequent;
- A high nation-wide toll of avoidable medical injury can be inferred; and
- Relatively few of the injured patients actually sued, leading to the notion that there is too little negligence litigation.

Some of the many problems with the study are:

- The reviewers often disagreed as to whether an adverse event was negligence;
- The study pooled all adverse events (e.g., a fall in the corridor was lumped with a surgical error);

L M. Newman: Department of Anesthesiology, Rush–Presbyterian–St. Luke's Medical Center, Chicago, Illinois 60612.

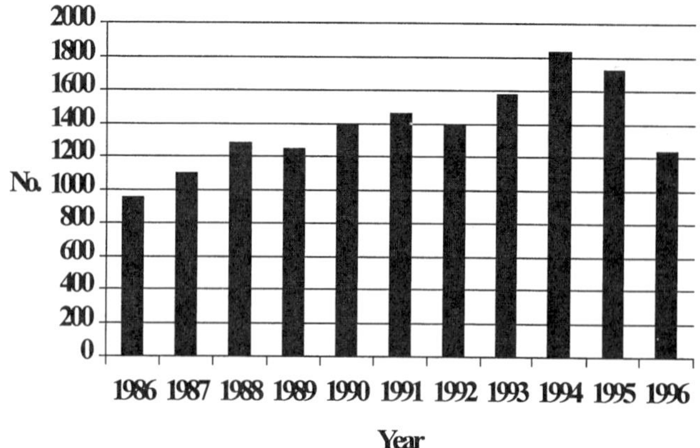

FIG. 1. The number of medical malpractice lawsuits from 1986 to 1996 in Cook County, Illinois.

- The majority of the events were minor or occurred within a short time of the death of a moribund patient; and
- The researchers did not find negligence in most cases in which actual claims were filed.

In summary:

> The study broadly defines negligent adverse events and then, premised on this inappropriate definition, concludes that too few lawsuits are filed. A physician need not even have been involved, let alone responsible. In fact, a separate team of Harvard reviewers was not even able to identify the same set of adverse outcomes, let alone medical negligence. It is troubling that such a study is so widely cited to prove that medical malpractice is common (10).

In 1996 Chadwick (11) published an update of the American Society of Anesthesiologists (ASA) Closed Claims Project analysis of obstetric anesthesia cases. Since 1985, the ASA has been investigating insurance company liability files that involve anesthesiologists. The files are no longer active (i.e., closed). The files are reviewed by practicing anesthesiologists and members of the ASA Closed Claims Committee and then entered into a database. By 1996, the cases included those closed before January 1995. They consisted of 3,533 obstetric and nonobstetric files from 35 companies. Some of the acknowledged limitations of the closed claims methods are:

TABLE 1. *Data from the 1994 report of the National Practitioner Data Bank*

	1993	1994
Number of claims	19,922	20,266
Total payments	$2,983,607,972	$3,257,213,944
Mean payment	$144,933[a]	$160,858[a]
Median payment		$60,000

[a]Statistically affected by the small number of large payments.
From ref. 4, with permission.

TABLE 2. *Number of guilty verdicts and awards for Cook County and the eight surrounding counties in Illinois for medical malpractice cases*

	Guilty verdicts	Not guilty verdicts	Guilty (%)	Awards
1988	31	70	30.7	$37,805,692
1989	48	96	33.3	$38,956,467
1990	65	93	41.1	$93,253,027
1991	78	121	39.2	$252,126,496
1992	32	78	29.1	$43,652,055
1993	42	78	35.0	$33,702,819
1994	48	97	34.1	$43,534,688
1995	40	82	32.8	$92,254,228
1970–1995	650	1,285	33.6	$859,831,613

- They provide no information about the incidence of claims filed;
- They provide no information about the incidence of adverse events;
- They include suits in which the adverse outcome or event was unrelated to anesthesia; and
- The interval from event to closing a claim may exceed 5 to 10 years. Thus closed-claims analysis provides little information about current anesthesia practice.

In spite of these limitations, closed claims data can help to address many questions:

- How do obstetric and nonobstetric claims compare?
- What injuries are more common in obstetric claims ?
- What leads to these injuries?
- Is there a relation between the anesthetic and the injury?
- Are more payments made in obstetric anesthesia claims than in nonobstetric claims? and
- Are the payments higher in obstetric anesthesia claims than in nonobstetric claims?

Of the 3,533 (12%) cases in the closed-claims study, 434 concerned obstetric anesthesia. Of these, 310 (72%) involved anesthesia for patients having a cesarean section, and 124 (28%) involved anesthesia for vaginal delivery (Table 3). Maternal mortality is 4 times greater in the patients receiving general anesthesia than in those who receive regional anesthesia ($p < 0.01$). Choice of anesthetic did not affect the incidence of suit for newborn brain damage or death (Table 4). Nerve damage, headache, back pain, and pain during anesthesia were principally associated with regional anesthesia (Tables 3 and 5). Headache accounted for 21% of claims involving regional anesthesia. Remarkably, headache was a claim in 2% of the cases done with general anesthesia. With the literature indicating that back pain is not causally related to regional anesthesia (12–15), we may see a decrease in the success of this type of claim in the future.

Closed-claim reviewers concluded that 46% of newborn brain-injury claims and 26% of newborn deaths were related to the anesthetic care. In contrast, 72% of the

TABLE 3. *The most common serious maternal injuries in the obstetric anesthesia file of the Closed Claims Project of the ASA*

	Obstetric files (n = 434)	Regional anesthesia (n = 290)	*p*	General anesthesia (n = 133)	Cesarean delivery (n= 310)	*p*	Vaginal delivery (n = 124)
Maternal Death	83 (19%)	31 (11%)	[a]	52 (39%)	71 (23%)	[a]	12 (10%)
Nerve Damage	43 (10%)	38 (13%)	[a]	5 (4%)	30 (10%)		13 (10%)
Maternal Brain Damage	32 (7%)	17 (6%)		14 (11%)	29 (9%)	[a]	3 (2%)
Aspiration Pneumonia	20 (5%)	2 (1%)	[a]	18 (14%)	16 (5%)		4 (3%)

Total n = 3,533.
[a]$p \leq 0.01$: Significance of differences between regional and general anesthesia and between cesarean and vaginal delivery.
From ref. 11, with permission.

injuries in both obstetric and nonobstetric cases were thought to be related to the anesthetic. Thus obstetric anesthesiologists are more likely to be named without cause in newborn injury claims than in other injuries. The payment rate for newborn brain damage (44%) and newborn death (41%) was lower than the obstetric (52%) and nonobstetric (59%) payment rates. Chadwick believes that this trend reflects recognition by the insurance and legal system of the lack of anesthetic involvement in newborn injury. Of the 36 cases of pain during regional anesthesia, 35 (97%) were during cesarean delivery. Thus pain during labor and vaginal delivery is rarely a source of liability risk in the United States.

Maternal claims contain a significantly greater proportion (47%) of relatively minor injuries (i.e., headache, back pain, emotional distress, and pain during anesthesia) than do nonobstetric claims (9%) (Table 6). The respiratory system was involved in 30% of the nonobstetric cases compared with 18% of the obstetric claims, but among the obstetric claims, respiratory events occurred in 6% of those involving regional anesthesia and in 47% of the claims involving general anesthesia. Difficult intubation (22%) and pulmonary aspiration (11%) were the main problems. Of the aspiration cases, three occurred during induction of anesthesia without cricoid pressure. An additional seven aspirations occurred during mask general anesthesia.

(I am reminded of a recent case in which a woman was to have a cesarean delivery, and the anesthesiologist induced general anesthesia without cricoid pressure. The patient vomited copious amounts of material and died within a day or two. In deposition, a nurse stated that Dr. X never used cricoid pressure during his rapid-sequence inductions for cesarean deliveries. This outcome was tragic enough; however, the husband was so distraught that he took his own life.)

Of the 38 claims for nerve injury, 21 (55%) of 38 were judged to be a consequence of the regional procedure (Table 7). Ischemic etiologies, such as epidural abscess, hypotension, or vascular insufficiency, are relatively uncommon. Obstetric cases accounted for 12% of the total claims for nerve injury and 14% of the total dollars expended (Table 8).

In addition to the dollars spent in legal and insurance fees, medical malpractice takes its toll on the physician being sued. St-Armand recounted his experience of a tragic case and needless trial (16). He reported a case of a young woman having an elective repeated cesarean delivery. He instituted an epidural block. Thirty minutes later, 10 minutes after skin incision, the patient experienced a massive amniotic fluid embolus. She was resuscitated and remained in a vegetative state. St-Armand recalled that for more than 4 years, he was the anesthetist that performed a "bad epidural." We cannot put a price on the cost to the individual who is being sued for something that is clearly not negligence, but we must weigh this against the cost to the patient who is seriously harmed by medical negligence. For every St-Armand, is there not a Dr. X?

In the field of obstetrics, concerns about medical malpractice have an additional cost (17). There is a positive association between malpractice claims and the rate of

TABLE 4. *The most common newborn injuries in the obstetric anesthesia file of the Closed Claims Project of the ASA*

	Obstetric files (n = 434)	Regional anesthesia (n = 290)	General anesthesia (n = 133)	Cesarean delivery (n = 310)	Vaginal delivery (n = 124)
Newborn brain damage	82 (19%)	51 (18%)	28 (21%)	52 (17%)	30 (24%)
Newborn death	27 (6%)	16 (6%)	8 (6%)	18 (6%)	9 (7%)

Total n = 3,533.
From ref. 11, with permission.

TABLE 5. *The most common less serious maternal injuries in the obstetric anesthesia file of the Closed Claims Project of the ASA*

	Obstetric files (n = 434)	Regional anesthesia (n = 290)	*p*	General anesthesia (n = 133)	Cesarean delivery (n = 310)	*p*	Vaginal delivery (n = 124)
Headache	64 (15%)	61 (21%)	a	2 (2%)	32 (10%)	a	32 (26%)
Nerve Damage	43 (10%)	38 (13%)	a	5 (4%)	30 (10%)		13 (10%)
Pain During Anesthesia	37 (9%)	36 (12%)	a	0 (0%)	35 (11%)	a	2 (2%)
Back Pain	36 (8%)	36 (12%)	a	0 (0%)	18 (6%)	b	18 (15%)
Emotional Distress	31 (7%)	23 (8%)		8 (6%)	23 (7%)		8 (6%)

Total n = 3,533.

[a]$p \leq 0.01$, [b]$p \leq 0.05$: Significance of differences between regional and general anesthesia and between cesarean and vaginal delivery.

From ref. 11, with permission.

TABLE 6. *Maternal injuries compared with similar injuries in the nonobstetric files*

	Maternal injury files (n = 356)		Nonobstetric files (n = 3,099)
Death	83 (12%)	a	1,111 (36%)
Nerve damage	43 (12%)	b	523 (17%)
Brain damage	32 (9%)	b	403 (13%)
Aspiration pneumonitis	20 (6%)	b	58 (2%)
Pain during anesthesia	37 (10%)	a	27 (1%)
Back pain	34 (10%)	a	27 (1%)
Emotional distress	31 (9%)	a	115 (4%)
Headache	64 (18%)	a	50 (2%)

[a]$p < 0.01$, [b]$p < 0.05$: Significance of the differences between obstetric and nonobstetric similar injuries.

From ref. 11, with permission.

TABLE 7. *Causes of regional block–related injuries*

Likely Cause	n (total = 21)
Needle or catheter trauma	11 (52%)
Neurotoxicity	4 (19%)
Ischemia	3 (14%)
Other identified causes	2 (10%)
Undetermined	1 (5%)

From ref. 11, with permission.

TABLE 8. *Payment data from the ASA closed claims study*

	Nonobstetric files (n = 3,099)	*p*	Obstetric files (n = 424)	Obstetric regional (n = 290)	*p*	Obstetric general (*n* = 133)
No payment	1,018 (33%)	a	171 (39%)	129 (44%)	b	37 (28%)
Payments made	1,814 (59%)	a	224 (52%)	130 (45%)	b	88 (66%)
Median payment	$100,000	b	$200,000	$77,500	b	345,426
Range	$15–$23.3 million		$675–$6.8 million	$675–$6.8 million		$750–$6 million

[a]$p \leq 0.05$, [b]$p \leq 0.01$: Statistical differences for the differences between obstetric and nonobstetric claims, as well as between obstetric regional and obstetric general anesthesia.

From ref, 11, with permission.

cesarean delivery. A physician with a higher malpractice insurance premium (New York City) is 3 times as likely to do a cesarean delivery as is a physician with a lower malpractice premium (Upstate New York). Accordingly, malpractice claims may increase the cost of medicine by their effect on cesarean delivery rate.

Chadwick (11) concluded that the large proportion of relatively minor injuries may be attributed to patient dissatisfaction. These patients felt ignored, mistreated, or assaulted. Medical malpractice suits are attributable to death in 18% of the cases, major injuries in 19% of the cases, and 63% are filed for minor and emotional injuries (18). Three of four medical malpractice claims arise from a communication breakdown. The anesthesiologist entering a room, obtaining a minimal history, doing a block, and disappearing is a setup for the estrangement necessary for a lawsuit. The more you interact with the patient and the family, the less likely you are to be sued. There is no better or more joyful place for this contact to occur than in labor and delivery. Remember, although optimal communication may prevent lawsuits stemming from dissatisfaction, it will do nothing for those generated by negligence or the lack of an expected "perfect outcome."

Anesthesia is the sixth leading cause of pregnancy-associated maternal mortality (19). Maternal death and neonatal brain damage are the most common injuries that lead to a malpractice claim (11). Hawkins et al. (20) examined anesthesia-related deaths during obstetric delivery in the United States between 1979 and 1990. With data from the Centers for Disease Control and Prevention, maternal death certificates were matched with live-birth or fetal-death certificates. Deaths due to anesthesia, cause of death, type of delivery, and type of anesthesia were analyzed. Anesthesia-related maternal mortality decreased from 4.3 per million in 1979 through 1981 to 1.7 per million in 1988 through 1990. The frequency of deaths due to general anesthesia remained stable, although deaths related to regional anesthesia decreased fourfold. Despite some limitations (23), we can learn much from these data. They strongly suggest that increased use of regional anesthesia for cesarean delivery should decrease maternal mortality.

At Rush–Presbyterian Medical Center, the use of general anesthesia for cesarean delivery decreased from 28% to 10% during the years from 1988 to 1994. During this time, the use of labor epidural analgesia increased from 38% to 80% (21,22).

The Legal System

The United States legal system is adversarial, not inquisitorial in nature. That is, the judge and jury do not investigate the merits of the claims but rather make their decision based on the facts and arguments of the legal representatives of the involved parties. In a jury trial, the jury makes a decision on the facts of the case, and the judge decides the legal principles and standards that apply. Our legal system is derived from the common law (or case law) system of eighteenth century England. In consequence, the law lies primarily, but not exclusively, in the opinions of judges. Statutory law, enacted by legislative bodies, places certain limits on the processes and the decisions by the judges. Regulations from agencies such as the Food and Drug Administration (FDA) are taken as "the law" by some medical caregivers. This thinking is erroneous; FDA approval is merely a labeling approval and not physician use approval (24).

A tort is damage or injury done willfully or negligently. Medical malpractice is an example of a tort. To triumph in a tort, the claimant must prove four points (Table 9).

Duty is what is owed the patient. Duty arises out of an explicit or implicit agreement to provide anesthesia care and is confirmed by the act of providing anesthesia. We may refuse to accept a patient in a nonemergency situation, but in that setting, it would be prudent to refer the patient to another available anesthesia provider.

Breach of duty is deviation from or noncompliance with the accepted standard of care. Accepted medical practice (or standard of care) means the care provided by a physician of recognized knowledge, skill, and judgment in the same community at time the professional services were rendered (26). The "community," particularly for a specialist, is no longer a geographic region but is rather the practice of a reasonable specialist in the same field regardless of locality in the United States. Failure to meet the standard of care will lead to liability.

By using the ASA's Closed Claims Study data, Cheney et al. (27) attempted to examine the impact of the standard of care on payment. Practicing anesthesiologist reviewers judged the appropriateness of care. Payments were made in 80% of cases in which the care administered was considered substandard. Payment also was made in 40% of the cases in which the care was deemed suitable. Like juries, these physician reviewers were influenced by the severity of the injury. The reviewers judged care to be substandard in 8% of cases without injury, 23% for minor injuries, 51% for disabling injuries, and 70% if death occurred. When reviewers were presented with identical cases with only the outcomes changed, they were more likely to judge the care substandard in cases of permanent

TABLE 9. *The four elements a plaintiff must prove to prevail in a tort action*

Duty	The standard of care owed the patient by the physician
Breach of duty	Violation of the standard of care
Causation	The physician's acts caused the injury
Damages	Physical or emotional injuries or both

From ref. 25, with permission.

injury. Thus "standard of care" is not easily identified and is subject to multiple influences.

Levinson (28) delineated some of the factors that are involved in determining the appropriate standard of care. He listed credibility of expert witnesses, learned articles in books and journals, recommendations of government agencies, and standards and guidelines published by medical societies. Standards are rigid rules that are intended to be adhered to at all times. Guidelines are less rigid and need not always be followed. However, if we deviate from a guideline, it is probably prudent to note it and write a short explanation explaining the reason for the deviation.

One area in obstetric anesthesia in which issues of duty and breach of duty are common is neonatal resuscitation. Of 69 obstetric anesthesia lawsuits filed between 1985 and 1993, 12 (17.4%) involved neonatal-resuscitation claims against anesthesia personnel (29). The issues mentioned were delayed intubation, improper intubation, and failure to initiate neonatal advanced life support. There was a payment to the plaintiff in 10 (85%) of 12 of the cases.

The resuscitation of a neonate may be a Good Samaritan act or a duty. Good Samaritan law provides immunity for voluntarily providing emergency care. No immunity exists for an anesthesiologist who has an employment duty to the neonate or a preexisting doctor–patient relationship with the neonate. Caring for the mother does not automatically create a doctor–patient relationship with the neonate, and no duty is created just because a baby is born requiring resuscitation. If, however, such assistance is provided because the anesthesiologist is expressly or customarily required to do so, then a duty and hence liability exist. In the case of neonatal resuscitation, either be clearly designated as not responsible by the hospital's rules and regulations or maintain skill in that area, including certification in neonatal advanced life support.

Causation or proximate cause is the link between the breach of duty and the injury to the patient. Accordingly, it is the physician's acts or omissions that caused the patient's damage. Some examples of acts considered causal are the administration of the wrong drug or the initiation of a regional or general anesthetic. Examples of acts of omission are things such as not using cricoid pressure during a rapid-sequence induction of anesthesia, not responding to hypotension after a regional anesthetic in a timely and suitable manner, or not using uterine displacement in a parturient.

Injury is the last of the four points a claimant must prove for a successful suit. The injury may be either physical or mental. The injury may be minor, such as a headache or back pain, or as catastrophic as maternal death or neonatal brain damage.

Although the plaintiff has the burden of proving all of these for a victorious medical malpractice outcome, there is an exception: the doctrine of *res ipsa loquitur* or "the thing speaks for itself." The essence of this doctrine is that the fact the injury occurred is itself sufficient evidence that the medical practitioner was negligent and caused the injury. Thus if someone is completely normal before delivery, and after a regional anesthetic, she develops cauda equina syndrome, she may invoke the doctrine of *res ipsa loquitur.* This puts the burden of proof on the practitioner to demonstrate the absence of negligence. This doctrine is not accepted in all states and is not uniformly implemented.

Expert Witnesses

To clarify issues involving standards of care and causation, both plaintiffs and defendants employ expert witnesses (24,30,31). There are many influences on expert witnesses. Economics may play a role, because this can be a lucrative avocation, with some charging as much as $500/hour. Expert witnesses may be obtained from a broker who has a stable of experts willing to testify. Indeed, the expert testifying against you may not be an anesthesiologist. Other sources of bias may develop, such as an affinity for the plaintiff or defendant or an antipathy for one of the attorneys. These issues can and do reduce impartiality and introduce advocacy into the expert's testimony. Experts use their own, often unstated, criteria as the basis for their standard-of-care and causation decisions. Posner et al. (30) had pairs of anesthesiologists assess the appropriateness of the care in 103 closed anesthesia-malpractice claims. The reviewers classified the care as appropriate, less than appropriate, and impossible to judge. The raters agreed on the appropriateness of care in 62% of the cases. Whereas the agreement was better than chance, the statistical assessment of this level of agreement was in the poor-to-good range. Thus divergence of opinion is inherent in the system, not necessarily a reflection of bias on the part of the experts. The severity of injury can influence reviewers' assessment of the appropriateness of anesthesia care (32). Anesthesiologist reviewers are more likely to judge care as appropriate if the injury was temporary. Permanent injury more often led the reviewers to conclude that care was inappropriate or impossible to judge. Thus the variability inherent in the judgment process may, in part, explain some discordant expert opinions.

The ASA has published guidelines for expert witness qualifications and testimony. In brief, the expert witness should:

- Have a current, valid, and unrestricted license to practice medicine;
- Be board certified by the ABA or the equivalent; and
- Be familiar with the practice and be in clinical practice at the time of the event.

The guidelines for expert testimony are:

- Be accurate and impartial (i.e., the unchanged testimony could be used by the attorney for either the plaintiff or defendant),
- Evaluate the performance in light of generally accepted standards;
- Clearly distinguish between medical malpractice and adverse outcomes not related to negligence;
- Assess the relation of the alleged deviation from the standard to the patient's outcome;
- Charge fees on a time basis and never contingent on the outcome; and
- Be willing to submit the testimony for peer review.

Even with adherence to these guidelines, genuine disagreements between expert witnesses are expected.

Discovery, Deposition, and Trial

Discovery is the formal pretrial process by which each side attempts to find (discover) salient facts about the event. Discovery devices include depositions, interrogatories, requests for admissions, document production, and requests for inspection. The latitude of discovery is quite broad. Information reasonably calculated to lead to the discovery of admissible evidence is included.

- Interrogatories: written questions sent by one party to be answered by the other party, in writing, under oath;
- Deposition: witnesses, parties to the suit, or experts are asked to answer questions orally under oath before a court reporter. Attorneys for the plaintiff as well as those representing the defendant(s) are present;
- Request for admission: request that a party admit to certain facts. This covers basic issues that both parties agree on and thus do not have to be proven at trial. For example, both parties would agree that Ms. X was 39 weeks pregnant on a certain date, that she was admitted to hospital Y in labor, and so forth;
- Request for production of documents: office records, papers an expert may have written, curriculum vitae; and
- Requests for a physical examination: to determine the extent of the injury or state of health.

A subpoena is an order instructing a witness to appear at a deposition or in court. Failure to comply can lead to the party being held in contempt of court. Contempt of court is punishable by a fine or imprisonment or both. A subpoena is not an invitation that can be declined.

In the United States, about 90% of malpractice claims are resolved without a decision on the merits of the claim by a judge or jury. About one half of these are settled by a payment to the claimant (34). Failing a settlement, the case goes to trial. In the United States, neither trial-by-combat nor ordeal is used, but rather, the alternative of a jury trial is used to settle a claim. In a trial, the evidence is presented by both sides to a jury, whose selection is governed by the applicable local rules. After both parties present evidence, witnesses, and experts, the judge sums up the evidence and explains to the jury the law applicable in this case. The jury then retires and deliberates. They render a verdict and, if they find for the plaintiff, they can assess damages.

Damages are the financial compensation awarded to someone who suffered an injury or was harmed by negligence. Damages for medical malpractice are compensatory in nature. Compensatory damages are given to compensate the plaintiff for the loss due to the negligent acts of the defendant(s). Actual damages are those damages that are awarded to compensate for the loss or injuries that have actually occurred. Examples of such damages are loss of past and future income because of the injury and past and future medical expenses due to the injury. There are also noneconomic damages that can be awarded. These consist of damages for pain, suffering, loss of companionship, and loss of consortium. In some states, laws limit the amount of noneconomic damages.

Avoiding and Defending a Malpractice Suit (24,35,36)

Documentation and Record Keeping

Documentation must be accurate and complete. Avoid these common errors: subjective remarks, inconsistencies between other care providers (i.e., all times recorded should agree), pointing fingers, airing differences of opinion, not noting abnormal test results, improperly documenting late entries, and altering medical records. Late entries, made on a chart days to a week after the event and not recorded as such but made to appear as though entered on the day of the event, are surprisingly common. A copy of the original record may have been made by this time, and you will have very large problem trying to explain why a copy of the chart made on June 4 does not show an entry dated June 2. There is nothing wrong with a later addendum as long as you indicate the current date and time and then note what you remembered or forgot to include.

Make sure the chart or anesthesia record is accurate and complete. In the normotensive parturient, it is easier to defend a transient decrease of the blood pressure to 40 mm Hg systolic than it is to defend the use of ephedrine to treat a recorded blood pressure of 98 mm Hg. Be honest in your recording. One case of neonatal brain damage hinged on whether or not the anesthesia personnel used uterine displacement. The anesthesiologist stated they always used uterine displacement but did not record it. Remember: if it is not recorded, it was not done. Record informed consent for anesthesia, either on a specific form or elsewhere in the chart. Indicate that side effects and possible complications as well as other anesthetic approaches were discussed. A checked box for individual items will suffice; a sentence that says, "informed consent obtained" will not.

Reacting to an Adverse Event

Make sure that the documentation is complete and accurate. Often, writing a narrative in the body of the chart or as an addendum to the anesthetic record is the best approach. It is impossible to record everything on the anesthetic record during a critical event. Ranges of vital signs rather than specific recorded values every 5 minutes are more believable. As soon as you are able, contact your hospital's risk-management group or legal department and your malpractice insurer. Have frequent honest discussions with the patient and family members. Be open and frank and at the same time neither accept nor assign blame for the event. Obtain consultation from other physicians to aid you in the diagnosis and treatment of a complication. A note from a neurologist indicating that the loss of sensation in the postpartum patient's leg is an obstetric nerve palsy and not a result of the regional anesthetic used can save everyone a lot of time, money, and anguish. Remain calm, and remember that only one of 20 or fewer malpractice claims ever goes to trial.

Preparation of Your Defense

Once a claim is filed, notify your insurance carrier as well as the hospital legal group. Do NOT alter the patient's chart. Have no further contact or discussions with the patient or the family of the patient. Do not discuss the case with friends and colleagues. Do not suggest your friends or those who owe you favors as an expert witness. An academic anesthesiologist will often be the best person for you. All cases go through five phases:

- Answering the complaint: a statement by your attorney replying to the allegations in the complaint;
- Discovery: the gathering of evidence by both sides;
- Interrogatory: a list of questions that ought to be answered in consultation with your legal counsel. Never reply directly to the plaintiff's counsel without having consulted your legal representative;
- Deposition: a sworn statement given by the defendant(s) and witness(s) (there are no surprises in court *a la* Perry Mason); only information contained in the deposition may be introduced as evidence in court; and
- Negotiations and settlements.

Settlement is a very difficult area. A settlement is often financially and emotionally cheaper than a protracted lawsuit. If negligence is involved, it is often better and cheaper to settle rather than to rely on a jury. Remember, with the advent of the National Practitioner Data Bank in 1990, all malpractice awards paid (negotiated or tried) must be reported within 30 days. It should be noted that claims are not reported to the Data Bank, but only awards. The impact of this rule has yet to be assessed.

If you are deposed, keep the following in mind. Know the records and medical information. Listen to the questions carefully, and respond directly and to the point. Keep your answers short, and do not try to impress the attorney with your wit or wisdom. Disregard the theatrics, bluster, or body language, including facial expressions of the attorneys; remember that this is a scripted play that repeats over and over with only the name(s) changing. A lawsuit is not about you in the personal sense but about being right and triumphing. Be consistent, regardless of how many times and ways the same question is asked. Watch out for questions that start, "Is this a fair statement," or "Let me summarize your testimony as follows"; often the attorney is trying to make you agree with some slightly different interpretation of what you have already stated. Listen carefully and agree or disagree; often it is best to restate what you already said in response to the original question. Be careful of what you say and to whom during breaks. Solitude and silence are often the safest course.

Some tips for testifying at a trial. Speak to the jury; your answers are for them not the counsel asking the questions. Make your answers complete. Unlike in a deposition, you should take any and every opportunity to state your position and establish your expertise. If the counsel cuts you off during an answer, so be it: do not become flustered or upset. The attorney is working on his case, not yours. Be alert so the plaintiff's counsel does not twist your words and to make you agree with a statement that you never would have made. Take your time in answering the questions, and be sure you are clear. Do not contradict what you said in your deposition; your credibility is at stake. If you always tell the truth, there is no problem here or at deposition. Do not lose control of your emotions; remember this is not a personal attack. It may look and sound as if it is, but a well-crafted script is being enacted, and it would not matter one iota who was sitting there. Finally, if your attorney makes an objection, stop talking and listen carefully. Do not resume speaking until the judge has ruled on the objection.

Malpractice lawsuits are not unique to physicians. It seems that bringing a claim is the American way of life. From 1970 through 1995, in Cook County, Illinois, in addition to the 1,935 malpractice suits against physicians, there were 106 lawsuits against attorneys, 18 against accountants, 86 against bankers, 107 against insurance companies, 38 against real estate brokers, and 38 against architects/ engineers (2). Whereas physicians were found not guilty approximately two thirds of the time, other professional groups did not fare so well. Here, not guilty verdicts ranged from 20.9% to 50%. Attorneys were found guilty 57% of the time. So, short of changing our culture, we need to change our habits. "Increasingly, any complication which a patient relates to the period of anaesthesia is regarded as unacceptable, and may lead to allegations of negligence" (51).

Summary

We may be sued for real or imagined injury to a parturient, and it is imperative that we communicate, document, be clear, be honest, and be informative with our patients and their families. Enrolling the parturient and her family in the decision process and having them be responsible for their care may be helpful. These suggestions will not prevent all malpractice litigation, but they may reduce the incidence. Finally, as we have heard over and over in obstetric anesthesia meetings, regional, regional, and regional. If you must embark on a general anesthetic, have all in readiness for an airway problem. This is not the time to charge ahead, but rather is cause for a well-planned, careful, general anesthetic.

ETHICAL ISSUES

The American Heritage Dictionary of the English Language defines ethic(s) as:

- a. A set of principles of right conduct. b. A theory or a system of moral values;
- Ethics (used with a sing. verb). The study of the general nature of morals and of the specific moral choices to be made by a person; moral philosophy; and
- Ethics (used with a sing. or pl. verb). The rules or standards governing the conduct of a person or the members of a profession: medical ethics.

A discussion of ethics and ethical behavior is not intended to teach or inspire people to be moral beings. In fact, a significant degree of moral goodness is expected of physicians, and if not present, it will not be created by education (37). The purpose of this discussion is to bring into awareness the ethical issues we face and to reinforce the practice of our inherent moral goodness. Some potential examples of current anesthesia-related ethical issues are:

- The avoidance of regional anesthesia in an effort to save time, regardless of the benefit to the patient;
- The encouragement of the use of less-expensive and less-effective drugs; and
- Not accurately charting a hypotensive episode during an anesthetic.

Because ethics seeks to tie a "system of moral values" to the "principles of right conduct" (i.e., laws), we might expect our legal system, considered by some to embody the morals and ethics of the American people, to promote ethical behavior and to prohibit unethical behavior. Unfortunately, few issues are that simple. Both ethics and the law contain few absolute principles or rules. For example, our society deems killing both ethically and legally wrong. Yet wars are legal and often considered ethically correct, as they are waged to produce some greater good or to right some greater wrong. In some states, the penalty for first degree murder is execution: killing on the one hand, ethically and legally wrong, and on the other hand, a just and right punishment. Both ethical and legal principles also change with time. The paternalism of the nineteenth century gave way to the principles of equal rights and self determination in the twentieth century. We can only speculate about the guiding principles of the twenty-first century.

The four equally essential principles of bioethics are (Table 10):

- Respect for autonomy,
- Beneficence,
- Nonmaleficence, and
- Justice.

"An ethical dilemma occurs when any action taken will violate at least one of these principles" (38).

Autonomy is defined as the quality or condition of being self-governing or the right of self-government. Respect for autonomy mandates that an individual's freedom and sovereignty be preserved and, if lost, regained where possible. Indeed, Jackson et al. (38) suggested that it is a physician's foremost duty to respect patients and to help them retain or recover their autonomy. It is easy to see how a conflict can occur between the autonomy of a physician and the autonomy of a patient. Based on their ethical rights of autonomy, a competent adult may refuse any treatment for any reason.

We need to examine our own ethical values to help us in situations in which they may conflict with a patient's autonomy. Are we willing to participate in abortions? First trimester? Second trimester? If not, are there circumstances that would modify this view? Jeopardy to the mother's life? Are we willing to follow do-not-resuscitate (DNR) orders? Are we willing to administer anesthesia for procedures such as gastric tubes and central lines in patients with terminal diseases? The answers to these questions are up to the individual, but they must be formulated in advance. A final question is, Under what circumstances do a patient's desires take precedence over our moral objections? Can we withhold medical assistance because we are morally opposed to the procedure or circumstances? We can easily do so when someone else can do the procedure, but what if we are the only

TABLE 10. *The four essential principles of bioethics*

Autonomy	The right of self-choice of the patient
Beneficence	Physician's duty to work for the good of the patient
Nonmaleficence	Physician's duty to avoid doing harm
Justice	Giving people what they deserve (i.e., fairness)

available anesthesiologist? If we are morally opposed to doing a legally sanctioned procedure (i.e., a gastric feeding tube in a terminal patient), can we refuse? Easy and simple answers are not readily available for these difficult questions.

An issue related to autonomy is paternalism. Physicians have traditionally practiced from the position of knowing what is best for the patient and acting as a parent in making decisions for the patient. Often patients want us to be paternalistic and tell us, "You do what you think is best, Doctor." However, we must strive to keep our paternalism from interfering with a patient's autonomy. Properly informed patients can and should participate fully in the medical decision-making process. This counseling calls on us to identify our own biases and label them as such. Then we must respect and honor the autonomy of the patient.

Beneficence is the physician's duty to work for the benefit of the patient. *Nonmaleficence* means that the physician should do nothing intentionally or allow something hurtful or damaging to happen to the patient. The final canon is *justice.* This term is used to connote some kind of "fairness." There are myriad writings on the subjects of justice and fairness, but perhaps the best definition of these terms is the simple dictum, "Do unto others as you would have them do unto you."

The remainder of this chapter considers some specific issues that may pose ethical dilemmas for the obstetric anesthesiologist. Specifically, we examine informed consent, forced cesarean delivery, blood transfusion and the Jehovah's Witnesses, and considerations of human embryo donation. We use the principles of autonomy, beneficence, nonmaleficence, and justice to create a framework for approaching these potentially divisive issues.

Informed Consent

For a parturient to make an informed choice, she must satisfactorily complete the phases of disclosure, comprehension, and voluntary choice (39). Disclosure is the presentation of the information that a reasonable person would require to understand the problem. Comprehension is the process of weighing the various aspects, risks, and outcomes as elucidated by the caregivers. Finally, the patient needs to evidence a voluntary choice that is free of coercion and is not made with a diminished capacity (i.e., psychosis). The evidence of this decision is either a signed consent form or the documentation of the discussion by the appropriate caregiver.

Except in the case of an emergency, a physician must obtain a patient's agreement before any course of action. A physician must inform the patient of the nature and purpose of the treatment or procedure, its risks, its consequences, and alternative courses of treatment or alternative procedures (Table 11). Consent issues can be divided into those concerning a medical (anesthetic) procedure and those involving clinical research. The issue of informed consent has both legal and ethical implications.

TABLE 11. *Necessary elements of informed consent*

Diagnosis: Usually done by another member of the health care team (i.e., OB)
Nature and purpose of proposed anesthetic
Risks, complications, and consequences of proposed anesthetic
Alternatives: Other anesthetic courses (i.e., regional versus general)
Consequences if proposed anesthetic is refused
Benefits if proposed anesthetic is used
Conflicts of interest
Who will be providing the anesthetic

The legal issues surrounding informed consent in obstetric anesthesia are more imaginary than real. Fewer than 1% of cases in the closed-claims study indicated that informed consent was a crucial issue (40). Courts have held that the stress of labor does not prevent a parturient from giving informed consent for an anesthetic (41). Historically, courts have concluded that patient cooperation and a recorded note of a discussion about consent, including benefits and risks, implies consent. If a patient shows up at a hospital with a packed bag and says she is there to have a certain procedure, there is implicit consent. The only issue is how informed was the consent. Informed consent, *per se*, did not seem to be an issue in and of itself in the closed-claims study. The related but separate issues of honoring specific requests, discussing possible alternatives, and explicitly delineating risks that are relatively common or especially serious were the problem areas (40).

All informed consents should contain a discussion of the nature of the proposed anesthetic, pertinent complications, alternatives to the proposed anesthetic, and complications of the alternative anesthetic (42). What complications should be discussed? Certainly those that are more likely to occur, such as postdural puncture headache, pruritus with neuraxial opiates, and the transient harmless fetal bradycardia observed after initiation of labor analgesia in 2% to 6% of parturients. Should we discuss the extremely remote possibility of paralysis or death with obstetric regional anesthesia? I think not, other than to reassure our patients about the rarity of these events.

The primary ethical issue involved in informed consent is respect for autonomy. In the process of informed consent, the patient should become a participant in and responsible for the decisions regarding her medical care. Informed consent has two basic elements: information and consent. Present the information clearly and honestly. Recognize your biases, and acknowledge them. Present the complications in such a way as to inform but not to frighten the patient.

There is a subtle and difficult distinction between unacceptable coercion and ethically acceptable persuasion. Is it ethical to use a persuasive and rational argument to convince a patient that a particular anesthetic technique is in her best interest? Is it coercion to cite the increased morbidity and mortality associated with general anesthesia in an attempt to have the parturient consent to regional anesthesia? Does this approach fly in the face of the principle of autonomy? What if you then cannot do regional anesthetic or it fails? Now you face inducing general anesthesia in a patient who as just been told that it is a bad choice, which may disable or kill her. Coercion for our own purposes, aside from being dishonest, smacks of paternalism and violates the patient's autonomy. Learn to calm irrational fears (i.e., paralysis during regional anesthesia) while respecting a patient's preference for an alternate anesthetic plan (i.e., general anesthesia for elective cesarean section). Reassure the patient that, regardless of her choice, you will do your best to care for her. Do not question the capacity of a patient just because she disagrees with your treatment plan.

Another issue is that of obtaining consent for clinical studies. It is clearly unethical to assign patients to receive placebo versus active drug without their consent. However, keeping track of outcomes from different commonly used and accepted procedures does not present an ethical dilemma or a need for a special consent. There are five categories of consent: voluntary, involuntary, coerced, enforced, and partially voluntary (42). In clinical research, consent lies within the context of illness (or pain in the case of a laboring patient) or the doctor–patient relationship, and as such, it is substantially influenced and thus only partially voluntary. The researcher's duty is to ensure that this partially voluntary consent is adequately voluntary. In this situation, obtaining informed consent requires spending considerable time with the patient. Consent for labor-analgesia studies that include a placebo group may best be obtained before the patient experiences significant labor pain. Patients in pain may feel coerced into a study because they view participation as a prerequisite for obtaining analgesia. Obtaining consent earlier removes pain as a factor and helps ensure that a patient's participation is truly voluntary.

> Let us remember that a slower progress in the conquest of diseases would not threaten society, but that society would indeed be threatened by the erosion of those moral values whose loss, possibly caused by too ruthless a pursuit of scientific progress, would make its most dazzling triumphs not worth having (43).

Thus we must ethically conduct our investigations while informing our patients of their options.

Compelled Cesarean Delivery

Compelling or coercing a woman to have a cesarean delivery is an ethical and legal quagmire. The pregnant woman has autonomy-based rights to choose her own medical treatment, including when and if she desires surgical intervention. Until the point of fetal viability, and even perhaps thereafter, the mother has the right to decide about options of fetal testing and intervention. In short, the fetus is not autonomous and has no moral claims (39). Compelled cesarean delivery is most likely justified for fetal benefit after consideration of these circumstances:

- A high likelihood of serious consequences for the mother and fetus without treatment;
- A high level of diagnostic and prognostic accuracy;
- A high likelihood of treatment efficacy of the cesarean delivery;
- Low maternal risk;
- Attempts of disclosure and informed consent have been exhausted or the parental capacity is questioned; and
- Malevolent intent by the mother (least likely to emerge in this constellation of conditions).

Such compelled care must be of high benefit, low risk, and not experimental (39). Even within these circumstances, compelled cesarean section is problematic. Court-ordered cesarean deliveries have been sought but not performed, and the predicted dire consequences have not come to pass. Remember that a court-ordered cesarean delivery invades a woman's privacy, limits her autonomy, and takes away her right to informed consent (44). Fortunately this ethical problem does not occur often. Further, if the parents are in agreement, the courts will not step in, and there is no legal issue.

Jehovah's Witnesses and Blood Transfusions

Based on a literal interpretation of certain biblical passages, Jehovah's Witnesses refuse transfusion of blood and blood products. If they transgress the proscriptions of the Bible, they will not be granted eternal salvation on Judgment Day. In other words, if they take or are given blood or blood products, their life is worthless. As with many religious beliefs, there are varying degrees of interpretation of the prohibition of blood products. Thus this situation usually mandates a careful discussion with the patient and sometimes with her minister. Some will allow a retransfusion of scavenged blood, and some, the use of erythropoietin (which contains albumin) and blood patches (45,46). Rothenberg (38) listed therapies, such as crystalloid, synthetic colloid solutions, aprotinin, desmopressin, iron, and aminocaproic acid, that are acceptable to Jehovah's Witnesses. A frank, open discussion of the patient's requests and an examination of your feelings about this issue are necessary. Could you allow a competent adult, with no dependents, to die when you knew that the administration of blood would save the patient?

As previously stated, a competent adult may refuse any treatment for any reason. Certainly the refusal of blood products by Jehovah's Witnesses falls under this precept. Problems occur with the existence of minor dependents or a fetus, or when an emergency precludes a thorough advance discussion. These cases present both ethical and legal quandaries. In the case of a woman with children who refuses transfusion or a minor whose parents refuse transfusion, the law has held that the interest of the State supersedes the beliefs of the individual. In essence the courts have held that "parents may be free to become martyrs themselves, but it does not follow that they are free, in identical circumstances, to make martyrs of their children before they have reached the age of full and legal discretion when they can make that choice for themselves" (38).

This principle is applied to the children of Jehovah's Witnesses who need blood, a parent with dependent children, and the unborn fetus late in pregnancy. Thus from a legal point of view, the Jehovah's Witness who has severe intra- and postpartum bleeding can and "should" be given a transfusion. From the ethical point of view, we have a dilemma because we are clearly violating the principles of maternal autonomy and nonmaleficence while staunchly upholding the principle of beneficence. In these cases, seek guidance from your hospital's legal representatives, its ethics committee, and your conscience. In an emergency, in which the time and situation prevent discussions with the patient and family, most physicians will initiate transfusions. This choice is both ethically correct and legally sanctioned.

In obstetrics, we are rarely faced with a competent adult without minor dependents (including intrauterine) making decisions only for herself. Suppose a young, single woman with no minor dependents had an intrauterine fetal death. She clearly stated that she is a Jehovah's Witness and refused all blood products, even to save her own life. According to Rothenberg, you would be practicing the principle of beneficence by respecting the patient's autonomy, even if she dies due to lack of blood and blood products transfusions. I concur, and if we practice the principle of "first do no harm," in this setting, we may do great harm by denying this patient salvation.

Human Embryo Donation

As science breeches new frontiers, it poses more ethical problems than it solves. Such is the case with embryo donation. The need for donation arises when neither partner can produce healthy, viable gametes, and the woman has adequate uterine capacity to carry and deliver a baby. There are two ways to treat this circumstance: (a) obtain donor sperm and donor eggs and place the resulting embryos in the recipient's uterus; and (b) use embryos that a donor couple neither need nor want. Once a couple meets their reproductive goals, any remaining embryos can be destroyed, used for research, or donated.

Controversy surrounds the issue of using human embryos for research purposes. In 1994, a National Institutes of Health panel on embryo research attempted to address this issue. Arguments in support of human embryo research included:

- Significant promise of human benefit,
- Embryos do not have the same moral status as infants or children, and
- Funding (and the funding agency) would provide consistent ethical and scientific review of embryo research (47).

Arguments against human embryo research included:

- The potential adverse consequences of such research to liveborn children, women, and men;
- The respect due the preimplantation embryo;
- Concern for public sensitivities on highly controversial research; and
- Concern for the meaning of humanness, parenthood, and the succession of generations.

If the fetus is not autonomous and has no moral claims, what then is the status of a preimplanted embryo? The most widely held opinion is that the embryo is too rudimentary to have interests or rights and thus cannot be harmed or wronged when used in research (48). Does this position negate the embryo-research panel's guidelines? Whereas some advocate the use of left-over embryos, they disapprove of creating and discarding embryos solely for research purposes. These unresolved questions are currently being debated. While not advocating for or against embryo research, I am left with the feeling that the current guidelines are based on a shifting loose substrate.

Donor couples may view each embryo as a "new human life" and prefer that it be given a chance to live (49). Embryo donation is often referred to as embryo adoption, and although it raises the same kinds of issues that complicate postnatal adoption, the two are not equivalent. Embryo donation does not involve the rigorous social screening that accompanies postnatal adoption.

Two unique ethical issues accompany human embryo donation: the child born to a genetically unrelated couple and the question of payment. We assume that genetic parents have a moral and legal commitment to the well-being of their children. Whereas donated embryos are born to genetically unrelated individuals, the prenatal commitment of the parents is obvious and should overcome all the real and postulated postnatal problems.

> Embryo donation is ethically acceptable because it helps infertile couples and does not harm offspring. It enables a child who would not otherwise exist to be born in a situation in which the benefits of existence are likely to far outweigh the psychological and social uncertainties of being raised by gestation but nongenetic parents (49).

Disclosure to the child is a matter left to the discretion of the parents. However, the donor couple should decide whether they would permit later contact with the child, should that become an option.

A related issue involves mixing left-over embryos before implantation. It is not known whether this is done, but conceivably it could be used to increase the chances for pregnancy in a single cycle when only one or two embryos are available from a single source. This approach renders the genetic origin of the child uncertain, which could have implications for the child's future medical treatment.

The issue of monetary compensation of the donor couple raises another ethical issue. In the United States, sperm and egg donors are usually paid. However, the situation radically changes when we discuss embryos. If the infertile couple pays for the embryo, human life becomes a commodity to be bought and sold. If this payment reduced the cost to the donor couple, it could act as an inducement for donation. Both of these situations are ethically questionable. Some suggest that these ethical issues could be resolved by paying into a fund to subsidize in vitro fertilization for couples that cannot afford it (49).

Embryo donation also creates legal issues. Should this event be treated as a gamete donation or the adoption of a child? Few laws specifically address the issue of embryo donation. In Texas and Florida, the recipient and her spouse, not the donating couple, are the legal parents of the resulting child. This legal parental assignment is predicated on the recipients' written consent to the donation. Both donors and recipients may proceed with a reasonable, but not 100%, certainty that the donor's intentions to relinquish all rearing rights and duties and the recipients intentions to take on all rearing rights and duties will be honored and upheld. These intention-based rights are strongest for a married couple but also exist in the circumstances when the donation is to a single woman, an unmarried couple, or a same-sex couple.

Analgesia for Labor

Before briefly discussing the ethics involved in providing labor analgesia, I should make my bias clear. I believe that every woman has a right to as painless a childbirth as she desires. Epidural analgesia can safely and effectively relieve the pain of labor. Unfortunately, issues of time and money prevent some of our colleagues from providing this form of analgesia to the suffering parturient. No doubt it is difficult, when practicing in a small hospital, to provide both labor analgesia in the middle of the night and surgical anesthesia during the day. Still, as physicians, we have an obligation to relieve pain and suffering when we can. That said, it also is important to note that patients and insurers have an obligation to pay for this service.

Perhaps we need to embrace more current techniques and reexamine our criteria for the monitoring of analgesia to deliver this type of pain relief to all women. Maybe the anesthesiologist does not need to be present all night. Conceivably the registered nurse can deliver carefully designated boluses for pain. Someone other than an anesthesiologist can deliver neuraxial analgesia (i.e., an obstetrician or a family practice physician). Possibly the administration of an analgesic during the night could delay the start of the elective schedule. I do not have the answers to this question, but if we accept the proposition that effective analgesia is a woman's right, we may derive novel, appropriate, and workable solutions.

As far as issues of nonreimbursement go, no one other than the woman in labor has the right to make a decision about her need for analgesia. I would urge that lawsuits, similar to the one launched in Canada (1) against third-party carriers and managed health care organizations, be instituted by patients denied "epidural" analgesia. This denial of care is a form of rationing that is totally unacceptable. The issue of rationing needs to be explored and decided on by patients, health care professionals, and the financers of health care. Rationing may be necessary, but to deny a segment of the population pain relief is unconscionable. The argument that childbirth was always a natural and painful process is ridiculous. I have not yet heard of a third-party payer not reimbursing the anesthesiologist (i.e., effectively denying anesthesia to the patient) for a below-the-knee amputation because it used to be done with restraints and a fast surgeon. Under the principle of autonomy, a woman may opt for a "natural" (i.e., drugless childbirth), but to deny her this option is, in my opinion, unethical and cruel. To quote the ASA and the American College of Obstetricians and Gynecologists: "There is no other circumstance where it is considered acceptable for a person to experience severe pain, amenable to safe intervention, while under a physician's care" (50).

Summary

Except for court-ordered operative interventions, the ethical issues in obstetrics rarely involve anesthesiologists directly. There are no right or wrong answers to the dilemmas these issues pose. Finding the balance between personal beliefs and individual rights is often a difficult process requiring input from the legal system, medical ethics boards, and the individuals involved. It also is a dynamic process, in need of constant reassessment and rethinking. With an understanding of the legal and ethical issues accomplished, we can fully, openly, and without fear participate in the joy and wonder that is obstetric anesthesia.

REFERENCES

1. Lowry F. Pain during childbirth leads to $2.4-million lawsuit. *Can Med Assoc J* 1995;152:1115.
2. Kirkton JL, ed. *Cook County jury verdict reporter: 1995 calendar year summary and index of malpractice trials.* Law Bulletin Publishing Company, Chicago, IL, 1996.
3. Kirkton JL, ed. *Cook County jury verdict reporter- 1995 medical malpractice suit list index.* : Law Bulletin Publishing Company, Chicago, IL, 1996.
4. Heath Resources and Services Administration. *1994 annual report of the National Practitioner Data Bank.* Washington DC: PHS, 1935.
5. Johnson WG, Brennan TA, Newhouse JP, et al. The economic consequences of medical injuries: implications for a no-fault insurance plan. *JAMA* 1992;267:2487.

6. Localio AR, Lawthers AG, Brennan TA, et al. Relation between malpractice claims and adverse events due to negligence: results of the Harvard Medical Practice Study III. *N Engl J Med* 1991;325:245.
7. Leape LL, Brennan TA, Laird N, et al. The nature of adverse events in hospitalized patients: results of the Harvard Medical Practice Study II. *N Engl J Med* 1991;324:377.
8. Weiler PC, Newhouse JP, Hiatt HH. Proposal for medical liability reform. *JAMA* 1992;267:2355.
9. Brennan TA, Leape LL, Laird NM, et al. Incidence of adverse events and negligence in hospitalized patients: results of the Harvard Medical Practice Study I. *N Engl J Med* 1991;324:370.
10. Anderson RE. *An "epidemic" of medical malpractice: a commentary on the Harvard Medical Practice Study.* New York: The Manhattan Institute, Civil Justice Memo of the Doctors Company, 1996.
11. Chadwick HS. An analysis of obstetric anesthesia cases from the American Society of Anesthesiologists closed claims project database. *Int J Obstet Anesth* 1996;5:258.
12. Breen TW, Oriol NE. Incidence of late low back pain after childbirth is not influenced by anesthesia for labor or delivery. *Anesthesiology* 1992; 77:A1044.
13. Macarthur AJ, Macarthur C, Weeks S. Epidural anesthesia and postpartum back pain. *Anesthesiology* 1993;9:A973.
14. Clark VA, McQueen MA. Factors influencing backache following epidural analgesia in labour. *Int J Obstet Anesth* 1993;2:193.
15. Breen TW, Ransil BJ, Groves PA, Oriol NE. Factors associated with back pain after childbirth. *Anesthesiology* 1994;81:29.
16. St-Amand J. Medicolegal nightmare: a tragic case, a needless trial. *Can Med Assoc J* 1993;148:806.
17. Localio AR, Lawthers AG, Bengtson JM, et al. Relationship between malpractice claims and cesarean delivery. *JAMA* 1993;269:366.
18. Bartlett EE. What's up doc?—the patient and the malpractice suit. *Risk Manage* 1987;August:26.
19. Oriol NE. Maternal mortality: part B. In: Van Zundert A, Ostheimer GW, eds. *USA view:* pain relief and anesthesia in obstetrics. New York: Churchill Livingstone, 1996:745.
20. Hawkins JL, Koonin LM, Palmer SK, Gibbs CP. Anesthesia-related deaths during obstetric delivery in the United States, 1979-1990. *Anesthesiology* 1997;86:277.
21. Newman LM, Perez EC, Krolick T, Ivankovich AD. Labor analgesia, cesarean anesthesia, and cesarean delivery rates for 18,000 deliveries from 1988 through 1994. *Anesthesiology* 1995;83:A968.
22. Newman LM, McCarthy RJ, Ivankovich AD. Epidural or combined spinal-epidural labor analgesia does not affect the incidence of cesarean delivery for dystocia or malposition. *Anesthesiology* 1996;85:A857.
23. Chestnut DH. Anesthesia and maternal mortality [Editorial]. *Anesthesiology* 1997;86:273.
24. Knapp RM. Liability: part B. In: Van Zundert A, Ostheimer GW, eds. *USA view, pain relief and anesthesia in obstetrics.* New York: Churchill Livingstone, 1996:878.
25. Ferrari HA. Medical malpractice litigation, consultants and expert witnesses. *ASA Newsl* 1997;61:11.
26. Black HC. *Black's law dictionary.* St. Paul: West Publishing Company, 1979.
27. Cheney FW, Posner K, Caplan RA, Ward RJ. Standard of care and anesthesia liability. *JAMA* 1989;261:1599.
28. Levinson G. Avoiding obstetric lawsuits: relevant guidelines and standards. 48, 276. American Society of Anesthesiologist's Annual Refresher Course, 1997:10.
29. Heyman HJ. Neonatal resuscitation and anesthesiologist liability [Letter]. *Anesthesiology* 1994;81:783.
30. Posner KL, Caplan RA, Cheney FW. Variation in expert opinion in medical malpractice review. *Anesthesiology* 1996;85:1049.
31. Strelec SR. Confessions of an "expert witness." *ASA Newsl* 1997;61:13.
32. Caplan RA, Posner KL, Cheney FW. Effect of outcome on physician judgments of appropriateness of care. *JAMA* 1957;265:1957.
33. Anonymous. Guidelines for expert witness qualifications and testimony. Directory of Members. ASA, Park Ridge, IL, 1997:403.
34. Battaglia JM. Medical malpractice claims in the US legal system. *Int J Obstet Anesth* 1996;5:254.
35. Salvesen JC, Spielman FJ. Legal and ethical issues in obstetric anesthesia. In: Norris MC, ed. *Obstetric anesthesia.* Philadelphia: Lippincott, 1993:847.
36. Office of Legal Affairs. Aunt Ola's helpful hints. *Health Law Rep* 1997; 5:1.
37. Waisel DB, Truog RD. An introduction to ethics. *Anesthesiology* 1997; 87:411.
38. Jackson SH, Palmer SK, Van Norman G, et al. Ethical issues in anesthesia. *Adv Anesth* 1997;14:227.
39. Doukas DJ, Elkins TE. Compelled cesarean section: an ethical perspective [Review]. *Primary Care* 1993;20:721.
40. Caplan RA, Posner K. Informed consent in anesthesia liability. *ASA Newsl* 1995;59:9.
41. Knapp RM. Legal view of informed consent for anesthesia during labor [Letter]. *Anesthesiology* 1990;72:211.
42. Waisel DB, Truog RD. Informed consent. *Anesthesiology* 1997;87:968.
43. Hewlett S. Consent to clinical research—adequately voluntary or substantially influenced? *J Med Ethics* 1996;22:232.
44. Lindgren K. Maternal-fetal conflict: court-ordered cesarean section. *J Obstet Gynecol Neonatal Nurs* 1996;25:653.
45. Brimacombe J, Clarke G, Craig L. Epidural blood patch in the Jehovah's Witness. *Anaesth Intens Care* 1994;22:319.
46. Kanumilli V, Kaza R, Johnson C, Nowacki C. Epidural blood patch for Jehovah's Witness patient. *Anesth Analg* 1993;77:872.
47. Parens E. What research? What embryos? *Hastings Cent Rep* 1995; 25:36.
48. Robertson JA. Symbolic issues in embryo research. *Hastings Cent Rep* 1995;25:37.
49. Robertson JA. Ethical and legal issues in human embryo donation. *Fertil Steril* 1995;64:885.
50. Chestnut DH. Effect on the progress of labor and method of delivery. In: Chestnut DH, ed. *Obstetric anesthesia: principles and practice.* St. Louis: Mosby, 1994:403.

Appendices

Obstetric Anesthesia, second edition,
edited by Mark C. Norris.
Lippincott Williams & Wilkins, Philadelphia © 1999.

APPENDIX A

Guidelines for Regional Anesthesia in Obstetrics

(Approved by House of Delegates on October 12, 1988, and last amended on October 30, 1991)

These guidelines apply to the use of regional anesthesia or analgesia in which local anesthetics are administered to the parturient during labor and delivery. They are intended to encourage quality patient care but cannot guarantee any specific patient outcome. Because the availability of anesthesia resources may vary, members are responsible for interpreting and establishing the guidelines for their own institutions and practices. These guidelines are subject to revision from time to time as warranted by the evolution of technology and practice.

GUIDELINE I

REGIONAL ANESTHESIA SHOULD BE INITIATED AND MAINTAINED ONLY IN LOCATIONS IN WHICH APPROPRIATE RESUSCITATION EQUIPMENT AND DRUGS ARE IMMEDIATELY AVAILABLE TO MANAGE PROCEDURALLY RELATED PROBLEMS.

Resuscitation equipment should include, but is not limited to: sources of oxygen and suction, equipment to maintain an airway and perform endotracheal intubation, a means to provide positive pressure ventilation, and drugs and equipment for cardiopulmonary resuscitation.

GUIDELINE II

REGIONAL ANESTHESIA SHOULD BE INITIATED BY A PHYSICIAN WITH APPROPRIATE PRIVILEGES AND MAINTAINED BY OR UNDER THE MEDICAL DIRECTION[1] OF SUCH AN INDIVIDUAL.

Physicians should be approved through the institutional credentialing process to initiate and direct the maintenance of obstetric anesthesia and to manage procedurally related complications.

GUIDELINE III

REGIONAL ANESTHESIA SHOULD NOT BE ADMINISTERED UNTIL 1) THE PATIENT HAS BEEN EXAMINED BY A QUALIFIED INDIVIDUAL[2]; AND 2) THE MATERNAL AND FETAL STATUS AND PROGRESS OF LABOR HAVE BEEN EVALUATED BY A PHYSICIAN WITH PRIVILEGES IN OBSTETRICS WHO IS READILY AVAILABLE TO SUPERVISE THE LABOR AND MANAGE ANY OBSTETRIC COMPLICATIONS THAT MAY ARISE.

Under circumstances defined by department protocol, qualified personnel may perform the initial pelvic examination. The physician responsible for the patient's obstetrical care should be informed of her status so that a decision can be made regarding present risk and further management.[2]

GUIDELINE IV

AN INTRAVENOUS INFUSION SHOULD BE ESTABLISHED BEFORE THE INITIATION OF REGIONAL ANESTHESIA AND MAINTAINED THROUGHOUT THE DURATION OF THE REGIONAL ANESTHETIC.

GUIDELINE V

REGIONAL ANESTHESIA FOR LABOR AND/OR VAGINAL DELIVERY REQUIRES THAT THE PAR-

[1]The Anesthesia Care Team (approved by ASA House of Delegates on October 26th, 1982, and last amended on October 25, 1995).

[2]Guidelines for Perinatal Care (American Academy of Pediatrics and American College of Obstetricians and Gynecologists, 1988).

TURIENT'S VITAL SIGNS AND THE FETAL HEART RATE BE MONITORED AND DOCUMENTED BY A QUALIFIED INDIVIDUAL. ADDITIONAL MONITORING APPROPRIATE TO THE CLINICAL CONDITION OF THE PARTURIENT AND THE FETUS SHOULD BE EMPLOYED WHEN INDICATED. WHEN EXTENSIVE REGIONAL BLOCKADE IS ADMINISTERED FOR COMPLICATED VAGINAL DELIVERY, THE STANDARDS FOR BASIC ANESTHETIC MONITORING[3] SHOULD BE APPLIED.

GUIDELINE VI

REGIONAL ANESTHESIA FOR CESAREAN DELIVERY REQUIRES THAT THE STANDARDS FOR BASIC ANESTHETIC MONITORING[3] BE APPLIED AND THAT A PHYSICIAN WITH PRIVILEGES IN OBSTETRICS BE IMMEDIATELY AVAILABLE.

GUIDELINE VII

QUALIFIED PERSONNEL, OTHER THAN THE ANESTHESIOLOGIST ATTENDING THE MOTHER, SHOULD BE IMMEDIATELY AVAILABLE TO ASSUME RESPONSIBILITY FOR RESUSCITATION OF THE NEWBORN.[3]

The primary responsibility of the anesthesiologist is to provide care to the mother. If the anesthesiologist is also requested to provide brief assistance in the care of the newborn, the benefit to the child must be compared to the risk to the mother.

[3]Standards for Basic Anesthetic Monitoring (approved by ASA House of Delegates on October 21, 1986, and last amended on October 25, 1995).

GUIDELINE VIII

A PHYSICIAN WITH APPROPRIATE PRIVILEGES SHOULD REMAIN READILY AVAILABLE DURING THE REGIONAL ANESTHETIC TO MANAGE ANESTHETIC COMPLICATIONS UNTIL THE PATIENT'S POSTANESTHESIA CONDITION IS SATISFACTORY AND STABLE.

GUIDELINE IX

ALL PATIENTS RECOVERING FROM REGIONAL ANESTHESIA SHOULD RECEIVE APPROPRIATE POSTANESTHESIA CARE. FOLLOWING CESAREAN DELIVERY AND/OR EXTENSIVE REGIONAL BLOCKADE, THE STANDARDS FOR POSTANESTHESIA CARE[4] SHOULD BE APPLIED.

1. A Postanesthesia Care Unit (PACU) should be available to receive patients. The design, equipment, and staffing should meet requirements of the facility's accrediting and licensing bodies.
2. When a site other than the PACU is used, equivalent postanesthesia care should be provided.

GUIDELINE X

THERE SHOULD BE A POLICY TO ASSURE THE AVAILABILITY IN THE FACILITY OF A PHYSICIAN TO MANAGE COMPLICATIONS AND TO PROVIDE CARDIOPULMONARY RESUSCITATION FOR PATIENTS RECEIVING POSTANESTHESIA CARE.

ASA Member Directory 1997:405.

[4]Standards for Postanesthesia Care (approved by ASA House of Delegates on October 12, 1988, and last amended on October 1, 1994).

Obstetric Anesthesia, second edition,
edited by Mark C. Norris.
Lippincott Williams & Wilkins, Philadelphia © 1999.

APPENDIX B

ACOG and ASA Recommend Obstetric Anesthesia Goals

Joint Statement on the Optimal Goals for Anesthesia Care in Obstetrics

This joint statement was adopted by the American Society of Anesthesiologists (ASA) and the American College of Obstetricians and Gynecologists (ACOG), and was designed to address issues of concern to both specialties. Good obstetric care requires the availability of qualified personnel and equipment to administer general or regional anesthesia on either an elective or emergent basis.

Optimal Goals

The extent and degree to which anesthesia services are available varies widely among hospitals. However, for any hospital providing obstetric care, certain optimal anesthesia goals should be sought.

Availability of Personnel. A person qualified to administer an appropriate anesthetic should be available whenever necessary. For many women, regional anesthesia (spinal or epidural) will be the most appropriate anesthetic.

A person qualified to maintain support of vital functions in any obstetric emergency should be available.

Anesthesia and surgical personnel able to start emergency cesarean deliveries within 30 minutes of recognition of need should be available.

Qualifications for administering anesthesia. A qualified anesthesiologist responsible for all anesthetics administered should be appointed. In many obstetric units, obstetricians or obstetrician-supervised nurse anesthetists administer the anesthetics. The administration of general or regional anesthesia requires numerous medical judgments and technical skills. Nurse anesthetists are not trained as physicians and cannot be expected to make medical decisions. Obstetricians seldom have sufficient training or experience in administering anesthesia to allow them to properly supervise nurse anesthetists.

Persons administering or supervising obstetric anesthesia should be qualified to manage the infrequent but occasionally life-threatening complications of major regional anesthesia, such as respiratory and cardiovascular failure, toxic local anesthetic convulsions, or vomiting and aspiration. Mastering and retaining the skills and knowledge necessary to manage these complications require adequate training and frequent application.

To ensure the safest and most effective anesthesia for obstetric patients, the director of anesthesia services, with the approval of the medical staff, must develop and enforce written policies regarding provision of obstetric anesthesia. It is the responsibility of the director of anesthesia services and the medical staff to review each individual's qualifications and competence and to determine which agents and techniques may be used.

The obstetrician. A qualified obstetrician should be available during administration of anesthesia. Neither major conduction anesthesia (epidural, caudal, or spinal) nor general anesthesia should be administered until the patient has been examined and the fetal status and progress of labor have been evaluated by a qualified physician who is readily available to supervise the labor and to deal with any obstetric complications that may arise.

Equipment, facilities, and support personnel. Equipment, facilities, and support personnel equal to those provided in the surgical suite should be available. This should include the availability of a properly equipped and staffed recovery room capable of receiving and caring for all patients recovering from major regional or general anesthesia. Birthing facilities, when used for anesthesia, must be appropriately equipped to provide safe anesthetic care during labor and delivery and postanesthesia recovery care.

Resuscitation of the depressed newborn. Personnel other than the surgical team should be immediately available to assume responsibility for resuscitation of the depressed newborn. The surgeon and anesthesiologist are responsible for the mother and may not be able to leave her to care for the newborn even when a regional anesthetic is functioning adequately. Individuals qualified to perform neonatal resuscitation should demonstrate:

- Skills in rapid and accurate evaluation of the newborn condition, including Apgar scoring,
- Knowledge of the pathogenesis and causes of a low Apgar score (asphyxia, drugs, hypovolemia, trauma, anomalies, and infection), as well as specific indications for resuscitation, and
- Skills in airway management, laryngoscopy, endotracheal intubation, suctioning of airways, artificial ventilation, cardiac massage, and maintenance of thermal stability.

In larger maternity units and those functioning as high-risk centers, 24-hour in-house anesthesia and obstetric and neonatal specialists usually are necessary. Preferably, the obstetric anesthesia services should be directed by an anesthesiologist with special training or experience in obstetric anesthesia. These units will also frequently require the availability of more sophisticated monitoring equipment and specially trained nursing personnel.

Recommendations

A recent survey jointly sponsored by ASA and ACOG found that many hospitals in the United States have not yet achieved the aforementioned goals. Deficiencies were most evident in smaller delivery units. Some small delivery units are necessary because of geographic considerations. Currently, 54% of hospitals providing obstetric care perform fewer than 500 deliveries per year. Providing comprehensive care for obstetric patients in these small units is extremely inefficient, not cost-effective, and frequently impossible. Thus, the following recommendations would seem appropriate:

1. Whenever possible, small units should consolidate.[1]
2. When geographic factors require the existence of smaller units, these units should be part of a well-established perinatal regionalizations system.

The availability of the appropriate personnel to assist in the management of a variety of obstetric problems is a necessary feature of good obstetric care. The presence of a pediatrician at a high-risk cesarean section or that of an anesthesiologist at a breech delivery are examples. Frequently, these professionals spend a considerable amount of time waiting but eventually may not be required to perform the tasks for which they are present. Reasonable compensation for these standby services is justifiable and necessary.

A variety of other mechanisms have been suggested to increase the availability and quality of anesthesia services in obstetrics. Improved hospital design to place labor and delivery suites closer to the operating room would allow for more efficient supervision of nurse anesthetists. Anesthesia equipment in the labor and delivery area must be comparable to that in the operating room.

Finally, interpersonal relations between obstetricians and anesthesiologists could be improved. Joint meetings between the two departments should be encouraged. Anesthesiologists should recognize the special needs and concerns of the obstetrician, and obstetricians should recognize the anesthesiologist as a consultant in the management of pain and life support measures. Both should recognize the need to provide high-quality care for all patients.

ACOG Newsletter September 1988:9–10.

ACOG, Anesthesiologists Clarify Standards Issues for Obstetric Anesthesia

The joint statement adopted by ACOG and the American Society of Anesthesiologists, Inc. (ASA) on optimal goals for obstetric anesthesia (*ACOG Newsletter* September 1988:9–10), and the subsequent standards for conductive anesthesia published by ASA in December 1988, have been subject to misinterpretation. This has caused problems at the local institutional level.

Concern is primarily directed toward the portion of the document delineating responsibilities of the obstetrician, which states that anesthesia should not be administered until the patient has been examined and the fetal status and progress of labor evaluated by a qualified physician who is readily available to supervise the labor. The passage in question also appeared in ASA's *Standards for Conduction Anesthesia* as Standard III, reprinted below:

> Major conduction anesthesia should not be administered until the patient has been examined and the fetal status and progress of labor evaluated by a qualified physician who is readily available to supervise the labor and to deal with any obstetric complications that may arise.

Both ACOG and the ASA have responded to concerns over this standard with a clarification of intent. The intent of this standard is that the examination of the patient may be performed by the physician responsible for obstetric management or may be delegated to a qualified individual, who may be a nurse or midwife. Standard III has been referred back to ASA's Committee on Obstetrical Anesthesia and Standards for further study, with clarification and rewording to be done in conjunction with

[1] The National Foundation-March of Dimes, Committee on Perinatal Health. Toward improving the outcome of pregnancy—recommendations for the regional development of maternal and perinatal health services. New York: The National Foundation-March of Dimes, 1977.

ACOG. In the interim, this explanation is meant to clear up some of the confusion caused by its misinterpretation.

ACOG Newsletter December 1989:7.

Anesthesiologists Send Statement Back for Rewording

About 2 years ago, ACOG consulted with the American Society of Anesthesiologists (ASA) about issues pertaining to the availability and quality of obstetric anesthesia. Their findings were summarized in the joint statement, "Optimal Goals for Anesthesia Care in Obstetrics," published in the September 1988 *ACOG Newsletter* and in the December 1988 *ASA Newsletter* under the title, "Standards for Conduction Anesthesia in Obstetrics."

In the intervening time, concerns have been raised about a passage stating that major conduction anesthesia should not be administered "until the patient has been examined and the fetal status and progress of labor have been evaluated by a qualified physician who is readily available to supervise the labor and to deal with any obstetric complications that may arise." In the ASA version the same passage in incorporated under the first part of "Standard III."

The intent of the standard, ASA notes, "is that the examination of the patient may be performed by the physician responsible for obstetric management or may be delegated to a qualified individual who may be a nurse or midwife" (1). The statement has been referred to the ASA Committees on Obstetrical Anesthesia and Standard of Care for clarification and rewording.

ACOG Newsletter February 1990:9.

1. American Society of Anesthesiologists. Clarification of standards for conduction anesthesia in obstetrics. *ASA Newsletter* 1989;53:19.

Obstetric Anesthesia, second edition,
edited by Mark C. Norris.
Lippincott Williams & Wilkins, Philadelphia © 1999.

APPENDIX C

The Anesthesia Care Team

(Approved by House of Delegates on October 26, 1982, and last amended on October 25, 1995)

Anesthesiology is a recognized specialty of medicine. Anesthesia care personally performed or medically directed by an anesthesiologist, a physician who has completed an approved residency in anesthesiology, constitutes the practice of medicine. Certain aspects of anesthesia care may be delegated to other properly trained professionals. These professionals, medically directed by the anesthesiologist, comprise the Anesthesia Care Team.

Such delegation and direction should be specifically defined by the anesthesiologist director of the Anesthesia Care Team and approved by the hospital medical staff. Although selected functions of overall anesthesia care may be delegated to appropriate members of the Anesthesia Care Team, responsibility and direction of the Anesthesia Care Team rest with the anesthesiologist.

The Society believes that the involvement of an anesthesiologist in the care of every patient undergoing anesthesia is essential. This may be accomplished throught personal provision of anesthesia care or by medical direction of the anesthesia care team.

Members of the medically directed Anesthesia Care Team may include physicians and nonphysician personnel.

A. Those who assist in providing direct patient care during the perioperative period, for example:
   ANESTHESIOLOGY RESIDENT—a physician who is presently in an approved anesthesiology residency program.
   NURSE ANESTHETIST—a registered nurse who has satisfactorily completed an approved nurse anesthesia training program.
   ANESTHESIOLOGIST'S ASSISTANT—a graduate physician's assistant who has satisfactorily completed an approved anesthesiologist's assistant training program.
B. Others who have patient care functions during the perioperative period include:
   POSTANESTHESIA NURSE—a nurse who cares for patients recovering from anesthesia.
   CRITICAL CARE NURSE—a nurse who cares for patients in a special care area such as the intensive care unit.
   RESPIRATORY THERAPIST—an allied health professional who provides respiratory care to patients.
C. Support personnel whose efforts deal with technical expertise, supply, and maintenance, for example:
   Anesthesia technologists and technicians
   Anesthesia aides
   Blood gas technicians
   Respiratory technicians
   Monitoring technicians

In order to apply the Anesthesia Care Team concept in a manner consistent with the highest standards of patient care, the following essentials should be observed:

1. Medical direction.
   Anesthesia direction, management, or instruction provided by an anesthesiologist whose responsibilities include:
   a. Preanesthetic evaluation of the patient.
   b. Prescription of the anesthesia plan.
   c. Personal participation in the most demanding procedures in this plan, especially those of induction and emergence.
   d. Following the course of anesthesia administration at frequent intervals.
   e. Remaining physically available for the immediate diagnosis and treatment of emergencies.
   f. Providing indicated postanesthesia care.

An anesthesiologist engaged in medical direction should not personally be administering another anesthetic and should use sound judgment in initiating other concurrent anesthetic and emergency procedures.

2. Delegation of any part of anesthesia care by an anesthesiologist to a member of the Anesthesia Care Team under that anesthesiologist's medical direction should be fully disclosed to all concerned.
3. Exploitation of patients, institutions, Anesthesia Care Team members, colleagues, or payors is unethical.

ASA Member Directory 1998:453.

Obstetric Anesthesia, second edition,
edited by Mark C. Norris.
Lippincott Williams & Wilkins, Philadelphia © 1999.

APPENDIX D

Statement on Invasive Monitoring in Anesthesiology

(Approved by House of Delegates on October 17, 1984)

A major contribution to the current practice of medicine is made by the galaxy of monitoring equipment and techniques developed in the past two decades. They have played a vital role in improving our ability to prevent, recognize, and treat many conditions that previously contributed to morbidity and mortality.

These techniques, particularly those involving insertion of central venous pressure (CVP) monitoring lines, intraarterial catheters (A-lines), and Swan-Ganz catheters (PA lines), all carry with their application some varying degree of risk to the patient.

This statement attempts to minimize such risk by outlining our position on the provision of such procedures in the delivery of anesthesia care by Anesthesia Care Team personnel:

A. The decision to use invasive monitoring is a medical judgment and should, therefore, be made only by a qualified physician.
B. Invasive monitoring techniques should be prescribed by a physician. Depending upon its risk, each should be applied only by a competent and trained physician, or under the personal and immediate medical direction of such a competent and responsible physician.
C. Training and credentialing of nonphysician members of the Anesthesia Care Team who may perform invasive monitoring techniques should be approved at the local medical staff level by the anesthesia department and the active medical staff.
D. Some of the invasive monitoring tasks, namely the insertion of CVP lines placed via the upper extremity and of arterial lines (A-lines), may be delegated to properly trained and credentialed members of an Anesthesia Care Team. Performance, however, should be under the immediate and personal medical direction of the leader of the Team, preferably an anesthesiologist.
E. Insertion of pulmonary artery catheters is a relatively hazardous procedure and should only be done by a properly trained physician.

ASA Member Directory 1998:457.

Obstetric Anesthesia, second edition,
edited by Mark C. Norris.
Lippincott Williams & Wilkins, Philadelphia © 1999.

APPENDIX E

Statement on Regional Anesthesia

(Approved by House of Delegates on October 12, 1983)

There has been an increased interest in the question of whether nurse anesthetists and other nonphysicians should be trained and permitted to perform spinal and other regional anesthesia procedures. While the permissible scope of practice by nurses and other nonphysicians is a matter to be determined by appropriate licensing and credentialing authorities, the Committee on Anesthesia Care Team believes that it is appropriate for the Society, as an organization of physicians dedicated to enhancing the safety and quality of anesthesia care, to state its views concerning the responsibilities of anesthesiologists for patient care in anesthesia and the role of nonphysicians in participating in such care. The Committee believes that these views are well and adequately set forth in guidelines and policy statements adopted by the House of Delegates.

These guidelines and policy statements emphasize that anesthesiology is the practice of medicine and that anesthesia, in all its forms, should be administered by, or under the medical direction of, a physician who is trained in the administration of anesthesia, preferably an anesthesiologist. Accordingly, anesthesiologists should assume responsibility for all aspects of anesthesia care, including obstetric anesthesia, outpatient anesthesia, and anesthesia for emergency surgery. Spinal and other regional anesthesia procedures involve diagnostic assessment, indications, contraindications, the prescription of drugs, and the institution of corrective measures and treatment in response to complications, and are not merely technical parts of patient care. In common with other medical practices, these procedures require a sound basic science background and experienced medical judgment.

Regional anesthesia should be performed only by an anesthesiologist or other physician trained in the administration of anesthesia.

ASA Member Directory 1998:457.

Obstetric Anesthesia, second edition,
edited by Mark C. Norris.
Lippincott Williams & Wilkins, Philadelphia © 1999.

APPENDIX F

Basic Standards for Preanesthesia Care

(Approved by House of Delegates on October 14, 1987)

These standards apply to all patients who receive anesthesia or monitored anesthesia care. Under unusual circumstances, e.g., extreme emergencies, these standards may be modified. When this is the case, the circumstances shall be documented in the patient's record.

Standard I: An anesthesiologist shall be responsible for determining the medical status of the patient, developing a plan of anesthesia care, and acquainting the patient or the responsible adult with the proposed plan

The development of an appropriate plan of anesthesia care is based upon:

1. Reviewing the medical record.
2. Interviewing and examining the patient to:
   a. Discuss the medical history, previous anesthetic experiences and drug therapy.
   b. Assess those aspects of the physical condition that might affect decisions regarding perioperative risk and management.
3. Obtaining and/or reviewing tests and consultations necessary to the conduct of anesthesia.
4. Determining the appropriate prescription of preoperative medications as necessary to the conduct of anesthesia.

The responsible anesthesiologist shall verify that the above have been properly performed and documented in the patient's record.

ASA Member Directory 1998:438.

Obstetric Anesthesia, second edition,
edited by Mark C. Norris.
Lippincott Williams & Wilkins, Philadelphia © 1999.

APPENDIX G

Guidelines for Delegation of Technical Anesthesia Functions to Nonphysician Personnel

(Approved by House of Delegates on October 17, 1984)

I. Anesthesiology is the practice of medicine. Anesthesia, in all its forms, should be administered by a physician who is trained in the administration of anesthesia, preferably an anesthesiologist, a physician who has completed an approved residency in anesthesiology. Accordingly, an anesthesiologist should be personally responsible to each patient for all aspects of anesthesia care.

II. While optimal anesthesia care involves a one-to-one relationship between anesthesiologist and patient, a shortage of anesthesiologists may necessitate the utilization of nonphysician personnel to perform technical functions relating the administration of anesthesia under the personal direction of an anesthesiologist or other qualified physician.

III. Delegation of functions to nonphysician personnel should be based on specific criteria (i.e., the individual's education, training, and demonstrated skills) approved by the medical staff on the recommendation of the physician responsible for anesthesia care. Such criteria should include competence to follow the anesthesia plan prescribed by the anesthesiologist and the technical ability to:

A. Induce anesthesia under the direction of an anesthesiologist.

B. Maintain anesthesia at prescribed levels

C. Monitor and support life functions during the perioperative period.

D. Recognize and report to the anesthesiologist any abnormal patient responses during anesthesia.

ASA Member Directory 1998:444.

Obstetric Anesthesia, second edition,
edited by Mark C. Norris.
Lippincott Williams & Wilkins, Philadelphia © 1999.

APPENDIX H

Standards for Postanesthesia Care

(Approved by House of Delegates on October 12, 1988, and last amended on October 19, 1994)

These Standards apply to postanesthesia care in all locations. These Standards may be exceeded based on the judgment of the responsible anesthesiologist. They are intended to encourage quality patient care, but cannot guarantee any specific patient outcome. They are subject to revision from time to time as warranted by the evolution of technology and practice. *Under extenuating circumstances, the responsible anesthesiologist may waive the requirements marked with an asterisk (*); it is recommended that when this is done, it should be so stated (including the reasons) in a note in the patient's medical record.*

STANDARD I

ALL PATIENTS WHO HAVE RECEIVED GENERAL ANESTHESIA, REGIONAL ANESTHESIA, OR MONITORED ANESTHESIA CARE SHALL RECEIVE APPROPRIATE POSTANESTHESIA MANAGEMENT.[1]

1. A Postanesthesia Care Unit (PACU) or an area that provides equivalent postanesthesia care shall be available to receive patients after anesthesia care. All patients who receive anesthesia care shall be admitted to the PACU or its equivalent **except** by specific order of the anesthesiologist responsible for the patient's care.
2. The medical aspects of care in the PACU shall be governed by policies and procedures that have been reviewed and approved by the Department of Anesthesiology.
3. The design, equipment, and staffing of the PACU shall meet requirements of the facility's accrediting and licensing bodies.

[1] Refer to *Standards of Postanesthesia Nursing Practice 1992* published by ASPAN, for issues of nursing care.

STANDARD II

A PATIENT TRANSPORTED TO THE PACU SHALL BE ACCOMPANIED BY A MEMBER OF THE ANESTHESIA CARE TEAM WHO IS KNOWLEDGEABLE ABOUT THE PATIENT'S CONDITION. THE PATIENT SHALL BE CONTINUALLY EVALUATED AND TREATED DURING TRANSPORT WITH MONITORING AND SUPPORT APPROPRIATE TO THE PATIENT'S CONDITION.

STANDARD III

UPON ARRIVAL IN THE PACU, THE PATIENT SHALL BE REEVALUATED AND A VERBAL REPORT PROVIDED TO THE RESPONSIBLE PACU NURSE BY THE MEMBER OF THE ANESTHESIA CARE TEAM WHO ACCOMPANIES THE PATIENT.

1. The patient's status on arrival in the PACU shall be documented.
2. Information concerning the preoperative condition and the surgical/anesthetic course shall be transmitted to the PACU nurse.
3. The member of the Anesthesia Care Team shall remain in the PACU until the PACU nurse accepts responsibility for the nursing care of the patient.

STANDARD IV

THE PATIENT'S CONDITION SHALL BE EVALUATED CONTINUALLY IN THE PACU.

1. The patient shall be observed and monitored by methods appropriate to the patient's medical condition. Particular attention should be given to monitoring oxygenation, ventilation, circulation, and temperature. During recovery from all anesthetics, a

quantitative method of assessing oxygenation such as pulse oximetry shall be employed in the initial phase of recovery.* This is not intended for application during the recovery of the obstetric patient in whom regional anesthesia was used for labor and vaginal delivery.

2. An accurate written report of the PACU period shall be maintained. Use of an appropriate PACU scoring system is encouraged for each patient on admission, at appropriate intervals prior to discharge, and at the time of discharge.
3. General medical supervision and coordination of patient care in the PACU should be the responsibility of an anesthesiologist.
4. There shall be a policy to assure the availability in the facility of a physician capable of managing complications and providing cardiopulmonary resuscitation for patients in the PACU.

STANDARD V

A PHYSICIAN IS RESPONSIBLE FOR THE DISCHARGE OF THE PATIENT FROM THE POSTANESTHESIA CARE UNIT.

1. When discharge criteria are used, they must be approved by the Department of Anesthesiology and the medical staff. They may vary depending upon whether the patient is discharged to a hospital room, to the Intensive Care Unit, to a short stay unit or home.
2. In the absence of the physician responsible for the discharge, the PACU nurse shall determine that the patient meets the discharge criteria. The name of the physician accepting responsibility for discharge shall be noted on the record.

ASA Member Directory 1998:439–440.

Obstetric Anesthesia, second edition,
edited by Mark C. Norris.
Lippincott Williams & Wilkins, Philadelphia © 1999.

APPENDIX I

Standards for Basic Anesthetic Monitoring

(Approved by House of Delegates on October 21, 1986, and last amended on October 23, 1996[1])

These standards apply to all anesthesia care although, in emergency circumstances, appropriate life support measures take precedence. These standards may be exceeded at any time based on the judgment of the responsible anesthesiologist. They are intended to encourage high-quality patient care, but observing them cannot guarantee any specific patient outcome. They are subject to revision from time to time, as warranted by the evolution of technology and practice. They apply to all general anesthetics, regional anesthetics, and monitored anesthesia care. This set of standards addresses only the issue of basic anesthetic monitoring, which is one component of anesthesia care. In certain rare or unusual circumstances, (1) some of these methods of monitoring may be clinically impractical, and (2) appropriate use of the described monitoring methods may fail to detect untoward clinical developments. Brief interruptions of continual monitoring may be unavoidable. *Under extenuating circumstances, the responsible anesthesiologist may waive the requirements marked with an asterisk (*); it is recommended that when this is done, it should be so stated (including the reasons) in a note in the patient's medical record.* These standards are not intended for application to the care of the obstetric patient in labor or in the conduct of pain management.

- Note that "continual" is defined as "repeated regularly and frequently in steady rapid succession" whereas "continuous" means "prolonged without any interruption at any time."

STANDARD I

Qualified anesthesia personnel shall be present in the room throughout the conduct of all general anesthetics, regional anesthetics, and monitored anesthesia care.

OBJECTIVE
Because of the rapid changes in patient status during anesthesia, qualified anesthesia personnel shall be continuously present to monitor the patient and provide anesthesia care. In the event there is a direct known hazard, e.g., radiation, to the anesthesia personnel that might require intermittent remote observation of the patient, some provision for monitoring the patient must be made. In the event that an emergency requires the temporary absence of the person primarily responsible for the anesthetic, the best judgment of the anesthesiologist will be exercised in comparing the emergency with the anesthetized patient's condition and in the selection of the person left responsible for the anesthetic during the temporary absence.

STANDARD II

During all anesthetics, the patient's oxygenation, ventilation, circulation, and temperature shall be continually evaluated.

OXYGENATION

OBJECTIVE
To ensure adequate oxygen concentration in the inspired gas and the blood during all anesthetics.

METHODS
1. Inspired gas: During every administration of general anesthesia using an anesthesia machine, the concentration of oxygen in the patient breathing system shall be measured by an oxygen analyzer with a low oxygen concentration limit alarm in use.*
2. Blood oxygenation: During all anesthetics, a quantitative method of assessing oxygenation such as pulse oximetry shall be employed.* Adequate illumination and exposure of the patient is necessary to assess color.*

VENTILATION

OBJECTIVE
To ensure adequate ventilation of the patient during all anesthetics.

[1]To become effective July 1, 1997.

METHODS

1. Every patient receiving general anesthesia shall have the adequacy of ventilation continually evaluated. While qualitative clinical signs such as chest excursion, observation of the reservoir breathing bag, and auscultation of breath sounds may be adequate, quantitative monitoring of the carbon dioxide content and/or volume of expired gas is strongly encouraged.
2. When an endotracheal tube or laryngeal mask is inserted, its correct positioning must be verified by clinical assessment and by identification of carbon dioxide in the expired gas. Continual end-tidal carbon dioxide analysis, in use from the time of endotracheal tube/laryngeal mask placement, until extubation/removal or initiating transfer to a postoperative care location, shall be performed using a quantitative method such as capnography, capnometry, or mass spectroscopy.*
3. When ventilation is controlled by a mechanical ventilator, there shall be in continuous use a device that is capable of detecting disconnection of components of the breathing system. The device must give an audible signal when its alarm threshold is exceeded.
4. During regional anesthesia and monitored anesthesia care, the adequacy of ventilation shall be evaluated, at least, by continual observation of qualitative clinical signs.

CIRCULATION

OBJECTIVE

To ensure the adequacy of the patient's circulatory function during all anesthetics.

METHODS

1. Every patient receiving anesthesia shall have the electrocardiogram continuously displayed from the beginning of anesthesia until preparing to leave the anesthetizing location.*
2. Every patient receiving anesthesia shall have arterial blood pressure and heart rate determined and evaluated at least every 5 minutes.*
3. Every patient receiving general anesthesia shall have, in addition to the above, circulatory function continually evaluated by at least one of the following: palpation of a pulse, auscultation of heart sounds, monitoring of a tracing of intraarterial pressure, ultrasound peripheral pulse monitoring, or pulse plethysmography or oximetry.

BODY TEMPERATURE

OBJECTIVE

To aid in the maintenance of appropriate body temperature during all anesthetics.

METHODS

There shall be readily available a means to continuously measure the patient's temperature. When changes in body temperature are intended, anticipated, or suspected, the temperature shall be measured.

ASA Member Directory 1998:438–439.

Obstetric Anesthesia, second edition,
edited by Mark C. Norris.
Lippincott Williams & Wilkins, Philadelphia © 1999.

APPENDIX J

Documentation of Anesthesia Care

(Approved by the House of Delegates on October 12, 1988)

Documentation is a factor in the provision of quality care, and is the responsibility of an anesthesiologist. While anesthesia care is a continuum, it is usually viewed as consisting of preanesthesia, perianesthesia, and postanesthesia components. Anesthesia care should be documented to reflect these components and to facilitate review.

The record should include documentation of:

I. Preanesthesia evaluation[1]
   A. Patient interview to review:
      1. Medical history
      2. Anesthesia history
      3. Medication history
   B. Appropriate physical examination.
   C. Review of objective diagnostic data (e.g., laboratory, electrocardiogram, x-ray).
   D. Assignment of ASA physical status.
   E. Formulation and discussion of anesthesia plan with the patient and/or responsible adult.

II. Perianesthesia (time-based record of events)
   A. Immediate review prior to initiation of anesthetic procedures:
      1. Patient reevaluation
      2. Check of equipment, drugs, and gas supply
   B. Monitoring of the patient[2] (e.g., recording of vital signs).
   C. Amounts of all drugs and agents used, and times given.
   D. The type and amounts of all intravenous fluids used, including blood and blood products, and times given.
   E. The technique(s) used.
   F. Unusual events during the anesthesia period.
   G. The status of the patient at the conclusion of anesthesia.

III. Postanesthesia
   A. Patient evaluation on admission and discharge from the postanesthesia care unit.
   B. A time-based record of vital signs and level of consciousness.
   C. All drugs administered and their dosages.
   D. Type and amounts of intravenous fluids administered, including blood and blood products.
   E. Any unusual events including postanesthesia or postprocedural complications.
   F. Postanesthesia visits.

ASA Member Directory 1998:455.

[1] See Basic Standards for Preanesthesia Care.

[2] See Standard for Basic Intraoperative Monitoring.

Obstetric Anesthesia, second edition,
edited by Mark C. Norris.
Lippincott Williams & Wilkins, Philadelphia © 1999.

APPENDIX K

Policy Statement on Practice Parameters

(Approved by House of Delegates on October 13, 1993)

Practice parameters are developed to demonstrate indications and/or methods for diagnosis, management, and treatment of specific problems.

> **Practice parameters** include standards, guidelines, and other strategies.
>
> **Standards** are rules; e.g., minimum requirements for sound practice. They are generally accepted principles for patient management.
>
> **Guidelines** are recommendations for patient management that may identify a particular management strategy or a range of management strategies.

Variances from practice parameters may be acceptable based on the judgment of the responsible anesthesiologist. Practice parameters are intended to encourage quality patient care, but cannot guarantee any specific patient outcome. They are subject to revision from time to time as warranted by the evolution of technology and practice.

Practice parameters are recommended to the ASA Board of Directors and House of Delegates. Committees which develop practice parameters are not empowered to define interpretations for specific institutions, organizations, or practices.

Members of the Society are responsible for interpreting and applying practice parameters to their own institutions and practices. The practice parameters adopted by ASA are not necessarily the only evidence of appropriate care. An individual physician should have the opportunity to show that the care rendered, even if departing from the parameters in some respects, satisfies the physician's duty to the patient under all the facts and circumstances.

In addition to standards and guidelines, the ASA House of Delegates has approved a number of documents variously titled Statements, Positions, or Protocols. These documents represent expressions of view by the House on a variety of subjects, but have not necessarily been subjected to the same level of formal scientific review as Standards or Guidelines. Variances from the terms of these documents may also be acceptable based on sound judgment of the responsible anesthesiologist. Appearing on the following pages are the Standards, Guidelines, Positions, and Protocols.

References for each Practice Parameter appear below. Because of their length, ASA's Practice Parameters do not appear in this booklet. Copies may be obtained from the ASA Publications Department.

ASA Member directory 1998: 437.

Obstetric Anesthesia, second edition,
edited by Mark C. Norris.
Lippincott Williams & Wilkins, Philadelphia © 1999.

APPENDIX L

Guidelines for Patient Care in Anesthesiology

(Approved by House of Delegates on October 3, 1967, and last amended on October 23, 1996)

I. Definition of Anesthesiology:

Anesthesiology is a discipline within the practice of medicine specializing in:

A. The medical management of patients who are rendered unconscious and/or insensible to pain and emotional stress during surgical, obstetric, and certain other medical procedures (involves preoperative, intraoperative, and postoperative evaluation and treatment of these patients);
B. The protection of life functions and vital organs (e.g., brain, heart, lungs, kidneys, liver) under the stress of anesthetic, surgical, and other medical procedures;
C. The management of problems in pain relief;
D. The management of cardiopulmonary resuscitation;
E. The management of problems in pulmonary care;
F. The management of critically ill patients in special care units.

II. Anesthesiologist's Responsibilities:

Anesthesiologists are physicians who, after college, have graduated from an accredited medical school and have successfully completed an approved residency in anesthesiology and, in addition, may have had additional training in critical care medicine and pain management. Anesthesiologists' responsibilities to patients should include:

A. Preanesthetic evaluation and treatment;
B. Medical management of patients and their anesthetic procedures;
C. Postanesthetic evaluation and treatment;
D. On-site medical direction of any nonphysician who assists in the technical aspects of anesthesia care to the patient.

III. Guidelines for Anesthesia Care:

A. The same quality of anesthetic care should be available for all patients:
   1. 24 hours a day, 7 days a week;
   2. Emergency as well as elective patients;
   3. Obstetric, medical, and surgical patients.
B. Preanesthetic evaluation and preparation means that an anesthesiologist:
   1. Reviews the chart.
   2. Interviews the patient to:
      a. Discuss medical history, including anesthetic experiences and drug therapy.
      b. Perform any examinations that would provide information that might assist in decisions regarding risk and management.
   3. Orders necessary tests and medications essential to the conduct of anesthesia.
   4. Obtains consultations as necessary.
   5. Records impressions on the patient's chart.
C. Perianesthetic care means:
   1. Reevaluation of the patient immediately prior to induction.
   2. Preparation and check of equipment, drugs, fluids, and gas supplies.
   3. Appropriate monitoring of the patient.
   4. Selection and administration of anesthetic agents to render the patient insensible to pain during the procedure.
   5. Support of life functions under the stress of anesthetic, surgical, and obstetric manipulations.
   6. Recording the events of the procedure.
D. Postanesthetic care means:
   1. A member of the anesthesia care team remains with the patient as long as necessary.
   2. Availability of adequate nursing personnel and equipment necessary for safe postanesthetic care.

3. Informing personnel caring for patients in the immediate postanesthetic period of any specific problems presented by each patient.
4. Assurance that the patient is discharged in accordance with policies established by the Department of Anesthesiology.
5. The period of postanesthetic surveillance is determined by the status of the patient and the judgment of the anesthesiologist.

(Ordinarily, when a patient remains in the hospital postoperatively for 48 hours or longer, one or more notes should appear in addition to the discharge note from the postanesthesia care unit.)

IV. Additional Areas of Expertise:

A. Resuscitation procedures.
B. Pulmonary care.
C. Critical (intensive) care.
D. Diagnosis and management of pain.
E. Trauma and emergency care.

V. Quality Assurance:

The anesthesiologist should participate in a planned program for evaluation of quality and appropriateness of patient care and resolving identified problems.

ASA Member Directory 1998:451.

Subject Index

Page numbers followed by *f* indicate figures; those followed by *t* indicate tabular material.

C

M